Nephrology and Urology of Small Animals

Nephrology and Urology of Small Animals

Edited by

Joe Bartges, DVM, PhD, DACVIM (Small Animal Internal Medicine), DACVN
Professor of Internal Medicine and Nutrition
The Acree Endowed Chair of Small Animal Research
Department of Small Animal Clinical Sciences
College of Veterinary Medicine
The University of Tennessee
Knoxville, TN

David J. Polzin, DVM, PhD, DACVIM (Small Animal Internal Medicine)
Professor of Internal Medicine
Department of Veterinary Clinical Sciences
College of Veterinary Medicine
University of Minnesota
St. Paul, MN

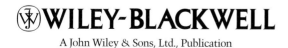

WILEY-BLACKWELL

A John Wiley & Sons, Ltd., Publication

Registered office: John Wiley & Sons Ltd, The Atrium, Southern Gate, Chichester, West Sussex, PO19 8SQ, UK

Editorial Offices: 2121 State Avenue, Ames, Iowa 50014-8300, USA
            The Atrium, Southern Gate, Chichester, West Sussex, PO19 8SQ, UK
            9600 Garsington Road, Oxford, OX4 2DQ, UK

For details of our global editorial offices, for customer services and for information about how to apply for permission to reuse the copyright material in this book please see our website at www.wiley.com/wiley-blackwell.

Disclaimer

Library of Congress Cataloging-in-Publication Data

Nephrology and urology of small animals / edited by Joe Bartges, David J. Polzin.
      p. ; cm.
   Includes bibliographical references and index.
   ISBN 978-0-8138-1717-0 (hardcover : alk. paper)   1. Veterinary nephrology.   2. Veterinary urology.
3. Pet medicine.   I. Bartges, Joe.   II. Polzin, David James.
   [DNLM: 1. Kidney Diseases–veterinary.   2. Cat Diseases.   3. Dog Diseases.   4. Urologic Diseases–veterinary.   SF 992.K53]
   SF992.K53N47 2011
   636.089′661–dc22

                                                                    2010026394

A catalogue record for this book is available from the British Library.

This book is published in the following electronic formats: ePDF 9780470958810; ePub 9780470958889

Set in 10.5/12.5pt Minion by Aptara® Inc., New Delhi, India
Printed and bound in Malaysia by Vivar Printing Sdn Bhd

1   2011

Dedications

To Carl Osborne, Del Finco, Don Low, and Ken Bovee, the "fathers" of Veterinary Nephrology and Urology. Their visions and efforts are responsible for the subspecialty as we know it today and have made this book possible.

To the book's contributors and the clinicians and researchers that generated the knowledge, expertise, and skills included in this book.

To the students, in school and out of school, who stimulate our pursuit of discovering new information that will improve the lives of dogs and cats with urinary diseases.

To the clients that we have worked with and their children whom they entrusted to our care.

And most importantly, to the dogs and cats that participated, some by giving their lives, in the many studies that have contributed to our knowledge, expertise, and skills in the field of veterinary nephrology and urology.

Joe Bartges dedicates this book:

- *To Joe Bartges, father:* "I've realized that I need him, when I look into my father's eyes" – "My Father's Eyes", *Eric Clapton*
- *To Garrick, son; Patrice, daughter; Lyn, sister; Richard, brother; Jacob, nephew, and all of the Bartges clan:* "And it goes on and on, watching the river run" – "Watching the River Run", *Loggins and Messina*
- *To Donna Raditic, friend, soul mate, and love:* "Have I told you lately that I love you? Fill my heart with gladness, take away my sadness, ease my troubles that's what you do" – "Have I Told You Lately?", *Van Morrison*
- *To the memory of Carol Bartges:* "Long ago, it must be, I have a photograph, preserve your memories" – "Old Friends", *Simon and Garfunkel*
- *For their love and support – and for putting up with me!*
- *To everyone who I am fortunate to call friend:* "To all the good friends I've known. . . And I'm gonna try to thank them all for the good times together" – "One of These Days", *Neil Young*; "No man is a failure who has friends." – *Clarence in "It's a Wonderful Life"*

David Polzin dedicates this book:

- *To my parents, Elmer and Patricia, who instilled in me the desire to learn*
- *To my wife Brenda, who has given me the joy and happiness needed to persevere*
- *To Kelsey and Elliot, my daughter and son, who are the future and make life interesting*
- *To my colleagues and friends that put life in perspective*
- *To the numerous pets in my life, that constantly remind me of the importance of what we do*

Contents

Contributors

Mark J. Acierno, MBA, DVM, DACVIM (Small Animal Internal Medicine)
Associate Professor of Internal Medicine
Dialysis Services Coordinator
Department of Veterinary Clinical Sciences
School of Veterinary Medicine
Louisiana State University
Baton Rouge, LA 70803

Larry G. Adams, DVM, PhD, DACVIM (Small Animal Internal Medicine)
Professor of Internal Medicine
Department of Veterinary Clinical Sciences
Purdue University
West Lafayette, IN 47907

Christopher A. Adin, DVM, DACVS
Assistant Professor of Surgery
Department of Veterinary Clinical Sciences
The Ohio State University
Columbus, OH 43210

Hasan Albasan, DVM, MS, PhD
Research Associate
Minnesota Urolith Center
Department of Veterinary Clinical Sciences
College of Veterinary Medicine
University of Minnesota
St. Paul, MN 55108

Kari L. Anderson, DVM, DACVR
Associate Clinical Professor of Medical Imaging
Department of Veterinary Clinical Sciences
College of Veterinary Medicine
University of Minnesota
St. Paul, MN 55108

Anne Bahr, DVM, DACVR, MS
Chief Radiologist
PetRays Teleradiology Consultants, PA
The Woodlands, TX 77380

Joe Bartges, DVM, PhD
DACVIM (Small Animal Internal Medicine), DACVN
Professor of Internal Medicine and Nutrition

The Acree Endowed Chair of Small Animal Research
Department of Small Animal Clinical Sciences
College of Veterinary Medicine
The University of Tennessee
Knoxville, TN 37996

Allyson Berent, DVM, DACVIM (Small Animal Internal Medicine)
Director, Interventional Endoscopy Services
Animal Medical Center
New York, NY 10065

Cathy A. Brown, VMD, PhD, DACVP (Anatomic Pathology)
Professor of Anatomic Pathology
Athens Veterinary Diagnostic Laboratory
College of Veterinary Medicine
University of Georgia
Athens, GA 30602

Scott Brown, VMD, PhD, DACVIM (Small Animal Internal Medicine)
Professor of Internal Medicine
Head, Department of Small Animal Medicine and Surgery
College of Veterinary Medicine
University of Georgia
Athens, GA 30602

Julie Byron, DVM, MS, MS, DACVIM (Small Animal Internal Medicine)
Assistant Professor of Internal Medicine
Department of Veterinary Clinical Medicine
College of Veterinary Medicine
University of Illinois
Urbana, IL 61802

Dennis Chew, DVM, DACVIM (Small Animal Internal Medicine)
Professor of Internal Medicine
Department of Veterinary Clinical Sciences
The Ohio State University
Columbus, OH 43210

Christina E. Clarkson, DVM, PhD
Assistant Professor
Department of Veterinary and Biomedical Sciences
College of Veterinary Medicine
University of Minnesota
St. Paul, MN 55108

Larry D. Cowgill, DVM, PhD, DACVIM
(Small Animal Internal Medicine)
Professor
Department of Medicine & Epidemiology
Co-Director, University of California Veterinary
    Medical Center-San Diego
School of Veterinary Medicine
University of California-Davis
Davis, CA 95616

Gregory B. Daniel, DVM, MS, DACVR
Professor of Radiology
Head, Department of Small Animal Clinical Sciences
Virginia-Maryland Regional College of Veterinary
    Medicine
Virginia Tech University
Blacksburg, VA 24061

Jonathan Elliott, MA, Vet MB, PhD, Cert SAC,
DECVPT, MRCVS
Professor of Clinical Pharmacology
Vice Principal - Research
Royal Veterinary College
Royal College Street
London, NW1 0TU, UK

Daniel A. Feeney, DVM, DACVR
Professor of Radiology
Department of Veterinary Clinical Sciences
College of Veterinary Medicine
University of Minnesota
St. Paul, MN 55108

Julie R. Fischer, DVM, DACVIM (Small Animal
Internal Medicine)
Associate
Veterinary Specialty Hospital of San Diego
San Diego, CA 92121

Thomas F. Fletcher, DVM, PhD
Professor
Department of Veterinary and Biomedical Sciences
College of Veterinary Medicine
University of Minnesota
St. Paul, MN 55108

Michael M. Fry, DVM, MS, DACVP
(Clinical Pathology)
Associate Professor of Clinical Pathology
Department of Pathobiology
College of Veterinary Medicine
The University of Tennessee
Knoxville, TN 37996

Corinne K. Goldman, DVM, MS, DACVIM
(Small Animal Internal Medicine)
Associate
South Carolina Veterinary Specialists
Columbia, SC 29210

Richard E Goldstein, DVM, DACVIM (Small Animal
Internal Medicine), DECVIM (Companion Animal)
Associate Professor of Medicine
Department of Clinical Sciences
College of Veterinary Medicine
Cornell University
Ithaca, NY 14853

Gregory F. Grauer, DVM, MS, DACVIM
(Small Animal Internal Medicine)
Professor of Internal Medicine
Jarvis Chair of Small Animal Internal Medicine
Department of Clinical Sciences
College of Veterinary Medicine
Kansas State University
Manhattan, KS 66506

Cheryl B. Greenacre, DVM, DABVP (Avian and Exotic
Companion Mammal)
Professor of Avian and Zoological Medicine
Department of Small Animal Clinical Sciences
College of Veterinary Medicine
The University of Tennessee
Knoxville, TN 37996

Silke Hecht, Dr Med Vet., DACVR, DECVDI
Assistant Professor of Radiology
Department of Small Animal Clinical Sciences
College of Veterinary Medicine
The University of Tennessee
Knoxville, TN 37996

Carolyn J. Henry, DVM, MS, DACVIM (Oncology)
Professor of Oncology
Director, Tom and Betty Scott Endowed Program in
    Veterinary Oncology
Faculty Facilitator, Mizzou Advantage One Health,
    One Medicine

Department of Veterinary Medicine and Surgery,
    College of Veterinary Medicine
and
Division of Hematology/Oncology, School of
    Medicine
University of Missouri
Columbia, MO 65211

George A. Henry, DVM, DACVR
Clinical Associate Professor of Radiology
Department of Small Animal Clinical
    Sciences
College of Veterinary Medicine
The University of Tennessee
Knoxville, TN 37996

**Katherine M. James, DVM, PhD, DACVIM
(Small Animal Internal Medicine)**
Veterinary Education Coordinator
Veterinary Information Network
Davis, CA 95616

**Marie E. Kerl, DVM, DACVIM (Small Animal
Internal Medicine), DACVECC**
Associate Teaching Professor
University of Missouri
Columbia, MO 65211

**Claudia A. Kirk, DVM, PhD, DACVN, DACVIM
(Small Animal Internal Medicine)**
Professor of Internal Medicine and Nutrition
Head, Department of Small Animal Clinical
    Sciences
College of Veterinary Medicine
The University of Tennessee
Knoxville, TN 37996

**John M. Kruger, DVM, PhD, DACVIM
(Small Animal Internal Medicine)**
Professor of Internal Medicine
Department of Small Animal Clinical Sciences
College of Veterinary Medicine
Michigan State University
East Lansing, MI 48824

**Mary Anna Labato, DVM, DACVIM
(Small Animal Internal Medicine)**
Clinical Professor of Internal Medicine
Section Head, Small Animal Medicine
Department of Clinical Sciences
Cummings School of Veterinary Medicine
Tufts University
North Grafton, MA 01536

**India F. Lane, DVM, MS, EdD, DACVIM
(Small Animal Internal Medicine)**
Associate Professor of Internal Medicine
Department of Small Animal Clinical Sciences
College of Veterinary Medicine
The University of Tennessee
Knoxville, TN 37996

**Cathy Langston, DVM, DACVIM (Small Animal
Internal Medicine)**
Head of Nephrology, Urology, and Hemodialysis Unit
Animal Medical Center
New York, NY 10065

**George E. Lees, DVM, MS, DACVIM (Small Animal
Internal Medicine)**
Professor of Internal Medicine
Department of Small Animal Clinical Sciences
College of Veterinary Medicine
Texas A&M University
College Station, TX 77843

Hervé P. Lefebvre, DVM, PhD, DECVPT
Professor of Physiology and Therapeutics
Department of Clinical Sciences
National Veterinary School of Toulouse
Toulouse, France

**Meryl P. Littman, VMD, DACVIM (Small Animal
Internal Medicine)**
Associate Professor of Internal Medicine
School of Veterinary Medicine
University of Pennsylvania
Philadelphia, PA 19104

**Jody P. Lulich, DVM, PhD, DACVIM (Small Animal
Internal Medicine)**
Professor of Internal Medicine
Minnesota Urolith Center
Department of Veterinary Clinical Sciences
College of Veterinary Medicine
University of Minnesota
St. Paul, MN 55108

Alexander G. MacLeod, DVM, DACVR
Staff Radiologist
Veterinary Specialty and Emergency Center
Langhorne, PA 19047

Roger K. Maes, DVM, MS, PhD
Professor, Department of Microbiology and Molecular
    Genetics
Section Chief, Virology

Diagnostic Center for Population and Animal Health
Michigan State University
East Lansing, MI 48910

Tomas Martin-Jimenez, DVM, PhD, DECVPT, DACVCP
Associate Professor of Pharmacology
Department of Comparative Medicine
College of Veterinary Medicine
The University of Tennessee
Knoxville, TN 37996

Mary B. Nabity, DVM, DAVCP (Clinical Pathology)
Clinical Assistant Professor of Clinical Pathology
Department of Pathobiology
College of Veterinary Medicine
Texas A&M University
College Station, TX 77843

Carl A. Osborne, DVM, PhD, DACVIM (Small Animal Internal Medicine)
Professor of Internal Medicine
Department of Veterinary Clinical Sciences
College of Veterinary Medicine
University of Minnesota
St. Paul, MN 55108

Jeffrey Phillips, DVM, PhD, DACVIM (Oncology)
Assistant Professor of Oncology
Department of Small Animal Clinical Sciences
College of Veterinary Medicine
The University of Tennessee
Knoxville, TN 37906

David J. Polzin, DVM, PhD, DACVIM (Small Animal Internal Medicine)
Professor of Internal Medicine
Department of Veterinary Clinical Sciences
College of Veterinary Medicine
University of Minnesota
St. Paul, MN 55108

Barrak M. Pressler, DVM, PhD, DACVIM (Small Animal Internal Medicine)
Assistant Professor of Internal Medicine
Department of Veterinary Clinical Sciences
School of Veterinary Medicine
Purdue University
West Lafayette, IN 47907

Margaret V. Root Kustritz, DVM, PhD, DACT
Associate Professor of Theiogenology
Department of Small Animal Clinical Sciences

College of Veterinary Medicine
University of Minnesota
St. Paul, MN 55108

Linda Ross, DVM, MS, DACVIM (Small Animal Internal Medicine)
Associate Professor of Internal Medicine
Department of Clinical Sciences
Cummings School of Veterinary Medicine
Tufts University
North Grafton, MA 01536

Sheri J. Ross, DVM, PhD, DACVIM (Small Animal Internal Medicine)
Clinical Faculty
Nephrology, Urology, and Hemodialysis
University of California Veterinary Medical
    Center
San Diego, CA 92121

Elizabeth Rozanski, DVM, DACVIM (Small Animal Internal Medicine), DACVECC
Assistant Professor of Internal Medicine and
    Emergency and Critical Care
Cummings School of Veterinary Medicine
Tufts University
North Grafton, MA 01536

Brian A. Scansen, DVM, MS, DACVIM (Cardiology)
Assistant Professor of Cardiology and Interventional
    Medicine
Department of Veterinary Clinical Sciences
College of Veterinary Medicine
The Ohio State University
Columbus, OH 43210

Gilad Segev, DVM, DECVIM (Companion Animal)
Clinical Lecturer in Internal Medicine
Head, Department of Small Animal Internal
    Medicine
Koret School of Veterinary Medicine
The Hebrew University of Jerusalem
Rehovot 76100, Israel

David F. Senior, BVSc, DACVIM (Small Animal Internal Medicine), DECVIM (Companion Animal)
Professor of Internal Medicine
Associate Dean of Advancement and Strategic
    Initiatives
School of Veterinary Medicine
Louisiana State University
Baton Rouge, LA 70810

Elizabeth A. Shull, DVM, DACVIM (Neurology), DACVB
Appalachian Veterinary Specialists and Gentle Pet Vet
Pet Wellness Center
Louisville, TN 37777

Andrea J. Sotirakopoulos, BVSc, MS
Small Animal Internal Medicine
San Diego, CA 92130

Rebecca L. Stepien, DVM, MS, DACVIM (Cardiology)
Clinical Professor of Cardiology
School of Veterinary Medicine
University of Wisconsin
Madison, WI 53706

Elizabeth Strand, LCSW, PhD
Clinical Associate Professor of Veterinary Social Work
Director, Veterinary Social Work
Department of Comparative Medicine
College of Veterinary Medicine
The University of Tennessee
Knoxville, TN 37996

Patricia A. Sura, MS, DVM, DACVS
Assistant Professor of Surgery
Department of Small Animal Clinical Sciences
College of Veterinary Medicine
The University of Tennessee
Knoxville, TN 37996

Harriet Syme, BSc, BVetMed, PhD, MRCVS, DACVIM (Small Animal Internal Medicine), DECVIM (Companion Animal)
Senior Lecturer in Internal Medicine
Department of Veterinary Clinical Sciences
Royal Veterinary College
University of London
Hatfield
Hertfordshire, AL9 7TA, UK

Karen M. Tobias, DVM, MS, DACVS
Professor of Surgery
Department of Small Animal Clinical Sciences
College of Veterinary Medicine
The University of Tennessee
Knoxville, TN 37996

Shelly L. Vaden, DVM, PhD, DACVIM (Small Animal Internal Medicine)
Professor of Internal Medicine
College of Veterinary Medicine
North Carolina State University
Raleigh, NC 27606

Jonathan Wall, BSc, PhD
Professor, Human Immunology and Cancer
    Program
Director, Preclinical and Diagnostic Molecular
    Imaging Laboratory
Graduate School of Medicine
The University of Tennessee
Knoxville, TN 37920

Jodi L. Westropp, DVM, PhD, DACVIM (Small Animal Internal Medicine)
Assistant Professor of Internal Medicine
Director, G. V. Ling Urinary Stone Analysis
    Laboratory
Department of Medicine and Epidemiology
School of Veterinary Medicine
University of California
Davis, CA 95616

Jacqueline C. Whittemore, DVM, PhD, DACVIM (Small Animal Internal Medicine)
Assistant Professor of Internal Medicine
Department of Small Animal Clinical Sciences
College of Veterinary Medicine
The University of Tennessee
Knoxville, TN 37996

Annabel G. Wise, DVM, MS, PhD
Academic Specialist in Virology
Diagnostic Center for Population and Animal Health
Michigan State University
East Lansing, MI 48910

Erik R. Wisner, DVM, DACVR
Professor of Radiology
Chair, Department of Surgical and Radiological
    Sciences
School of Veterinary Medicine
University of California
Davis, CA 95616

Preface

I will not use the knife, even upon those suffering from stones, but I will leave this to those who are trained in this craft.

> Original Hippocratic Oath ("*The Hippocratic Oath*". National Institute of Health. http://www.nlm.nih.gov/ hmd/greek/greek_oath.html. (accessed May 14, 2010))

The practice of urology is one of the oldest medical specialties and surgical removal of uroliths is one of the oldest surgical techniques known. The original Hippocratic Oath refers to the surgical removal of uroliths and obligates medical practitioners to leave such specialized procedures to specialists. In fact, the oldest known urolith was discovered in the body of a boy in Egypt dated approximately 4800 BC. Over the centuries, advances were made in the diagnosis and management of urinary diseases. From *Susruta* in India in 1000 BC through the uroscopists of the Middle Ages to hemodialysis, lithotripsy, and transplantation, the science and art of nephrology and urology grew. The field of veterinary nephrology and urology has also blossomed into a subspecialty including many practices and techniques performed in human medicine such as hemodialysis, lithotripsy, stent placement, and transplantation.

To say that the kidney produces urine is to say that Michelangelo produced marble chips.

> Anonymous

The urinary tract is truly an amazing system. The purpose of this book is to provide the best available compilation of the "state of the art and science" of the anatomy and physiology, diagnostic and therapeutic techniques, and the pathophysiology and management of diseases of the urinary system. It is divided into the following 11 sections:

- Anatomy and physiology
- Diagnostic testing
- Therapeutic techniques
- Clinical syndromes
- Upper urinary tract disorders
- Fluid, electrolyte, and acid–base disorders
- Systemic arterial hypertension
- Upper and lower urinary tract disorders
- Lower urinary tract disorders
- Urinary disorders of avian and exotic companion animals
- Counseling clients

With the expertise of 66 authors contributing 85 chapters, we intend this book to be a resource for veterinary students, house officers, general practitioners, and specialists. Our goal is to provide a readily accessible resource providing information ranging from basic to advanced, and to cover all aspects of nephrology and urology. We acknowledge that scientific information is dynamic and that some information contained herein may already be outdated by the date of publication. We ask the reader to inform us of errors and discrepancies.

In addition to the time and effort put forth by the authors, whom we thank, we also appreciate the efforts that Nancy Simmerman of Wiley-Blackwell expended in helping us to complete the book.

Section 1
Anatomy and physiology

1

Anatomy of the kidney and proximal ureter

Christina E. Clarkson and Thomas F. Fletcher

The kidney removes waste via blood filtration followed by tubular reabsorption and secretion. This chapter highlights renal anatomy of the dog and cat, including anatomy of the renal pelvis and proximal ureter.

Gross anatomy

Kidney topography and surface features

The kidneys of the dog and cat are similar in structure and relative size. They are paired, bean-shaped, and located dorsally in the abdominal cavity. Kidneys are retroperitoneal, dorsal to the peritoneal cavity, and covered by parietal peritoneum only. The surface facing laterally is convex; the medial surface is concave, with an indented region called the hilus (hilum) where vessels, nerves, and the ureter enter/exit the kidney. The right kidney is positioned cranial to the left, with its cranial pole situated within a recess of the caudate lobe of the liver.

In the dog, the right kidney is more firmly attached to the dorsal body wall than the left kidney. Thus, the location of the right kidney is more predictable, extending from vertebrae T_{13} to L_2. The left kidney is approximately half a kidney length caudal to the right (Osborne et al. 1972); its looser attachment can result in movement during respiration or body positioning. In the cat, both kidneys are pendulous, moveable, and more caudally located than in the dog. The feline right kidney is positioned at the level of vertebrae L_1 to L_4, left kidney at the level of L_2 to L_5 (Nickel et al. 1973).

The kidney develops embryologically from discrete lobes that fuse for the most part in the dog and cat. The carnivore kidney is classified as unilobar. It is devoid of lobe demarcations externally, presenting a smooth sur-

face encased within a fibrous capsule. Sectioning the kidney reveals an outer layer of dark-colored, highly vascular cortex, surrounding a lighter colored medulla (Figure 1.1).

Renal cortex and medulla

The cut surface of the renal cortex has a relatively rough texture due to collections of capillary tufts (glomeruli) and a labyrinth of tubules (cortical labyrinth). Medullary rays, smooth striations that appear to be radiating out of the medulla toward the periphery of the cortex, are scattered throughout the cortex.

The renal medulla is composed of renal pyramids that fuse to form a central ridge called the renal crest. The pyramids, wedges of medulla separated by interlobar vessels, are apparent in marginal planes of the section. Each pyramid has an apex (papilla) directed toward the renal pelvis. (Renal pyramids are remaining evidence of embryonic lobation.) The medulla contains papillary ducts that open onto the renal crest surface.

Renal pelvis and proximal ureter

Urine collects in the renal pelvis, a dilatation of the proximal end of the ureter. The pelvis is located within the renal sinus, a fat-containing, medial recess situated at the hilus. In the carnivore, the funnel-shaped renal pelvis has irregular margins due to reflection around interlobar vessels. The scalloped outpockets between vessels are referred to as pelvic recesses (Figure 1.1).

The ureter is an extension of the renal pelvis. It runs retroperitoneally along the dorsal wall of the abdominal cavity and through the lateral ligament of the bladder. The pelvis and ureter are lined by transitional epithelium and have smooth muscle walls. Peristaltic contraction waves initiated in the wall of the renal pelvis travel down

Nephrology and Urology of Small Animals. Edited by Joe Bartges and David J. Polzin. © 2011 Blackwell Publishing Ltd.

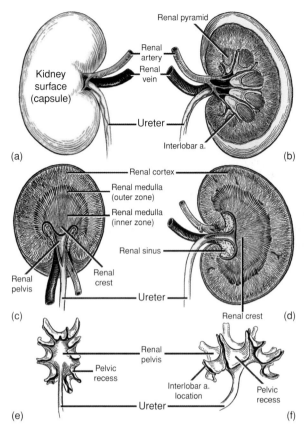

Figure 1.1 Anatomy of the canine kidney, pelvis, and ureter. (a) The intact kidney appears unilobar and enclosed in a fibrous capsule. Vessels and the ureter connect at the hilus of the kidney. (b) When sliced marginally on a sagittal plane, the cut surface reveals a fibrous capsule, a continuous renal cortex, and a medulla segregated into renal pyramids by interlobar arteries. The papilla of each pyramid is within a recess of the renal pelvis. (c) When sliced transversely, inner and outer zones of medulla can be seen surrounded by cortex. Along the midline, renal pyramids have fused into a renal crest located above the renal pelvis. (d) A mid-sagittal slice of kidney reveals renal crest rather than pyramids. Renal pelvis and fat occupy a space designated renal sinus. (e) External view of an isolated renal pelvis and ureter. (f) Side view of an isolated renal pelvis and ureter. The wall of the renal pelvis is scalloped, divided into pelvic recesses by wall projections around interlobar arteries (modified from Evans, 1993).

the ureter, conveying urine into the bladder. (The distal ureter is discussed in chapters on the lower urinary tract.)

Renal vessels

In most cases, a single renal artery divides into dorsal and ventral rami before entering the renal hilus (Marques-Sampaio et al. 2007). Further branching gives rise to interlobar arteries that enter kidney parenchyma. Arcuate arteries are branches of interlobar arteries at the corticomedullary junction. Interlobular arteries (cortical radial arteries) arise from arcuate arteries and run

radially through the cortex toward the kidney surface, some extending into the capsule (Nickel et al. 1973). In the cat, additional small branches from renal artery rami travel along the periphery of the kidney to supply the cortical surface and renal capsule (Fuller and Huelke 1973).

Interlobular arteries give off afferent arterioles. Each afferent arteriole gives rise to a ball of capillary loops, called a glomerulus. Glomerular capillaries unite to form an efferent arteriole that feeds a second capillary network surrounding renal tubules. The kidney is unusual in having two capillary beds connected by an arteriole, and thus an arterial portal system. The glomerulus constitutes the first capillary bed.

Efferent arterioles from glomeruli located peripherally in the cortex supply peritubular capillaries around cortical tubules, whereas efferent arterioles from juxtamedullary glomeruli supply peritubular capillaries around medullary tubules (Figure 1.2). In the medulla,

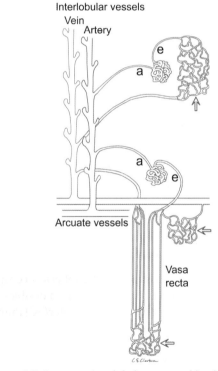

Figure 1.2 From an interlobular artery, blood flows to the glomerulus via an afferent arteriole (a). The glomerulus constitutes the first capillary network within the kidney. Efferent arterioles (e) convey blood to a second capillary bed that supplies the renal tubules, peritubular capillaries (arrows). Efferent arterioles from peripheral glomeruli (upper corpuscle) form a capillary network around cortical tubules; efferent arterioles from juxtamedullary glomeruli (lower corpuscle) form capillary networks around tubules located in the medulla. Medullary vessels (vasa recta) are closely associated with the loop of Henle. Peritubular capillaries drain via venules primarily into the interlobular veins.

the peritubular capillary network forms between descending efferent arterioles and venules that ascend back toward the cortex. These more or less straight vessels and their connections are referred to as vasa recta. They participate in an important countercurrent exchange between vessels and tubules. (Less commonly, peritubular capillaries arise from afferent arterioles or arcuate arterial branches (Christensen 1952; Nickel et al. 1973).)

Kidney veins are generally satellites of arteries. Venules arise from capillary beds surrounding cortical and medullary tubules. Veins travel with arterial branches, emptying into interlobular, arcuate, interlobar, and finally renal veins. A subcapsular venous system drains the renal capsule. In the cat, these veins are located within or immediately under the capsule (capsular veins); in the dog, the veins are deeper within the cortex (stellate veins) (Yadava and Calhoun 1958; Nickel et al. 1973). The cat's prominent capsular veins continue around the kidney periphery to the hilar region where they drain directly into the renal vein (Fuller and Huelke 1973). In the dog, the stellate veins drain into cortex and eventually into the renal vein (Christensen 1952). (The canine renal vein may also receive a direct contribution from stellate veins near the hilus (Fuller and Huelke 1973).)

Microscopic renal anatomy

Nephron

The nephron (renal corpuscle plus renal tubules) is the functional unit of the kidney. Urine produced within the nephron is further modified as it travels through the collecting duct system. (The term "uriniferous tubule" refers to the nephron plus its associated collecting duct.)

Nephron: renal corpuscle

The renal corpuscle is composed of a spherical complex of capillaries (glomerulus) surrounded by a double-wall capsule (Bowman's capsule). Arterioles enter/exit the corpuscle at its vascular pole, and ultrafiltrate exits at the opposite end of the corpuscle, the urinary pole.

Renal corpuscles are typically scattered throughout the cortex, although there is a small region immediately below the capsule where they are absent in the canine (Sherwood et al. 1969; Bulger et al. 1979). The number of corpuscles per kidney varies with species: 400,000–600,000 in the dog (Horster et al. 1971; Finco and Duncan 1972; Eisenbrandt and Phemister 1979) and approximately 200,000 in the cat (Kunkel 1930).

The glomerulus is formed by an afferent arteriole that gives rise to a ball of capillary loops, which then coalesce, into an efferent arteriole. The diameter of the affer-

ent arteriole is usually larger than that of the efferent. Arteriolar size is autoregulated to maintain a consistent glomerular filtration rate over a wide range of systemic arterial pressures. Intraglomerular mesangial cells and matrix occupy the spaces between capillary loops within the glomerulus (see below).

The blind-ended beginning of the renal tubule, called Bowman's capsule, surrounds the glomerulus. The capsule is cup-shaped, with inner and outer layers separated by a cavity, the urinary space. The outer layer of the capsule, called the parietal layer, is continuous with the epithelial cells of the proximal tubule at the urinary pole of the renal corpuscle. The inner layer of the cup, called the visceral layer, is composed of specialized cells called podocytes.

Podocytes have elaborate primary and secondary processes (foot processes) that interdigitate with processes of neighboring podocytes. Podocytes cover glomerular endothelial cells and intraglomerular mesangial cells. An intervening glomerular basement membrane (GBM) separates podocytes from endothelial cells and intraglomerular mesangial cells. The GBM is formed by fusion of podocyte and endothelial cell basal laminae (Figure 1.3a) (Abrahamson 1987).

Mesangial cells are found among glomerular capillaries (intraglomerular) and also outside the glomerulus near its vascular pole (extraglomerular). The latter are associated with the juxtaglomerular apparatus (described below). Mesangial cells function to maintain a "clean" GBM for blood filtration, by extending cytoplasmic processes between the GBM and endothelial cells for phagocytosis of debris. Additionally, mesangial cells secrete

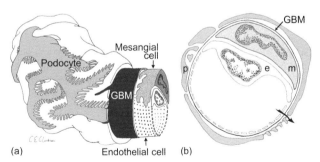

Figure 1.3 A segment of glomerular capillary loop is drawn to demonstrate cellular relationships among endothelial cells (e), glomerular basement membrane (GBM), mesangial cells (m), and podocytes (p). (a) Several podocytes (one shaded) wrap around a portion of glomerular capillary loop. The GBM, endothelium, and mesangial cells are revealed deep to the podocytes. (b) End view of a capillary surrounded by podocytes (shaded). An arrow indicates flow from blood to urinary space, passing through capillary pores, GBM, and between podocyte foot processes. A slit diaphragm spans the spaces between podocyte foot processes.

a variety of biologically active molecules and proliferate in response to glomerular injury. The mesangium (mesangial cells and associated matrix) provides physical support for the glomerulus (Sakai and Kriz 1987). Glomerular endothelial cells and mesangium together are surrounded by the GBM.

Renal "filter"

Urine formation begins as an ultrafiltrate within the urinary space of the renal corpuscle. The three major components of the renal "filter" are as follows (Figure 1.3b):

1. Endothelial cells of the glomerulus
2. GBM
3. Podocytes of the visceral layer of Bowman's capsule

Endothelial cells possess large fenestrations (pores); however, negatively charged material occupies much of this space. This represents the first barrier to filtration (Rostgaard and Qvortrup 2002). The GBM is thought to be the main filtration barrier to cells and large molecules. The GBM is also negatively charged. Podocyte foot processes form a discontinuous covering on the urinary space side of the GBM. Spaces between apposing foot processes are referred to as filtration slits. Filtration of smaller molecules is blocked by the presence of a thin negatively charged membrane within the filtrations slits (slit diaphragm) (Rodewald and Karnovsky 1974).

Taken together, passage through the renal "filter" is dependent on molecular size and charge. Blood cells and most proteins are too large to pass through endothelial fenestrations, and negatively charged macromolecules are repelled by negatively charged components of the "filter."

Nephron: tubular components

In addition to the renal corpuscle, the nephron has the following renal tubules: proximal convoluted tubule, loop of Henle, and distal convoluted tubule (Figure 1.4).

Proximal convoluted tubule

Ultrafiltrate within the urinary space travels first into the proximal convoluted tubule (PCT). This highly coiled tubule is the major tubule type of the cortical labyrinth. PCT cells feature apical intercellular tight junctions that limit intercellular (paracellular) movement of molecules from the lumen to the intercellular compartment. The PCT contains the only renal tubular epithelial cells with intercellular gap junctions (evidence of intercellular com-

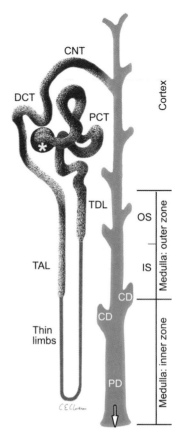

Figure 1.4 A drawing of one feline uriniferous tubule (nephron plus collecting duct). Glomerular ultrafiltrate flows into the urinary space in Bowman's capsule (*) and then through the following tubules: proximal convoluted tubule (PCT), loop of Henle (i.e., thick descending limb (TDL), thin limbs, and thick ascending limb (TAL)), distal convoluted tubule (DCT), connecting tubule (CNT), and collecting ducts (CD). Urine exits the kidney at the papillary duct opening (arrow). The cortex contains convoluted tubules. The outer zone of the medulla may be subdivided into outer stripe (OS) and inner stripe (IS) based on the presence of thick descending limbs of Henle's loop in the outer stripe. The inner zone of the medulla contains only thin limbs of Henle's loop and collecting ducts.

munication). The following cellular features exhibited by simple cuboidal epithelium of the PCT may be present to varying degrees on other renal tubular epithelial cells:

- *Microvilli (brush border)*: An apical membrane modification that provides increased surface area for absorption, modification, and intracellular transport of luminal material.
- *Basolateral intercellular interdigitations*: They are extensive and serve to increase available cell membrane for transcellular transport of materials.
- *Mitochondria*: They provide energy for the extensive reabsorption that occurs within the tubule. Vertically oriented mitochondria are closely associated with

infoldings of the basolateral cell membrane, producing a striated appearance. This close association provides energy for intramembranous transport pumps.

Loop of Henle

The loop of Henle is a straight tubular loop that initially descends from cortex into the medulla and then ascends back to the cortex. It is composed of a thick descending limb, thin limbs of the loop, and a thick ascending limb:

- The thick descending limb of Henle's loop is often described with proximal tubules and referred to as the proximal straight tubule. This segment is lined by simple cuboidal epithelium. It has less extensive cellular modifications than the PCT (shorter microvilli, fewer cellular interdigitations, and smaller mitochondria).
- The descending and ascending thin limb of Henle's loop begins with an abrupt change to simple squamous epithelium. This thin segment descends into the medulla and then abruptly turns to ascend toward the cortex. Ultrastructural characterization of this epithelium reveals a heterogeneous cellular population that varies with species, length of loop, and specific region. Microvilli and lateral interdigitations are underdeveloped or absent, and organelles are sparse in most thin limb regions. The thin limbs of Henle's loop in combination with its surrounding vascular network (vasa recta) play an important role in concentrating urine and maintaining a medulla high in solute concentration.
- The thick ascending limb (TAL) of Henle's loop (distal straight tubule) is the last segment of the loop of Henle. Its simple cuboidal epithelium is similar to the PCT but with less developed microvilli. The TAL ascends into the cortex to the vicinity of the vascular pole of its glomerulus of origin. TAL epithelial cells in the vicinity of the afferent arteriole will become a specialized group of cells called the macula densa, a component of the juxtaglomerular apparatus (described below).

Ultrafiltrate within Henle's loop travels next into the distal convoluted tubule (DCT). This tubule is shorter in length and has less developed microvilli than the PCT. Similar to PCT cells, there are many basolateral interdigitations; differing from the PCT, DCT has an even higher concentration of mitochondria.

Connecting tubule

The connecting tubule (CNT) runs from the DCT to a cortically located collecting duct within a medullary ray. The classification of this tubule as part of the nephron (i.e., derived from the nephrogenic ridge) or as part of the collecting duct (i.e., ureteric bud derivation) is open to debate. Interestingly, it has been shown in a variety of mammalian species (rats, rabbits, and humans) that CNTs pass in close proximity to the afferent arteriole, feeding the glomerulus of origin (Barajas et al. 1986; Vio et al. 1988; Dorup et al. 1992). There is evidence of paracrine signaling occurring between CNTs and afferent arterioles, a feedback arrangement. The epithelium of the CNT is simple cuboidal with less mitochondria and less intercellular interdigitations than PCT epithelium.

Collecting duct system

Nephrons (including CNTs) drain into a collecting duct system. Several nephrons join the same collecting duct and several collecting ducts unite to form a papillary duct. The renal medulla contains collecting ducts, papillary ducts, and the loops of Henle. Papillary ducts open onto the renal crest surface. There is a progressive change from cuboidal to columnar epithelium along the collecting duct system.

Collecting ducts have two cell types: principal and intercalated cells. The principal cells (collecting duct cells, light cells) are cuboidal, with short microvilli. These cells have distinct lateral borders that are noninterdigiting. Additionally, the cell base is filled with infoldings that displace organelles and create a visibly lighter zone. The darker appearing intercalated cells (dark cells) are most frequently found in collecting ducts, although low numbers can occur in the DCT and CNT. Several subtypes of intercalated cells exist with differing roles in acid or bicarbonate secretion. The intercalated cell has many mitochondria, but basal infoldings are absent.

Tubular organization gives rise to regions within the renal medulla (see Figure 1.4):

- Distinct inner and outer zones of the medulla are due to a difference in renal tubular segments.
- The inner zone of the medulla contains only thin limbs of Henle's loop, collecting ducts, vasa recta, and a relatively large component of interstitium. (Collecting ducts originate in a medullary ray of the cortex.)
- The outer zone of the medulla is where the thick limbs of the loop of Henle are located. It is subdivided generally into an inner stripe and an outer stripe (except in the dog). The junction of the inner and outer stripes correlates with the transition from thick tubules to thin segments of the descending limb of Henle's loop. In the cat and most species, this transition occurs within the outer zone. In the dog, this transition occurs at or near the corticomedullary junction, and therefore the outer stripe is absent (Bulger et al. 1979).
- The cat and dog normally have long loops of Henle. Even peripherally located corpuscles have loops of

Henle that extend all the way to the inner zone of the medulla (Beeuwkes and Bonventre 1975; Bulger et al. 1979). (In most mammals, the length of Henle's loop is variable and related to the position of its associated corpuscle within the cortex. Peripherally located corpuscles have shorter loops of Henle, only reaching the outer medulla, and juxtamedullary corpuscles have long loops of Henle, extending deep into the medulla (Schmidt-Nielsen and O'Dell 1961).)

Juxtaglomerular apparatus

The juxtaglomerular apparatus (JGA) is an anatomically distinct region at the vascular pole of the glomerulus. The JGA has three components: juxtaglomerular cells, macula densa cells, and extraglomerular mesangial cells (Figure 1.5).

Juxtaglomerular cells are modified smooth muscle cells in the walls of afferent and rarely efferent arterioles. The cells contain renin granules and may be referred to

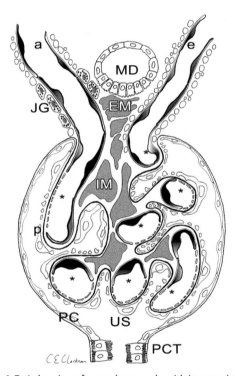

Figure 1.5 A drawing of a renal corpuscle with its associated juxtaglomerular apparatus (JGA): juxtaglomerular cells (JG), macula densa (MD), and extraglomerular mesangial cells (EM). The JGA is located at the vascular pole of the glomerulus between the afferent arteriole (a) and efferent arteriole (e). Several capillary profiles (*) are evident. Extraglomerular mesangial cells of the JGA are continuous with intraglomerular mesangial cells (IM). Bowman's capsule consists of the parietal epithelial cells (PC) and the layer of podocytes (p). Ultrafiltrate within the urinary space (US) flows into the proximal convoluted tubule (PCT).

as granular cells. The release of renin in response to signals from the macula densa cells generates a cascade of reactions leading to increased systemic blood pressure, thus increasing glomerular perfusion pressure.

The macula densa is a specialization of epithelial cells in the TAL of Henle's loop near the afferent and efferent arterioles. The cells are tall columnar versus the adjacent cuboidal epithelium. Cells of the macula densa detect changes in luminal sodium chloride concentration. In response, they generate paracrine signals that result in changes in arteriolar resistance and renin release by juxtaglomerular cells.

Extraglomerular mesangial cells are interposed between the two arterioles and macula densa cells. The cells are continuous with intraglomerular mesangial cells. A key feature of extraglomerular cells is the gap junctions they form with neighboring cells including juxtaglomerular cells, normal smooth muscle cells, and other mesangial cells (but not with macula densa cells). Although their entire role is unclear, the cells are thought to take part in coordinating JGA activities through gap junction communication. Also, because of their observed cytoskeletal "bridging" within the juxtaglomerular region, they are thought to help structurally reinforce this region.

Renal interstitium, lymphatics, and nerves

The interstitium—a composite of fibers, matrix, and cells—provides structural support for the kidney. The major cell type is the fibroblast, functioning to produce stroma and maintain structural connections to other cells, nerves, and epithelial basement membranes (Kaissling et al. 1996). Dendritic cells are also present, playing a role in immune regulation within the kidney (Dong et al. 2005). Macrophages and rarely lymphocytes may be present under normal conditions (Kaissling et al. 1996).

Lymphatic vessels are located within the renal cortex in association with vessels, encircling corpuscles and tubules and penetrating the renal capsule. The renal medulla lacks lymph vessels (Albertine and O'Morchoe 1980; Eliska 1984). Connective tissue sheaths surrounding vessels and tubules may serve as an avenue for lymph to move out of the medulla.

Sympathetic nerves typically travel along periarterial connective tissue sheaths (Barajas 1978) and innervate vascular smooth muscle (Fourman 1970). Tubules in close proximity to the arteries may be under a direct neuronal influence (Barajas 1978). Efferent innervation is still not completely understood and even less is known about the afferent innervation of the kidney.

References

Abrahamson, D.R. (1987). Structure and development of the glomerular capillary wall and basement membrane. *Am J Physiol* **253**(5 Pt 2): F783–F794.

Albertine, K.H. and C.C. O'Morchoe (1980). An integrated light and electron microscopic study on the existence of intramedullary lymphatics in the dog kidney. *Lymphology* **13**(2): 100–106.

Barajas, L. (1978). Innervation of the renal cortex. *Fed Proc* **37**(5): 1192–1201.

Barajas, L., et al. (1986). Immunocytochemical localization of renin and kallikrein in the rat renal cortex. *Kidney Int* **29**(5): 965–970.

Beeuwkes, R., III and J.V. Bonventre (1975). Tubular organization and vascular-tubular relations in the dog kidney. *Am J Physiol* **229**(3): 695–713.

Bulger, R.E., et al. (1979). Survey of the morphology of the dog kidney. *Anat Rec* **194**(1): 41–65.

Christensen, G.C. (1952). Circulation of blood through the canine kidney. *Am J Vet Res* **13**(47): 236–245.

Dong, X., et al. (2005). Antigen presentation by dendritic cells in renal lymph nodes is linked to systemic and local injury to the kidney. *Kidney Int* **68**(3): 1096–1108.

Dorup, J., et al. (1992). Tubule-tubule and tubule-arteriole contacts in rat kidney distal nephrons. A morphologic study based on computer-assisted three-dimensional reconstructions. *Lab Invest J Tech Methods Pathol* **67**(6): 761–769.

Eisenbrandt, D.L. and R.D. Phemister (1979). Postnatal development of the canine kidney: quantitative and qualitative morphology. *Am J Anat* **154**(2): 179–193.

Eliska, O. (1984). Topography of intrarenal lymphatics. *Lymphology* **17**(4): 135–141.

Evans, H.E. (1993). *Miller's Anatomy of the Dog*, 3rd edition. Philadelphia, PA: WB Saunders.

Finco, D.R. and J.R. Duncan (1972). Relationship of glomerular number and diameter to body size of the dog. *Am J Vet Res* **33**(12): 2447–2450.

Fourman, J. (1970). The adrenergic innervation of the efferent arterioles and the vasa recta in the mammalian kidney. *Experientia* **26**(3): 293–294.

Fuller, P.M. and D.F. Huelke (1973). Kidney vascular supply in the rat, cat and dog. *Acta Anat* **84**(4): 516–522.

Horster, M., et al. (1971). Intracortical distribution of number and volume of glomeruli during postnatal maturation in the dog. *J Clin Invest* **50**(4): 796–800.

Kaissling, B., et al. (1996). Morphology of interstitial cells in the healthy kidney. *Anat Embryol* **193**(4): 303–318.

Kunkel, P.A. (1930). The number and size of glomeruli in the kidney of several mammals. *Bull Johns Hopkins Hosp* **47**: 285–291.

Marques-Sampaio, B.P., et al. (2007). Dog kidney: anatomical relationships between intrarenal arteries and kidney collecting system. *Anat Rec* **290**(8): 1017–1022.

Nickel, R., et al. (1973). Urinary organs. In: *The Viscera of the Domestic Mammals*. Berlin; New York: Springer.

Osborne, C., et al. (1972). Applied anatomy of the urinary system. In: *Canine and Feline Urology*. Philadelphia, PA: WB Saunders.

Rodewald, R. and M.J. Karnovsky (1974). Porous substructure of the glomerular slit diaphragm in the rat and mouse. *J Cell Biol* **60**(2): 423–433.

Rostgaard, J. and K. Qvortrup (2002). Sieve plugs in fenestrae of glomerular capillaries—site of the filtration barrier? *Cells Tissues Organs* **170**(2–3): 132–138.

Sakai, T. and W. Kriz (1987). The structural relationship between mesangial cells and basement membrane of the renal glomerulus. *Anat Embryol* **176**(3): 373–386.

Schmidt-Nielsen, B. and R. O'Dell (1961). Structure and concentrating mechanism in the mammalian kidney. *Am J Physiol* **200**: 1119–1124.

Sherwood, T., et al. (1969). Renal magnification angiograms in the dog. Observations on responses to vasodilators and surgical trauma. *Br J Radiol* **42**(496): 241–246.

Vio, C.P., et al. (1988). Anatomical relationship between kallikrein-containing tubules and the juxtaglomerular apparatus in the human kidney. *Am J Hypertens J Am Soc Hypertens* **1**(3 Pt 1): 269–271.

Yadava, R.P. and M.L. Calhoun (1958). Comparative histology of the kidney of domestic animals. *Am J Vet Res* **19**(73): 958–968.

2

Physiology of the kidneys

Scott Brown

Homeostatic role of the kidneys

The kidneys act as the sum of the functions of individual nephrons (approximately 200,000 per kidney in cats and 500,000 per kidney in dogs) (Brown et al. 1990; Brown and Brown 1995) and their primary overall function is regulation of the composition of extracellular fluid. In doing so, the kidneys play a major role in the regulation of blood volume, extracellular fluid volume, systemic arterial blood pressure, hematocrit, acid–base balance, and plasma concentrations of electrolytes, minerals, and metabolic waste products.

Specific renal functions and their control

Renal blood flow

In dogs and cats, the kidneys receive approximately 25% of cardiac output, despite the fact that they account for only about 0.5% of total body weight, providing a flow of 4 mL/min/g of kidney weight (Brown et al. 1990; Brown and Brown 1995). This high flow exceeds that of other vascular beds, including brain, heart, and active skeletal muscle. Although formation of urine represents a metabolic energy requirement, hemodynamic rather than oxygen demands are apparently the determining factors for this high perfusion rate.

Cortical blood flow is considerably greater than medullary. Inert gas washout studies in anesthetized dogs demonstrated that blood flow in the cortex averaged 4.6 mL/min/g of kidney tissue, 0.7 mL/min/g in the outer medulla, and 0.1 mL/min/g kidney in the inner medulla (Bovee and Webster 1972). Approximately 90% of renal blood flow traverses the cortex, 10% perfuses the outer medulla, and 1% the medulla and papilla

Blood flow to the kidney is equivalent to perfusion pressure (systemic arterial pressure) divided by renal vascular resistance. Afferent and efferent arteriolar tone provide the bulk of renal vascular resistance and these vessels exert predominant control over renal blood flow (Carmines et al. 1987). When assessed by micropuncture techniques, pre- and postglomerular resistances are approximately equal in normal dogs and cats (Brown et al. 1990; Brown and Brown 1995).

Glomerular filtration

Formation of glomerular filtrate occurs as a result of Starling forces in the glomerular capillary bed; these determinants of glomerular filtration have been quantitatively evaluated in dogs and cats (Table 2.1) (Brown et al. 1990; Brown and Brown 1995). The filtration barrier is composed of three layers: fenestrated endothelium, anionic basement membrane, and podocyte slit diaphragm. Recent advances in our understanding of podocyte biology and molecular structure (e.g., discovery of nephrin) emphasize its previously underappreciated importance in health and disease (Barisoni et al. 2009; Hauser et al. 2009). Although plasma protein concentration averages 6–8 g/100 mL, the filtration barrier is believed to result in a protein content of filtrate that rarely exceeds 10 mg/100 mL, and the colloid osmotic pressure within the filtrate is so small that its contribution to the filtration process is negligible. Recently, it has been suggested that filtrate may contain more protein then previously thought, though this hypothesis remains unproven (Comper et al. 2008). The process of glomerular filtration is still generally accepted as being driven by glomerular capillary hydrostatic pressure and opposed by both plasma colloid osmotic pressure and Bowman's capsule hydrostatic pressure.

Nephrology and Urology of Small Animals. Edited by Joe Bartges and David J. Polzin. © 2011 Blackwell Publishing Ltd.

Table 2.1 Representative values for forces controlling renal fluid and solute movement in cats (Brown and Brown 1995)

Glomerular filtration	
Hydrostatic pressures (mmHg):	
Glomerular capillary pressure	59
Bowman's space	18
Difference (ΔP; favors filtration)	41
Colloid osmotic pressures (mmHg):	
Glomerular	22
Bowman's space	0
Difference ($\Delta\pi$; opposes filtration)	22
Mean filtration pressure	
$\Delta P - \Delta\pi = (41 - 22)$ mmHg $= 19$ mmHg	
Tubular reabsorption	
Hydrostatic pressures (mmHg):	
Peritubular capillary pressure	10
Interstitial space	(−5)
Difference (ΔP; opposes reabsorption)	15
Colloid osmotic pressures (mmHg):	
Peritubular capillary	35
Interstitial space	5
Difference ($\Delta\pi$; favors reabsorption)	30
Mean reabsorptive pressure	
$\Delta\pi - \Delta P = (30 - 15)$ mmHg $= 15$ mmHg	

Mechanisms controlling renal blood flow and glomerular filtration

The driving force for glomerular filtration rate, glomerular capillary hydrostatic pressure, is controlled by the relative resistance of the afferent and efferent arterioles (Carmines et al. 1987). While constriction of either type of arteriole tends to reduce renal blood flow, afferent arteriolar constriction tends to reduce glomerular capillary pressure and filtration rate and efferent arteriolar constriction tends to increase glomerular capillary pressure and thus glomerular filtration rate. As glomerular capillary pressure drives the formation of glomerular filtrate, the relative tone of these arterioles can contribute to the regulation of glomerular filtration rate. The relative tone of the afferent and efferent arterioles affects the proportion of glomerular plasma that is filtered, referred to as the filtration fraction. On a whole organ basis, filtration fraction is equal to glomerular filtration rate divided by renal plasma flow, and it averages 0.25–0.35 in normal dogs and cats. For example, a decline in efferent arteriolar tone will increase renal plasma flow but may decrease glomerular filtration rate, causing a decrease in filtration fraction. However, the relationship between arteriolar tone and filtration fraction is complex (Carmines et al.

1987). Most vasoactive compounds affecting renal blood flow and glomerular filtration rate act by altering the relative or absolute tone of these arterioles.

Beyond effects of changes in arteriolar tone, additional local control of the filtration process is provided by glomerular mesangial cells, which possess actin and myosin contractile filaments (Ennulat and Brown 1997). The main effect of mesangial cellular contraction is believed to be a reduction in the glomerular capillary surface area and/or the glomerular wall's permeability to water, which reduces glomerular filtration rate. The mesangial cells contract in response to several hormones and other vasoactive substances, such as angiotensin II.

A central concept of renal hemodynamics is that renal blood flow and glomerular filtration rate tends to remain constant despite variations in mean systemic arterial pressure between 75 and 160 mmHg in dogs and cats (Brown et al. 1995). This capacity is referred to as renal autoregulation because it occurs in the denervated, isolated perfused kidney and is thus an intrinsic property of the kidney. Whole kidney and single nephron glomerular filtration rate and glomerular capillary pressure are also autoregulated. The tone of preglomerular vessels alters glomerular capillary pressure and perfusion rate similarly and thus the vascular site primarily responsible for autoregulatory adjustments is the afferent arteriole.

Tubular reabsorption

Due to the formation of glomerular filtrate, there is a large decrease in hydrostatic pressure and increase in oncotic pressure in the peritubular capillary (Table 2.1). Physical factors play an important role in regulating total solute and water reabsorption. For example, extracellular fluid volume expansion causes fluid to accumulate in the interstitium, thereby lowering interstitial colloid osmotic pressure and raising interstitial hydrostatic pressure. Both changes act to inhibit tubular solute and water reabsorption, with the resultant diuresis and natriuresis returning extracellular fluid volume toward normal. Conversely, volume contraction (e.g., dehydration) has the opposite effects, appropriately enhancing renal reabsorption of salt and water.

Although more than 100 L of glomerular filtrate is formed daily by the average normal dog, less than 1% of this ultimately becomes urine. Due to the large quantity of water and electrolytes in the filtrate, tubular reabsorption is essential for the maintenance of homeostasis (Table 2.2). The reabsorptive process is arranged axially along the nephrons, with proximal reabsorptive processes occurring in an isotonic manner without regard to body needs utilizing high-capacity, low-affinity transport systems. As fluid progresses along the length of

Table 2.2 Renal solute and water handling[a]

Molecule	Sites of transport (normal renal handling)	Factors affecting renal handling
Conserved solutes		
Glucose	Proximal tubule (>99% reabsorption)	Glucosuria results from filtered load exceeding tubular transport maximum.
		Plasma glucose concentration at which glucosuria first occurs is referred to as the renal threshold for glucosuria, which is approximately 180–200 mg/100 mL in normal dogs and 290 mg/100 mL in normal cats.[25]
		Glucosuria due to reduced tubular transport capacity may be acquired or congenital and may be selective (renal glucosuria) or associated with generalized proximal tubular reabsorptive defects (e.g., Fanconi syndrome).
Amino acids	Proximal tubule (>99% reabsorption)	Family of transporters
		Aminoaciduria almost always due to reduced transport capacity, which may be selective (e.g., cystinuria) or generalized (e.g., Fanconi syndrome).
		Felininuria is normal in cats.
Balanced solutes[b]		
Sodium	Proximal and distal tubule, loop of Henle (>99% reabsorption)	2/3 reabsorbed in proximal tubule without regard to body needs.
		Na–K–2Cl cotransport in loop, inhibited by loop diuretics, contributes to medullary hypertonicity.
		Distal reabsorption enhanced by aldosterone.
		Proximal reabsorption enhanced by angiotensin II and inhibited by atrial natriuretic factor.
Potassium	Proximal and distal tubule (60–90% reabsorption)	2/3 reabsorbed in proximal tubule without regard to body needs.
		Distal secretion enhanced by aldosterone, diuresis, and the presence of anions (e.g., bicarbonate).
Phosphate	Proximal tubule (80–90% reabsorption)	Proximal reabsorption inhibited by parathyroid hormone.
Calcium	Proximal tubule (>90% reabsorption; widely variable, according to body needs)	Only ionized and chelated fractions are freely filtered (~50% of total plasma calcium); remainder is protein bound.
		Reabsorption enhanced by parathyroid hormone.
		Reabsorption inhibited by loop diuretics, enhanced by thiazide diuretics.
Bicarbonate	Proximal tubule (>99% reabsorption)	Proximal tubule reabsorption in accordance with body needs; reabsorption generally complete in dogs and cats on an animal protein diet; vegetable protein diet and/or dietary alkalinization may lead to appropriate bicarbonaturia and alkaluria.
Protons	Distal tubule and collecting duct (widely variable, according to body needs)	Secreted in proximal and distal tubule
		Proximal secretion leads to bicarbonate reabsorption.
		Distal proton secretion alters final urine pH and results in formation of titratable acid (combination with phosphate) or ammonium ion.

Table 2.2 *(Continued)*

Molecule	Sites of transport (normal renal handling)	Factors affecting renal handling
Excreted Solutes		
Uremic toxins	Variable	Most are freely filtered unless protein bound.
		Tubular reabsorption and/or secretion occurs for some.
Creatinine	Proximal tubule in dogs	Freely filtered
		Some proximal tubular secretion in dogs, especially males or dogs with kidney disease.
		No tubular transport in cats.
Urea	Loop of Henle and collecting duct	Tubular reabsorption and secretion occur.
		Renal excretion directly related to tubular flow rate.
Organic molecules	Proximal tubule	Family of transporters
		Net secretion
Renal water handling		
Water	All tubular segments (>99% reabsorption)	Water is freely filtered.
		Dramatic excess is filtered (3–4 mL/min/kg or approximately 5 L/kg per day).
		Reabsorption of 85% of filtered load is obligate, without regard to body need, occurring in the proximal tubule, loops of Henle, and early distal tubule.
		Reabsorption of remaining 15% is regulated by antidiuretic hormone (ADH), whose release is controlled primarily (90% of control) by extracellular fluid osmolarity and secondarily (10% of control) by blood volume.
		ADH causes insertion of aquaporin-2 water channels in the luminal membrane of epithelial cells in the late distal tubule and principal cells of the collecting ducts.
		Water is reabsorbed by osmosis, dependent on high medullary interstitial concentrations of Na, Cl, and urea.
		Chronic ADH stimulation causes increased expression of urea transporters in the distal collecting duct, enhancing interstitial urea concentration and maximal urinary concentrating capacity.

[a]All listed solutes and water are freely filtered, unless protein bound.
[b]For balanced solutes, normal reabsorptive rates vary according to body balance.

the tubule, reabsorption occurs in accordance with body needs through low-capacity, high-affinity transport processes. For conserved solutes, such as glucose and amino acids, this entire process of reabsorption occurs in the proximal tubule, and all (>99%) of the filtered solute is normally removed from the tubular fluid. For other solutes, such as sodium, the bulk (2/3) of filtered solute is reabsorbed in the proximal tubule, with the amount present in the urine being adjusted according to body needs in the distal tubule and collecting duct. Many hormones have effects on these tubular reabsorptive processes.

The fraction of the filtered solute that ultimately appears in urine is termed the fractional excretion (%), or fractional clearance, of a solute: (Brown et al. 1995)

$$\text{Fractional excretion (\%)} = \frac{100 \times \text{urine volume} \times [\text{solute}]u}{\text{GFR} \times [\text{solute}]p}$$

Here, $[\text{solute}]p$ and $[\text{solute}]u$ represent the concentrations of solute in plasma and urine, respectively, and GFR is the glomerular filtration rate. Some freely filtered solutes, glucose and amino acids, require metabolic energy to produce and these are conserved in the kidney, with near complete reabsorption of filtered load (>99%) by the end of the proximal tubule. Thus, for glucose and amino acids, the fractional excretion is normally <1% (Kruth and Cowgill 1982). Normal fractional excretion values for balanced solutes depend on body needs for maintenance of homeostasis. For example, if a dog's ration were switched from a low-salt (e.g., 0.2% sodium) to a normal-salt (e.g., 0.6% sodium) diet, urinary fractional excretion for sodium would be expected to increase threefold in order to maintain balance. This would be a normal homeostatic response, not a defect in the reabsorption of sodium. Hence, interpretation of values for fractional excretion rates for balanced solutes (i.e., sodium, potassium, calcium, phosphate, magnesium, and bicarbonate) requires knowledge of the animal's solute balance, which can be profoundly affected by dietary intake, fluid therapy, and other factors.

Some clinical utility may be obtained from calculation of fractional excretion of a given solute obtained from a single urine sample, according to the following formula:

$$\text{Fractional excretion } (\%)$$
$$= \frac{100 \times [\text{creatinine}]p \times [\text{solute}]u}{[\text{creatinine}]u \times [\text{solute}]p}$$

However, there are several limitations to the single sample or spot determination of fractional excretion. Because of variations in normal values for plasma creatinine concentration, plasma creatinine concentration provides only a crude reflection of glomerular filtration rate. Fluctuations in urinary excretion of solutes related to food intake or circadian rhythms are generally not time averaged by such single sample determinations.

Renal contribution to acid–base homeostasis

Bicarbonate freely passes the filtration barrier and reabsorption is according to body needs for maintenance of acid–base homeostasis. Bicarbonate reabsorption in the proximal tubule can be inhibited by volume expansion, alkalemia, parathyroid hormone, and carbon dioxide. It is stimulated by potassium depletion, elevated luminal pH, and increased glomerular filtration rate. Bicarbonate reabsorption in the proximal tubule of normal dogs and cats fed an animal protein diet is complete (>99%) and, unlike most electrolytes, there are several mechanisms contributing to control of bicarbonate reabsorption in the proximal tubules.

Although the addition of alkalinizing agents (e.g., sodium bicarbonate, potassium citrate, or calcium carbonate) or the ingestion of a vegetable- or cereal-based diet may have a net alkalinizing effect, cats and dogs ingesting a meat-based diet must usually generate acidic urine to maintain acid–base balance. Proton secretion by the distal tubules and collecting ducts is responsible for the final adjustment urine pH and maintenance of body acid–base balance. Protons secreted into the distal tubular lumen combine with ammonia and phosphate, which act as urinary buffers resulting in the production of the ammonium ion and titratable acid (phosphate), two nonreabsorbed solutes.

Abnormalities of renal acid–base handling occur in a variety of renal diseases. Because dogs and cats usually ingest a diet that leads to metabolic generation of acid, renal diseases are more commonly associated with acidosis than alkalosis in these species. Renal acidosis may be due to a tubular defect in bicarbonate reabsorption (proximal renal tubular acidosis), tubular defect in proton secretion (distal renal tubular acidosis), or a reduced overall capacity for proton secretion due to loss of functional renal mass (uremic acidosis) (DiBartola 2000).

Water reabsorption—the urine concentrating mechanism

Extracellular fluid volume and plasma osmolality are regulated by the kidneys. This regulation is dependent upon control of renal water excretion in accordance with body needs (Table 2.2). The loop of Henle plays a vital role in water homeostasis. In particular, the thick portion of the ascending limb reabsorbs solute via luminal Na–K–2Cl cotransport driven by the Na electrochemical gradient created by the Na–K ATPase in the basolateral membrane (Boone and Deen 2008; Halperin et al. 2008). This solute reabsorption causes a progressive decrease in tubular fluid tonicity and leading to tubular fluid hypotonicity in the early distal tubule. Urea also contributes to the urine concentrating mechanism by passively concentrating in the medullary interstitium under the influence of antidiuretic hormone. Urea movement through various portions of the nephron is facilitated by diffusion through carriers belonging to a family of urea transporters (Bagnasco 2005).In the absence of further water transport, dilute (hypotonic) urine is produced. Distal tubular fluid is more hypotonic in normal canine kidneys and, thus, can produce a more maximally dilute urine than in cats.However, if antidiuretic hormone is released from the posterior pituitary in response to an increase in plasma osmolarity or a low extracellular fluid volume as detected by low pressure baroreceptors, it will bind to receptors on the basolateral membrane of principal cells of the distal tubule and collecting duct and stimulate adenyl cyclase enzyme activity. This effect of antidiuretic hormone increases intracellular levels of cyclic adenosine monophosphate, which subsequently enhances water permeability through the incorporation of aquaporin-2 water channels in the luminal membrane (Boone and Deen 2008; Halperin et al. 2008). In the presence of antidiuretic hormones, water will be passively reabsorbed along the osmotic gradient provided by the medullary hypertonicity. Antidiuretic hormones also upregulate urea transporter activity in the distal collecting duct. This effect is gradual, requiring days to be fully manifest, and its absence contributes to the loss of urinary concentrating ability associated with chronic polyuria with low ADH levels.

Renal endocrine functions

The kidney is responsible for secretion of a variety of autocrine, paracrine, and endocrine factors and is responsive to many of these factors as well as other hormones. These play a vital role in renal regulation of extracellular fluid.

Renin–angiotensin–aldosterone system (Lefebvre et al. 2007; Fyhrquist and Saijonmaa 2008)

Renin is released into afferent arteriolar plasma from the granular cells of the juxtaglomerular apparatus in response to various stimuli, including a decline in systemic arterial pressure and direct sympathetic stimulation. Renin cleaves a ten amino acid fragment from angiotensinogen (a globulin produced by the liver, which is also known as renin substrate). This peptide fragment is termed angiotensin I. Angiotensin-converting enzyme, present on the surface of vascular endothelial cells and elsewhere, cleaves a terminal two amino acid fragment from angiotensin I, converting it to angiotensin II. The latter two compounds (angiotensin I and II) have short half-lives, generally <1 min.

There are other cleavage products (i.e., the heptapeptides angiotensin III and IV), but angiotensin II is generally held to be the most important product and is a potent vasoconstrictor for systemic arterioles that increases renal vascular resistance in efferent (preferentially) and afferent arterioles. Although there is a family of cell membrane receptors, the type 1 receptor (AT1) mediates most known effects of angiotensin II (Aplin et al. 2009). Angiotensin II also augments proximal tubular reabsorption of sodium and release of aldosterone from the adrenal cortex, which subsequently enhances distal tubular sodium reabsorption. Overall effects of angiotensin II include an increase in systemic arterial blood pressure (secondary to the increase in total peripheral resistance and blood volume) and an increase in glomerular capillary pressure (secondary to the increases in efferent arteriolar tone and systemic arterial blood pressure). Angiotensin II may decrease, increase, or have little effect on the glomerular filtration rate, depending on the pre-existing physiological state of the animal. The kidney, as well as several other tissues of the body, contains all of the components necessary to generate angiotensin II locally. This local rennin–angiotensin system may be more important than the classic systemic rennin–angiotensin system, as measurement of angiotensin II concentrations have suggested that intrarenal levels of this compound may exceed systemic concentrations by 1,000-fold.

Erythropoietin

Erythropoietin is essential for the growth of erythroid stem cells and the rate of red blood cell production is largely determined by serum erythropoietin concentrations. The primary (90%) site of erythropoietin production in adult animals is the kidney, largely renal cortical peritubular fibroblasts. In the adult, erythropoietin production is inversely related to oxygen availability in the kidney. Hypoxia-inducible factors (HIFs), which are constitutively expressed transcription factors, are modified and degraded in the presence of oxygen (Nangaku and Eckardt 2007). When renal cortical oxygen tension is reduced, accumulated HIFs activate a signaling cascade that leads to enhanced erythropoietin production and release. Erythropoietin production is affected by a variety of kidney diseases, including those with complete or localized renal ischemia (enhanced production) and chronic kidney diseases (Cowgill et al. 1998) with generalized loss of functional renal tissue (reduced production). There are a variety of commercially available preparations that permit administration of exogenous erythropoietin as well as related erythropoiesis stimulating agents with longer half-lives, such as darbopoietin and continuous erythropoietin receptor activator (CERA). Besides their effect to enhance red blood cell production, erythropoietin and related compounds have a variety of other functions, including a supportive effect on cellular metabolism, positive effects on angiogenesis and vascular tone, and a neuroprotective effect. The effect on vascular tone may raise blood pressure in animals receiving exogenous erythropoietin and erythropoietin-like compounds.

Renal eicosanoids

Eicosanoids (prostaglandins, thromboxanes, and leukotrienes) are derived locally from cell membrane phospholipids and have many effects on the renal vasculature. Vasodilatory prostaglandins (prostaglandins E2 and I2) are opposed by the vasoconstrictive effects of thromboxane A2 and leukotrienes (Brown et al. 2000; Giovanni and Giovanni 2002). Although apparently having unimportant effects on renal function in normal animals, vasodilatory prostaglandins can be important for the maintenance of renal blood flow and glomerular filtration rate when renal hemodynamics are compromised. These are referred to as high-renin states, which include dehydration, anesthesia, renal failure, converting enzyme inhibition, and urinary tract obstruction. Both normal and diseased kidneys contain constitutively expressed cyclooxygenase-1 and cyclooxygenase-2 activities, explaining why cyclooxygenase-nonselective and cyclooxygenase-2 selective agents can have effects

Table 2.3 Homeostatic renal functions

Function	Important regulatory mechanisms
Volume regulation	Antidiuretic hormone controls extracellular fluid osmolarity by regulating water excretion via urinary concentrating mechanism.
Blood pressure regulation	Changes in blood pressure are opposed by altering NaCl excretion (pressure natriuresis)
	Renin–angiotensin–aldosterone, controlled by intrarenal mechanisms, contributes to blood pressure regulation through vasoconstriction and enhancement of sodium reabsorption in proximal (angiotensin II-mediated) and distal (aldosterone-mediated) sites.
Red cell production	Erythropoietin release regulated in response to changes in intrarenal oxygen tension.
Acid–base balance	Bicarbonate reabsorption (proximal tubule) and proton secretion (distal tubule) regulated in accordance with acid–base status of animal.
Electrolyte and mineral homeostasis	Total body content and extracellular fluid concentration of Na, Cl, K, Mg, and P controlled by renal mechanisms with hormonal influences.
	Calcium homeostasis is regulated by interactions of intestinal tract, vitamin D, parathyroid hormone, and the kidney.
	See Table 2.2.
Excretion of metabolic wastes	Uremic toxin removal is dependent on glomerular filtration and tubular reabsorption.
	High tubular flow rates enhance excretion of many of these molecules by limiting reabsorption.

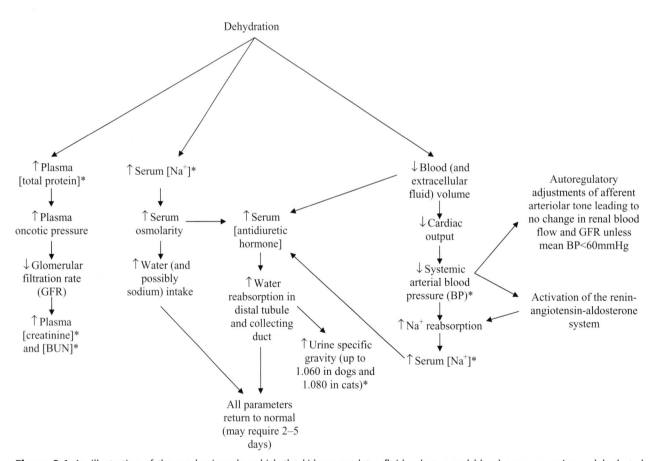

Figure 2.1 An illustration of the mechanisms by which the kidney regulates fluid volumes and blood pressure, using a dehydrated patient as an example. The rennin–angiotensin–aldosterone system also helps to sustain systemic arterial blood pressure through vasoconstrictive effects, though this is a temporary effect that does not act to return other altered parameters to normal. See text for further explanation. *Parameters that may be readily assessed in a clinical patient.

on renal function during high-renin states (Giovanni and Giovanni 2002).

Renal innervation

Both nonmyelinated and myelinated nerve fibers are found in the kidneys, which are predominantly alpha-adrenergic sympathetic fibers. These fibers enter the renal parenchyma with the renal arterial branches and innervate the renal arterioles, tubular epithelium, and juxtaglomerular apparatus. In a normal dog or cat at rest, renal nerves are believed to have only a small influence on glomerular filtration rate and renal blood flow. During extreme exercise or pathophysiological states (e.g., congestive heart failure or systemic hypotension), increased sympathetic nerve activity may be responsible for a decrease in renal blood flow and glomerular filtration rate and enhanced release of renin. Renal nerve activity may also be important in the genesis and/or maintenance of systemic hypertension through a variety of tubular and vascular effects, (Blankestijn 2007) though little is known about this phenomenon in dogs and cats.

Other renal hormones

Two compounds, endothelin and endothelium derived relaxing factor (nitric oxide or a related compound), are released by vascular endothelial cells to produce either marked, prolonged contraction (endothelin) (Barton 2008) or relaxation (endothelium derived relaxing factor) (McCarthy et al. 2008) of vascular smooth muscle, with particularly important effects on the renal arterioles. Atrial natriuretic factor, a peptide released from atrial myocytes in response to distention, causes an increase in renal blood flow, glomerular filtration rate, and urinary sodium excretion. Vasodilatory effects of atrial natriuretic factor apparently occur at the afferent arteriole.

Renal homeostatic functions

The individual renal functions described above permit the kidney to regulate blood volume, extracellular fluid volume, systemic arterial blood pressure, hematocrit, acid–base balance, and plasma concentrations of electrolytes, minerals, and metabolic waste products (Table 2.3). Of particular importance in clinical patients, the kidney regulates blood and extracellular fluid volume indirectly through a complex interaction of renal sodium and water handling and glomerular filtration that involves a central role for antidiuretic hormone (Figure 2.1).

References

Aplin, M., M.M. Bonde, et al. (2009). Molecular determinants of angiotensin II type 1 receptor functional selectivity. *J Mol Cell Cardiol* **46**: 15–24.

Bagnasco, S.M. (2005). Role and regulation of urea transporters. *Pflugers Arch* **450**: 217–226.

Barisoni, L., H.W. Schnaper, et al. (2009). Advances in the biology and genetics of the podocytopathies: implications for diagnosis and therapy. *Arch Pathol Lab Me* **133**: 201–216.

Barton, M. (2008). Reversal of proteinuric renal disease and the emerging role of endothelin. *Nat Clin Pract Nephrol* **4**: 490–501.

Blankestijn, P.J. (2007). Sympathetic hyperactivity–a hidden enemy in chronic kidney disease patients. *Perit Dial Int* **27**: S293–S297.

Boone, M. and P.M. Deen (2008). Physiology and pathophysiology of the vasopressin-regulated renal water reabsorption. *Pflugers Arch* **456**: 1005–1024.

Bovee, K.C. and G.D. Webster (1972). Values for intrarenal distribution of blood flow using xenon 133 in the anesthetized dog. *Am J Vet Res* **33**: 501–510.

Brown, S., D. Finco, et al. (1990). Single nephron adaptations to partial renal ablation in dogs. *Am J Physiol* **258**: F495–F503.

Brown, S.A. and C.A. Brown (1995). Single nephron adaptations to partial renal ablation in cats. *Am J Physiol* **269**: R1002–R1008.

Brown, S.A., C. Brown, et al. (2000). Effect of dietary fatty acid supplementation in early renal insufficiency in dogs. *J Lab Clin Med* **135**: 275–286.

Brown, S.A., D.R. Finco, et al. (1995). Impaired renal autoregulatory ability in dogs with reduced renal mass. *J Am Soc Nephrol* **5**: 1768–1774.

Carmines, P.K., et al. (1987). Effects of preglomerular and postglomerular vascular resistance alterations on filtration fraction. *Kidney Int* **31**: S229–S235.

Comper, W.D., B. Haraldsson, et al. (2008). Normal glomeruli filter nephrotic levels of albumin. *J Am Soc Nephrol* **19**: 427–432.

Cowgill, L.D., K.M. James, et al. (1998). Use of recombinant human erythropoietin for management of anemia in dogs and cats with renal failure. *J Am Vet Med Asso.* **212**: 521–528.

DiBartola, S.P. (2000). Clinical approach and laboratory evaluation of renal disease. In: *Textbook of Veterinary Internal Medicine*, edited by S.J. Ettinger and E. Feldman. Philadelphia: Saunders, pp. 1600–1614.

Ennulat, D. and S.A. Brown (1997). Effects of growth factors on canine and equine mesangial cell proliferation. *Am J Vet Res* **58**: 1308–1313.

Fyhrquist, F. and O. Saijonmaa (2008). Renin-angiotensin system revisited. *J Intern Med* **264**: 224–236.

Giovanni, G. and P. Giovanni (2002). Do non-steroidal anti-inflammatory drugs and COX-2 selective inhibitors have different renal effects? *J Nephrol* **15**: 480–488.

Halperin, M.L., K.S. Kamel, et al. (2008). Mechanisms to concentrate the urine. *Curr Opin Nephrol Hypertens* **17**: 416–422.

Hauser, P.V., F. Collino, et al. (2009). Nephrin and endothelial injury. *Curr Opin Nephrol Hypertens* **18**: 3–8.

Kruth, S.A. and L.D. Cowgill (1982). Renal glucose transport in the cat. *Proceedings*, American College of Veterinary Internal Medicine Scientific Forum, San Diego, p. 78 (abstract).

Laing, C.M. and R.J. Unwin (2008). Renal tubular acidosis. *J Nephrol* **19**: S46–S52.

Lefebvre, H., S. Brown, et al. (2007). Angiotensin-converting enzyme inhibitors in veterinary medicine. *Curr Pharm Des* **13**: 1347–1361.

McCarthy, H.O., J.A. Coulter, et al. (2008). Gene therapy via inducible nitric oxide synthase: a tool for the treatment of a diverse range of pathological conditions. *J Pharmacol* **60**: 999–1017.

Nangaku, M. and K.U. Eckardt (2007). Hypoxia and the HIF system in kidney disease. *J Mol Med* **85**: 1325–1330.

3

Anatomy of the lower urogenital tract

Thomas F. Fletcher and Christina E. Clarkson

The lower urinary tract consists of the urinary bladder and urethra plus the caudal segment of each ureter. The three functional components of the lower urinary tract are determined ultimately by innervation (Fletcher et al. 2010):

- *Detrusor muscle*, which expels urine, is the smooth muscle coat of the bladder apex and body.
- *Smooth muscle sphincter* (internal urethral sphincter) consists of the muscle coat of the bladder neck and cranial urethra.
- *Striated urethral sphincter* (external urethral sphincter) is the urethralis muscle that encircles the caudal urethra.

Blood supply to the lower urinary tract is delivered by the internal iliac artery. One of its branches, the umbilical artery, supplies cranial vesical arteries to the apex of the bladder. Another branch, the internal pudendal artery, terminates in the vestibule/penis. Before terminating, the artery gives off a vaginal/prostatic branch that supplies blood to the bladder (caudal vesical arteries) and urethra (Evans 1993).

Urinary bladder

The position of the urinary bladder depends on its volume. An empty contracted bladder may be tucked into the pelvic cavity. A full bladder can extend cranially to the level of the umbilicus. The bladder is coated by visceral peritoneum. Three ligaments run from the bladder surface to parietal peritoneum: The ventral median ligament connects along the ventral midline of the abdominal wall as far cranially as the umbilicus; in the neonate, it con-

tains the urachus or its remnant. The lateral ligament of the urinary bladder is bilateral. The ureter and umbilical artery run in the lateral ligament.

Three urinary bladder regions are defined (Figure 3.1):

- The *apex* is the cranial blind end.
- The *neck* is the funnel-shaped region located between ureter openings and the urethra.
- The *body* is the region situated between the neck and apex.

Each ureter passes obliquely through the bladder wall and terminates in a slit opening at the cranial margin of the vesical neck. The oblique intramural passage plus intramural tension produced by intravesical pressure combine to close the terminal ureter to preclude urine reflux. The muscle coat of the ureter is mainly circular but inner and outer longitudinal fascicles are augmented in the terminal ureter. Outer fascicles are contributed by the bladder. Inner longitudinal muscle bundles continue into the bladder trigone.

The bladder trigone is evident as triangular smooth mucosa on the dorsal internal wall of the bladder neck. The trigone attaches ureters to the bladder neck and urethra. The cranial border of the trigone is formed by longitudinal muscle fascicles from each ureter crossing the midline. The lateral borders and apex are formed by the ureter's longitudinal muscle that continues caudally into the urethral crest (Figure 3.2).

Like the ureter, the urinary bladder is lined by transitional epithelium. The epithelium is bacteriostatic by virtue of a glycosaminoglycan secretion that impairs bacterial adhesion to the epithelium (Gasser and Madsen 1993). A rich capillary plexus is present immediately deep to the transitional epithelium in the lamina propria region of the mucosa. The presence of a muscularis mucosae between lamina propria and submucosa is

Nephrology and Urology of Small Animals. Edited by Joe Bartges and David J. Polzin. © 2011 Blackwell Publishing Ltd.

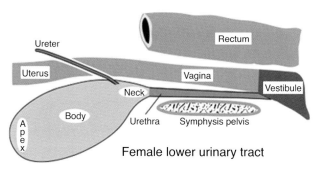

Figure 3.1 Cartoon of a female lower urinary tract and related pelvic viscera. The urinary bladder has three regions: apex, body, and neck. The urethra conveys urine from the bladder to the floor of the vestibule.

inconsistent. When empty, bladder mucosa and submucosa exhibits folds that disappear during distension.

The smooth muscle coat of the apex and body of the bladder constitutes the detrusor muscle. Its muscle fascicles are variably organized rather than arranged in consistent layers. As the bladder distends, the muscle coat becomes thinner and individual muscle fascicles shift their positions relative to one another. With major distension, the general direction of detrusor fascicles shifts from an encompassing orientation toward a tangential one. As a result, the detrusor loses mechanical advantage for generating intravesical pressure as bladder volume expands and wall tension becomes tangential.

In contrast to the detrusor, the bladder neck has a sphincter function. The submucosa of the bladder neck is relatively rich in elastic fibers. Excepting longitudinal fascicles of the trigone, the muscle coat of the neck is composed predominantly of circular fascicles. The circular muscle fascicles of the neck continue into the urethra. Oblique muscle fascicles of the detrusor run onto the bladder neck in order to open it.

Female urethra

Unlike male urethrae, female urethrae are anatomically similar in dogs and cats (Cullen et al. 1981a, 1983b). The female urethra runs from the internal urethral orifice at the bladder neck to the external urethral orifice in the vestibule. The external orifice opens on the floor of the cranial vestibule in a urethral tubercle (dog) or as a groove (cat). The apparent vesicourethral junction can shift slightly because of funneling differences associated with different intravesical pressures.

Transitional epithelium lining the urethral lumen is 2–3 cells thick, thinner than in the bladder. Urethral epithelium gradually becomes stratified cuboidal in the middle of the urethra and stratified squamous at the terminal end of the urethra. The submucosa contains elastic fibers, more than in the bladder, and a stratum spongiosum (venous sinuses) that becomes more plentiful from cranial to caudal along the urethra (Figure 3.3).

The urethral muscle coat is smooth muscle in the cranial, two-thirds of the urethra and striated muscle in the caudal third. The muscle types overlap in the canine mid-urethra and further caudally in the cat. Urethral

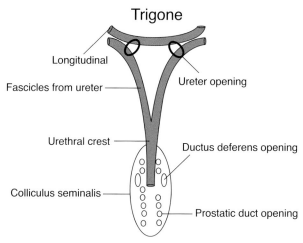

Figure 3.2 Schematic diagram of longitudinal muscle fascicles from the ureters giving rise to the trigone and urethral crest in a male. The muscle fascicles anchor the ureters to the bladder neck and urethra. The trigone is located on the inner surface of the dorsal wall of the bladder neck and the colliculus seminalis is located in the dorsal wall of the prostatic urethra.

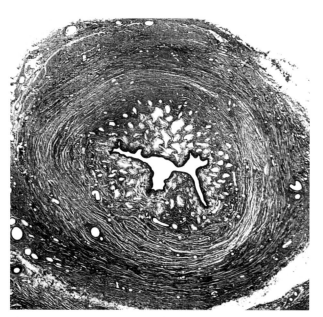

Figure 3.3 Transverse section through the caudal urethra of a bitch. The urethra was fixed by perfusion, so stratum spongiosum is clearly evident within the submucosa, which is surrounded by striated urethralis muscle. (From Cullen 1981a).

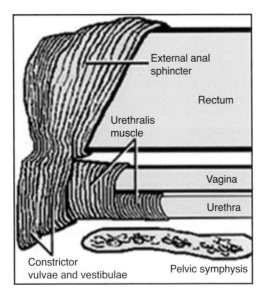

Figure 3.4 Cartoon showing that urethralis muscle initially encircles only the urethra but further caudally it encircles both urethra and vagina. (From Fletcher 1996).

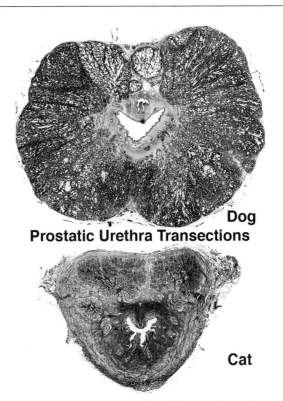

Figure 3.5 Transverse sections through prostatic urethrae of a dog (top) and a cat (below). In both cases, the prostate is bilobed, but it is smaller and restricted to the dorsal surface in the cat. Smooth muscle is significant only within trabeculae enclosing gland lobules. Fascicles of striated urethralis muscle are present ventrally in the feline section. (From Cullen 1981b and Cullen 1981a).

smooth muscle is predominantly circular in orientation, like the bladder neck. Longitudinal fascicles are significant only within the urethral crest. The crest is a dorsal submucosal ridge that typically runs the length of the female urethra.

Striated urethralis muscle (external urethral sphincter) entirely replaces smooth muscle in the distal third of the urethra. Urethralis muscle is relatively longer and thicker in the bitch than in the queen. The striated muscle completely encircles the urethra, and further caudally it encircles urethra and vagina together (Figure 3.4). By encircling both, the muscle effectively anchors the caudal end of the urethra to the more massive genital tract providing sphincter stability.

Male feline pelvic urethra

The urethra of the male cat runs through the pelvic canal (pelvic urethra) and continues into the penis (penile urethra). A small bi-lobed prostate gland is positioned in the middle of the pelvic urethra. The body of the prostate gland is a landmark for dividing the pelvic urethra into preprostatic, prostatic, and postprostatic divisions.

The preprostatic urethra extends from the bladder neck to the prostate gland and resembles the cranial half of the female urethra. The smooth muscle coat is mainly circular, like the bladder neck. Longitudinal fascicles from the trigone are evident dorsally in the urethral crest.

The prostatic urethra is ventral to the body of the prostate gland. The submucosa is rich in elastic fibers but generally deficient in smooth muscle. A bilateral opening

of each ductus deferens and numerous prostatic ducts are visible on the colliculus seminalis, a dorsal region of thickened submucosa (Figure 3.2).

The feline prostate gland consists of dorsally positioned bilateral lobes (Figure 3.5); each lobe is composed of lobules partitioned by trabeculae. Smooth muscle is present within trabeculae and as a thin coat on the surface of the prostate but smooth muscle does not surround the submucosa and lumen of the prostatic urethra. Postprostatic striated muscle fascicles coat the ventral surface of the prostatic urethra.

The postprostatic urethra runs from the body of the prostate gland to the root of the penis where paired bulbourethral glands are present in the cat. The postprostatic submucosa features a rich stratum spongiosum and disseminated glandular tissue (which stains like bulbourethral gland (Cullen et al. 1983a). Entirely replacing smooth muscle, the striated urethralis muscle forms a thick muscle coat encircling urethral submucosa. Striated fascicles also cover each bulbourethral gland, as bulboglandularis muscle (Martin et al. 1974).

Male canine pelvic urethra

The pelvic urethra of the male dog has two divisions: prostatic and postprostatic (membranous). A large bi-lobed prostate gland completely encircles the prostatic urethra (Figure 3.5). Within the prostate, the urethral lumen appears enlarged and a prominent colliculus seminalis occupies the dorsal submucosa.

The prostatic submucosa is rich in elastic fibers but lacks encircling smooth muscle (except for a short distance at the cranial edge of the prostatic urethra). Smooth muscle is associated principally with trabeculae that partition prostate lobules; it is sparse on the outer capsule of the prostate. Thus, in the prostatic urethra, smooth muscle is not structured for a urethral sphincter role; instead, it is designed to contract prostatic lobules. Thus, the smooth muscle sphincter in male dogs is restricted primarily to the bladder neck (Cullen et al. 1981a).

The canine postprostatic urethra features a thick coat of striated urethralis muscle. The muscle fascicles overlap the caudal surface of the prostate gland and they contact bulbospongiosus muscle at the ischial arch. There is not significant smooth muscle in the postprostatic urethra. Within the submucosa, islands of disseminate prostate gland are evident and a rich stratum spongiosum surrounds the urethral lumen (Cullen et al. 1981b).

Innervation

Although the ureter receives autonomic innervation, it is not functionally dependent on innervation. The bladder and urethra, however, require innervation to function effectively. They are innervated via bilateral pelvic plexuses (Oliver et al. 1969). Part of each pelvic plexus spills onto the caudal bladder as a vesical plexus. Nerves in the bladder wall are tortuous to accommodate distension.

Autonomic ganglia within pelvic plexuses contain both sympathetic and parasympathetic postganglionic neurons, predominantly the latter. Postganglionic axons are nonmyelinated. Their terminal branches have preterminal and terminal varicosities (enlargements) that contain synaptic vesicles (Fletcher et al. 1969). The vesicles release neurotransmitter molecules that diffuse variable distances and bind to receptors on myocytes. Distinct neuromuscular junctions are not evident.

Parasympathetic innervation to the detrusor muscle begins with preganglionic neurons located in intermediate gray matter of the sacral spinal cord (S_{1-3}). Axons reach the pelvic plexus via the pelvic nerve, which is a branch of the sacral portion of the lumbosacral plexus (Figure 3.6). Postganglionic neurons are within pelvic ganglia. Parasympathetic nerves release acetylcholine which leads to detrusor contraction.

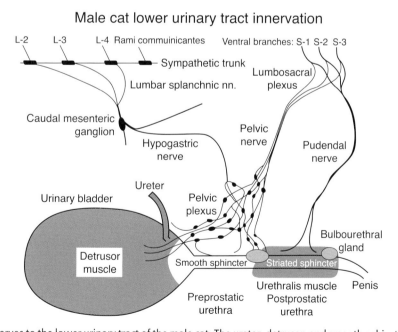

Male cat lower urinary tract innervation

Figure 3.6 Diagram of nerves to the lower urinary tract of the male cat. The ureter, detrusor, and smooth sphincter are supplied bilaterally by a pelvic plexus. Sympathetic innervation from the lumbar spinal cord reaches the plexus via the hypogastric nerve. Parasympathetic innervation from the sacral spinal cord reaches the plexus via the pelvic nerve. The striated urethralis muscle is innervated by axons of sacral somatic neurons that run in the pudendal nerve.

Sympathetic innervation to the bladder and urethra originates with preganglionic neurons located in the intermediolateral nucleus of the lumbar spinal cord (L_{2-4}). The preganglionic axons travel through lumbar splanchnic nerves to the caudal mesenteric ganglion where the majority synapse. The continuing pathway involves right/left hypogastric nerve and pelvic plexus. Sympathetic postganglionic axons release norepinephrine, which leads to contraction of smooth muscle in the bladder neck and urethra but inhibition of the detrusor (Janig and McLachlan 1987).

Somatic innervation of the urethralis muscle involves motor nuclei in the ventral horn of the sacral spinal cord ($S_{2,3}$). The axons travel through the sacral part of the lumbosacral plexus and pudendal nerve to release acetycholine at neuromuscular junctions of the urethralis muscle, as well as striated muscles of the anal canal and root of the penis. Somatic afferent activity from these muscles and from genitalia, anal canal, and skin of the perineum is also conveyed by the pudendal nerve.

Visceral afferent innervation starts with bladder free nerve endings and mostly nonmyelinated axons. The sensation of pain is conveyed by afferent axons with endings in the submucosa (Uemura et al. 1975). The axons travel through hypogastric nerves to the lumbar spinal cord. Pain afferents synapse on dorsal horn projection neurons that generally receive somatic afferent input also. Thus, bladder pain may be interpreted as coming from the body surface (referred pain). The spinothalamic tract is the ascending pain pathway.

The sense of bladder fullness that leads to micturition is conveyed by thin C and A-delta axons associated with slowly adapting mechanoreceptors within the muscle coat. The axons travel through the pelvic nerve to the sacral spinal cord where they synapse on projection neurons that send axons ventrally in the lateral funiculus to the midbrain, hypothalamus, and thalamus. (The same primary afferent neurons synapse on interneurons responsible for sympathetic spinal reflexes involving the smooth muscle sphincter.)

Several brain structures are concerned with micturition. In the dorsal pons, a medial pontine micturition center enables micturition by dispatching a descending pontospinal pathway through the ipsilateral ventral funiculus. Pathway axons excite parasympathetic preganglionic neurons that supply the detrusor and inhibit sphincter neurons. More lateral in the pons, a pontine continence center gives rise to axons that descend in the dorsal half of the lateral funiculus. The axons activate the striated urethral sphincter and pelvic diaphragm (Holstege et al. 1986).

Midbrain periaqueductal gray matter receives spinal input and forebrain input and communicates with pontine centers. The limbic system, including the hypothalamus, septum, amygdala, and cingulate cortex becomes involved because micturition timing is influenced by emotional status. Finally, the medial frontal cortex ultimately decides whether to urinate or not and so notifies the pons via the midbrain (Blok and Holstege 2001).

References

Blok, B.F.M. and G. Holstege (2001). The neural control of micturition and urinary continence. In: *The Urinary Sphincter*, edited by J. Corcos and E. Schick. New York: Marcel Dekker, pp. 89–99.

Cullen, W.C., et al. (1981a). Histology of the canine urethra. I. morphometry of the female urethra. *Anat Rec* **199**: 177–186.

Cullen, W.C., et al. (1981b). Histology of the canine urethra. II. morphometry of the male pelvic urethra. *Anat Rec* **199**: 187–195.

Cullen, W.C., et al. (1983a). Morphometry of the male feline pelvic urethra. *J Urol* **129**: 186–189.

Cullen, W.C., et al. (1983b). Morphometry of the female feline urethra. *J Urol* **129**: 190–193.

Evans, H.E. (1993). *Anatomy of the Dog*, 3rd edition. Philadelphia, PA: WB Saunders.

Fletcher, T.F. (1996). Applied anatomy and physiology of the feline lower urinary tract. In: *Veterinary Clinics of North America: Small Animal Practice*. Philadelphia, PA: WB Saunders, pp. 181–195.

Fletcher, T.F., et al. (1969). Nerve endings in the urinary bladder of the cat. *J Comp Neur* **136**: 1–20.

Fletcher, T.F., et al. (2010). *Lower Urinary Tract*. Available at: http://vanat.cvm.umn.edu/lut/.

Gasser, T.C. and P.O. Madsen (1993). Influence of urologic irrigation fluids on urothelial bacterial adherence. *Urol Res* **21**(6): 401–405.

Holstege, G., et al. (1986). Anatomical and physiological observations on supraspinal control of bladder and urethral sphincter muscles in the cat. *J Comp Neur* **250**: 449–461.

Janig, W. and E.M. McLachlan (1987). Organization of lumbar spinal outflow to distal colon and pelvic organs. *Physiol Rev* **67**(4): 1332–1400.

Martin, W.D., et al. (1974). Perineal musculature in the cat. *Anat Rec* **180**: 3–14.

Oliver Jr, J.E., et al. (1969). Spinal cord representation of the micturition reflex. *J Comp Neur* **137**: 329–346.

Uemura, E., et al. (1975). Distribution of lumbar and sacral afferent axons in submucosa of cat urinary bladder. *Anat Rec* **183**: 579–588.

Section 2
Diagnostic testing

4

Historical information and physical examination

Joe Bartges and David Polzin

The urinary system consists of kidneys, ureters, urinary bladder, and urethra, and is intimately associated with the genital system. The upper urinary tract comprises the kidneys and ureters; the lower urinary tract comprises the bladder and urethra. Diseases of the urinary tract are common in dogs and cats and may involve individual parts, multiple sites, or the entire urinary system. Diagnostic evaluation of dogs and cats with urinary tract diseases begins with historical data collection and physical examination.

History and signalment

The historical evaluation should include information on frequency of urination, volume of urine produced, changes in water intake, appearance and odor of urine, and the presence or absence of polysystemic signs of disease. General information should also be gathered including vaccination and heartworm status, possible exposure to infectious agents or toxins, appetite, energy level, changes in behavior, etc.

Polydipsia is defined as excessive thirst and is more easily recognized by owners than is polyuria. Polyuria is defined as passage of abnormally large quantity of urine. Asking owners to measure intake can be attempted, but is usually unsuccessful because animals may consume water not observed by owners such as out of toilets or sinks, puddles outside, or even their own urine. Normally, water consumption is 5–30 mL/kg per day; however, it is dependent on composition of diet (i.e., dry versus canned diet, salt content of diet, etc.). Polydipsia is defined as water intake of greater than 100 mL/kg per day including water from food and water that is directly consumed. Owners

may recognize polyuria by decreased color or odor of urine, increased time while voiding, or larger clumps of litter in boxes. Normal urine production is 10–60 mL/kg per day; cats consuming dry formulated diets often urinate 5–10 mL/kg per day. Polyuria is defined as urine production exceeding 50 mL/kg per day (see Chapter 42).

Pollakiuria refers to excessively frequent urination and must be differentiated from polyuria (see Chapter 47). Pollakiuria is often associated with other signs of lower urinary tract disease such as stranguria (slow and painful urination) and dysuria (difficult urination). Pollakiuria must also be differentiated from constipation where attempts at defecation are mistaken for attempts at urination. Anuresis (inability to pass urine) may result from urinary outflow obstruction or to inability of the urinary bladder to contract, and may also be confused with constipation. Periuria is defined as urinating in inappropriate locations (i.e., outside of the litter box, on the carpet, etc.). It may occur with polyuric states or with lower urinary tract disease. Enuresis refers to urinary incontinence especially occurring at night or during periods of relaxation. It may occur with or independent of periuria. Hematuria refers to red blood cells (hemorrhage) in urine, and can be present with many diseases of the upper and lower urinary tract (see Chapter 46).

Collection of historical information from owners should include information on diet fed, frequency of feeding, possible exposure to toxins, and medications administered. Many owners do not consider over-the-counter medications as "drugs" or nutriceuticals or supplements as potentially harmful, although some may be, particularly if given inappropriately (e.g., ibuprofen to dogs).

Signalment of the animal may help suggest more likely diagnoses and direct diagnostic evaluation. Congenital anatomic disease (see Chapters 56 and 80) is more

Nephrology and Urology of Small Animals. Edited by Joe Bartges and David J. Polzin. © 2011 Blackwell Publishing Ltd.

common in pediatric or young adult animals, whereas neoplasia occurs more commonly in older animals. Renal failure (see Chapter 48) occurs more commonly in older animals, but nephrotic syndrome occurs more commonly in young to middle-aged adult animals. Bacterial urinary tract infections occur more commonly in female dogs than in male dogs, and occur uncommonly in cats (see Chapters 71 and 72). Prostatomegaly in a dog that has been castrated more than six months prior to discovery suggests neoplasia, whereas benign prostatic hypertrophy is more likely if the dog is reproductively intact (see Chapters 78 and 79).

Physical examination

A complete physical examination is a routine part of patient evaluation. With suspected or confirmed urinary tract disease, the physical examination should also include a rectal examination and an ocular fundic examination. Hydration status is evaluated using skin turgor, mucous membrane moistness, and a comparison of current body weight to recent body weight as rapid changes in body weight often reflect changes in hydration status. The presence of subcutaneous edema or ascites may be associated with proteinuria and nephrotic syndrome. Examine the oral cavity for halitosis, pale mucous membrane color, ulcers, or necrosis of tongue tip that may be present in patients with uremia. Examine ocular fundus for edema, detachment, hemorrhage, or vascular tortuosity that may be associated with systemic arterial hypertension. In young dogs and cats with congenital renal failure, fibrous osteodystrophy ("rubber jaw") may be present. Palpate the mandible and maxilla for swelling, pain, deformity, and ability to bend abnormally. In animals with urinary incontinence, a thorough neurological and musculoskeletal examination is performed including evaluation of the lumbosacral area. Rectal temperature may be increased with infectious disease.

Kidneys and ureters

Palpate the abdomen for renal location, size, shape, consistency, and pain. Canine kidneys are bean shaped, while feline kidneys are more spherical. In dogs, the right kidney is located level with the first three lumbar vertebrae and situated almost entirely under the ribs, while the left kidney is more caudal at the level of the second through fourth lumbar vertebrae. In cats, the right kidney is located ventral to the first through fourth lumbar vertebrae and the left kidney is located more caudally. In dogs, usually only the left kidney is palpable and occasionally the caudal pole of the right kidney, while in cats,

both kidneys are palpable and easily moveable. Ureters are normally not palpable.

Urinary bladder

The urinary bladder can be palpated in most dogs and cats unless it is empty or the animal is obese. It is easiest to palpate while the animal is standing using one hand placed on the caudal ventral abdomen with the thumb positioned on one side of the caudal ventral abdomen and the fingers positioned on the other side. Gently squeeze thumb and fingers together and slide them forward and backwards. The urinary bladder is evaluated for position in the abdomen, degree of distension, evidence of pain, thickness of wall, the presence of intramural masses (i.e., neoplasms) or intraluminal masses (i.e., calculi). A full bladder has a spherical and taut shape and may be situated more cranially than expected. The presence of a full bladder with pain and dehydration may indicate a urethral obstruction; heart rate may be lower than expected in a stressed animal due to hyperkalemia-induced bradycardia. The presence of a full bladder in a dehydrated animal without urethral obstruction suggests polyuria. A moderately distended bladder will be more pliable and less spherical, and more caudally situated. A bladder that is empty may not be palpable or may be small and firm.

Urethra

The urethra is examined as well. This is difficult in male and female cats with sedation or anesthesia, but can be performed in most awake male and female dogs.

In male dogs, extrude the penis and examine the urethral orifice at the tip of the penis in addition to the preputial sheath. Palpate along the length of the urethra especially at the base of the os penis, which is a common site for urethral obstruction due to calculi. The perineal and penile urethra cannot be palpated, per se, but the course of the urethra is palpated for abnormalities such as masses or calculi. Rectal examination should be performed in all male dogs regardless of age or reproductive status. The urethra can be palpated on midline dorsal to the pubic symphysis and the prostate may be palpable cranial to the cranial edge of the pelvis. Transrectal palpation of the prostate may be facilitated by using the other hand to push upwards on the caudal ventral abdomen, which "pushes" the prostate toward the finger inserted rectally. In female dogs, the urethra can be palpated transrectally as described before. Vaginal palpation should also be considered and vaginoscopy using an otoscope and cone or vaginascope may be performed usually without sedation or anesthesia.

In cats, examination of the urethra usually requires sedation or anesthesia unless the animal is obtunded. In male cats, the penis should be extruded and examined visually and by palpation. Rectal palpation of the urethra can also be done in male and female cats, and should be performed in cats with signs of lower urinary tract disease that are sedated or anesthetized.

Additional diagnostic testing

Additional diagnostic testing depends on clinical signs, results of historical and physical examination, and required diagnostic work-up. Collection of urine for analysis is a routine part of a minimum database and should be performed in all cases of urinary tract disease (see Chapter 7). Complete blood cell counts and serum or plasma biochemical analysis may be performed as part of the minimum database, particularly in the cases where renal disease, nephrotic syndrome, or urinary obstruc-

tion is suspected. Aerobic bacteriological urine culture is performed when bacterial or fungal urinary tract infections may be present (see Chapter 9). Indirect arterial blood pressure determination and ocular fundic examination is performed in all cases of renal disease (see Chapter 13). Other testing may include screening for systemic infectious disease (i.e., leptospirosis or rickettsia; see Chapter 27), imaging (i.e., radiography, ultrasonography, contrast radiography or computed tomography or magnetic resonance imaging; see Chapters 15–17), visualization (i.e., endoscopy, laparoscopy, or surgical exploration; see Chapters 19–21), biopsy of one or more areas of the urinary tract (see Chapters 23, 25, and 26), endocrinological testing (i.e., adrenal gland disease, etc.), or urinary function testing (i.e., determination of glomerular filtration rate, tubular function, or urodynamic testing; see Chapters 14 and 22).

5

The ins and outs of urine collection

Carl A. Osborne, Jody P. Lulich, and Hasan Albasan

Overview

Collection of urine is an integral part of urinalysis. The method of collection and the collection container itself may influence test results and their interpretation. Patients should be protected from iatrogenic complications associated with collection techniques, including trauma to the urinary tract and urinary tract infection. The sample being collected should be one whose in vitro characteristics are similar to its in vivo characteristics. The collection container should be selected with care. Since drugs may alter laboratory test values by a variety of pharmacologic, physical, and/or chemical mechanisms, urine samples collected for diagnostic purposes should be collected prior to the administration of diagnostic or therapeutic agents. Withholding the administration of fluids prior to sample collection is especially important since oral or parenteral fluids may significantly alter the specific gravity of urine. The significance of sterile urine bacterial cultures obtained from a patient that has been receiving antibiotics should be ascertained. Erroneous conclusions formulated on the basis of erroneous laboratory data may lead to an incorrect diagnosis (Osborne 1985).

Collection containers

Disposable and reusable containers (designed specifically for collection of urine from humans) may be obtained from a variety of medical supply houses. We routinely use disposable plastic cups which are clean, readily available, inexpensive, and have tight-fitting lids. They may be sterilized with ethylene oxide gas. Use of containers improvised by owners is not recommended since they often contain contaminants (detergents, food, cosmetics, etc.) that may interfere with reagent strip tests. Use of transparent containers, made of glass or plastic, facilitates observation of macroscopic characteristics of urine. However, if urinalysis cannot be performed within 30 minutes following collection, opaque containers should be considered to minimize photochemical degradation of urine constituents by bright light (Osborne and Stevens 1981).

Urine obtained for bacterial culture must be collected in sterilized syringes or sterilized containers with tight-fitting lids. Sterilized containers may be obtained by (1) sterilizing disposable plastic cups in ethylene oxide gas, (2) sterilizing glass or metal drinking cups in an autoclave, and (3) purchasing them from commercial manufacturers.

Collection techniques

Urine may be collected from the urinary bladder by using several methods: natural voiding, manual compression of the urinary bladder, transurethral catheterization, or cystocentesis. The method used should minimize iatrogenic trauma to the urethra and bladder. Proper techniques must be used to prevent iatrogenic urinary tract infection. Urine samples voided early in the morning are likely to be highly concentrated. Since consumption of water is likely to be greatest during the daytime, samples voided throughout the day are less likely to be concentrated. Knowledge about the level of urine concentration provides important information about the status of renal function. Red and white blood cells will lyse in dilute urine (i.e., urine with a specific gravity below approximately 1.007.) Voiding of large volumes of dilute urine tends to reduce the concentration of all substances present in the sample. Therefore, the significance of debris, cells, or microscopic organisms

Nephrology and Urology of Small Animals. Edited by Joe Bartges and David J. Polzin. © 2011 Blackwell Publishing Ltd.

in urine sediment should be interpreted with knowledge of the method of urine-specific gravity. This should be recorded on the form used to record urinalysis results.

Normal voiding

The primary advantage of this technique is that it is not associated with any risk of patient complications. The primary disadvantages of this method are (1) samples may be contaminated with cells and bacteria located in distal urethra, genital tract, and/or on the skin and hair, (2) samples may be contaminated by substances in the collection container and the external environment, and (3) the patient (the collectee) will not always void at the will of the collector. Voided samples are satisfactory for routine urinalysis which is obtained to screen patients for abnormalities of the urinary tract and other body systems. Depending on specific circumstances, however, it may be necessary to repeat the analysis on a subsequent sample collected by cystocentesis.

Voided samples are also satisfactory for serial evaluation of various chemical tests (glucose, ketones, bilirubin, etc.). Comparing abnormal results in voided urine samples with urinalysis results collected by cystocentesis or catheterization, may aid in localizing the underlying cause(s) of abnormal results (e.g., is the disorder proximal and/or distal to the urinary bladder). When possible, the first portion of the urine stream should be excluded from the sample submitted for analysis as it is often contaminated due to contact with the genital tract, skin, and hair. In order to do this, two cups may be used to collect the sample. The portion of the sample collected in the second cup, will represent a mid-stream sample. The sample in the first cup may be discarded or used to help localize hemorrhage or inflammatory disease to the urethra or genital tract. If technical difficulties prevent collection of the sample in two cups, the sample in the first cup is still available for analysis.

Manual compression of the urinary bladder

Induction of micturition (by application of digital pressure to the urinary bladder through the bladder wall) may be used to collect urine samples from dogs and cats. The primary advantages of this procedure are (1) the risk of iatrogenic lower urinary tract infection and iatrogenic trauma is minimal, and (2) urine samples may be collected from patients (collectees) with distended urinary bladders at the convenience of the collector. The primary disadvantages of this procedure are (1) the urinary bladder may be traumatized if excessive digital pressure is used. Not only is this detrimental to the patient, but the associated hematuria may interfere with interpretation of the results; (2) the urinary bladder may not contain

sufficient volume of urine to facilitate this technique; (3) samples may be contaminated with cells, bacteria, and other debris located in the genital tract, or on the skin and hair. Therefore, they are unsatisfactory for bacterial culture; (4) micturition may be difficult to induce in some patients, especially male cats; (5) bladder urine contaminated or infected with bacteria may be forced into the prostate gland, ureters, renal pelves, and kidneys (Feeney et al. 1983). Unlike normal micturition (where detrusor contraction is associated with a coordinated relaxation of voluntary and involuntary urethral sphincters), manual compression of the bladder increases intravesical pressure, but may not be associated with simultaneous relaxation of the urethral sphincters. Application of digital pressure to the urinary bladder for a prolonged period is associated with a greater risk of reflux than application of digital pressure for a transient period; and (6) it is unsatisfactory for use during the immediate postoperative phase of cystotomies.

Another technique is to outline the urinary bladder by abdominal palpation. Generally, this will not be successful in the conscious patient unless the bladder contains at least 10–15 mL of urine. The patient may be in a standing or recumbent position. The technique requires gradual exertion of moderate digital pressure over as large an area of the bladder as possible, with the fingers and thumb of one hand or with the fingers of both hands (Figure 5.1). Digital pressure should be directed toward the neck of the urinary bladder. A gradual but steady increase

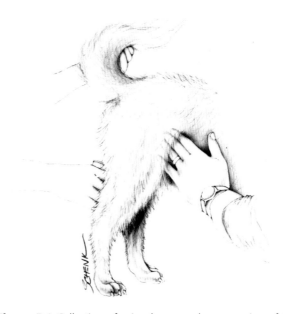

Figure 5.1 Collection of urine by manual compression of the urinary bladder. The fingers of both hands are used to gradually exert moderate digital pressure over as large an area of the bladder as possible.

in pressure should be applied rather than forced intermittent squeezing motions. Vigorous palpation and/or excessive pressure should be avoided since the latter is invariably associated with iatrogenic hematuria caused by trauma. Moderate digital pressure should be sustained until the urethral sphincters relax and urine is expelled from the bladder. Several minutes of digital pressure may be required before micturition is induced. If the bladder is overdistended with urine because of partial obstruction to the urine flow, caution must be excercised so as not to rupture the bladder or urethra.

Diuretics (such as furosemide) are recommended by some investigators to facilitate collection of urine samples by increasing urine formation. However, a notable drawback of this procedure is that it results in alteration of the specific gravity values of urine. Use of diuretics to enhance urine collection by augmenting urine flow is therefore best suited for serial urine sample collections when quantitative information about urine specific gravity, and semi-quantitative information about chemical tests and structures found in urine sediment, are not significant. If voiding does not occur following application of digital pressure to the urinary bladder, return the patient (cat) to the ward with a container of plastic litter, or walk the patient (dog) outside (Lees and Osborne 1984). If the bladder contains a sufficient volume of urine, the patient will often voluntarily void it at that time.

Collection of table-top urine samples

Patients with a lower urinary tract disease often have reduced bladder capacity and urge incontinence. As a result, collection of urine into a cup during the voiding phase of micturition, or by cystocentesis, is difficult. Frequently, small quantities of urine are voided before they can be collected. Collection of urine for analysis from smooth clean table-tops by aspiration through a needle into a syringe may be facilitated by the use of two rectangular microscope slides. The goal is to use the edges of the microscopic slides to form a deeper pool of urine that can more readily be aspirated. The long edges of two microscopic slides should be placed flat on the table surface so that the small sample of urine is between them. The slides should be parallel to each other, and tilted away from the urine sample at an angle. With the edges of the slides in close contact with the table, the slides should be advanced toward each other. This will cause the urine to pool along the edges of the slides. During this time, an assistant with a syringe and needle should aspirate the urine as it pools in front of the microscope slides. When the slides meet, they will form a V-shaped trough, from which most of the voided urine may be collected. Urine samples collected in this fashion are satisfactory for screening urinalysis provided they are analyzed soon after collection. The value of the results will be influenced by the cleanliness of the table from which the sample was collected. To determine if disinfectant solutions agents used to clean table tops will interfere with reagent-strip tests, evaluate results of a urinalysis performed before and after exposure to the disinfectant.

Transurethral catheterization

Avoid unnecessary catheterization! If selected, the goal of catheterization should be to use an atraumatic and aseptic technique by persons familiar with correct procedure. Due to the risks of trauma and bacterial urinary tract infection, it is not a technique that should be conducted by inadequately trained personnel who are unaware of the consequences. Indications for transurethral catheterization of the urinary bladder may be categorized as diagnostic or therapeutic (Table 5.1). The purpose(s) of catheterization largely determines which of the three general types of catheterization will be most appropriate.

Table 5.1 Indications for transurethral catheterization of the urinary bladder

Diagnostic
    Collection of a urine sample for analysis or bacterial culture
    Collection of accurately timed volumes of urine for renal function studies
    Measurement of urine output
    Measurement of postmicturition residual urine volume
    Instillation of contrast material for radiographic studies of the bladder, urethra, or prostate gland
    Verification and localization of urethral obstruction
    Catheter aspiration biopsy of urethral, prostatic, or bladder lesions
Therapeutic
    Relief of urethral obstruction to urine flow
    Relief of urine retention
    Instillation of medications into the urinary bladder
    Facilitation of surgery of the bladder, urethra, or surrounding structures

Single brief catheterization is appropriate when the need for a catheter is a few hours or less. However, when need for catheterization spans longer periods, intermittent or indwelling catheterization is required. Size, composition, and types of catheters should be carefully considered.

Size

The Fr scale of measurement (commonly abbreviated as F) is most often used for calibrating the diameter of catheters. Each Fr unit is equivalent to 1/3 mm. and hence, Fr units may be converted to millimeters by dividing by 3. A 9 F catheter has an external diameter of 3 mm. Catheters are available in a variety of diameters and lengths.

Composition

Urinary catheters are fabricated from a variety of materials including rubber, plastic, metal, nylon, latex, and woven silk. Catheters impregnated with radiopaque material are of value when used in conjunction with radiographic evaluation of the urinary system. Catheters impregnated with antimicrobial agents have been recommended to minimize iatrogenic infection.

Types (Figure 5.2)

A wide variety of catheters are available for use in human and veterinary medicine and each is designated to serve a particular need (Figure 5.2). The openings adjacent

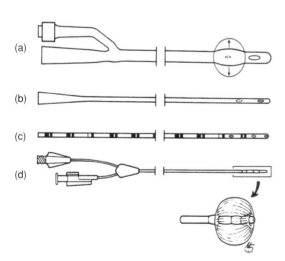

Figure 5.2 Drawings of catheters used for retrograde contrast urethrocystography, retrograde contrast vaginography, and various types of collection of urine from the urinary bladder. Key: (a) pediatric Foley catheter. Air injected through the upper arm of the catheter will inflate the balloon (arrows); (b) polypropylene urethral catheter with two eyes; (c) whistle-tip ureteral catheter; (d) Swan–Ganz flow-directed balloon catheter. Air injected into the valve (lower arm) will inflate the balloon (insert).

to the tips of the catheters are commonly called "eyes." Catheters may have as few as one, or as many as six, or more, eyes. The edges of the eyes of polypropylene catheters are sometimes rough and, as a consequence, may irritate the mucosa of the bladder and urethra. On the basis of the site of their insertion, human catheters are classified as urethral or ureteral catheters. Human urethral catheters are usually too large (and sometimes too short) for routine use in veterinary medicine. Human ureteral catheters have been commonly used to catheterize male and female dogs. Urethral catheters with inflatable balloons located at the tip are called (Thomas) Foley catheters (Figure 5.2)[1]. By inflating the balloon following insertion of the catheter into the bladder, the tip of the catheter cannot migrate out of the bladder lumen. Foley catheters are designed to be used as indwelling (or self retention) catheters. Foley catheters are sometimes used for retrograde contrast urethrography and retrograde vaginography. Angiographic catheters with inflatable balloons (Swan–Ganz flow-directed balloon catheters) may be used for retrograde urethrocystography (Figure 5.2)[2].

Canine urinary catheters

Flexible plastic[3] and rubber[4] catheters, similar in diameter and length, to human ureteral catheters may be used to catheterize male or female dogs. As they are relatively inflexible, polypropylene catheters frequently traumatize the urethra of male dogs as they curve around the ischial arch. Metal catheters designed for use in female dogs are not recommended because their rigid structure is frequently the cause of iatrogenic trauma to the mucosa of the urethra and urinary bladder. Swan–Ganz flow-directed balloon catheters designed for human angiography are very useful for collection of quantitative urine specimens from dogs (and cats) (Figure 5.2). (Garner and Laks 1976)

Feline urinary catheters

Disposable polypropylene tomcat catheters (3 1/2 to 5 F) are available from commercial manufacturers[5]. Infant feeding tubes and polyethylene tubing may also be used to catheterize cats. Minnesota olive tip feline urethral catheters[6] are often used to remove plugs from the distal urethra of male cats. They are too short to reach the lumen of the bladder. Rigid metal tomcat catheters should not be used since they often cause trauma to the urethral and bladder mucosa. Wysong urethral catheters[7] constructed of a silicone elastomer are designed for indwelling use in male cats (Wysong 1983). Jackson cat catheters[8] are also designed for indwelling use in male cats. However, their relatively rigid construction may cause trauma to the urinary bladder vertex as it contracts.

Filiforms and followers

Filiforms and followers are instruments commonly used in human medicine to locate and dilate ureteral strictures. Filiforms are solid structures made of pliable synthetic material. They have a variety of different types of tips (i.e., coude and corkscrew). Followers may be solid or hollow. Hollow followers permit catheterization.

Sounds

Sounds are special instruments made of solid metal that may be used to explore the urethral lumen for stenoses and to dilate the urethra and the bladder neck. Sounds are available in a wide variety of designs. Human textbooks of urology provide specific details about filiforms, followers, and sounds.

It is useful to designate a special drawer in the hospital as a catheter drawer (analogous to an auto mechanics tool box). Sterilized catheters of all sizes, composition, and types should be stored in this drawer so that they are readily available when needed. Speculums and light sources may also be stored in the catheter drawer.

Care of urinary catheters

Only sterilized catheters that are in excellent condition should be used. Catheters that have been weakened during use or abuse may break apart while in the patient. The "eye" is the weakest part of flexible catheters. Catheters that have a rough external surface may traumatize the mucosa of the urethral and urinary bladder. Not only are they detrimental to the patient, iatrogenic hematuria may interfere with interpretation of the urinalysis. Pre-sterilized catheters are recommended. Non-sterilized catheters should be individually packaged prior to use. The use of transparent packages that may be sterilized with ethylene oxide[9] enable storage and selection, since they permit visualization of the catheter. Unsterilized catheters should not be used because they may cause iatrogenic infection of the urinary system. Also, they may contaminate urine that is collected for bacterial culture.

Sterilization

Catheters must be thoroughly cleaned prior to sterilization. Cleansing solutions should be completely rinsed from the surface of catheters since they may interfere with enzymatic and chemical tests. Repeated autoclaving of nonmetal catheters may reduce their longevity. Ethylene oxide sterilization is an excellent method.

A technique that uses microwave ovens to sterilize urinary catheters has been described (Douglas et al. 1990). Basically, this technique involves putting flexible urinary catheters in reusable freezer bags and placing them in a microwave oven. In addition to the catheter, a beaker with water must be placed in the oven to absorb excessive heat. The microwave oven is set at 12 minutes (high power). The authors emphasized the need to avoid "cold areas" in the microwave oven. It is recommended that this procedure be validated with each hospital's microwave before using it to sterilize urinary catheters. This may be accomplished by culturing contaminated urinary catheters for bacteria before and after microwaving them.

Chemical sterilizing solutions containing quaternary ammonia compounds may be used, but these are less effective than sterilization by autoclaving or ethylene oxide gas. If residual antiseptic solutions are not thoroughly rinsed from catheters, they may irritate the mucosa of the urethra or urinary bladder, interfere with growth of bacteria, and/or alter chemical and enzyme tests. Disposable catheters which are prepackaged in sterilized wrappers may be obtained from commercial manufacturers.

Potential complications of transurethral catheterization

Urinary catheters may produce two general types of adverse effects: (1) trauma to the urinary tract – during insertion or continued presence of the catheter, and (2) initiation of bacterial urinary tract infection (UTI). The risk of these adverse effects varies from patient to patient as is it caused by numerous factors.

Status of the urinary tract

Among the key variables that affect the risk of catheter-induced complications is the physical and functional status of the patient's urinary tract (especially the urethra and bladder) during and following catheterization.

When diseases of the urinary tract make catheterization mechanically difficult, bacterial contamination and urinary tract trauma are likely.

Local urinary tract defense mechanisms are usually compromised by urinary tract diseases. Thus, animals with urinary tract disorders have a greater risk of catheter-induced complications. Unfortunately, it is these very patients for whom catheterization is required most often.

Patient profile

The risks of catheter-induced complications are also dependent on factors such as species, sex, size, temperament, and general health status. Cats are generally more difficult to catheterize than dogs. However, dogs are more susceptible to UTI than cats. Regardless of species, males are more easily catheterized than females. Perhaps this, and other sex-related risk factors, are associated with the greater risk of catheter-induced UTI in female dogs as compared to male dogs.

As veterinary patients vary greatly in size and cooperativeness, the equipment and techniques that work optimally for some patients are less satisfactory for others. It is detrimental to use methods that are not appropriate for the particular patient. Catheter-induced UTI can lead to episodes of bacteremia, particularly when a catheter is removed from an infected urinary tract.

General health status and concomitant disorders can influence the risk of catheter associated complications. Dogs with Cushing's syndrome, diabetes mellitus, and renal failure have higher susceptibility to UTI. Patients with valvular cardiac disease have increased risk of developing bacterial endocarditis as a result of such bacteremia.

Techniques

Techniques of catheterization influence the frequency and nature of adverse sequela. Abrasions, contusions, lacerations, and even puncture of the urethra and bladder can occur during catheterization. Prevention of these undesirable outcomes is dependent on the selection and careful use of an appropriate catheter. The frequency and duration of catheterization also influences the risk of catheter-induced complications; iatrogenic infection is least likely to occur as a consequence of a single brief catheterization. Studies of repeated intermittent brief catheterization have revealed that the risk of inducing infection is similar following each catheterization. Thus, the cumulative risk of catheter-induced UTI is proportional to the number of catheterizations. Risk of iatrogenic infection is greatest during indwelling catheterization, especially when the portion of catheter protruding from the urethra is not connected to a receptacle (i.e., it is open) (Lees et al. 1981; Lees and Osborne 1984). In general, the risk of infection during indwelling catheterization is proportional to the duration of catheterization (Lees et al. 1981; Lees and Osborne 1984; Barsanti et al. 1985). When there is need for long-term catheterization, intermittent catheterization is often safer because it is less likely to induce UTI than indwelling catheterization. Indwelling catheters may cause continuous trauma to the urinary tract, and may elicit a foreign body reaction in surrounding tissue (Lees et al. 1980). In some situations, however, the higher risk of urethral trauma caused by repeated insertion of a catheter makes indwelling catheterization the safer alternative. Due to the risk of inducing infection of the bladder as a result of catheterization, indiscriminate use of this technique is not recommended. However, this generality must be kept in perspective. When necessary for diagnostic or therapeutic purposes, transurethral catheterization of the urinary bladder should be performed carefully and with appropriate caution.

Axioms

1. Avoid unnecessary catheterization, especially in patients with increased risk of bacterial UTI and its sequela. This includes patients with urinary disease, especially of the lower urinary tract; hyperadrenocorticism; diabetes mellitus; and polyuria.
2. Urinary catheterization should only be performed by properly trained personnel.
3. If the need for catheterization spans more than a few hours, intermittent catheterizations as well as indwelling catheterization should be considered. If a single brief catheterization is required for a high-risk patient, consider an antibiotic excreted in high concentration in urine and administer it 8–12 hours before and 8–12 hours after catheterization.
4. To minimize damage to bladder mucosa, avoid overinsertion of catheters.
5. If indwelling urethral catheters are required, strive to maintain a closed system.
6. Select indwelling urethral catheters which are constructed of materials least likely to cause irritation and inflammation of the adjacent mucosa.
7. Consider administering antibiotics during indwelling urethral catheterization only if evidence of infection is detected. This minimizes the likelihood of infection with bacteria resistant to antimicrobial agents. If catheter-induced infection develops and remains asymptomatic, treat the infection following removal of the catheter. Periodically perform urinalysis and bacterial culture during the period of indwelling urethral catheterization, and at the time the catheter is removed.

Technique—generalities for male and female dogs and cats

Regardless of the specific procedure being employed, meticulous aseptic and gentle "feather touch" technique should be used to prevent damage to the delicate tissues of the genital tract, urethra, and urinary bladder. Only well-trained individuals who comprehend the potential consequences of iatrogenic trauma and UTI should be given the responsibility to catheterize the urethra and urinary bladder. Conscious patients should be restrained by an assistant in order to minimize contamination of the catheter as well as trauma to the urethra. Animals should be gently restrained in a comfortable position in order to minimize the possibility of sudden unexpected movement which may result in contamination of the catheter or trauma to the urinary tract. Some types of sedation may be required for male cats and is usually required for female cats. Appropriate caution should be exercised so as not to use a drug that alters the diagnostic, physical, or chemical composition of urine. Use the smallest diameter catheter that will permit the objective of catheterization. Few patients will tolerate the passage of large catheters without some form of sedation.

Catheters with flared ends are recommended, particularly if the length of the catheter is similar to the length of the urethra. If the end is not flared, the catheter may migrate into the urethra to a point where it cannot then be manually removed. In this event, insertion of a Swan–Ganz flow-directed balloon catheter inside the lumen of the damaged catheter, followed by distention of the balloon, will be needed to withdraw it. Many commercially prepared catheters have flared ends which accommodate the tip of a syringe. If a stylet is used, it should be lubricated before it is inserted into the lumen of the catheter. If the stylet is not lubricated, it may be difficult to remove it after the catheter is placed in the patient (especially male dogs). If necessary, structures adjacent to the external urethral orifice should be cleansed with germicidal soap, water, and sterilized sponges. The soap and water mixture should be thoroughly removed by rinsing to prevent contamination of the urine sample. Soapy water may (a) impart a cloudy appearance to the sample, (b) inhibit bacterial growth, (c) cause lysis of cells, and/or (d) interfere with chemical and enzyme tests. The distance from the external urethral orifice to the beginning of the lumen of the bladder lumen should be estimated and mentally transposed to the catheter. This step will reduce the likelihood of traumatizing the bladder mucosa due to over-insertion of the catheter. It will also prevent the catheter from reentering the urethral lumen. The tip of the catheter and the adjacent area should be liberally lubricated with sterilized aqueous lubricant. Proper lubrication of the catheter will minimize discomfort to the patient and reduce catheter-induced trauma to the urethra. Local anesthesia may be induced with a topical anesthetic such as lidocaine hydrochloride[9].

Asepsis must be maintained throughout the procedure. The catheter should not be allowed to come in contact with the hair or skin of the patient or clinician. The catheter may be manipulated (1) through the packaging material in which it is contained, (2) with the aid of a sterilized pediatric hemostat, (3) with sterilized surgical gloves, and (4) by holding the distal end only. The catheter should never be forced through the urethra. If difficulty is encountered in inserting the catheter through the urethra, withdraw the catheter for a short distance and insert it again with a gradual rotating motion. If difficulty persists, the diameter of the catheter should be reevaluated.

Injection of a sterilized mixture of aqueous lubricant, whose viscosity has been diluted with sterilized water or saline, through the lumen of the catheter may be effective. If these steps are unsuccessful, a catheter with a smaller diameter should be used. The tip of the catheter should be positioned so that its eyes are located just beyond the junction of the neck of the bladder with the urethra. In most instances, this may be accomplished by inserting the catheter approximately one inch beyond the point at which urine flows through the catheter lumen. This position may be verified by injection of a known quantity of air through the catheter into an otherwise empty bladder lumen. Inability to remove most of the air indicates improper positioning of the catheter. The catheter should be repositioned until the quantity of air injected into the bladder lumen can be readily aspirated into the syringe. Proper positioning of catheters facilitates removal of all the urine from the bladder and minimizes the possibility of catheter-induced trauma. Urine may be aspirated from the bladder with the aid of a syringe. Aspiration must be gentle in order to prevent trauma to the bladder or urethral mucosa as a result of sucking it into the eyes of the catheter. An attempt to force urine through the catheter by application of digital pressure to the bladder is not the recommended routine procedure since it increases the likelihood of catheter-induced damage to the bladder mucosa. Use of a two-way or three-way valve minimizes inadvertent injection of bacteria into the bladder. Unless specifically required for a study, the first several milliliters of urine obtained via the catheter should be discarded since it may be contaminated with bacteria and cells from the genital tract and urethra. In patients who run a high risk of developing iatrogenic infection as a result of catheterization, sterilized solutions of antimicrobial drugs may be injected into the bladder lumen as a prophylactic measure. However, local instillation of antimicrobial agents should not be used as a substitute for orally or parenterally administered antimicrobial agents if the risk of iatrogenic bacterial UTI warrants antimicrobial therapy. Follow-up urinalyses or bacterial cultures should be considered several days later in order to detect iatrogenic infection at a subclinical stage.

Transurethral catheterization of the urinary bladder of male dogs (Figure 5.3)

Reference should be made to the general discussion about catheterization. The length and diameter of the catheter varies with the size of the patient. Four to ten Fr catheters are satisfactory for most dogs. The length of human ureteral and veterinary ureteral catheters usually does not vary. The external urethral orifice should be exposed by reflecting the prepuce away from the penis. To retract the

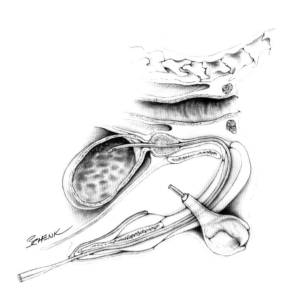

Figure 5.3 Proper position of the tip of the flexible catheter in the lumen of the urinary bladder of a male dog. Rigid plastic catheters are often unsatisfactory because they may cause trauma and pain during passage through the curved portion of the perineal urethra.

prepuce, apply caudal pressure with the index finger at the point where the prepuce reflects onto the ventral abdominal wall. Grasp the penis through the prepuce with the other hand, and push it cranially. Once exposed, the tip of the penis and the external urethral orifice should be thoroughly cleansed with soap and water. Once reflected, the prepuce must not be allowed to contact the catheter as it is being advanced through the urethral lumen. Difficulty in advancing the catheter through the urethral lumen may be encountered at the level of the os penis and at the site where the urethra curves around the ischial arch. Resistance encountered at the level of the os penis may be minimized by grasping the penis through the prepuce and pushing it forward along the ventral body wall. Resistance of the catheter at the ischial arch may be minimized by application of digital pressure over the top of the catheter as it is slowly advanced. Care must be taken not to insert an excessive length of the catheter because it may follow the curvature of the bladder wall, double back on itself, and reenter the urethral lumen. As the catheter is withdrawn, the loop of the catheter becomes progressively smaller until the point where the wall of the catheter bends. The catheter often bends at the eye since it is the weakest point of the catheter wall. As the bent catheter is withdrawn, it usually lodges at the caudal end of the os penis. If a catheter gets lodged in the wall of the urethra as a result of bending itself, the following procedures, which are listed in order of priority, should be considered (Osborne et al. 1972) (a) Advance

the catheter back into the bladder lumen with the objective of releasing the tight bend in the catheter wall, (b) Apply a liberal quantity of sterilized lubricant to the outside wall of the catheter, and inject a dilute solution (2 parts lubricant to 1 part water) of sterilized lubricant into the catheter lumen. Apply gentle, steady traction to the catheter with the objective of dilating the urethral lumen ventral to the os penis thereby enabling the catheter to be withdrawn. The force of the traction being applied should be carefully monitored as extra force could tear the urethral mucosa, and (c) If the catheter cannot be removed by steady traction, a liberal quantity of dilute sterilized aqueous lubricant should be injected through and around the catheter. An assistant should then occlude the lumen of the pelvic urethra by applying digital pressure against the ischium through the ventral wall of the rectum (refer to the chapter describing the technique of retrograde urohydropropulsion). Next, a catheter of appropriate size with an attached syringe (loaded with sterilized saline) should be placed in the penile urethra via the external urethral orifice. Using digital pressure, the external urethral orifice should be compressed around the both catheters. As a result of these maneuvers, a portion of the urethra, from the external urethral orifice to the bony pelvis, becomes a closed system. Saline should then be injected into the urethra until a definite rebound is perceived through the syringe plunger. This rebound should be associated with a palpable increase in the diameter of the pelvic urethra. At this point, another assistant should grasp the bent catheter and attempt to remove it with gentle but steady pressure. If the portion of the urethral lumen ventral to the os penis dilates sufficiently, the catheter may be removed from the uretha. If the catheter cannot be removed by these maneuvers, aqueous contrast agent should be injected into and around the catheter with the objective of visualizing the exact nature of the problem via contrast radiography. Anesthetize the patient and repeat step (b) or (c). Stretching the urethral lumen with the catheter is likely to induce a lesser degree of injury than a urethrotomy. If all of the above steps are unsuccessful, consider removing the catheter by urethrotomy.

Transurethral catheterization of the urinary bladder of female dogs (Figures 5.4–5.7)

Equipment

Flexible veterinary urethral or human ureteral catheters, identical to those used for male dogs, are recommended. Rigid metal catheters are not recommended for routine use as they have a tendency to traumatize the mucosa of the vagina, urethra, and urinary bladder. A variety of endoscopes may be used in the vagina to aid

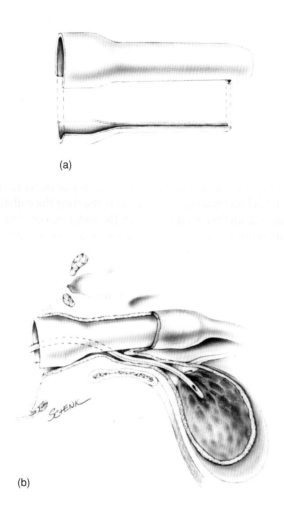

(a)

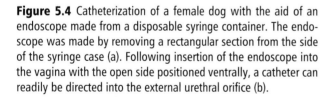

(b)

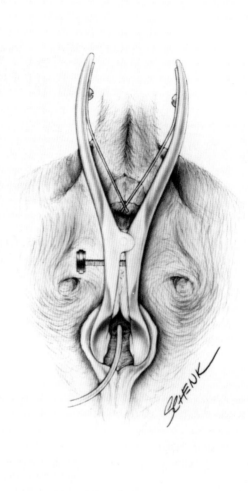

Figure 5.5 Preferred position of nasal speculum used as a vaginal endoscope to permit visualization of the external urethral orifice of female dogs.

Figure 5.4 Catheterization of a female dog with the aid of an endoscope made from a disposable syringe container. The endoscope was made by removing a rectangular section from the side of the syringe case (a). Following insertion of the endoscope into the vagina with the open side positioned ventrally, a catheter can readily be directed into the external urethral orifice (b).

visualization of the external urethral orifice, including (1) human nasal specula, (small size Figure 5.5), (2) specula fashioned from disposable syringe cases (Figure 5.4), (3) pyrex test tubes from which the end has been removed and the edge fire-polished (4) otoscope cones, (5) laryngoscopes, (6) cystoscope sheaths, and (7) transilluminator (Welch–Allen) light sources for otoscopes. If necessary, remove excessive hair from around the vulva. Cleanse the perivulvar skin and vulva with germicidal soap, water, and sterilized sponges. If required, flush the lumen of the vagina with sterilized water or saline injected through a syringe. Lidocaine jelly may be injected into the distal lumen of the vagina. The external urethral ori-

fice is located on a small tubercle in the ventral wall of the vagina. In mature, small to medium-sized dogs, the external urethral orifice is approximately 3–5 cm cranial to the ventral commissure of the vulva. The clitoral fossa lies just caudal to the external urethral orifice. Catheters and endoscopes inserted into the vagina must be carefully directed above and past this structure.

Catheterization via endoscopy

Restraint, a good light source, and a comfortable position for both patient and clinician are important considerations. Having the dog in a standing position is recommended as it facilitates the anatomical orientation required to locate the external urethral orifice (Figure 5.5). Ideally, the speculum must be large enough to remove the folds of the vaginal wall by distending

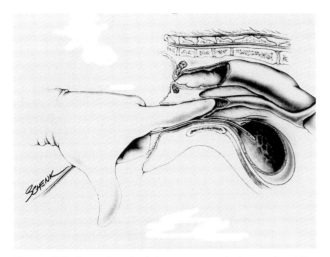

Figure 5.6 Illustration depicting correct techniques of guiding a flexible catheter into the external urethral orifice of a female dog. Keeping the patient in a standing position aids in anatomical orientation during blind digital palpation of the vaginal lumen.

its lumen. Injection of air into the vagina sometimes enables dilatation of the lumen.

Foley catheter technique

For patients who are too small to permit visualization of the external urethral orifice with the aid of an endoscope, an 8–10 F Foley catheter may permit catheterization. Insert the Foley catheter into the vagina as far as possible and inflate the balloon. Insert a small nasal speculum into the vagina and open the blades. Gently pull the Foley catheter outward. The urethral orifice may be visualized as a small opening in the ventral midline of the vaginal floor. Insertion of the urethral catheter is usually not hindered by the Foley balloon. If it is, however, the balloon should be deflated.

Digital technique (Figure 5.6)

Female dogs that are large enough to permit digital palpation of the vaginal lumen may be catheterized without the requirement for direct visualization. However, this technique is more likely to be associated with bacterial contamination of the urinary tract, than the use of endoscopy to directly visualize the external urethral orifice. The dog should be standing as this facilitates anatomical orientation. The external urethral orifice is located on the ventral midline of the vaginal floor. Using sterilized disposable surgery gloves, an index finger should be lubricated and gently inserted into the vagina. A sterilized flexible catheter should be inserted into the lumen of the vagina, dorsal to the clitoral fossa, and guided along the midline of the vaginal floor toward the external urethral orifice. Although the external urethral orifice cannot be palpated, entry of the catheter into the urethra can be determined when the tip of the catheter disappears into the floor of the vagina. The most common error caused by lack of experience with this technique, is over-insertion of the catheter into the vaginal lumen. Those inexperienced with this technique should first place a catheter into the urethra with the aid of an endoscope and light source. After the catheter is in place, remove the endoscope. Thereafter, insert a gloved index finger into the vaginal lumen and palpate the catheter at the site of the external urethral orifice. Next, pull the catheter out just enough so that the tip of the catheter is just distal to the external urethral orifice. Practice reinserting the catheter into the urethra with the aid of the index finger. This is somewhat reminiscent of learning how to swim or how to ride a bicycle, once you become familiar with the technique, you will never forget how to do it.

Blind catheterization (Figure 5.7)

This technique is more difficult than the methods described above. Blind catheterization is useful when visualization or digital palpation of the external urethral orifice is not feasible as patients may be uncooperative, have a small vulva, or have vaginal strictures. The position of the portion of the catheter within the vaginal lumen cannot be visualized, hence caution must be exercised to prevent trauma to the genital tract. The patient should be standing to facilitate anatomical orientation. The lips of the vulva should be parted. A sterilized, lubricated

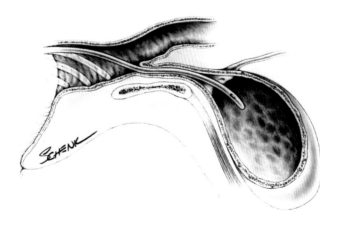

Figure 5.7 Schematic drawing illustrating the proper direction and curvature of a flexible catheter during blind advancement through the vaginal lumen into the external urethral orifice of a female dog.

catheter should be inserted into the vagina and directed above the clitoral fossa. With the long axis of the catheter directed in a cranioventral direction with respect to the long axis of the vagina, the tip of the catheter should be slowly advanced along the ventral midline of the vaginal floor. Detection of increased resistance to advancement of the catheter indicates that it has encountered the vaginal fornix. In this situation, the catheter should be withdrawn to a position just cranial to the clitoral fossa and the procedure should be repeated. Successful entry into the bladder is ascertained at the point where there is a lack of resistance to advancement of the catheter, and/or by passage of urine through the lumen.

Transurethral catheterization of the urinary bladder of male cats (Figure 5.8)

Commercially prepared flexible catheters that are 3–5 F in diameter are usually appropriate for this process. Catheters made from polyethylene tubing may be prepared by cutting one end at a 45° angle, and flaring the other end with heat (using a Bunsen burner, a match, etc.). Rigid metal catheters should be avoided for transurethral catheterization of the urinary bladder as they often induce trauma to the mucosal lining of the urethral and bladder. Although manual restraint by an assistant is usually adequate, sedation may be required for uncooperative cats. Appropriate caution should be taken in the selection of sedatives, in order to prevent alterations in the diagnostic, physical, and chemical components of urine. Extend the penis from the preputial sheath by pulling it in a caudal direction. Wash the end of the

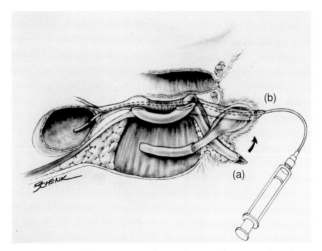

Figure 5.8 Catheterization of a male cat. The penis has been extended from the preputial sheath by pulling it in a caudal position (a). The natural curvature of the caudal portion of the urethra is then minimized by displacing the extended penis in a dorsal direction with the objective of aligning the long axis of the urethra with the long axis of the vertebral column (b).

penis with germicidal soap, water, and sterilized sponges. Displace the extended penis in a dorsal direction until the long axis of the urethra is approximately parallel to the vertebral column. This maneuver will facilitate atraumatic catheterization by reducing the natural curvature of the caudal portion of the urethra. Gently insert the tip of the catheter into the external urethral orifice and advance it to the lumen of the urinary bladder. Variable degrees of resistance may be encountered in normal cats because of the curvature of the urethra adjacent to the bony pelvis, and/or voluntary contraction of skeletal muscle that surrounds the distal urethra. Resistance may be minimized by advancing the catheter with a gradual rotating motion. Injecti a small quantity of sterilized isotonic fluid to distend the urethral lumen (caution: injection of fluids may alter test results). Use care not to over-insert the catheter into the bladder lumen.

Transurethral catheterization of the urinary bladder of female cats

Flexible catheters used for catheterization of male cats are suitable. Otoscope cones provide satisfactory vaginal endoscopes. Some form of pharmacologic restraint is often required. Carefully insert the tip of the catheter into the slit-like external urethral orifice located in the midline of the vaginal floor, and advance it to the lumen of the urinary bladder.

Indications for indwelling transurethral catheters

Indwelling catheters should generally be used only during intensive care of critically ill patients when continuous measurement of urine production is required, and during the initial management period following relief of urethral obstruction. In this situation, the purpose of the catheter is to assure urethral patency and prevent continued urine retention. The three main situations where indwelling catheters are used following the initial relief of urethral obstruction are (1) lack of a relatively normal urine stream, (2) persistence of intraluminal material or extraluminal compression likely to cause re-obstruction, and (3) loss of detrusor muscle contractility and over distention of the bladder that has resulted in ineffective micturition despite urethral patency. If these abnormalities do not exist following relief of urethral obstruction, indwelling catheterization is usually unnecessary and should be avoided.

If indwelling catheters are employed, closed drainage systems should be used. Even if an antimicrobial drug is administered, UTI may still develop. Therefore, the catheter should be removed as soon as it has served its purpose and bacterial urine culture should then be obtained to detect iatrogenic infection. Urine retention caused by neurogenic disorders of urinary tract function (e.g., spinal cord disease, reflex dyssynergia, etc.) is optimally managed by manual compression of the bladder to expel the urine, or by intermittent catheterization. Indwelling catheterization is the least desirable method of combating urine retention in these situations because of the likelihood of iatrogenic infection and trauma.

Cystocentesis (Figures 5.9 and 5.10)

Cystocentesis is a form of paracentesis, consisting of needle puncture of the urinary bladder for the purpose of removing a variable quantity of urine by aspiration. Extensive clinical experience has revealed that correctly performed cystocentesis is of great diagnostic and therapeutic value. This technique is usually associated with a lesser risk of iatrogenic infection than catheterization and is often better tolerated by patients (especially cats and female dogs) than catheterization.

Diagnostic cystocentesis may be the best way to prevent contamination of urine samples with bacteria, cells, etc. from the lower urogenital tract, to aid in localization of hematuria, pyuria, and bacteriuria, and to minimize iatrogenic UTI caused by catheterization, especially in patients with diseases that predispose them to bacterial UTI. Therapeutic cystocentesis may be employed to provide temporary decompression of the excretory pathway

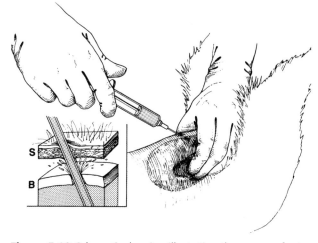

Figure 5.10 Schematic drawing illustrating the escape of urine through the bladder wall adjacent to the needle tract as a result of excessive digital pressure used to localize and immobilize the bladder. S represents skin of the abdominal wall, and B represents the wall of the urinary bladder.

of the urinary system, when urethral obstruction or herniation of the urinary bladder prevents normal micturition. It is frequently used to decompress the urinary tract of obstructed male cats and dogs prior to reverse flushing or other nonsurgical techniques designed to restore patency of the urethral lumen.

Contraindications

The main contraindications to cystocentesis are: (a) an insufficient volume of urine in the urinary bladder, and (b) the patient's resistance to restraint and abdominal palpation. Blind cystocentesis performed without digital localization and immobilization of the urinary bladder is usually unsuccessful, and may cause damage to the bladder or adjacent structures. Cystocentesis of patients with recent cystotomy incisions should be performed with appropriate caution. In our experience, collection of urine by cystocentesis from patients with bacterial UTI has not been associated with a detectable spread of infection outside the urinary tract. In fact, collection of a urine sample for bacterial culture that has not been contaminated by passage through the urethra and genital tract is a frequent reason for performing cystocentesis. The major diagnostic limitation of cystocentesis is that it is frequently associated with varying degrees of microscopic hematuria. The magnitude of hematuria induced by cystocentesis is greatest in patients with inflammation and/or congestion of the urinary bladder. Therefore, cystocentesis is not recommended for monitoring remission of microscopic hematuria originating from the urinary bladder following diagnosis.

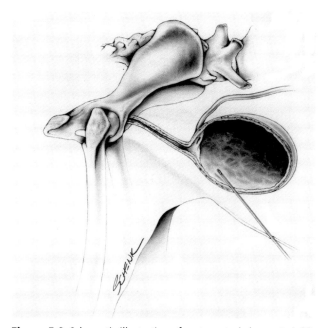

Figure 5.9 Schematic illustration of cystocentesis in a cat. A 22-gauge 3-in. spinal needle has been inserted through the ventral wall of the urinary bladder at an oblique angle. The point of insertion is several centimeters cranial to the junction of the bladder with the urethra.

Equipment

We routinely use 22-gauge needles. Depending on the size of the patient and the distance of the ventral bladder wall from the ventral abdominal wall, 1.5-in. hypodermic or 3-in. spinal needles can be used. Small-capacity (~2–12 mL) syringes are usually employed for diagnostic cystocentesis, while large-capacity (20–60 mL) syringes, separated from the hypodermic needle by an intravenous extension set and a two-way or three-way valve, are used for therapeutic cystocentesis.

Site

The risk to the patient can be minimized by careful planning of the site and direction of the needle puncture of the bladder wall. Some clinicians recommend insertion of the needle into the dorsal wall of the bladder to minimize gravity-induced leakage of urine into the peritoneal cavity following withdrawal of the needle. However, we recommend that the needle be inserted *in the ventral or ventrolateral* wall of the bladder in order to minimize the chance of trauma to the ureters and major abdominal vessels (Figure 5.9). If therapeutic cystocentesis is to be performed, we recommend insertion of the needle a short distance cranial to the junction of the bladder with the urethra, rather than at the vertex of the bladder. This will permit removal of the urine and decompression of the bladder without the need for reinsertion of the needle into the bladder lumen. If the needle is placed in, or adjacent to, the vertex of the bladder, it may not remain within the bladder lumen as the bladder progressively decreases in size following aspiration of urine. We also recommend that the needle be directed through the bladder wall at an angle of approximately 45° so that an oblique needle tract is created (Figure 5.9). By directing the needle through the bladder wall in an oblique fashion, the elasticity of the vesical musculature and the interlacing arrangement of individual muscle fibers will provide better sealing of the small pathway created by the needle when it is removed. In addition, subsequent distension of the bladder wall (as the lumen refills with urine) tends to force the walls of the needle tract into apposition in a fashion somewhat analogous to the flap valve of the ureterovesical junction.

Precystocentesis considerations

Insertion and withdrawal of a 22-gauge needle through the walls of the abdomen and bladder cause only marginal discomfort. Hence, tranquilization, general anesthesia, and local anesthesia are rarely required for diagnostic or therapeutic cystocentesis. If the urinary bladder does not contain a sufficient volume of urine to permit digital localization and immobilization, the patient may be given oral fluids or a diuretic. Although diuretics such as furosemide may be used to facilitate collection of urine-samples by increasing urine formation, alteration of urine specific gravity and urine pH are notable drawbacks of this procedure. Even the quantity of bacteria per milliliter of urine may be significantly reduced, thereby altering the results of quantitative urine cultures. Use of diuretics to enhance urine collection by augmenting urine flow is therefore best suited for serial urine sample collection in situations where information about urine specific gravity, urine pH, and semi-quantitative evaluation of routine test components is not significant.

Techniques of cystocentesis

In order to minimize the risk to the patient, careful planning of the site and direction of needle puncture is essential. The bladder must contain a sufficient volume of urine to permit immobilization and localization by palpation. Excessive hair should be removed with scissors or clippers. The ventral abdominal skin penetrated by the needle should be cleansed with an antiseptic solution each time cystocentesis is performed. Surgical preparation of the skin is usually unnecessary. Appropriate caution should be taken to avoid iatrogenic trauma and/or infection of the urinary bladder and surrounding structures.

In cats, it is usually easiest to perform the procedure with the patient in lateral or dorsal recumbancy. In large dogs, the procedure may also be performed when the patient is standing. In order to enhance recovery of crystalline material that may have gravitated to the dependent portion of the bladder lumen, urine within the bladder may be gently agitated via abdominal palpation just prior to cystocentesis. Elevating the rear of the dog by lifting with the legs (wheelbarrow position) may help. Following localization and immobilization of the urinary bladder, the needle should be inserted through the ventral abdominal wall and advanced to the caudoventral aspect of the bladder. The precise location of entry of the needle into the bladder wall is not critical. The needle should be inserted through the bladder wall at an oblique angle. If a large quantity of urine is to be aspirated, the needle should be directed so that it will enter the bladder lumen a short distance cranial to the junction of the bladder with the urethra. While the needle and bladder are immobilized, urine should be gently aspirated into the syringe. Excessive digital pressure should not be applied to the bladder wall while the needle is in its lumen, in order to prevent urine from being forced around the needle into the peritoneal cavity (Figure 5.10). When the ventral surface of the bladder wall is more than 1–1.25 in. from the ventral abdominal wall, the use of a 3-in. spinal needle rather than a 1.5-in. hypodermic needle facilitates immobilization of the urinary bladder without pulling it toward the ventral abdominal wall. An appropriate quantity of urine for analysis and/or bacterial culture should be aspirated into the syringe. If disease of the bladder wall or virulence of urinary pathogens are likely risks for complications associated with loss of urine into the peritoneal cavity, the bladder should be emptied as completely as is consistent with atraumatic technique. These potential complications have not been a problem in our patients.

Postcystocentesis considerations

The need for prophylactic antibacterial therapy following cystocentesis must be determined on the basis of the status of the patient and retrospective evaluation of the technique. In most instances, it is not required. In order to minimize contamination of the peritoneal cavity with urine, unnecessary digital pressure should not be applied to the urinary bladder immediately following cystocentesis.

Postcystocentesis complications

Other than hematuria, we have not observed antemortem complications. Potential complications include damage to the bladder wall or adjacent structures with the needle, local or generalized peritonitis, vesicoperitoneal fistulas, adhesion of adjacent structures to the bladder wall, and sudden collapse (Koch et al. 2001). We have encountered a few instances in which penetration of a loop of intestine by the needle has resulted in false-positive significant bacteriuria. Varying degrees of microscopic hematuria are expected for a short period of time following cystocentesis, especially if the needle passes through an area of active inflammation.

Samples for quantitative versus qualitative analysis

Urine samples collected without considering the rate of urine formation (i.e., number of milliliters per unit of time) are only suitable for qualitative and semi-quantitative evaluation of substances, because the concentration of any solute will vary with the quantity of water being excreted at that time. Samples for routine analysis are usually collected in this fashion.

Collection of urine specimens during a specified period of time is required for quantitative analysis. Quantitative renal function tests (glomerular filtration rate, clearances of various analytes, etc.) require collection of all urine formed during a known period of time. A metabolism cage is frequently used to collect all urine formed during a 24-hour interval, in order to determine the quantity of electrolytes or hormones (cortisol metabolites, etc.) excreted per day. For the best results, two or more 24-hour collections should be performed after the patient has had one or more days to adapt to the metabolism cage. Also, the urinary bladder should be emptied with the aid of a urinary catheter at the beginning and at the end of each timed collection period. Oral or parenteral administration of appropriate antimicrobial agents at least 8 hours prior to catheterization and for 2–3 days following catheterization, will minimize the likelihood of catheter-induced bacterial urinary tract infections.

Normal 24-hour urine volume is variable. It is influenced by water consumption, dietary moisture, dietary ingredients that affect urine concentrating capacity, environmental conditions, and activity of the patient. Normal dogs produce approximately 12–30 mL of urine per pound of body weight every 24 hours. Normal cats produce approximately 4.5–9.0 mL of urine per pound of body weight every 24 hours.

Endnotes

1. Available from Rusch, Inc., 2450 Meadowbrook Parkway, Duluth, Georgia 30136.
2. Available from Baxter-Edwards Laboratories, Inc., P.O. Box 11150, Santa Ana, California 92711.
3. Polypropylene catheters, Sherwood Medical Industries, Inc., St. Louis, Missouri 63103.
4. Sterile disposable feeding tube and urethral catheter, Sherwood Medical Industries, Inc., St. Louis, Missouri 63103.
5. Tomcat catheter, Sherwood Medical Industries, Inc., St. Louis, Missouri 63103.
6. Available from Ejay International, Inc., P.O. Box 1835, Glendora, California 91740.
7. Available from Wysong Medical Corporation, 4925 Jefferson Ave., Midland, Michigan 48640.
8. Available from Arnold's Veterinary Products Ltd., 14 Tessa Road, Richfield Avenue, Reading, England RG1 8NF.
9. Anestacon, Conal Pharmaceuticals, Inc., Chicago, Illinois 60640. Xylocaine 2% Jelly, Astra Pharmaceutical Products, Inc., Westborough, Massachusetts 01581. Uro-Jet Delivery System (2% lidocaine HC1 Jelly), International Medications Systems Ltd., 1886 Santa Anita Ave., South Elmonte, California 91733.

References

Barsanti, J.A., et al. (1985). Urinary tract infection due to indwelling bladder catheters in dogs and cats. *J Am Vet Med Assoc* **187**: 384–388.

Douglas, C., et al. (1990). Microwave: practical cost-effective method for sterilizing urinary catheters in the home. *Urology* **35**: 219–222.

Feeney, D.A., et al. (1983). Vesicoureteral reflux induced by manual compression of the urinary bladder of dogs nod cats. *J Am Vet Med Assoc* **182**: 795–797.

Garner, D. and M.M. Laks (1976). Technique for the performance of repeatable urine clearances in the conscious male dog. *Nephron* **16**: 143–147.

Koch, A.J., et al. (2001). Severe bradyarrhythmia in a patient with Alzheimer's disease and a patient with cerebral ischemia, both induced by acute distension of the bladder. *Int J Clin Pract* **55**: 323–325.

Lees, G.E. and C.A. Osborne (1984). Use and misuse of indwelling urinary catheters in cats. *Vet Clin North Am* **14**: 599–608.

Lees, G.E., et al. (1980). Adverse effects caused by polypropylene and polyvinyl feline urinary catheters. *Am J Vet Res* **41**: 1836–1840.

Lees, G.E., et al. (1981). Adverse effects of open indwelling urethral catheterization in normal male cats. *Am J Vet Res* **42U**: 825–833.

Osborne, C.A. (1985). Techniques of urine collection and preservation. In: *Canine and Feline Nephrology and Urology*, edited by C.A. Osborne and D.R. Finco. Baltimore, MD: Williams and Wilkins, pp. 100–121.

Osborne, C.A., et al. (1972). *Canine and Feline Urology*. Philadelphia, PA: WB Saunders.

Osborne, C.A. and J.B. Stevens (1981). *Handbook of Canine and Feline Urinalysis*. St. Louis, MO: Ralston Purina Co.

Wysong, R.L. (1983) A new indwelling tomcat urethral catheter. *Vet Med Small Anim Clin* **78**: 703–708.

6

Nephropyelocentesis and antegrade pyelography

Silke Hecht

Dilatation of the renal pelvis can result from obstruction, or it can be related to a variety of nonobstructive disorders including pyelonephritis (Pugh et al. 1994; Felkai et al. 1995; Confer and Panciera 2001). Imaging-guided interventional procedures (nephropyelocentesis and antegrade pyelography) may be considered in cases where a diagnosis of pyelonephritis or obstructive pyelectasia cannot be achieved by other means. In initial descriptions of these techniques, fluoroscopy was utilized to guide a needle into a dilated renal pelvis following excretory urography (Ling et al. 1979; Ackerman et al. 1980). Disadvantages of this method include the need for intravenous administration of contrast medium and associated risks of adverse effects, radiation exposure of the examiner, and the presence of iodinated contrast material in the sample obtained from the renal pelvis. With increasing use of ultrasonography in the diagnosis of urinary tract disorders, ultrasound-assisted interventional procedures have become commonplace (Penninck and Finn-Bodner 1998; Nyland et al. 2002; D'Anjou 2008).

Nephropyelocentesis

It is beneficial to perform laboratory analysis and (bacterial) culture on samples obtained directly from a dilated renal pelvis especially in cases of chronic or therapy resistant urinary tract infections. Ultrasound-guided nephropyelocentesis can usually be performed under sedation, although general anesthesia might be required in some animals. On the basis of the examiner's preference, the animal is positioned in dorsal or lateral recumbency, and the skin is clipped and aseptically prepared.

A sterile 2.5–3.5-inch (6.4–8.9 cm), 22–25-gauge spinal needle is advanced into the renal pelvis at a 45° angle through the greater curvature of the renal parenchyma, opposite the renal hilus (Ling et al. 1979; Figure 6.1).

The procedure can be performed freehand. Use of a biopsy guide attached to the transducer is preferred by some as it allows visualization of the needle path prior to insertion of the needle. After successful positioning of the needle tip in the renal pelvis, the stylet is removed, a syringe or a syringe equipped with an extension set is attached to the needle, and fluid is aspirated from the renal pelvis.

A technique for ultrasound-guided drainage for treatment of pyelonephritis (pyonephrosis) in dogs is described below (Szatmári et al. 2001). After administration of a broad-spectrum antibiotic to prevent puncture-associated sepsis, a large-bore (18-gauge or larger) IV catheter or pigtail catheter is inserted percutaneously using the trocar or Seldinger technique. For the trocar technique, the trocar pigtail catheter is introduced percutaneously and advanced to the correct depth under ultrasound guidance. The inner stylet is removed, and the catheter is deployed by advancing the catheter over the outer stylet. The outer stylet is then removed, and the catheter is secured. For the Seldinger technique, a needle is introduced into the renal pelvis under ultrasound guidance, a working wire is passed through the needle, and the needle is removed. The drainage catheter and stiffener are then advanced over the wire, the catheter is deployed, the stylet and wire are removed, and the catheter is secured. After as much pus as possible has been aspirated from the renal pelvis, a 1:9 solution of povidone iodine in 0.9% NaCl is injected into the renal pelvis using the same catheter and then the catheter is removed. The volume of lavage solution should be approximately 50–60% of the volume aspirated during nephropyelocentesis. The lavage procedure is repeated until the solution appears

Nephrology and Urology of Small Animals. Edited by Joe Bartges and David J. Polzin. © 2011 Blackwell Publishing Ltd.

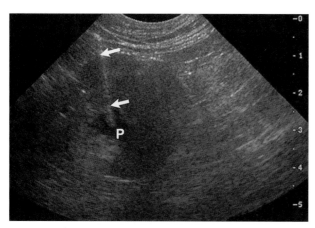

Figure 6.1 Ultrasound-guided pyelocentesis in a cat. Note the placement of the needle (arrows) in the dilated renal pelvis (P). (From D'Anjou 2008. Reprinted with permission.)

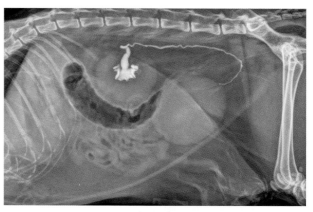

Figure 6.2 Antegrade pyelography of the left kidney in a cat to rule out ureteral obstruction. Moderate dilation of renal pelvis and proximal ureter and irregularity/tortuosity of the ureter are consistent with pyelonephritis and ureteritis and/or ureteral scarring/fibrosis. There is no evidence of ureteral obstruction. (Note the small size of the right kidney due to chronic renal disease.)

grossly clear. Following the procedure, the catheter is removed. Ultrasound-guided drainage and lavage of the renal pelvis should be repeated daily until the renal pelvis is so small that it can no longer be punctured.

Antegrade pyelography

Differentiating obstructive from nonobstructive pyelectasia is important, since obstructive uropathies require early intervention to prevent progressive deterioration of renal function (Fink et al. 1980; Andren-Sandberg 1983). Several imaging modalities have been described to aid in the diagnosis of ureteral obstruction in dogs and cats. Survey radiographs may show a ureteral calculus, but do not give information about the presence or degree of ureteral obstruction (Kyles et al. 2005). Excretory urography may show dilatation of renal pelvis and ureter proximal to the obstructive lesion, but opacification of the affected kidney and ureter can be poor if renal function is decreased (Hardie and Kyles 2004). Ultrasonography has a high sensitivity for the detection of pyelectasia and obstructive ureteral calculi but lacks diagnostic information regarding renal function or ureteral patency (Felkai et al. 1995; Kyles et al. 2005). Initial studies investigating diuretic renal scintigraphy in dogs and cats with ureteral obstruction have been promising (Hecht et al. 2006; Hecht et al. 2010), but the procedure is limited to specialty hospitals with nuclear medicine equipment, and studies investigating accuracy of this procedure are lacking.

Ultrasound-guided antegrade pyelography has been used in the diagnosis and localization of ureteral obstruction in dogs and cats (Rivers et al. 1997; Adin et al. 2003). The procedure has the advantage of good contrast-medium filling of renal pelvis and ureter while minimiz-

ing risk of adverse reactions to contrast medium, which is beneficial especially in patients with preexisting renal insufficiency (Fox et al. 1993). The procedure should be performed under general anesthesia. Patient preparation and needle placement in the dilated renal pelvis are performed as described above. Nephropyelocentesis is performed until the transverse diameter of the renal pelvis is reduced to approximately 50% of its original diameter. A volume of aqueous, iodinated contrast media equal to one-half of the aspirated volume of urine is then infused under direct ultrasonographic visualization (Rivers et al. 1997). Lateral and ventrodorsal radiographs are obtained immediately and 15 minutes after injection of contrast medium (Figure 6.2).

The most common complication of this procedure is leakage of contrast material from the retroperitoneal space or renal pelvis, preventing proper filling of the ureter and potentially rendering a nondiagnostic study. Other potential complications include laceration of the renal pelvis, subcapsular hemorrhage, hemorrhage into the renal pelvis, and ureteral obstruction with blood clot following the procedure (Rivers et al. 1997; Adin et al. 2003).

References

Ackerman, N., et al. (1980). Percutaneous nephropyelocentesis and antegrade ureterography: a fluoroscopically assisted diagnostic technic in canine urology. *Vet Radiol* **21**(3): 117–122.

Adin, C.A., et al. (2003). Antegrade pyelography for suspected ureteral obstruction in cats: 11 cases (1995–2001). *J Am Vet Med Assoc* **222**(11): 1576–1581.

Andren-Sandberg, A. (1983). Permanent impairment of renal function demonstrated by renographic follow-up in ureterolithiasis. *Scand J Urol Nephrol* **17**(1): 81–84.

Confer, A.W. and R.J. Panciera (2001). The urinary system. In: *Thomson's Special Veterinary Pathology*, edited by M.D. McGavin, W.W. Carlton, and J.F. Zachary, 3rd edition. St. Louis, MO: Mosby, pp. 235–277.

D'Anjou, M.A. (2008). Kidneys and ureters. In: *Atlas of Small Animal Ultrasonography*, edited by D.G. Penninck and M.A. d'Anjou. Ames, IA: Blackwell Publishing, pp. 339–364.

Felkai, C., et al. (1995). Lesions of the renal pelvis and proximal ureter in various nephro-urological conditions: an ultrasonographic study. *Vet Radiol Ultrasound* **36**(5): 397–401.

Fink, R.L., et al. (1980). Renal impairment and its reversibility following variable periods of complete ureteric obstruction. *Aust N Z J Surg* **50**(1): 77–83.

Fox, L.E., et al. (1993). Urinary obstruction secondary to a retroperitoneal carcinoma in a dog. *Vet Radiol Ultrasound* **34**(3): 181–184.

Hardie, E.M. and A.E. Kyles (2004). Management of ureteral obstruction. *Vet Clin North Am Small Anim Pract* **34**(4): 989–1010.

Hecht, S., et al. (2006). ^{99m}Tc-DTPA diuretic renography in dogs with urolithiasis (abstract). *IVRA/ACVR/ECVDI Scientific Meeting*, August 7–11, 2006, Vancouver, Canada.

Hecht, S., et al. (2010). ^{99m}Tc-DTPA diuretic renal scintigraphy in cats with nephroureterolithiasis. *J Fel Med Surg* **12**(6): 423–430.

Kyles, A.E., et al. (2005). Clinical, clinicopathologic, radiographic, and ultrasonographic abnormalities in cats with ureteral calculi: 163 cases (1984–2002). *J Am Vet Med Assoc* **226**(6): 932–936.

Ling, G.V., et al. (1979). Percutaneous nephropyelocentesis and nephropyelostomy in the dog: a description of the technique. *Am J Vet Res* **40**(11): 1605–1612.

Nyland, T.G., et al. (2002). Urinary Tract. In: *Small Animal Diagnostic Ultrasound*, edited by T.G. Nyland and J.S. Mattoon, 2nd edition. Philadelphia, PA: WB Saunders, pp. 158–195.

Penninck, D.G. and S.T. Finn-Bodner (1998). Updates in interventional ultrasonography. *Vet Clin North Am Small Anim Pract* **28**(4): 1017–1040.

Pugh, C.R., et al. (1994). Iatrogenic renal pyelectasia in the dog. *Vet Radiol Ultrasound* **35**(1): 50–51.

Rivers, B.J., et al. (1997). Ultrasonographic-guided, percutaneous antegrade pyelography: technique and clinical application in the dog and cat. *J Am Anim Hosp Assoc* **33**: 61–68.

Szatmári, V., et al. (2001). Ultrasound-guided percutaneous drainage for treatment of pyonephrosis in two dogs. *J Am Vet Med Assoc* **218**(11): 1796–1799.

7

Urinalysis

Michael M. Fry

"Urinalysis is the best bargain in veterinary medicine."

Dr. Jeanne W. George

Introduction

The aim of this chapter is to provide a concise overview of routine urinalysis in dogs and cats, with an emphasis on the most important analytical aspects. The chapter will also consider preanalytical sample variables that may influence urinalysis results, as well as preanalytical patient variables other than those related to disease. Sampling techniques, expected urinalysis results with various diseases, other tests performed on urine, and recommended therapy are covered elsewhere in this text. Excellent resources are available to readers who want more comprehensive information about urinalysis in small animals (Osborne and Stevens 1999; Osborne and Stevens 2006; Wamsley and Alleman 2007).

Together with a complete blood count and a serum or plasma biochemical profile, urinalysis is considered part of the laboratory "minimum database". Routine urinalysis provides information about renal concentrating ability, glomerular permeability, other processes involving the urinary system (e.g., crystalluria, inflammation, infection, hemorrhage, and tubular damage), and processes involving other body systems (e.g., carbohydrate metabolism, intravascular hemolysis, rhabdomyolysis, and acid–base disturbances). Urinalysis is indicated *to help determine a diagnosis* in virtually all ill patients, *to monitor progression of disease and/or response to therapy* in patients with known disease, and *to screen asymptomatic individuals* for underlying disease (e.g., as part of preanesthetic evaluation or annual wellness examination or in individuals with a genetic or environmental predisposition to diseases with urinary manifestations). Although this chapter is not intended as an interpretive guide, the reader is asked to keep in mind that full, accurate interpretation of urinalysis results requires the clinician to integrate these findings with all the available patient data, including history, physical examination, clinical signs, and results of other diagnostic tests.

In-house versus send-out testing

It makes sense for most veterinary practices to do urinalysis in-house, from the standpoint of both practice economics and quality of care. The test requires only basic laboratory supplies (Table 7.1), and can be performed easily by clinic technical staff if they are properly trained—thus, it is an inexpensive and technically feasible test to perform (Table 7.2). By doing urinalysis in-house rather than sending samples to a commercial diagnostic laboratory, practices can offer the test at an affordable cost to the client and still make a reasonable profit. In-house testing is also preferred because of the faster turnaround time and greater accuracy of results, since delayed analysis is a potential source of introduced error (see *Preanalytical sample variables*, below). Another advantage of in-house testing is that results can be correlated more easily with the rest of the patient's clinical picture.

Preanalytical sample variables

Ideally, a urine sample submitted for analysis will be free of any contaminants, collected in a clean, opaque, airtight and sterile container and analyzed within 60 minutes of collection. However, as this is not always the case, the clinician should consider the influence of preanalytical sample (i.e., nonbiologic) variables when interpreting urinalysis results. The most important of these variables are the *collection method* and, if the sample is not analyzed immediately, the *storage time and conditions*. The collection method is particularly relevant with regard to

Nephrology and Urology of Small Animals. Edited by Joe Bartges and David J. Polzin. © 2011 Blackwell Publishing Ltd.

Table 7.1 Urinalysis supplies

Equipment
- Centrifuge
- Refractometer—preferably a temperature-compensated veterinary model with a feline-specific scale for urine-specific gravity
- Microscope—set to optimize contrast for unstained samples
- +/- Automated dipstick reader (optional)

Disposables
- Specimen container—should be clean, opaque, air-tight, sterile
- Disposable pipettes
- Conical centrifuge tubes
- Urine dipsticks
- Glass slides and coverslips
- +/- Sediment stain (optional)

potential contamination of the urine sample. For example, samples collected by cystocentesis typically have a small amount of iatrogenic blood contamination; voided samples often contain contaminants from the lower urogenital tract (e.g., bacteria, epithelial cells, spermatozoa, and blood) or the environment (e.g., bacteria, plant material, and debris); samples obtained by urinary catheterization may contain lower urogenital tract contaminants or iatrogenic hemorrhage; and samples obtained from the floor or examination table or from a litter box lined with nonabsorbent material are often contaminated with microbes and debris. Storage time and conditions may also affect urinalysis results. For example, refrigeration may promote crystal formation; prolonged storage of samples at room temperature may result in degeneration of cells and casts, altered crystal formation, or bacterial overgrowth and resultant secondary artifacts (e.g., altered pH and decreased glucose concentration); and exposure to light or air may alter the composition of the sample as a result of photodegradation, oxidation or evaporation.

Preanalytical patient variables

Other chapters in this text discuss the influence of disease on urinalysis results. This chapter's mention of the influence of preanalytical patient (i.e., biologic) variables on urinalysis results will be limited to common *physiologic variables* or *introduced variables* related to treatment or diagnosis. Physiologic variables that commonly affect urinalysis results include diet, time of day, and reproductive factors. For example, diet may influence urine pH or crystal formation; samples collected first thing in the morning tend to be more concentrated, and may have altered cellular morphology or microbial viability; and estrus or recent breeding may influence microscopic findings. Introduced patient variables that commonly affect urinalysis results include administration of drugs, fluids, or other exogenous agents. For example, corticos-

teroids and diuretics interfere with renal concentrating ability; corticosteroids may cause proteinuria; antimicrobials may mask urinary tract infections or form crystals; hydroxyethyl starch interferes with measurement of specific gravity; and radiographic contrast agents may interfere with measurement of specific gravity or biochemical analytes or may form crystals.

Components of routine urinalysis

Basic components of routine urinalysis include description of *gross appearance* and odor of the urine (odor is typically not reported by commercial laboratories), measurement of urine *specific gravity* using a refractometer, measurement of urine *biochemistry* using a commercial multi-analyte dipstick, and *microscopic examination* of urine sediment. Table 7.2 provides a step-by-step procedural guide to urinalysis, and Figure 7.1 provides a sample reporting form. Each component of urinalysis is discussed in more detail below.

Gross appearance and odor of urine

The gross appearance of urine provides subjective information about the composition of the sample. Normal urine is very pale yellow (virtually colorless) to dark yellow in color, and transparent to faintly cloudy. Highly concentrated urine is darker than more dilute urine, although color is not a reliable indicator of renal concentrating ability. High number of cells or bacteria may impart turbidity, and blood, free hemoglobin, myoglobin, or bilirubin may impart discoloration. Urine odor may also provide clues about pathology–for example, an ammoniacal odor suggests the presence of urease-producing bacteria, and a fruity odor suggests the presence of ketones–but odor is considered a nonspecific and generally an unreliable diagnostic indicator of disease.

Table 7.2 Urinalysis procedure

Sample submission
- Make sure the specimen identification matches the request/reporting form(s).
- The specimen container should be labeled with the patient's name or number and the date.
- The request/reporting form(s) should include the following information
  - The patient's name or ID number and signalment.
  - The date.
  - The time and method of urine collection.
  - Any current or recent therapeutic or diagnostic agents (e.g., drugs, radiographic contrast agents).
- If the same sample is to be used for urine culture, the portion for culture should be removed first into a sterile container (after gently mixing the sample) to avoid subsequent contamination.

Analysis
- General
  - Record the time the urinalysis is performed.
  - Record whether the sample has been refrigerated—if so, allow it to reach room temperature before proceeding.
  - Gently mix the sample by inverting the container at least 5 times.
  - Transfer 5 mL well-mixed urine to a clear conical centrifuge tube, saving the remainder of the sample for any further testing that may be indicated; if there is <5mL, then transfer the entire available volume to the conical tube.
  - Record the gross appearance of the urine in the conical tube.
- Dipstick biochemistry
  - Individuals performing urinalysis should read the dipstick package insert for details of the recommended procedure for that particular product. These instructions assume that dipstick results will be evaluated by direct visual inspection. If using an automated dipstick analyzer, consult the manufacturer for the recommended procedure.
  - Immerse all dipstick reagent pads in the well-mixed urine uncentrifuged sample, remove the dipstick immediately, start timing the reaction, and drag the edge of the reagent strip against the rim of the tube to remove any excess urine and help prevent cross-contamination of reagents (which may cause erroneous results).
  - Allow the specified time to elapse, then immediately read the results by using the color key provided by the dipstick manufacturer. Typically, the incubation time and the color key are printed on the dipstick container label.
  - Record dipstick results for the following tests:
    - Protein
    - pH
    - Blood
    - Glucose
    - Ketones
    - Bilirubin
    - (The following dipstick tests are either unreliable, inferior to other tests that are part of urinalysis, or of little clinical significance in dogs and cats and should not be recorded: specific gravity, leukocytes, nitrite, urobilinogen.)
  - If the sample is grossly bloody or highly turbid, repeat dipstick analysis using the supernatant from a centrifuged sample (see below for centrifugation instructions).
- Specific gravity
  - Use a refractometer, preferably a temperature-compensated instrument with a separate specific gravity scale for feline samples.
  - If the urine is clear (i.e., not turbid), use a well-mixed uncentrifuged sample. If the urine is turbid, use the supernatant from a centrifuged sample (see below for centrifugation instructions).
  - Record the specific gravity of the urine.
- Urine sediment examination
  - Centrifuge the 5 mL sample in the conical tube. The centrifuge should be set for 5 minutes at 1,500–2,000 rpm (or relative centrifugation force of 450).
  - Remove the supernatant by decanting or using a disposable transfer pipette, saving the supernatant for any further testing that may be indicated.
  - Re-suspend the sedimented "pellet" in 0.5-1 mL supernatant, mixing the re-suspension with a disposable transfer pipette or by flicking the tube with a finger. If <5 mL urine is centrifuged, then re-suspend the sediment in a proportionally smaller amount of supernatant (e.g., if 3 mL is centrifuged, re-suspend in 0.3-0.6 mL).
  - Using a disposable pipette, transfer a small drop of the re-suspension to a clean glass microscope slide and place a glass coverslip over it. There should be enough fluid to fill the area of the coverslip, but not enough to make it float.
  - The microscope should be set up to optimize contrast. This can be accomplished easily by closing the condenser diaphragm (if the microscope has one) or by lowering the condenser. Phase contrast microscopy also works well.
  - Survey the entire slide at low power (10x objective), then examine representative fields at high power (40x–60x objective) to verify and enhance observations made at lower power and to detect any bacteria.
  - Record the results of microscopic examination of the urine sediment.
  - If clinically significant crystalluria is noted in a sample that has been refrigerated, or stored for more than several hours under any conditions, microscopic examination should be repeated on a fresh, unrefrigerated sample.

Date: _____

Patient information

    Animal's name/Owner's name

    _____
    _____
    _____
    _____

    Patient ID#: _____

    Age: _____

    Species: _____

    Breed: _____

    Sex: _____

    Intact/neutered: _____

    Recent therapeutic or diagnostic agents administered?

    _____
    _____
    _____
    _____

Sample information

    Time of collection: _____

    Method of collection: _____

    Was the sample refrigerated? _____

    Sample also submitted for culture? _____

    Gross appearance: _____

    Odor: _____

Dipstick results

    pH _____

    Protein _____

    Blood _____

    Glucose _____

    Ketones _____

    Bilirubin _____

Refractometer specific gravity: _____

Sediment examination (# per 40× to 60× field)

    Cells

        RBCs _____

        WBCs _____

        Epithelial cells _____

    Crystals/type(s) _____

    Casts _____

    Organisms _____

    Other (lipid, sperm, debris) _____

Figure 7.1 Example urinalysis reporting form.

Urine-specific gravity

Urine-specific gravity (USG) is an index of concentration—the higher the USG, the more concentrated the urine—and is measured using a refractometer (see Chapter 41). Refractometers are not all the same, and will not all yield identical results (George 2001). Calibration scales for USG are different for humans and animals, and notably so for cats. If a refractometer with a scale calibrated for human urine is used for cat urine, the measured value will be falsely increased; the more concentrated the urine, the more pronounced the difference. Although the magnitude of the difference is not great, it is potentially of clinical significance, especially when the USG is near the threshold value for determining full concentrating ability. A feline urine sample with a USG of 1.034 will be measured as 1.040 using a human scale, which potentially could lead a clinician to misinterpret the result as evidence of full concentrating ability. Any laboratory or veterinary practice that performs urinalysis on feline samples should have a refractometer with a separate USG calibration scale for feline samples (Figure 7.2). As of 2001, only two refractometers had a separate scale for feline USG: the Vet 360 manufactured by Misco Corp., and the Vet 360 manufactured by Leica (George 2001). Temperature-compensated refractometers are preferred to those that are not temperature-compensated and

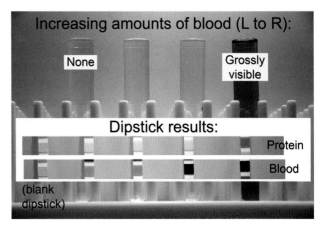

Figure 7.3 Urine dipstick results are semi-quantitative estimates based on the degree of color change in the reagent pads. This image illustrates the greater sensitivity of the blood reagent pad compared to the protein reagent pad: the sample in the second tube from the right is negative for protein, but strongly positive for blood.

which underestimate USG as ambient temperature increases above 68°F.

Marked proteinuria or glycosuria will cause a slight overestimation of urine concentration. For every gram per deciliter present in the urine, protein will add approximately 0.003–0.005, and glucose will add approximately 0.004–0.005, to the USG value (Stockham and Scott 2008). Intravenous administration of hetastarch in dogs causes a false increase in USG that is presumably transient (Smart et al. 2009).

Urine biochemistry

Urine biochemistry is routinely evaluated using the dipstick method. The degree of the color change on the dipstick reagent pad correlates with the concentration of the analyte (Figure 7.3). Results are evaluated semi-quantitatively, usually as negative, trace and 1+ to 4+; the concentration ranges that correlate with the semi-quantitative values are not identical for all dipsticks (Stockham and Scott 2008). Results may be obtained either by visual inspection of the dipstick or by an instrument that scans the dipstick automatically. A recently published study comparing visual and automated evaluation methods found them similar in terms of results, ease of use, and turnaround time (Bauer et al. 2008). The study noted that a clear advantage of the automated method is the ability to transmit results electronically to the laboratory information system, which not only saves time but reduces the probability of postanalytical (i.e., transcriptional) error.

In general, it is advisable to perform the urine dipstick test on a well-mixed uncentrifuged sample, since

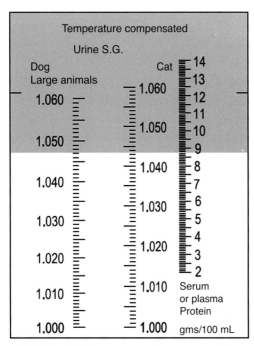

Figure 7.2 It is advisable to use a refractometer with a separate urine specific gravity scale for feline samples. This is from a Reichert VET 360 model. (Used with permission by Reichert Technologies, Depew, NY.)

cells or particles may not be present in the supernatant of a centrifuged sample. Usually, it does not make much difference whether dipstick assays are performed on a well-mixed uncentrifuged sample or supernatant of a centrifuged sample. The dipstick method is inexpensive, easy to use, and quite a reliable means of detecting some urine abnormalities. Note that false-negative or false-positive dipstick results may occur under some conditions and pigmenturia (abnormal urine color) may interfere with interpretation of dipstick results. Readers are strongly advised to consult the package insert for the urine dipstick used in their practice, and to familiarize themselves with recommended protocol and recognized interferents. The most common urine dipstick analytes are listed below.

pH

The dipstick method is an unreliable means of measuring pH. If accurate measurement of urine pH is important, a pH meter should be used—relatively inexpensive handheld instruments are commercially available (Johnson et al. 2007). Inaccuracy of the dipstick method is most likely to be of clinical significance when the urine pH is close to neutral. A recently published study in dogs found that the dipstick method tended to overestimate pH, in some cases yielding an alkaline result for a sample that had a mildly acidic urine as determined by the reference method (Johnson et al. 2007).

Glucose

The dipstick method is a reasonably accurate means of detecting glucose in the urine (glycosuria). Glycosuria occurs whenever the renal tubular reabsorption threshold is exceeded due to hyperglycemia, even if only transiently, and may also occur due to defective renal tubular function.

Bilirubin

The dipstick method is a reasonably accurate means of detecting conjugated bilirubin in the urine. Trace to mild bilirubinuria (1+ or occasionally higher in highly concentrated urine) is within normal limits in dogs, most commonly in male dogs, but otherwise bilirubinuria is a pathologic finding. Bilirubinuria is expected in any patient with abnormally high plasma concentration of bilirubin in the plasma (hyperbilirubinemia).

Ketones

The dipstick method is a common means of detecting ketoacidosis. A positive result is always an abnormal finding. However, false negatives may occur because the dipstick reagent reacts only with certain ketones (acetoacetate and acetone, but not β-hydroxybutyrate).

Specific gravity

The dipstick method is an unreliable means of measuring specific gravity. Refractometry is the method of choice (see above).

Blood (sometimes known as "blood protein", "occult blood", or "heme", or "heme protein")

The dipstick reagent for blood reacts with heme, and therefore yields a positive test result in cases of hematuria (erythrocytes lyse in contact with the reagent pad), hemoglobinuria, or myoglobinuria—thus, it is important to correlate dipstick results with microscopic urine sediment findings and with the gross appearance of the urine and plasma (see Chapter 46). This dipstick test is very sensitive, that is, it takes very little of any of these heme-containing substances to produce a positive result. It is much more sensitive than the regular protein dipstick test (see below). In the absence of any other abnormal protein in the urine, it typically takes a strongly positive blood result to cause a weakly positive regular protein result, so it is common to have a positive result for the former and a negative result for the latter (Figure 7.3).

Protein

The dipstick method is quite a reliable means of detecting protein in the urine. The dipstick reagent reacts strongly with albumin, which is usually the predominant type of protein in the urine in cases of clinically significant proteinuria, but does not react with some globulins (e.g., Bence Jones proteins). Some evidence indicates that false-positive results occur with alkaline urine, but at least one recent study suggests that this occurs infrequently (Welles et al. 2006). Trace to 1+ proteinuria may be found incidentally in dogs with USG of ≥ 1.020 (but may also occur due to pathology); however, proteinuria is otherwise an abnormal finding in dogs and is always an abnormal finding in cats.

For many years, most laboratories have included another semi-quantitative method, the sulfasalicylic acid (SSA) precipitation test, as a component of routine urinalysis, to verify urine dipstick protein findings. A recently published study found the dipstick method to be a more sensitive means of detecting proteinuria in dogs and cats than the SSA method, using a quantitative microprotein assay as the basis for comparison. The overall specificity of the dipstick and SSA tests were comparable, although the dipstick was more likely to yield a falsely low value (trace or 1+) compared to the quantitative method (Welles et al. 2006). On the basis of these findings, a similar study was done in our laboratory, comparing protein values obtained using a dipstick method (Bayer Multistix 10 SG, Bayer Corporation, Elkhart, IN) or the SSA method with those obtained using a quantitative method on our automated chemistry analyzer (Hitachi 911 analyzer; Roche Urinary/CSF Protein reagent) and found the dipstick method to have higher sensitivity than and equal specificity to the SSA method in dogs and cats (unpublished data). We no longer use the SSA test in our laboratory for canine or feline urine samples. Our recommendation is to do a quantitative urine protein measurement and urine protein to creatinine ratio in any patient suspected of having clinically significant proteinuria (see Chapter 8).

Recently, commercially available microalbuminuria assays have become widely available for dog and cats. The microalbuminuria assay detects urinary albumin in concentrations below the detection limits of the dipstick and SSA methods—and it has been suggested that the microalbuminuria assay may be appropriate for use as a screening test (Whittemore et al. 2006, 2007). At present, however, a clear rationale for incorporating this assay into the "minimum database" is lacking. (See Chapter 8 in this book for additional information on urine protein testing.)

Urobilinogen

This test is of little clinical value.

Nitrite

The dipstick method is an unreliable means of detecting bacteria in urine and is of little clinical value.

Leukocytes

The dipstick method is an unreliable means of detecting leukocytes in the urine, especially in cats. Microscopic examination of the urine sediment is the method of choice (see below).

Urine sediment evaluation

Much information can be gained from microscopic examination of the urine sediment. Urine sediment stains, stains that are mixed with urine sediment before applying a drop of the resuspension to a glass slide and coverslipping it, are commercially available, and novice microscopists often find it easier to examine stained rather than unstained "wet-mounted" preparations. A good rule of thumb is to always look at the unstained sediment first. It is the author's experience that most

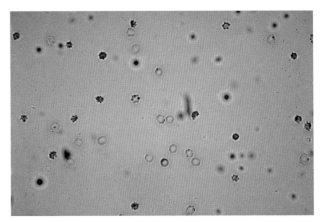

Figure 7.4 Normal and crenated RBCs in unstained urine sediment. (Osborne and Stevens 1999. Used with permission.)

clinical pathologists and medical technologists prefer to examine unstained urine sediment, and with a properly set up microscope, this is no more technically demanding than examining stained preparations. A rationale offered for this preference is that the disadvantages of using a urine sediment stain, especially the introduced variation (dilution, variable staining quality, potential stain precipitation or contamination) outweigh the advantages. However, there is evidence that a different type of staining technique helps with detection of bacteriuria: a blinded prospective study comparing routine unstained wet-mounted preparations and air-dried modified Wright-stained preparations of urine sediment with results of quantitative urine culture found that this staining method improved sensitivity, specificity, positive predictive value, and test efficiency (Swenson et al. 2004). This principle is illustrated in Figure 7.7. Rapid stains commonly used in the practice setting (e.g., Diff-Quik

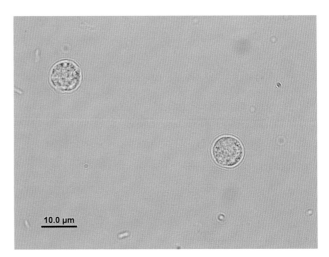

10.0 μm

Figure 7.5 WBCs and bacterial rods in unstained urine sediment (the rods are in a slightly different focal plane and are out of focus in this image).

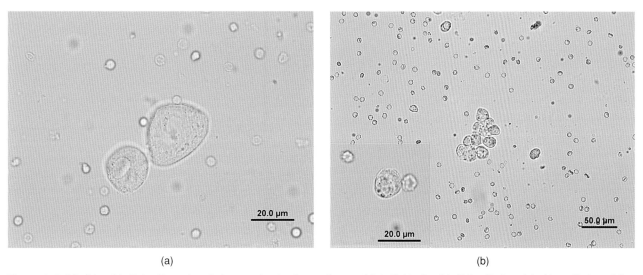

Figure 7.6 (a), (b) Epithelial cells and RBCs in unstained urine sediment: (a) Individual epithelial cells found incidentally in a feline sample; (b) Clustered epithelial cells found in a canine sample (further testing may be indicated to evaluate for possible urinary tract neoplasia or other underlying disease).

or Camco) would be likely to confer a similar benefit. Another approach to staining urine sediment is to use a microhematocrit tube to introduce new methylene blue under the coverslip of a wet mount by capillary action. Stained and unstained preparations can be placed side-by-side on the same slide, allowing for a direct "before and after" comparison.

Erythrocytes (Figure 7.4)

It is within normal limits to see low numbers (5/hpf) of erythrocytes (red blood cells, RBCs) in urine, or more in samples obtained by cystocentesis (iatrogenic contami-

nation) or in females in estrus. RBCs in increased numbers in the urine (hematuria) are indicative of a hemorrhage. It is within normal limits for RBCs in urine to have a crenated morphology.

Leukocytes (Figure 7.5)

It is within normal limits to see low numbers (5/hpf) of leukocytes (white blood cells, WBCs) in urine. WBCs in increased numbers in the urine (pyuria) indicate inflammation. Mildly increased numbers of WBCs in the urine may also occur as a result hematuria, but the increase is

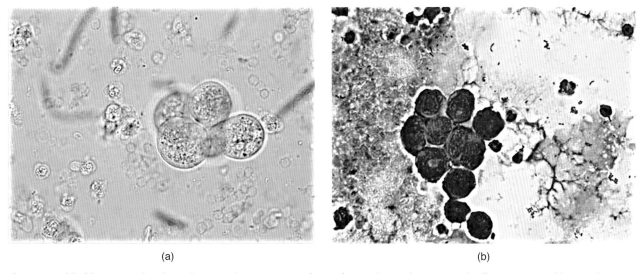

Figure 7.7 (a), (b) Unstained and Wright-stained preparations of urine from a dog with transitional cell carcinoma and bacterial cystitis. Staining helps with detection of bacteriuria.

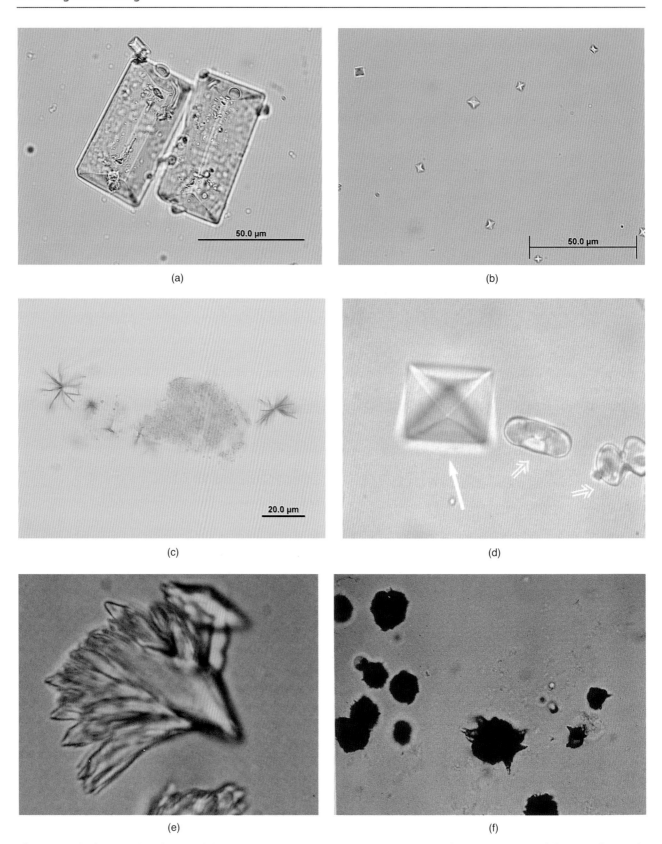

(a)

(b)

(c)

(d)

(e)

(f)

Figure 7.8 (a–f), Examples of some of the more commonly encountered crystals in urine (unstained sediment) from small animals: (a) struvite; (b) calcium oxalate dihydrate; (c) bilirubin; (d) calcium oxalate dihydrate (closed arrow) and monohydrate (open arrows); (e) calcium oxalate monohydrate; (f) ammonium urate. (df: Osborne and Stevens 1999. Used with permission.) Readers are advised to consult other references (Osborne and Stevens 1999; Osborne and Stevens 2006) for more comprehensive crystalluria images, including images of rarely-encountered crystals.

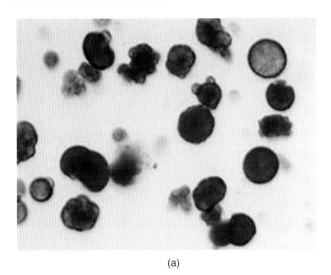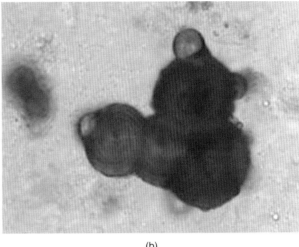

(a)   (b)

Figure 7.9 (a), (b) Low power (a) and 400x power (b) images of melamine-cyanuric acid crystals in unstained urine sediment from a cat. (Images courtesy of Dr. Brent Hoff, Animal Health Laboratory, University of Guelph. Used with permission.)

generally undetectable because the proportion of WBCs is so low compared to RBCs.

Epithelial cells (Figures 7.6 and 7.7)

It is within normal limits to see low numbers of epithelial cells in urine samples. Normal epithelial cells include transitional cells (urothelium) in samples obtained by cystocentesis, transitional cells and/or squamous epithelial cells in voided samples or samples obtained by catheter, and even rare renal tubular cells in any type of sample. Large, atypical epithelial cells, or high numbers of any type of epithelial cells, are an abnormal finding, and may indicate further testing to evaluate for possible urinary tract neoplasia or other underlying disease (see Chapter 79).

Crystals (Figures 7.8 and 7.9)

Urine crystals may be seen as an incidental finding (e.g., struvite) or pathologic finding (e.g., calcium oxalate monohydrate in ethylene glycol toxicity, ammonium biurate in patients with portosystemic shunts, etc.). Crystalluria does not correlate highly with urolithiasis (see Chapter 69). Some of the more commonly encountered crystals in dogs and cats are shown in Figure 7.8. However, it is worth keeping in mind that previously unreported crystals may occur, as was the case with the recent outbreak of melamine and cyanuric acid contamination of pet food (Figure 7.9).

Organisms (Figures 7.5, 7.7, and 7.10)

It is within normal limits to see low numbers of bacteria in voided samples (especially cocci) or samples obtained

from the floor, table, or litter box (mixed bacteria). It is not normal to see organisms in samples obtained by cystocentesis. Pyuria is expected in cases of UTI (see Chapters 71), but not always found, especially in immunocompromised patients. Not seeing any bacteria does not exclude the possibility of a urinary tract infection (UTI). A culture is a more sensitive means of detection (see Chapter 9). Fungi or parasite eggs may rarely be found in urine samples as pathogens or contaminants (see Chapters 72 and 74).

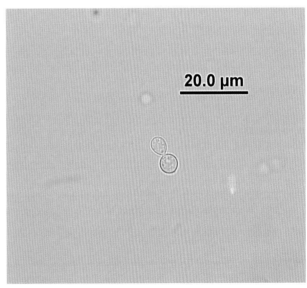

Figure 7.10 Budding yeast in unstained urine sediment from a dog. *Cryptococcus neoformans* was cultured from this sample. The organism's characteristic narrow-based budding is evident, but its characteristic capsule is not apparent in this preparation.

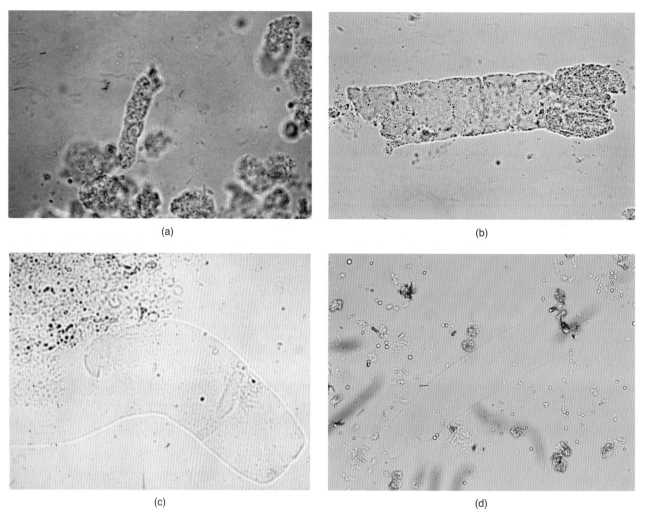

Figure 7.11 (a–d) Examples of casts in unstained urine sediment: (a) mixed granular cast containing what appears to be a cell and surrounding granular epithelial cells; (b) mixed granular and waxy cast; (c) hyaline cast and amorphous debris; (d) bilirubin-stained waxy cast with surrounding bilirubin crystals, fat droplets, and occasional cells. (a–c: Osborne and Stevens 1999. Used with permission.)

Casts (Figure 7.11)

Casts are cylinder-shaped forms that literally are casts of the renal tubules (the tubular lumen acts as a mold); the presence of casts in the urine is sometimes called cylinduria. Casts are composed mainly of a mucoprotein (Tamm-Horsfall protein) secreted by cells lining certain parts of the nephron, and often have cells incorporated within them. Casts are classified as cellular (individual cells are discernible), granular (cells have partially disintegrated), waxy (cells have disintegrated and the casts have a smooth, waxy texture), or hyaline (casts are acellular, clear, and colorless). The presence of rare hyaline or granular casts is considered within normal limits; otherwise, cylinduria indicates urinary tract (usually tubular) pathology.

Lipid (Figure 7.12)

Fat droplets are occasionally noted in urine, most often in cats, and are usually an incidental finding. They may be confused with bacterial cocci, but typically are of more variable size than organisms.

Debris (Figures 7.11c and 7.12)

Amorphous to granular debris is commonly seen in urine as an incidental finding.

Spermatozoa (Figure 7.12)

Spermatozoa are often present in urine from intact males (even in samples obtained by cystocentesis), and are occasionally noted in females after breeding.

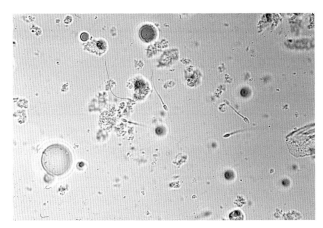

Figure 7.12 Other common findings in urine sediment include lipid droplets, amorphous granular debris, and/or spermatozoa, all of which are present in this image. (Osborne and Stevens 1999. Used with permission.)

References

Bauer, N., S. Rettig, et al. (2008). Evaluation of the Clinitek status trade mark automated dipstick analysis device for semi-quantitative testing of canine urine. *Res Vet Sci* **85**(3): 467–472.

George, J. (2001). The usefulness and limitations of hand-held refractometers in veterinary laboratory medicine: a historical and technical review. *Vet Clin Pathol* **30**: 201–210.

Johnson, K., J. Lulich, *et al.* (2007). Evaluation of the reproducibility and accuracy of pH-determining devices used to measure urine pH in dogs. *J Am Vet Med Assoc* **230**: 364–369.

Osborne, C.A. and J.B. Stevens. (1999). *Urinalysis: A Clinical Guide to Compassionate Patient Care.* Shawnee Mission, Kansas: Bayer Corporation.

Osborne, C.A. and J.B. Stevens. (2006). *Urine Sediment Reference Guide.* Shawnee Mission, Kansas: Bayer Corporation.

Smart, L., K. Hopper, *et al.* (2009). The effect of hetastarch (670/0.75) on specific gravity and osmolality of urine in the dog. *J Vet Intern Med* **23**: 388–391.

Stockham, S.L. and M.A. Scott. (2008). Urinary system. In: *Fundamentals of Veterinary Clinical Pathology*, edited by S.L. Stockham and M.A. Scott, 2nd edition. Ames, IA: Blackwell, pp. 415–494.

Swenson, C., A. Boisvert, *et al.* (2004). Evaluation of modified Wright-staining of urine sediment as a method for accurate detection of bacteriuria in dogs. *J Am Vet Med Assoc* **224**: 1282–1289.

Wamsley, H. and R. Alleman. (2007). Complete urinalysis. In: *BSAVA Manual of Canine and Feline Nephrology and Urology*, edited by J. Elliott and G.F. Grauer, 2nd edition. Waterwells, UK: British Small Animal Veterinary Association, pp. 87–116.

Welles, E., E. Whatley, *et al.* (2006). Comparison of Multistix PRO dipsticks with other biochemical assays for determining urine protein (UP), urine creatinine (UC) and UP:UC ratio in dogs and cats. *Vet Clin Pathol* **35**: 31–36.

Whittemore, J., V. Gill, *et al.* (2006). Evaluation of the association between microalbuminuria and the urine albumin-creatinine ratio and systemic disease in dogs. *J Am Vet Med Assoc* **229**: 958–963.

Whittemore, J., Z. Miyoshi, *et al.* (2007). Association of microalbuminuria and the urine albumin-to-creatinine ratio with systemic disease in cats. *J Am Vet Med Assoc* **230**: 1165–1169.

8

Urine protein and microalbuminuria

Mary B. Nabity

Normal urine should contain little protein, since the glomerulus prevents large proteins from entering the urine filtrate and the tubules reabsorb most small proteins that pass through. In addition, tubules only secrete a small amount of protein. Thus, protein normally present in urine is not detectable with common screening methods (urine dipstick, SSA; see Chapter 7) (Table 8.1). When the dipstick is positive for proteinuria it is abnormal, and the next steps are to (1) confirm proteinuria if it is a trace or 1+ reaction (many advocate the SSA or microalbuminuria test as confirmatory tests), and (2) determine the origin of the protein. Before additional specific testing of the proteinuria is performed, it should be localized to the kidney (rule out prerenal and postrenal causes of proteinuria), and the sediment should ideally be inactive (absence of hematuria, particularly gross hematuria, and pyuria). However, if a large degree of proteinuria is found with an active sediment, it could indicate renal disease (Vaden et al. 2004). In this case, the proteinuria should be re-evaluated after the sediment is cleared, if possible.

Quantitative evaluation of proteinuria

Once the source of the protein has been localized to the kidney, the degree of proteinuria should be quantified (Table 8.1) since the magnitude of proteinuria appears to correlate with worse disease and a poorer prognosis in dogs and cats with chronic renal disease (see Chapters 43 and 53) (Jacob et al. 2005; Syme et al. 2006). Proteinuria is classically defined as excretion of >15–20 mg protein/kg per day in dogs and cats based on a 24-hour urine collection (Lulich and Osborne 1990) (Monroe, 1989; Adams, 1992). However, the most convenient method to quantify proteinuria is the urine protein/creatinine ratio (UPC).

Currently, the UPC is considered abnormal if >0.5 in an adult dog and >0.4 in an adult cat, although the UPC is generally <0.2 in most healthy adult animals (Lees et al. 2005; Grauer et al. 1985). The UPC can be measured by most reference laboratory chemistry analyzers. A bench top chemistry analyzer is now available to the general practitioner.[1] In addition, semi-quantitative urine dipsticks can be used to estimate the UPC in dogs (Welles et al. 2006).

Serial UPC measurements are recommended to establish persistence of proteinuria (defined as proteinuria detected on three separate occasions ≥ 2 weeks apart) and to assess progression and treatment of renal disease. When monitoring the UPC in dogs, one study suggests that in order to determine if a value has changed from baseline (when the baseline is between 0.5 and 12), it must increase or decrease by a minimum of 35–80% with a higher percent change required at lower UPC values (Nabity et al. 2007).

Qualitative evaluation of proteinuria

Qualitative evaluation of proteinuria refers to identification of specific proteins in the urine or patterns of proteins (as identified by proteomics techniques) rather than the magnitude of proteinuria. These proteins and protein patterns can help determine whether tubular and/or glomerular disease is present. Qualitative proteinuria can also be informative when monitoring both acute renal injury and chronic renal disease, although additional studies in veterinary medicine are required.

Glomerular proteinuria refers to the presence of intermediate ($\sim$60–90 kD, e.g., albumin) to large ($\geq$100 kD, e.g., IgG) molecular weight proteins due to a compromised filtration barrier. Tubular proteinuria refers to the predominance of low molecular weight (LMW) proteins (<60 kD) (Zini et al. 2004). The proteins present with

Nephrology and Urology of Small Animals. Edited by Joe Bartges and David J. Polzin. © 2011 Blackwell Publishing Ltd.

Table 8.1 Methods for measuring urine protein

	Test type	Methodology of protein measurement	Protein type measured	Lower limit of detection	False-negative	False-positive	Comments
Semi-quantitative							
urine dipstick	Colorimetric	Indicator dye[a] binds amino groups; pad buffered at pH3	Mostly albumin; others to lesser extent	15–30 mg/dL	Dilute urine, proteins other than albumin	Highly concentrated urine, extreme alkaluria, quaternary ammonium salts, chlorhexidine	Good initial screening tool; must take into account SG
Sulfo salicylic acid test (SSA)	Turbidometric	Acid denatures protein resulting in precipitation	All protein	5–10 mg/dL	Dilute urine, alkaluria	Turbid urine, radiographic contrast agent, some antibiotics, crystal precipitation	Confirmatory test for dipstick; must account for SG
E.R.D.-HealthScreen™ (dipstick)[b]	Immunoassay	Monoclonal antibody against albumin	Albumin	1 mg/dL	Proteins other than albumin	Reportedly 100% specific	Standardized by SG; species-specific
Quantitative							
UPC[c]	Colorimetric	CBB[d], PVD[e], PS[f]	All protein	5 mg/dL	Dependent on methodology	Dependent on methodology	Not affected by urine volume and concentration
24-hour collection	Colorimetric	Same as for UPC	All protein	5 mg/dL	Dependent on methodology	Dependent on methodology	Gold-standard, cumbersome (metabolic cage or catheter)
ERD™ test[g]	Immunoassay	Monoclonal antibody against albumin	Albumin	1 mg/dL	Proteins other than albumin	Reportedly 100% specific	Standardized by SG, species-specific

[a]Tetrabromphenol blue.
[b]Heska, Ft. Collins, CO.
[c]Creatinine measured by amidohydrolase, iminohydrolase, or alkaline picrate method.
[c]UPC = Urine protein/creatinine ratio.
[d]Coomassie brilliant blue.
[e]Pyrocatechol violet dye.
[f]Ponceau S.
[g]Antech Diagnostic Laboratories.

tubular proteinuria can originate from two main sources: (1) damaged tubular cells, and (2) plasma. The proteins originating from the plasma are LMW and appear in the urine secondary to decreased reabsorption due to tubular injury and/or overload. Many tubular proteins have shown promise in the detection and monitoring of acute and chronic renal disease (Table 8.2).

Microalbuminuria

Microalbuminuria (MA) is defined as albumin present between 1–30 mg/dL when the specific gravity (SG) is normalized to 1.010. The standard urine dipstick does not reliably detect this small degree of albumin, and MA may be a significant indicator of renal disease even in the absence of a positive dipstick or an increased UPC. MA is associated with renal disease progression and increased mortality in humans (Basi and Lewis 2006), and it has been associated with underlying disease in both dogs and cats (Whittemore et al. 2006, 2007). It may also precede overt proteinuria in dogs with hereditary glomerular disease that leads to renal failure (Vaden et al. 2001; Lees et al. 2002). However, while persistent MA is considered an abnormal finding, it does not always indicate

Table 8.2 A sampling of urinary proteins that may be promising indicators of renal tubular damage

Protein	Origin	Evaluated in cats or dogs (if known)
Decreased presence in urine:		
Cauxin	Proximal tubules	Cats
Tamm-Horsfall protein	Distal tubules	Dogs
Increased presence in urine:		
α_1-microglobulin	Plasma	Dogs
β_2-microglobulin	Plasma	Dogs
Clusterin	Proximal tubules	
Cystatin C	Plasma	
Cysteine-rich protein 61	Proximal tubules	
γ-glutamyl transferase	Proximal tubules	Dogs and cats
Glutathione-s-transferase	Tubules	
Interleukin 18	Tubules	
Kidney injury molecule 1	Proximal tubules	
Lysozyme	Plasma and tubules	Dogs
N-acetyl-β-D-glucosaminidase	Proximal tubules	Dogs and cats
Neutrophil gelatinase-associated lipocalin	Plasma and tubules	Dogs
Pap X 5C10 antigen	Papillary collecting ducts	
Retinol-binding protein	Plasma	Dogs and cats
Transthyretin	Plasma	Dogs
Vitamin D-binding protein	Plasma	Dogs

progressive or clinically significant renal disease. Prognostic studies are still needed in veterinary medicine, and the list of causes for MA is extensive and includes a variety of extra-renal diseases as well as renal diseases. Therefore, a patient should be thoroughly evaluated for both systemic disease and renal disease when MA is detected.

The available tests to detect MA in dogs and cats are normalized to SG 1.010 to account for urine concentration (Table 8.1). They use a species-specific monoclonal antibody so only those tests designed specifically for the cat or dog should be used. If MA is detected a follow-up UPC is recommended to quantify the proteinuria. Although there is reasonably good positive correlation between UPC and MA concentration, one does not always predict the results of the other. In fact, some cats with a negative MA test had an increased UPC (Mardell and Sparkes 2006). MA can be useful to confirm proteinuria when results for conventional tests are equivocal or conflicting. However, in general, it is not worthwhile to test for microalbuminuria when the UPC > 2, since most of the protein in that case should be albumin.

Endnote

1. *VetTest® Chemistry Analyzer, IDEXX Laboratories, Inc.

References

Adams, L. et al. (1992). Correlation of urine protein/creatinine ratio and twenty-four-hour urinary protein excretion in normal cats and cats with surgically induced chronic renal failure. *J Vet Intern Med* **6**(1): 36–40.

Basi, S. and J. Lewis (2006). Microalbuminuria as a target to improve cardiovascular and renal outcomes. *Am J Kidney Dis* **47**(6): 927–946.

Grauer, G., et al. (1985). Estimation of quantitative proteinuria in the dog, using the urine protein-to-creatinine ratio from a random, voided sample. *Am J Vet Res* **46**(10): 2116–2119.

Jacob, F., et al. (2005). Evaluation of the association between initial proteinuria and morbidity rate or death in dogs with naturally occurring chronic renal failure. *Am J Vet Res* **226**(3): 393–400.

Lees, G., et al. (2005). Assessment and management of proteinuria in dogs and cats: 2004 ACVIM forum consensus statement (small animal). *J Vet Intern Med* **19**(3): 377–385.

Lees, G., et al. (2002). Persistent albuminuria precedes onset of overt proteinuria in male dogs with X-linked hereditary nephropathy. *J Vet Intern Med* **16**(3): 353A.

Lulich, J. and C. Osborne (1990). Interpretation of protein-creanine ratios in dogs with glomerular and nonglomerular disorders. *Comp Cont Ed Pract Vet* **12**(1): 59–72.

Mardell, E. and A. Sparkes (2006). Evaluation of a commercial in-house test for the semi-quantitative assessment of microalbuminuria in cats. *J Feline Med Surg* **8**(4): 269–278.

Monroe, W. et al. (1989). Twenty-four hour urinary protein loss in healthy cats and the urinary protein-creatinine ratio as an estimate. *Am J Vet Res* **50**(11): 1906–1909.

Nabity, M., et al. (2007). Day-to-day variation of the urine protein:creatinine ratio in female dogs with stable glomerular proteinuria caused by X-linked hereditary nephropathy. *J Vet Intern Med* **21**(3): 425–430.

Syme, H., et al. (2006). Survival of cats with naturally occurring chronic renal failure is related to severity of proteinuria. *J Vet Intern Med* **20**(3): 528–535.

Vaden, S., et al. (2001). Longitudinal study of microalbuminuria in soft-coated wheaten terriers. *J Vet Intern Med* **15**(3): 300A.

Vaden, S., et al. (2004). Effects of urinary tract inflammation and sample blood contamination on urine albumin and total protein concentration in canine urine samples. *Vet Clin pathol* **33**(1): 14–19.

Welles, E., et al. (2006). Comparison of multistix PRO dipsticks with other biochemical assays for determining urine protein, urine creatinine, and UP:UC ratio in dogs and cats. *Vet Clin Pathol* **35**(1): 31–36.

Whittemore, J., et al. (2006). Evaluation of the association between microalbuminuria and the urine albumin-creatinine ratio systemic disease in dogs. *J Am Vet Med Assoc* **229**(6): 958–963.

Whittemore, J., et al. (2007). Association of microalbuminuria and the urine albumin-to-creatinine ratio with systemic disease in cats. *J Am Vet Med Assoc* **230**(8): 1165–1169.

Zini, E., et al. (2004). Diagnostic relevance of qualitative proteinuria evaluated by use of sodium dodecyl sulfate-agarose gel electrophoresis and comparison with renal histologic findings in dogs. *Am J Vet Res* **65**(7): 964–971.

9

Urine culture

Joe Bartges

Urinary tract infections (UTIs) develop when a temporary or permanent breach in host defense mechanisms allows virulent microbes to adhere, multiply, and persist within the urinary tract (see Chapters 71, 72, and 73). UTIs are most commonly caused by bacteria although fungi and viruses may also infect the urinary tract. Analysis of urine for infection (urine culture and antimicrobial susceptibility testing) is an important part of diagnosing and treating bacterial UTIs.

Urine collection

Ideally, urine samples submitted for culture should be collected by cystocentesis (see Chapter 5). In animals with severe clinical signs of lower urinary tract disease, collection of urine by this method may be difficult because of frequent voiding. In these patients it may be necessary to collect urine by catheterization or, less desirably, voiding. Urine collection by catheterization requires cleansing of the pet's external genitalia prior to catheterization and the perivulvar fur may require clipping to prevent contamination. Although urinary catheterization of male dogs is usually accomplished without chemical restraint, many female dogs and all cats require sedation or anesthesia. A sterile catheter and collection container (a syringe or a collection cup with a tight-fitting lid) should be used. Urine samples collected during natural voiding should ideally be "mid-stream," thus avoiding bacterial contamination that may result from initial flushing out of resident flora in the distal urethra and external genitalia. If the results of quantitative culture of urine samples obtained by catheterization or mid-stream voiding are equivocal after culture (Table 9.1), urine should be collected by cystocentesis.

Urine culture

As already mentioned, urine culture is the gold standard for diagnosis of bacterial UTI. A diagnosis of UTI based solely on clinical signs or urinalysis findings of hematuria and/or urinary tract inflammation may result in a misdiagnosis, as it does not allow precise identification of the infecting organism or determination of sensitivity to various antimicrobials, and thus possibly inadequate or inappropriate treatment. Under some circumstances, antimicrobial therapy may be considered without first obtaining the results of urine culture; however, samples for urine culture should be collected before drug therapy is started. If antimicrobial therapy has occurred, it should be discontinued for 3–5 days prior to collection of urine for urine culture to minimize in vitro inhibition of microbial growth.

Following collection of urine, samples should be preserved and transported so as to avoid bacterial contamination, proliferation, or death (Padilla et al. 1981). Urine specimens for aerobic bacterial culture should be stored and transported in sealed, sterilized containers, and processing should begin as soon as possible. A variety of sterile containers can be used which do not contain preservatives or inhibitors; these are suitable only when samples are immediately transported and processed by microbiology laboratories, as they will not prevent bacterial proliferation (thus, falsely increasing the number of colony-forming units [CFU] per milliliter of urine) or eventual death (thus resulting in false-negative results). When these standard transport containers are used and laboratory processing is delayed by more than 30 minutes, urine specimens should be refrigerated at 4°C (Ling 1984; Lees 1996). Bacterial counts may double every 20–45 minutes at room temperature (Lees and Osborne 1979). Multiplication or destruction of bacteria may occur within 1 hour of collection.

Nephrology and Urology of Small Animals. Edited by Joe Bartges and David J. Polzin. © 2011 Blackwell Publishing Ltd.

Table 9.1 Interpretation of quantitative urine cultures in dogs and cats[a]

Sample type	Significant		Suspicious		Contaminant	
	Dogs	Cats	Dogs	Cats	Dogs	Cats
Cystocentesis	≥1,000	≥1,000	100–1,000	100–1,000	≤100	≤100
Catheterization	≥10,000	≥1,000	1,000–10,000	100–1,000	≤1,000	≤100
Mid-Stream voiding	≥100,000[b]	≥10,000	10,000–90,000	1,000–10,000	≤10,000	≤1,000
Manual compression	≥100,000[b]	≥10,000	10,000–90,000	1,000–10,000	≤10,000	≤1,000

Source: From Lulich and Osborne (1999).
[a]Values are given in colony-forming units per milliliter of urine (CFU/mL). Data represent generalities. Occasionally, bacterial UTI may be detected with fewer organisms (i.e., false-negative results).
[b]Due to the contamination level of mid-stream samples may be 10,000 CFU/mL or higher (i.e., false-positive result), these samples should not be used for routine diagnostic culture.

If samples cannot be processed immediately for urine culture, several alternatives are available. In-clinic urine cultures allow immediate processing of urine and may also decrease cost to owners by allowing veterinarians to select only positive samples for species identification and sensitivity testing by outside laboratories. Blood agar and MacConkey's agar plates may be inoculated and incubated for 24–48 hours. A calibrated bacteriologic loop or a microliter mechanical pipette that delivers exactly 0.01 or 0.001 mL of urine to the culture plates should be used to estimate CFU per mL, and urine should be streaked over the plates by conventional methods (Figure 9.1).

Blood agar supports the growth of most aerobic bacterial uropathogens, and MacConkey's agar provides mor-phologic information that aids in the identification of bacteria and prevents "swarming" of Proteus spp. Plates are incubated or placed under an incandescent light (Figure 9.2) (Saunders et al. 2002).

If bacterial growth is noted within 48 hours, the plates may be submitted for identification and determination of antimicrobial sensitivities (Figure 9.3) (Blanco et al. 2001; Saunders et al. 2001). If no growth occurs after 48–72 hours, the plates may be discarded.

Commercially available urine culture collection tubes containing preservative, which may or may not be combined with refrigeration, may be used to preserve

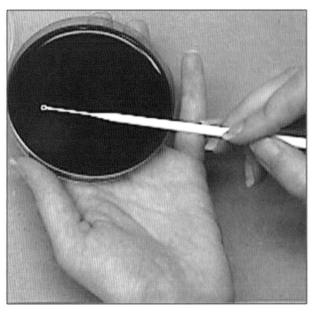

Figure 9.1 Use of a calibrated loop for inoculation of urine on a blood agar culture plate.

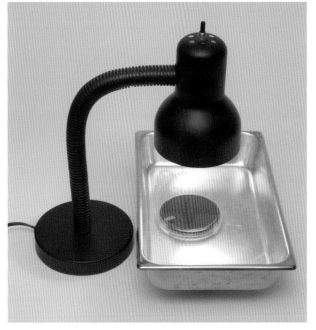

Figure 9.2 Incubation of an inoculated blood agar plate using a 60-watt incandescent light bulb to maintain a surface temperature on the culture plate of 38°C.

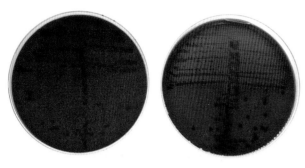

Figure 9.3 Blood agar plate with microbial growth after inoculation with a calibrated loop and incubation under an incandescent light bulb for 24 hours.

specimens for up to 72 hours before processing occurs (Allen et al. 1987). The advantage of these preservative tubes is that they allow veterinarians to delay submission of samples for urine culture until results of other diagnostic tests, such as urinalysis, become available. Innoculation of urine into an "enrichment" media (such as thioglycollate) may allow detection of low numbers of bacteria; this is most useful when urine culture during antimicrobial therapy cannot be avoided.

Qualitative urine culture

Qualitative urine culture refers to isolation and identification of bacteria in urine without precise quantification of bacterial numbers. Although urine in the bladder is normally sterile, urine that passes through the distal urogenital tract often becomes contaminated with resident microflora (see Table 9.2).

Therefore, the presence of bacteria in urine collected by catheterization or voiding may be difficult to interpret, even with quantification of bacteria. For this reason, purely qualitative urine cultures are not recommended, and a diagnostic urine culture should include quantitation of bacterial numbers in addition to precise identification of the infecting organism and antimicrobial susceptibility testing.

Quantitative urine culture

A quantitative urine culture includes isolation and identification of the infecting organism and determination of the number of bacteria (i.e., CFU per unit volume). Quantitation allows interpretation of the significance of bacteria present in a urine sample. Suggested ranges for number of CFU per mL of urine that likely indicate true infection have been suggested for each method of urine collection, and differ in dogs versus cats (Table 9.1); in cats, significant bacteriuria requires lower numbers of organisms because this species is more resistant to UTI than dogs. The presence of bacteria, even in low numbers,

Table 9.2 Commensal bacterial genera in the urogenital tract of normal dogs

Genus	Distal urethra of males	Prepuce	Vagina
Acinetobacter		+	+
Bacteroides			+
Bacillus		+	+
Citrobacter			+
Corynebacterium	+	+	+
Enterococcus			+
Enterobacter			+
Escherichia	+	+	+
Flavobacterium	+	+	+
Haemophilus	+	+	+
Klebsiella	+	+	+
Micrococcus			+
Moraxella		+	+
Mycoplasma	+	+	+
Neisseria			+
Pasteurella		+	+
Proteus		+	+
Pseudomonas			+
Staphylococcus	+	+	+
Streptococcus	+	+	+
Ureaplasma	+	+	+

Source: From Barsanti (2006).

in urine collected aseptically by cystocentesis indicates a UTI. Although urine obtained from most dogs without a UTI by any method is usually sterile or contains less than 10,000 CFU/mL, counts of 100,000 CFU/mL, or higher nevertheless occur with sufficient frequency to make collection of urine by mid-stream voiding or manual expression unsatisfactory in most cases (Barsanti 2006).

Antimicrobial susceptibility testing

Antimicrobial drugs are the cornerstone of treatment for UTI. The antimicrobial agent selected should be (1) easy to administer, (2) associated with few, if any, adverse effects, (3) inexpensive, (4) able to attain urine concentrations (and tissue concentrations in the event of kidney or prostatic infection) that exceed the minimum inhibitory concentration (MIC) for the uropathogen by at least fourfold, and (5) unlikely to affect the animal's resident gastrointestinal flora adversely. In most cases the antimicrobial agent chosen should be based on susceptibility testing of the uropathogen.

Agar disk diffusion technique

Antimicrobial susceptibility testing is often performed using agar disk diffusion (i.e., Kirby-Bauer technique), which is adequate for most bacterial UTIs. This method consists of Mueller-Hinton agar plates that have been inoculated with a standardized suspension of a single uropathogen isolated from the patient's urine. Paper disks impregnated with different antimicrobial drugs are placed on the plate. After 18–24 hours' inoculation at 38°C, antimicrobial susceptibility is estimated by measuring zones of inhibition of bacterial growth surrounding each disk. The zones of inhibition are then interpreted in light of established standards and reported as "resistant," "susceptible," or "intermediate susceptibility." Due to differences in the ability of various antimicrobials to diffuse through agar, the antimicrobial disk surrounded by the largest zone of inhibition is not necessarily the drug most likely to be effective. Also, because

the concentration of most antimicrobial drugs in the paper disks is comparable to the typical serum concentration of the drug, drugs that are found to have intermediate susceptibility by the agar disk diffusion method may still be effective in the urinary tract if they are excreted in high concentrations in urine (e.g., ampicillin, cephalexin).

Antimicrobial dilution technique

Antimicrobial dilution susceptibility testing determines the minimum concentration of an antimicrobial drug that will inhibit the growth of the uropathogen (i.e., the minimum bacteriostatic concentration, or MIC). After inoculation and incubation of uropathogens into

Table 9.3 Mean concentrations of selected antimicrobial agents in canine (D) or feline (C) urine

Drug	Daily dosage (mg/kg)	Route of administration	Mean urine concentration ($\pm$ SD)
Amikacin	5	SQ	342 $\pm$ 143 μg/mL (D)
Amoxicillin	11	PO	202 $\pm$ 93 μg/mL (D)
Ampicillin	26	PO	309 $\pm$ 55 μg/mL (D)
Cefovecin	8 (q15 d)	SQ	12 hours post: 9 $\pm$ 6.5 μg/mL (D)
			12 hours post: 66 $\pm$ 37 μg/mL (C)
			15 days post: 0.9 $\pm$ 0.7 μg/mL (D)
			15 days post: 3 $\pm$ 1.6 μg/mL (C)
Cephalexin	18	PO	500 μg/mL (D)
Chloramphenicol	33	PO	124 $\pm$ 40 μg/mL (D)
Difloxacin	5	PO	0.3 μg/mL (D)
Doxycycline	5	PO	53 $\pm$ 24 μg/mL (D, C)
Enrofloxacin	5	PO	40 $\pm$ 10 μg/mL (D)
Gentamicin	2	SQ	107 $\pm$ 33 μg/mL (D)
Hetacillin	26	PO	300 $\pm$ 156 μg/mL (D)
Ibafloxacin	15	PO	36–85 μg/mL (C)
Kanamycin	4	SQ	530 $\pm$ 151 μg/mL (D)
Marbofloxacin	2.75	PO	14 μg/mL (D)
Meropenem	20	IV, SQ	1296 μg/mL (D)
Nitrofurantoin	4.4	PO	100 μg/mL (D)
Norfloxacin	5	PO	34 $\pm$ 15 μg/mL (D)
	20	PO	57 $\pm$ 18 μg/mL (D)
Penicillin G	36,700 U/kg	PO	295 $\pm$ 211 μg/mL (D)
Penicillin V	26	PO	148 $\pm$ 99 μg/mL (D)
Sulfasoxazole	22	PO	1466 $\pm$ 832 μg/mL (D)
Tetracycline	18	PO	139 $\pm$ 65 μg/mL (D)
	20	PO	145 $\pm$ 39 μg/mL (D, C)
Trimethoprim/sulfadiazine	13	PO	55 $\pm$ 19 μg/mL (D)
Tobramycin	2.2	SQ	66 $\pm$ 39 μg/mL (D)
Vancomycin	15	IV	24 $\pm$ 15 μg/mL (D)

Source: Adapted from Ling (1984).
SD, Standard deviation; SQ, subcutaneous; PO, per os (by mouth); D, dog; C, cat.

Table 9.4 In vitro antimicrobial susceptibility testing

Antimicrobial susceptibility testing for urinary pathogens in dogs and cats is often reported as susceptible (S), intermediate susceptibility (I), or resistant (R), and is based on standardized methods published by the National Committee for Clinical Laboratory Standards (NCLS). The criteria and interpretations are based on studies from human beings, but can be extrapolated to dogs and cats. Using the SIR system:

- S indicates that the infection due to the identified organism may be appropriately treated with the dosage of antimicrobial agent recommended.
- I indicates that the response rates may be lower than those for susceptible isolates of the identified organism. This category implies that drugs that achieve high concentrations in urine may still be used and effective.
- R indicates clinical efficacy of this antimicrobial agent has not been reliable or is unlikely to be effective.

Antimicrobial agents against Gram negative bacteria (except *Pseudomonas spp*)

Antimicrobial		MIC (μg/mL) Interpretation		
		S	I	R
Penicillins				
P	Penicillin G	N/A	N/A	N/A
P/O	Ampicillin	≤ 8	16	≥ 32
O/P	Amoxicillin			
P	Ticarcillin	≤ 16	32–64	≥ 128
P	Mezlocilin	≤ 16	32–64	≥ 128
P	Piperacillin	≤ 16	32–64	≥ 128
O	Amoxicillin/clavulanate	≤ 8	16	≥ 32
O	Ampicillin/sulbactam			
P	Piperacillin/tazobactam	≤ 16	32–64	≥ 128
P	Ticarcillin/clavulanate	≤ 16	32–64	≥ 128
Cephalosporins				
P	Cepholothin	≤ 8	16	≥ 32
O	Cephalexin			
O	Cefadroxil			
P	Cephapirin			
O	Cefaclor			
P	Ceftiofur	≤ 8	16	≥ 32
P	Cefazolin	≤ 8	16	≥ 32
P	Cefoxitin	≤ 8	16	≥ 32
P	Ceftazidime	≤ 8	16	≥ 32
P	Cefepime	≤ 8	16	≥ 32
P	Cefotaxime	≤ 8	16–32	≥ 64
O	Cefpodoxime	≤ 2	4	≥ 8
P	Ceftriaxone	≤ 8	16–32	≥ 64
O	Cefuroxime axetil	≤ 4	8–16	≥ 32
P	Cefixime	≤ 1	2	≥ 4
Carbapenems				
P	Imipenem	≤ 4	8	≥ 16
P	Meropenem	≤ 4	8	≥ 16
Monobactams				
P	Aztreonam	≤ 8	16	≥ 32
Aminoglycosides				
P	Gentamicin	≤ 4	8	≥ 16
P	Amikacin	≤ 16	32	≥ 64
P	Tobramycin	≤ 4	8	≥ 16
P	Netilmycin	≤ 8	16	≥ 32
P	Kanamycin	≤ 16	32	≥ 64

Table 9.4 (*Continued*)

Antimicrobial		MIC (μg/mL) Interpretation		
		S	I	R
Quinolones				
O/P	Enrofloxacin	$\leq$0.5	1–2	$\geq$4
O	Orbifloxacin	$\leq$1	2–4	$\geq$8
O	Difloxacin	$\leq$0.5	1–2	$\geq$4
O	Marbofloxacin	$\leq$1	2	$\geq$4
Tetracyclines				
P	Tetracycline	$\leq$4	8	$\geq$16
P	Doxycycline			
	Minocycline			
Other				
P	Trimethorprim/sulfa	$\leq$2/38		$\geq$4/76
P	Nitrofurantoin	$\leq$32	64	$\geq$128
P	Chloramphenicol	$\leq$8	16	$\geq$32
P	Fluphenicol			
Antimicrobial agents against *Staphylococcus spp.*				
Penicillins				
P	Penicillin G	$\leq$0.12		$\geq$0.25
P/O	Ampicillin	$\leq$0.25		$\geq$0.5
O/P	Amoxicillin			
P	Oxacillin	$\leq$8		$\geq$16
O	Amoxicillin/clavulanate	$\leq$4		$\geq$8
O	Ampicillin/sulbactam			
P	Piperacillin/tazobactam	$\leq$8		$\geq$16
P	Ticarcillin/clavulanate	$\leq$8		$\geq$16
Cephalosporins				
P	Cepholothin	$\leq$8	16	$\geq$32
O	Cephalexin			
O	Cefadroxil			
P	Cephapirin			
O	Cefaclor			
P	Ceftiofur	$\leq$8	16	$\geq$32
P	Cefazolin	$\leq$8	16	$\geq$32
P	Cefoxitin	$\leq$8	16	$\geq$32
P	Ceftazidime	$\leq$8	16	$\geq$32
P	Cefepime	$\leq$8	16	$\geq$32
P	Cefotaxime	$\leq$8	16–32	$\geq$64
O	Cefpodoxime	$\leq$2	4	$\geq$8
P	Ceftriaxone	$\leq$8	16–32	$\geq$64
O	Cefuroxime axetil	$\leq$4	8–16	$\geq$32
Carbapenems				
P	Imipenem	$\leq$4	8	$\geq$16
P	Meropenem	$\leq$4	8	$\geq$16

(*Continued*)

Table 9.4 (*Continued*)

Antimicrobial		MIC (μg/mL) Interpretation		
		S	I	R
Aminoglycosides				
P	Gentamicin	≤4	8	≥16
P	Amikacin	≤16	32	≥64
P	Tobramycin	≤4	8	≥16
P	Netilmycin	≤8	16	≥32
P	Kanamycin	≤16	32	≥64
Quinolones				
O/P	Enrofloxacin	≤0.5	1–2	≥4
O	Orbifloxacin	≤1	2–4	≥8
O	Difloxacin	≤0.5	1–2	≥4
O	Marbofloxacin	≤1	2	≥4
Tetracyclines				
P	Tetracycline	≤4	8	≥16
P	Doxycycline			
	Minocycline			
Macrolides				
P	Erythromycin	≤2	4	≥8
P	Azithromycin			
P	Clorithromycin			
Lincosamides				
P	Clindamycin	≤0.5	1–2	≥4
P	Lincomycin			
Other				
P	Trimethorprim/sulfa	≤2/38		≥4/76
P	Nitrofurantoin	≤32	64	≥128
P	Chloramphenicol	≤8	16	≥32
P	Fluphenicol			

MIC, minimum inhibitory concentration; O, oral; P, parenteral (intravenous, subcutaneous, or intramuscular); S, susceptible; I, intermediate susceptibility; R, resistant.
Source: Used with permission from Aucoin (2007).

wells containing serial two-fold dilutions of antimicrobial drugs at concentrations achievable in tissues and urine, the MIC is defined as the lowest antimicrobial concentration (or highest dilution) that prevents visible bacterial growth. The MIC is usually several dilutions lower than the minimum bactericidal concentration of drugs. In general, the antimicrobial agent is likely to achieve bactericidal concentrations within urine if a concentration four times that of the MIC can be achieved (Table 9.3) (Ling 1984). Many antimicrobial drugs that are renally excreted reach concentrations in urine that are 10–100 times greater than the serum concentration. Guidelines for interpretation of antimicrobial susceptibility testing is provided in Table 9.4.

References

Allen, T.A., et al. (1987). Microbiologic evaluation of canine urine: direct microscopic examination and preservation of specimen quality for culture. *J Am Vet Med Assoc* **190**(10): 1289–1291.

Aucoin, D. (2007). Target: the antimicrobial reference guide to effective treatment. Port Huron, MI: North American Compendiums Inc.

Barsanti, J.A. (2006). Genitourinary infections. In: *Infectious Diseases of the Dog and Cat*, edited by C.E. Greene, 3rd edition. St. Louis, MO: Elsevier Saunders, pp. 935–961.

Blanco, L.J., et al. (2001). Evaluation of blood agar plates as a transport medium for aerobic bacterial urine cultures [abstract]. *J Vet Intern Med* **15**(3): 303.

Lees, G.E. (1996). Bacterial urinary tract infections. *Vet Clin North Am Small Anim Pract* **26**(2): 297–304.

Lees, G.E. and C.A. Osborne (1979). Antibacterial properties of urine: a comparative review. *J Am Anim Hosp Assoc* **15**: 125–132.

Ling, G.V. (1984). Therapeutic strategies involving antimicrobial treatment of the canine urinary tract. *J Am Vet Med Assoc* **185**(10): 1162–1164.

Lulich, J.P. and C.A. Osborne (1999). Bacterial urinary tract infections. In: *Textbook of Veterinary Internal Medicine*, edited by S.J. Ettinger and E.C. Feldman, 4th edition. Philadelphia, PA: WB Saunders, pp. 1775–1788.

Padilla, J., et al. (1981). Effects of storage time and temperature on quantitative culture of canine urine. *J Am Vet Med Assoc* **178**(10): 1077–1081.

Saunders, A.B., et al. (2002). Evaluation of blood agar plates and incandescent lighting for aerobic bacterial urine cultures [abstract]. *J Vet Intern Med.* **16**(3): 379.

10

Urinary enzyme activity for detection of acute kidney injury

Richard Goldstein

Successful prevention, recognition, and treatment of acute kidney injury (AKI) should be at the forefront of our efforts to successfully limit eventual non-reversible or progressive kidney disease. Once the damage has been propagated and is evident on routine biochemical testing, or even worse by clinical signs of uremia, it is often too late to intervene successfully. This chapter will focus on one aspect of early detection—the excess leakage of urinary enzymes and other biomarkers and their activity as measured in the urine. The enzymatic activity used as a marker for AKI belongs to enzymes that are found within the renal tubular cells. These enzymes are too large to be filtered through a normal glomerulus, and so in the absence of profound glomerular disease, a rise in the urinary activity of such enzymes is typically caused by acute damage to the tubules and leakage from the tubular cells. Other urinary markers of AKI such as urinary electrolyte concentrations, as well as urinary glucose and protein will be discussed elsewhere in the text.

The use of urinary enzyme activity as a marker for AKI has been studied in humans, and rodent models of kidney injury since the 1960s and 1970s (Ceriotti et al. 1970; Wright and Plummer 1974). At the same time, studies were also performed in domestic animals mostly as models for humans. Such early studies included, among others, assessing urinary psi-glutamyl transpeptidase in sheep (Shaw 1976), and N-acetyl-β-glucosaminidase (NAG) in dogs (Ellis et al. 1973) as markers for AKI induced by mercuric chloride toxicity. These studies, as well as other similar ones, showed a rise in the concentrations of these enzymes following induc-

tion of experimental kidney injury, typically, via 24-hour urine collection. More recently, in the 1980s, studies were initiated in companion animal veterinary medicine to assess the values of monitoring urinary enzymes in more clinically relevant models of AKI. In 1985, Greco et al. assessed urinary gamma-glutamyl transpeptidase (GGT) activity in dogs with gentamicin-induced nephrotoxicity. In this study, urinary GGT increased prior to development of azotemia and was considered a more sensitive and reliable method of detecting AKI induced by gentamicin than serum creatinine concentrations or 24-hour endogenous creatinine clearance (Greco et al. 1985). Since that time a number of additional studies have been performed focusing on 24-hour urinary excretion and urine enzyme activity to creatinine ratios for GGT and NAG in experimental models (Grauer et al. 1995; Rivers et al. 1996) as well as naturally occurring kidney disease in dogs (Sato et al. 2002a) and cats (Sato et al. 2002b). Similarly, a recent study assessing human patients in an ICU setting showed that urinary enzymes such as GGT and NAG detected AKI from 12 hours to 4 days prior to the development of azotemia (Westhuyzen et al. 2003).

The practical use of urinary enzyme activity in naturally occurring disease

A few things appear to be clear from the literature reviewed above:

1. Urinary enzymes, GGT, and NAG are the most commonly used and most practical enzymes to assess urinary activity. NAG is found within the proximal tubular lysosomes and GGT with the proximal tubule brush border. The activity of these enzymes is a sensitive method of detecting acute tubular kidney

Nephrology and Urology of Small Animals. Edited by Joe Bartges and David J. Polzin. © 2011 Blackwell Publishing Ltd.

injury, more sensitive than changes in glomerular filtration rate, serum biochemistry (azotemia), and clinical signs.

2. Changes in urinary enzyme concentrations, GGT, and NAG, can be estimated by enzyme to creatinine ratios on spot urine samples, deeming 24-hour urine collections not absolutely necessary.

3. Normal or baseline values vary greatly from study to study and likely from assay to assay making the determination of a healthy reference range very difficult. Thus, the ideal method to use this tool today appears to be when a baseline value can be determined in an individual case and then a two and threefold increase in the GGT or NAG to creatinine ratio indicates an early sign of acute tubular injury. This is most feasible when a dog or cat has either very recently been exposed or will be exposed to a known renal toxin and a baseline can still be established. Examples of such cases include the use of renal toxic chemotherapeutic agents, the use of aminoglycosides, a very recent overdose of a nonsteroidal anti-inflammatory drug (NSAID), or the use of an NSAID in a renal compromised patient.

The following is a case example where the use of urinary enzymes was of value

Red is a 2 year old male neutered Irish setter who was presented to the Cornell University Hospital for Animals Emergency Service within a few hours of eating a large, toxic amount of a veterinary approved non-steroidal anti-inflammatory medicine. Red had no relevant past history and was completely nonclinical on presentation. Following induced emesis, the decision was made to treat Red with intravenous fluids as well as additional medications to try and prevent gastrointestinal and renal toxicity associated with an NSAID overdose. The following plan for monitoring Red was devised:

1. Baseline and then daily serum chemistry panel, complete blood count and urinalysis including urine cytology for casts and a urine GGT and creatinine assays for the calculation of a urine GGT/creatinine.

2. The plan was to continue high rates of fluids for 48 hours unless signs of AKI were identified. A two fold rise in urine GGT/creatinine ratio from baseline was determined to be significant.

Results

Red's urine creatinine and GGT concentrations over time during his hospitalization and therapy (Table 10.1) and GGT/creatinine ratio in graphic form (Figure 10.1).

Table 10.1 Serial urine creatinine and gamma-glutamyl transpeptidase (GGT) concentrations from a 2 year old, castrated male, Irish setter after ingesting a toxic quantity of a nonsteroidal anti-inflammatory drug (NSAID)

Day	1	2	3	4	5
Urine creatinine mg/dL	24	38	51.2	38.2	60
Urine GGT U/L	5	12	28	13	16
GGT/creatinine U/mg	0.02	0.032	0.054	0.034	0.027

In this case, the clinicians used the doubling of the GGT to creatinine ratio as an early indicator of AKI and continued aggressive fluid therapy until the value returned to baseline. No other changes were noted in the chemistry panel, complete blood count, or urinalysis during the same time period.

Another excellent example for the use of this method is to monitor urine GGT/creatinine or NAG/creatinine every other day or twice a week during aminoglycoside therapy. This should be done in addition to urinalysis (searching for changes in specific gravity, proteinuria, glucosuria, and casts) and serum chemistry panels. A doubling of the urinary enzyme to creatinine ratio should be seen as a possible sign of early AKI and discontinuation of the aminoglycoside should be considered.

Conclusions

It is clear that AKI is best managed and severe kidney injury leading to renal death or chronic kidney disease is best avoided when caught early. Insensitive methods of

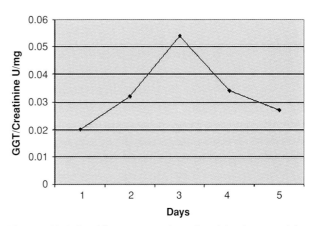

Figure 10.1 Graphic representation of serial urine creatinine and gamma-glutamyl transpeptidase (GGT) concentrations from a 2 year old, castrated male, Irish setter after ingesting a toxic quantity of a nonsteroidal anti-inflammatory drug (NSAID).

identifying AKI such as clinical signs and azotemia are insufficient for this purpose. Thus, whenever possible, either following acute toxicity or during known exposure to a renal toxin, measuring urinary enzymes can have substantial added value in allowing early detection of AKI. Today, GGT and NAG can easily be measured in the urine by commercial laboratories and a urinary GGT or NAG to creatinine ratio calculated. Although reference ranges are not available, a doubling of the ratio should lead the clinician to suspect AKI. In the future, additional biomarkers may also become available in veterinary medicine.

References

Ceriotti, G., et al. (1970). Human urinary alpha-glucosidase as an index of kidney tubular damage. *Clin Chim Acta* **27**(3): 415–419.

Ellis, B.G., et al. (1973). The effect of tubular damage by mercuric chloride on kidney function and some urinary enzymes in the dog. *Chem Biol Interact* **7**(2): 101–113.

Grauer, G.F., et al. (1995). Estimation of quantitative enzymuria in dogs with gentamicin-induced nephrotoxicosis using urine enzyme/creatinine ratios from spot urine samples. *J Vet Intern Med* **9**(5): 324–327.

Greco, D.S., et al. (1985). Urinary gamma-glutamyl transpeptidase activity in dogs with gentamicin-induced nephrotoxicity. *Am J Vet Res* **46**(11): 2332–2335.

Rivers, B.J., et al. (1996). Evaluation of urine gamma-glutamyl transpeptidase-to-creatinine ratio as a diagnostic tool in an experimental model of aminoglycoside-induced acute renal failure in the dog. *J Am Anim Hosp Assoc* **32**(4): 323–336.

Sato, R., et al. (2002a). Clinical availability of urinary N-acetyl-beta-D-glucosaminidase index in dogs with urinary diseases. *J Vet Med Sci* **64**(4): 361–365.

Sato, R., et al. (2002b). Urinary excretion of N-acetyl-beta-D-glucosaminidase and its isoenzymes in cats with urinary disease. *J Vet Med Sci* **64**(4): 367–371.

Shaw, F.D. (1976). The effect of mercuric chloride intoxication on urinary psi-glutamyl transpeptidase excretion in the sheep. *Res Vet Sci* **20**(2): 226–268.

Westhuyzen, J., et al. (2003). Measurement of tubular enzymuria facilitates early detection of acute renal impairment in the intensive care unit. *Nephrol Dial Transplant* **18**(3): 543–551.

Wright, P.J. and D.T. Plummer. (1974). The use of urinary enzyme measurements to detect renal damage caused by nephrotoxic compounds. *Biochem Pharmacol* **23**(1): 65–73.

11

Diagnosis of uroabdomen

Michael M. Fry

Uroabdomen, also known as uroperitoneum, means presence of urine in the peritoneal cavity—that is outside of the urinary tract. The condition occurs most often due to trauma (see Chapters 59 and 82). Recognized specific causes of uroabdomen include vehicular or other blunt trauma, urinary catheterization, traumatic palpation or manual expression of the bladder, urinary tract obstruction, surgery, neoplasia, and (especially in foals) parturition. Leakage may occur anywhere throughout the urinary tract (Aumann et al. 1998; Weisse et al. 2002; Hamilton et al. 2006); leakage from the upper urinary tract may result in uroretroperitoneum (Weisse et al. 2002; Rieser 2005). In a study of 26 cases of uroabdomen in cats, blunt trauma was most likely to result in leakage from the urinary bladder, and catheterization was most likely to result in leakage from the urethra (Aumann et al. 1998). Neither ability to urinate nor a palpable urinary bladder rules out the possibility of a patient having uroabdomen (Aumann et al. 1998). Although uroabdomen often can be diagnosed on the basis of laboratory findings, identification of the site of leakage requires contrast-enhanced diagnostic imaging or surgical exploration.

Dogs and cats with uroabdomen typically have azotemia and other serum or plasma biochemical abnormalities, but definitive laboratory diagnosis of uroabdomen requires paired testing of time-matched peritoneal fluid and serum or plasma samples. In patients with uroabdomen, analytes that are normally excreted in urine are expected to be present in higher concentration in peritoneal fluid than in plasma. The most clinically useful of these analytes are creatinine and potassium. Creatinine does not diffuse as readily as urea, and is therefore slower to equilibrate between peritoneal fluid

and blood (Stockham and Scott 2008). This principle was illustrated in a study of experimentally-induced rupture of the urinary bladder in dogs, in which in creatinine concentrations in peritoneal fluid and blood were markedly different, but urea concentrations were not (Burrows and Bovee 1974). Measurement of potassium is also likely to be useful in cases of suspected uroabdomen. A retrospective study in dogs (13 animals with uroabdomen, 8 with nonurinary peritoneal effusion) found that a creatinine peritoneal fluid:blood ratio of >2:1 had 100% specificity and 86% sensitivity, and a potassium peritoneal fluid:blood ratio of >1.4:1 had 100% specificity and 100% sensitivity, for diagnosing uroabdomen (Schmiedt et al. 2001). A retrospective study in cats found increased peritoneal fluid:serum ratios for both analytes (mean values of 2:1 and 1.9:1, respectively) in 4/5 animals, and decreased peritoneal fluid:serum ratios in 1/5 animals (Aumann et al. 1998). Suggested guidelines for interpreting the results of paired testing are shown in Table 11.1.

Even in the absence of prior clinical suspicion of uroabdomen, finding of an unexplained nonseptic inflammatory peritoneal effusion with a low protein concentration should raise the possibility of uroabdomen. Urine which is free in the peritoneal cavity acts as a chemical irritant and elicits an inflammatory response, and routine fluid analysis and cytologic examination of peritoneal fluid typically shows a mildly increased total nucleated cell count comprised predominantly of neutrophils and a normal to mildly increased protein concentration. The fluid is usually sterile (provided there was no urinary tract infection prior to leakage), but the neutrophils often have poor morphologic preservation, presumably because of the harsh chemical environment (Alleman 2003).

Nephrology and Urology of Small Animals. Edited by Joe Bartges and David J. Polzin. © 2011 Blackwell Publishing Ltd.

Table 11.1 Suggested guidelines for interpreting results of paired (time-matched) testing of peritoneal fluid and serum or plasma in dogs and cats with suspected uroabdomen. In all cases, but particularly in the case of equivocal findings (the "Suspicious for uroabdomen" category below), these results should be interpreted along with all of the available clinical data

Results of paired testing	Interpretation
Creatinine concentration of peritoneal fluid $\geq 2\times$ higher than creatinine concentration of serum or plasma	Diagnostic for uroabdomen
Creatinine concentration of peritoneal fluid $< 2\times$ higher than creatinine concentration of serum or plasma AND	Suspicious for uroabdomen—measure potassium concentration
Potassium concentration of peritoneal fluid $>$ potassium concentration of serum or plasma OR	Supports diagnosis of uroabdomen (the higher the ratio, the more strongly supportive)
Potassium concentration of peritoneal fluid $\leq$ potassium concentration of serum or plasma	Does not support diagnosis of uroabdomen
Creatinine concentration of peritoneal fluid $\leq$ creatinine concentration of serum or plasma	No evidence of uroabdomen (does not exclude the possibility of uroabdomen, but no evidence to support the diagnosis)

References

Alleman, A.R. (2003). Abdominal, thoracic, and pericardial effusions. *Vet Clin North Am Small Anim Pract* **33**(1): 89–118.

Aumann, M., et al. (1998). Uroperitoneum in cats: 26 cases (1986–1995). *J Am Anim Hosp Assoc* **34**(4): 315–324.

Burrows, C.F. and K.C. Bovee. (1974). Metabolic changes due to experimentally induced rupture of the canine urinary bladder. *Am J Vet Res* **35**(8): 1083–1088.

Hamilton, M.H., et al. (2006). Traumatic bilateral ureteric rupture in two dogs. *J Small Anim Pract* **47**(12): 737–740.

Rieser, T.M. (2005). Urinary tract emergencies. *Vet Clin North Am Small Anim Pract* **35**(2): 359–373.

Schmiedt, C., et al. (2001). Evaluation of abdominal fluid:peripheral blood creatinine and potassium ratios for diagnosis of uroperitoneum in dogs. *J Vet Emerg Crit Care* **11**(4): 275–280.

Stockham, S.L. and M.A. Scott. (2008). *Fundamentals of Veterinary Clinical Pathology*, 2nd edition. Ames, IA: Blackwell Publishing.

Weisse, C., et al. (2002). Traumatic rupture of the ureter: 10 cases. *J Am Anim Hosp Assoc* **38**(2): 188–192.

12

Urinary saturation testing

Joe Bartges

Urolith formation

Overview

Urolith formation, dissolution, and prevention involves complex physical processes. Major factors include (1) supersaturation resulting in crystal formation, (2) effects of inhibitors of crystallization and inhibitors of crystal aggregation and growth, (3) crystalloid complexors, (4) effects of promoters of crystal aggregation and growth, and (5) effects of noncrystalline matrix (Coe and Parks 1988; Brown and Purich 1992; Brown et al. 1994; Bartges et al. 1999).

Concept of urine saturation (Figure 12.1)

An important driving force behind stone formation is the saturation state of urine with calculogenic substances (Coe et al. 1992). When a solution such as urine is saturated, it refers to the maximal amount of a substance, such as calcium oxalate, that can be completed dissolved. This point is termed the *thermodynamic solubility product*. When calcium oxalate is present in urine at a concentration less than the solubility point, the urine is *undersaturated* with calcium oxalate and calcium oxalate completely dissociates and dissolves. When calcium oxalate is present in urine at a concentration that is equal to the solubility point, the urine is *saturated* with calcium oxalate and calcium oxalate begins to precipitate. When calcium oxalate is present in urine at a concentration above the solubility point, the urine is *supersaturated* with calcium oxalate and calcium oxalate precipitates.

Urine contains ions and proteins that interact and/or complex with calcium and oxalic acid so as to allow them to remain in solution. This explains why calcium and oxalic acid in urine do not normally precipitate to form calcium oxalate crystals. Urine is normally supersaturated with respect to calcium and oxalic acid, but energy is required to maintain this state of calcium and oxalic acid solubility; therefore, the urine must constantly "struggle" energetically to maintain calcium and oxalic acid in solution. Thus, urine is described as being *metastable*, implying varying degrees of instability with respect to the potential for calcium oxalate crystals to form. In this metastable state, new calcium oxalate crystals will not precipitate, but if already present, crystals will be maintained and grow in size. If the concentration of calcium and oxalic acid is increased, a threshold is eventually reached at which urine cannot hold more calcium and oxalic acid in solution. The urine concentration at which this occurs is the formation point of calcium oxalate. Above the *thermodynamic formation product*, urine is *oversaturated* and unstable with respect to calcium and oxalic acid; thus, calcium oxalate crystals will spontaneously precipitate, grow in size, and aggregate.

Medical dissolution of certain types of uroliths is achieved by inducing a state of undersaturation with respect to the calculogenic minerals. Medical prevention is achieved by inducing a state of undersaturation or low to mid metastability as long as there is no mechanism for heterogeneous nucleation present. Urinary supersaturation with calculogenic minerals represents an increased risk toward urolith formation and is required for urolith formation, but other factors are important.

Assessment of urolith formation

Overview

Various factors involved with urolith formation may be evaluated by several methods including (1) epidemiological studies performed at urolith centers and designed to identify risk and protective factors, (2) measuring urine

Nephrology and Urology of Small Animals. Edited by Joe Bartges and David J. Polzin. © 2011 Blackwell Publishing Ltd.

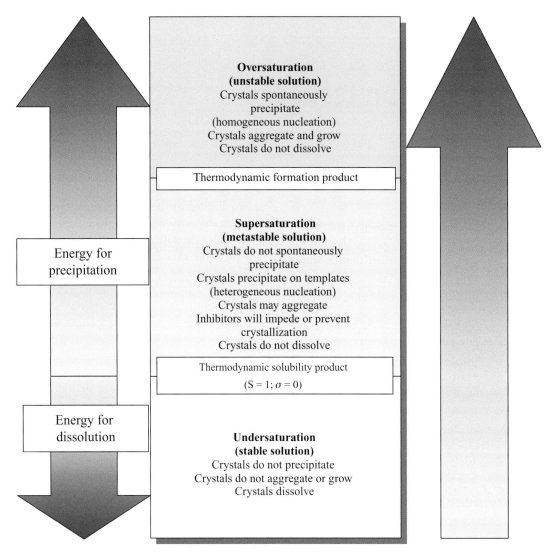

Figure 12.1 States of saturation. *S* represents the supersaturation ratio and σ represents the relative supersaturation.

concentrations of calculogenic substances, (3) evaluating the influence of urine pH on crystal formation, and (4) measuring the degree of undersaturation, supersaturation, and/or oversaturation of urine with crystallogenic substances. Determination of urinary biochemical parameters and urinary saturation can only be done in patients that are "stone free" because active urolith disease results in depletion of calculogenic compounds in urine that alters results (Laube et al. 2003).

Supersaturation

In solution chemistry, the difference in chemical potential of two states ($\Delta\mu$) is dependent on the activities of the crystallizing salt in the supersaturated solution (*a*) and in the solution when it has come to equilibrium (a_{eq}): $\Delta\mu = RTln(a/a_{eq})$ where *R* is the universal

gas constant and *T* is the absolute temperature (Kelvin). The activity of the crystallizing salt is represented by the activity product (AP) for that salt where the activities of the ions comprising that salt are multiplied. The term "activity" of a mineral is an index of the likelihood that the mineral will combine with other substances in urine, and is determined by multiplying the concentration of the ion by the activity coefficient for similarly charged molecules. For example, the activity of calcium is determined by multiplying the concentration of calcium in solution (molarity) by the activity coefficient for a doubly charged molecule since calcium carries a "2+" charge. The "activity" of a mineral is dependent on several factors including (1) the urine concentration of that mineral, (2) the urine concentrations of other substances such as sodium, potassium, calcium, etc., (3) the quantity and functional state of nonmineral or nonmeasured mineral inhibitors and promoters of crystal formation, growth, and aggregation, (4) urine pH, and (5) temperature of urine. Thus, a and a_{eq} represent the AP's for the salt in supersaturated solution and the solution at equilibrium, respectively. Furthermore, the supersaturation ratio $(S) = a/a_{eq}$; therefore, $\Delta\mu/RT = ln(S)$ (Werness et al. 1985). For practical purposes, S is expressed as concentrations (molarities) or activities (a). For example, for calcium oxalate:

$$S = \text{APcaox} = [Ca^{2+}] \times [Ox^{2-}]$$
$$\text{APcaox}_{eq}[Ca^{2+}_{eq}] \times [Ox^{2-}_{eq}]$$

where "[]" represents the activities or concentrations of the ions, calcium (Ca^{2+}) or oxalate (Ox^{2-}). Usually, the relative supersaturation (σ) is used rather than S, where $\sigma = S$–1 (Finlayson and Miller 1969; Finlayson 1978; Werness et al. 1985; Brown et al. 1994; Kavanagh 2006).

Crystallization involves nucleation, growth, and aggregation. Nucleation may be heterogeneous (where a foreign substance provides a nucleation catalyst for crystal formation) or homogeneous (where no foreign substance is used). Supersaturation required for homogeneous nucleation is much higher than that required for heterogeneous nucleation. There is still a supersaturation barrier that must be overcome before nucleation can occur (Figure 12.1). Growth of crystals may occur through enlargement of existing crystals by direct incorporation of solution species into the solid crystal lattice or by aggregation of crystals. The rate of crystal growth is described by second-order kinetics: $G = k\sigma^2$, where G is the growth rate and k is the rate constant (Kavanagh 2006). Aggregation can also result in enlargement of the crystal mass, and occurs through the net result of crystals colliding and either dispersing or consolidating, with the outcome being dependent on an efficiency factor. As consolidation is achieved by crystal bridges that fuse the lattice structures of individual crystals, aggregation is also dependent on supersaturation (David et al. 2001; Hounslow et al. 2001).

Relative supersaturation

Determining the relative supersaturation (RSS) of a urolith-forming substance in a patient's urine is one technique used to assess risk of urolith formation (Pak et al. 1977; Brown and Purich 1992). RSS is determined by measuring urine concentrations of several analytes including ammonium, calcium, chloride, citrate, hydrogen (pH), magnesium, oxalate, phosphate, potassium, and sodium (and possibly cystine, sulfate, uric acid and other compounds) in urine. These values are then entered into a computer program (EQUIL or SUPERSAT), which calculates the activity coefficients for the various ions

and combines the relevant ion concentrations and activity coefficients to produce the activity product (AP). For example, the AP of calcium oxalate is calculated as the mathematical product of the activity of calcium and activity of oxalic acid. The AP for each urolith-forming compound is divided by its known thermodynamic solubility product (SP) and the resultant RSS produced.

RSS = ion AP of the patient's urine/ion SP

Relative supersaturation is related to the energy available for crystal nucleation and growth; however, RSS values are limited by the fact that the thermodynamic solubility products used for these calculations have not been measured in the patient's urine. This is of concern because it is probable that different macromolecules, including inhibitors and promoters of crystal formation, growth and aggregation, in the patient's urine have a pronounced influence on free ion concentrations. By using calculations measured in urine from healthy human beings, RSS may overestimate SPs and APs of different minerals, and thus tend to underestimate the risk of urolith formation. Another technical problem in evaluating dogs and cats is that the computer program used to calculate RSS involves the comparison of the pet's urine values to standardized values based on the composition of human urine.

Activity product ratios

Activity product ratios (APR) also are designed to express the degree of supersaturation of solutions with calculogenic minerals. APR's are obtained by calculating the ion AP in the patient's urine samples before and after equilibrium with various seed crystals such as calcium oxalate.

APR = ion AP of patient's urine before incubation with seed crystals
ion AP of patient's urine after incubation with seed crystals

In determining the APR, the patient's urine is incubated with preformed seed crystals composed of pure urolith-forming mineral of interest (e.g., calcium oxalate). Following incubation for 48 hours with the seed crystals, the urine concentration of the same analytes are measured. The postincubation concentrations of analytes are then used to calculate a "post-incubation" AP. Dividing the "pre-incubation" AP by the "post-incubation" AP gives the APR for that patient's urine sample.

An exact measurement of supersaturation is not obtained by determining APR, but the method provides useful information about the relative increase or decrease of the ion AP in the patient's urine that results from seed crystal growth or seed crystal dissolution. An APR less than one represents undersaturation of urine with the mineral being evaluated An APR equal to one represents saturation of the patient's urine sample. An APR greater than one indicates that the patient's urine sample is supersaturated.

APRs can be calculated for any calculogenic mineral as long as pure seed crystals for that type of mineral are available. Use of APR methodology will not eliminate errors associated with the effect of unknown factors such as crystallization inhibitors or promoters of ion activities; however, since the same urine sample obtained from the patient is analyzed before and after equilibration with seed crystals (such as calcium oxalate), the same type of error occurs in evaluation of both analyses and therefore the errors cancel. Whereas calculation of RSS can overestimate supersaturation, saturation, and undersaturation, the APR method overestimates undersaturation, underestimates supersaturation, and correctly measures saturation, provided that a sufficient amount of seed crystals have been used. One limitation of APR determination is the assumption that urine has reached the SP for the salt following 48 hours of incubation, which has been shown to be a false assumption in some cases (Robertson et al. 2002). Urine may not reach true equilibrium saturation level, particularly if coming from a supersaturated level, presumably due to presence of various inhibitors of crystal growth that slow down the approach to equilibrium. In this instance, when the true RSS is measured following 48 hours of seed incubation, the AP achieved at that point may be 2-3 times higher than the thermodynamic solubility product. The APR calculated at this point, therefore, systematically underestimates the actual level of supersaturation since the denominator (AP/SP) is too large. The opposite may occur when the urine is undersaturated.

Bonn risk index

A newer method for evaluating risk of calcium oxalate urolith formation in human beings is the use of the Bonn Risk Index (BRI) (Laube et al. 2000; Laube et al. 2001; Laube et al. 2004). Supersaturation of urine with respect to a urolith-forming salt is a fundamental prerequisite of salt precipitation as supersaturation is the thermodynamic driving force behind the process; however, supersaturation alone is not sufficient to induce pathologic salting-out. The BRI uses the ratio calculated from the urinary concentration of ionized calcium and the amount of ammonium oxalate that is titrated to the urine in order to induce a precipitation of calcium oxalate salts. A high BRI value indicates low risk of urolith formation (whereas a low RSS indicates low risk) and a low BRI indicates a high risk of urolith formation (whereas a high RSS indicates high risk). BRI has been shown to correlate with RSS (Laube et al. 2001). For crystallization to occur in

the urinary tract, the existence of a correct combination of supersaturation and of factors that inhibit/promote the nucleation process is necessary. To what extent this propensity for crystallization actually relates to the risk of urolith formation also depends on factors that regulate steps leading from a crystal to a urolith. An advantage of BRI is the fact that all urinary components contribute their effects in their native ratio to the determination. Thus, the BRI includes an imbalance between promoters and inhibitors in the individual's urine, if an imbalance is present; however, the BRI is a nonspecific method with respect to urinary constituents as only the concentration of ionized calcium is measured. Additional urinary chemistry determination may be necessary to fully evaluate the metabolic status of a patient. This technique has not been tested in animals, and the instrument (Urolizer, Raumedic Ag, Munchberg, Germany) is not available in the United States.

Use of urinary saturation testing in dogs and cats

Limited studies utilizing urine saturation testing has been performed in veterinary medicine, particularly in animals that have formed uroliths (Table 12.1). Despite the number of studies, very few have been performed on dogs or cats that are urolith-formers and no studies exist that compare estimates of urinary saturation with recurrence rates of uroliths. In dogs, calcium oxalate urolith formation typically occurs when urinary relative supersaturation for calcium oxalate is greater than 10; the metastable zone lies between a relative supersaturation value for calcium oxalate of 1 and 10–14 (Stevenson and Rutgers 2006). In cats, calcium oxalate urolith formation typically occurs when urinary relative supersaturation for calcium oxalate is greater than 12; the metastable zone lies between a relative supersaturation value for calcium oxalate of 1 and approximately 12 (Houston and Elliott 2008). Sterile struvite urolith formation in cats typically occurs when urinary relative supersaturation for struvite is greater than 2.5; the metastable zone lies between a relative supersaturation value for struvite of 1 and approximately 2.5 (Houston and Elliott 2008). Data presented in the Table 12.1 supports these numbers, although there are exceptions. Urinary supersaturation represents a risk for urolith formation, but as in human beings, there is an overlap in values between urolith-forming animals and healthy, nonurolith-forming animals (Robertson et al. 1968; Kavanagh 2006); therefore, other factors are important. Use of urinary saturation studies can provide further information on mechanisms of urolith formation, screening of animals at risk for urolith formation and monitoring efficacy of urolith management.

Table 12.1 Summary of studies utilizing relative supersaturation or activity product ratio estimates of urinary saturation in dogs and cats. Data, when available, is presented as average (standard deviation)

	Health status[a]	Treatment group[b]	Test and results[c]	Reference
Dogs	Healthy Labrador retrievers Healthy miniature schnauzers	Maintenance dry dog food	RSScaox = 4.60 (1.66) RSSbr = 0.47 (0.23) RSScaox = 5.31 (1.62) RSSbr = 1.22 (0.31)	(Stevenson and Markwell 2001) EQUIL[d]
Dogs	Healthy miniature schnauzers, beagles, Labrador retrievers	Adult maintenance canned diet Control diet + liquid potassium citrate Control diet + potassium citrate tablet	RSScaox = 1.42 (0.63) RSSmap = 2.59 (1.40) RSScaox = 1.68 (0.83) RSSmap = 3.55 (3.43) RSScaox = 1.24 (0.53) RSSmap = 3.44 (2.63)	(Stevenson et al. 2000) SUPERSAT[e]
Dogs	Healthy beagles	Canned ultra-low protein, alkalinizing diet (0.24% DM) Above diet + 1.2% NaCl DM	RSScaox = 4.02 (2.43) RSScaox = 2.83 (2.25)	(Lulich et al. 2005) EQUIL
Dogs	Healthy Labrador retrievers Healthy miniature schnauzers	Maintenance dry dog food Maintenance dry dog food + water Maintenance dry dog food + 0.05 g NaCl/100 kcal Maintenance dry dog food + 0.2 g NaCl/100 kcal Maintenance dry dog food + 0.3 g NaCl/100 kca Maintenance dry dog food Maintenance dry dog food + water Maintenance dry dog food + 0.05 g NaCl/100 kcal) Maintenance dry dog food + 0.2 g NaCl/100 kcal Maintenance dry dog food + 0.3 g NaCl/100 kcal	RSScaox = 11 (6) RSScaox = 9 (7) RSScaox = 9 (4) RSScaox = 5 (3) RSScaox = 3 (3) RSScaox = 14 (3) RSScaox = 9 (5) RSScaox = 15 (9) RSScaox = 10 (6) RSScaox RSS = 6 (3)	(Stevenson et al. 2003) SUPERSAT[e]
Dogs	Healthy cairn terriers and miniature schnauzers	Low calcium (0.18), low oxalate (10) dry diet Low calcium (0.18), medium oxalate (17.5) dry diet Low calcium (0.18), high oxalate (25) dry diet Moderate calcium (0.45), low oxalate (10) dry diet Moderate calcium (0.45), moderate oxalate (17.5) dry diet High calcium (0.75), low oxalate (10) dry diet High calcium (0.75), high oxalate (25) dry diet g/100 kcal	RSScaox = 2.5 (0.5) RSScaox = 5.2 (4) RSScaox = 4.3 (1) RSScaox = 4 (2) RSScaox = 4 (2) RSScaox = 6 (5.5) RSScaox = 5.8 (3)	(Stevenson et al. 2003) SUPERSAT

(Continued)

Table 12.1 (*Continued*)

	Health status[a]	Treatment group[b]	Test and results[c]	Reference
Dogs	Various	Stone-formers Nonstone-formers Variable diets	RSScaox = 21.4 (15.8) RSScaox = 4.1 (2.0)	(Stevenson et al. 2003) SUPERSAT
Dogs	Various	Stone formers—baseline 1 month 12 months Normal—baseline 1 month Baseline = variable diets 1–12 months = canned oxalate prevent diet	RSScaox = 21.4 (15.8) RSScaox = 7.8 (7.1) RSScaox = 5.1 (2.9) RSScaox = 4.1 (2.0) RSScaox = 2.4 (1.4)	(Stevenson et al. 2002; Stevenson et al. 2004) SUPERSAT
Dogs	Healthy beagles	Adult Maintenance canned diet Ultra-low protein, canned diet	APRua = 0.05 (0.04) APRnau = 0.04 (0.03) APRau = 0.14 (0.07) APRua = 0.005 (0.003) APRnau = 0.004 (0.003) APRau = 0.03 (0.03)	(Bartges et al. 1995b) EQUIL
Dogs	Healthy beagles	Ultra-low protein, canned diet with casein (10.4% DM) Ultra-low protein, canned diet with casein (20.8% DM)	APRua = 0.005 (0.003) APRnau = 0.005 (0.003) APRau = 0.03 (0.009) APRua = 0.02 (0.01) APRnau = 0.03 (0.02) APRau = 0.13 (0.10)	(Bartges et al. 1995c) EQUIL
Dogs	Healthy beagles	Canned diet, casein-based (10.8% protein DM) Dry diet, egg-based (9.2% protein DM) Canned diet, chicken-based (11.1% protein DM) Canned diet, chicken and liver-based (10.7% protein DM)	APRua = 0.007 (0.006) APRnau = 0.015 (0.012) APRau = 0.036 (0.028) APRua = 0.033 (0.026) APRnau = 0.50 (0.28) APRau = 0.44 (0.33) APRua = 0.007 (0.007) APRnau = 0.042 (0.002) APRau = 0.052 (0.046) APRua = 0.008 (0.006) APRnau = 0.064 (0.075 APRau = 0.15 (0.15)	(Bartges et al. 1995a) EQUIL
Dogs	Healthy beagles	Ultra-low protein, canned diet + allopurinol (15 mg/kg PO q12 h) Week 4 Week 8	APRua = 0.01 (0.006) APRnau = 0.02 (0.013) APRau = 0.32 (0.27) APRxan = 0 (0) APRua = 0.003 (0.003) APRnau = 0.004 (0.002)	(Bartges et al. 1994) EQUIL

Table 12.1 (*Continued*)

	Health status[a]	Treatment group[b]	Test and results[c]	Reference
			APRau = 0.03 (0.02)	
			APRxan = 0.26 (0.09)	
			APRua = 0.005 (0.003)	
			APRnau = 0.009 (0.004)	
			APRau = 0.088 (0.051)	
			APRxan = 0.27 (0.12)	
Dogs Cats	Healthy beagles and Labrador retrievers Healthy DSH cats	Maintenance dry dog food Maintenance canned cat food	RSScaox = 1.21 (0.03) S	(Robertson et al. 2002) SUPERSAT AND EQUIL
			RSScaox = 1.52 (0.03) E	
			RSSmap = 1.48 (0.25) S	
			RSSmap = 6.61 (1.17) E	
			RSScaox = 0.97 (0.03) S	
			RSScaox = 1.14 (0.03) E	
			RSSmap = 1.35 (0.15) S	
			RSSmap = 5.74 (0.58) E	
Cats	Healthy	Whiskas low pH canned Waltham feline pH control canned	RSSmap = 0.16 (0.14)	(Markwell et al. 1999) EQUIL
			RSScaox = 0.37 (0.24)	
			RSSmap = 0.58 (0.18)	
			RSScaox = 0.45 (0.16)	
Cats	Healthy	RC veterinary cats young adult dry PD feline c/d dry Hill's hariball control dry Eukanuba low pH/O dry	APRcaox = 1.11 (0.19)	(Devois et al. 2000) EQUIL
			APRmap = 0.72 (0.28)	
			APRcaox = 1.20 (0.23)	
			APRmap = 0.32 (0.06)	
			APRcaox = 1.21 (0.23)	
			APRmap = 0.66 (0.34)	
			APRcaox = 1.25 (0.22)	
			APRmap = 0.91 (0.2)	
Cats	Various—stone formers	Diet on which stone formed Canned oxalate preventative diet	RSScaox = 14.3 (8.4)	(Lulich et al. 2004) EQUIL
			APRcaox = 3.86 (1.59)	
			RSScaox = 5.9 (1.9)	
			APRcaox = 2.01 (0.59)	
Cats	Healthy	Adult maintenance canned diet with 0.4% Na Adult maintenance canned diet with 0.8% Na Adult maintenance canned diet with 1.2% Na	RSScaox = 4.04 (2.04)	(Xu et al. 2006) EQUIL
			APRcaox = 6.30 (13.69)	
			RSSmap = 0.06 (0.04)	
			APRmap = 1.26 (0.51)	
			RSScaox = 2.97 (2.04)	
			APRcaox = 4.76 (3.69)	
			RSSmap = 0.06 (0.04)	
			APRmap = 1.13 (0.51)	
			RSScaox = 2.52 (2.04)	
			APRcaox = 4.20 (3.69)	
			RSSmap = 0.1 (0.04)	
			APRmap = 0.79 (0.51)	

(*Continued*)

Table 12.1 (*Continued*)

	Health status[a]	Treatment group[b]	Test and results[c]	Reference
Cats	Healthy DSH	Adult maintenance, dry diet Diet with hydrochlorothiazide (1 mg/kg PO q12 h)	RSScom = 3.48 (1.12) RSScod = 1.49 (0.46) RSSmap = 3.82 (2.30) RSScom = 1.12 (0.70) RSScod = 0.48 (0.30) RSSmap = 1.35 (0.05)	(Hezel et al. 2007) EQUIL
Cats	Healthy DSH	Adult maintenance, dry diet Diet with prednisolone (2.2 mg/kg PO q24 h)	RSScom = 0.36 (0.33) RSScod = 0.47 (0.38) RSSmap = 0.38 (0.32) RSScom = 0.62 (0.42) RSScod = 0.49 (0.40) RSSmap = 1.59 (0.88)	(Geyer et al. 2007) EQUIL
Cats	Healthy DSH	Commercial adult maintenance, dry foods: A B C D E F G H I	RSScaox = 2.96 (0.68) RSSmap = 19.12 (5.42) RSScaox = 5.66 (0.91) RSSmap = 4.08 (1.36) RSScaox = 5.40 (0.91) RSSmap = 3.22 (1.23) RSScaox = 6.52 (1.9) RSSmap = 2.85 (1.43) RSScaox = 2.88 (1.69) RSSmap = 2.98 (2.22) RSScaox = 1.30 (0.52) RSSmap = 1.63 (1.14) RSScaox = 3.68 (2.09) RSSmap = 0.85 (0.69) RSScaox = 3.47 (1.59) RSSmap = 12.18 RSScaox = 2.32 (1.15) RSSmap = 0.75 (0.37)	(Smith et al. 1998) EQUIL
Cats	Healthy	Purified adult maintenance diet Purified diet with 0.45% MgCl Purified diet with 0.45% MgOxide Adult maintenance canned diet Adult struvite preventative canned diet	$pSAP_{calc}$ = 9.18 (0.83) $pSAP_{EQUIL}$ = 10.76 (0.65) $pSAP_{calc}$ = 11.40 (0.24) $pSAP_{EQUIL}$ = 12.10 (0.24) $pSAP_{calc}$ = 7.80 (0.91) $pSAP_{EQUIL}$ = 10.21 (0.60) $pSAP_{calc}$ = 10.78 (0.38) $pSAP_{EQUIL}$ = 11.61 (0.28) $pSAP_{calc}$ = 10.11 (0.66) $pSAP_{EQUIL}$ = 11.32 (0.38)	(Buffington et al. 1990) Hand calculated or EQUIL

Table 12.1 (*Continued*)

	Health status[a]	Treatment group[b]	Test and results[c]	Reference
Cats	Healthy	Dry diet with 29% protein DM corn gluten and fish meal Dry diet with 55% protein DM corn gluten and fish meal	pSAP = 9.07 (0.34) pSAP = 9.91 (0.34)	(Funaba et al. 1996) Hand calculated
Cats	Healthy	Dry diet with 32.6% protein as meat meal Dry diet with 32.5% protein as corn gluten meal	pSAP = 10.17 (0.34) pSAP = 10.11 (0.34)	(Funaba et al. 2002) Hand calculated
Cats	Healthy	Adult dry diet with 39% protein DM as meat meal Adult dry diet with 39% protein DM as chicken meal Adult dry diet with 39% protein DM as corn gluten meal	pSAP = 9.27 (0.31) pSAP = 9.20 (0.31) pSAP = 9.61 (0.52)	(Funaba et al. 2005) Hand calculated
Cats	Healthy	Dry diet (72% protein, 7.5% fat, 14% NFE, 0.4% fiber DM) Dry diet (52% protein, 9% fat, 32% NFE, 0.8% fiber DM) Dry diet (52% protein, 14% fat, 25% NFE, 3.3% fiber DM) Diets as above, but daily intake normalized for protein Dry diet (72% protein, 7.5% fat, 14% NFE, 0.4% fiber DM) Dry diet (52% protein, 9% fat, 32% NFE, 0.8% fiber DM) Dry diet (52% protein, 14% fat, 25% NFE, 3.3% fiber DM)	pSAP = 9.45 (0.38) pSAP = 9.04 (0.55) pSAP = 9.29 (0.42) pSAP = 9.48 (0.39) pSAP = 9.05 (0.45) pSAP = 8.99 (0.39)	(Funaba et al. 2004) Hand calculated
Cats	Healthy	Adult dry diet with 29% protein DM Adult dry diet with 55% protein DM Adult dry diet with 29% protein DM Same diet with 1.5% ammonium chloride Same diet with 0.75% sodium chloride	pSAP = 9.08 (0.68) pSAP = 9.71 (0.63) pSAP = 8.81 (0.45) pSAP = 9.00 (0.73) pSAP = 10.56 (0.66)	(Funaba et al. 2003) Hand calculated
Cats	Healthy	Adult maintenance dry diet Diet with 1% D,L-methionine Diet with 2% D,L-methionine Experimental diet with 27% protein DM Experimental diet with 1.5% ammonium chloride	pSAP = 9.71 (1.13) pSAP = 9.46 (1.13) pSAP = 10.61 (1.13) pSAP = 8.43 (3.04) pSAP = 9.65 (3.04)	(Funaba et al. 2001) Hand calculated
Cats	Healthy	Adult maintenance canned diet Diet + 0.1 mg/BWkg takushya Diet + 0.5 mg/BWkg choreito	RSSmap = 5.70 (4.74) pSAPmap = 9.52 (0.44) RSSmap = 3.47 (2.02) pSAPmap = 9.76 (0.45) RSSmap = 2.53 (2.56) pSAPmap = 9.92 (0.44)	(Buffington et al. 1997) EQUIL

(*Continued*)

Table 12.1 (*Continued*)

	Health status[a]	Treatment group[b]	Test and results[c]	Reference
Cats	Healthy	Adult maintenance canned diet	pSAP = 8.5 (0.3)	(Buffington et al. 1992)
		Same diet with 0.25 gm/BWkg chorieto	pSAP = 8.9 (0.3)	
		Same diet with 0.5 gm/BWkg chorieto	pSAP = 9.2 (0.6)	
		Same diet with 1 gm/BWkg chorieto	pSAP = 9.2 (0.6)	
		Same diet with 2 gm/BWkg chorieto	pSAP = 9.3 (0.4)	
		Same diet with 4 gm/BWkg chorieto	pSAP = 9.4 (0.2)	
Cats	Healthy	Adult maintenance dry struvite preventive diet	APRmap = 0.47 (0.31)	(Bartges et al. 1998)
			APRcaox = 2.51 (1.15)	
		Adult maintenance canned struvite preventative diet	APRmap = 0.68 (0.29)	
			APRcaox = 1.43 (1.27)	
		Adult maintenance dry high fiber diet	APRmap = 0.84 (0.49)	
			APRcaox = 2.21 (0.90)	
		Adult maintenance canned high fiber diet	APRmap = 1.98 (0.96)	
			APRcaox = 0.52 (0.30)	

[a]Healthy—non-urolith-forming animals; DSH, domestic short-hair.

[b]NFE, nitrogen free extract.

[c]RSScaox, relative supersaturation for calcium oxalate; APRcaox, activity product ratio for calcium oxalate; RSSmap, relative supersaturation for struvite (magnesium ammonium phosphate); APRmap, activity product ratio for struvite; RSScom, relative supersaturation for calcium oxalate monohydrate; RSScod, relative supersaturation for calcium oxalate dihydrate; RSSbr, relative supersaturation for brushite; APRua, activity product ratio for uric acid; APRnau, activity product ratio for sodium urate; APRau, activity product ratio for ammonium urate; APRxan, activity product ratio for xanthine; pSAP, negative logarithm of struvite activity product where pSAP is negatively related to struvite crystal formation.

[d]EQUIL, EQUIL program (various versions), College of Medicine, University of Florida.

[e]SUPERSAT, SUPERSAT program by Dr. W.G. Robertson. Values are approximate based on figure in manuscript; results were not included in table in text.

References

Bartges, J.W., et al. (1994). Influence of chronic allopurinol administration on urine activity product ratios of uric acid, sodium urate, ammonium urate and xanthine. *J Vet Intern Med* **8**: 168A.

Bartges, J.W., et al. (1995a). Influence of four diets containing approximately 11% protein (dry weight) on uric acid, sodium urate, and ammonium urate urine activity product ratios of healthy beagles. *Am J Vet Res* **56**(1): 60–65.

Bartges, J.W., et al. (1995b). Diet effect on activity product ratios of uric acid, sodium urate, and ammonium urate in urine formed by healthy beagles. *Am J Vet Res* **56**(3): 329–333.

Bartges, J.W., et al. (1995c). Influence of two amounts of dietary casein on uric acid, sodium urate, and ammonium urate urinary activity product ratios of healthy beagles. *Am J Vet Res* **56**(7): 893–897.

Bartges, J.W., et al. (1998). Comparison of struvite activity product ratios and relative supersaturations in urine collected from healthy cats consuming four struvite management diets. St. Louis, MO: Ralston Purina Nutrition Symposium.

Bartges, J.W., et al. (1999). Methods for evaluating treatment of uroliths. *Vet Clin North Am Small Anim Pract* **29**(1): 45–57.

Brown, C., et al. (1994). EQUIL 93: a tool for experimental and clinical urolithiasis. *Urol Res* **22**: 119–126.

Brown, C. and D. Purich (1992). Physical-chemical processes in kidney stone formation. In: *Disorders of Bone and Mineral Metabolism*, edited by F. Coe and M. Favus. New York: Raven Press, pp. 613–624.

Buffington, C.A., et al. (1992). Effect of choreito on struvite solubility in cats. *Feline Pract* **20**(6): 13–17.

Buffington, C.A., et al. (1997). Effects of choreito and takushya consumption on in vitro and in vivo struvite solubility in cat urine. *Am J Vet Res* **58**(2): 150–152.

Buffington, C.A., et al. (1990). Effect of diet on struvite activity product in feline urine. *Am J Vet Res* **51**(12): 2025–2030.

Coe, F. and J. Parks (1988). *Nephrolithiasis: Pathogenesis and Treatment*. Chicago, IL: Year Book Medical Publishers Inc.

Coe, F.L., et al. (1992). The pathogenesis and treatment of kidney stones. *N Engl J Med* **327**(16): 1141–1152.

David, R., et al. (2001). Developments in the understanding and modelling of the aggregation of suspended crystals in crystallization from solution. *KONA Powder and Particle* **21**: 40–46.

Devois, C., et al. (2000). *Struvite and Oxalate Activity Product Ratios and Crystalluria in Cats fed Acidifying Diets*. Capetown, South Africa: Urolithiasis, pp. 821–822.

Finlayson, B. (1978). Physiochemical aspects of urolithiasis. *Kidney Int* **13**: 344–360.

Finlayson, B. and G.H.J. Miller (1969). Urine ion equilibria: a numerical approach demonstrated by application to antistone therapy. *Invest Urol* **6**(4): 428–440.

Funaba, M., et al. (1996). Effects of a high-protein diet on mineral metabolism and struvite activity product in clinically normal cats. *Am J Vet Res* **57**(12): 1726–1732.

Funaba, M., et al. (2001). Effect of supplementation of dry cat food with D,L-methionine and ammonium chloride on struvite activity product and sediment in urine. *J Vet Med Sci* **63**(3): 337–339.

Funaba, M., et al. (2002). Comparison of corn gluten meal and meat meal as a protein source in dry foods formulated for cats. *Am J Vet Res* **63**(9): 1247–1251.

Funaba, M., et al. (2003). Effects of a high-protein diet versus dietary supplementation with ammonium chloride on struvite crystal formation in urine of clinically normal cats. *Am J Vet Res* **64**(8): 1059–1064.

Funaba, M., et al. (2004). Evaluation of effects of dietary carbohydrate on formation of struvite crystals in urine and macromineral balance in clinically normal cats. *Am J Vet Res* **65**(2): 138–142.

Funaba, M., et al. (2005). Evaluation of meat meal, chicken meal, and corn gluten meal as dietary sources of protein in dry cat food. *Can J Vet Res* **69**(4): 299–304.

Geyer, N., et al. (2007). Influence of prednisolone on urinary calcium oxalate and struvite relative supersaturation in healthy young adult female domestic shorthaired cats. *Vet Ther* **8**(4): 239–246.

Hezel, A., et al. (2007). Influence of hydrochlorothiazide on urinary calcium oxalate relative supersaturation in healthy young adult female domestic shorthaired cats. *Vet Ther* **8**(4): 247–254.

Hounslow, M.J., et al. (2001). A micro-mechanical model for the rate of aggregation during precipitation from solution. *Chem Eng Sci* **56**: 2543–2552.

Houston, D.M. and D.A. Elliott (2008). Nutritional management of feline lower urinary tract disorders. In: *Encyclopedia of Feline Clinical Nutrition*, edited by P. Pibot, V. Biourge, and D.A. Elliott. Aimargues, France: Anawa SAS-Royal Canin, pp. 285–321.

Kavanagh, J. P. (2006). Supersaturation and renal precipitation: the key to stone formation? *Urol Res* **34**(2): 81–85.

Laube, N., et al. (2000). A new approach to calculate the risk of calcium oxalate crystallization from unprepared native urine. *Urol Res* **28**(4): 274–280.

Laube, N., et al. (2001). Testing the predictability of the relative urinary supersaturation from the Bonn-Risk-Index for calcium oxalate stone formation. *Clin Chem Lab Med* **39**(10): 966–969.

Laube, N., et al. (2003). Influence of urinary stones on the composition of a 24-hour urine sample. *Clin Chem* **49**(2): 281–285.

Laube, N., et al. (2004). Determination of the calcium oxalate crystallization risk from urine samples: the BONN-Risk-Index in comparison to other risk formulas. *J Urol* **172**(1): 355–359.

Lulich, J.P., et al. (2004). Effects of diet on urine composition of cats with calcium oxalate urolithiasis. *J Am Anim Hosp Assoc* **40**(3): 185–191.

Lulich, J.P., et al. (2005). Effects of dietary supplementation with sodium chloride on urinary relative supersaturation with calcium oxalate in healthy dogs. *Am J Vet Res* **66**(2): 319–324.

Markwell, P.J., et al. (1999). A non-invasive method for assessing the effect of diet on urinary calcium oxalate and struvite relative supersaturation in the cat. *Anim Tech* **50**(2): 61–67.

Pak, C.Y.C., et al. (1977). Estimation of the state of saturation of brushite and calcium oxalate in urine: A comparison of three methods. *J Lab Clin Med* **89**(4): 891–901.

Robertson, W.G., et al. (2002). Predicting the crystallization potential of urine from cats and dogs with respect to calcium oxalate and magnesium ammonium phosphate (struvite). *J Nutr* **132**(6 Suppl 2): 1637S–1641S.

Robertson, W.G., et al. (1968). Activity products in stone-forming and non-stone forming urine. *Clin Sci* **34**: 579–594.

Smith, B.H., et al. (1998). Urinary relative supersaturations of calcium oxalate and struvite in cats are influenced by diet. *J Nutr* **128**(12 Suppl): 2763S–2764S.

Stevenson, A.E. and C. Rutgers (2006). Nutritional management of canine urolithiasis. In: *Encyclopedia of Canine Clinical Nutrition*, edited by P. Pibot, V. Biourge, and D.A. Elliott. Aimargues, France: Aniwa SAS-Royal Canin, pp. 284–315.

Stevenson, A.E. and P.J. Markwell (2001). Comparison of urine composition of healthy Labrador retrievers and miniature schnauzers. *Am J Vet Res* **62**(11): 1782–1786.

Stevenson, A.E., et al. (2000). Effects of dietary potassium citrate supplementation on urine pH and urinary relative supersaturation of calcium oxalate and struvite in healthy dogs. *Am J Vet Res* **61**(4): 430–435.

Stevenson, A.E., et al. (2002). The effect of diet on calcium oxalate urinary relative supersaturation (RSS) of stone-forming (SF) and normal (N) dogs. *J Vet Intern Med* **16**(3): 377.

Stevenson, A.E., et al. (2003). Effect of dietary moisture and sodium content on urine composition and calcium oxalate relative supersaturation in healthy miniature schnauzers and Labrador retrievers. *Res Vet Sci* **74**(2): 145–151.

Stevenson, A.E., et al. (2003). Risk factor analysis and relative supersaturation as tools for identifying calcium oxalate stone-forming dogs. *J Small Anim Pract* **44**(11): 491–496.

Stevenson, A.E., et al. (2003). The relative effects of supplemental dietary calcium and oxalate on urine composition and calcium oxalate relative supersaturation in healthy adult dogs. *Res Vet Sci* **75**(1): 33–41.

Stevenson, A.E., et al. (2004). Nutrient intake and urine composition in calcium oxalate stone-forming dogs: comparison with healthy dogs and impact of dietary modification. *Vet Ther* **5**(3): 218–231.

Werness, P.G., et al. (1985). Equil 2: a basic computer program for the calculation of urinary saturation. *J Urol* **134**: 1242–1244.

Xu, H., et al. (2006). Effect of dietary sodium on urine characteristics in healthy adult cats (abstract). *J Vet Intern Med* **20**(3): 738.

13

Blood pressure determination

Rebecca L. Stepien

"Systemic hypertension" refers to a sustained increase in blood pressure (BP) (Brown et al. 2007) and has been documented as a cause of progressive renal damage in dogs and cats (see Chapters 48 and 68) (Mathur et al. 2002; Jacob et al. 2003; Finco 2004; et al. 2002). Accurate measurement and effective management of elevated systemic BP is a critical component in managing renal disease in dogs and cats, decreasing proteinuria, (Brown et al. 1993; Grauer et al. 2000) and prolonging survival (Jepson et al. 2007; Wehner et al. 2008). Additionally, successful therapy of systemic hypertension may circumvent critical target organ damage (TOD) in the eyes, brain, kidneys, and heart (Kyles et al. 1999; Maggio et al. 2000; Brown et al. 2007; Jepson et al. 2007).

Indications for blood pressure determination

Blood pressure assessment is indicated when there is evidence of TOD or when diseases known to be associated with systemic hypertension are documented or suspected. Blood pressure measurement in normal, healthy young animals is not recommended unless evidence of TOD is present, but "screening" older feline patients with yearly BP measurements may be useful since renal disease and hyperthyroidism are prevalent in elderly cats. If elevated BP is detected in a patient without signs of TOD, a repeat measurement occasion should be scheduled within several hours to 7 days to confirm the abnormal measurement.

Evidence of target organ damage

Target organs most frequently affected by systemic hypertension include the eyes, brain, kidneys, and heart (Brown et al. 2007). When there is evidence of TOD, BP should be measured at the earliest possible occasion to confirm or rule out systemic hypertension as the cause of clinical signs. Other diagnostic testing is recommended based on clinical presentation (Table 13.1). Detection of compatible ocular or central nervous system signs in the presence of elevated BP measurements is considered an emergency and therapy should begin as soon as hypertensive status is detected.

Presence of systemic disease causally associated with systemic hypertension

Certain systemic diseases (Table 13.2) are known to cause systemic hypertension in some affected dogs and cats (Anderson and Fisher 1968; Cowgill and Kallet 1983; Gilson et al. 1994; Ortega et al. 1996; Barthez et al. (1997); Struble et al. 1998; Rapoport and Stepien 2001; Syme et al. 2002; Syme and Elliott 2003; Brown et al. 2007). Screening BP measurements are indicated in patients with these diagnoses or in patients who are suspected to have these diagnoses. If signs of TOD are present in patients with these diagnoses, systemic hypertension is a likely cause of the signs of TOD and BP should be measured immediately.

At present, renal diseases represent the most common cause of systemic hypertension in both dogs and cats, and all renal patients should undergo BP screening as soon as their renal disease is recognized. Prevalence of systemic hypertension in chronic renal disease patients with or without proteinuria is variable but high with a rate of 9–93% (most studies report rates of 60–80%) in dogs (Cowgill and Kallet 1983; Cortadellas et al. 2006) and 20–65% in cats (Kobayashi et al. 1990; Syme et al. 2002).

Nephrology and Urology of Small Animals. Edited by Joe Bartges and David J. Polzin. © 2011 Blackwell Publishing Ltd.

Table 13.1 Clinical signs of target organ damage and additional recommended testing

Target organs affected	Associated clinical findings	Recommended diagnostic testing
Eyes	Acute blindness due to retinal detachment or severe hyphema Retinal hemorrhage Retinal vascular narrowing or tortuosity Focal retinal transudates Focal retinal ischemic degeneration Partial/complete retinal detachment Papilledema	Complete fundoscopic examination (multiple examinations may be required) Assessment for coagulopathies may be indicated in patients with hyphema or retinal hemorrhage
Brain	Seizures (focal facial or grand mal) "Stroke-like" intracranial neurologic deficits Decreased mentation Photophobia Nystagmus	Complete neurologic examination Additional imaging (e.g., MRI)
Kidneys	Proteinuria Microalbuminuria Progressive decrease in function	Serum BUN and creatinine Complete urinalysis Quantitation of proteinuria/microalbuminuria Advanced renal testing (e.g., GFR)
Heart	LV concentric hypertrophy Arrhythmia Gallop rhythm Systolic heart murmur Increased sensitivity to fluid loading (unexpected acute heart failure after fluid administration) Epistaxis	Auscultation Thoracic radiographs Echocardiography Doppler echocardiography may be required to rule out other causes of LV hypertrophy (e.g., subaortic stenosis)

Note: Recommended testing list is not exhaustive, additional testing may be indicated in individual patients.
BUN, blood urea nitrogen; GFR, glomerular filtration rate; LV, left ventricle.

Table 13.2 Diseases causally associated with systemic hypertension in dogs and cats

Both species	
Renal disease (acute or chronic, proteinuric, or nonproteinuric) Diabetes mellitus Pheochromocytoma Hyperaldosteronism	
Dogs	Cats
Above plus: Hyperadrenocorticism	Above plus: Hyperthyroidism

Prevalence of systemic hypertension is variable among diseases and between species and some reports are anecdotal.
See references for more specific information. In some cases, the cause of systemic hypertension may not be clear (i.e., "idiopathic hypertension").

Prevalence of systemic hypertension in acute renal failure in dogs is also high (Francey and Cowgill 2004). Some renal patients may develop systemic hypertension after initially having had normal BP (Jacob et al. 2003), so renal patients with normal initial BP values should have BP assessed at regular intervals after their renal diagnosis.

Methods of measuring blood pressure

Commonly available methods to assess BP in dogs and cats include direct measurement (via arterial puncture or arterial cannulation) or indirect (noninvasive) methods, including Doppler sphygmomanometry (DS) and oscillometry (OSC). More recently, high-definition oscillometry (HDO) has been used to measurement BP noninvasively, but results may be not comparable to other methods and repeatable measurements may be difficult to obtain in cats (Jepson et al. 2005). "Standard" OSC is recommended for clinical use until more comparative information is available.

No matter which method is used, three rules of BP measurement apply (1) the patient should be unsedated but calm (5–10 minutes of acclimatization in a quiet area is recommended before clinical BP measurement), (2) 3–5 replicates are obtained and the mean value is used for analysis, and (3) since diastolic BP measured by indirect methods is somewhat unreliable, systolic BP is typically used for clinical decision-making.

Direct BP measurement

Direct measurement of BP by arterial puncture or arterial cannulation provides a "gold standard" assessment of blood pressure, but is more time-consuming and requires an increased level of clinical skill for daily use. In addition, use of more peripheral arteries for puncture or cannulation (e.g., dorsal pedal artery versus proximal femoral artery) will, due to the elastic properties of arterial walls, deliver higher systolic and lower diastolic pressures than more central arteries. Acute arterial puncture is not recommended in cats; if direct BP measurement is required, a femoral arterial catheter may be inserted with use of a local anesthetic.

Prior to measurement, a clinical pressure monitor or measurement system with print capabilities should be calibrated according to manufacturer's instructions. A pressure transducer is attached to the monitor with stiff and relatively short connection tubing and the needle (22-gauge, 1-inch needles are typically used for arterial puncture) is attached directly to the transducer (Figure 13.1a). The transducer, tubing, and needle are carefully flushed with heparinized saline to eject any air bubbles

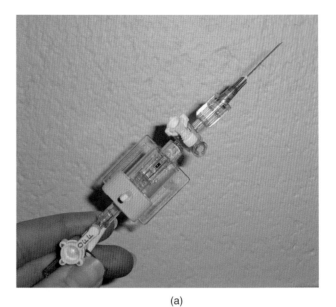

(a)

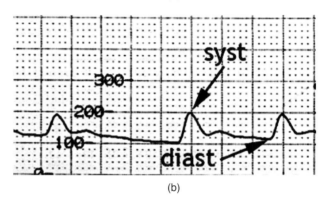

(b)

Figure 13.1 (a) A disposable pressure transducer attached to a 22-gauge, 1-inch needle for acute arterial puncture. The transducer, needle, and attached tubing are flushed with heparinized saline prior to use, to eject any air bubbles. (b) An arterial pressure trace from a femoral artery puncture in a dog. The pressure scale in mmHg appears on the left. This dog's blood pressure is approximately 200/100 mmHg. Syst refers to systolic blood pressure and diast refers to diastolic blood pressure.

and the transducer is zeroed to room air at the level of the sternum in the laterally recumbent patient.

For most dogs, direct arterial puncture is most easily performed with the patient gently restrained in lateral recumbency. The femoral arterial pulse is palpated in the femoral triangle, on the most proximal portion of the inner thigh. The area over the artery is clipped and approximately 0.5–1 cc of local anesthetic (lidocaine hydrochloride, 2% solution) is injected subcutaneously. After several minutes, the artery is again palpated and the needle advanced into the artery until a waveform is detected on the monitor. A paper trace of the pressure waveform is printed (Figure 13.1b) and the needle is withdrawn with immediate firm pressure applied to the artery at the level of the puncture to prevent hemorrhage. Manual pressure should be maintained on the puncture site for approximately 5 minutes with close monitoring thereafter to avoid possible hematoma development.

Arterial catheterization may be used for BP monitoring over time in patients during anesthesia or in critical care situations. "Over-the-needle" or cephalic catheters are typically placed in the dorsal pedal artery in the awake animal. The area over the palpable dorsal pedal arterial pulse is clipped and prepped for catheter placement and an appropriately-sized catheter (20–23-gauge based on patient size) is placed with a technique similar to cephalic catheter placement. A flushed transducer/tubing apparatus is zeroed to room air at the level of the patient's atria (the thoracic inlet in the sternal patient and the sternum in the lateral patient). Once the arterial catheter is in place and secured, a flushed transducer/tubing apparatus is attached and the pressure waveform is read and printed off the patient monitor. Note that the catheter must be at the approximate level of the heart and transducer when BP is recorded.

Indirect (noninvasive) BP measurement

DS or oscillometric BP measurement systems use a BP cuff wrapped around a forelimb, hindlimb, or tailhead and a manual (DS) or automated (OSC) inflation/deflation cycle to detect the pressure required to occlude a peripheral artery.

Doppler sphygmomanometry

Using DS methods to measure BP requires a BP cuff (premeasured and sized such that the width of the cuff is approximately 40% of the circumference of the limb or tail at the level of cuff placement), a Doppler probe with coupling gel attached to an audio amplifier, and an inflation bulb with pressure dial (sphygmomanometer, Figure 13.2). In dogs and cats, the forelimb is the most common measurement site with the animal in lateral recumbency or sitting. The cuff is placed at mid-antebrachium and attached to the sphygmomanometer. The probe (with coupling gel) is held or taped in place over an artery distal to the cuff (usually the palmar arterial arch) and the position is adjusted until a clear pulsatile signal can be detected. The cuff is inflated to approximately 20–40 mmHg past the point at which the sound of blood flow is occluded and then slowly deflated. The pressure at which the sound signal reappears is recorded as the systolic BP. As the cuff is further deflated, the audio signal will become muffled—this pressure may be recorded as diastolic BP, but is less reliable than the systolic BP recorded by this method.

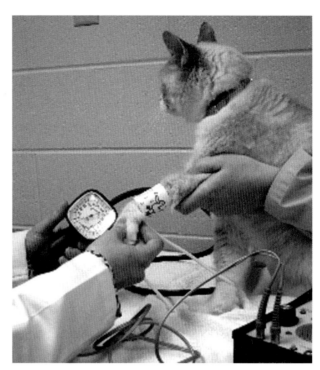

Figure 13.2 A Doppler sphygomomanometric technique is used to measure blood pressure in a sitting cat. Note that the cuff is wrapped around the mid-level radius and the limb is gently held in extension with the cuff at the level of the heart during measurement.

Oscillometry

Oscillometric BP devices deliver systolic, diastolic, and mean BP values as well as heart rate. These systems are most reliable in cats when a tailhead cuff is used in unrestrained sternal recumbency (Figure 13.3a), but forelimb (radial level), hindlimb (metatarsal level *or* proximal to hock in recumbent animal, Figure 13.3b), or tailhead (in standing or recumbent animals) cuffs may be used in dogs. The cuff width is chosen similarly to the DS technique. The cuff is positioned with the bladder of the cuff squarely over the artery and secured. The OSC machine is set to read BP at approximately 1-minute intervals. Mean values of five replicates are used as representative values, with any obvious erroneous or outlying values discarded. OSC equipment may be unable to read BP accurately at high heart rates (>180 bpm) or if an arrhythmia is present.

Record keeping

Each individual measurement plus the averages should be recorded in the patient record along with heart rate and assessment of patient demeanor during the exam. In addition, the technique, cuff size, and cuff position should be recorded so that the same technique and

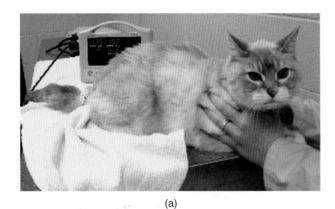

(a)

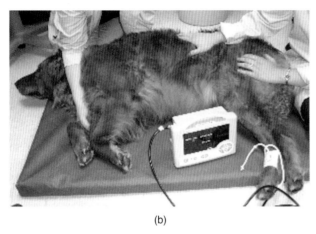

(b)

Figure 13.3 (a) A sternally recumbent cat with oscillometric blood pressure measurement using a tail cuff. The cat is minimally restrained after a period of calming prior to measurement. (b) A dog with oscillometric blood pressure assessment using a distal hindlimb cuff at the level of the metatarsals. The dog is relaxed and minimally restrained on a comfortable surface, with the cuff at the level of the sternum in the laterally recumbent dog.

equipment can be used at the next measurement. This information increases the reliability of measurements and can be used as future measurements are compared to measurements already recorded.

References

Anderson, L.J. and E.W. Fisher (1968). The blood pressure in canine interstitial nephritis. *Res Vet Sci* **9**: 304–313.

Barthez, P.Y., et al. (1997)). Pheochromocytoma in dogs: 61 cases (1984–1995). *J Vet Intern Med* **11**: 272–278.

Brown, S.A., et al. (1993). Long-term effects of antihypertensive regimens on renal hemodynamics and proteinuria. *Kidney Int* **43**: 1210–1218.

Brown, S., et al. (2007). Guidelines for the identification, evaluation and management of systemic hypertension in dogs and cats. *J Vet Intern Med* **21**: 542–558.

Cortadellas, O., et al. (2006). Systemic hypertension in dogs with leishmaniasis: prevalence and clinical consequences. *J Vet Intern Med* **20**: 941–947.

Cowgill, L.G. and A.J. Kallet (1983). Recognition and management of hypertension in the dog. In: *Current Veterinary Therapy VIII: Small Animal Practice*, edited by R.W. Kirk and J.D. Bonagura. Philadelphia, PA: WB Saunders, pp. 1025–1028.

Finco, D.R. (2004). Association of systemic hypertension with renal injury in dogs with induced renal failure. *J Vet Intern Med* **18**: 289–294.

Francey, T. and L.D. Cowgill (2004). Hypertension in dogs with severe acute renal failure (abstract). *J Vet Intern Med* **18**: 418.

Gilson, S.D., et al. (1994). Pheochromocytoma in 50 dogs. *J Vet Int Med* **8**(3): 228–232.

Grauer, G.F., et al. (2000). Effects of enalapril versus placebo as a treatment for canine idiopathic glomerulonephritis. *J Vet Intern Med* **14**: 526–533.

Jacob, F., et al. (2003). Association between initial systolic blood pressure and risk of developing a uremic crisis or of dying in dogs with chronic renal failure. *J Am Vet Med Assoc* **222**(3): 322–329.

Jepson, R.E., et al. (2005). A comparison of CAT Doppler and oscillometric Memoprint machines for non-invasive blood pressure measurement in conscious cats. *J Feline Med Surg* **7**: 147–152.

Jepson, R.E., et al. (2007). Effect of control of systolic blood pressure on survival in cats with systemic hypertension. *J Vet Intern Med* **21**: 402–409.

Kobayashi, D.L., et al. (1990). Hypertension in cats with chronic renal failure or hyperthyroidism. *J Vet Intern Med* **4**: 58–62.

Kyles, A.E., et al. (1999). Management of hypertension controls postoperative neurologic disorders after renal transplantation. *Vet Surg* **28**: 436–441.

Maggio, F., et al. (2000). Ocular lesions associated with systemic hypertension in cats: 69 cases (1985–1998). *J Am Vet Med Assoc* **217**: 695–702.

Mathur, S., et al. (2002). Effects of the calcium channel antagonist amlodipine in cats with surgically induced hypertensive renal insufficiency. *Am J Vet Res* **63**(6): 833–839.

Ortega, T.M., et al. (1996). Systemic arterial blood pressure and urine protein/creatinine ratio in dogs with hyperadrenocorticism. *J Am Vet Med Assoc* **209**(10): 1724–1729.

Rapoport, G.S. and R.L. Stepien (2001). Direct arterial blood pressure measurement in 54 dogs presented for systemic hypertension screening 1998–2001 (abstract). *Proc 11th Congress, European Society of Veterinary Internal Medicine*, Dublin, Ireland.

Struble, A.L., et al. (1998). Systemic hypertension and proteinuria in dogs with diabetes mellitus. *J Am Vet Med Assoc* **213**(6): 822–825.

Syme, H.M., et al. (2002). Prevalence of systolic hypertension in cats with chronic renal failure at initial evaluation. *J Am Vet Med Assoc* **220**(12): 1799–1804.

Syme, H.M. and J. Elliott (2003). The prevalence of hypertension in hyperthyroid cats at diagnosis and following treatment (abstract). *Proc 13th Congress, European Society of Veterinary Internal Medicine, Uppsala, Sweden.*

Wehner, A., et al. (2008). Associations between proteinuria, systemic hypertension and glomerular filtration rate in dogs with renal and non-renal diseases. *Vet Rec* **162**: 141–147.

14

Renal function testing

Hervé P. Lefebvre

The interpretation of tests of renal function in dogs and cats requires specific knowledge of renal physiology (see Chapter 2) and information, when available, about intra- and inter-individual variability, analytical factors of variation, and specificity/sensitivity. Glomerular function is generally considered as the best indicator of renal function. Indirect tests are used for practical reasons, but direct testing is more sensitive and should be encouraged.

Testing glomerular function

Indirect tests

Azotemia is defined as an increased plasma urea and/or creatinine concentration. Assessment of the azotemic status is essential in the diagnosis, prognosis, and follow-up of patients with chronic kidney disease or acute renal injury.

Creatinine

Plasma creatinine concentration is currently considered as the best indirect marker of GFR and is also used by the International Renal Interest Society (IRIS) to stage canine and feline CKD (see Chapter 48). Creatinine is produced by degradation of creatine and creatine phosphate in skeletal muscles. The normal daily input into plasma is about 45 and 65 mg/kg BW in dogs and cats, respectively. Creatinine is distributed in the body water, filtered by the glomeruli, not reabsorbed and not or negligibly secreted. The plasma half-life of creatinine is about 3 hours in healthy dogs and cats (Watson et al. 2002; Le Garreres et al. 2007). The major preanalytical, analytical and physiological factors of variations are listed in Tables 14.1 and 14.2 (Braun et al. 2003).

Rationally established reference intervals for dogs have paradoxically not been published in a peer-reviewed journal. The upper limit of the reference interval for most analyzers, generally ranges from 1.3 to 1.6 mg/dL. However plasma creatinine is higher in dogs with BW>25 kg (upper limit: 1.7–1.8 mg/dL) than in dogs with BW<10 kg (upper limit: 0.9 mg/dL) (Craig et al. 2006). Basal plasma creatinine is higher in the cat, and also increases slightly with body weight. The reference interval in domestic short-haired cats is 1.0–2.3 mg/dL (Reynolds et al. 2008).

An abnormally high plasma creatinine value is assumed to indicate the loss of at least 65–75% of the renal functional mass. However, sensitivity (or specificity) is not very high in dogs (Gleadhill, 1994; Braun and Lefebvre, 2005). Subtle changes in renal function can be detected by repeating plasma creatinine measurements over time under well-standardized conditions (Lees, 2004). The critical difference, that is, minimal difference between two consecutive measurements in the same individual which may be an increase or a decrease, is about 0.4 mg/dL in healthy dogs (Jensen and Aes, 1993). The inverse curvilinear relationship existing between plasma creatinine and GFR in dogs (Finco et al. 1995) should be taken into account for clinical interpretation (Figure 14.1).

A decrease in plasma creatinine has been reported in portosystemic shunts in dogs and hyperthyroidism in cats. Thus, the sensitivity of plasma creatinine to detect CKD in such patients is decreased.

Urea

Urea is the main form in which nitrogen is eliminated from the body and its metabolism is presented in Figure 14.2.

Plasma/serum urea concentration (1 mmol/L = 6 mg/dL) can also be expressed as blood urea nitrogen

---

Nephrology and Urology of Small Animals. Edited by Joe Bartges and David J. Polzin. © 2011 Blackwell Publishing Ltd.

Table 14.1 Preanalytical and analytical factors of variation of plasma/serum creatinine in dogs

Factor of variation	Comment
Specimen	Differences between serum and plasma creatinine are negligible.
Stability	Creatinine is stable for up to 4 days in canine whole blood at 4°C, and in serum/heparinized plasma at room temperature.
Analytical techniques	Enzymatic procedures, used by veterinary analyzers, are preferred to the nonspecific Jaffé reaction because the analytical interference is less.
Between-laboratory variation	Differences may exist from analyzer to analyzer, and from laboratory to laboratory. The same analyzer/laboratory should be used to follow-up renal function.

(BUN) or serum urea nitrogen (BUN (mg/dL) $\times$ 2.14 = Plasma urea (mg/dL)). The stabilities of urea and creatinine in blood or plasma are very similar. The upper limit for plasma urea is generally about 55–65 mg/dL (i.e., 25–30 mg/dL for BUN). Plasma urea and creatinine are both similarly affected by age and meals. Plasma urea is increased in renal failure but is not a good indirect indicator of GFR because of its tubular re-absorption. Moreover multiple extrarenal factors of variation exist (Figure 14.2). The sensitivity and specificity of plasma urea in renal dysfunction diagnosis is unknown. The estimated critical difference for plasma urea in dogs is 14.4 mg/dL (i.e., BUN = 6.7 mg/dL) for a mean value of 30.0 mg/dL (i.e., BUN = 14.0 mg/dL) (Jensen and Aes, 1993). Although the clinical relevance of the plasma urea to creatinine ratio remains questionable (Finco and Duncan, 1976), it may be increased during excessive protein catabolism or early prerenal azotemia, as observed in dogs with heart disease (Nicolle et al. 2007). Inversely it may be decreased by severe protein malnutrition.

Cystatin C

This small constitutive protein is synthesized by all nucleated cells and has been proposed as an indirect marker

of GFR in dogs. No advantage of plasma cystatin C over plasma creatinine has been evidenced in dogs (Almy et al. 2002).

Assessment of glomerular filtration rate

Definition, clearance concept and GFR markers

Glomerular filtration rate (GFR) is considered as the best indicator of overall renal function. It is defined as the volume of ultrafiltrate produced by glomerular filtration per unit of time. GFR can be calculated from the urinary/plasma clearance of appropriate markers. Clearance is a proportionality constant, describing the relationship between the rate of transfer of a substance (amount per unit of time) and its concentration in urine and/or plasma.

A GFR marker should satisfy the following criteria: it must be freely filtered by the glomeruli, not be reabsorbed or secreted by the renal tubule, not be metabolized or produced by the kidney and not alter the GFR value. The marker should also be totally cleared by the kidneys when a plasma clearance approach is used. The main GFR markers in dogs and cats are presented in Table 14.3.

Table 14.2 Physiological factors of variations of plasma/serum creatinine and specific recommendations

Factor	Comment
Breed/muscle mass	A breed effect (e.g., higher plasma creatinine in Greyhound dog or Birman cat), due or not, to differences in muscle mass, exists in dogs and cats.
Food intake	Plasma creatinine may increase after meals (Watson et al. 1981). Blood samples should be taken from fasting animals.
Age	Plasma creatinine decreases in the first days of life, but then increases to normal adult values from the age of 2 months up to 1 year (Wolford et al. 1988). Plasma creatinine is then relatively stable.
Hydration status	Hydration status should be checked as plasma creatinine can be moderately increased by dehydration.
Physical exercise	Effect of physical exercise on serum/plasma creatinine is variable. Blood sampling in animals after strenuous exercise should be avoided.

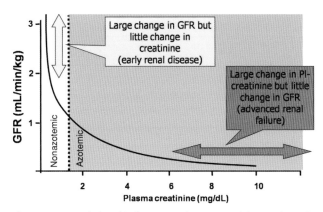

Figure 14.1 Relationship between plasma creatinine and GFR in dogs (according to Finco et al. 1995). In early stages of CKD, the change in plasma creatinine is very limited whereas the decrease in GFR is pronounced. Inversely, in end-stage CKD, a large decrease in plasma creatinine (e.g., after fluid therapy) may be associated with a minimal concomitant increase in GFR. The dashed line represents the upper limit of the reference interval (1.5 mg/dL), above which the dog is declared azotemic.

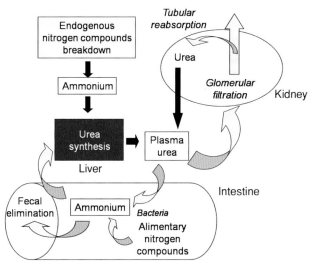

Figure 14.2 Metabolism of urea. Urea is synthesized in the liver from ammonia. Ammonia is produced from nitrogen (essentially from digestion of alimentary proteins and breakdown of endogenous tissue proteins). Urea is filtered by the kidneys and excreted in urine, but also reabsorbed from the collecting tubule. Urea reabsorption increases when the urine tubular flow decreases (e.g., in animals with hypovolemia or decreased renal perfusion). Urea is also excreted in the intestinal lumen where it is converted to amino acids and ammonium, and consequently recycled. Plasma urea may increase with increased protein catabolism (e.g., starvation) or digestion (gastrointestinal haemorrhage, high-protein diet), and may decrease in dogs on low-protein diet, with hepatic failure or portosystemic shunt, or when treated with anabolic steroids.

Clearance methods

The urinary (or renal) clearance of the GFR marker is equal to the amount of marker excreted in urine (the product of the urine concentration of the marker and the flow of urine collected over a given period of time) divided by its average plasma concentration. The urinary clearance of exogenous creatinine (Finco et al. 1991) is currently the method best documented in dogs and cats. However, the accurate and tedious collection of urine and the required bladder emptying by urethral catheterization are major issues with this approach. A more practicable alternative is the plasma clearance approach which does not require urine collection and is simply based on repeated blood sampling (Figure 14.3).

Clinical use and interpretation

GFR determination is pivotal in evaluating the severity and course of renal disease. (Table 14.4)

A decrease in GFR may be the first sign of chronic kidney disease. Most published normal values of GFR are between 2 and 5 mL/minute per kg in dogs and cats irrespective of technique or marker (Heiene and Moe, 1998). A GFR value below 1.5 mL/minute per kg is generally assumed to be abnormal in average-sized dogs. This cut-off value would be 2.1 mL/minute per kg for dogs with a BW<10 kg and about 1.2 mL/minute per kg for dogs with a BW>45 kg (Lefebvre et al. 2006). The GFR value can only be interpreted in terms of renal function under standardized conditions, that is, in normohydrated (dehydration may decrease GFR), fasted (because of potential postprandial increase), and awake animals (anesthetic or sedative agents may alter GFR) in stable clinical conditions. The GFR may change from hour to hour in dogs or cats with acute renal injury. GFR does not seem to be affected by repeated renal biopsies in dogs (Groman et al. 2004).

Testing tubular function

Urine specific gravity

The urine concentration is evaluated from the urine specific gravity (USG) (i.e., ratio of the weight of a given volume of urine to the same volume of water) measured by refractometry. USG reflects the ability of the renal tubules to concentrate or dilute urine according to the body water requirements (Watson, 1998) (Table 14.5). USG is generally decreased in chronic renal disease. However, because of the large variability of USG (van Vonderen et al. 1997), and to reliably indicate renal dysfunction,

Table 14.3 Major markers of glomerular filtration rate (GFR) used in dogs and cats

Marker	Comment
Inulin	Urinary inulin clearance is considered as the gold standard method for GFR measurement. Plasma inulin clearance has also been proposed but inulin can be cleared by extrarenal route. Assay is not readily available.
Creatinine	Creatinine is an appropriate marker for both urinary and plasma clearance approaches. Urine and plasma assays can be easily performed and are not expensive. Medical grade creatinine formulation is not commercially available.
Iohexol	Iohexol, an iodinated radiocontrast medium, offers an interesting alternative for GFR testing using plasma clearance. However, the two stereoisomers, endo- and exo-iohexol, have different plasma clearances. Assay is performed by HPLC.
Radiolabelled markers	Radiolabelled markers (e.g., ^{99m}Tc-DTPA)) have been used for GFR assessment, but require special licensing and equipment (see Chapter 18).

abnormally low USG values must be confirmed on repeated samples.

In acute renal injury, USG is generally increased in prerenal azotemia (>1.035 (dog) or 1.045 (cat)), decreased in renal azotemia (USG from 1.008 to 1.028 (dog) or 1.035 (cat)), and variable in postrenal azotemia.

USG may also be useful to interpret results from urinalysis. For example, 2+ proteinuria represents a more substantial loss in dilute urine (e.g., USG 1.015) than in concentrated urine (e.g., USG 1.060) (see Chapter 8). Falsely elevated USG values may be induced by glucose or proteins in the urine.

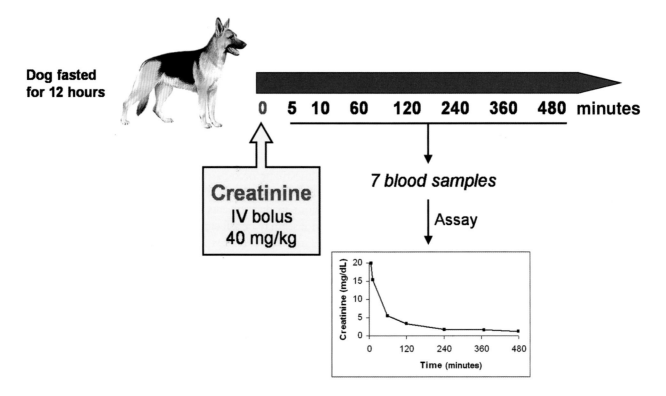

GFR = Dose/area under the curve

Figure 14.3 Principle of plasma clearance test for evaluation of glomerular filtration rate (GFR). The plasma exogenous creatinine clearance test is illustrated here. A bolus of creatinine (40 mg/kg) is injected intravenously. Blood is sampled at different times postinjection (here, 5, 10 minutes, 1, 2, 4, 6, and 8 hours). Plasma creatinine is then assayed. The area under the plasma creatinine vs time curve (AUC) is determined by pharmacokinetic approach. The plasma clearance (i.e., the GFR estimate) is calculated by dividing the injected dose by the AUC. (For details concerning the calculation, see Watson et al. 2002).

Table 14.4 Indications for GFR testing

Suspected renal dysfunction which cannot be confirmed by other tests, for example, polyuria/polydipsia without azotemia, or persistent moderate azotemia without any other clinical/pathological signs
Presence of asymptomatic renal lesions (e.g., evidenced by renal ultrasonography)
Presence of extrarenal disease with potential adverse effects on renal function, such as cardiovascular disease (e.g., heart failure and systemic arterial hypertension), endocrine disease (e.g., hypothyroidism in dogs and hyperthyroid cat after treatment), or infectious disease (e.g., pyometra and leishmaniasis)
Dosage adjustments for drugs essentially cleared by the kidney and with a low therapeutic index
Assessment of renal function in kidney donor

Water deprivation tests (WDT)

WDT (see Chapter 42) are recommended in small animal patients with polyuria/polydipsia to distinguish between nephrogenic diabetes insipidus, psychogenic polydipsia and central diabetes insipidus. The principle of WDT is, that the increased plasma osmolality will increase ADH secretion, and thereby the urine concentration (i.e., USG or urine osmolality). Administration of synthetic ADH analogues (vasopressin or desmopressin) should not produce a further increase in urine concentration in patients with primary polydipsia. During WDT the USG does not increase in patients with central diabetes insipidus but, does so after vasopressin administration. No response to vasopressin is observed in patients with primary nephrogenic diabetes insipidus. In secondary nephrogenic diabetes insipidus, the response may be equivocal and very difficult to interpret (for details, see Syme, 2007). WDT should be performed only when all other causes of polyuria/polydipsia have been ruled out. They are contraindicated in patients with azotemia and/or dehydration, or with identified renal dysfunction. WDT are particularly tedious and require well-trained staff.

Fractional excretion of electrolytes

The fractional excretion (FE) of a given electrolyte is defined as the fraction of filtered solute that is excreted into urine. It also corresponds to the ratio (also called fractional clearance) of the renal clearance of the electrolyte to the GFR, which can be determined from the urinary endogenous creatinine clearance.

An alternative to clearance methods is the spot sample approach based on Equation 14.1:

$$FE = \frac{Ue \times Pcreat}{Pe \times Ucreat} \tag{14.1}$$

Table 14.5 Physiological and clinical interpretation of urine specific gravity

USG value	<1.008	1.008–1.012	1.013–1.029 (dog) 1.013–1.034 (cat)	>1.029 (dog) >1.034 (cat)
Terminology	Hyposthenuria	Isosthenuria	Hypersthenuria	
Physiological interpretation	Renal tubules can dilute urine by active metabolic work	No dilution, no concentration of the urine by the renal tubules	Urine is minimally concentrated by the tubules	Urine is normally concentrated by the tubules
Clinical interpretation	Multiple causes can induce hyposthenuria: hyperadrenocorticism, pyometra, diabetes insipidus, etc. Renal dysfunction is possible in dehydrated and/or azotemic dogs/cats	Renal dysfunction is possible, and should be highly suspected in the dehydrated and/or azotemic animal. Isosthenuria may be observed in overhydration or after recent and copious water intake	See isosthenuria	Chronic kidney disease may exist as some animals (especially cats) are able to maintain their concentrating ability. In young animals, USG is higher than in adults

Only "spot" samples of urine and plasma are required. Spot determinations have given inaccurate values in cats and dogs. FE exhibits large inter-individual and intra-individual variability. Also, as FE values do not remain fixed but vary as needed to maintain homeostasis, no reference interval can be defined. FE values should always be interpreted in the light of plasma electrolyte concentration and clinical findings. FE are generally <1% for sodium and <25% for potassium. FE tests have been used to diagnose Fanconi's syndrome in dogs (see Chapter 55), but their clinical relevance is generally limited (for details, see Lefebvre et al. 2008).

References

Almy, F.S., et al. (2002). Evaluation of cystatin C as an endogenous marker of glomerular filtration rate in dogs. *J Vet Intern Med* **16**: 45–51.

Braun, J.P. and H.P. Lefebvre (2005). Early detection of renal disease in the canine patient. *Eur J Companion Anim Pract* **15**: 59–64.

Braun, J.P., et al. (2003). Creatinine in the dog: a review. *Vet Clin Pathol* **32**: 162–179.

Craig, A.J., et al. (2006). Refining the reference interval for plasma creatinine in dogs: effect of age, gender, body weight, and breed. American College of Veterinary Internal Medicine. 24th Annual Forum, Louisville, USA, May 31–June 3, 2006, p. 740.

Finco, D.R. and J.R. Duncan (1976). Evaluation of blood urea nitrogen and serum creatinine concentrations as indicators of renal dysfunction: a study of 111 cases and a review of related literature. *J Am Vet Med Assoc* **168**: 593–601.

Finco, D.R., et al. (1991). Exogenous creatinine clearance as a measure of glomerular filtration rate in dogs with reduced renal mass. *Am J Vet Res* **52**: 1029–1032.

Finco, D.R., et al. (1995). Relationship between plasma creatinine and glomerular filtration rate in dogs. *J Vet Pharmacol Ther* **18**: 418–421.

Gleadhill, A. (1994). Evaluation of screening tests for renal insufficiency in the dog. *J Small Anim Pract* **35**: 391–396.

Groman, R.D., et al. (2004). Effects of serial ultrasound-guided renal biopsies on kidneys of healthy adolescent dogs. *Vet Radiol Ultrasound* **45**: 62–69.

Heiene, R. and L. Moe (1998). Pharmacokinetic aspects of measurement of glomerular filtration rate in the dog: a review. *J Vet Intern Med* **12**: 401–412.

Jensen, A.L. and H. Aes (1993). Critical difference of clinical chemical parameters in blood from dogs. *Res Vet Sci* **54**: 10–14.

Lees, G.E. (2004). Early diagnosis of renal disease and renal failure. *Vet Clin North Am Small Anim Pract* **34**: 867–885.

Lefebvre, H.P., et al. (2006). GFR in the dog: breed effects. European College of Veterinary Internal Medicine, *16th Congress*, Amsterdam, The Netherlands, September 14–16, 2006, p. 61.

Le Garreres, A., et al. (2007). Disposition of plasma creatinine in non-azotemic and moderately azotemic cats. *J Feline Med Surg* **9**: 89–96.

Lefebvre, H.P., et al. (2008). Fractional excretion tests: a critical review of methods and application in domestic animals. *Vet Clin Pathol*, **37**: 4–20.

Nicolle, A.P., et al. (2007). Azotemia and glomerular filtration rate in dogs with chronic valvular disease. *J Vet Intern Med* **21**: 943–949.

Reynolds, B.S., et al. (2008). Determination of reference intervals for plasma biochemical values in clinically normal adult domestic shorthair cats by use of a dry-slide biochemical analyzer. *Am J Vet Res* **69**: 471–477.

Syme, H.M. (2007) Polyuria and polydipsia. In: *BSAVA Manual of Canine and Feline Nephrology and Uroloy*, edited by J. Elliott and Gregory F. Grauer, 2nd edition. Gloucester, UK: British Small Animal Veterinary Association, pp. 8–25.

van Vonderen, I.K., et al. (1997). Intra- and inter-individual variation in urine osmolality and urine specific gravity in healthy pet dogs of various ages. *J Vet Intern Med* **11**: 30–35.

Watson, A.D.J., et al. (1981). Postprandial changes in plasma urea and creatinine concentration in dogs. *Am J Vet Res* **42**: 1878–1880.

Watson, A.D. (1998). Urine specific gravity in practice. *Aust Vet J* **76**: 392–398.

Watson, A.D.J., et al. (2002). Plasma exogenous creatinine clearance test in dogs: comparison with other methods and proposed limited sampling strategy. *J Vet Intern Med* **16**: 22–23.

Wolford, S.T., et al. (1988). Effect of age on serum chemistry profile, electrophoresis and thyroid hormones in Beagle dogs two weeks to one year of age. *Vet Clin Pathol* **17**: 35–42.

15

Radiographic imaging in urinary tract disease

Daniel A. Feeney and Kari L. Anderson

Introduction

Indications for urinary tract imaging

The urinary and genital tracts are in relatively close abdominopelvic proximity and share common pathways to exit the body including the urethra in the male and the vestibule in the female. Therefore, it must be recognized that diseases affecting one of the systems may well affect the others as well. This generality applies to both naturally occurring diseases such as infections or tumors as well as iatrogenic problems such as ovariohysterectomy-induced invasive uterine stump granulomas affecting the bladder or inadvertent ureteral ligation during ovariohysterectomy. These relationships must be considered in the approach to diagnoses. Urinary organ clinical signs range from those suggestive of upper urinary disease (e.g., polyuria and paraspinal pain) through those indicative of lower urinary disease (e.g., pollakiuria and dysuria) and those associated with genital disease (e.g., vaginal discharge and urethral discharge) (see Chapters 4 and 41–47). The relative roles of the urogenital parenchymal organs (i.e., kidneys, prostate gland, and ovaries) to those of the tubular organs (i.e., ureters, bladder, urethra, uterus, and vagina) in these clinical signs must be continually addressed to assure that an erroneous and/or myopic clinical approach is avoided. In addition, the embryologic origins of the various urogenital organs cannot be forgotten. An anomaly in one system may create a clinical problem or a related anomaly in the other. The key to the analysis of either pathoanatomy or dysfunction between these two organ systems is to expeditiously include or exclude organs and conditions where possible using a combination of pertinent history, physical examination, risk analysis, serum biochemical, urine and hematologic analyses, and survey radiographs. Following critical assessment of the results from these routinely available tests, more sophisticated (and costly) procedures such as contrast radiographic procedures, ultrasonography, computed tomography, and nuclear scintigraphy can be justified. The goal of this chapter is to foster a predictable and organized approach to the imaging aspects of urinary tract disease evaluation.

Dilemmas in urinary imaging choices

The integration of the likelihood of specific conditions (e.g., breed-specific hereditary disorders, post surgical problems, age, and gender-adjusted disease likelihood) with a complete physical examination including abdominal, vaginal, and rectal palpation is of paramount importance. Imaging procedures have specific yields under certain circumstances. An inappropriate choice of imaging procedure may at best yield no information and at worst may induce needless patient morbidity and/or client expenditures. In general, radiography-based imaging procedures provide morphologic information. However, qualitative insight into functional problems (incontinence, relative renal function) can also be garnered with appropriate choices and judicious interpretation of selected procedures. Before choosing any imaging procedure, a specific decision must be made about what the procedure will predictably yield compared to the costs incurred and the morbidity induced. The most applicable procedure may be different depending on the suspected diagnosis. If the goal is only regional organ geometry like size, shape, location, surface character, number, or degree/extent of organ affliction or organ opacity (e.g., gas, fluid, mineral and metal), retrograde contrast imaging or ultrasound may be adequate. However, if the goal is qualitative assessment of function (e.g., relative renal

Nephrology and Urology of Small Animals. Edited by Joe Bartges and David J. Polzin. © 2011 Blackwell Publishing Ltd.

function and urethral sphincter competence) or physiologic organ distension (ureters or bladder), more serial or dynamic procedures such as excretory urography or voiding urethrography may be indicated. Acknowledging that glomerular filtration and tubular modification occur at the kidney, most of the urinary tract is either a storage compartment or a conduit between other urinary and/or genital structures. As clinical problems are associated with leakage, obstruction, irritation, inflammation, infiltration, displacement, or malpositioning, the chosen imaging procedure must enable the identification and localization of these problems. Depending on the clinical circumstances, survey radiographs may be adequate (e.g., end-stage kidney and cystoliths). If the utilization of a contrast radiographic procedure is clinically justified, there are further considerations including: the goal of the study (e.g., organ localization, organ distension, propulsion analysis, leakage detection, foreign body identification, organ connections, distinguish urinary from other organs/masses, etc.), the effects of iodinated contrast medium administered systemically versus via external orifice, the potential for air embolism from retrograde administration of negative contrast medium (room air), and the risk–benefit considerations of nonionic compared to ionic iodinated contrast media.

Background deliberations before urinary imaging

As patients with urinary disease can be nauseous, weak, in pain, or dehydrated as well as suffering from the numerous side-effects of clinical urinary problems including sepsis, electrolyte and acid–base abnormalities, and abdominal distension, a balance between what is optimal for imaging and what is practical and humane for the patient must be determined. The following questions may facilitate decisions regarding type of procedure and/or the risk:benefit of additional procedures: What is the status and demeanor of the patient (septic, coagulopathic, acutely painful, fear biter)? Is sedation necessary/indicated (balance between patient compliance and patient physiology)? Has the animal been appropriately prepared for the procedure under consideration, if applicable? Are there appropriately placed personnel body monitors? Is it necessary to physically hold the patient? Are appropriate personnel shielding devices being used (e.g., aprons, gloves, eye shields, and/or thyroid shields). REMEMBER: KEEP POTENTIAL RADIATION EXPOSURE (including scatter as well as primary beam) AS LOW AS IS REASONABLY ACHIEVABLE!!!!!!

Applicable special procedures

Standard views

Initial radiographic investigation of the urinary tract should begin with routine survey orthogonal views. The right lateral is the authors' preference as this recumbency generally allows improved visualization of the right and left kidneys through increased separation (Feeney et al. 1982a). The ventrodorsal (VD) view is the orthogonal view of choice and is the view used for measurement of the kidneys (Figures 15.1 and 15.2).

When obtaining survey views of the urinary tract, it is important to include the entire urinary tract, from the kidneys through the urethra, on both views. In large dogs, this may require obtaining two lateral and VD views (of the cranial and the caudal half of the patient). The rear limbs should be extended caudally in order to best evaluate the bladder and proximal urethra. In the male canine patient, particularly if presenting with signs referable to the urethra, an additional view with the rear limbs pulled cranial to the os penis allows improved visualization of the penile urethra.

Ideally, radiographs will be made prior to any intervention such as cystocentesis or urinary catheterization. Additionally, it is helpful to have a distended urinary bladder when evaluating the lower urinary tract; thus, do not allow the patient to urinate immediately before the procedure. While the authors' acknowledge that for general abdominal imaging we recommend making radiographs of the patient without any manipulation in order to see the patient in the natural state, an evacuated colon is important for optimal visualization of the urinary tract, particularly when evaluating for uroliths. This may necessitate withholding food for 18–24 hours and performing a cleansing enema prior to the radiographic procedure. If not done prior to initial examination, radiographs may need to be retaken after this type of patient preparation, thus increasing costs and radiation exposure.

Horizontal-beam views/special views

In general, horizontal views are not performed when imaging the urinary tract. However, horizontal beam radiography may be useful in certain circumstances. A standing lateral view may allow for ventral migration of the intestines to improve visualization of the retroperitoneal space and kidneys. Additionally, standing lateral views can be useful in identifying small opaque cystic calculi or sand, because the material will form layers in the dependent portion of the urinary bladder, thereby increasing their opacity (Steyn and Lowry 1991; Burk and Feeney 2003).

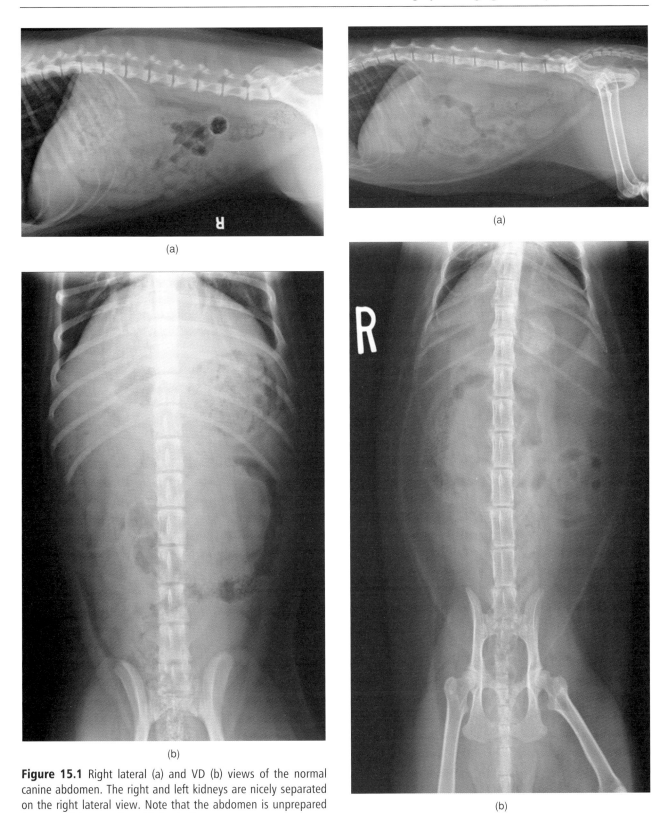

Figure 15.1 Right lateral (a) and VD (b) views of the normal canine abdomen. The right and left kidneys are nicely separated on the right lateral view. Note that the abdomen is unprepared (postprandial stomach and full colon).

Figure 15.2 Right lateral (a) and VD (b) views of the normal feline abdomen. The right and left kidneys are nicely separated on the right lateral view. Note that the abdomen is unprepared (full colon).

One special view which is quite helpful, is a view in which a radiolucent paddle or wooden spoon is used to apply regional compression. The compression effectively separates adjacent organs to minimize confusion due to overlying structures (such as intestines) by displacing them away from the kidneys or bladder and decreases patient thickness (and therefore scatter radiation) which both lead to improved visualization and detail. During application of compression, the thickness of the area of interest decreases and adjustment of technique is necessary from that used to obtain the noncompression view of the abdomen (Carrig and Mostosky 1976). In general, decreasing the mAs by 50% (Burk and Feeney 2003) or the kVp by 15% (Graham et al. 2007) results in an appropriately exposed view in the region of interest. Compression technique is easily performed, inexpensive, well tolerated by the patient and provides additional diagnostic information in selected cases (Armbrust et al. 2000). Compression can also be used with contrast procedures of the upper and lower urinary tracts (Carrig and Mostosky 1976; Biery 1981). Contraindications include enlarged organs which could rupture (e.g., severely enlarged uterus or splenic mass), diaphragmatic hernia or severe respiratory distress.

Patient preparation

For any of the urinary tract contrast procedures the patient must be fasted for 18–24 hours and a cleansing enema should be performed two to three hours before the procedure. An exception is made with the urgent/emergent patient (e.g., a trauma patient or a patient with lower urinary tract obstruction). Survey radiographic views must always be obtained on the day of the procedure, even if radiographs were obtained previously. Survey views determine if the procedure is necessary, evaluate the patient in the "natural state" for comparison with the contrast views (abnormalities on survey views may be obscured by contrast, as with radiopaque urinary calculi), assessment of proper preparation of the patient for the study, and selection of the appropriate radiographic technique. Heavy sedation or general anesthesia is required for cystourethrogram and vaginogram contrast procedures. Intravenous catheter access is required for the excretory urogram. Finally, as part of routine preparation, one should collect any urine samples needed prior to administering contrast which can have effects on the urinalysis and culture (Feeney et al. 1980a; Ruby et al. 1983).

Excretory urogram

The excretory urogram is useful for defining morphology of the upper urinary tract as well as providing a quali-

tative assessment of global and individual renal function (Feeney and Johnston 2007). The excellent visualization and assessment of the renal parenchyma and collecting system is due to the fact that the iodinated contrast compounds are excreted almost entirely by glomerular filtration, with a small percentage excreted by the liver and small intestine. Indications for excretory urogram include (1) to visualize the size, shape, and location of a kidney not seen on survey radiographic views, (2) to visualize the size, shape, and position of the portions of the upper urinary tract not normally seen on survey radiographic views and (3) to obtain qualitative information regarding renal function (Biery 1981). Numerous protocols for the excretory urogram have been previously described (Lord et al. 1974; Ackerman 1974; Kneller 1974; Feeney et al. 1979; Biery 1981; Feeney and Johnston 2007). The excretory urogram can be performed safely in azotemic and non-azotemic patients as long as the patients are well hydrated (Thrall and Finco 1976; Feeney and Johnston 2007). Side effects are rare, with the most common side effects being transient retching or vomiting. Rarely, are other side effects, such as, anaphylactoid reaction, hypotension, contrast-induced renal failure, urticaria, or bronchospasm, seen. The basic toxicity is related to the hyperosmolality of the contrast media. The most well-accepted contraindication to an excretory urogram in the veterinary patient is dehydration.

Contrast media, dose and route of administration

The first choice is to determine which type of water-soluble iodinated contrast should be used in the patient. Choices in general include ionic or nonionic preparations. Ionic preparations are generally quite hyperosmolar to blood and in general have more potential complications (although complications are rare). Nonionic preparations are closer in osmolarity to blood, and potential complications are fewer; however, these preparations are more expensive. In our practice, we tend to use the ionic preparations in young, healthy patients and the nonionic preparations in older or sick patients or patients with preexisting diseases such as renal disease, cardiac disease, or seizures.

The second important factor is the determination of dose. A typical dose in our practice will range from 400 to 800 mg iodine/lb body weight, and we will not exceed 800 mg iodine/lb body weight in one or multiple consecutive doses. Some authors have recommended 330–440 mg iodine/lb body weight (Ackerman 1974; Feeney et al. 1979; Feeney et al. 1982a) for a general dose. The low end of the dose (400 mg iodine/lb body weight) is administered to patients with normal renal function and urine concentration ability. The upper end of the dose (800 mg iodine/lb body weight) is administered to patients with poor renal function and/or urine concentration ability. Increasing the contrast dose generally allows improved visualization of the urinary tract in patients with poorer renal function. It has been suggested that if the serum creatinine is 3.5 mg/dL and rising, the intravenous urogram will not likely provide adequate visualization of the upper urinary tract (Biery 1981); although it has been shown that the BUN should not be used as a prognostic parameter for the quality of the study, nor should the presence of an elevated BUN alone preclude performance of the study (Thrall and Finco 1976). Valuable information from the excretory urogram can be obtained in certain cases such as when the patient has obstructive uropathy (Thrall and Finco 1976) or when the renal function is static or improving (Biery 1981).

It must be emphasized that the clinician must know the concentration of iodine in the chosen contrast preparation in order to determine the appropriate volume to inject. The iodine concentration in commercially available products can vary significantly. For example, Conray 400 has a concentration of 400 mg iodine/mL, whereas Conray 60 has a concentration of 282 mg iodine/mL.

The contrast should be administered through a peripheral intravenous catheter as a bolus over several seconds. We recommend a short, large bore intravenous catheter. For larger patients to whom a large volume of contrast is administered, the authors recommend the placement of two intravenous catheters for simultaneous injection of the contrast divided between two syringes. Contrast, especially the ionic preparations, is very viscous and injection can be relatively slow.

Radiographic views and filming sequence

In our practice, we use the following protocol: VD view immediately and at 5, 20, and 40 minutes; right lateral view at 5, 20, and 40 minutes. In cases of poor concentration ability or ureteral obstruction, VD and right lateral views made at 90 and 120 minutes may add useful information. In patients with suspected ectopic ureters, we obtain oblique views of the distal ureters and bladder at 10 minutes as well as at 20 minutes. It is important to include the entire perineal region to assess for vaginal pooling or perineal staining. If available, these patients are also imaged using digital fluoroscopy. In incontinent patients, we also recommend obtaining a postvoiding lateral view after the 40 minute time point. This allows for evaluation of complete emptying of the bladder and for detection of pooling of contrast in the vagina. Some authors recommend the routine use of abdominal compression during the initial portion of the study to block the ureters, interfere with ureteral peristalsis, and distend the collecting renal collecting system to improve filling and visualization for a more accurate assessment of these structures (Kneller 1974; Carrig and Mostosky 1976; Ackerman 1974; Biery 1981). We do not recommend abdominal compression because of the variability that it produces and the lack of any proven efficacy to facilitate diagnosis.

Contrast cystourethrogram

The contrast cystourethrogram generally consists of a study of the bladder (cystogram) and of the urethra (urethrogram) combined together to provide useful information regarding the anatomic structures of the lower urinary tract. The procedure is simple, quick, relatively inexpensive, safe, and rewarding. A decision to perform cystourethrography can be driven by clinical signs (e.g., intermittent or chronic hematuria, dysuria, stranguria, pollakiuria, chronic/recurrent urinary tract infections, or suspected trauma/rupture of the lower urinary tract) or by radiographic abnormalities (e.g., abnormal position, shape, size, or opacity of the lower urinary tract; nonvisualization of the bladder, particularly in a trauma patient; or evaluation of caudal abdominal masses in the region of or adjacent to the bladder). Numerous protocols for the contrast cystogram and urethrogram have been previously described (Ticer et al. 1980; Park 1981; Johnston et al. 1982; Essman 2005; Park and Wrigley 2007; Pechman 2007). As stated above, the procedure has only infrequent complications, if performed properly. Poor catheterization techniques may lead to trauma, perforation, or infection (Johnston et al. 1982; Johnston et al. 1983). Catheters can become kinked or knotted (Park and Wrigley 2007). Bladder distention itself can increase the likelihood of iatrogenic infection (Barsanti et al. 1981). Macroscopic hematuria is a common complication seen in dogs and cats after cystourethrography (Barsanti et al. 1981; Johnston et al. 1982; Johnston et al. 1983). With overdistention, mural dissection of contrast or even bladder rupture may occur (Johnston et al. 1982; Johnston et al. 1983). The most significant complication reported is the development of an air embolism in dogs and cats during negative contrast administration (Ackerman et al. 1972; Zontine and Andrews 1978). This rare but fatal complication can generally be avoided by utilizing a more soluble negative contrast agent (e.g., carbon dioxide) in patients with visible hematuria.

A complete contrast cystourethrogram includes a negative cystogram (pneumocystogram), a double contrast cystogram, a positive contrast cystogram, and a positive contrast urethrogram. In certain circumstances (e.g., to distinguish a stricture from poor filling) it can be helpful to perform both a retrograde as well as an antegrade (or voiding) urethrogram. For most diagnostic procedures, a complete study should be obtained as we have noted that some lesions are only demonstrated on one of the portions of the procedure (and not always the expected portion). When the aim of the study is to determine position or integrity of the lower urinary tract, a complete study may not be necessary.

The pneumocystogram is a cheap and simple means to localize the bladder and may also have the ability to demonstrate some radiolucent stones or masses. The positive contrast cystogram is also an excellent means to demonstrate bladder position and can often demonstrate mural lesions; particularly ones that lead to focal nondistensible regions of the wall (e.g., wall fibrosis or infiltrative neoplasia). The positive contrast cystogram or urethrogram should always be chosen if the aim of the study is to demonstrate lack of integrity, as the demonstration of free air in the peritoneal cavity after a pneumocystogram can be challenging. For the best evaluation of the mucosa, wall thickness, and luminal filling defects, the double contrast cystogram is the study of choice.

The patient should be heavily sedated or anesthetized for the procedure. A urinary catheter is placed using aseptic technique. We prefer to use a balloon-tip catheter in dogs and a red rubber catheter in cats. As mentioned above, any urine samples should be obtained prior to the administration of contrast. The bladder is completely emptied prior to the start of the procedure.

Contrast media, dose, and route of administration

Any commercially available water-soluble ionic or nonionic iodinated contrast preparation can be used for the positive and double contrast portion of the bladder or urethral study. The concentration of the iodine solution should be approximately 20% (Park and Wrigley 2007) for the positive contrast cystogram. We generally use a concentration of approximately 150 mg iodine/mL. A relatively high concentration of iodine (200 mg iodine/mL) should be used for the puddle in the double contrast cystogram. An in vitro study showed that this concentration was the best for detection and enumeration for uroliths (Weichselbaum et al. 1999). Another in vitro study demonstrated the ability to differentiate the composition of various uroliths using different concentrations of iodine (Weichselbaum et al. 1998 [a and b]); however, we currently do not use this technique clinically. For urethrography a 10–15% solution of iodine is used (Ticer et al. 1980). Negative contrast agents include room air, oxygen, nitrous oxide, and carbon dioxide (ascending order of solubility in the blood). Carbon dioxide is

the safest agent to choose (and should always be used in patients with hematuria) as it is 20 times more soluble in blood than room air and has the least possibility of gas embolism. Although we have used room air in thousands of patients with no to little complication, our current standard operating procedure is to choose carbon dioxide as the negative contrast agent.

The volume of contrast to inject for the pneumocystogram and the positive contrast cystogram can be based upon the capacity of the bladder (10 mL/kg body weight [Park and Wrigley 2007]). However, a diseased bladder may have less distensibility, and therefore we base our administered volume on several factors: the amount of urine removed from the bladder at the beginning of the study, turgidity of the bladder upon palpation and any back pressure felt during injection. A radiograph can always be obtained to assess bladder distention. The aim is to have moderate bladder distention as complete or severe distention of the bladder may mask mild mucosal irregularities or mild increases in bladder wall thickness (Mahaffey et al. 1989).

For the double contrast cystogram, the bladder is first distended with negative contrast and then a small puddle of positive contrast is administered. The volume is dependent upon the size of the patient. One recommendation is 0.5–1.0 mL for a cat, 1.0–3.0 mL for a dog weighing less than 25 lb, and 3.0–6.0 mL for dogs weighing more than 25 lb (Park and Wrigley 2007). We recommend 0.75 mL for a cat or similar size dog, 1–2 mL for a small dog, 2–3 mL for a medium dog, and 3–4 mL for a large dog. It is important to make sure that administered contrast does not provide too deep a puddle, which may mask certain uroliths (Weischelbaum and Feeney 1998). After administration of the contrast puddle, the patient should be rotated in order to coat the entire mucosa.

The retrograde urethrogram can be performed with or without bladder distention. There may be fewer potential complications when performed without bladder distention (Barsanti et al. 1981); however, without moderate distention of the urinary bladder there may not be sufficient intraluminal pressure to ensure maximum distention of the proximal portion of the urethra (Johnston et al. 1982). The recommended volume is 10–15 mL in dogs and 5–10 mL in cats. Exposure should be made while the last couple milliliter are injected (Pechman 2007); and contrast should be injected with each subsequent view. No additional contrast is needed during a voiding urethrogram, although the bladder must contain positive contrast.

Radiographic views and filming sequence

In our practice, we perform the complete study in the following order: pneumocystogram, double contrast cystogram, positive contrast cystogram, positive contrast urethrogram. We generally perform both a retrograde and an antegrade (voiding) urethrogram. In general, obtain at least orthogonal views of each portion of the study. Ideally, right and left lateral and VD views (or right ventral-45° left dorsal oblique and left ventral-45° right dorsal oblique views) of the double contrast portion are obtained for more complete evaluation of the bladder mucosa and wall (Scrivani et al. 1997). In the male dog, a right ventral-45° left dorsal oblique view is obtained instead of a VD view to avoid superimposition of the proximal and distal urethra.

Vaginography

The vagina is usually amenable to direct palpation and visualization utilizing endoscopic equipment; however, at times, contrast imaging may be the only method of viewing the area cranial to the vestibule. Positive contrast vaginography is the retrograde filling of the vestibule and vagina. For discussion on the urinary tract, we find that vaginography can be useful to demonstrate morphology in the incontinent female dog if used as an adjunct to the cystourethrogram or excretory urogram. Positive contrast vaginography has been used to demonstrate various abnormalities of the vagina associated with lower urinary tract signs and disease such as vestibulovaginal stenosis (Kyles et al. 1996; Crawford and Adams 2002), vaginal septa (Root et al. 1995), and ectopic ureter (Levéillé and Atilola 1991). Several authors have described the protocol of contrast vaginography (Levéillé and Atilola 1991; Rivers and Johnston 1991; Root et al. 1995; Feeney and Johnston 2007).

Contrast media, dose, and route of administration

Any commercially available water-soluble ionic or non-ionic iodinated preparation can be used for the positive contrast vaginogram. We use a final concentration of 150 mg iodine/mL. Suggested doses range from 1 (Rivers and Johnston 1991) to 5 mL/kg body weight (Root et al. 1995). Contrast should be administered to fully distend the vaginal vault. If more contrast is administered beyond vaginal distention, a retrograde urethrogram will also be obtained. Contrast is administered through a balloon-tip catheter which is placed within the vestibule caudal to the urethral orifice. Often, the vulva must be clamped with atraumatic forceps in order to prevent contrast leakage during the procedure.

Radiographic views and filming sequence

Lateral and VD views should be obtained with the vagina and vestibule at maximal distention. Radiographs should be obtained at the end of injection.

Integrative overview

Considerations in urinary imaging

With the background issues discussed above given appropriate consideration, the next step is clinically applicable interpretive principles. First, urinary disease should be classified as one or more of the following: filtration failure (generalized low GFR, functional parenchymal loss) and/or inadequate post filtration processing (renal tubular dysfunction, destruction, or obstruction) (Thrall and Finco 1976; Barber and Finco 1979; Brace 1980; Caywood et al. 1980; Senior 1980; Feeney et al. 1982 [a and b], Feeney and Johnston 2007; Tarr and DiBartola 1985; Lulich et al. 1988; Neuwirth et al. 1993; Cuypers et al. 1997; Burk and Feeney 2003; Agut et al. 2004; Lyons et al. 2004; Zatelli and D'Ippolito 2004; Bryan et al. 2006; Westropp et al. 2006; Holloway and O'Brien 2007; Ross et al. 2007; Valdes-Martinez et al. 2007) (Figures 15.3–15.5) conduit failure (renal pelvic, ureteral, or urethral leakage or obstruction (Rose and Gillenwater 1974; Johnston et al. 1977; Faulkner et al. 1983; Klausner and Feeney 1983), storage failure (bladder leakage, dysmotility, outflow obstruction, capacity compromise [masses, uroliths, fibrosis, herniation]

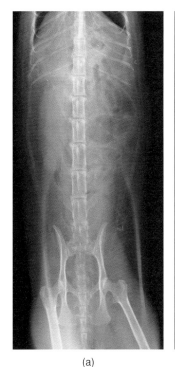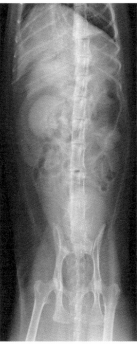
(a)   (b)

Figure 15.3 VD survey (a) and 5 minutes postinjection excretory urogram (b) views in which there is a urolith medial to the shrunken and irregular left kidney. There is a partial ureteral obstruction due to the urolith, defined to be in the proximal left ureter, but the left kidney is sufficiently small to be classified as end-stage. The right kidney and ureter are normal. Final diagnosis: end-stage left kidney with proximal left ureteral stone.

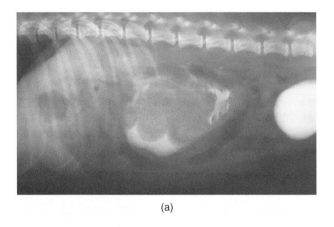

(a)

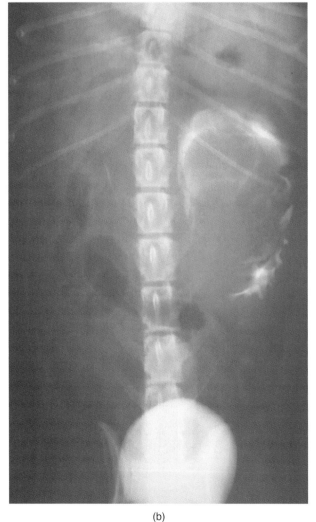

(b)

Figure 15.4 Lateral (a) and VD (b) views of an excretory urogram performed because of an enlarged left kidney. There is a mass which is surrounded by concentrated (pyelographic) contrast medium indicating that the mass arose in the left renal pelvis and created both a mass effect in and partial outflow obstruction therein. Final diagnosis: left renal pelvic tumor.

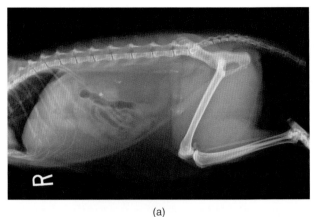

(a)

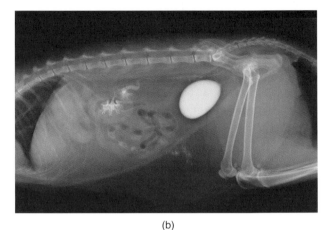

(b)

Figure 15.5 Lateral survey (a) and lateral (b) views of an excretory urogram performed to clarify the functional relevance of the retroperitoneal opacities in the cranial and caudal retroperitoneal space seen on the survey views. There is a high-grade partial obstruction of the left ureter at the level of the transverse plane of L4 and additional partial obstructive effect due to the "sand" in the left distal ureter. The right kidney and ureter are normal. Final diagnosis: urolith-induced left ureteral partial obstruction and hydronephrosis.

(Figures 15.6 and 15.7); urethral sphincter dysfunction) (Figure 15.8), single/multiple urinary organ inflammation/infection (pyelonephritis, cystitis, urethritis) (Figures 15.9 and 15.10), or congenital or heritable renal and ureteral diseases (Finco 1973; Johnston et al. 1977; Faulkner et al. 1983; Owen 1983; Hayes 1984; Davenport et al. 1986; Hager and Blevins 1986; Holt and Moore 1995; Lees 1996; Greco 2001; Lautzenhiser and Bjorling 2002; Eisele et al. 2005; Esterline et al. 2005; Hamilton et al. 2006). The intent of this classification is to encompass and define the diagnostic possibilities based on the distribution of the abnormality within the urinary tract.

It is imperative that the shortcomings of serum biochemical assessments, urinalysis (see Chapter 7), and

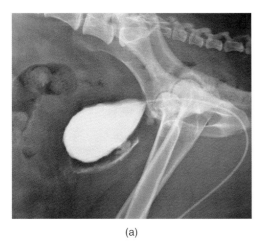
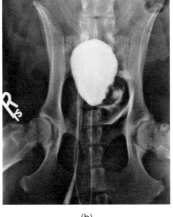
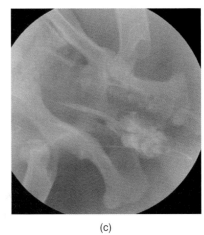

(a)   (b)   (c)

Figure 15.6 Right lateral (a) and VD (b) views of a positive contrast cystogram in a male dog presenting for painful abdomen one day after cystocentesis. Note the leakage of contrast from the left ventral bladder wall. VD view (c) of a positive contrast retrograde urethrogram in a male dog with retroperitoneal and perineal swelling after vehicular trauma. Note the leakage of contrast from the membranous urethra. A right coxofemoral luxation and sacral fracture are also present.

urine culture (see Chapter 9) be clearly understood due to the functional redundancy and common excretory pathways of the paired kidneys and ureters. Part of the role of imaging is to localize the disease recognized using clinical or laboratory techniques to one or both halves of the upper urinary tract versus the lower urinary tract. A further role for contrast radiographic imaging is to estimate the functional significance of clinical (incontinence) or survey radiographic (ureterolith) observations (Figure 15.5). A clear understanding of anatomic relationships is also important in the interpretation of urinary organ abnormalities like bladder trigone mass and ureteral obstruction, their distinction from genital organ abnormalities (i.e., urinary bladder distension versus prostatomegaly), and the regional manifestations of suspected urinary abnormalities such as peritoneal fluid

accumulation in urinary bladder rupture. Acknowledging that the kidneys, most of the ureteral length, as well as the distal membranous urethra are retroperitoneal, is paramount. The recognition of potential urinary tract organ roles in and the contrast radiographic assessment of body cavity fluid collections are based on this anatomic principle. The serial continuity of the urinary tract is also an important concept. In short, obstruction downstream affects everything upstream including not only the organ's size but also its function. In short, as urinary bladder pressure increases beyond some critical point, ureteral peristalsis becomes ineffective, renal pelvic pressure rises, glomerular filtration decreases and azotemia develops.

In addition to localizing a disease process to a region of the urinary tract, it is also important to characterize the

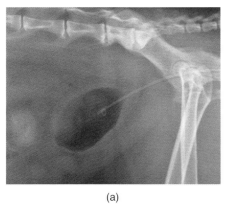
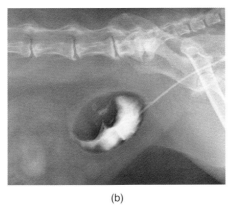
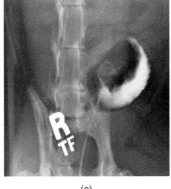

(a)   (b)   (c)

Figure 15.7 Right lateral pneumocystogram (a) and right lateral (b) and right ventro-left dorsal oblique (c) double contrast cystogram in a 13-year-old neutered male cat presenting for recurrent lower urinary tract signs. There is a large sessile mass arising from the right dorsal bladder wall seen as a soft tissue opacity on the pneumocystogram and a filling defect on the double contrast cystogram. Final diagnosis: bladder tumor, presumed transitional cell carcinoma.

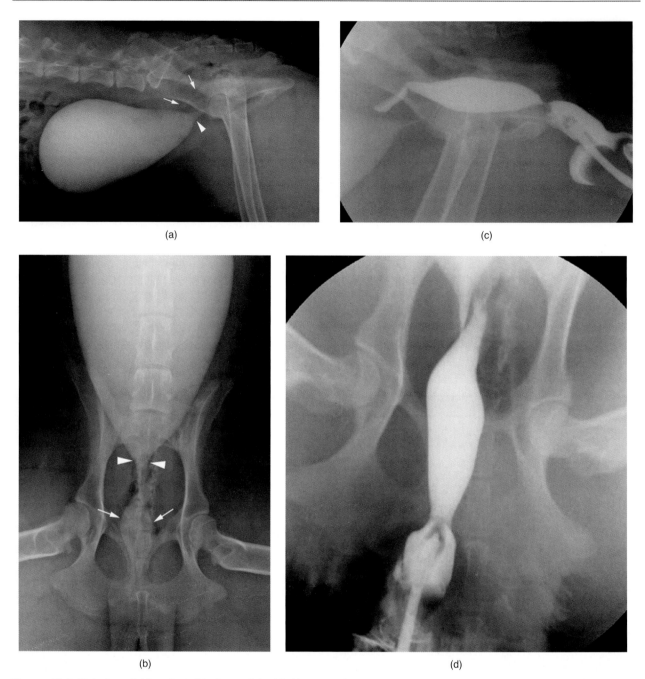

(a)

(c)

(b)

(d)

Figure 15.8 Right lateral (a) and VD (b) views of the bladder seen during excretory urography in a 1-year-old spayed female dog presenting for 6-month history of incontinence. The neck of the bladder is elongated with urine in the proximal urethra (arrowhead) demonstrating urethral sphincter incompetence. Additionally, contrast is pooling in the vagina (arrows). Right lateral (c) and VD (d) views of the vaginogram performed in the same patient. There is a severe stricture at the vestibulovaginal junction.

abnormality as originating outside the organ (e.g., uterine stump granuloma invading the urinary bladder or urinary bladder incarceration in a hernia), in the wall or parenchyma of the organ (e.g., tumor, hematoma, granuloma, fibrosis or stricture), or in the lumen of the organ (e.g., urolith, blood clot, matrix plug or foreign body). For the assessment of luminal lesions, the normal renal pelvic and ureteral width is usually less than 2–3 mm (Feeney et al. 1979, 1982). For common mural lesions, the urinary bladder wall thickness is usually approximately 1 mm (Mahaffey et al. 1984). Kidney measurements (most commonly, the length) are usually scaled according to the length of the second lumbar vertebral body (L2) (Barrett and Kneller 1972; Finco 1971; Feeney et al. 1979,

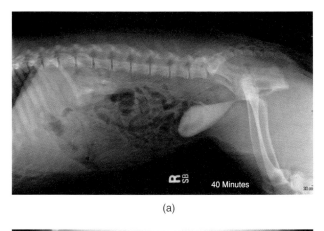

(a)

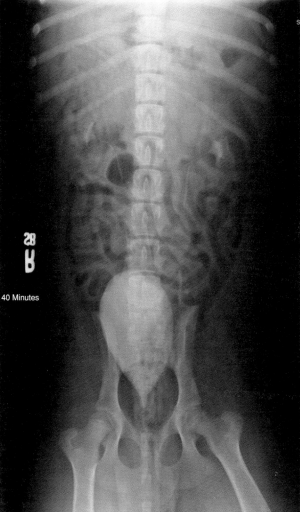

(b)

Figure 15.9 Lateral (a) and VD (b) views made 40 minutes after contrast medium for excretory urography in which a dilated left renal pelvis with a lack of proportional dilation of the left pelvic recesses can be seen. The right kidney is normal. Final diagnosis: chronic pyelonephritis, left kidney.

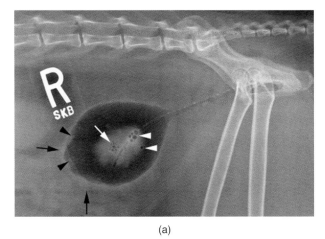

(a)

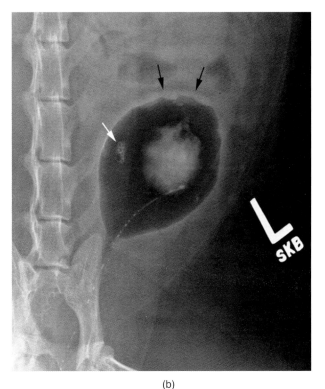

(b)

Figure 15.10 Right lateral (a) and right ventro-left dorsal oblique (b) double contrast cystogram in a 6-year-old neutered male cat presenting for multiple bouts of lower urinary tract obstruction. The study demonstrates multiple adhered calculi (white arrows) and irregular cranioventral bladder wall thickening (black arrows) with mucosal ulceration (black arrowheads) consistent with ulcerative cystitis. Air bubbles are also present as filling defects on the lateral view (white arrowheads).

1982 [a and b]; Shiroma et al. 1999). For dogs, the range is usually 2.5 to 3.5 L2 increments. For cats, the range is between 2 and 3 L2 increments with measurements between 2.1 and 2.4 L2 increments considered acceptable only in middle-aged to older neutered cats.

A consistent approach and a complete imaging dataset improves the odds of success in urinary tract radiographic imaging. In short, any and all urinary tract procedures should be preceded by survey radiographs of sufficient quality to assure that available information can be appropriately garnered. It is desirable to withhold food for 24 hours (but water ad lib) and to perform 1–2 cleansing enemas prior to searching for uroliths. While this is often not necessary because of the size and opacity of most uroliths, one cannot predict which patients will have small, minimally opaque uroliths (sand-like) that may be obscured by ingesta and fecal material. Clinical judgment has to be exercised regarding the benefit to urinary imaging garnered from the enema and the loss of baseline information for other body systems, particularly the alimentary tract due to the enema. In general, we recommend withholding food for alimentary imaging only because of the effects of enema on small bowel appearance. The goal here is to get the most out of the survey radiographs including any germane information about other parenchymal organs, the peritoneal and retroperitoneal spaces and the alimentary tract as well as the urinary and genital tracts. In addition, it is important to ensure that the entire urinary tract is covered by the survey radiographs. As mentioned above, this may require more than one lateral and or more than one VD view. Similarly, VD views are preferable to DV views, because the relative magnification of the kidneys compared to the L2 increments mentioned above were derived using VD not DV positions. The decision about patient sedation is based on a composite judgment including the need for restraint to assure diagnostic quality views and patient/handler safety, as well as the need to limit needless "re-take" views which contribute to patient and personnel exposure. These considerations must be balanced against the risk to the patient and the physiologic effects of the drugs on potentially relevant aspects of the imaging procedure (e.g., sphincter continence, blood pressure and GFR). In general, endoscopic procedures (see Chapter 19) are limited to intraluminal urinary bladder disease with visible mucosal abnormalities and then only in patients where the equipment is suitable for transurethral access and the operator skills exist to justify its consideration. By comparison, radiographic procedures, particularly positive contrast procedures, are superior for intraluminal, intramural, transmural and extramural disease characterization and are adequate for mucosal assessment.

It is also important to have perspective on the relationship between radiography-based urinary tract imaging and more costly and focused imaging techniques such as ultrasonographic (see Chapter 16), computed tomographic (CT), and magnetic resonance scans (see Chapter 17). In general, survey radiographs are a mainstay in urinary imaging because they are readily available, cost-effective, and provide a reasonable "overview" of the regional anatomy. For imaging relevant to qualitative assessment of renal function and urethral sphincter continence, the excretory urogram is the most practical and predictable. To visualize the distended urethral lumen, the urethrogram, by whichever method it is executed, (retrograde or voiding) is the most utilitarian approach. The ureters, bladder, and kidneys have broader applications among other imaging procedures. For example, if the specific focus is on the presence or absence of ectopic ureters, contrast-enhanced computed tomography is quite effective and may be more accurate than excretory urography (Rozear and Tidwell 2003; Samii et al. 2004). It is also more expensive and requires heavy sedation or general anesthesia. Ultrasound has a debatable role in the diagnosis of ectopic ureters. While a detailed search for the ureteral jets (urine ejected from the ureteral opening into the urinary bladder trigone) has been recommended in the diagnosis of ectopic ureters (Lamb and Gregory 1998), its applicability varies with the information sought. Failure to identify both ureteral jets may raise the suspicion of ectopic ureters (assuming both kidneys are present and functioning), but it does not determine where the ureteral termination is and whether there may be multiple terminations (e.g., bladder and urethra or vagina for the same ureter). We, therefore, prefer excretory urography as our first-line diagnostic technique in incontinent animals because it also provides information on urethral sphincter continence in unsedated patients. Deliberate decisions must be made on individual patients regarding the use of intravenously-administered, iodinated contrast medium and the radiation exposure for either CT or excretory urography. Some circumstances may favor ultrasonography. Similarly, if the specific focus is on the urinary bladder, both contrast cystography and ultrasonography provide useful information about the presence or absence of masses as well as cystoliths and on wall thickness. The advantage of the ultrasonographic procedure is that sedation is generally not necessary. However, if the urinary bladder is insufficiently distended, over-estimation of wall thickness and over or under-estimation of cystoliths and/or masses can result. With the contrast cystographic procedure, the degree of distension is under the control of the person overseeing the procedure. The caveat there is over-distension and subsequent rupture. This is particularly worrisome in postcystotomy or post-trauma patients.

The size and shape of a urinary organ can provide some insight about the underlying abnormality. Size (and to varying degrees the shape) of an organ or segment thereof is governed by several factors including muscle tone (particularly the ureters but to some degree the urinary bladder), downstream or outflow resistance (such as sphincter dysfunction, strictures or any obstruction), wall pliability (such as fibrosis or cellular infiltrates), wall thickness or parenchymal organ mass-effect (e.g., tumor, granuloma or abscess), upstream delivery of materials (glomerular and tubular function), and the influence of drugs on everything from renal function through sphincter continence. It is imperative that radiographic interpreters understand the interplay between the functional renal parenchyma and the upper as well as lower urinary collecting and storage systems. An increase in bladder or ureteral pressure can cause the renal pelvis to enlarge which will eventually influence kidney size. On the other hand, focal, multifocal or diffuse renal parenchymal processes will influence both the size and the shape of the kidney as well as its functional capacity to deliver urine to the collecting and storage systems.

Survey radiographs provide useful information regarding renal size and shape, but this translates to only a modicum of information about the underlying pathophysiology or pathoanatomy. It is then the purview of additional imaging procedures to provide further insight. The applicable radiographic procedure is the excretory urogram (nephrographic phase) (Feeney et al. 1982, Feeney and Johnston 2007; Burk and Feeney 2003). However, we prefer ultrasonography performed on multiple planes as a first-line diagnostic approach to problems creating renal size or shape abnormalities or for screening the kidneys for architecture or echotexture change that might explain renal dysfunction. The negative aspect of nephrographic imaging (opacification of the renal parenchyma during an excretory urogram) is that anything that creates a local-regional renal parenchymal architectural disruption (mass, infarct, cyst, abscess) will not opacify as will functional renal parenchyma (Burk and Feeney 2003; Feeney and Johnston 2007). This limits interpretive capacity to differentiate among these possibilities. For regional staging of renal masses (or any retroperitoneal mass), the excretory urogram is a distant second to ultrasonography, computed tomography, or magnetic resonance imaging. The decision regarding which of these procedures is applicable is based on both the judicious interpretation of the survey radiographs and the combination of cost and availability. From our perspective, ureteral and urethral size and status are best imaged using the excretory urogram and the positive contrast urethrogram, respectively. Keep in mind that ascending infection by some organisms limits ureteral peristaltic capacity and may cause mild ureteral dilation directly or compound the effects of partial downstream obstruction. Similarly, the degree of ureteral dilation identified must be considered as a composite result

of pressure, duration, infection, and autonomic function (e.g., dysautonomia) (Rose and Gillenwater 1974; Faulkner et al. 1983; Jakovljevic et al. 1998; Neuwirth et al. 1993; Burton et al. 1994; Reichle et al. 2003; Eisele et al. 2005). The urinary bladder is generally more accessible for ultrasound imaging. However, unless a definable etiology (e.g., trigone mass) is found, the bladder may be very large but not directly as a result of bladder disease and the specific problem is not sonographically apparent. Therefore, enlarged urinary bladder can be due to things outside the bladder including urethral obstruction, dysynergia, neurologic disease, and even behavioral problems. Some insight may be gained by examining regional structures such as disk spaces, retroperitoneal lymphadenopathy, prostatic size shape and opacity, regional bony reaction (vertebrae and pelvis), as well as the presumed course of the urethra (for suspicious opacities that might be urethroliths). Our first-line for all but the simplest urinary bladder-related case involves a sequence of survey radiographs (right lateral and VD), pneumocystogram, double contrast cystogram, positive contrast cystogram, and either voiding or retrograde positive contrast urethrogram. If there is visible hematuria, we use carbon dioxide as the negative contrast agent to limit the likelihood of fatal air embolism. Keep in mind that urethral diameter at imaging is a function of the bladder pressure upstream and the infusion pressure downstream (at the catheter, usually a balloon catheter). Our approach is to have the bladder palpably turgid to assure reasonable filling and then perform the urethrogram with radiographic exposures made during the retrograde injection on both the lateral and VD oblique views (Burk and Feeney 2003). This limits the need for equivocation regarding ill-defined narrowings or intraluminal filling defects in the urethra.

Variances in the intraluminal appearance of urinary tract organs are subdivided into those that are "free" (moveable with changes in body position) and those that are "attached" (not moveable with changes in body position) (Park 1981; Burk and Feeney 2003; Westropp et al. 2006). Attached filling defects range from mucosal irregularity due to cystitis, through inflammatory polyps to sessile mucosal/mural processes that are usually urothelial origin neoplasms. Blood clots can either be free or attached. In general, the more the mucosal irregularity and the more sessile appearing the filling defect, the more similar to urothelial-origin cancer. Biopsy is however mandatory to differentiate among the various causes of these problems (e.g., pyogranulomatous cystitis/urethritis versus transitional cell carcinoma). Uroliths on occasion are attached (embedded in mucosal reaction) but are usually free. Variances in recumbency during radiographic views facilitates differentiation of free versus attached intraluminal processes, particularly on double contrast cystography. The caveats are numerous, including the need for sufficient room to define mobility. For instance, a urolith in the renal pelvis, ureter, or urethra may not be mobile because it is lodged in a specific position. Other caveats include air bubbles (usually more smooth and symmetric than blood clots, tumor fragments, or uroliths) and blood clots (which can be irregular like tumors or uroliths and which can gravitate to the dependent position in a double contrast "puddle" like uroliths) (Feeney et al. 1982; Burk and Feeney 2003). Typically, surface tension promotes air bubble migration to the periphery of a contrast puddle whereas uroliths and blood clots fall to the deepest part of the puddle (usually the geographic center). The renal pelvic lumen shape is a relevant determinant of disease beyond the presence or absence of filling defects that may be disruptive (tumor) or obstructive (uroliths, urothelial-origin tumors). To keep it simple, when interpreting the pyelographic phase of the excretory urogram, the appearance of a mildly dilated intra-renal collecting system (renal pelvis and pelvic recesses) must be categorized as symmetrical (the pelvic recesses dilate proportionally with the pelvis) or asymmetrical (the pelvic recesses are shortened and blunted in a less than proportionate distension compared to the renal pelvis itself) dilation (Barber and Finco 1979; Burk and Feeney 2003; Feeney and Johnston 2007). The former is seen with physiologic diuresis and early hydronephrosis (Figure 15.5). The latter is seen with pyelonephritis (Figure 15.9). In our hands, this is more specific for the diagnosis of pyelonephritis than are ultrasonographic findings although a mildly dilated renal pelvis containing "complex" urine is a suspicious ultrasonographic finding, particularly when paired with a positive urine culture.

One of the major goals of an imaging study that involves uroliths (see Chapter 69), particularly cystoliths, is whether the uroliths found can be medically eliminated (struvite) or must be surgically eliminated (Osborne et al. 1996; Ross et al. 1999; Weichselbaum et al. 2001). In addition, in the case of asymptomatic uroliths, medical management to prevent enlargement may also be germane. Radiographic, but not ultrasonographic appearance coupled with consideration of age and breed predisposition can facilitate this differentiation (Clark 1966; Weaver 1970; Brown et al. 1977; Osborne et al. 1996, 1999; Thumchai et al. 1996; Ling et al. 1998 [a and b], 2003; Weichselbaum et al. 1998 [a and b], 2001; Lulich et al. 1999; Ross et al. 1999; Houston et al. 2004; Cannon et al. 2007). In general, canine urocystoliths > 10 mm in any dimension were over 90% likely to be struvite. Smooth, blunt-edged or faceted, and pyramidal canine urocystoliths were usually also struvite. Jackstone shapes were almost always silica. Botryoidal (grape-like clusters) urocystoliths were likely to be oxalates in dogs. The more opaque a stone is, the more likely it is a calcium-based, with oxalate being the most common. Breeds commonly afflicted with urocystoliths include: Bichon Frise, Dalmatian, English Bulldog, Miniature Schnauzer, Pekingese, Pug, Shih Tzu, Welsh Corgi, and West Highland Terrier. Details of the predominate types of uroliths seen in these breeds is beyond the scope of this chapter, but is available elsewhere. Over 90% of urocystoliths produced in female or spayed female dogs are struvite whereas males and neutered males had a greater assortment but with a relatively high frequency of oxalate uroliths. In addition, younger dogs are more commonly afflicted with struvite (females), urate (males), or cystine (males) than with the other stone types. By comparison, overall, oxalate uroliths are slightly more common in cats than struvite, but the odds slightly favor oxalate in males and struvite in females. The exceptions to this are the penile matrix plugs which are predominately struvite.

Iodinated contrast media are used to promote identification of urinary tract problems. They are usually administered via intravenous injection for excretory urography and retrograde catheterization for urethrocystography or vaginography. There are several germane considerations regarding contrast medium use and misuse. First, for an excretory urogram to be diagnostic, there must be sufficient renal function to filter and concentrate the contrast medium from the blood. Second, the concentration of iodinated contrast medium used for retrograde studies can have an effective atomic number (Z_{eff}) similar to that of specific uroliths rendering them invisible (Weichselbaum et al. 1998 [a and b]). In general, uroliths isopaque in contrast medium solutions approximating 23.5 mgI_2/mL are most likely ammonium urate or sodium urate. Uroliths isopaque in contrast medium solutions between 23.5 mgI_2/mL and 44.4 mgI_2/mL are probably magnesium ammonium phosphate, cystine, or silica. Uroliths isopaque in solutions approximating 80 mgI_2/mL almost always contain calcium (most commonly either calcium oxalate monohydrate or dihydrate). Third, intravenous or intra-arterial iodinated contrast medium should not be administered to dehydrated patients, patients with a history of previous contrast medium reactions or patients with suspected serum or urine protein disorders that might result in renal tubular dysfunction or obstruction including diabetes-induced renal dysfunction (Feeney et al. 1980b; Katzberg et al. 1986; Ihle and Kostolich 1991; Briguori and Marenzi 2006; Mehran et al. 2006; Benko et al. 2007). Fourth, iodinated contrast medium by virtue of its osmolarity and biochemical structure can influence assessments of urine concentrating capacity, urine sediment cytology, and urine culture results (Hurt 1960; Narins and Chase 1971; Constantinou et al. 1974; Barry et al. 1978; McClennan et al. 1978; Feeney et al. 1980; Fischer et al. 1982; Ruby et al. 1983; Smith et al. 1983; Dawson and Howell 1985; Shanahan et al. 1985; Andriole et al. 1989; Sewell 1996). This is usually more profound with the ionic than nonionic contrast media, but it is still best to complete such assessments either before or at least 48 hours after contrast medium administration.

Although there are numerous personalized approaches to radiographic interpretation of any body system, the urinary tract is well suited to a common sense check list in addition to the usual Roentgen Sign approach (e.g., size, shape, location, surface characteristics [margination], opacity, and function) (Burk and Feeney 2003; Feeney and Johnston 2007). We suggest the following questions be considered to avoid over or under-interpretation. Are there unexpected or disproportionate regions of urinary organ enlargement? Can the enlargement be specifically differentiated from genital or even alimentary organ enlargement? Are there unexplained persistent opacities that do not move with time (as would be expected with opacities in the alimentary tract)? Is the material that might be causing the distension radiographically opaque (i.e., dystrophic tumor mineralization, some foreign bodies and uroliths) and is it of sufficient size and in the appropriate location (e.g., punctate retroperitoneal opacities that may be ureteroliths) to create the presumed obstruction? Is there any evidence of segmental or regional luminal distortion/dilation or wall rigidity? Is the serosal contrast good or bad in the area of the possible urinary organ abnormality? Is there a mass in the area of the urinary organ and, if so, is the urinary organ displaced by, invaded by, or potentially the source of the mass? Is there any free fluid in the peritoneal or retroperitoneal cavities? Is the etiology of the urinary problem obvious? If not, what type of cost-effective and predictable procedures ranging from vaginoscopy through contrast urinary procedures, are necessary for clarification?

To facilitate the interpretation of urinary imaging techniques, the authors advocate two approaches. The first is the gamut approach (Reeder and Felson 1975) in which the radiographic signs are listed and specific thought is given to what pathophysiologic or pathoanatomic causes could be associated with those findings. The findings are then ranked in descending order of likelihood based on risk modifiers including clinical history, age, gender (and in the case of animals, species and breed). To foster defining the possible gamuts, another approach referred to by the acronym DAMNIT, which is basically a list of pathologic conditions that can be used to trigger possible etiologies or diagnoses, is helpful. These include

degenerative/developmental, anomalous, metabolic, nutritional/neoplastic, infectious (bacterial, fungal, viral)/infesting (parasitic)/inflammatory/immune-mediated, and toxic/teratogenic. Judicious use of these options limits the likelihood of a diagnosis being missed because that etiologic possibility was not included in the gamuts.

Kidneys and upper ureter

Functional morphology

The excretory urogram (EU) has had different names including intravenous pyelogram (IVP) and intravenous urogram (IVU). The procedure was used in human urologic imaging before veterinary imaging so much of what happened in veterinary medicine relied on the human experience and then generally adopted the human terminology. There have been differing philosophies regarding the use of this procedure including using intravenously-administered, iodinated contrast medium to outline the upper urinary collecting system (pyelogram) without regard to imaging the functional parenchyma (nephrogram). This procedure was referred to as the IVP. As contrast media became less toxic and doses (in $mgI_2/\#$ of body weight) were increased to improve the quality (radiopacity) of the study, the opacification of the nephrogram became an integral part of the study (IVU). The underlying need for adequate renal function balanced against the need for even higher doses of iodinated contrast medium became a decision point regarding the applicability of the procedure in patients with significant renal compromise. This led to the gradual adoption of the term excretory urogram in veterinary medicine. Simply, it was a constant reminder that this was a physiologic excretory procedure that depended on both glomerular filtration and tubular concentration to produce interpretable results.

In its current status, the EU is both a functional assessment as well as a morphologic procedure (Feeney et al. 1979, 1982 [a and b], 2007; Burk and Feeney 2003). The morphologic aspects are the geometry of the renal parenchyma (nephrographic morphology) and the upper urinary collecting system (pyelographic morphology) which includes the renal pelvis, the renal pelvic recesses, and the ureter. The functional aspects, although only qualitative, include the degree and chronology of overall nephrographic opacification and the degree of the pyelographic opacification. The underlying physiology of the EU is a sequence of events that includes the availability of filterable iodinated agents in the blood (plasma concentration of the radiocontrast agent) → the timely filtration of the iodinated products from the blood (glomerular filtration rate) → the concentration of the filtered iodinated agent in the renal tubular system (tubular concentration) → excretion of the concentrated iodinated agent into a low-resistance reservoir (renal pelvis) → continuous evacuation of that reservoir by ureteral activity resulting in delivery of the concentrated iodinated agent to the urinary bladder. The diagnostic quality as well as the interpretation of the radiographic findings rely on the effective and orderly nature of each of these processes (Barber and Finco 1979; Feeney et al. 1982a, 2007; Burk and Feeney 2003). For interpretive purposes, the nephrogram has two phases. First is the vascular nephrogram which is basically a "blush" of opacity in the kidney due to the effect of the unfiltered iodinated agent in the renal parenchymal vessels (basically a nonselective angiogram). The second phase is the parenchymal nephrogram which is the opacification of the kidney from the filtered and partially concentrated iodinated agent in the renal tubules (dominated by the proximal convoluted tubule). The early nephrogram (usually 30–60 seconds after intravenous administration of the iodinated agent) therefore may have a modestly more cortical than medullary opacity, but this rapidly fades to an even opacity if everything is normal. The normal nephrogram is most opaque shortly after intravenous injection and progressively fades to the same comparative opacity as seen on survey radiography over the ensuing 30–90 minutes depending on the dose of contrast administered and the renal functional capacity (Feeney et al. 1979, 1982 [a and b]). The pyelogram does not have specific phases, but it does have a varying appearance of its components. The first component to opacify is the renal pelvis (usually 2–3 minutes after intravenous contrast medium administration) followed almost immediately by the opacification of the ureter. The normal ureter is an actively peristaltic structure which literally "milks" the renal pelvis. Therefore, the normal ureter is visualized in chronologically varying linear segments instead of just a tube connecting the renal pelvis with the urinary bladder. The renal pelvic recesses are basically extensions of the renal pelvis around the interlobar renal vessels. These recesses (which have been called diverticula in earlier literature) are embryologic remnants of the multiple segments of paired renal papillae and calices which were precursors to the current canine and feline fused renal papillae referred to as the renal crest. The exit of concentrated iodinated agent from the renal collecting system occurs along the edge of the renal crest and not into the recesses. The recesses now simply serve as a buffer between the delivery rate of urine to the pelvis from the nephrons and the evacuation rate of the urine from the pelvis by the ureter. How well and when the recesses can be recognized in dogs depends on the dose of iodinated agent, the renal func-

tion, the ureteral peristaltic capacity, and the resistance encountered at the distal end of the ureter. Therefore, in normal dogs and cats, renal pelvic recess opacity is usually limited to seeing predictably spaced, paired thin pillars of opacity extending away from the renal pelvis into the renal medulla. These pillars are normally thinner than the renal pelvis and can extend to almost the cortiomedullary junction. The nonopacified linear structures between the paired recesses are the interlobar vessels. In the normal dog, the pelvis recesses are best visualized in the later phases of the EU (e.g., 20–40 minutes after intravenous injection). In the normal cat, they are readily visualized almost simultaneously with the renal pelvic opacification.

Practical radiographic observations

The interpretation of the renal and proximal ureteral status is fostered by the integration of the sequential physiologic processes outlined above and the knowledge of the pathologic possibilities defined using the DAMNIT system mentioned earlier. In short, anything that interferes with delivery of the iodinated agent to the kidney can affect the onset (delayed is abnormal), duration (prolonged is abnormal), opacification sequence (normal initial peak opacity followed by gradual return to survey radiographic opacity), and general opacity (minimally opacified is abnormal) of nephrographic opacification. Influential factors include the plasma concentration of the iodinated agent (proportional to dose and intravenous [versus perivascular extravasation] delivery rate), the glomerular filtration rate, the tubular concentrating activity (can be affected by hydration), and the uninhibited delivery into the renal pelvis (can be affected by renal pelvic pressure from downstream resistance or obstruction). The visualization of the renal parenchymal opacification depends on functional renal parenchyma being present in the region of interest. Therefore, not only is the overall opacity of the kidney affected by regional physiologic factors, the intra-renal opacity can vary depending on factors such as segmental vascular occlusion (parenchymal infarct) or any space-occupying entity that does not contain functional nephrons (e.g., cysts, tumors or abscesses). Because the renal pelvis (including the pelvic recesses) is an intermediate, low-resistance reservoir between the renal parenchyma and the ureter, it is also influenced by renal physiologic capacity to excrete the iodinated agent (pelvic opacity), the ureteral capacity to evacuate it, and regional, intraluminal, mural, and extraluminal space-occupying entities (e.g., stones, masses, scarring, parenchymal pressure) (Figures 15.4 and 15.5). The third component of the upper urinary tract is the ureter. The ureteral appearance

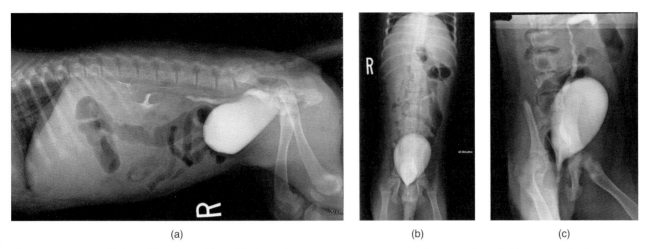

(a)   (b)   (c)

Figure 15.11 Lateral (a), VD (b), and VD oblique (c) views of an excretory urogram exposed at approximately 40 minutes after intravenous injection of sterile iodinated contrast medium. There is a dilated left ureter with a distal termination just beyond the urinary bladder trigone. The left renal pelvis is dilated with blunted pelvic recesses indicating pyelonephritis. Final diagnosis: left ectopic ureter with left pyelonephritis.

is influenced by the rate of delivery of urine to the pelvis (iodinated contrast media have varying degrees of osmotic diuretic activity), the ureteral peristaltic capacity (affected by toxins from some bacteria), the status of the ureteral mural and luminal segments (e.g., regional fibrosis, stones, masses), the ureteral integrity (leaks), and the resistance created by the ureteral termination site (Figure 15.11). The latter is normally the urinary bladder trigone which can be affected by bladder stones, regional tumors, surgical intervention, and trauma. In the case of ectopic ureters, there may be both increased resistance and a higher probability of ascending infection depending on where the ureter actually ends (e.g., urethra, vagina, urethra, etc.).

Spectrum of disease

The process of interpretation of survey radiographic and excretory urographic techniques must be dominated by the inter-relationships of the upper urinary organs. The process that affects renal parenchyma may also affect the renal pelvis downstream and renal blood flow upstream. Interpretation must incorporate general renal physiology including the physiology of iodinated contrast agents, the radiographic findings (defined by the geometric Roentgen signs) and the age, gender, species, and breed-associated risk factors for upper urinary tract disease. Like any interpretive exercise, things are made simpler if broken down into understandable components. There are many goals of the EU, including to differentiate reversible from irreversible renal or ureteral disease as well as to determine if surgical intervention versus medical management is appropriate. For the EU, these are first the nephrographic morphology including

specifically kidney size, shape, and uniformity of nephrographic opacity (Feeney et al. 1979, 1982, 2007). This combination of morphologic descriptors encompasses most renal parenchymal abnormalities. At one end of the spectrum are compensatory hypertrophy and infiltrative renal disease (including amyloidosis, glomerulonephritis, and round cell neoplasia) which appear as normal to large smooth kidneys with uniform but varying quality of nephrographic opacity. In the middle of the spectrum are the focal or multifocal renal masses including primary or metastatic tumors (Figure 15.4), the focal or multifocal renal abscesses or cysts, and the dilated renal pelvis which appear as normal to large irregularly shaped kidneys with nonuniform nephrographic opacity. The distribution of the variations in nephrographic opacity provide clues as to which of these possibilities are more likely e.g., geographically central or hilar loss of nephrographic opacity and be associated with hydronephrosis. At the other end of the spectrum are the chronic (inflammatory or circulatory disease) (Figure 15.3) and the breed-associated dysplastic renal diseases. Next are the overall sequences of nephrographic opacification and fade-out (Feeney et al. 1982). Circulatory and glomerular diseases tend (on a basis relative to normal expectations) to slow the onset of peak opacity and delay the return to survey radiographically equivalent opacity. By comparison, acute toxic processes including acute contrast-induced renal disease and acute tubular necrosis tend to have a prompt peak, but a persistence of the increased opacity beyond that is normally expected. Finally, conditions that compromise overall renal function (e.g., glomerulonephritis, end-stage kidney) tend to have poor but prompt nephrographic opacity with slow fading. Obstructive disease has a spectrum of nephrographic opacification wherein acute obstructions may have fair and prompt opacification nephrographic with delayed fading while chronic obstructions may have very delayed (hours or even next day) and poor nephrographic opacity, if they opacify at all. Readers are directed elsewhere for more details (Barber and Finco 1979; Feeney et al. 1982, 2007; Burk and Feeney 2003).

As mentioned above, the integrated nature of the parenchymal (nephrographic) with the collecting and transport (pyelographic) aspects must influence EU interpretation. For example, a ureteral obstruction will influence the nephrographic opacity (hilar opacity void ↔ thin rim of residual opacity), the nephrographic opacification timing, and the appearance of the pyelogram. As for the nephrographic morphology, the interpretation of pyelographic abnormalities are focused on size, shape, and uniformity of pyelographic opacity (Thrall and Finco 1976; Barber and Finco 1979; Burk

and Feeney 2003, Feeney and Johnston 2007). This combination of morphologic descriptors encompass most renal collecting system abnormalities. At one end of the spectrum is the diffuse dilatory disease (usually renal pelvic or ureteral obstruction leading to hydronephrosis) in which the renal pelvis and pelvic recesses are dilated proportionally. Depending on the severity, the overall renal size may also be enlarged, but usually smooth. In the middle of the spectrum is pyelonephritis in which the renal pelvis is mildly dilated and somewhat irregular (chronic), but the pelvic recesses are blunted and distorted (Figure 15.9). At the far end of the spectrum are "filling defects" that involve the renal pelvic and/or ureteral lumina and either displace or obstruct the flow of the iodine-laden urine. These include stones (Figures 15.5 and 15.12), strictures, and regionally invasive masses (including those extending from the kidney as well as the occasional mass that originates from

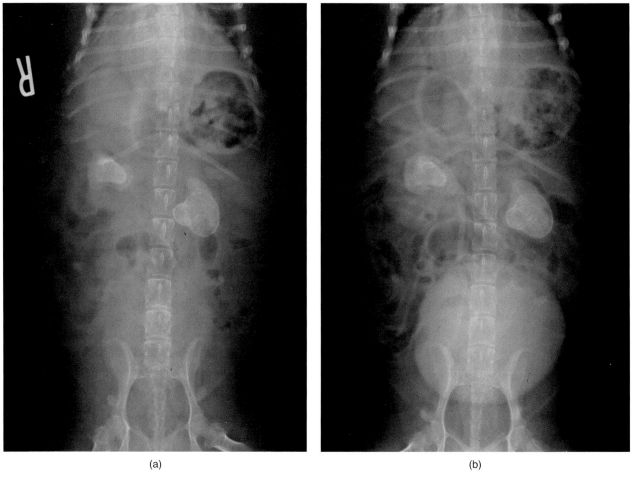

(a)   (b)

Figure 15.12 VD survey (a) and VD (b) views of an excretory urogram performed to clarify the presence of functional renal parenchyma (nephrogram) and the degree of obstruction (pyelogram) as a result of the laminated bilateral renal pelvic stones. There is limited opacification of any renal parenchyma around the left renal stone, but reasonable parenchymal opacification around the right renal stone. Neither renal pelvic is dilated beyond the confines of the intrapelvic stone. Final diagnosis: bilateral renal pelvic stones with negligible pelvic outflow obstruction but limited residual functional renal parenchyma on the left.

the renal pelvic or ureteral epithelium) (Figure 15.4). The distribution of the variations in pyelographic opacity provide clues as to which of these possibilities are more likely (e.g., geographically central voids in pyelographic opacity can be associated with hydronephrosis whereas eccentric filling defects may indicate tumor). Pyelographic opacity sequences are simpler than nephrographic opacity sequences (Thrall and Finco 1976; Barber and Finco 1979; Burk and Feeney 2003; Feeney and Johnston 2007). Basically, poor renal function (from any cause in the sequence of events defined earlier) yields poor or even absent pyelographic opacification. Partial downstream obstructions can cause delayed pyelographic opacification while complete downstream obstructions effectively block urine flow so no urine containing the iodinated agent can get to the pelvis. In general, if there is poor nephrographic opacity, there will also be poor pyelographic opacity. Pyelographic opacity is a function of both the dose of iodinated agent administered intravenously coupled with the filtration and concentration capacity of the renal parenchyma. Poor pyelographic opacity can be seen with a normal nephrogram in polyuric states. However, usually poor pyelographic opacity implies poor, often irreversible renal concentrating capacity.

Distal ureter and ureterovesical junction

Functional Morphology

The underlying renal physiology that contributes to the opacification of the ureter has been described above. In this part of the discussion we will focus on the ureter as an entity including its role as an effective conduit for urine from the renal pelvis to the urinary bladder. The ureter is an urothelial-lined, muscular tube capable of rhythmic longitudinally-directed peristalsis (from the kidney toward the bladder). This peristalsis can increase in frequency as a response to dilation which in the physiologic sense is increased urine volume delivery from the kidney (diuretic effect). Because of its peristaltic capacity, there are segments of the normal ureter that are not visible at any segment in time. Therefore, visualization of a continuously opacified ureter from the renal pelvis to the urinary bladder should not be expected and usually indicates some abnormality (Feeney et al. 1979, 1982a). Normally, both ureters terminate in the dorsal aspect of the urinary bladder just proximal to the urethral outflow tract. Because of the three conduits entering/exiting the urinary bladder at this region, it is referred to as the bladder trigone. Ureteral termination is morphologically characterized as a linear dissection through the various bladder layers. This is the basis of the antire-

flux mechanism that limits or prevents urine from the bladder going back up the ureter. As the intravesicle pressure increases, the intramural portion of the distal ureter near the trigone collapses essentially forming a one-way valve that only allows urine to flow toward the bladder and then primarily as a result of ureteral peristalsis. There are times during canine adolescence that this antireflux mechanism is rendered somewhat ineffective predisposing them to ascending infection (Goulden 1968; Christie 1971; Lenaghan 1972 [a and b]; Klausner and Feeney 1983). Vesicoureteral reflux can result in retrograde flow of urine up the ureter during voiding (requires a specific but impractical radiographic procedure) but can also be induced (presumed to be artifactual not specifically pathologic) by manual bladder compression to the point of voiding (Klausner and Feeney 1983).

Practical radiographic observations and spectrum of disease

Ureteral and ureterovesical abnormalities can be identified and characterized relatively simply (Rose and Gillenwater 1974; Johnston et al. 1977; Faulkner et al. 1983; Owen 1983; Hayes 1984; Hager and Blevins 1986; Moroff et al. 1991; Burton et al. 1994; Holt and Moore 1995; Jakovljevic et al. 1998; Lautzenhiser and Bjorling 2002; Moores et al. 2002; Weisse et al. 2002; Burk and Feeney 2003; Reichle et al. 2003; Samii et al. 2004; Worth and Tomlin 2004; Eisele et al. 2005; Esterline et al. 2005; Kyles et al. 2005; Hamilton et al. 2006; Feeney and Johnston 2007). First, mild diffuse ureteral dilation is usually associated with ascending infection (look for renal pelvic signs of pyelonephritis) or partial obstruction at the ureteral termination (look for ectopic ureter or small trigone-related abnormalities [stones, tumors]). Second, severe diffuse ureteral dilation is usually associated with near complete obstruction at the ureteral termination (look for large trigone-related abnormalities [stones, tumors, severe ectopic ureters]). Keep in mind that a chronic and complete ureteral obstruction will not allow urine laden with the iodinated agent to flow into the ureter (may not opacify because of already being filled with stagnant urine). On occasion, delayed opacification (hours to next day) may occur. Third, segmental ureteral dilation is usually a function of some downstream narrowing (stricture, entrapment/ligation) or obstruction (stone, tumor polyp) (Figure 15.5). If urine can flow, the ureter will dilate proximal to the site of the problem. Segmental ureteral dilation without specific obstruction can be due to developmental anomalies such as ureterocele which is a dilation of the intramural portion of the ureter in the urinary bladder wall at the trigone region.

This can present as either a bladder outflow problem or an incontinence problem depending upon its effect on the proximal urethral sphincter mechanism (as well as any possibly associated developmental urethral sphincter abnormalities). Fourth, anomalous ureteral termination (aka. ectopic ureter) (Figure 15.11) can present a number of abnormalities including dilated ureter, termination of the ureter at some point other than the bladder trigone (i.e., vagina, urethra, uterus), opacification of urogenital structures distal to the urethral sphincter without actively voiding (e.g., vaginal opacification), and dilation and distortion of the renal pelvis and pelvic recesses typical of pyelonephritis (Figure 15.9). Finally, the ureter must not leak. Ureteral leaks are usually not spontaneous, instead, are due to endogenous (stone) or exogenous (blunt external trauma or surgical disruption) causes. The primary suspicion for ureteral (or the very rare renal pelvic) leak is the presence of retroperitoneal fluid on a survey radiograph. As both a pelvic urethral leak and a ureteral leak can cause the accumulation of retroperitoneal fluid, clinical judgments must be made about the choice of procedure (urethrogram or excretory urogram). A decision is usually facilitated by the circumstances surrounding the patient, such as fractured pelvis increasing the likelihood of urethral trauma. As the ureter is not normally visualized in its entirety from the renal pelvis to the bladder trigone, sequential radiographic (or optimally fluoroscopic) assessment is necessary to check for both the repeated absence of a segment of the opacified ureter as well as the insidious increase in regional retroperitoneal opacity created by the leaking of urine laden with the iodinated agent (Figure 15.13).

Urinary bladder

Anatomic considerations and functional morphology

The bladder is a hollow, distensible, musculomembranous organ which varies in form, size, and position, depending upon the amount of urine it contains. In general, the bladder lies along the ventral body wall in the caudal abdomen or within the ventral aspect of the pelvic canal. The bladder is arbitrarily divided into the vertex (apex), the body and the neck, which connects with the urethra. The trigone is a triangular region near the bladder neck where the apex of the trigone is at the urethral orifice and the base is indicated by a line connecting the ureteral openings (Evans and Christensen 1993). The mucosa of the bladder consists of transitional epithelium containing folds when the bladder is empty but these mucosal folds disappear with distention. The bladder is held loosely in place by three ligaments (middle bladder ligament and two lateral bladder ligaments) which are formed by peritoneal reflections (Evans and Christensen 1993). Because of the loose ligaments, the bladder can be easily displaced to the left or the right by adjacent bowel or other structures. The majority of the bladder is a peritoneal structure; the bladder neck and urethra are retroperitoneal. The significance of this is that a caudal bladder or urethral tear will result in retroperitoneal effusion.

The bladder, along with the urethra, functions as a reservoir for urine and as a conduit and excretory organ for urine expulsion (Park 1981). It must be noted that it is inappropriate to evaluate bladder function based solely upon bladder size, as the degree of distention

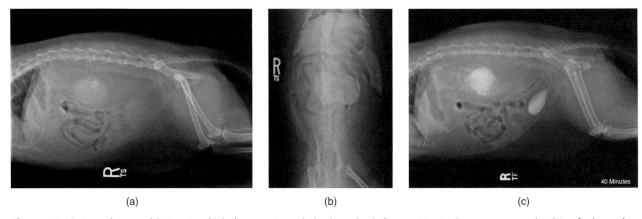

(a)   (b)   (c)

Figure 15.13 Lateral survey (a) view in which there are irregularly-shaped calcific opacities in the common renal pelvis of a horseshoe kidney and some loss of retroperitoneal clarity around the kidney. Immediate postinjection VD (b) and 40 minutes lateral (c) excretory urographic views in which the fused kidney parenchymal regions are defined and the leakage of concentrated contrast medium around the kidney can be seen (primarily on the lateral view) indicative of renal pelvic or proximal ureteral leakage. Final diagnosis: horseshoe kidney with presumed pelvic urolith-related proximal pyelographic leak.

often reflects when the patient last had an opportunity to void; however, when the patient history is correlated to the bladder size, some functional information can be gleaned from the radiograph (e.g., a distended bladder in a patient straining to urinate suggests obstruction) (Burk and Feeney 2003).

Practical radiographic observations and spectrum of disease

The bladder is a well-defined, uniformly soft tissue structure within the caudal abdomen and varies in size depending upon the amount of urine it contains. The shape of the bladder in the dog is usually oval to teardrop, but becomes more ellipsoid with distention; whereas the feline bladder is almost always ellipsoid (Park and Wrigley 2007). Cranially, the apex is blunt, the body is rounded, and the neck is long and gradually tapering in the female dog and cats, but shorter and more abruptly tapering in male dogs (Burk and Feeney 2003). In the dog, the bladder is generally located immediately cranial to the pubis in the female and immediately cranial to the pubis and prostate in the male. In the cat, the bladder is generally more cranial (2–3 cm) to the pubis than in the dog (Park 1981) (Figures 15.1 and 15.2). When the bladder is completely empty it may be partially or wholly located in the pelvic canal. The bladder is easily identifiable because of the adjacent omental and peritoneal fat; but visualization may be compromised by insufficient abdominal fat, inadequate bladder distention, or superimposed opacities (e.g., small intestines, colon, peritoneal effusion) (Park and Wrigley 2007).

Survey views are generally limited for evaluation of bladder diseases. Interpretation should include evaluation for the Roentgen signs of opacity, size, shape, position, margination, and number. Any change in opacity is abnormal and generally easy to detect. The bladder should be evaluated for mineralization, which is most commonly due to uroliths, but may be due to dystrophic mineralization of the wall or of a tumor. Generally, uroliths are dependent and will be within the central portion of the bladder on recumbent orthogonal views; however, uroliths may be adherent and thus in an unexpected location. Mineral in unexpected locations (e.g., at the bladder neck or trigone) should raise the index of suspicion for a neoplastic or chronic inflammatory condition with dystrophic mineralization. Radiolucencies in the bladder are due to gas (iatrogenic from catheterization/cystocentesis or pathologic from emphysematous cystitis). Gas in the lumen will appear as a smooth, round lucency in the center of the bladder shadow; whereas gas in the wall will be linear following the wall contour or will

be multiple coalescing bubbles in the wall (Park 1981). Additionally, one must differentiate changes in bladder opacity from overlying opacities (e.g., colon, small intestine, nipples, prepuce, fur debris), which may necessitate additional views, compression views, or special procedures. As previously mentioned, bladder size is very dependent upon when the patient last voided, and the clinical signs must be correlated to the radiographic findings or other diagnostics methods to determine clinical significance. If the bladder extends cranial to the umbilicus, this is likely pathologic and may be due to congenital defects, lower urinary tract obstruction (due to neoplasia, uroliths, blood clots or stricture), neurologic disease, or trauma (to the spine or pelvis) (Park 1981). A small bladder is generally normal but may be secondary to rupture, disease leading to lack of distensibility, or lack of urine formation. An alteration in bladder shape is rarely seen and can be normal (caused by extraluminal pressure of adjacent structures) or may be abnormal (e.g., patent urachus, urachal diverticulum, loss of tone, bladder spasm, bladder trauma, infiltrating neoplasm) (Park 1981; Burk and Feeney 2003). Displacement of the bladder generally indicates pathology in adjacent structures. Cranial displacement is caused by prostatomegaly, uteromegaly, or pelvic mass. Ventral displacements can be caused by colonic or rectal diseases, uteromegaly, lymphadenopathy, retroperitoneal masses, or inguinal hernia. Caudal displacements can be caused by abdominal masses, perineal hernias, or congenital defects (e.g., short urethra or ectopic ureter) (Park 1981).

The various cystographic special procedures will elucidate much more information regarding the bladder. When evaluating the cystogram, one must pay careful attention to shape, location, and integrity; thickness and regularity of the wall and mucosa; and presence or absence of luminal material. It can also be helpful to classify abnormalities as mucosal, mural, filling defects and contrast projections from the normal confines of the bladder. Shape is generally best defined with the positive contrast cystogram; although alterations in shape can also be seen on the other portions of the study. The bladder should fill uniformly and have a regular shape; abnormalities may include focal areas of rigidity/nondistensibility (e.g., neoplastic or inflammatory infiltrate) (Figure 15.14), regions of contrast projecting outside the normal limit but still confined within the urinary tract (e.g., persistent urachal remnant or urachal or other diverticulum), or extramural compressions on the bladder from adjacent structures (these will be even more apparent with incomplete bladder distention).

Bladder wall changes (mural lesions) and mucosal changes are the most common cystographic abnormality

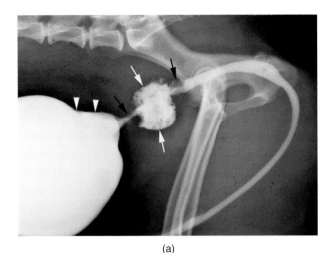

(a)

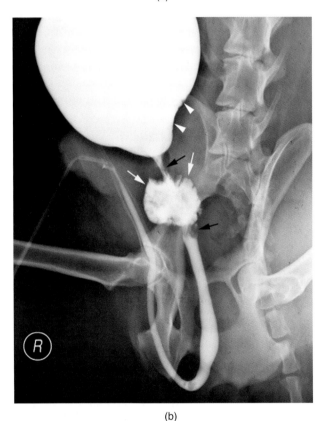

(b)

Figure 15.14 Right lateral (a) and left ventro-right dorsal oblique (b) retrograde cystourethrogram views in a 13-year-old neutered male dog unable to urinate. The study demonstrates mural lesions in the urethra (black arrows) and bladder trigone (white arrowheads) secondary to transitional cell carcinoma. In addition, abnormal retrograde filling of the prostatic ducts is seen secondary to prostatic involvement (white arrows).

and are best demonstrated with the double contrast cystogram. The bladder wall thickness is approximately 1 mm regardless of distention (Mahaffey et al. 1984) and the wall and mucosa should be smooth. The location and appearance of the lesion can provide distinguishing criteria for various diseases but final diagnosis requires cytology or histopathology (Burk and Feeney 2003). Cystitis generally causes thickening and irregularity in the cranioventral portion of the bladder (Figure 15.10); and although the entire circumference may be thick and irregular secondary to chronic inflammation, a diffuse neoplastic process may also have this appearance. Polypoid cystitis is a rare inflammatory disease which has multiple smooth polypoid or pedunculated masses generally arising from a thickened cranioventral bladder wall and projecting into the lumen (Martinez et al. 2003). Neoplastic infiltrate is generally focal and commonly presents as sessile masses projecting into the lumen on both the positive contrast and double contrast cystogram (Figure 15.7). Mucosal ulceration is recognized as regions of mucosa with clumps of adherent contrast (Park 1981) and can be seen with chronic cystitis, polypoid cystitis, and neoplasia (more severe with epithelial neoplasia than with mesenchymal neoplasia) (Figure 15.10). Trauma to the wall can result in contrast projecting outside the normal limit but still contained within the urinary tract (mural dissection of contrast) or contrast extravasation into the peritoneal or occasionally the retroperitoneal space (bladder wall rupture) (Figure 15.6). Filling defects are caused by anything in the lumen which alters the normal contrast filling pattern on positive contrast or double contrast cystography; and it is important to observe size, shape, number, contour, position, and attachment (Park 1981). Free luminal filling defects will remain in the contrast puddle with positional changes. Air bubbles will show as smooth, round filling defects at the periphery of the puddle (Figure 15.10). Uroliths are generally small and irregular and remain in the most dependent portion of the puddle, unless adhered to the bladder wall (Figure 15.10). Blood clots may be round, wedge-shaped, or irregularly shaped filling defects with smooth distinct borders, generally larger than most uroliths, and remain in the most dependent portion of the puddle (Burk and Feeney 2003). Mucus causes thin, linear filling defects. Cellular debris presents as small, amorphous filling defects. Foreign bodies (such as pellets, fragments of catheters, or migrating plant awns) are rare. Adhered luminal filling defects will only be demonstrated with specific positions, although contrast will often cling to the lesion and still be visible outside the contrast puddle. For differentiation, assess the shape, size, number, contour, base and associated wall, and mucosa. Neoplasia generally has a broad base with an irregular mucosal surface, while polyps generally have a narrow stalk and a smooth mucosal surface (Figure 15.7). Other adhered filling defects include uroliths, blood clots, and wall hematomas.

Interpretation of the bladder is simplified through the use of Roentgen sign description in combination with the DAMNIT scheme and gamut approach. This thought process should foster a logical approach to evaluation of the study and the generation of a list of possible diagnoses that is not inappropriately narrowed to two or three conditions. The clinical presentation of the case will aid in inclusion and exclusion of the list of likely possibilities. As previously stated, disease can be categorized into storage failure (i.e., bladder leakage, dysmotility, or outflow obstruction) or capacity compromise (namely, masses, uroliths, fibrosis, and herniation). Refining the classification to characterize it as extramural (regional masses or herniation), mural (inflammatory [cystitis, polypoid cystitis, emphysematous cystitis], neoplastic, fibrotic, trauma/tear, atony, or diverticula) or intraluminal (uroliths, blood clots, cellular debris, air bubbles, or foreign bodies) is useful not only for narrowing the list of possible/likely diagnoses but also for determining what diagnostic or therapeutic approaches should be considered next.

Urethra

Anatomic considerations and functional morphology

The urethra is a hollow organ which connects the urinary bladder to the outside environment. It serves as a conduit for urine and a sphincter. The male urethra in the dog consists of the prostatic, the membranous, and the penile urethra. The prostatic portion passes through the prostate gland and is made up of various longitudinal mucosal folds; the dorsally located urethral crest does not obliterate when distended (Evans and Christensen 1993). The male urethra in the cat consists of the membranous and the penile urethra. The membranous urethra ends at approximately the caudal aspect of the ischium in both the dog and cat (Pechman 2007). The female urethra corresponds to that portion of the male urethra that lies cranial to the prostatic utricle (Evans and Christensen 1993). The female urethra enters the genital tract just caudal to the vaginovestibular junction. The vagina is a dilatable canal, limited cranially by the fornix just ventral and cranial to the cervix, and terminating just cranial to the urethral opening. Longitudinal folds allow for great expansion in diameter (Evans and Christensen 1993). The vestibule is the space connecting the vagina with the external genital opening and is the common opening for both the urinary and the genital tracts.

Practical radiographic observations and spectrum of disease

The normal urethra is not radiographically visible in either species. Survey radiography is generally limited for evaluation of urethral diseases with the exception of radiopaque calculi. Radiopaque calculi may be located anywhere along the urethra but are most commonly lodged at the ischial arch, base of the os penis in the male dog, urethral papilla in the female dog, and distal penile urethra in the male cat (Burk and Feeney 2003). Rarely, is a distended or irregularly shaped proximal urethra evident on survey views (urethral obstruction or neoplastic infiltrate). Regional tissues should be evaluated for evidence of trauma (retroperitoneal effusion) or neoplasia (medial iliac lymphadenopathy or lytic/proliferative vertebral or pelvic lesions).

The normal vagina is not visible on survey radiographs. Unless quite large, lesions affecting the vagina will not be seen on survey views.

The urethrogram is instrumental in defining urethral disease. During evaluation, pay careful attention to shape, location, and integrity; thickness and regularity of the wall and mucosa; and presence or absence of luminal material. As with the bladder, it can be helpful to classify abnormalities as mucosal, mural, filling defects, and contrast projections from the normal confines of the urethra. In male dogs, the normal urethral width varies depending upon the degree of bladder distention and volume and pressure of injection; the male urethra may be uniform except for slight narrowing at the pelvic brim, bladder neck, and ischial arch or may be nonuniform with a wider prostatic portion (Burk and Feeney 2003). A dorsal filling defect within the prostatic portion of the urethra may be at the level of the colliculus seminalis. With adequate intravesicular pressure, the normal male cat urethra has a continuous and uniformly smooth luminal surface with some variation in the normal urethral luminal diameter; the maximum diameter of the penile urethra occurs at the level of the ischiatic arch, after which the diameter becomes progressively smaller toward the external urethral orifice (Johnston et al. 1982). The urethra of the female dog and cat is short and wide with tapering toward the external sphincter; the diameter varies depending upon bladder fullness and volume and pressure of injection (Burk and Feeney 2003). Urethral wall lesions include mucosal irregularity (neoplasia, granulomatous urethritis) and rupture (traumatic [including iatrogenic], tearing by calculi) (Figures 15.6c and 15.14). Urethral narrowing can be caused by periurethral fibrosis from trauma, rupture, surgery, or inflammation. This should be documented on two views or on two contrast injections to rule-out urethral spasm (Burk and Feeney

2003). Filling defects are common. Calculi tend to be irregularly shaped and may distort the urethral lumen if large; they will generally not move in position with contrast injection. Air bubbles are usually smooth and round or oval and will not distend the urethral lumen; they will generally move in position with contrast injection. Neoplasia can cause a filling defect; careful inspection will demonstrate a lesion arising from the wall with a broad base. Increased urethral diameter may be due to chronic obstruction or congenital lesions. Another condition described in female dogs which may lead to incontinence and pelvic bladder is a congenital short urethra.

The distended vagina and vestibule should be uniform with smooth mucosal margins. There is generally a mild narrowing at the vestibulovaginal junction (Rivers and Johnston 1991). When the vagina is distended sufficiently, contrast will reflux into the urethra. Vaginal wall lesions include mucosal irregularity (e.g., inflammation and neoplasia) and narrowing (i.e., vaginal stricture, inflammation, or neoplasia) (Figure 15.8). Filling defects include vaginal septum, persistent hymen, and vaginal masses. Vaginography cannot differentiate between inflammatory and neoplastic conditions. Contrast extending beyond the confines of the normal vagina may be due to rupture (such as after traumatic breeding), rectovaginal fistula, or ectopic ureter.

Interpretation of urethral lesions is also simplified through the use of Roentgen sign description in combination with the DAMNIT scheme and gamut approach. This thought process should foster a logical approach to evaluation of the study and the generation of a list of possible diagnoses that it not inappropriately narrowed to too few of conditions. The clinical presentation of the case will aid in inclusion and exclusion of the list of likely possibilities. As previously mentioned, urethral disease can be categorized as conduit failure (urethral leakage or obstruction), outflow obstruction (due calculi, neoplasia, granulomatous urethritis or stricture), or urethral sphincter dysfunction (incontinence, reflex dysnergia or upper motor neuron). Refining the classification to characterize it as extramural (regional masses), mural (inflammatory, neoplastic, fibrotic, trauma/tear) or intraluminal (calculi, blood clots or air bubbles) is useful not only for narrowing the list of possible/likely diagnoses but also for determining what diagnostic or therapeutic approaches should be next considered.

Integrated approach to urinary tract syndromes

Hematuria

The definition of hematuria is blood in the urine. When approaching a patient presenting for hematuria, it is important to rule out nonurinary tract causes (such as thrombocytopenia and coagulopathy) and to determine that the reported color change of the urine is truly blood in the urine and not other causes (such as myoglobinuria, bilirubinuria, false hematuria [redness of urine due to food or drugs containing pigment]). The role of imaging is to define potential urinary morphologic abnormalities leading to the hematuria. This covers a broad spectrum of disorders including cystitis/urethritis/vaginitis, prostatic disease (benign prostatic hypertrophy, prostatitis, neoplasia), feline lower urinary tract syndrome, uroliths anywhere in the upper or lower urinary tract, neoplasia anywhere in the upper or lower urinary tract, or essential renal hematuria. The correlation of hematuria and voiding may be helpful to locate the source of the hematuria (Park 1981). Hematuria at the initiation of voiding is usually localized to the urethra; hematuria during the terminal portion of voiding is potentially related to the prostate, prostatic urethra, or trigone; and hematuria present throughout the voiding process is localized to either the bladder or the upper urinary tract. Initial work-up of the patient presenting for hematuria should include a physical examination (including rectal palpation), urinalysis, serum chemistry analysis (e.g., to evaluate for liver disease), and complete blood cell count (particularly to evaluate for thrombocytopenia and anemia). If the patient is young, the initial work-up may include only a physical examination and urinalysis. If the urinalysis reveals infection, treatment with repeat urinalysis at the end of treatment would be appropriate. If the patient is older, and the urinalysis doesn't reveal a cause for the hematuria or if the hematuria is chronic, diagnostic imaging is recommended.

The initial radiographic procedure in investigation of hematuria is the survey radiograph looking for mineral opacities such as calculi or dystrophic mineralization (particularly concerning in the prostate or in an abnormal location in the bladder for carcinoma) as well as enlarged or abnormally shaped urogenital organs and regional lymphadenopathy. Depending upon the survey radiographic findings (as well as the history, physical examination, serum biochemical, hematologic, and urinalysis data) and correlation with the clinical presentation a decision about excretory urography, cystourethrography or ultrasonography can be made. In our practice, the next likely diagnostic step would be ultrasonography to evaluate both the upper urinary and lower urinary tract (including prostate), unless the hematuria has been localized to the urethra (in which case retrograde urethrography should be pursued). Ultrasonography is useful for detecting parenchymal abnormalities of the kidneys and prostate, nephroliths, mural lesions of the bladder (e.g., cystitis, inflammatory polyps and neoplasia) and intraluminal lesions of the bladder (such as calculi and blood clots). It is important to remember that sonography will not adequately evaluate the entire urethra, ureters, or vagina. If the ultrasound examination is negative, one must consider a retrograde urethrogram in order to completely evaluate the lower urinary tract.

The choice of imaging procedure is important to assure that the disease is predictably detected (sensitivity) and that the disease that is not present is confidently excluded (specificity). In light of the fiscal realities of many clients, consideration must also be given to procedural costs. As there is no single imaging procedure that will confidently evaluate the entire urinary tract, it is important to thoroughly evaluate all pertinent available information, as well as weigh the pros and cons of each procedure (cost, risk, availability) before taking the next diagnostic step.

Dysuria

Dysuria is painful or difficult urination. This sign should localize the lesion to the lower urinary tract. The role of imaging is to define any morphologic abnormalities leading to dysuria. This covers a broad spectrum of disorders including inflammatory (e.g., interstitial cystitis, feline lower urinary tract disease, and granulomatous urethritis), infectious (e.g., cystitis, urethritis, prostatitis, vaginitis), uroliths anywhere in the lower urinary tract, neoplasia anywhere in or adjacent to the lower urinary tract, or structural abnormalities of the urethra (such as fibrosis and stricture). Initial work-up of the patient should include physical examination (including rectal palpation) and urinalysis. If the urinalysis does not reveal a potential cause for the dysuria, or if the signs are not consistent with simple infection, diagnostic imaging is recommended.

As with other signs referable to the urogenital tract, survey radiography is the mainstay of initial investigation. The survey radiographs are evaluated for mineral opacities such as calculi or dystrophic mineralization (particularly concerning in the prostate or in an abnormal location in the bladder for carcinoma) as well as enlarged or abnormally shaped urogenital organs and regional lymphadenopathy. Urine retention or a distended bladder is particularly suggestive of outflow obstruction. Depending upon the survey radiographic findings (as well as the history, physical examination, serum biochemical, hematologic, and urinalysis data) and correlation with the clinical presentation a decision about cystourethrography or ultrasonography can be made. Ultrasonography can be utilized to evaluate parenchymal changes of the prostate, mural lesions of the bladder (cystitis, inflammatory polyps, neoplasia) and intraluminal lesions (calculi). As previously mentioned, sonography will not adequately evaluate the entire urethra. If the ultrasound examination is negative, a retrograde urethrogram is essential to completely evaluate the lower urinary tract. One consideration would be an imaging package that includes a positive contrast retrograde urethrogram followed by ultrasonography of the bladder (and prostate). As always, the determination of the choice of imaging procedure must take into consideration all pertinent available patient information, as well as weigh the relative pros and cons of each procedure (namely, cost, risk, availability and technical expertise).

Polyuria

Polyuria is the passage of a large volume of urine in a given period. The first step when confronted with the history of polyuria is to confirm. It is suggested to have the client collect a urine sample in the home environment to exclude the possibility of water being withheld prior to the trip to the veterinarian; the truly polyuric patient will almost always have urine specific gravity <1.012 (Feldman 2005). Next, it is important to rule out nonurinary tract causes (e.g., diabetes mellitus, hyperadrenocorticism, hypercalcemia, pyometra, hepatic insufficiency, iatrogenic, and rarely psychogenic polydipsia or central diabetes insipidus) before determining the appropriate diagnostic approach to urinary causes of polyuria. The role of imaging is to define potential urinary morphologic abnormalities leading to polyuria. This covers a broad spectrum of disorders including numerous causes of acute or chronic renal failure, pyelonephritis, glomerular diseases, and rarely nephrogenic diabetes insipidus. Initial work-up should include a physical examination, urinalysis (to confirm polyuria), serum chemistry analysis (to include renal causes and exclude nonrenal causes), and complete blood cell count (to help distinguish infection and differentiate acute from chronic renal disease). Once polyuria is confirmed and nonurinary tract causes are ruled out, further investigation of the urinary tract can be undertaken.

The mainstay for evaluation of polyuria is the survey radiographic examination to evaluate size, shape, margination, and opacity of the kidneys. Of particular importance is that if the kidneys are shrunken and irregular shaped (chronic diseases including chronic pyelonephritis or renal dysplasia) or large and regularly or irregularly shaped (acute disease including acute pyelonephritis or glomerulonephritis). Also evaluate for renal mineralization which can be seen with a variety of diseases having associated polyuria. Depending upon the survey radiographic findings (as well as the history, physical examination, serum biochemical, hematologic, and urinalysis data) and correlation with the clinical presentation a decision about excretory urography or ultrasonography, if indicated at all, can be made. While ultrasonography can be helpful in evaluating renal parenchymal abnormalities and can guide fine needle or core biopsy sampling of the renal parenchyma or pelvis (generally needed for definitive diagnosis of renal causes of polyuria), it must be remembered that ultrasonography will provide limited information regarding renal function. We recommend excretory urography if the goal of the study is to determine qualitive renal function or assess for pyelonephritis. In cases where survey radiographs reveal enlarged kidneys, our first recommendation would be ultrasonography, which can be useful to distinguish between infiltrative diseases (e.g., neoplasia, FIP), polycystic kidney disease, perirenal pseudocysts, acute pyelonephritis, and hydronephrosis, as well as guide sampling. A word must be said regarding the diagnostic work-up of chronic kidney disease. Imaging beyond the survey radiographs is likely of limited value unless assessing for chronic pyelonephritis (recommend excretory urogram), comorbid conditions (urinary tract infection, urolithiasis, urinary obstruction) or qualitative renal function (excretory urogram), or presented with a patient having an acute crisis superimposed over chronic kidney disease.

The choice of imaging procedure, if at all, is important in cases of polyuria. One must consider the goals of the study, the cost of the procedures, the risk to the patient, the availability (including technical expertise) of the procedure, and the information that can be garnered from the procedure. For example, if the goal of the procedure is to obtain biopsy samples, ultrasound is the procedure of choice; whereas if the goal of the procedure is to evaluate for chronic pyelonephritis, we recommend an excretory urogram. Unfortunately, in cases of polyuria, imaging procedures may provide limited information as to the underlying cause and the client must be made aware of this fact before proceeding.

Recurrent Infection

Recurrent urinary tract infection usually implies the presence of some morphologic predisposition, a nidus of infection that is not completely cleared, a condition of immuno-incompetence, or some metabolic or pharmacologic effect that fosters organism growth. The role of imaging, usually radiographic, is to define potential morphologic problems or potential sources of recurrent urinary tract infections (Barber and Finco 1979; Burk and Feeney 2003; Agut et al. 2004; Feeney and Johnston 2007). This covers a broad spectrum of disease including tumors anywhere in the upper or lower urinary tract, uroliths anywhere in the upper or lower urinary tract, upper or lower urinary tract anomalies (most commonly

ectopic ureter), "dead space" (herniated, retroflexed, or atonic bladder, urethral strictures, bladder or urethral diverticula), lower male genital tract conditions including prostatitis, abscesses or tumors, and female genital tract conditions including uterine stump granulomas, vaginal anomalies (most commonly strictures), recurrent vaginitis, and vaginal tumors. The clinical findings of urethral or vaginal discharge, dysuria, paraspinal pain, incontinence, azotemia, polakyuria, abdominal wall, or perineal distortion (hernias) may provide insight into the initial choice of imaging procedure.

The radiographic mainstay of urinary tract infection investigations are survey radiographs looking for opacities such as stones or dystrophic mineralization (particularly worrisome in the prostate for carcinoma) as well as enlarged, obviously shrunken or distorted urogenital organs and regional lymphadenopathy. Depending on the survey radiographic findings (as well as the history, physical examination, serum biochemical, hematologic, and urinalysis data) and their comparison with the clinical presentation, a decision can be made whether excretory urography, retrograde urethrocystography, or ultrasonography should be the next approach. A word about ultrasonography is in order here even though it is addressed in another segment of this text. Ultrasonography is a noninvasive tool to characterize parenchymal lesions, particularly the kidney and the prostate gland. It has been reported as a potential tool for investigation of ectopic ureters (Lamb and Gregory 1998), but in our hands it lacks sufficient predictability and characterization to be acceptable. It has the advantage of not requiring sedation (cystography does require it) or the use of systemic iodinated agents (excretory urography does require them). However, it provides little functional information other than the potential for identification of residual urine after voiding. It has a role in the assessment of bladder masses and bladder wall thickening due to cystitis, but is not applicable for urethral, ureteral, or vaginal investigations. Our approach is that if the most likely clinical problem is something that can be confidently identified and adequately characterized by ultrasound, we use it. Otherwise, we recommend excretory urography (useful for identification of pyelonephritis, small or lucent upper urinary tract stones or ectopic ureter, qualitative characterization of relative renal and ureteral function and integrity, physiologic [no drugs or lower urinary catheters] assessment of urethral sphincter-based incontinence and the identification of postvoiding vaginal urine pooling [which can be mistaken for sphincter incontinence)], retrograde urethrocystography (useful for morphologic identification of lower urinary tract stones not detected by survey radiography, characterization of bladder or urethral wall or luminal abnormalities including polyps, foreign bodies and neoplasms as well as any bladder, prostatic, or urethral diverticula or communicating cavitations), or retrograde vaginography (useful for characterization of vaginal stricture and other anomalies, staging of vaginal tumors [if computed tomographic or magnetic resonance are unavailable], and occasionally for odd ectopic ureter assessment).

The choice of imaging procedure is important to ansure that disease that is present is predictably detected (sensitivity) and that disease that is not present is confidently excluded (specificity). These considerations must be combined with procedural costs, procedural risks (e.g., systemic contrast media administration and chemical restraint), and the timely availability of nonradiographic imaging instrumentation (e.g., computed tomography, ultrasonography, magnetic resonance imaging). These criteria influence our decisions particularly in the first choice of ultrasonography versus contrast radiography. We do not operate on the assumption that if nothing is found in an ultrasound the client can automatically afford additional procedures and we do not assume that because an ultrasound was done and nothing was found that this always constitutes due diligence.

Uroliths

Survey radiography is the imaging mainstay for urolith assessment. Implied in this assessment is the combination of finding the stone, predicting the predominant mineral type (aids in determining dietary management and surgical considerations), and assessing the physiologic relevance of the stone (e.g., present but not obstructing, potentially obstructive, obviously obstructive) particularly in the renal pelvis, ureter, and urethra. In complicated cases wherein the stones may be small or radiolucent, upper or lower urinary tract contrast procedures may be indicated, if the identification of the urolith and/or the assessment of its effects on urine flow will influence the management plan. The role of ultrasound for urolith detection is only one of detection and not characterization (Weichselbaum et al. 2001). Therefore, only in specific circumstances is it indicated and then only for the kidney or urinary bladder. Excretory urography is the procedure of choice to find survey radiographically occult upper urinary tract stones and to determine the physiologic effect of a renal or ureteral stone unless there is a high probability of near complete obstruction wherein ultrasonography is adequate. On occasion, we use ultrasound-guided positive contrast pyelography wherein iodinated contrast agent is injected directly into the renal pelvis and followed with radiographs to see if the iodinated agent can pass the suspected obstruction (usually an ureterolith seen on survey radiography coupled

with ipsilateral renal pelvic dilation at ultrasonography) (Rivers et al. 1997). Double contrast cystography followed by positive contrast urethrography is the sequence of choice to identify and characterize survey radiographically occult lower urinary tract stones.

So far, we have addressed the considerations for urolith detection and assessment of the regional physiologic effects. The other aspect of radiographic evaluation is the prediction of predominant mineral type (Weichselbaum et al. 1998 [a and b], 2001). While urolith radiographic appearance is not always correlated with mineral composition, this assessment is complementary to both the available urolith occurrence data and the characterization of the crystals in the urine sediment. Under the considerations in the Urinary Imaging section earlier in this chapter, some information was presented on the comparison between the concentration of the iodinated radiographic agent and the perceived relative opacity (including the potential for obscuring) uroliths. Using dilutions of ≥ 100 mgI$_2$/mL for retrograde double contrast cystography or positive contrast urethrography, procedures are unlikely to obscure stones because it will almost always be more opaque than even the calcium-based stones. One should, however, be cautious not to have the depth of contrast medium over 5–6 mm because it can overwhelm and obscure small stones. The use of the mgI$_2$ per milliliter in contrast solutions as a diagnostic tool to predict urolith mineral type is not practical. The use of surface characteristics (particularly faceted, randomly irregular, or speculated [jackstone]), size, and relative opacity have some clinical utility in the assessment of predominate mineral type particularly in bladder and urethral stones. In general, the combination of species, breed risk, gender, age, and radiographic appearance can provide clinically relevant information to facilitate the decision to manage the patient medically (antibiotics and/or diet) and recheck versus prompt surgical intervention (to remove stones that won't dissolve or pass) (Clark 1966; Weaver 1970; Brown et al. 1977; Osborne et al. 1996, 1999; Thumchai et al. 1996; Ling et al. 1998 [a and b], 2003; Weichselbaum et al. 1998 [a and b], 2001; Lulich et al. 1999; Ross et al. 1999; Houston et al. 2004; Cannon et al. 2007). Female dogs are more likely to have struvite stones; male dogs are more likely to have oxalate stones. Cats follow a similar, but less predictable trend. Overall trends in stone occurrence in both dogs and cats are somewhat dynamic and this change is presumably unintended consequence of dietary formulation and genetic selection for phenotypic characteristics that are further complicated by hereditary breed predispositions. Across both dogs and cats, uroliths that approach or exceed the opacity of the ilial shaft are more likely to be calcium-based with oxalate being the predominate mineral type. Readers faced with this decision are referred to other chapters in this text as well as these references (Weichselbaum et al. 1998 [a and b], 2001).

Incontinence

Urinary incontinence is a multifaceted condition (Banks et al. 1991; Silverman and Long 2000; Burk and Feeney 2003; Feeney and Johnston 2007). It can be due to hormonal deficiencies, it can be due to morphologic abnormalities of the lower urogenital tract and it can be due to neurophysiologic abnormalities of the urethral sphincter. In our opinion, hormonal deficiencies should be ruled out first because they can be approached, at least initially, with therapeutic trials instead of expensive imaging procedures. Assuming that the hormonal etiology was either unlikely or the intervention was ineffective, imaging procedures become very germane. The next questions to be answered before choosing an imaging procedure are whether the apparent incontinence is accompanied by dysuria or hematuria and what are the relative likelihoods of a morphologic anomaly (e.g., ectopic ureter), sphincter-based incontinence, chronic infection, or bladder/urethral/prostatic tumor as the basis for the problem? If there is any question about the role of the lower female genital tract (e.g., anomaly, vaginal pooling, or tumor), a detailed vaginoscopic examination is indicated before an imaging decision is made. The goal here would be to identify vaginal anomalies that might predispose to vaginal pooling (e.g., stricture) and which might be associated with other lower urinary abnormalities (e.g., ectopic ureter, sphincter-based incontinence, or tumor invasion).

While the specific and complete diagnosis may not be made without imaging (including vaginography or even computed tomography) at least some assessment of risk and likelihood of successful outcome can be made. If there is no evidence of dysuria, hematuria, or pollakiuria, the intravenous excretory urogram is probably the best first imaging choice because of its capability to detect sphincter incontinence based on the absence of other abnormalities and the elongated appearance of the dysfunctional urethra (Figure 15.8a,b). The expectation is that iodine-laden urine will show up in places where it should not (outside the kidney, ureter, and bladder) during the procedure to constitute a morphologic diagnosis of the underlying etiology. The excretory urogram physiologically fills the bladder and there should not be distal leakage in a normal bitch or dog (Feeney et al. 1979, 1982, 2007; Burk and Feeney 2003). In female dogs, we use an additional technique which is to prevent the bitch from urinating during the 40 minute EU procedure. Once the bladder is full, spontaneous void-

ing is encouraged and followed immediately with survey radiographs. This facilitates the assessment of vaginal pooling as the cause of presumed incontinence and initiates the discussion of surgical vaginal alteration. If there is evidence of dysuria, hematuria, or pollakiuria, the retrograde contrast cystourethrogram is probably the best choice because of its capability to detect abnormal bladder position (retroflexed bladder, herniated bladder and, pelvic bladder [all pelvic bladders are not directly associated with incontinence, however]), urethral and/or bladder tumors. In addition, this technique enables the identification of both the compression and/or distortion effects of prostatic disease (most likely carcinoma, but possibly abscess) on the prostatic portion of the urethra and the abnormal degree of urethroprostatic reflux (not specific for the type of disease, but indicative of clinically relevant disease). Ultrasound then becomes an effective complementary procedure for further assessment of the prostate gland.

It should be apparent that every incontinence case is not the same and that preimaging assessment should minimize the expense and morbidity associated with procedures that have limited differentiating capacity for the patient in question. The integral roles of both survey radiography (for identification of masses [acknowledging that urethral, vaginal, and bladder masses will not be differentiated by this technique], stones, lymphadenopathy) and a detailed physical examination (including digital vaginal and rectal examinations as well as a vaginoscopic examination, if applicable), cannot be over-emphasized. Remember, the intent of incontinence investigation is to cost-effectively determine if the problem is treatable surgically with the assumption that applicable medical management treatment protocols have failed. In fairness to the owner, if an anomaly (e.g., vaginal stricture) with the potential for multiple other problems (e.g., sphincter-based incontinence) can be identified without an expensive imaging procedure, they can then decide how far they are willing to pursue the problem. Both the owners and the attending clinician can chart a course for the patient based on what further diagnostic techniques will yield and whether or not surgery is an option based on the probable case complexity, the estimated cost, and likely outcome.

References

Ackerman, N. (1974). Intravenous pyelography. *J Am Anim Hosp Assoc* **10**: 277–280.

Ackerman, N. (1974). Intravenous pyelography-interpretation of the study. *J Am Anim Hosp Assoc* **10**: 281–284.

Ackerman, N., et al. (1972). Fatal air embolism associated with pneumourethrography and pneumocystography in a dog. *J Am Anim Hosp Assoc* **160**(12): 1616–1618.

Agut, A., et al. (2004). Left perinephric abscess associated with nephrolithiasis and bladder calculi in a bitch. *Vet Rec* **154**(18): 562–565.

Andriole, G.L., et al. (1989). Effect of low osmolar, ionic and nonionic, contrast media on the cytologic features of exfoliated urothelial cells. *Urol Radiol* **11**(3): 133–135.

Armbrust, L.J., et al. (2000). Compression radiography: an old technique revisited. *J Am Anim Hosp Assoc* **36**: 537–541.

Banks, S.E., et al. (1991). Urinary incontinence in a bitch caused by vaginoureteral fistulation. *Vet Rec* **128**(5): 108.

Barber, D.L. and D.R. Finco (1979). Radiographic findings in induced bacterial pyelonephritis in dogs. *J Am Vet Med Assoc* **175**(11): 1183–1190.

Barrett, R.B. and S.L. Kneller (1972). Feline kidney measurement. Acta Radiol *(Stockh)* **319**(suppl): 279.

Barry, J.M., et al. (1978). The influence of retrograde contrast medium on urinary cytodiagnosis: a preliminary report. *J Urol* **119**(5): 633–634.

Barsanti, J.A., et al. (1981). Complications of bladder distention during retrograde urethrography. *Am J Vet Res* **42**(5): 819–821.

Benko, A., et al. (2007). Canadian association of radiologists: consensus guidelines for the prevention of contrast-induced nephropathy. *Can Assoc Radiol J* **58**(2): 79–87.

Biery, D.N. (1981). Upper urinary tract. In: *Radiographic Diagnosis of Abdominal Disorders in the Dog and Cat*, edited by T.R. O'Brien. Davis, CA: Covell Park Vet Company, pp. 481–542.

Brace, J.J. (1980). Perirenal cysts (pseudocysts) in the cat. In: Current Veterinary Therapy VIII, edited by R.W. Kirk. Philadelphia, PA: WB Saunders, pp. 980–981.

Briguori, C. and G. Marenzi *(2006). Contrast-induced nephropathy: pharmacological prophylaxis. Kidney Int Suppl* **100**: S30–S38.

Brown, N.O., et al. (1977). Canine urolithiasis: retrospective analysis of 438 cases. *J Am Vet Med Assoc* **170**(4): 414–418.

Bryan, J.N., et al. (2006). Primary renal neoplasia of dogs. *J Vet Intern Med* **20**(5): 1155–1160.

Burk, R.L. and D.A. Feeney (2003). The Abdomen. In: *Small Animal Radiology and Ultrasonography*, 3rd edition, edited by Burk, R,L, and D.A. Feeney. Philadelphia, PA: WB Saunders, pp. 249–476.

Burton, C.A., et al. (1994). Ureteric fibroepithelial polyps in 2 dogs. *J Small Animal Pract* **35**: 593.

Cannon, A.B., et al. (2007). Evaluation of trends in urolith composition in cats: 5,230 cases (1985–2004). *J Am Vet Med Assoc* **231**(4): 570–576.

Carrig, C.B. and U.V. Mostosky (1976). The use of compression in abdominal radiography of the dog and cat. *J Am Vet Radiol Soc* **17**(5): 178–181.

Caywood, D.D., et al. (1980). Neoplasms of the canine and feline urinary tracts. In: *Current Veterinary Therapy VII*, edited by R.W. Kirk. Philadelphia, PA: WB Saunders, pp. 1203–1212.

Christie, B.A. (1971). Incidence and etiology of vesicoureteral reflux in apparently normal dogs. *Invest Urol* **9**(3): 184–194.

Clark, W.T. (1966). Urolithiasis in the dog. IV. Diagnosis. *J Small Anim Pract* **7**(8): 553–556.

Constantinou, C.E., et al. (1974). Effects of radiopaque contrast media on the dynamic characteristics of ureteral function. *Urol Int* **29**(6): 401–413.

Crawford, J.T. and W.M. Adams. (2002). Influence of vestibulovaginal stenosis, pelvic bladder, and recessed vulva on response to treatment for clinical signs of lower urinary tract disease in dogs: 38 cases (1990–1999). *J Am Vet Med Assoc* **221**(7): 995–999.

Cuypers, M.D., et al. (1997). Renomegaly in dogs and cats: differential diagnosis. *Compend Contin Educ Pract Vet* **19**: 1019.

Davenport, D.J., et al. (1986). Familial renal disease in the dog and cat. *Cont Issues Small Anim Pract* **4**: 137.

Dawson, P. and M. Howell (1985). Misleading urine tests after using contrast media. *Br J Radiol* **58**(692): 785.

Eisele, J.G., et al. (2005). Ectopic ureterocele in a cat. *J Am Anim Hosp Assoc* **41**(5): 332–335.

Essman, S.C. (2005). Contrast cystography. *Clin Tech Small Anim Pract* **20**(1): 46–51.

Esterline, M.L., et al. (2005). Ureteral duplication in a dog. *Vet Radiol Ultrasound* **46**(6): 485–489.

Evans, H.E. and G.C. Christensen (1993). The urogenital system. In: *Miller's Anatomy of the Dog*, edited by H.E. Evans, 3rd edition. Philadelphia, PA: WB Saunders, pp. 494–558.

Faulkner, R.T., et al. (1983). Canine and feline ureteral ectopia. In: *Current Veterinary Therapy VIII*, edited by R.W. Kirk. Philadelphia, PA: WB Saunders, pp. 1043–1048.

Feeney, D.A., et al. (1982a). The excretory urogram: I. Techniques, normal radiographic appearance and misinterpretation. II. Interpretation of abnormal findings. *Compend Contin Educ Pract Vet* **4**: 233–240, 321–329.

Feeney, D.A., et al. (1982b). Functional aspects of the nephrogram in excretory urography: a review. *Vet Radiol* **23**: 42.

Feeney, D.A. and G.R. Johnston (2007). The kidneys and ureters. In: *Textbook of Veterinary Diagnostic Radiology*, edited by D.E. Thrall. St. Louis, MO: Missouri, Saunders, pp. 693–707.

Feeney, D.A. and G.R. Johnston (2007). The uterus, ovaries and testes. In: *Textbook of Veterinary Diagnostic Radiology*, edited by D.E. Thrall. St. Louis, MO: Missouri, Saunders, pp. 738–749.

Feeney, D.A., et al. (1980a). Effects of radiographic contrast media on results of urinalysis, with emphasis on alteration in specific gravity. *J Am Vet Med Assoc* **176**(12): 1378–1381.

Feeney, D.A., et al. (1980b). Effect of multiple excretory urograms on glomerular filtration of normal dogs: a preliminary report. *Am J Vet Res* **41**(6): 960–963.

Feeney, D.A., et al. (1979). Normal canine excretory urogram: effects of dose, time, and individual dog variation. *Am J Vet Res* **40**(11): 1596–1604.

Feldman, E.C. (2005). Polyuria and Polydipsia. In: *Textbook of Veterinary Internal Medicine*, 6th edition. St. Louis, MO Elsevier Saunders, pp. 102–105.

Finco, D.R. (1973). Congenital and inherited renal disease. *J Am Anim Hosp Assoc* **9**: 301.

Finco, D.R., et al. (1971). Radiologic estimation of kidney size in the dog. *J Am Vet Med Assoc* **159**: 995.

Fischer, S., et al. (1982). Increased abnormal urothelial cells in voided urine following excretory urography. *Acta Cytol* **26**(2): 153–158.

Graham, J.P., et al. (2007). Technical issues and interpretation principles relating to the canine and feline abdomen. In: *Textbook of Veterinary Diagnostic Radiology*, edited by D.E. Thrall, 5th edition. St. Louis, MO: Missouri, Saunders, pp. 626–644.

Goulden, B.E. (1968). Vesico-ureteral reflux in the dog. *N Z Vet J* **16**(12): 167–175.

Greco, D.S. (2001). Congenital and inherited renal disease of small animals. *Vet Clin North Am Small Anim Pract* **31**: 393.

Hager, D.A. and W.E. Blevins (1986). Ectopic ureter in a dog: extension from the kidney to the urinary bladder and to the urethra. *J Am Vet Med Assoc* **189**(3): 309–310.

Hamilton, M.H., et al. (2006). Traumatic bilateral ureteric rupture in two dogs. *J Small Anim Pract* **47**(12): 737–740.

Hayes, H.M. (1984). Breed associations of canine ectopic ureter: a study of 217 female cases. *J Small Anim Pract* **25**: 501.

Holloway, A. and R. O'Brien (2007). Perirenal effusion in dogs and cats with acute renal failure. *Vet Radiol Ultrasound* **48**(6): 574–579.

Holt, P.E. and A.H. Moore (1995). Canine ureteral ectopia: an analysis of 175 cases and comparison of surgical treatments. *Vet Rec* **136**(14): 345–349.

Houston, D.M., et al. (2004). Canine urolithiasis: a look at over 16 000 urolith submissions to the Canadian Veterinary Urolith Centre from February 1998 to April 2003. *Can Vet J* **45**(3): 225–230.

Hurt, R. (1960). The effect of radiographic contrast media on urinalysis. *Am J Med Technol* **26**: 122–124.

Ihle, S.L. and M. Kostolich (1991). Acute renal failure associated with contrast medium administration in a dog. *J Am Vet Med Assoc* **199**(7): 899–901.

Jakovljevic, S., et al. (1998). Ureteral diverticula in two dogs. [review] [35 refs]. *Vet Radiol Ultrasound* **39**(5): 425–429.

Johnston, G.R., et al. (1982). Urethrography and cystography in cats. I. Techniques, normal radiographic anatomy, and artifacts. II. Abnormal radiographic anatomy and complications. *Comp Cont Ed Pract Vet* **4**(10): 823–835, 931–946.

Johnston, G.R., et al. (1977). Familial ureteral ectopia in the dog. *J Am Anim Hosp Assoc* **13**: 168.

Johnston, G.R., et al. (1983). Complications of retrograde contrast urethrography in dogs and cats. *Am J Vet Res* **44**(7): 1248–1256.

Katzberg, R.W., et al. (1986). Effects of contrast media on renal function and subcellular morphology in the dog. *Invest Radiol* **21**(1): 64–70.

Klausner, J.S. and D.A. Feeney (1983). Vesicoureteral reflux. In: *Current Veterinary Therapy VIII*, edited by R.W. Kirk. Philadelphia, PA: WB Saunders, pp. 1041–1043.

Kneller, S.K. (1974). Role of the excretory urogram in the diagnosis of renal and ureteral disease. *Vet Clin North Am* **4**(4): 843–861.

Kyles, A.E., et al. (2005). Clinical, clinicopathologic, radiographic, and ultrasonographic abnormalities in cats with ureteral calculi: 163 cases (1984–2002). *J Am Vet Med Assoc* **226**(6): 932–936.

Kyles, A.E., et al. (1996). Vestibulovaginal stenosis in dogs: 18 cases (1987–1995). *J Am Vet Med Assoc* **209**(11): 1889–1893.

Lamb, C.R. and S.P. Gregory (1998). Ultrasonographic findings in 14 dogs with ectopic ureter. *Vet Radiol Ultrasound* **39**: 218–223.

Lautzenhiser, S.J. and D.E. Bjorling (2002). Urinary incontinence in a dog with an ectopic ureterocele. *J Am Anim Hosp Assoc* **38**(1): 29–32.

Lees, G. (1996). Congenital renal diseases. *Vet Clin North Am Small Anim Pract* **26**: 1379.

Lenaghan, D., et al. (1972a). Long-term effect of vesicoureteral reflux on the upper urinary tract of dogs. II. with urethral obstruction. *J Urol* **107**(5): 758–761.

Lenaghan, D., et al. (1972b). Long-term effect of vesicoureteral reflux on the upper urinary tract of dogs. I. without urinary infection. *J Urol* **107**(5): 755–757.

Levéillé, R. and M.A.O. Atilola (1991). Retrograde vaginocystography: a contrast study for evaluation of bitches with urinary incontinence. *Compend Contin Educ Pract Vet* **934**(13): 934–941.

Ling, G.V., et al. (1998a). Renal calculi in dogs & cats: prevalence, mineral type, breed, age, and gender interrelationships. *J Vet Int Med* **12**: 11.

Ling, G.V., et al. (1998b). Urolithiasis in dogs. I. Mineral prevalence and interrelations of mineral composition, age, and sex. *Am J Vet Res* **59**(5): 624–629.

Ling, G.V., et al. (2003). Changes in proportion of canine urinary calculi composed of calcium oxalate or struvite in specimens analyzed from 1981 through 2001. *J Vet Intern Med* **17**(6): 817–823.

Lord, P.F., et al. (1974). Intravenous urography for evaluation of renal diseases in small animals. *J Am Anim Hosp Assoc* **10**: 139–152.

Lulich, J.P., et al. (1999). Epidemiology of canine calcium oxalate uroliths. Identifying risk factors. *Vet Clin North Am Small Anim Pract* **29**(1): 113–122.

Lulich, J.P., et al. (1988). Feline idiopathic polycystic kidney disease. *Compend Contin Educ Pract Vet* **10**: 1030–1041.

Lyons, L.A., et al. (2004). Feline polycystic kidney disease mutation identified in PKD1. *J Am Soc Nephrol* **15**(10): 2548–2555.

Mahaffey, M.B., et al. (1984). Simultaneous double-contrast cystography and cystometry in dogs. *Vet Radiol* **25**(6): 254–259.

Mahaffey, M.B., et al. (1989). Cystography: effect of technique on diagnosis of cystitis in dogs. *Vet Radiol* **30**(6): 261–267.

Martinez, I., et al. (2003). Polypoid cystitis in 17 dogs (1978–2001). *J Vet Intern Med* **17**(4): 499–509.

Mehran, R. and E. Nikolsky ((2006). Contrast-induced nephropathy: definition, epidemiology, and patients at risk. *Kidney Int Suppl* **100**: S11–S15.

McClennan, B.L., et al. (1978). The effect of water soluble contrast material on urine cytology. *Acta Cytol* **22**(4): 230–233.

Moores, A.P., et al. (2002). Urinoma (para-ureteral pseudocyst) as a consequence of trauma in a cat. *J Small Anim Pract* **43**(5): 213–216.

Moroff, S.D., et al. (1991). Infiltrative ureteral disease in female dogs; 41 cases (1980–1987). *J Am Vet Med Assoc* **199**: 247.

Narins, D.J. and R.M. Chase Jr (1971). The effect of hypaque upon urine cultures. *J Urol* **105**(3): 433–435.

Neuwirth, L., et al. (1993). Comparison of excretory urography and ultrasonography for detection of experimentally induced pyelonephritis in dogs. *Am J Vet Res* **54**(5): 660–669.

Osborne, C.A., et al. (1999). Analysis of 77000 canine uroliths. Perspectives from the Minnesota Urolith Center. *Vet Clin North Am Small Anim Pract* **29**(1): 17–38.

Osborne, C.A., et al. (1996). Diagnosis, medical treatment, and prognosis of feline urolithiasis. [review] [42 refs]. *Vet Clin North Am Small Anim Pract* **26**(3): 589–627.

Owen, R.R. (1983). Canine ureteral ectopia. *J Small Anim Pract* **14**: 407.

Park, R.D. and R.H. Wrigley (2007). The urinary bladder. In: *Textbook of Veterinary Diagnostic Radiology*, edited by D.E. Thrall. St. Louis, MO: Missouri, Saunders, pp. 708–724.

Park, R.D. (1981). Radiology of the urinary bladder and urethra. In: *Radiographic Diagnosis of Abdominal Disorders in the Dog and Cat*, edited by T.R. O'Brien. Davis, CA: Covell Park Vet Company, pp. 543–614.

Pechman, R.D. (2007). The urethra. In: *Textbook of Veterinary Diagnostic Radiology*, edited by D.E. Thrall. St. Louis, MO: Saunders, pp. 725–728.

Reeder, M.M. and B. Felson (1975). *Gamuts in Radiology: Comprehensive Lists of Roentgen Differential Diagnosis*. Cincinnati, OH: Audiovisual of Cincinnati.

Reichle, J.K., et al. (2003). Ureteral fibroepithelial polyps in four dogs. *Vet Radiol Ultrasound* **44**: 433.

Rivers, B. and G.R. Johnston (1991). Diagnostic imaging of the reproductive organs of the bitch. *Vet Clin North Am Small Anim Pract* **21**(3): 437–466.

Rivers, B.J., et al. (1997). Ultrasonographic-guided, percutaneous antegrade pyelography: technique and clinical application in the dog and cat. *J Am Anim Hosp Assoc* **33**(1): 61–68.

Root, M.V., et al. (1995). Vaginal septa in dogs: 15 cases (1983–1992). *J Am Vet Med Assoc* **206**(1): 56–58.

Rose, J.G. and J.Y. Gillenwater (1974). Effects of obstruction and infection upon ureteral function. *Invest Urol* **11**: 471.

Ross, S.J., et al. (2007). A case-control study of the effects of nephrolithiasis in cats with chronic kidney disease. *J Am Vet Med Assoc* **230**(12): 1854–1859.

Ross, S.J., et al. (1999). Canine and feline nephrolithiasis. Epidemiology, detection, and management. *Vet Clin North Am Small Anim Pract* **29**(1): 231–250.

Rozear, L. and A.S. Tidwell (*2003*). Evaluation of the ureter and ureterovesicular junction using helical computed tomographic excretory urography in healthy dogs. *Vet Radiol Ultrasound* **44**(2): 155–164.

Ruby, A.L., et al. (1983). Effect of sodium diatrizoate on the in vitro growth of three common canine urinary bacterial species. *Vet Radiol* **24**(5): 222–225.

Samii, V.F., et al. (2004). Digital fluoroscopic excretory urography, digital fluoroscopic urethrography, helical computed tomography and cystoscopy in 24 dogs with suspected ureteral ectopia. *J Vet Int Med* **18**: 271.

Scrivani, P.V., et al. (1997). The effect of patient positioning on mural filling defects during double contrast cystography. *Vet Radiol Ultrasound* **38**(5): 355–359.

Senior, D.F. (1980). Parasites of the urinary tract. In: *Current Veterinary Therapy VII*, edited by R.W. Kirk. Philadelphia, PA: WB Saunders, pp. 1141–1143.

Sewell, A.C. (1996). Urinary crystals due to X-ray contrast medium. *Nephron* **72**(3): 487–488.

Shanahan, J.C., et al. (1985). Misleading urine tests after hexabrix IVU. *Br J Radiol* **58**(688): 389.

Shiroma, J.T., et al. (1999). Effect of reproductive status on feline renal size. *Vet Radiol Ultrasound* **40**(3): 242–245.

Silverman, S. and C.D. Long (2000). The diagnosis of urinary incontinence and abnormal urination in dogs and cats. [review] [9 refs]. *Vet Clin North Am Small Anim Pract* **30**(2): 427–448.

Smith, C., et al. (1983). Effect of X-ray contrast media on results for relative density of urine. *Clin Chem* **29**(4): 730–731.

Steyn, P.F. and J. Lowry (1991). Postional radiography as an aid to diagnose sand-like uroliths in the urinary bladder of feline urologic syndrome in cats. *Feline Pract* **19**(5): 21–23.

Tarr, M.J. and S.P. DiBartola (1985). Familial amyloidosis in Abyssinian cats: a possible model for familial Mediterranean fever and pathogenesis of secondary amyloidosis. *Lab Invest* **52**: 67a.

Thrall, D.E. and D.R. Finco (1976). Canine excretory urography: is quality a function of BUN? *J Am Anim Hosp Assoc* **12**(4): 446–450.

Thumchai, R., et al. (1996). Epizootiologic evaluation of urolithiasis in cats: 3498 cases (1982–1992). *J Am Vet Med Assoc* **208**(4): 547–551.

Ticer, J.W., et al. (1980). Positive contrast retrograde urethrography: a useful procedure for evaluating urethral disorders in the dog. *Vet Radiol* **21**(1): 2–11.

Valdes-Martinez, A., et al. (2007). Association between renal hypoechoic subcapsular thickening and lymphosarcoma in cats. *Vet Radiol Ultrasound* **48**(4): 357–360.

Weaver, A.D. (1970). Canine urolithiasis: incidence, chemical composition and outcome of 100 cases. *J Small Anim Pract* **11**(2): 93–107.

Weichselbaum, R.C., et al. (1999). Urocystolith detection: comparison of survey, contrast radiographic and ultrasonographic techniques in an in vitro bladder phantom. *Vet Radiol Ultrasound* **40**(4): 386–400.

Weichselbaum, R.C., et al. (1998a). in vitro evaluation of contrast medium concentration and depth effects on the radiographic appearance of specific canine urolith mineral types. *Vet Radiol Ultrasound* **39**(5): 396–411.

Weichselbaum, R.C., et al. (2001). An integrated epidemiologic and radiographic algorithm for canine urocystolith mineral type prediction. *Vet Radiol Ultrasound* **42**(4): 311–319.

Weichselbaum, R.C., et al. (1998b). Evaluation of the morphologic characteristics and prevalence of canine urocystoliths from a regional urolith center. *Am J Vet Res* **59**(4): 379–387.

Weisse, C., et al. (2002). Traumatic rupture of the ureters: 10 cases. *J Am Anim Hosp Assoc* **38**: 188.

Westropp, J.L., et al. (2006). Dried solidified blood calculi in the urinary tract of cats. *J Vet Intern Med* **20**(4): 828–834.

Worth, A.J. and S.C. Tomlin (2004). Post-traumatic paraureteral urinoma in a cat. *J Small Anim Pract* **45**: 413.

Zatelli, A. and P. D'Ippolito (2004). Bilateral perirenal abscesses in a domestic neutered shorthair cat. J Vet Intern Med **18**(6): 902–903.

Zontine, W.J. and L.K. Andrews (1978). Fatal sir embolization as a complication of pneumocystography in two cats. *J Am Vet Rad Soc* **19**(1): 8–11.

16

Ultrasonography of the urinary tract

Silke Hecht and George A. Henry

Ultrasound examination is an integral tool in the thorough evaluation of the urinary system. Ultrasound is a noninvasive, nonpainful, and economical procedure that provides valuable information concerning morphology, vascular status, and luminal contents usually with little or no sedation in most patients. Abdominal fluid, perirenal fluid, or emaciation are not limiting factors for ultrasound imaging as they are for survey radiography (see Chapter 15). Ultrasound is superior to survey radiographs in detecting smaller renal parenchymal masses, renal pelvic and ureteral dilation, renal blood flow abnormalities, urinary bladder masses, and differentiating solid masses from cavitations and cystic lesions. Ultrasound-guided interventional procedures increase the accuracy and safety of percutaneous aspirates, biopsies (see Chapter 23), pyelocentesis (see Chapter 6), and antegrade pyelography (see Chapter 6) for diagnostic and therapeutic purposes.

Limitations of ultrasonographic evaluation of the urinary tract include difficulty in imaging due to body conformation, overlying bowel, sonographer skill level, and inability to provide renal functional information other than blood flow. Additional limitations include inability to visualize normal ureters and inability to examine the entire length of the urethra due to intrapelvic position. Survey radiography is often superior for localization of radiopaque uroliths in nondilated ureters and the urethra. Excretory urography or positive contrast cystourethrography allow visualization of the entire length of ureters and urethra, respectively, and are considered superior in the evaluation of trauma-induced urine leakage.

Ultrasound examination, interpretation, and artifacts

Patient preparation is performed in a routine manner. A complete discussion of the principles of ultrasound imaging is beyond the scope of this chapter, and the reader is referred to pertinent references (Kremkau 1995, Kremkau 2002). However, a short overview over pertinent ultrasound artifacts is provided, since these must be recognized for correct interpretation of the ultrasound findings. Acoustic shadowing, reverberation artifact, distal acoustic enhancement, slice thickness artifact, grating or side-lobe artifact, edge refraction or edge shadowing artifact, mirror image artifact, and twinkle artifact may be encountered when investigating the urinary tract (Douglass and Kremkau 1993; Kirberger 1995; Barthez et al. 1997; Penninck 2002; Louvet 2006; d'Anjou 2008; Sutherland-Smith 2008).

Acoustic shadowing occurs due to mineral or air interfaces causing loss of echo intensity deep to the interface. Fat within the renal hilus may occasionally cause mild attenuation of the deep tissues and must not be confused with a renal calculus. Mineral interfaces such as uroliths typically cause strong distal hypoechoic to anechoic shadows. An anechoic (dark) acoustic shadow is more evident with larger uroliths and higher frequency transducers. Air interfaces typically cause echogenic ("dirty") distal shadows due to concurrent reverberation artifact. This artifact may be encountered when gas is present within bladder lumen or wall. The smooth surfaces of catheters and wires may also produce reverberation artifact when perpendicular to the sound beam.

Distal acoustic enhancement is due to passage of sound through an area of decreased attenuation, resulting in higher echo intensity from tissues deep to the area compared with surrounding tissues at the same depth. This artifact is typically seen with fluid filled structures such as cysts.

Nephrology and Urology of Small Animals. Edited by Joe Bartges and David J. Polzin. © 2011 Blackwell Publishing Ltd.

Slice thickness, side-lobe, and grating-lobe artifacts may cause the appearance of echoic material within anechoic areas. These can give the false impression of echogenic material within the urine of the bladder or other fluid-filled structures and must be recognized to prevent erroneous interpretation.

Edge refraction artifact is due to refraction of the ultrasound beam, resulting in the apparent loss of a margin. If this artifact involves a curved fluid-filled structure (bladder) surrounded by fluid (abdominal effusion) it will cause the impression of a defect in the bladder wall. Edge shadowing is similar to edge refraction artifact but is seen associated with curved margins of structures that cause refraction of the sound, resulting in a dark line or shadow in the tissues distal to the structure. Edge shadowing caused by arcuate vessel walls in the kidneys should not be mistaken for small renal calculi.

Mirror image artifacts occur when strongly reflective interfaces reflect scattered ultrasound waves back to the transducer, resulting in erroneous display of anatomic Structures. Although this artifact is relatively rare when examining the urinary tract, it may be encountered when the colon is filled with a large amount of gas and/or feces, resulting in display of dual urinary bladder.

Twinkling artifact is a color Doppler artifact that occurs behind strongly reflective interfaces such as those produced by urinary tract stones or parenchymal calcifications. It appears as a quickly fluctuating mixture of Doppler signals with an associated spectrum of noisy appearance and can be utilized to differentiate mineral structures from other hyperechoic material.

Kidneys and ureters

Normal sonographic anatomy

The kidneys are symmetrical in size and shape in the dog and cat. Canine kidneys are typically more bean shaped, and the right kidney is located more cranial than the left. Feline kidneys are more oval shaped and are both located in the mid abdomen.

Cats have more uniform renal size with normal length reported to vary from 3.0 to 4.3 cm in length (Walter et al. 1987a). A study investigating feline renal size on radiographs found significantly smaller kidneys in neutered versus intact cats (Shiroma et al. 1999), which should be taken into consideration when examining feline patients. The large variation in canine body weight and conformation present a wide range of renal measurements. Normal values for the dog using body weight and conformation as variables have been reported (Barr et al. 1990). A recently described method using a ratio of kidney length to aortic luminal diameter gives a range in the dog of 5.5–9.1

(Mareschal et al. 2007). Renal volume can be calculated based on ultrasonographic measurements (Nyland et al. 1989; Felkai et al. 1992); however, this is not commonly performed. While measurements of renal size may be helpful in some cases especially with repeated examinations over a period of time, small deviations from the reported ranges do not necessarily indicate clinical disease.

The renal cortex, medulla, collecting system, and vasculature may be observed with ultrasound imaging in dogs and cats (Konde et al. 1984; Walter et al. 1987a). The cortex is the outer rim of tissue and is normally hyperechoic to the more central hypoechoic medulla. The renal cortex is typically isoechoic to hypoechoic to the liver and hypoechoic to the spleen (Churchill et al. 1999; Drost et al. 2000a; Nyland et al. 2002a). However, in some dogs and cats, the renal cortex may be hyperechoic to the liver even without clinical evidence of renal disease (Drost et al. 2000a; Ivancić and Mai 2008). One study found an increase in echogenicity of the renal cortex in dogs when using a high frequency transducer (7.5 MHz) compared with a lower frequency transducer (5 MHz) (Hartzband et al. 1991). Increased echogenicity can be seen in cats due to accumulation of fatty vacuoles in the renal cortex (Yeager and Anderson 1989). Because of these variations of normal, care must be taken not to over-interpret mild variations of renal cortical echogenicity.

The medulla is divided by interlobular vessels and renal recesses of the collecting system with a single longitudinally oriented renal crest extending into the renal pelvis. The interlobar vessels are often seen as two short parallel hyperechoic lines traversing the medulla to the corticomedullary junction, and arcuate vessels characterized by bright walls are seen at the level of the corticomedullary junction. Using color Doppler or power Doppler ultrasound, interlobular vessels can be visualized extending from the corticomedullary junction into the cortex (Figure 16.1). As stated earlier, edge shadowing from these vessels should be differentiated from renal calculi or mineralization. The renal artery and vein can be followed from the kidneys to the aorta and caudal vena cava, respectively. There are usually one renal artery and vein although duplicate arteries and veins have been reported (Bouma et al. 2003; Cáceres 2008).

The renal pelvis is sometimes seen in normal animals, especially after induction of diuresis, if receiving fluid therapy or if the urinary bladder is distended (Pugh et al. 1994; d'Anjou 2008). It is best evaluated on transverse view and appears as a V-shaped anechoic area adjacent to the renal crest.

The ureters exit from the center of the renal hilus and extend medially for a short distance, then turn caudally and travel in the retroperitoneal tissues to the dorsal

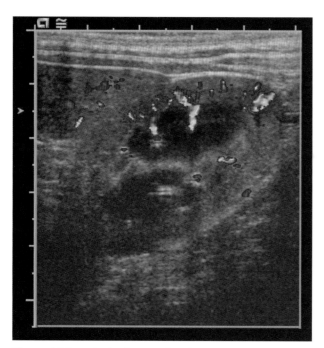

Figure 16.1 Sagittal color Doppler ultrasound image of the left kidney in a dog. The interlobar arteries are seen traversing the hypoechic medulla and branching into arcuate vessels at the level of the corticomedullary junction. Flow signals in the medium echogenic renal cortex correspond to interlobular vessels.

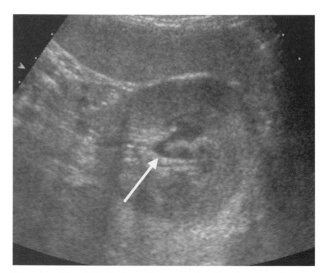

Figure 16.2 Mild dilation of the renal pelvis (pyelectasia) in a dog receiving intravenous fluid therapy. The renal pelvis (arrow) appears as V-shaped anechoic area adjacent to the renal crest.

wall of the bladder at the trigone. Normal ureters are not visible on ultrasonographic examination. However, ureteral abnormalities (wall thickening, abnormal contents, ureteral dilation) increase conspicuity and allow ultrasonographic assessment. Imaging in a transverse plane from the right or left dorsolateral abdominal wall is best for following a visible ureter from the kidney to the bladder. Peristaltic contractions of the ureters can be observed in some cases.

Renal pelvic and ureteral dilation

Renal pelvic dilation is commonly seen during ultrasonographic examination and—dependent on degree and etiology—may be incidental or clinically significant. The term "pyelectasia" is used for mild to moderate dilation of the renal pelvis without evidence of obstruction of the urinary outflow tract, while the term "hydronephrosis" is used to describe renal pelvic dilation secondary to obstruction of renal pelvis and/or ureter (Pugh et al. 1994). Mild dilation of the renal pelvis is best observed on transverse image and manifests as widening of the typically thin (<2 mm) triangular anechoic area around the renal crest (Figure 16.2). Moderate dilation is easily observed in transverse and sagittal plane. With progressive filling, the dilated pelvis becomes more rounded and the renal pelvic diverticula are clearly recognized. In severe pelvic dilation, there is enlargement of the kidney, with progressive thinning and ultimately complete atrophy of the renal parenchyma (Figure 16.3).

Mild dilation of the renal pelvis may be an incidental finding encountered after fluid therapy, administration of diuretics, or secondary to back pressure from a distended urinary bladder (Pugh et al. 1994; d'Anjou 2008). Possible pathologic reasons include inflammatory disorders (pyelonephritis or ureteritis), increased diuresis due to renal insufficiency, congenital malformations, and early

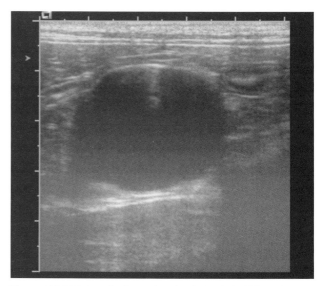

Figure 16.3 Severe hydronephrosis of the right kidney in a cat secondary to chronic ureteral obstruction. The renal parenchyma is atrophied, and the renal pelvis is severely distended with anechoic fluid. Note hyperechogenicity in the far field, consistent with distal enhancement artifact.

or partial renal pelvic and/or ureteral obstruction. Moderate dilation may be encountered in pyelonephritis (see Chapter 49) or obstructive uropathy (see Chapter 70), and severe hydronephrosis is usually indicative of renal pelvic or ureteral obstruction (d'Anjou 2008).

Obstruction of the renal pelvis can occur at the level of the pelvicoureteral junction (renal calculi, sediment, congenital malformation, neoplasia), the ureter (ectopia, calculi, sediment, strictures, iatrogenic, masses, retroperitoneal disease), or the bladder (infiltrative mass at the level of the trigone). Regardless of degree of renal pelvis dilation seen on ultrasonographic examination, care must be taken to thoroughly evaluate renal pelvis, ureters, and bladder for any indication of obstruction. If findings are equivocal for obstructive hydronephrosis, recheck ultrasound, excretory urography, and antegrade pyelography with injection of positive contrast material into the dilated renal pelvis under ultrasound guidance, or advanced imaging procedures should be considered to further assess, since persistent obstruction will result in irreversible damage to the renal parenchyma (Fink et al. 1980). Resistive index measurements utilizing Doppler measurements are utilized in humans to distinguish ureteral obstruction from pyelonephritis, and, however, are only of limited value in the diagnosis of ureteral obstruction in dogs (Nyland et al. 1993).

Ureteral dilation is a relatively common finding on ultrasound and may be related to obstruction or nonobstructive disorders. Ureteral obstruction may be caused by ureteral calculi, ureteral, cystic or retroperitoneal mass lesions, blood clots, inflammatory products, fibrosis, or inadvertent ligation during ovariohysterectomy. Nonobstructive dilation of the ureter may be related to vesicoureteral reflux, trauma, infection, or congenital anomalies (Felkai et al. 1995; Lamb 1998; Confer and Panciera 2001). Ultrasonographically, the dilated ureter appears as tubular and often tortuous anechoic structure extending from the renal pelvis distally. Concurrent pyelectasia or hydronephrosis is common. Dependent on underlying etiology, hydroureter can be focal or affect the entire length of the ureter. Color Doppler ultrasound can occasionally be helpful in distinguishing a dilated ureter from abdominal vessels. If a dilated ureter is identified, it should be traced distally to confirm or rule out an obstructive lesion (Figure 16.4). However, even if a lesion such as a ureteral calculus or a bladder mass at the level of the trigone is identified, a definitive diagnosis of complete obstruction can be difficult to achieve (Lamb 1998). Recheck ultrasound or other imaging techniques such as percutaneous antegrade pyelography may be necessary to achieve a definitive diagnosis (Rivers et al. 1997; Adin et al. 2003; Hardie and Kyles 2004).

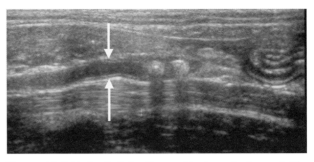

Figure 16.4 Ureteral obstruction and hydroureter in a cat. The ureter (arrows) appears as anechoic tubular structure of approximately 3 mm diameter proximal to two ureteral calculi, which are characterized by a strongly hyperechoic interface and distal shadowing. The ureter is not visible distal to the calculi.

Congenital renal and ureteral disorders

Reports on imaging findings in congenital renal (see Chapter 56) and ureteral diseases in small animals are scarce with the exception of ectopic ureters (see Chapter 58).

Congenital renal disorders

Renal agenesis is rare but may occasionally be encountered, sometimes as incidental finding in animals with appropriate renal function. The contralateral kidney may undergo compensatory hypertrophy and appear larger than expected for a given animal (Diez-Prieto et al. 2001). Major differential diagnosis for a missing kidney is previous nephrectomy, which in most cases is easily ruled out by obtaining a proper history. Other reasons for inability to identify a kidney on ultrasound include conformation of the patient (deep-chested dogs) and failure to achieve sufficient depth on ultrasonographic examination, kidney in abnormal position (renal ectopia, herniation), and kidneys that are abnormally small and/or have abnormal architecture (renal hypoplasia/dysplasia, end-stage renal disease). Renal agenesis is often associated with ipsilateral ureteral agenesis. Ureteral agenesis may also take the form of segmental absence of the ureter or lack of the lumen, resulting in ureteral obstruction (Lamb 1998).

Renal hypoplasia is characterized by small renal size and may occur uni- or bilaterally. If only one kidney is affected, the other kidney may be enlarged due to compensatory hypertrophy. Renal architecture and echogenicity are usually within normal limits.

Renal dysplasia is a congenital disease, which has been reported in the Alaskan Malamute, Chow Chow, Golden Retriever, Lhasa Apso, Shi Tzu, Miniature Schnauzer, Soft-coated Wheaten terrier, and Standard Poodle (DiBartola 2000a). Ultrasonographically, both

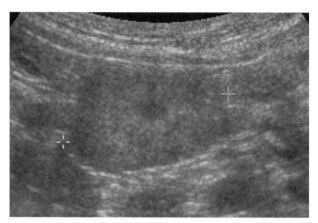

Figure 16.5 Renal dysplasia in a 1-year-old Boxer (presumptive). Both kidneys are small (<4 cm) (left kidney seen between cursors) and diffusely hyperechoic, with loss of corticomedullary distinction.

kidneys appear small and often slightly irregular in shape, the renal cortex is usually diffusely hyperechoic, and the corticomedullary distinction may be decreased (Figure 16.5). Although these ultrasonographic changes can be caused by other renal diseases, renal dysplasia should strongly be considered in a young animal presented with renal insufficiency and small kidneys.

Renal ectopia and renal fusion are associated with failure of the fetal metanephric kidneys to appropriately separate and/or migrate from their original position in the pelvic region. They may be found in a pelvic, iliac, or abdominal position, on the same or opposite side of the abdomen. Renal ectopia has been described in cats and dogs (Lulich et al. 1987; Finco 1995), but ultrasonographic reports are rare. Pelvic position of the left kidney as an incidental finding in a 4-year-old cat has been reported (Hecht et al. 2005). The kidney was small but had maintained normal architecture, and the animal had no laboratory evidence of renal disease. Crossed renal ectopia with fusion was reported in a cat with ultrasound showing two renal crests and pelvises (Allworth and Hoffmann 1999). Although ectopic kidneys are commonly structurally and functionally normal, the short ureter may be kinked, predisposing to obstruction and secondary hydronephrosis or pyelonephritis (Maxie 1993; Gleason et al. 1994).

Congenital ureteral disorders

Ureteral ectopia is a congenital abnormality of the terminal segment of one or both ureters, in which the ureteral orifice is located distal to the trigone of the urinary bladder. Common sites of ectopically displaced ureteral orifices include the bladder neck, proximal, middle, or distal urethra, vagina, or uterus (McLoughlin and Chew 2000).

Extramural ectopic ureters completely bypass the urinary bladder without anatomic attachment, while intramural ectopic ureters attach on the dorsal or dorsolateral surface of the urinary bladder but fail to open in the normal anatomic position at the tip of the trigone. Female dogs are more commonly affected than male dogs, and concurrent abnormalities of other parts of the urogenital tract are possible. A variety of techniques, including contrast radiographic procedures, computed tomography, ultrasonography, and cystoscopy, can be used for the diagnosis of ectopic ureters. One study comparing ultrasonography and contrast radiography found them to be similarly sensitive in the detection of ectopic ureters (91%) (Lamb and Gregory 1998). Dilation of renal pelvis and ureter are common in ureteral ectopia, allowing identification of the ureter and facilitating examination from pelvicoureteral junction to site of termination. A diagnosis of ectopic ureter can be made when the ureter can be followed past the trigone to the point of termination or to the entrance into the pelvic canal (Oglesby and Carter 2003). Although ultrasonography is potentially useful in the diagnosis of ectopic ureters, it has to be stressed that it may be difficult to visualize a ureter that is minimally dilated, particularly if image quality is limited by use of a low-frequency transducer or patient factors such as obesity (Lamb 1998). Additionally, the ureterovesicular junctions are small structures that may be difficult to identify, and reflux from the urethra into the bladder may be mistaken for a ureteral jet, which may result in false-positive and false-negative diagnosis, respectively (Lamb and Gregory 1998).

Ureterocele refers to dilation of the submucosal portion of the distal ureter (McLoughlin et al. 1989; Stiffler et al. 2002). The opening of the ureterocele may be close to the normal ureterovesicular junction and may not produce clinical signs ("orthotopic" ureterocele). If the ureterocele is located more caudally (within bladder neck or urethra), it is referred to as "ectopic" ureterocele, which may be associated with incontinence or stranguria due to obstruction of the bladder neck (McLoughlin et al. 1989; Osborne et al. 1995). Ultrasonographically, ureterocele appears as a rounded anechoic structure with a thin hyperechoic wall associated with the lumen of or impinging on the wall of the urinary bladder (Nyland et al. 2002a; Takiguchi et al. 1997) (Figure 16.6). Connection to the ipsilateral ureter may be evident in case of concurrent ureteral dilation (Lamb 1998).

Ureteral duplication has been reported in the dog as a dilated tubular fluid-filled structure extending caudally from the left kidney to a blind end lateral to the bladder. The dog had associated mild hydronephrosis and hydroureter of the patent left ureter (Esterline et al. 2005).

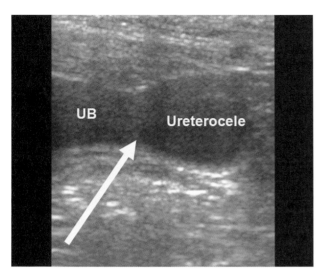

Figure 16.6 Ureterocele in a dog. Transverse image of the caudal abdomen shows focal dilation of the left ureter (ureterocele), with impingement on the urinary bladder (UB). The septum between ureterocele and UB is indicated by the arrow.

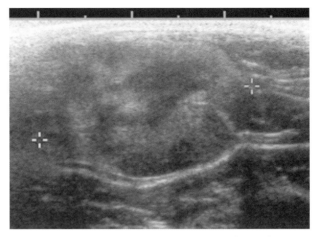

Figure 16.7 End stage renal disease in a cat. The kidney (between cursors) is small (2.3 cm length), irregular, diffusely hyperechoic, with decreased corticomedullary distinction. Histopathologic examination revealed marked, chronic glomerulonephritis with glomerulosclerosis, interstitial fibrosis, and tubular necrosis.

Acquired renal disorders

Renal disorders can be subdivided into abnormalities in renal size, diffuse parenchymal abnormalities, focal or multifocal renal parenchymal abnormalities, abnormalities of the renal collecting system, and vascular abnormalities, which can be encountered as isolated findings or in combination. Evaluation of renal size and diffuse cortical changes is difficult. Ultrasonographic changes, especially in acute renal disease, may be minimal; variations in renal size and echogenicity often hamper an unequivocal diagnosis of "abnormal"; and degenerative renal changes are often encountered in older animals with maintained appropriate renal function. The ultrasonographer has to be aware of these limitations, and results of ultrasonographic examination have to be judged in light of patient signalment, history, clinical and laboratory findings, and other ultrasonographic findings that might support a specific diagnosis. Recheck ultrasonography to monitor renal changes in a given patient or further imaging, such as excretory urography and interventional procedures (fine-needle aspiration or biopsy of the kidney, pyelocentesis), might be needed to achieve a definitive diagnosis.

Abnormalities in renal size

Although normal renal size (see Chapter 45) has been reported for dogs and cats, the diagnosis of enlarged or small kidneys is often subjective. Decrease in renal size may be seen in congenital/developmental disorders such as hypoplasia or dysplasia (see above) as well as in chronic degenerative and end-stage renal disease.

Small size of the kidneys due to chronic renal disease is a common finding in especially older dogs and cats. Concurrent ultrasound findings may include irregular shape of the kidneys, hyperechoic cortices, and decreased corticomedullary distinction (Figure 16.7). Dilation of the renal pelvis due to polyuria, previous or current pyelonephritis, and renal mineralization/ nephrolithiasis are also commonly seen. Depending on underlying etiology and duration of the disease process, one or both kidneys may be affected.

An increase in renal size may be related to a variety of disorders. Many diseases resulting in renomegaly on radiographs such as hydronephrosis, perinephric pseudocysts, and renal mass lesions (cyst(s), abscess, granuloma, focal neoplasm) are easily distinguished by means of ultrasonography (Cartee et al. 1980; Konde et al. 1985; Konde et al. 1986). Diffuse increase in renal size may be seen in acute inflammatory renal diseases (interstitial nephritis, glomerulonephritis, pyelonephritis), acute toxic nephropathy, metabolic nephropathy, congenital portosystemic shunts, and diffuse infiltrative neoplastic processes (lymphoma). Concurrent echogenicity changes of the kidney and other ultrasonographic findings may allow a presumptive diagnosis; however, fine-needle aspiration or biopsy is often needed for a definitive diagnosis.

Diffuse parenchymal abnormalities

Diffuse increase in cortical echogenicity is a common finding. Variations of normal, fat deposition, and ultrasound machine settings (transducer frequency) may result in diffuse hyperechogenicity of the renal cortices, and the diagnosis of pathologically increased renal cortical echogenicity is often difficult. Developmental diseases, inflammatory diseases, toxic and metabolic diseases, diffuse renal mineralization (nephrocalcinosis), and diffuse infiltrative neoplastic disorders all can result in diffuse increase in renal cortical echogenicity (Walter et al. 1987b, Walter et al. 1988).

Inflammatory renal diseases (interstitial nephritis, glomerulonephritis, and pyelonephritis) may result in increased cortical echogenicity, often associated with a decrease in corticomedullary distinction (Figure 16.7). Possible concurrent findings include change in renal size, renal pelvis dilation, and perinephric fluid accumulation. While renomegaly may be seen in acute inflammation, decreased renal size is common in animals with chronic nephritis. A larger degree of renal pelvis dilation would be expected for pyelonephritis than for other inflammatory renal diseases. However, overlap between the categories exists, since pyelectasia may also result from polyuria, intravenous fluid therapy, or back pressure from a distended bladder. Mild perinephric fluid accumulation may be noted in acute inflammatory renal diseases. It is important to note that nephritis can be present without observable changes, and other diseases such as toxic nephropathy may result in similar ultrasonographic findings.

Animals with toxic nephropathies (due to ingestion of ethylene glycol, lilies in cats and grapes or raisins in dogs) are usually presented at an acute stage (see Chapter 49). Imaging findings are similar to acute nephritis (hyperechoic cortices, renomegaly, perinephric fluid accumulation), and differentiation may be difficult especially if no complete history is provided. A hyperechoic band paralleling the cortex within the renal medulla ("medullary rim sign") due to intratubular calcium oxalate crystal deposition has been described in dogs with ethylene glycol intoxication (Adams et al. 1989; Biller et al. 1992). However, this finding may be seen in other renal diseases in dogs, such as hypercalcemic nephropathy (Barr et al. 1989), leptospirosis, and chronic interstitial nephritis (Biller et al. 1992), and may even be present in canine kidneys without evidence of renal dysfunction (Mantis and Lamb 2000). A wider (0.5–1.0 cm diameter) medullary band of increased echogenicity has been described in dogs with leptospirosis (Forrest et al. 1998). The medullary rim sign is a common finding in normal cats and is attributed to nonpathologic mineral deposition within the lumen of medullary tubules (Yeager and Anderson 1989).

Nephrocalcinosis may be seen in hyperadrenocorticism, chronic renal disease, hypervitaminosis D, and nephrotoxicity (Kealy and McAllister 2005). Diffuse hyperechogenicity of the kidneys is the most common finding, although distinct pinpoint mineral foci may be observed.

Many neoplastic diseases of the kidneys result in uni- or bilateral mass lesions that are easily depicted (see Chapter 57). However, renal lymphosarcoma can result in diffuse increase in renal cortical echogenicity in cats, usually with concurrent increase in renal size. Typically, both kidneys are affected (Gabor et al. 1998). Hypoechoic subcapsular thickening is occasionally seen in feline renal lymphosarcoma and appears to be a fairly specific finding, although it has been described in other renal diseases such as undifferentiated malignant neoplasia, renal anaplastic carcinoma, and feline infectious peritonitis (FIP) (Valdés-Martínez et al. 2007).

Diffuse hypoechogenicity of the renal cortices is rarely encountered. In theory, diffuse parenchymal diseases such as nephritis or metabolic nephropathies might cause decrease instead of increase of renal cortical echogenicity, but supporting evidence is not found in the Veterinary literature.

Focal parenchymal abnormalities

Renal nodules/mass lesions

Renal nodules or masses are most commonly neoplastic in etiology. In dogs, primary renal neoplasms are less common than metastases to the kidneys and include tubular cell carcinoma, transitional cell carcinoma, and transitional cell papilloma (Klein et al. 1988). Other less common renal tumors include anaplastic carcinoma, anaplastic sarcoma, fibroma, hemangiosarcoma, lymphoma, nephroblastoma, cystadenocarcinoma, mast cell tumor, and histiocytic diseases (disseminated histiocytic sarcoma, malignant fibrous histiocytoma) (Lium and Moe 1985; Klein et al. 1988; Ramirez et al. 2002; Cruz-Aeambulo et al. 2004; Sato and Solano 2004; Locke and Barber 2006; Knapp 2007). Most renal tumors are unilateral; however, metastases, lymphoma, mast cell disease, disseminated histiocytic sarcoma, and renal tubular cell carcinoma can affect both kidneys. In general, renal neoplasms manifest as masses of variable echogenicity (hyperechoic, isoechoic, hypoechoic, homogenous, or mixed echogenic) (Figure 16.8). Different tumor types cannot be differentiated based on their ultrasonographic appearance (Konde et al. 1985). An unusual syndrome reported in German shepherd dogs consists of uni- or bilateral renal cystadenocarcinomas, dermal fibrosis, and uterine tumors in affected females (Lium and Moe 1985; Knapp 2007). These tumors have a cystic component that can be identified by means of ultrasonography. Renal hemangiosarcoma usually has a lacy cavitary appearance on ultrasound (Figure 16.9) and is commonly associated with retroperitoneal effusion/hemorrhage

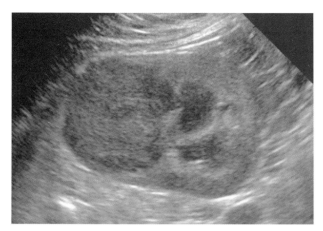

Figure 16.8 Renal mass in a 1-year-old dog. The cranial pole of the right kidney contains a hypoechoic and relatively homogenous mass. A similar mass was found in the left kidney (not shown). Fine needle aspiration yielded a diagnosis of lymphoma.

(Locke and Barber 2006). However, vascular invasion or rupture of tumor with hemorrhage can occur with other renal tumors and is not pathognomonic for hemangiosarcoma.

Lymphosarcoma is the most common renal tumor in cats (Knapp 2007). Unlike in dogs, feline renal lymphosarcoma commonly results in diffuse renal changes rather than focal masses.

Nonneoplastic focal renal masses such as abscesses, solid hematomas, or granulomas (fungal, FIP) are rare but cannot be distinguished from malignant lesions by ultrasonography alone (d'Anjou 2008). Fine-needle aspiration or biopsy of the kidney is needed to establish a definitive diagnosis of a malignant versus benign renal

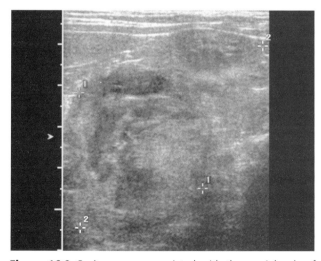

Figure 16.9 Cavitary mass associated with the cranial pole of the left kidney in a 12-year-old Yorkshire Terrier. Histologic diagnosis was hemangiosarcoma. Concurrent retroperitoneal effusion (hemorrhage) is common in these tumors.

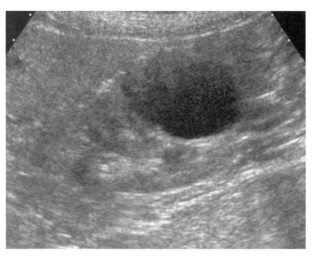

Figure 16.10 Large renal cyst associated with the caudal pole of the left kidney as an incidental finding in a 9-year-old Siberian Husky. The cyst appears as well-circumscribed round anechoic area.

mass lesion and to determine the exact tumor type in case of neoplasia.

Renal cysts and polycystic kidney disease

Renal cysts manifest as round to ovoid anechoic structures with a thin hyperechoic lining. They can be single or multiple, uni- or bilateral, and are usually associated with distal acoustic enhancement and edge shadowing (Figure 16.10). Renal cysts can be completely incidental or can be associated with chronic degenerative renal disease (d'Anjou 2008). With increasing size, they can result in distortion of the renal margin. On occasion, renal cysts may appear complex and show septation or echogenic contents due to accumulation of necrotic debris. In these instances, it may be difficult to distinguish a cyst from a renal abscess or a cystic/cavitary renal mass such as cystadenocarcinoma or hemangiosarcoma.

Polycystic renal disease has been reported in Persian cats, Cairn Terriers, Bull terriers, and West Highland white terriers (see Chapter 56) (DiBartola 2000a). Affected kidneys are often enlarged and significantly distorted, with numerous variable sized cysts mostly associated with renal cortex and corticomedullary junction (Reichle et al. 2002).

Chronic renal infarcts

Chronic infarcts are a relatively frequent finding especially in older animals and are usually considered incidental. They appear as sharply marginated, homogenous linear, or wedge-shaped hyperechoic areas associated with the renal cortex perpendicular to the renal capsule, often

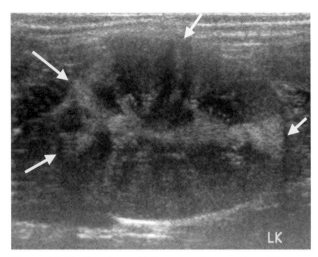

Figure 16.11 Chronic renal infarcts in a 6-year-old cat. There are numerous well-circumscribed and homogenous linear or wedge-shaped hyperechoic areas associated with the renal cortex perpendicular to the renal capsule (arrows). The cranial pole of the kidney is blunted.

with concurrent concave indentation of the renal surface (Figure 16.11) (d'Anjou 2008).

Focal renal mineralization/nephrolithiasis

Mineral foci due to metastatic or dystrophic mineralization and nephroliths are common. They appear as strongly hyperechoic structures of variable size, often associated with distal shadowing (Figure 16.12). They may or may not be of clinical significance and have to be judged in light of clinical presentation of the patient.

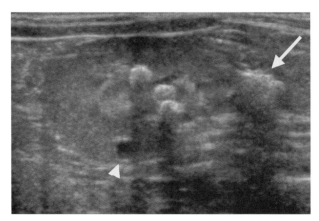

Figure 16.12 Nephrolithiasis in a dog. There are three rounded strongly hyperechoic structures associated with the kidney, at least two of which show distal shadowing. The irregular hyperechoic area caudal to the kidney represents part of the gastrointestinal tract (arrow). A small cortical cyst is noted in the far field (arrowhead).

Renal pelvis disorders

Disorders of the renal pelvis include dilation (see above) and abnormal content.

Pyelonephritis

Infection of the renal collecting system (pyelonephritis) is relatively common in dogs and cats and is usually associated with urinary bladder and/or ureteral infection. The major ultrasonographic findings in acute pyelonephritis are renal pelvic dilatation, usually with proximal ureteral dilatation, and a hyperechoic mucosal margin line within the renal pelvis, proximal portion of the ureter, or both (Neuwirth et al. 1993). Other common findings include generalized hyperechoic renal cortex, focal hyperechoic areas within the medulla, focal hyperechoic or hypoechoic cortical lesions, and increased echogenicity of urine within the renal pelvis due to increased cell and protein content. In chronic pyelonephritis, the pelvis and diverticula can become distorted and blunted, and additional renal parenchymal changes and/or mineralization of the renal collecting system are common (d'Anjou 2008). One study found ultrasonography to be 82% sensitive and 100% specific for the detection of mild to moderate pyelonephritis (Neuwirth et al. 1993). Since false-negative results are possible especially in early and mild cases, recheck ultrasound should be considered if a clinical suspicion of pyelonephritis persists despite initial negative ultrasound examination. Since renal pelvic fluid accumulation may be observed under a variety of circumstances other than pyelonephritis (Pugh et al. 1994; d'Anjou 2008), false-positive results of ultrasonographic examination are possible in our experience. Retroperitoneal abscess and regional cellulitis have been reported as sequelae of pyelonephritis and appear as fluid-filled areas in the vicinity of the kidneys and the urinary bladder, containing a mixture of anechoic, hypoechoic, and hyperechoic components (Hylands 2006).

Renal pelvic luminal abnormalities

Renal calculi, inflammatory sediment, and blood clots can be found associated with the renal collecting system, with or without renal pelvic dilation (Felkai et al. 1995).

Renal calculi can reach considerable size (see Chapter 69). They are characterized by a strongly hyperechoic interface with distal sound beam attenuation, with or without concurrent renal pelvic dilation (Felkai et al. 1995) (Figure 16.12).

Inflammatory sediment as seen in pyelonephritis, and blood clots found in animals following trauma, secondary to renal hematuria, or bleeding renal tumors occur as mixed echogenic material within the renal pelvis, often associated with renal pelvic dilation.

Other renal and perirenal disorders

Renal parasites

Dioctophyma renale is a parasitic nematode of fish-eating mammals, which can be found in dogs (see Chapter 74) (Low 1995). Ultrasonographic findings in a dog with two parasites residing in the right kidney have been described (Soler et al. 2008). The affected kidney was enlarged and deformed, and there were multiple ring-like structures in the pelvis of the right kidney measuring between 5 and 10 mm in diameter. These structures had a double-layer wall: the outer was hyperechoic and the inner hypoechoic, containing internal echos. In the longitudinal plane, these ring-like structures were visualized as bands, with alternating hypo- and hyperechoic layers. The kidney was outlined by a thin hyperechoic rim.

Perinephric pseudocysts

Large anechoic fluid filled cystic structures are occasionally seen in cats (Essman et al. 2000) and rarely in dogs (Miles and Jergens 1992). Clinical signs are variable, but renal dysfunction is common (Beck et al. 2000). These cases are usually easily differentiated from retroperitoneal or abdominal effusion on ultrasound due to an echogenic capsule surrounding the anechoic fluid (Figure 16.13).

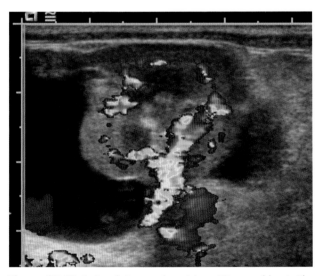

Figure 16.13 Perinephric pseudocyst in a 13-year-old cat. The kidney is smaller than normal but otherwise of normal architecture. A well-circumscribed anechoic area with a thin hyperechoic lining is seen surrounding the kidney.

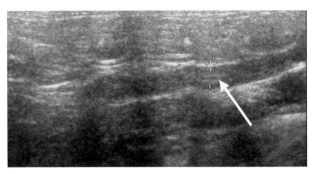

Figure 16.14 Ureteritis in a dog with chronic urinary tract infection. The ureter (between cursors) is thickened (total thickness 0.37 cm including both walls and lumen). The lumen contains a minimal amount of urine (arrow).

Acquired ureteral disorders

Ureteral calculi are a relatively common problem especially in cats (see Chapter 58) (Kyles et al. 2005). They may be difficult to identify on ultrasonographic evaluation alone, especially if they are small and nonobstructive, or if overlying colonic contents hamper evaluation. When combining radiography and ultrasonography, the sensitivity to detect ureterolithiasis in cats has been reported to reach 90% (Kyles et al. 2005). Ultrasonographically, ureteroliths appear as rounded to irregular hyperechoic luminal structures (Figure 16.4). Distal shadowing is seen if the calculus is large enough and if a high frequency transducer is used. Several migrating ureteroliths may be present, necessitating a detailed examination of the entire region of each ureter, from renal pelvis to the level of the bladder (d'Anjou 2008). Concurrent dilation of the ureter proximal to the calculus and hydronephrosis suggest obstructive ureterolithiasis; however, differentiation between partial or intermittent and complete obstruction may be difficult.

Inflammation of the ureters (ureteritis) is seldom recognized except in association with infections involving other portions of the urinary tract (Polzin and Jeraj 1980). Infections may descend from the kidneys or ascend from the urinary bladder. Ureteritis may result in decreased ureteral peristalsis and functional or mechanical ureteral obstruction (Polzin and Jeraj 1980; Crawford and Turk 1984). Ultrasonographically, fluid accumulation within the ureters or wall thickening may occasionally be seen, although are rare in our experience (Figure 16.14). Concurrent changes compatible with pyelonephritis and/or cystitis may be present.

Ureteral neoplasia is very rare. Ultrasound findings in ureteral fibroepithelial polyps have been reported in four older dogs. Findings included renal pelvis and ureteral dilation proximal to the level of an intraluminal mass (Reichle et al. 2003). Ureteral lymphoma has been described in a cat that appeared as a large irregular hypoechoic mass (d'Anjou 2008).

Ureteral rupture is most commonly seen following abdominal trauma. Although ultrasonography may demonstrate signs of renal pelvic and ureteral dilation and retroperitoneal fluid accumulation, it is considered inferior to excretory urography due to inability to distinguish hemorrhage or inflammatory exudate from extravasated urine and inability to identify exact site of rupture (Nyland et al. 2002a; Weisse et al. 2002).

A paraureteral pseudocyst ("urinoma") is a mass formed by encapsulation of extravasated urine secondary to blunt trauma, surgery, or obstruction (McInerney et al. 1977). Imaging findings in a case of a paraureteral urinoma in a dog have been reported. The animal is presented with a palpable mass in the right flank following ovariohysterectomy. Ultrasonographically, a sharply marginated anechoic mass with ipsilateral hydronephrosis and hydroureter was detected caudal to the right kidney (Tidwell et al. 1990).

Retroperitoneal fluid accumulation

Retroperitoneal fluid accumulation is a nonspecific finding and may be encountered in urine leakage, hemorrhage, abscessation, neoplasia, and renal disorders (Stoneham et al. 2004). While larger volumes appear as anechoic or hypoechoic areas in the vicinity of the kidneys, smaller volumes may appear as thin anechoic or hypoechoic striations within hyperechoic retroperitoneal fat. Dependent on the underlying disease process and the amount of effusion, fluid can be found unilaterally or bilaterally. If urine leakage due to kidney or ureteral rupture is of concern, excretory urography is indicated to identify the lesion. Retroperitoneal hemorrhage may be found after trauma, in animals with coagulopathy or due to a bleeding retroperitoneal tumor (renal, ureteral, adrenal). Renal and other retroperitoneal abscesses can rupture and result in accumulation of inflammatory exudate in the retroperitoneal space. Retroperitoneal neoplasms can result in effusion either due to hemorrhage, ureteral obstruction, or interference with lymphatic drainage of the retroperitoneal space. Perinephric fluid accumulation has been described in dogs and cats with acute renal failure due to nephrotoxicity, leptospirosis, ureteral obstruction, renal lymphoma, ureteronephrolithiasis, prostatic urethral obstruction, and interstitial nephritis and ureteritis (Holloway and O'Brien 2007). Perirenal fluid developing in acute renal failure is thought to be an ultrafiltrate associated with tubular back-leak into the renal interstitium, which overwhelms lymphatic drainage within the perirenal and retroperitoneal connective tissues although obstruction to urine flow may also play a role.

Urinary bladder and urethra

Normal sonographic anatomy

The urinary bladder is found in the caudoventral abdomen and can vary greatly in normal size due to distention with urine. An empty bladder may be difficult to find in some cases, and mild to moderate distention is desirable for examination of the bladder. The bladder can be located on the ventral midline or along either side of the caudal abdomen depending on the position of the patient, distention of the bladder, and colon. The colon lies dorsal or dorsolateral to the bladder and often indents the bladder wall when the bladder is not fully distended. The bladder wall becomes thinner as the bladder distends, and wall thickness should be measured when the bladder is adequately distended. Normal wall thickness should be less than 2 mm in normal dogs, with larger dogs having a slightly thicker wall than smaller dogs (Geisse et al. 1997). Normal bladder wall thickness varies from 1.3 to 1.7 mm in cats (Finn-Bodner 1995). Wall thickness measurements of an empty bladder are significantly thicker and are not reliable. Lower frequency transducers show the bladder wall as a single echogenic line; however, current high frequency transducers typically show three distinct bladder wall layers. The normal wall is seen as two echogenic layers separated by a hypoechoic layer. The trigone is not observably different than the remainder of the bladder wall. Normal ureteral papillae may be seen in some bladders as small focal smooth thickening of the dorsal wall and should not be confused with abnormal wall thickening or a bladder mass (Douglass 1993). Ureteral "jetting" of urine may on occasion be observed and helps identifying the ureteral openings (Figure 16.15). The position of the neck of the bladder varies with individual anatomy and degree of distension of the bladder. Position of the bladder neck within the pelvic canal in some dogs makes complete evaluation difficult due to overlying bone and colon.

Normal dog and cat urine is typically anechoic. Echogenic debris seen in the urine may be due to crystals, protein, cells, cellular debris, calculi, or fat droplets, and urinalysis is necessary for evaluation of the clinical significance.

The urethra extends from an ill-defined juncture with the bladder neck into the pelvic canal as a hypoechoic tubular structure that can be viewed in transverse and longitudinal planes. The urethra of the cat typically extends further cranial in the abdomen. Normally, the lumen of the urethra does not contain observable fluid.

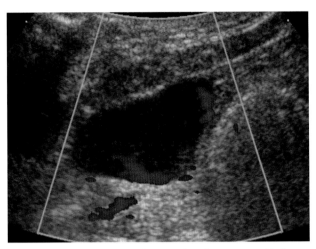

Figure 16.15 Transverse color Doppler ultrasonographic image of the bladder in a young dog demonstrating "jetting" of urine from both ureteral papillae.

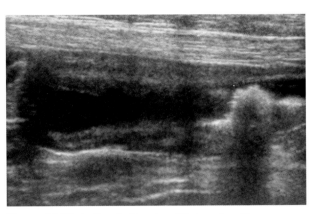

Figure 16.16 Cystic calculi and cystitis in a dog. There are several irregular marginated uroliths with distal shadowing associated with the bladder neck. Although distension of the bladder is less than usually desired for evaluation of wall thickness, severe wall thickening (7 mm) and irregularity of the mucosal surface is consistent with cystitis.

The entire intrapelvic urethra is not usually visualized due to overlying pelvic bone and shadowing from rectal contents. The pelvic urethra may be observable through the obturator foramen in some cases. Transrectal imaging of the urethra can be performed but requires expensive specialized transducers. In male dogs, the prostatic and penile urethra may be evaluated from a perineal and/or ventral approach. Although the mucosal margin of the urethra is best assessed by positive contrast urethrography, ultrasound offers complementary information and can be used to assess urethral thickness and echogenicity (Hanson and Tidwell 1996).

Disorders of the urinary bladder and urethra

Congenital disorders

Congenital disorders of the urinary bladder include patent urachus and bladder (urachal) diverticulum (see Chapter 80) (Confer and Panciera 2001). While patent urachus is uncommon in small animals, urachal diverticula are occasionally found. These occur due to incomplete closure of the bladder musculature during postpartum regression of the urachus, resulting in an outpouching of the cranioventral aspect of the urinary bladder wall. Urine stasis in this diverticulum can occur, predisposing the animal to cystitis or urinary calculi. Ultrasonographically, a urachal diverticulum appears as thin-walled convex outpouching of the bladder wall at the level of the apex, although a thick and irregular wall may be noted in cases of chronic cystitis (Sutherland-Smith 2008). A case of a bladder diverticulum at the level of the trigone has been reported in a 14-month-old dog with chronic recurrent urinary tract infection and emphysematous cystitis (Lobetti and Goldin 1998).

Acquired disorders

Cystitis and urethritis

Cystitis (see Chapter 71) is common in dogs and cats. In early or mild cases, the ultrasonographic examination may be unremarkable. In chronic and more severe cases, diffuse thickening of the urinary bladder wall is the most common finding, which is most severe in the cranioventral portion of the bladder (Léveillé 1998). Additional findings might include echogenic urine due to presence of inflammatory products and/or hemorrhage, mineral sediment, or cystic calculi (Figure 16.16).

Polypoid cystitis is a rare disease of the urinary bladder in dogs characterized by inflammation, epithelial proliferation, and development of a polypoid to pedunculated mass or masses without histopathologic evidence of neoplasia (Martinez et al. 2003; Takiguchi and Inaba 2005). Concurrent cystic calculi are common. Most of the masses are located cranioventrally in the bladder as opposed to transitional cell carcinoma, which has a predilection for the bladder neck or trigone area. However, since bladder neoplasia cannot be excluded based on ultrasonographic appearance, biopsy may be warranted to establish a definitive diagnosis.

Emphysematous cystitis due to infection with gas-producing bacteria such as *Escherichia coli* or Clostridium species is most commonly seen in dogs with diabetes mellitus but may affect other animals. Ultrasonographically, gas inclusions in the wall appear as multifocal hyperechoic areas with distal reverberation artifacts (Petite et al. 2006) (Figure 16.17). Care must be taken to distinguish these pathologic gas accumulations from intraluminal gas introduced during cystocentesis, catheterization, or endoscopy. This can be accomplished by repositioning

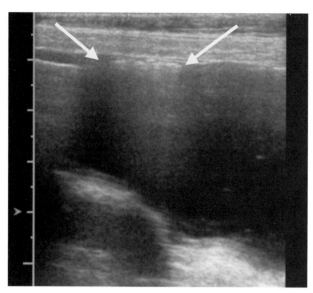

Figure 16.17 Emphysematous cystitis in a 13-year-old dog with chronic urinary tract infection. There are numerous hyperechoic foci associated with the bladder wall (arrows), which show distal reverberation artifacts ("dirty shadowing").

the dog; while free luminal gas will move with change in patient position, gas within the wall will remain static (Sutherland-Smith 2008).

Urethritis is uncommon in small animals and is usually associated with cystitis, prostatitis, or vaginitis (Polzin and Jeraj 1980). Granulomatous urethritis results in diffuse and irregular thickening of the urethra and may mimic urethral neoplasia (Moroff et al. 1991).

Calculi

Cystic calculi (see Chapter 69) are common in small animals, and various mineral types can be encountered (struvite, calcium oxalate, urate, cystine, silica, calcium phosphate, and mixed) (Lulich et al. 2000; Osborne et al. 2000). Bladder stones appear as single or multiple strongly hyperechoic structures of variable size and shape (Figure 16.16). Dependent on size of the calculus and transducer frequency, distal shadowing may be present (Weichselbaum et al. 2000). Sensitivity of ultrasonographic examination for the detection of cystic calculi is high and similar to double contrast cystography if using a high-frequency (7.5 MHz or above) transducer. However, if a lower frequency (5 MHz or lower) transducer is used, false-negative results are common especially with small stones (Weichselbaum et al. 1999). Possible concurrent findings in animals with bladder stones include bladder wall thickening, uroliths associated with kidneys, ureters, or urethra, and inflammatory renal changes (pyelectasia, hyperechogenicity of renal cortices, etc.).

Urinary calculi may become lodged in the urethra and result in partial or complete urethral obstruction. If the calculus is located in the intraabdominal portion of the urethra or in the penile urethra in male dogs, it can usually be visualized by means of ultrasonography. Distension of the visible portion of the urethra and failure to visualize an obstructive lesion necessitates further imaging (positive contrast urethrography), since the entire length of urethra cannot be reliably investigated by means of ultrasonography.

Neoplasia

Transitional cell carcinoma is the most common bladder tumor (see Chapter 79) (Knapp 2007). Other epithelial tumors include transitional cell papillomas, squamous cell carcinomas, adenocarcinomas, and undifferentiated carcinomas. Mesenchymal tumors are less common and include fibromas, fibrosarcomas, leiomyomas, leiomyosarcomas, rhabdomyosarcomas, lymphosarcomas, hemangiomas, and hemangiosarcomas (Confer and Panciera 2001). Cystic transitional cell carcinomas are usually sessile, irregularly shaped masses of variable echogenicity (Léveillé et al. 1992). They are most commonly located at the level of the trigone but may be found in any location. Dependent on size and location, uni- or bilateral ureteral obstruction or urethral obstruction may be present (Figure 16.18). Diffuse infiltration of the bladder wall instead of formation of a distinct mass is less common but possible (Sutherland-Smith 2008).

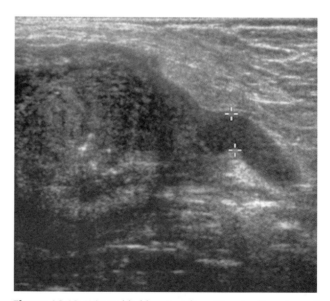

Figure 16.18 Urinary bladder mass (transitional cell carcinoma) in an 11-year-old Shetland sheepdog. There is a large mixed echogenic mass occupying almost the entire lumen of the urinary bladder and resulting in obstruction of the left ureter (between cursors).

Metastases to regional lymph nodes (medial iliac lymph nodes) or vertebral bodies of the lumbar spine may be present at time of diagnosis, and thorough evaluation of these structures is important if bladder neoplasia is suspected. Smooth muscle tumors of the urinary bladder have been reported as smoothly marginated hypoechoic or heterogeneous masses (Heng et al. 2006; Sutherland-Smith 2008). Lymphoma of the urinary bladder wall causes masses of variable echogenicity, size, and location (Benigni et al. 2006). Concurrent ureteral obstruction and lymphadenopathy are common, and differentiation from other tumor types is not possible by means of ultrasonography. Hemangiosarcoma of the bladder has been reported to appear as a large potentially cavitary mass of mixed echogenicity in the caudal abdomen, the origin of which might be difficult to determine (Liptak et al. 2004; Sutherland-Smith 2008). Fibrosarcoma of the urinary bladder in a young dog appeared as a focal multilobulated thickening of the urinary bladder wall. The solid mass originated from the area of the ureteral papillae and bulged into the lumen of the bladder neck (Olausson et al. 2005). A mast cell tumor of the bladder wall has been described as a highly vascular pedunculated mixed echogenic mass (Sutherland-Smith 2008).

Most urethral tumors are malignant epithelial tumors (transitional cell carcinoma or squamous cell carcinoma); smooth muscle tumors are less frequently reported (Davies and Read 1990). Transitional cell carcinoma results in hypoechogenicity and irregular thickening of the urethra, with a hyperechoic line along the epithelial surface (Hanson and Tidwell 1996) (Figure 16.19). Possible concurrent findings include abnormalities of bladder and prostatic gland, hydronephrosis, and medial iliac lymph node enlargement. A case of urethral hemangiosarcoma has been reported in a dog (Mellanby et al. 2004). Ultrasonographic examination revealed a

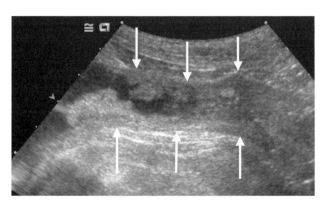

Figure 16.19 Urethral mass (transitional cell carcinoma) in an 11-year-old Schnauzer. The sagittal image of the urethra (between arrows) demonstrates mural thickening and severe mucosal irregularity, with numerous variably sized urethral nodules and masses.

4×4 cm mass within the pelvic canal. An extraskeletal osteosarcoma of the penile urethra was described in a dog, which appeared as a hyperechoic mass with distal shadowing (Sutherland-Smith 2008). Neoplasms of structures bordering the urethra, such as prostate, os penis, or vagina/uterus, may involve the urethra (Mirkovic et al. 2004; Suzuki et al. 2006; Winter et al. 2006), and origin of the disease process may not be obvious in some cases.

Since there is overlap in the ultrasonographic appearance of various bladder/urethral tumors as well as tumors and inflammatory conditions (polypoid cystitis/granulomatous urethritis), biopsy is necessary for a definitive diagnosis.

Mural and luminal hemorrhage

Numerous causes of hematuria (see Chapter 46) have been described in dogs and cats, including trauma, urolithiasis, neoplasia, inflammatory disorders, parasites, coagulopathy, renal infarction, renal pelvic hematoma, and vascular malformation (DiBartola 2000b). Regardless of the underlying cause, urine will appear more echogenic than normal, and sedimentation of echogenic particles may be noted. Luminal blood clots are generally hyperechoic to surrounding urine and range from thin linear structures to large masses (Sutherland-Smith 2008). Color Doppler examination is helpful in distinguishing blood clots from inflammatory or neoplastic masses. Diffuse thickening of the bladder wall secondary to mural hemorrhage has been described in dogs with systemic bleeding disorders (O'Brien and Wood 1998). Focal wall thickening can be encountered in case of focal hematomas, for example, following cystocentesis. Since intraluminal and intramural hemorrhage are variable in appearance and may mimic inflammatory as well as neoplastic conditions, recheck ultrasonographic examination may be indicated to confirm suspicion of hemorrhage and rule out concurrent or underlying abnormalities.

Rupture

Although the use of contrast cystosonography has been described as a sensitive tool for bladder rupture (see Chapter 82), positive contrast cystography provides more information on location of the rupture than ultrasound (Côté et al. 2002; Nyland et al. 2002a). Similarly, urethrography is considered superior to ultrasonography for the diagnosis of urethral rupture.

Foreign bodies

While cystic foreign bodies in humans are not uncommon and are usually self-inflicted (Kochakarn and

Pummanagura 2008), they are very rare in animals. Potential causes include migration of foreign material from other organs (Morshead 1983; Houston and Eaglesome 1999; Wyatt et al. 1999), bullets or BBs (Nyland et al. 2002a), and urinary catheter fragments after catheter failure.

Ultrasound-assisted interventional procedures

The use of ultrasound guidance has become routine for many interventional procedures of the urinary tract assisting in accurate placement of devices and sample sites. Fine-needle aspirations using 20- to 25-gauge needles can usually be performed with minimal sedation and with minimal risk of complications (see Chapter 26). Core biopsy of the kidneys using 16- to 18-gauge automated needles usually requires general anesthesia and is associated with a higher rate of complications (see Chapter 23). Complication rates of 9% in dogs and 15% in cats have been reported. Hemorrhage is the most common complication (Vaden et al. 2005). Larger needle sizes provide better samples but are associated with higher risk of hemorrhage (Rawlings et al. 2003). Increased risk of complications has been observed in older dogs and dogs with severe azotemia (Vaden et al. 2005). No measurable change in renal functions was detected following renal biopsy in healthy cats and dogs (Drost et al. 2000b; Groman et al. 2004). Neoplasia such as lymphoma in cats can often be diagnosed with cytologic specimens from fine-needle aspirations. Fine-needle aspirates of infectious diseases may help identify the presence of organisms and provide culture samples. For chronic inflammatory or degenerative changes of the kidneys, biopsy is usually necessary to obtain sufficient tissue for evaluation.

Ultrasound guided cystocentesis (see Chapter 5) is routinely performed and is especially helpful in obese patients or for obtaining samples from mildly distended bladders. Fine-needle aspiration of a dilated renal pelvis (see Chapter 6) may provide samples for evaluation as well as means of infusing radiopaque water-soluble organic iodine contrast media (antegrade pyelography) for subsequent evaluation by radiography in cases where routine excretory urography is not possible or a diagnosis of ureteral obstruction cannot be achieved by other means (Rivers et al. 1997; Adin et al. 2003).

Fine-needle aspirates of cavitary lesions such as cysts or abscesses may be performed to provide diagnostic samples as well as for therapeutic purposes (Ochoa et al. 1999; Szatmári et al. 2001; Agut et al. 2008).

Samples of bladder or urethral masses can be obtained by means of traumatic catheterization ("suction biopsy") instead of percutaneous fine-needle aspiration or biopsy (Lamb et al. 1996). This method is preferred by many

investigators, since needle tract implantation of transitional cell carcinoma has been reported to occur after percutaneous fine-needle aspiration (Nyland et al. 2002b; Vignoli et al. 2007).

References

Adams, W.H., R.L. Toal, et al. (1989). Early renal ultrasonographic findings in dogs with experimentally induced ethylene glycol nephrosis. *Am J Vet Res* **50**(8): 1370–1376.

Adin, C.A., E.J. Herrgesell, et al. (2003). Antegrade pyelography for suspected ureteral obstruction in cats: 11 cases (1995–2001). *J Am Vet Med Assoc* **222**(11): 1576–1581.

Agut, A., M. Soler, et al. (2008). Imaging diagnosis—ultrasound-guided ethanol sclerotherapy for a simple renal cyst. *Vet Radiol Ultrasound* **49**(1): 65–67.

Allworth, M.S. and K.L. Hoffmann (1999). Crossed renal ectopia with fusion in a cat. *Vet Radiol Ultrasound* **40**(4): 357–360.

Barr, F.J., M.W. Patteson, et al. (1989). Hypercalcemic nephropathy in three dogs: sonographic appearance. *Vet Radiol Ultrasound* **30**(4): 169–173.

Barr, F.J., P.E. Holt, et al. (1990). Ultrasonographic measurements of normal renal parameters. *J Small Anim Pract* **31**(4): 180–184.

Barthez, P.Y., R. Leveille, et al. (1997). Side lobes and grating lobes artifacts in ultrasound imaging. *Vet Radiol Ultrasound* **38**(5): 387–393.

Beck, J.A., C.R. Bellenger, et al. (2000). Perirenal pseudocysts in 26 cats. *Aust Vet J* **78**(3): 166–171.

Benigni, L., C.R. Lamb, et al. (2006). Lymphoma affecting the urinary bladder in three dogs and a cat. *Vet Radiol Ultrasound* **47**(6): 592–596.

Biller, D.S., G.A. Bradley, et al. (1992). Renal medullary rim sign: ultrasonographic evidence of renal disease. *Vet Radiol Ultrasound* **33**(5): 286–290.

Bouma, J.L., L.R. Aronson, et al. (2003). Use of computed tomography renal angiography for screening feline renal transplant donors. *Vet Radiol Ultrasound* **44**(6): 636–641.

Cáceres, A.V., A.L. Zwingenberger, et al. (2008). Characterization of normal feline renal vascular anatomy with dual-phase, C.T. angiography. *Vet Radiol Ultrasound* **49**(4): 350–356.

Cartee, R.E., B.A. Selcer, et al. (1980). Ultrasonographic diagnosis of renal disease in small animals. *J Am Vet Med Assoc* **176**(5): 426–430.

Churchill, J.A., D.A. Feeney, et al. (1999). Effects of diet and aging on renal measurements in uninephrectomized geriatric bitches. *Vet Radio Ultrasound* **40**(3): 233–240.

Confer, A.W. and R.J. Panciera. (2001). The urinary system. In: Thomson's Special Veterinary Pathology, *3rd ed*, edited by M.D. McGavin, W.W. Carlton, and J.F. Zachary. St. Louis, MO: Mosby, pp. 235–277.

Côté, E., M.C. Carroll, et al. (2002). Diagnosis of urinary bladder rupture using ultrasound contrast cystography: in vitro model and two case-history reports. *Vet Radiol Ultrasound* **43**(3): 281–286.

Crawford, M.A. and M.A. Turk. (1984). Ureteral obstruction associated with proliferative ureteritis in a dog. *J Am Vet Med Assoc* **184**(5): 586–588.

Cruz-Arámbulo, R., R. Wrigley, et al. (2004). Sonographic features of histiocytic neoplasms in the canine abdomen. *Vet Radiol Ultrasound* **45**(6): 554–558.

D'Anjou, M.A. (2008). Kidneys and ureters. In: *Atlas of Small Animal Ultrasonography*, edited by D.G. Penninck and M.A. d'Anjou. Ames, IA: Blackwell Publishing, pp. 339–364.

Davies, J.V, and H.M. Read. (1990). Urethral tumours in dogs. *J Small Anim Pract* **31**(3): 131–136.

DiBartola, S.P. (2000a). Familial renal disease in dogs and cats. In: Textbook of Veterinary Internal Medicine, *5th ed*, Vol. 2, edited by S.J. Ettinger, and E.C. Feldman. Philadelphia, PA: WB Saunders, pp. 1698–1703.

DiBartola, S.P. (2000b). Clinical approach and laboratory evaluation of renal disease. In: Textbook of Veterinary Internal Medicine, *5th ed*, Vol.2, edited by S.J. Ettinger, and E.C. Feldman. Philadelphia, PA: WB Saunders, pp. 1600–1614.

Diez-Prieto I., M.B. García-Rodríguez, et al. (2001). Diagnosis of renal agenesis in a beagle. *J Small Anim Pract* **42**(12): 599–602.

Douglass, J.P. and F.W. Kremkau. (1993). Ultrasound corner—the urinary bladder wall hypoechoic pseudolesion. *Vet Radiol Ultrasound* **34**(1): 45–46.

Douglass, J.P. (1993). Ultrasound corner—bladder wall mass effect caused by the intramural portion of the canine ureter. *Vet Radiol Ultrasound* **34**(2): 107.

Drost, W.T., G.A. Henry, et al. (2000a). Quantification of hepatic and renal cortical echogenicity in clinically normal cats. *Am J Vet Res* **61**(9): 1016–1020.

Drost, W.T., G.A. Henry, et al. (2000b). The effects of a unilateral ultrasound-guided renal biopsy on renal function in healthy sedated cats. *Vet Radiol Ultrasound* **41**(1): 57–62.

Essman, S.C., W.T. Drost, et al. (2000). Imaging of a cat with perirenal pseudocysts. *Vet Radiol Ultrasound* **41**(4): 329–334.

Esterline, M.L., D.S. Biller, et al. (2005). Ureteral duplication in a dog. *Vet Radiol Ultrasound* **46**(6): 485–489.

Felkai, C.S., K. Voros, et al. (1992). Ultrasonographic determination of renal volume in the dog. *Vet Radiol Ultrasound* **33**(5): 292–296.

Felkai C., K. Vörös, et al. (1995). Lesions of the renal pelvis and proximal ureter in various nephro-urological conditions: an ultrasonographic study. *Vet Radiol Ultrasound* **36**(5): 397–401.

Finco, D.R. (1995). Congenital, inherited and familial renal diseases. In: *Canine and Feline Nephrology and Urology*, edited by C.A. Osborne, and D.R. Finco. Baltimore: Williams & Wilkins, pp. 471–483.

Fink, R.L., D.T. Caridis, et al. (1980). Renal impairment and its reversibility following variable periods of complete ureteric obstruction. *Aust N Z J Surg* **50**(1): 77–83.

Finn-Bodner, S.T. (1995). The urinary bladder. In: *Practical Veterinary Ultrasound*, edited by R.E. Cartee, B.A. Selcer, J.A. Hudson, et al. Philadelphia, PA: Lea and Febiger, pp. 210–235.

Forrest, L.J., R.T. O'Brien, et al. (1998). Sonographic renal findings in 20 dogs with leptospirosis. *Vet Radiol Ultrasound* **39**(4): 337–340.

Gabor, L.J., R. Malik, et al. (1998). Clinical and anatomical features of lymphosarcoma in 118 cats. *Aust Vet J* **76**(11): 725–732.

Geisse, A.L., J.E. Lowry, et al. (1997). Sonographic evaluation of urinary bladder wall thickness in normal dogs. *Vet Radiol Ultrasound* **38**(2): 132–137.

Gleason, P.E., P.P. Kelalis, et al. (1994). Hydronephrosis in renal ectopia: incidence, etiology and significance. *J Urol* **151**(6): 1660–1661.

Groman, R.P., A. Bahr, et al. (2004). Effects of serial ultrasound-guided renal biopsies on kidneys of healthy adolescent dogs. *Vet Radiol Ultrasound* **45**(1): 62–69.

Hanson, J.A. and A.S. Tidwell. (1996). Ultrasonographic appearance of urethral transitional cell carcinoma in ten dogs. *Vet Radiol Ultrasound* **37**(4): 293–299.

Hardie, E.M. and A.E. Kyles. (2004). Management of ureteral obstruction. *Vet Clin North Am Small Anim Pract* **34**: 989–1010.

Hartzband, L.E., A.S. Tidwell, et al. (1991). Relative echogenicity of the renal cortex and liver in normal dogs (abstract). *Br J Radiol* **64**: 654.

Hecht, S., R.J. McCarthy, et al. (2005). What is you diagnosis? Ectopic kidney in a cat. *J Am Vet Med Assoc* **227**(2): 223–224.

Heng, H.G., J.E. Lowry, et al. (2006). Smooth muscle neoplasia of the urinary bladder wall in three dogs. *Vet Radiol Ultrasound* **47**(1): 83–86.

Holloway, A. and R. O'Brien. (2007). Perirenal effusion in dogs and cats with acute renal failure. *Vet Radiol Ultrasound* **48**(6): 574–579.

Houston, D.M. and H. Eaglesome. (1999). Unusual case of foreign body-induced struvite urolithiasis in a dog. *Can Vet J* **40**(2): 125–126.

Hylands, R. (2006). Veterinary diagnostic imaging. Retroperitoneal abscess and regional cellulitis secondary to a pyelonephritis within the left kidney. *Can Vet J* **47**(10): 1033–1035.

Ivancić, M. and W. Mai. (2008). Qualitative and quantitative comparison of renal vs. hepatic ultrasonographic intensity in healthy dogs. *Vet Radiol Ultrasound* **49**(4): 368–373.

Kealy, J.K. and H. McAllister. (2005). The abdomen. In: Diagnostic Radiology & Ultrasonography of the Dog and Cat, *4th ed*, edited by J.K. Kealy and H. McAllister. St. Louis, MO: Elsevier Saunders, pp. 21–172.

Kirberger, R.M. (1995). Imaging artifacts in diagnostic ultrasound: a review. *Vet Radiol Ultrasound* **36**(4): 297–306.

Klein, M.K., G.L. Cockerell, et al. (1988). Canine primary renal neoplasms: a retrospective review of 54 cases. *J Am Anim Hosp Assoc* **24**: 443–452.

Knapp, D.W. (2007). Tumors of the urinary system. In: Small Animal Clinical Oncology, *4th ed*, edited by S.J. Withrow and D.M. Vail. St. Louis: Saunders Elsevier, pp. 649–658.

Kochakarn, W. and W. Pummanagura. (2008). Foreign bodies in the female urinary bladder: 20-year experience in Ramathibodi Hospital. *Asian J Surg* **31**(3): 130–133.

Konde, L.J., R.H. Wrigley, et al. (1984). Ultrasonographic anatomy of the normal canine kidney. *Vet Radiol* **25**(4): 173–178.

Konde, L.J., R.H. Wrigley, et al. (1985). Sonographic appearance of renal neoplasia in the dog. *Vet Radiol* **26**(3): 74–81.

Konde, L.J., R.D. Park, et al. (1986). Comparison of radiography and ultrasonography in the evaluation of renal lesions in the dog. *J Am Vet Med Assoc* **188**(12): 1420–1425.

Kremkau, F.W. (1995). *Doppler Ultrasound—Principles and Instruments*, *2nd ed*. Philadelphia, PA: WB Saunders.

Kremkau, F.W. (2002). Diagnostic Ultrasound—Principles and Instruments, *6th ed*. Philadelphia, PA: WB Saunders.

Kyles, A.E., E.M. Hardie, et al. (2005). Clinical, clinicopathologic, radiographic, and ultrasonographic abnormalities in cats with ureteral calculi: 163 cases (1984–2002). *J Am Vet Med Assoc* **226**(6): 932–936.

Lamb, C.R., N.D. Trower, et al. (1996). Ultrasound-guided catheter biopsy of the lower urinary tract: technique and results in 12 dogs. *J Small Anim Pract* **37**(9): 413–416.

Lamb, C.R. and S.P. Gregory. (1998). Ultrasonographic findings in 14 dogs with ectopic ureter. *Vet Radiol Ultrasound* **39**(3): 218–223.

Lamb, C.R. (1998). Ultrasonography of the ureters. *Vet Clin North Am Small Anim Pract* **28**(4): 823–848.

Léveillé, R., D.S. Biller, et al. (1992). Sonographic investigation of transitional cell carcinoma of the urinary bladder in small animals. *Vet Radiol Ultrasound* **33**(2): 103–107.

Léveillé, R. (1998). Ultrasonography of urinary bladder disorders. *Vet Clin North Am Small Anim Pract* **28**(4): 799–821.

Liptak, J.M., W.S. Dernell, et al. (2004). Haemangiosarcoma of the urinary bladder in a dog. *Aust Vet J* **82**(4): 215–217.

Lium, B. and L. Moe. (1985). Hereditary multifocal renal cystadenocarcinomas and nodular dermatofibrosis in the German shepherd dog: macroscopic and histopathologic findings. *Vet Pathol* **22**(5): 447–455.

Lobetti, R.G. and J.P. Goldin. (1998). Emphysematous cystitis and bladder trigone diverticulum in a dog. *J Small Anim Pract* **39**(3): 144–147.

Locke, J.E. and L.G. Barber. (2006). Comparative aspects and clinical outcomes of canine renal hemangiosarcoma. *J Vet Intern Med* **20**(4): 962–967.

Louvet, A. (2006). Twinkling artifact in small animal color-Doppler sonography. *Vet Radiol Ultrasound* **47**(4): 384–390.

Low, D.G. (1995). Parasites of the upper and lower urinary tract of dogs and cats. In: *Canine and feline nephrology and urology*, edited by C.A. Osborne and D.R. Finco. Philadelphia, PA: Williams and Wilkins, pp. 917–921.

Lulich, J.P., C.A. Osborne, et al. (1987). Urologic disorders of immature cats. *Vet Clin North Am Small Anim Pract* **17**(3): 663–696.

Lulich, J.P., C.A. Osborne, et al. (2000). Canine lower urinary tract diseases. In: Textbook of Veterinary Internal Medicine, *5th ed, Vol. 2*, edited by S.J. Ettinger and E.C. Feldman. Philadelphia, PA: WB Saunders, pp. 1747–1781.

Mantis, P. and C.R. Lamb. (2000). Most dogs with medullary rim sign on ultrasonography have no demonstrable renal dysfunction. *Vet Radiol Ultrasound* **41**(2): 164–166.

Mareschal, A., M.A. d'Anjou, et al. (2007). Ultrasonographic measurement of kidney-to-aorta ratio as a method of estimating renal size in dogs. *Vet Radiol Ultrasound* **48**(5): 434–438.

Martinez, I., J.S. Mattoon, et al. (2003). Polypoid cystitis in 17 dogs (1978–2001). *J Vet Intern Med* **17**(4): 499–509.

Maxie, M.G. (1993). The urinary system. In: *Pathology of Domestic Animals*, 4th ed, edited by K.V.F. Jubb, P.C. Kennedy and N. Palmer. San Diego: Academic Press, pp. 447–538.

McInerney, D., A. Jones et al. (1977). Urinoma. *Clin Radiol* **28**(3): 345–351.

McLoughlin, M.A., J.G. Haupman, et al. (1989). Canine ureteroceles: a case report and literature review. *J Am Anim Hosp Assoc* **25**: 699–706.

McLoughlin, M.A. and D.J. Chew. (2000). Diagnosis and surgical management of ectopic ureters. *Clin Tech Small Anim Pract* **15**(1): 17–24.

Mellanby, R.J., J.C. Chantrey, et al. (2004). Urethral haemangiosarcoma in a boxer. *J Small Anim Pract* **45**(3): 154–156.

Miles, K.G. and A.E. Jergens. (1992). Unilateral perinephric pseudocyst of undetermined origin in a dog. *Vet Radiol Ultrasound* **33**(5): 277–281.

Mirkovic, T.K., C.L. Shmon, et al. (2004). Urinary obstruction secondary to an ossifying fibroma of the os penis in a dog. *J Am Anim Hosp Assoc* **40**: 152–156.

Moroff, S.D., B.A. Brown, et al. (1991). Infiltrative urethral disease in female dogs: 41 cases (1980–1987). *J Am Vet Med Assoc* **199**(2): 247–251.

Morshead, D. (1983). Submucosal urethral calculus secondary to foxtail awn migration in a dog. *J Am Vet Med Assoc* **182**(11): 1247–1248.

Neuwirth, L., M. Mahaffey, et al. (1993). Comparison of excretory urography and ultrasonography for detection of experimentally induced pyelonephritis in dogs. *Am J Vet Res* **54**(5): 660–669.

Nyland, T.G., B.M. Kantrowitz, et al. (1989). Ultrasonic determination of kidney volume in the dog. *Vet Radiol* **30**(4): 174–180.

Nyland, T.G., P.E. Fisher, et al. (1993). Diagnosis of urinary tract obstruction in dogs using duplex Doppler ultrasonography. *Vet Radiol Ultrasound* **34**(5): 348–352.

Nyland, T.G., J.S. Mattoon, et al. (2002a). Urinary tract. In: *Small Animal Diagnostic Ultrasound*, 2nd ed, edited by T.G. Nyland and J.S. Mattoon. Philadelphia, PA: WB Saunders, pp. 158–195.

Nyland, T.G., S.T. Wallack, et al. (2002b). Needle-tract implantation following us-guided fine-needle aspiration biopsy of transitional cell carcinoma of the bladder, urethra, and prostate. *Vet Radiol Ultrasound* **43**(1): 50–53.

O'Brien, R.T. and E.F. Wood. (1998). Urinary bladder mural hemorrhage associated with systemic bleeding disorders in three dogs. *Vet Radiol Ultrasound* **39**(4): 354–356.

Ochoa, V.B., S.P. DiBartola, et al. (1999). Perinephric pseudocysts in the cat: a retrospective study and review of the literature. *J Vet Intern Med* **13**(1): 47–55.

Olausson, A., S.M. Stieger, et al. (2005). A urinary bladder fibrosarcoma in a young dog. *Vet Radiol Ultrasound* **46**(2): 135–138.

Oglesby, P.A. and A. Carter. (2003). Ultrasonographic diagnosis of unilateral ectopic ureter in a Labrador dog. *J S Afr Vet Assoc* **74**(3): 84–86.

Osborne, C.A., G.R. Johnston, et al. (1995). Ectopic ureters and ureteroceles. In: *Canine and Feline Nephrology and Urology*, edited by C.A. Osborne and D.R. Finco. Baltimore: Williams and Wilkins, pp. 608–622.

Osborne, C.A., J.M. Kruger, et al. (2000). Feline lower urinary tract diseases. In: *Textbook of Veterinary Internal Medicine*, 5th ed., Vol. 2., edited by S.J. Ettinger and E.C. Feldman. Philadelphia, PA: WB Saunders, pp. 1710–1747.

Penninck, D.G. (2002). Artifacts. In: *Small Animal Diagnostic Ultrasound*, 2nd ed., edited by T.G. Nyland and J.S. Mattoon. Philadelphia, PA: WB Saunders Company, pp. 19–29.

Petite, A., V. Busoni, et al. (2006). Radiographic and ultrasonographic findings of emphysematous cystitis in four nondiabetic female dogs. *Vet Radiol Ultrasound* **47**(1): 90–93.

Polzin, D.J. and K. Jeraj. (1980). Urethritis, cystitis, and ureteritis. *Vet Clin North Am Small Anim Pract* **9**(4): 661–678.

Pugh, C.R., C.G. Schelling, et al. (1994). Iatrogenic renal pyelectasia in the dog. *Vet Radiol Ultrasound* **35**(1): 50–51.

Ramirez, S., J.P. Douglass, et al. (2002). Ultrasonographic features of canine abdominal malignant histiocytosis. *Vet Radiol Ultrasound* **43**(2): 167–170.

Rawlings, C.A., H. Diamond, et al. (2003). Diagnostic quality of percutaneous kidney biopsy specimens obtained with laparoscopy versus ultrasound guidance in dogs. *J Am Vet Med Assoc* **223**(3): 317–321.

Reichle, J.K., S.P. DiBartola, et al. (2002). Renal ultrasonographic and computed tomographic appearance, volume, and function of cats with autosomal dominant polycystic kidney disease. *Vet Radiol Ultrasound* **43**(4): 368–373.

Reichle, J.K., R.A. Peterson, et al. (2003). Ureteral fibroepithelial polyps in four dogs. *Vet Radiol Ultrasound* **44**(4): 433–437.

Rivers, B.J., P.A. Walter, et al. (1997). Ultrasonographic-guided, percutaneous antegrade pyelography: technique and clinical application in the dog and cat. *J Am Anim Hosp Assoc* **33**: 61–68.

Sato, A.F. and M. Solano. (2004). Ultrasonographic findings in abdominal mast cell disease: a retrospective study of 19 patients. *Vet Radiol Ultrasound* **45**(1): 51–57.

Shiroma, J.T., J.K. Gabriel, et al. (1999). Effect of reproductive status on feline renal size. *Vet Radiol Ultrasound* **40**(3): 242–245.

Soler, M., L. Cardoso, et al. (2008). Imaging diagnosis-dioctophyma renale in a dog. *Vet Radiol Ultrasound* **49**(3): 307–308.

Stiffler, K.S., M.A.M. Stevenson, et al. (2002). Intravesical ureterocele with concurrent renal dysfunction in a dog: a case report and proposed classification system. *J Am Anim Hosp Assoc* **38**: 33–39.

Stoneham, A.E., T.E. O'Toole, et al. (2004). Retroperitoneal effusion in dogs and cats. *J Vet Emerg Crit Care* **14**(S1): S1–S17.

Sutherland-Smith, J. (2008). Bladder and urethra. In: *Atlas of Small Animal Ultrasonography*, edited by D.G. Penninck and M.A. d'Anjou. Ames TA: Blackwell Publishing, pp. 365–384.

Suzuki, K., K. Nakatani, et al. (2006). Vaginal rhabdomyosarcoma in a dog. *Vet Pathol* **43**(2): 186–188.

Szatmári, V., Z. Osi, et al. (2001). Ultrasound-guided percutaneous drainage for treatment of pyonephrosis in two dogs. *J Am Vet Med Assoc* **218**(11): 1796–1799, 1778–1779.

Takiguchi, M., J. Yasuda, et al. (1997). Ultrasonographic appearance of orthotopic ureterocele in a dog. *Vet Radiol Ultrasound* **38**(5): 398–399.

Takiguchi, M. and M. Inaba. (2005). Diagnostic ultrasound of polypoid cystitis in dogs. *J Vet Med Sci* **67**(1): 57–61.

Tidwell, A.S., S.L. Ullman, et al. (1990). Urinoma (para-ureteral pseudocyst) in a dog. *Vet Radiol Ultrasound* **31**(4): 203–206.

Vaden, S.L., J.F. Levine, et al. (2005). Renal biopsy: a retrospective study of methods and complications in 283 dogs and 65 cats. *J Vet Intern Med* **19**(6): 794–801.

Valdés-Martínez, A., R. Cianciolo, et al. (2007). Association between renal hypoechoic subcapsular thickening and lymphosarcoma in cats. *Vet Radiol Ultrasound* **48**(4): 357–360.

Vignoli, M., F. Rossi, et al. (2007). Needle tract implantation after fine needle aspiration biopsy (FNAB) of transitional cell carcinoma of the urinary bladder and adenocarcinoma of the lung. *Schweiz Arch Tierheilkd* **149**(7): 314–318.

Walter, P.A., G.R. Johnston, et al. (1987a). Renal ultrasonography in healthy cats. *Am J Vet Res* **48**(4): 600–607.

Walter, P.A., D.A. Feeney, et al. (1987b). Ultrasonographic evaluation of renal parenchymal diseases in dogs: 32 cases (1981–1986). *J Am Vet Med Assoc* **191**(8): 999–1007.

Walter, P.A., G.R. Johnston, et al. (1988). Applications of ultrasonography in the diagnosis of parenchymal kidney disease in cats: 24 cases (1981–1986). *J Am Vet Med Assoc* **192**(1): 92–98.

Weichselbaum, R.C., D.A. Feeney, et al. (1999). Urocystolith detection: comparison of survey, contrast radiographic and ultrasonographic techniques in an in vitro bladder phantom. *Vet Radiol Ultrasound* **40**(4): 386–400.

Weichselbaum, R.C., D.A. Feeney, et al. (2000). Relevance of sonographic artifacts observed during in vitro characterization of urocystolith mineral composition. *Vet Radiol Ultrasound* **41**(5): 438–446.

Weisse, C., L.R. Aronson, et al. (2002). Traumatic rupture of the ureter: 10 cases. *J Am Anim Hosp Assoc* **38**: 188–192.

Winter, M.D., J.E. Locke, et al. (2006). Imaging diagnosis—urinary obstruction secondary to prostatic lymphoma in a young dog. *Vet Radiol Ultrasound* **47**(6): 597–601.

Wyatt, K.M., A.M. Marchevsky, et al. (1999). An enterovesical foreign body in a dog. *Aust Vet J* **77**(1): 27–29.

Yeager, A.E. and W.I. Anderson. (1989). Study of association between histologic features and echogenicity of architecturally normal cat kidneys. *Am J Vet Res* **50**(6): 860–863.

17

Computed tomography and magnetic resonance imaging of the urinary tract

Alexander G. MacLeod and Erik R. Wisner

The use of computed tomography (CT) and magnetic resonance (MR) imaging in veterinary medicine continues to increase as more specialists and general practitioners gain direct or referral access to these technologies. Radiologists and other specialists have accordingly developed the technical skills and knowledge necessary to interpret these studies in order to determine appropriate therapy and prognosis. Although initially primarily used for neuroimaging, CT and, to a lesser extent, MR are now routinely used for body imaging as well. The urinary tract is particularly suited to CT and MR imaging because of its fixed anatomic position, imaging characteristics, and potential for quantitative and qualitative functional imaging due to predominantly renal excretion of the commonly used CT and MR contrast agents.

Ultrasound imaging (see Chapter 16) has supplanted many but not all survey and contrast radiographic studies of the urinary tract (see Chapter 15). An advantage of ultrasound over radiography is the ability to discriminate the internal architecture of parenchymal organs such as the kidneys and the luminal contents and mural characteristics of hollow viscera, inclusive of the ureters, urinary bladder, and urethra, without the need for intravenous or intraluminal contrast media. However, utility of ultrasound is limited in certain anatomic sites such as the intrapelvic urethra, and it is not possible to qualitatively or quantitatively assess renal function. For reasons such as these, excretory urography and retrograde urethrography continue to be useful for diagnosis and prognosis and for surgical planning.

CT image generation follows the same principles as conventional radiography in that X-rays and iodinated contrast media are used to acquire images. Therefore, comparable contrast radiographic procedures of the urinary tract can be performed and, due to the superior contrast resolution and anatomic detail provided by CT, the specificity and sensitivity of lesion detection and diagnosis are often improved. Because of cost, availability, and inherent challenges to image production, such as respiratory and cardiac motion, MR imaging of the urinary tract has not been used to the same extent as CT. However, MR imaging also has great potential to provide functional and internal anatomic information relating to the urinary tract. A distinct advantage of both CT and MR is the consistency and reproducibility with which diagnostic studies can be produced as compared to ultrasound in which the quality of an imaging study is highly dependent on the expertise of the individual performing the scan. CT and MR images are often easier to interpret than ultrasound images because the relative anatomic relationships are more clearly demonstrated, particularly when imaging data is manipulated by reformatting into other anatomic planes, redefined by using techniques such as maximum intensity projection (MIP) display or rendered as three-dimensional anatomic representations. In conjunction with ultrasound, survey and contrast radiography, and nuclear medicine, CT and MR increase the specificity and sensitivity for a number of urologic disorders. In our experience, CT and MR are most beneficial for refining a presumptive diagnosis and for surgical planning and postoperative evaluation.

Image formation and technical considerations

In almost all cases, the patient is maintained under general anesthesia for the imaging study to facilitate positioning, minimize patient motion, and to allow for

Nephrology and Urology of Small Animals. Edited by Joe Bartges and David J. Polzin. © 2011 Blackwell Publishing Ltd.

cardiac and/or respiratory gating (MR) or forced breath-hold to eliminate respiratory motion (CT). For both CT and MR imaging, standard imaging protocols should generally include both pre- and postcontrast acquisitions. This is particularly important in CT imaging to distinguish parenchymal or luminal mineral opacities that might be evident on precontrast images from increased density due to soft tissue or luminal contrast enhancement.

Computed tomography

In CT imaging, the patient is placed on a moving table that passes through the CT gantry as X-rays are transmitted through the patient from a rotating X-ray tube to a detector array. The differential X-ray attenuation from multiple tube positions is collected and processed to form a cross-sectional image of the patient. Because ionizing radiation is the basis for image production, radiation safety precautions must be taken to minimize exposure to both the patient and personnel. As with conventional radiographs, because X-ray photons are used for CT image acquisition, image opacity is directly related to tissue or organ density. The light intensities of pixels that form a digital CT image displayed on a monitor or on print film reflect the underlying tissue densities of the anatomical structures represented on the image. Low-density materials such as air and fat are often referred to as hypodense or hypoattenuating, whereas high-density materials such as bone and contrast-enhancing soft tissues are referred to as hyperdense or hyperattenuating. Because these terms are relative, they are typically used to compare a given structure to a material of neutral density, such as fluid or soft tissue, or used to compare the density of one tissue to an adjacent tissue or structure. Conventional iodinated contrast medium is used for contrast-enhanced CT studies and, as with conventional contrast radiography, results in an increase in tissue density in those structures in which it concentrates. Although both ionic and nonionic iodinated media can be used for CT contrast enhancement, nonionic CT contrast media is recommended if the patient has cardiac or renal insufficiency because it will result in less osmotic hypervolemia. In addition, nonionic contrast agents have been shown to be associated with fewer adverse reactions than ionic agents and should be considered as part of a standard CT imaging protocol even in patients without identified risk factors.

Certain image acquisition parameters can be modified to extract more diagnostic information from the imaging examination. With both CT and MR, decreasing image collimation (decreasing "slice thickness") increases image resolution and reduces partial volume averaging though this may come at the expense of increased radiation exposure (CT) or increased acquisition time (MR) to maintain adequate image quality (Bushberg et al. 2001). Most CT scanners currently being used today are helical scanners in which the imaging data is acquired with the patient moving through the CT gantry at a constant rate as the X-ray tube rotates continuously around the patient. Older single slice helical scanners and newer multiple slice scanners are now in use with the latter, providing faster scan times and better spatial resolution of reformatted images. Within limits, the table movement can be increased while maintaining a given image collimation thickness to increase the volume of anatomy scanned in a single acquisition. This is particularly useful in larger patients in which the entire urinary tract is to be imaged. The relationship of table travel to X-ray tube rotation is referred to as pitch. As pitch increases, larger lengths of anatomy can be imaged with a given number of images of fixed collimation thickness. For example, when imaging the urinary system of a larger dog, one can increase either the slice thickness or the pitch to obtain images from the cranial aspect of the right kidney to the most caudal aspect of the urethra. On the basis of this initial study, more thinly collimated images can be acquired over a specific site to better define a specific organ or structure (Figure 17.1).

CT and MR both provide improved contrast resolution and internal architectural detail when compared to conventional radiography and fluoroscopy (Figure 17.2). Additionally, sequential CT imaging of the kidneys following the administration of iodinated contrast media (CT intravenous pyelogram, [IVP]) allows for a subjective or quantitative assessment of renal function (Figure 17.3). As with conventional IVP, CT image acquisitions can be timed to result in vascular, nephrogram, and pyelogram phases (Figure 17.4). Contrast-enhanced CT images can also reveal or more accurately delineate changes within the renal parenchyma that result in altered blood flow. Qualitative assessment of renal function is made by evaluating the rapidity and degree to which the kidneys contrast enhance and by evaluating the transit of contrast medium through the collecting system. An advantage of CT over conventional IVP is that iodinated contrast medium concentration is linearly related to image density as measured in CT units and therefore a quantitative estimation of glomeruler filtration can be made. However, CT underestimates GFR when compared to plasma clearance and scintigraphy, which is thought to be due to the effects of anesthetic hypotension and possible effects of contrast media on nephron function (O'Dell-Anderson et al. 2006).

Although the spatial resolution of CT is less than that of conventional radiography, the tomographic image

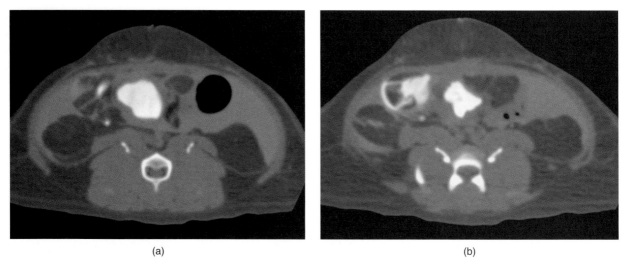

(a)   (b)

Figure 17.1 Four-year-old spayed cat with uroabdomen. (a) 3 mm collimated transverse plane CT image acquired with the patient in dorsal recumbency and following intravenous contrast administration. In addition to the presence of moderate free peritoneal fluid, contrast medium is present in the urinary bladder lumen, the right ureter, and within the right caudal abdomen. (b) 1-mm collimated images were acquired at the level of the urinary bladder to better localize the source of urine leakage. These images show a larger amount of contrast medium in the right caudal peritoneal cavity. Diagnosis: right ureterovesicular avulsion and uroabdomen.

improves characterization of anatomy by minimizing the superimposing effect of adjacent anatomic structures. This, in combination with IV contrast administration, allows for the visualization of small structures such as the ureters and urethra as contrast medium accumulates in the collecting system (Figure 17.5). In normal animals, optimal ureteral opacification with ionic iodinated contrast medium occurs 3–60 minutes following intravenous contrast administration of 400–800 mg iodine/kg (Barthez et al. 1998).

There are relatively few reports on the use of CT for diagnosis of urinary tract disorders. A specific CT protocol has been described for detection and characterization of supernumerary renal blood vessels as a screening test for feline renal donors (Bouma et al. 2003). CT has also been used to characterize hereditary multifocal renal cystadenomas (Moe and Lium 1997) and tumors such as renal carcinoma and nephroblastoma (Figure 17.6) (Yamazoe et al. 1994). In the paper on multifocal renal cystadenomas, intravenously administered contrast medium was found to increase the detection of small solid renal nodules (Moe and Lium 1997).

Magnetic resonance imaging

In MR imaging, the patient is placed within the core of the MR scanner, which generates a strong constant magnetic field. The hydrogen atoms within the body align with this magnetic field. Temporary disruption of proton alignment is induced with a series of radiofrequency (RF) waves pulsed into the patient using prede-

fined sequences. As the protons come back into realignment, they generate their own characteristic RF signals that are in turn detected by the MR scanner. The strength and character of the returning RF signals depend on the proton concentration and the specific chemical characteristics of the tissues from which the RF waves emanate. The RF response is mapped to produce a cross-sectional image, which has excellent soft tissue contrast resolution. The most commonly used pulse sequences result in T1-weighted or T2-weighted images. The characteristic appearance of common anatomical structures using these sequences is presented in Table 17.1. The light intensities of pixels that form a digital MR image displayed on a monitor or on print film reflect the underlying RF responses of the anatomical structures represented on the image. Black or dark grey structures are referred to as hypointense, whereas light grey or white structures are referred to as hyperintense. As with the comparable CT terminology, these terms reflect signal intensity relative to other structures in an image. Unlike CT, the signal intensity of a given tissue may change depending on the specific pulse sequence used to generate the image, and the relative intensity differences between tissues may change or even become inverted with the use of different sequences. The most commonly used MR contrast media are small molecular gadolinium agents that increase the signal intensity of contrast-enhancing structures on T1-weighted images. Although the patient is not exposed to ionizing radiation, the high magnetic field environment can pose a risk to both the patient and personnel, and appropriate safety precautions should be taken.

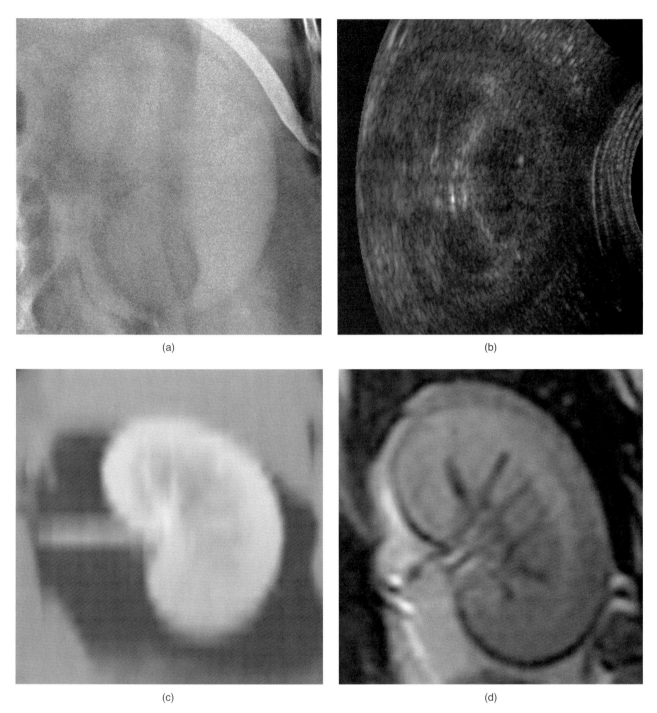

(a)

(b)

(c)

(d)

Figure 17.2 Comparison of the kidney evaluated using four different imaging modalities. (a) image from a ventrodorsal radiograph of the abdomen of a dog. The shape, size, contour, and soft tissue opacity of the kidney can be assessed. (b) Ultrasound image of the left kidney. In addition to the previously listed characteristics, the internal architecture of the kidney, including the renal pelvis, the pelvic recesses, and the cortico-medullary junction, can be identified. (c) Dorsal plane reformatted image of the left kidney from a 3 mm collimated contrast-enhanced CT examination. This image was obtained during the late nephrogram/early pyelogram phase. There is differential contrast enhancement of the renal cortex and medulla. (d) Dorsal plane T2-weighted MR image of the right kidney. The medulla is hypointense relative to the cortex. The connective tissue of the pelvic recesses is hypointense. The pelvic and retroperitoneal fat is hyperintense.

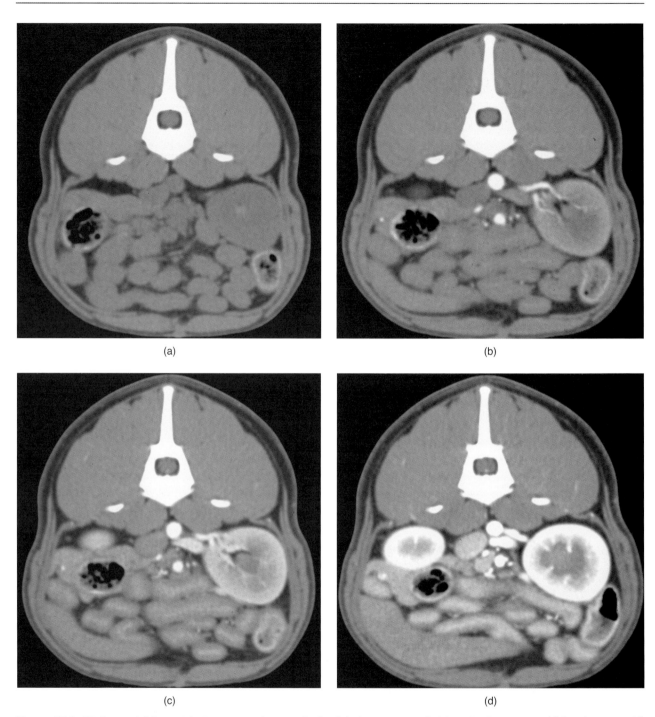

(a)

(b)

(c)

(d)

Figure 17.3 CT. Sequential 3 mm "cine" transverse images obtained during contrast administration in a 1-year-old female Boxer with recurrent urinary tract infections and hematuria. No abnormalities were detected on CT urography. The patient is in sternal recumbency. (a) Precontrast. (b) 15 s postcontrast, arterial vascular phase. There is strong enhancement of the aorta, cranial mesenteric, and left renal artery. The dorsal and ventral branches and some interlobar arteries can be seen. There is early enhancement of the renal cortex. (c) 24 s postcontrast. Early nephrogram phase. There is enhancement of the arteries, renal cortex, and renal vein. (d) 38 s postcontrast. Later nephrogram phase. There is strong enhancement of the renal cortex, arteries, and veins, and moderate enhancement of the vena cava. The caudal pole of the right kidney can be seen due to respiratory motion. (e) 4 m postcontrast, 7 mm transverse image. Pyelo-ureterogram phase. There is strong contrast enhancement of the renal pelvis and both ureters, which appear as small hyperdensities on either side of the great vessels. Because of volume averaging, a longitudinal segment of the proximal left ureter is within the imaging plane.

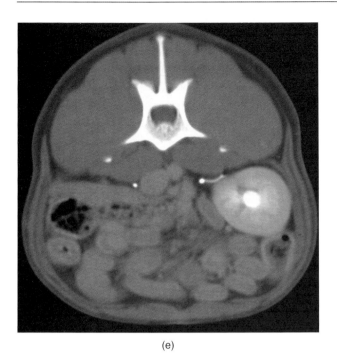

(e)

Figure 17.3 (*Continued*)

To date, abdominal MRI has seen limited use in veterinary medicine (Muleya et al. 1997; Newell et al. 2000; Yamada et al. 2005). This is due to the relatively high cost and lower availability of MRI, the need for prolonged anesthesia, advances and increased use of abdominal ultrasound and CT, and technical hurdles such as the effect of respiratory and visceral motion on image

quality. With the use of respiratory gating, the excellent soft tissue contrast resolution of MR can be employed to characterize disorders of the kidneys and the collecting system (Figure 17.7). However, if trends in human medicine are any indication, CT will likely continue to be the imaging modality of choice for abdominal imaging when compared to MR for most clinical conditions.

T1, T2, and postcontrast T1-weighted sequences in the transverse and dorsal planes are recommended to best define the normal anatomy and any pathology. Paramedian plane images may also prove useful, although in this plane, the anatomic symmetry is lost within each image. Excellent anatomical detail and the characteristic signal intensities of fluid, blood, and vascular and avascular tissues on different MR pulse sequences may be used to characterize many urinary tract disorders though biopsy is still most often required for definitive diagnosis (Figure 17.8).

Postacquisition image processing

Postacquisition image processing technology has increased in quality and availability in recent years. Commonly available image processing tools allow the clinician or technician to reformat a series of images into different imaging planes (multiplanar reformatting), create three-dimensional images (surface rendering or volume rendering), or create a maximum- or minimum-intensity projection (MIP) in which an image is created from the highest or lowest CT numbers or MR intensity values

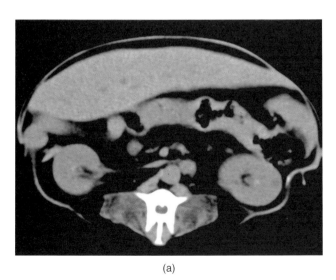

(a)

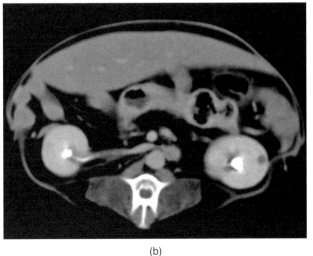

(b)

Figure 17.4 Seventeen-year-old male Poodle cross with hepatic and splenic masses. Five millimeter collimated transverse CT images acquired with the patient in dorsal reumbency. (a) Precontrast image. A faint, round hypodensity is identified in the lateral left renal cortex. The spleen is enlarged. (b) Postcontrast image. There is enhancement of the renal cortices and filling of the renal pelvises with contrast media. The previously identified hypodensity is now well delineated due to the cortical contrast enhancement. Although the cyst is evident on both pre- and postcontrast images, the lesion is most conspicuous on the postcontrast CT image due to the absence of enhancement within thin the cyst. Diagnosis: renal cortical cyst.

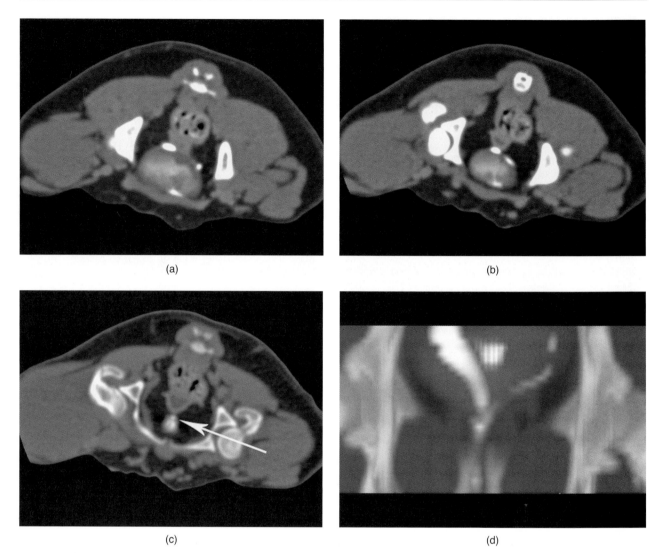

(a)

(b)

(c)

(d)

Figure 17.5 Six-month-old female Bichon Frise with urinary incontinence. One millimeter collimated transverse CT images at the level of the urinary bladder trigone acquired with the patient in sternal recumbency and following intravenous contrast administration. (a) Both ureters are filled with contrast medium and are identified at the dorsal aspect of the urinary bladder. The right ureter is dilated. There is contrast within the urinary bladder lumen. The urinary bladder wall is thickened and irregular. (b) and (c) More caudally, the left ureter inserts normally and the right ureter tunnels through the dorsal urinary bladder and urethral wall (arrow). Contrast media is present within the urethral lumen. (d) Maximum intensity projection (MIP) image of the pelvic canal, demonstrating the dilated right ureter extending caudally adjacent to the urethra. Diagnosis: right ectopic ureter.

in an "anatomical slab" of imaging data. These forms of postacquisition image processing facilitate surgical planning and can provide a more cohesive representation of a complex structure or lesion (Figures 17.5d and 17.9).

Upper urinary tract

Kidneys

General considerations

When evaluating the kidneys, the location, size, shape, contour, and density (CT) or tissue signal intensity (MR)

should be assessed. The stages of contrast enhancement in the normal kidneys on CT are shown in Figure 17.3. A precontrast CT examination should always be performed prior to a contrast-enhanced CT study to detect tissue mineralization or uroliths that can often be obscured following contrast medium administration. In order to image the entire urinary tract, a complete abdominal examination with breath hold is recommended. The right kidney should be well-seated in the renal fossa of the caudate lobe of the liver. The left kidney should be just caudal to the head of the spleen, and the lateral cortical aspect may be slightly ventral to the renal pelvis if the patient

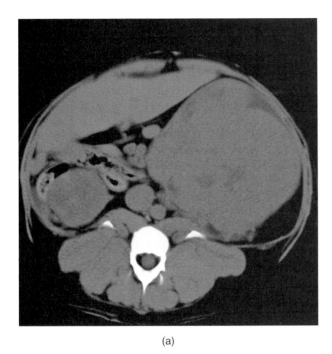

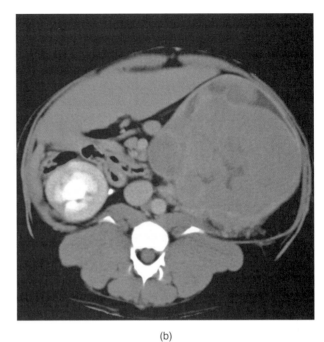

(a)   (b)

Figure 17.6 Two-year-old male castrated Doberman Pinscher with hematuria, dorsal recumbency. (a) 7 mm collimated transverse plane CT image at the level of the left kidney. There is a large, lobular, mildly heterogeneous left midabdominal mass with well-delineated margins. The right kidney is of near-normal size but has slightly irregular margins and faint wedge-shaped cortical hyperdensities which distort the renal contour. (b) Following intravenous contrast administration, there is nonuniform contrast enhancement of the left renal mass. Wedge-shaped enhancement defects are identified in the right renal cortex and the right renal pelvis is dilated. The left renal pelvis and ureter were not identified. Diagnoses: nephroblastoma of the left kidney, right renal cortical infarcts, and pelvic dilation.

is in sternal recumbency. The renal pelves should be at approximately the same level as the abdominal vena cava. Displacement of the kidneys can be due to retroperitoneal or peritoneal fluid or mass effect, traumatic avulsion or herniation, or surgical intervention.

Images reformatted (CT) or acquired (MR) in the dorsal plane are helpful to fully evaluate the size, shape, and contour of both kidneys. On CT images, in the absence of contrast enhancement, the corticomedullary junction is not apparent, and the kidneys are of soft-

tissue density, measuring 30–40 CT Units. The hypo-attenuating pelvic fat will be clearly defined forming a "Y" shape on transverse plane images around the renal

Table 17.1 Typical appearance of common anatomical structures on T1- and T2-weighted MR images

	T1-weighted image[a]	T2-weighted image
Air	Black	Black
Fluid (urine, transudative ascites)	Dark gray	White
Fat	Light gray/white	Light gray
Cortical bone	Black	Black
Bone marrow	Light gray	Light gray
Solid viscera (liver, spleen, kidney)	Medium gray	Variable gray

[a]Appearance on noncontrast enhanced T1 images. The administration of MR contrast medium results in increased signal intensity (increased image whiteness) of tissues containing a high contrast concentration.

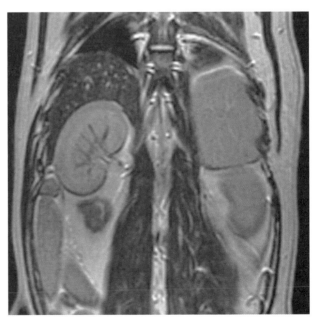

Figure 17.7 T2-weighted MR image of the right kidney acquired in the dorsal plane.

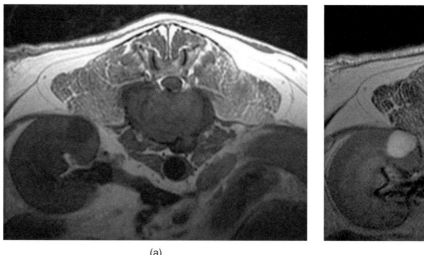

(a)   (b)

Figure 17.8 Thirteen-year-old male castrated Bassett Hound with pelvic limb paralysis and lumbar pain. Sternal recumbency. (a) T1-weighted MR image of the right kidney acquired in the transverse plane. There is a round, well-margined, hypointense structure mildly distorting the capsular margin in the dorsal cortex of the kidney. (b) T2-weighted MR image at the same site. The round structure is well-delineated and markedly hyperintense. These imaging characteristics are consistent with a fluid-filled cyst. Diagnosis: incidental finding of a renal cortical cyst.

papilla and surrounding the renal vasculature and ureter. Abnormal renal densities include mineralization, which will be hyperattenuating compared to adjacent renal parenchyma, and fluid accumulation, which appears mildly hypoattenuating compared to renal parenchyma. Abnormal mineralization may be due to dystrophic mineralization of renal tissue, mineralization within the collecting system (nephrolithiasis), or mineralization

within a mass lesion such as a neoplasia, granuloma, or hematoma. Abnormal fluid density may be due to cyst formation or renal pelvic dilation (hydronephrosis) or may result from a mass of high fluid content when intraparenchymal (Figure 17.10). Intravenously administered contrast medium allows for more definitive identification of cysts and renal pelvic distortion since contrast accentuates the definition between contrast-enhancing tissue and noncontrast-enhancing fluid (Figure 17.4) (Reichle et al. 2002).

Renal cysts

Renal cysts may form as the result of developmental disorders such as of polycystic kidney disease or may be acquired (see Chapter 56) (Figures 17.4 and 17.8). These cysts are most often identified in the cortex, but can be seen in the medulla or at the corticomedullary junction. The clinical significance of acquired cysts is unknown; they are often incidental findings in patients without biochemical abnormalities associated with renal disease, although they are thought to be a component of chronic renal disease in some cases.

Figure 17.9 Adult male castrated DLH cat with acute renal failure. This is a dorsal plane maximal intensity projection (MIP) image generated from overlapping 2 mm transverse plane CT images of the caudal half of the left kidney and the proximal ureter. The kidney is enlarged and focal mineralized density is present within the proximal left ureter, which is also mildly dilated proximally. Diagnosis: left ureterolithiasis with obstruction.

Vascular disorders

Thromboembolic insult to the kidney, or renal infarct, is recognized in both acute and chronic stages. An acute infarct may be difficult to identify on precontrast CT images, but will appear as a discrete, wedge-shaped

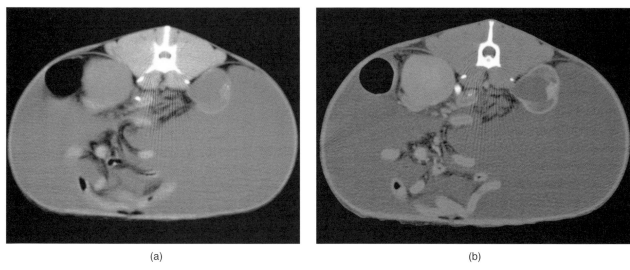

(a)   (b)

Figure 17.10 Five-year-old female spayed DSH cat with azotemia. (a) 7 mm collimated transverse plane precontrast CT image with the patient in sternal recumbency. There is a large volume of ascites causing abdominal distension. There is marked left-sided hydronephrosis with only a thin layer of renal cortex remaining. An obstructing ureterolith was identified caudal to this level (not pictured). The caudal pole of the right kidney can be seen. There is a focal mineralization evident in the right ureter. The small focal densities within the ventral paraspinal musculature are the vertebral transverse processes and should not be mistaken for ureteral calculi or contrast medium. (b) 2 mm postcontrast transverse CT image acquired at approximately the same level. There is mild enhancement of the right renal cortex and no appreciable contrast enhancement of the thin left cortex. Contrast medium can be seen in the right ureter lateral to the previously described ureterolith. Diagnosis: bilateral ureteroliths resulting in chronic obstructive hydronephrosis, degenerative disease, and reduced renal function. Marked ascites.

enhancement defect following contrast administration. The shape of the kidney is often not affected by the presence of an acute infarct (Figure 17.11). Eventually, the cortical tissue that does not reperfuse will atrophy and result in a wedge-shaped area of decreased contrast

enhancement with an associated focal capsular contour depression (Figure 17.6b). Multiple infarcts are often detected and may represent either a component of primary nephropathy or secondary to systemic thromboembolic disorders such as neoplasia, sepsis, or coagulopathy.

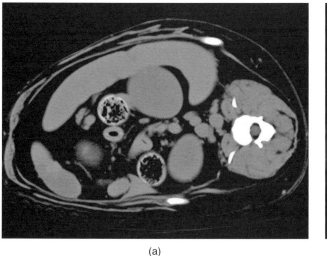   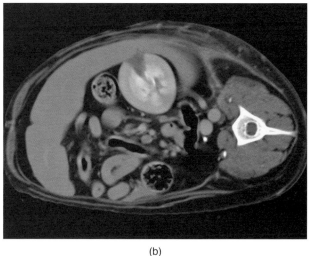

(a)   (b)

Figure 17.11 Seven-year-old female spayed Labrador Retriever with a body wall mass. (a) 5 mm collimated transverse plane precontrast CT image at the level of the left kidney with the patient positioned in right lateral recumbency. There is subcutaneous density consistent with edema or cellulitis. (b) Postcontrast image acquired at the same level. A wedge-shaped contrast enhancement defect is present in the lateral cortex and medulla of the left kidney. Note that this lesion is not recognized on the precontrast image. Diagnosis: acute renal infarct.

MR appearance of renal infarcts has not been described in the veterinary literature.

Inflammatory disorders

Inflammatory renal disease is generally accurately characterized using ultrasound, and CT and MR are not necessary for diagnosis. However, pyelonephritis (see Chapters 49 and 71) may be present in association with other disorders of the urinary tract and typical imaging findings should be recognized. The general imaging characteristics of pyelonephritis include renal pelvic dilation, blunting of diverticula, and dilation of the pelvic recesses and ureter (Figure 17.12). These findings may also be present with obstructive disease, but in the absence of an obstructive lesion, ascending pyelonephritis should be suspected when there is a diffuse dilation of the collecting system. Additional abnormalities, such as bladder wall thickening suggestive of cystitis or diffuse thickening of the ureteral wall may increase the index of suspicion for pyelonephritis.

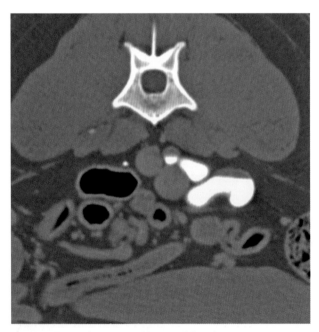

Figure 17.12 Three-year-old spayed female Bernese Mountain Dog with a urinary tract infection diagnosed on urinalysis. 2 mm collimated transverse plane postcontrast image at the level of the ureters with the patient positioned in sternal recumbency. There is moderate left ureteral dilation consistent with ureteral obstruction. There is a congenital vascular anomaly in which the caudal vena cava is positioned to the left of the aorta with the left ureter coursing dorsal to the vena cava, resulting in extramural compression and partial ureteral obstruction. Additional images acquired caudal to this figure reveals contrast material in the distal aspect of the left ureter, indicating persisting patency and urine flow within the ureter.

Neoplasia

Although a presumptive diagnosis of renal neoplasia (see Chapter 57) is often made from clinical radiographic and ultrasound findings, CT and MR can be useful in determining the character and extent of renal tumors, due to their excellent soft tissue contrast resolution (Figure 17.6). CT and MR are most helpful in precisely delineating primary tumor margins and local or regional extension as part of preoperative planning or postoperative assessment.

Degenerative disease

Imaging findings of chronic degenerative renal disease may include reduced size, abnormal shape, renal pelvic dilation, and decreased contrast enhancement due to reduced renal blood flow (Figure 17.13).

Ureters

General considerations

CT can be used to document a wide range of ureteral disorders, including obstruction and developmental malformations such as ureteral ectopia and ureteral duplication (Esterline et al. 2005). Following intravenous contrast administration, one can readily identify the renal pelvis, the ureters, and the ureterovesicular junction (Rozear and Tidwell 2003). The normal ureter should be less than 1–2 mm in diameter and have a relatively uniform appearance throughout its length. Normal peristaltic activity, however, may result in a segmental contrast voids in the normal ureter. Normal dynamic segmental contractions can be differentiated from strictures or other causes of obstruction by reacquiring images of the region of concern.

Ureteral obstruction

Ureteral obstruction (see Chapters 58 and 70) can be due to intraluminal, mural, or extramural causes. Ureterolithiasis is most common and is often seen in cats. Ureteroliths can be seen on precontrast CT images as a focal mineral density in the region of the normally fluid-dense ureter. Thinly collimated images are recommended to best characterize ureteroliths and nephroliths as to number and specific location (Figure 17.14). Although ureteroliths can often be identified with conventional radiographs and ultrasound, CT is sometimes more sensitive for lesion detection and is helpful for surgical planning.

In instances of acute obstruction and in most cases of chronic obstruction, the renal pelvis is dilated and

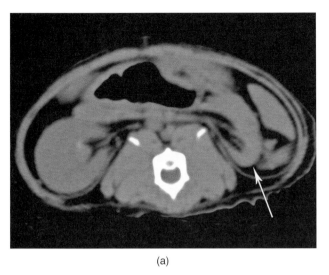
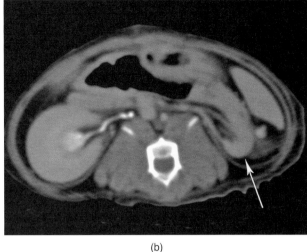

(a)   (b)

Figure 17.13 Seven-year-old female spayed DSH cat with chronic urinary obstruction due to a pelvic mass. (a) 7 mm collimated transverse plane precontrast CT image with the patient in dorsal recumbency. The right kidney is large with faint mineralization in the margin of the renal papilla. The left kidney is small (arrow). (b) Postcontrast 3 mm collimated transverse image at approximately the same level. There is contrast enhancement of the right renal cortex, renal pelvis, and ureter. There is no contrast enhancement of the left renal structures. These findings are consistent with a nonfunctional atrophic or end-stage left kidney with compensatory right renal hypertrophy.

the ureter is dilated cranial to the site of obstruction. In patients with obstructive urolithiasis, the kidneys, urinary bladder, and urethra are also fully evaluated for the presence of additional uroliths. Mural causes for ureteral obstruction are rare, but smooth muscle or epithelial neoplasia and polyps of the ureters have been reported (Reichle et al. 2003). Extramural causes of ureteral obstruction include sarcomas, hemorrhage, or lipomas of the retroperitoneal or intrapelvic spaces, which result in ureteral obstruction by mass effect or invasion.

Developmental anomalies

Contrast CT urography is used for diagnosis of ectopic ureters (see Chapter 58) and often proves to be superior for definitive diagnosis as compared to other approaches such as excretory urography/double contrast cystography (Samii et al. 2004) and ultrasound. If thinly collimated images are acquired, the route of the ectopic ureter can often be more clearly defined, particularly when the distal aspect of the abnormal ureter courses intramurally before exiting. A 2 mm dilation of the renal pelvis and 3 mm or greater dilation of the ureter is consistent with hydronephrosis and hydroureter, respectively, and though nonspecific is routinely seen in patients with ureteral ectopia. A diagnosis of ectopia can be made if the ureter can be followed caudal to the ureterovesicular junction. Often, the termination of the ureter can be definitively identified caudal to the junction. If the ureter

apposes the bladder for more than 9 mm, a diagnosis of ureteral intramural tunneling can be made (Samii 2005). In normal dogs, the degree of bladder distention does not affect the location of the ureterovesicular junction and should therefore not affect interpretation of the location of ureteral termination (Rozear and Tidwell 2003). Reformatting transverse images into a dorsal or sagittal plane and using MIP projections can often best define the path of the ureters (Figure 17.5d). Often, multiple image acquisitions are necessary to fully evaluate the ureters when ureteral peristalsis results in segmentation of the intraluminal ureteral contrast column.

Lower urinary tract

General considerations

CT and MR are best utilized in lower urinary tract imaging for preoperative planning to delineate masses or diffuse disease involving the urethra and urinary bladder. The bones surrounding the pelvic canal can impede radiographic and sonographic imaging of the caudal urinary bladder, urethra, and prostate. CT can be used in these cases to evaluate not only the relationships between the soft tissues of the pelvic canal, but also the extent and margins of disease and changes in the sublumbar lymph nodes, distal ureters, and lower urinary tract. Subtle skeletal changes such as periosteal reaction or nondisplaced fractures may also be identified more clearly on CT than on radiographic examination.

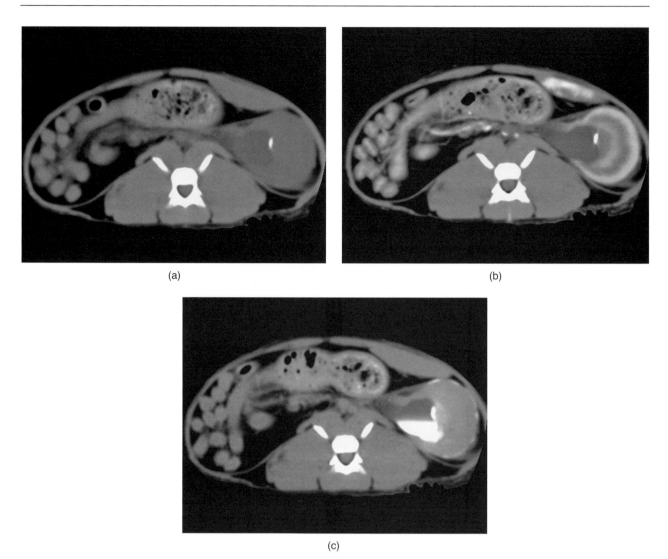

(a)   (b)

(c)

Figure 17.14 Seven-year-old spayed female cat with azotemia, a small right kidney, and enlarged left kidney. Dorsal recumbency. (a) 7 mm collimated transverse plane precontrast image at the level of the left kidney with the patient positioned in dorsal recumbency. The left renal pelvis is moderately dilated and contains a focal mineralized density (nephrolith). The margins of the kidney are irregular, consistent with subcapsular fluid accumulation. (b) 5 mm transverse plane image acquired 10 minutes following intravenous contrast medium administration. There is marked enhancement of the renal cortex, indicating a persistence of the nephrogram phase of the study. There is also enhancement of the tail of the spleen seen on this image. (c) 2 mm transverse plane image acquired 20 minutes following intravenous contrast medium administration. There is pooling of contrast medium within the dependent part of the dilated left renal pelvis. Subcapsular contrast enhancement can also be seen peripherally. These findings are consistent with left ureteral obstruction resulting in hydronephrosis, hydroureter, and subcapsular fluid accumulation.

The urinary bladder wall is variable in thickness depending on bladder distension but mural thickness should generally be less than 1 mm and uniform in width. Regardless of the degree of bladder distension, if the trigone is caudal to the pubis, a diagnosis of pelvic bladder should be considered (Samii et al. 2004). Normal urine density is similar to that of water having a CT value approaching 0. On MR images, normal urine will appear dark gray or black on T1-weighted images and white on T2-weighted images. Following renal filtration, contrast medium will distribute into the dependent part of the urinary bladder after exiting the ureters due to the density of the iodinated (CT) or gadolinium (MR) agent, resulting in a stratified appearance to the bladder. Although gadolinium agents generally produce increased signal intensity on T1-weighted images, the highly concentrated agent within the urinary bladder produces a paradoxical decrease in signal intensity on postcontrast T1-weighted images. An inverted contrast medium-urine layering in the bladder will also occasionally be seen on

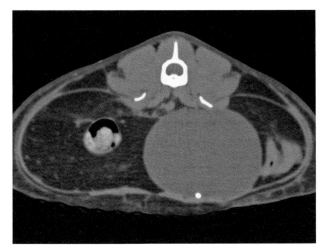

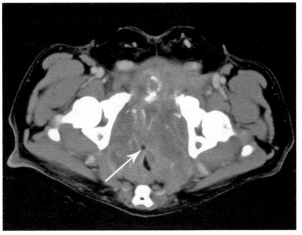

Figure 17.15 Seven-year-old spayed female cat with renal failure. Two millimeter collimated transverse plane precontrast CT image of the urinary bladder with the patient in sternal recumbency. A solitary mineralized body is identified in the dependent urinary bladder lumen. Diagnosis: cystolithiasis.

Figure 17.16 Ten-year-old spayed female mixed breed dog with stranguria. Seven millimeter collimated transverse plane postcontrast CT image of the pelvic canal with the patient positioned in dorsal recumbency. There is a partially mineralized, peripherally and heterogeneously contrast enhancing soft tissue mass filling the pelvic canal. There is bone destruction of the pubis with associated disorganized bone production. A urinary catheter is in place and can be seen in cross section in the urethra as a round lucency (arrow). Presumptive diagnosis: primary bone tumor of the pubis.

CT and is thought to be due to increased urine-specific gravity in the dependent urinary bladder (Samii 2005).

Urolithiasis

Cystolithiasis (see Chapter 69) may be a clinically significant or incidental finding on abdominal CT examination. Mineralized bodies may be solitary or numerous and should be dependently located (Figure 17.15). The urinary tract should be evaluated in its entirety to rule out other sites of urolithiasis and possible obstruction.

Neoplasia and other mass lesions

Tumors of the urinary bladder and urethra (see Chapter 79) have been well described using ultrasound and contrast radiography, and these principles can be applied to CT and MR imaging of the lower urinary tract. Tumors arising from the bones of the pelvis or the soft tissues of the pelvic canal can result in secondary urethral obstruction or urinary bladder compression. Nonneoplastic mass lesions such as paraprostatic cysts or proliferative callus from pelvic fractures can result in similar clinical signs. CT or MR imaging provides excellent imaging of this area of the body and allows for thorough preoperative planning. In these cases, passage of a urinary catheter is helpful to clearly define the position and path of the urethra before scanning (Figure 17.16).

The most common site for transitional cell carcinomas is the urinary bladder, but may also arise in the ureters (Hanika and Rebar 1980), the prostate (Nyland et al. 2002), and the urethra (Figure 17.17) (Moroff et al. 1991). CT and MR can be used to effectively image urethral

masses that would otherwise be difficult to characterize with radiography or ultrasound (Figure 17.18). The CT or MR examination should extend cranially to the level of the origin of the iliac vessels in order to assess regional lymph nodes.

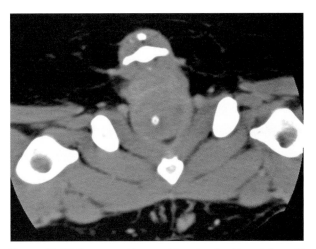

Figure 17.17 Ten-year-old spayed female mixed breed dog with diarrhea and pollakiuria. Three millimeter transverse plane postcontrast CT image acquired at the level of the vestibule with the patient in dorsal recumbency. A radiodense urinary catheter is in place and is used to document urethral position. There is a heterogeneously contrast-enhancing soft tissue mass surrounding the urethra. Histopathologic diagnosis: urethral transitional cell carcinoma.

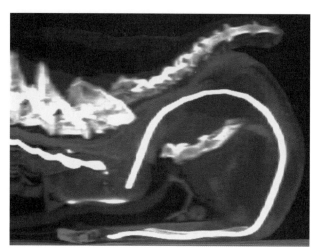

Figure 17.18 Four-year-old castrated male Doberman Pinscher with dyschezia and stranguria. Sagittal plane maximal intensity projection (MIP) from 5 mm collimated postcontrast transverse plane images of the pelvic canal. A urinary catheter is in place that defines the path of the urethra. A small amount of contrast medium is present in the dependent urinary bladder. The ureters are dilated and superimposed and can be seen craniodorsal to the urinary bladder. A peripherally contrast enhancing mass is present surrounding the membranous and proximal penile urethra. CT diagnosis: hematoma or neoplasia of the corpus cavernosum. Histopathologic diagnosis: lipoma with hemorrhage and fibrovascular tissue.

Conclusion

Computed tomography and magnetic resonance imaging offer certain advantages to contrast radiography and ultrasound of the urinary tract. These advantages included excellent soft tissue contrast resolution and the ability to recognize and characterize small structures such as the ureters and urethra. Tomographic imaging provides an excellent visual representation of complex anatomy and is particularly well suited for preoperative planning and postoperative case management. These sophisticated imaging modalities complement and supplement imaging findings of radiography (see Chapter 15), ultrasonography (see Chapter 16), and scintigraphy (see Chapter 18), often leading to more accurate diagnosis and staging of urinary tract disorders.

References

Barthez, P.Y., D. Begon, et al. (1998). Effect of contrast medium dose and image acquisition timing on ureteral opacification in the normal dog as assessed by computed tomography. *Vet Radiol Ultrasound* **39**: 524–527.

Bouma, J.L., L.R. Aronson, et al. (2003). Use of computed tomography renal angiography for screening feline renal transplant donors. *Vet Radiol Ultrasound* **44**: 636–641.

Bushberg, J.T., J.A. Seibert, et al. (2001). *The Essential Physics of Medical Imaging*. Philadelphia, PA: Lippincott Williams and Wilkins.

Esterline, M.L., D.S. Biller, et al. (2005). Ureteral duplication in a dog. *Vet Radiol Ultrasound* **46**: 485–489.

Hanika, C. and A.H. Rebar (1980). Ureteral transitional cell carcinoma in the dog. *Vet Pathol* **17**: 643–646.

Moe, L. and B. Lium (1997). Computed tomography of hereditary multifocal renal cystadenocarcinomas in German shepherd dogs. *Vet Radiol Ultrasound* **38**: 335–343.

Moroff, S.D., B.A. Brown, et al. (1991). Infiltrative urethral disease in female dogs: 41 cases (1980–1987). *J Am Vet Med Assoc* **199**: 247–251.

Muleya, J.S., Y. Taura, et al. (1997). Appearance of canine abdominal tumors with magnetic resonance imaging using a low field permanent magnet. *Vet Radiol Ultrasound* **38**: 444–447.

Newell, S.M., J.P. Graham, et al. (2000). Quantitative magnetic resonance imaging of the normal feline cranial abdomen. *Vet Radiol Ultrasound* **41**: 27–34.

Nyland, T.G., S.T. Wallack, et al. (2002). Needle-tract implantation following us-guided fine-needle aspiration biopsy of transitional cell carcinoma of the bladder, urethra, and prostate. *Vet Radiol Ultrasound* **43**: 50–53.

O'Dell-Anderson, K.J., R. Twardock, et al. (2006). Determination of glomerular filtration rate in dogs using contrast-enhanced computed tomography. *Vet Radiol Ultrasound* **47**: 127–135.

Reichle, J.K., S.P. DiBartola, et al. (2002). Renal ultrasonographic and computed tomographic appearance, volume, and function of cats with autosomal dominant polycystic kidney disease. *Vet Radiol Ultrasound* **43**: 368–373.

Reichle, J.K., R.A. Peterson II, et al. (2003). Ureteral fibroepithelial polyps in four dogs. *Vet Radiol Ultrasound* **44**: 433–437

Rozear, L. and A.S. Tidwell (2003). Evaluation of the ureter and ureterovesicular junction using helical computed tomographic excretory urography in healthy dogs. *Vet Radiol Ultrasound* **44**: 155–164.

Samii, V.F. (2005). Inverted contrast medium-urine layering in the canine urinary bladder on computed tomography. *Vet Radiol Ultrasound* **46**: 502–505.

Samii, V.F., M.A. McLoughlin, et al. (2004). Digital fluoroscopic excretory urography, digital fluoroscopic urethrography, helical computed tomography, and cystoscopy in 24 dogs with suspected ureteral ectopia. *J Vet Intern Med* **18**: 271–281.

Yamada, K., K. Miyahara, et al. (2005). Optimizing technical conditions for magnetic resonance imaging of the rat brain and abdomen in a low magnetic field. *Vet Radiol Ultrasound* **36**: 523–527.

Yamazoe, K., F. Ohashi, et al. (1994). Computed tomography on renal masses in dogs and cats. *J Vet Med Sci* **56**: 813–816.

18

Renal scintigraphy

Gregory B. Daniel

Renal anatomy and physiology

Renal scintigraphy is used to evaluate renal function and renal morphology. To understand the principles of renal scintigraphy, a brief review of normal anatomy and physiology is in order. The kidneys are paired organs located in the retroperitoneal space that function to rid the body of waste material and to control the volume and composition of body fluid (Evans and Christensen 1993). The kidneys perform these functions by filtering the plasma and removing substances from the filtrate. The kidney can be divided into the outer cortical regional and the inner medulla.

The functional unit of the kidney is the nephron, which is composed of a glomerular capsule that leads into the proximal tubule (Evans and Christensen 1993; Thrall and Ziessman 1995; Daniel et al. 1999; Guyton and Hall 2006). The glomerular capsule is invaginated by a spherical rete of blood capillaries, the glomerulus. There are a million or more of these functional units in a normal kidney (Guyton and Hall 2006). The kidney receives about 25% of the cardiac output (Thrall and Ziessman 1995). The average renal plasma flow is 15 mL/min/kg of body weight. About 20% of this is filtered through the glomerulus, but the percentage changes as a result of autoregulatory mechanisms (Thrall and Ziessman 1995; Guyton and Hall 2006). The remaining plasma that is not filtered enters the peritubular fluid and is actively secreted by the tubular epithelial cells into the renal tubules (Guyton and Hall 2006). Autoregulatory mechanisms can maintain glomerular filtration rate (GFR) in the face of decreased renal blood flow (RBF) or a decrease in systemic blood pressure. Blood pressure within the glomerulus determines GFR, and the pressure within the glomerulus is controlled by vasoconstriction of the afferent or efferent arteriole. In times of decreased blood pressure or decreased RBF, the efferent arteriole will constrict, thus increasing the pressure within the glomerulus, resulting in an increase in GFR (Mazze 1986).

The kidney can be imaged by a variety of modalities. Survey radiographs (see Chapter 15) are used to evaluate renal size, shape, margination, and opacity (Feeney and Johnson 2007). Administration of intravenous contrast can be used to evaluate space-occupying lesion in the renal cortex and subsequent contrast accumulation within renal collecting system, allowing the visualization of the renal recess, renal pelvis, and proximal ureter. Changes in the pattern of renal–cortical opacification can be used as qualitative assessment of renal function. (Feeney and Johnson 2007) Ultrasound (see Chapter 16) provides morphologic information, such as renal size, shape, and internal architecture, even in patients with poor renal function (Nyland et al. 2002). Doppler ultrasound permits assessment of additional indices related to blood flow.

Renal scintigraphy is a nuclear medicine procedure that is performed after intravenous injection of a radiopharmaceutical. The radiopharmaceutical is a chemical compound, that has certain biologic properties, labeled with a radionuclide (Thrall and Ziessman 1995). By using different radiopharmaceuticals, which are selectively filtered or undergo tubular secretion, quantification of GFR and effective renal plasma flow (ERPF) is possible (Thrall and Ziessman 1995). Other radiopharmaceuticals localize in renal tubules and provide morphologic information about the kidney.

The radionuclide is the portion of the radiopharmaceutical that emits a gamma ray. The gamma ray is detected by either a gamma camera, making a scintigraphic image, or a well detector that would quantify the amount of the radionuclide in a sample of blood. The

Nephrology and Urology of Small Animals. Edited by Joe Bartges and David J. Polzin. © 2011 Blackwell Publishing Ltd.

equipment needed for detection of gamma rays is limited to a selected referral centers, large equine practices, and various veterinary teaching hospitals. In addition, state and federal offices regulate the handling of the radionuclide and release of the patient (Berry and Daniel 2006b). In most cases, an animal injected with a radionuclide is held overnight in a specially designated area of the hospital. As such, renal scintigraphy is rarely an outpatient procedure. Because of these limitations, renal scintigraphy is not as commonly performed as radiography and ultrasound.

Nuclear scintigraphy is used primarily to evaluate renal function (Daniel et al. 1999; Twardock and Bahr 2006). A variety of functional indices such as GFR or ERPF mean that renal transit time and renal clearance rates can be derived from nuclear medicine procedures. This chapter focuses on methods to measure GFR and to evaluate for postrenal obstruction.

Measuring glomerular filtration

GFR is considered the best single parameter for assessing renal function as it is directly proportional to the number of functional nephrons. Measurement of GFR is based on the clearance of an indicator that does not bind to plasma proteins, does not enter red blood cells, and is cleared from the plasma by glomerular filtration with no extrarenal uptake and no tubular reabsorption or secretion (Peter 2004). GFR can be measured by a variety of markers including inulin, ^{51}Cr-EDTA, ^{125}I-iothalamate, and radiographic contact agents, such as iothalamate (Conray®) or iohexol (Omnipaque®) (Peter 2004). The radiopharmaceutical used for measuring GFR is ^{99m}Tc-*Diethylene Triamine Pentaacetic Acid* (^{99m}Tc-DTPA), also know ^{99m}Tc-pentetate (Thrall and Ziessman 1995). Today, most radiopharmacuticals are purchased from a nuclear pharmacy. The nuclear pharmacy prepares the radiopharmaceutical by injecting pertechnetate ($Na^{99m}TcO_4$) into commercially prepared vials containing lyophilized chemicals in a nitrogen atmosphere. Most of these commercially available kits use stannous chloride to reduce the ^{99m}Tc to a valance state that will bind to the DTPA molecule. While preparing the kit, care must be taken not to introduce room air or moisture into the reaction vial before the addition of pertechnetate (Kowalsky 2006). Oxidation of the kit results in the formation of radiochemical impurities that will alter distribution of radiopharmaceutical within the body. Free pertechnetate localizes in the thyroid gland, salivary gland, and gastric mucosa, and there would be prolonged blood pool activity and slower clearance by the kidney. Radiocolloid impurities concentrate within the liver and spleen. If the radiopharmaceutical is pre-

pared by a nuclear pharmacy, they will assess for these radiochemical impurities using thin-layer chromatography (Thrall and Ziessman 1995; Daniel 2006).

^{99m}Tc-DTPA is a vascular agent that quickly equilibrates with the extracellular fluid space. ^{99m}Tc-DTPA is a small-molecular weight (492 Da)(Nilsson et al. 1997) compound that is permeable to the glomerular membrane. Following glomerular filtration, there is no tubular absorption or secretion. Uptake of ^{99m}Tc-DTPA within the kidney or clearance from the plasma is directly proportional to GFR.

The suitability of ^{99m}Tc-DTPA to measure GFR varies among animal species. If a portion of the injected dose of ^{99m}Tc-DTPA becomes bound to plasma proteins, then it will not be available for glomerular filtration and will falsely decrease the measured GFR. In dogs, there is a minimal amount (6–7%) of protein binding of ^{99m}Tc-DTPA, which does not significantly influence the measured GFR (Krawiec et al. 1986). Protein binding can be a problem in other species. For example, in green iguanas, nearly 50% of the ^{99m}Tc-DTPA is protein bound (Greer et al. 2005). In corn snakes, approximately 30% of the ^{99m}Tc-DTPA is protein bound (Sykes et al. 2006). In these species, the image quality of the kidney is poor and GFR cannot be quantified using ^{99m}Tc-DTPA.

Approximately 20% of the ^{99m}Tc-DTPA is normally removed from the plasma by the kidney on each circulatory pass, resulting in a rapid blood clearance. In human beings, biologic half-life for ^{99m}Tc-DTPA is 2.5 hours with 95% of the ^{99m}Tc-DTPA within the urine by 24 hours (Kim et al. 1996). These values are not known in dogs and cats, but normal clearance rates of 3–4 mL/min/kg should produce a similar biologic clearance.

Clearance of ^{99m}Tc-DTPA is measured using a gamma camera. The gamma camera is a large radiation detector which creates two-dimensional (conventional study) or three-dimensional (spect) images showing distribution of the radionuclide within the body (Berry and Daniel 2006a). If properly calibrated, the gamma camera can quantify the amount of the radionuclide in areas of the body by drawing regions of interest (ROI) and determining activity with these ROIs. By applying these ROI to a series of images taken sequentially over time, a time–activity plot can be generated.

Imaging studies

Renal scintigraphy is a quick, noninvasive method to evaluate GFR. Another important advantage of renal scintigraphy is that the individual kidney function can be determined from the uptake of ^{99m}Tc-DTPA by each kidney. The relative blood flow to the kidneys can be determined by the first-pass analysis of the renogram curve. Finally, kidney morphology can be determined along with patency of the renal collecting system and ureters.

Dynamic renal scintigraphy with ^{99m}Tc-DTPA

The only patient preparation for dynamic renal scintigraphy is placement of an intravenous catheter. The animal must remain motionless in lateral or dorsal recumbency for a minimum of 3 minutes. If needed, sedation can be used to prevent patient movement during acquisition. There is no significant effect of commonly used sedative protocols on measured GFR values (Newell et al. 1997; Winter et al. 2007). Dynamic renal scintigraphy can be completed within 15–20 minutes including setup time, with results available in an additional 15 minutes.

Depending on the method of analysis, it may be necessary to quantify the amount of radioactivity administered to the animal. This is done by placing the dose of ^{99m}Tc-DTPA (typically, 3–4 mCi or 111–148 Mbq) at a fixed distance (26 cm) above the center of the gamma camera. The exact distance is not critical since the sensitivity of a parallel hole collimator varies little with distance (Young et al. 1997). The gamma camera should be fitted with a low energy all purpose (LEAP)-parallel hole collimator. A preinjection syringe count is made and expressed in counts per minute (cpm). Following the image acquisition, the residual activity within the syringe and injection apparatus is imaged again using the same setup parameters (Twardock et al. 1991). Correction of radioactivity decay will be necessary if the time from the pre- to postinjection images was greater than 20 minutes. Radioactive decay of ^{99m}Tc will be less that 5% in 20 minutes.

The animal is positioned with the gamma camera centered dorsal to the kidneys. The image acquisition is controlled by the imaging computer and is initiated simultaneously with injection. The duration of the acquisition may vary, but for GFR analysis the acquisition must last for at least 3 minutes. A variety of frame rates may be used. The most common frame rate is 1 frame every 6 seconds. The images are stored as a $128 \times 128 \times 16$-digital matrix. After the dynamic acquisition, the camera is positioned lateral to the abdomen by moving the camera head, leaving the animal in the recumbent position. A single static image is obtained from which kidney depth is measured. The syringe and injection apparatus is imaged as described above to determine residual activity.

Image analysis

The injected dose is equal to the difference in the pre- and postinjection syringe counts and is expressed in cpm. ROI are drawn around both kidneys. Planar nuclear medicine images are two-dimensional images of a three-dimensional object. When an ROI is placed over an organ in the image field, the radioactivity recorded includes the radioactivity within the organ plus the entire radioactivity above and below the organ. Background radioactivity will produce significant errors in quantification, as it can account for as much as 50% of the total counts recorded in an ROI. Some basic terms regarding background correction are as follows. *Gross counts* are the total numbers of counts that have not been corrected for background within an ROI. *Net counts* are the total numbers of counts that have been corrected for background radioactivity within an ROI. A background ROI is drawn around the kidney ROI. The background region is usually 1 or 2 pixels away from the kidney ROI. The background ROI does not have to be a ring encircling the kidney ROI. Other methods include drawing a semicircular or rectangular ROI on cranial and caudal to the kidney ROI. The mean count density of the background ROI is determined and this value is subtracted from each pixel of the target ROI using the following formula.

$$\text{Net kidney counts} = \text{Gross kidney counts} - \left(\left(\frac{\text{BKD count}}{\text{no. of BKD pixels}} \right) \times \text{no. of kidney pixels} \right)$$

Some of the radioactivity originating within the kidney will be absorbed by the soft tissues before it reaches the gamma camera to be recorded. Each centimeter of soft tissue absorbs approximately 15% of the gamma rays emitted by ^{99m}Tc. In dogs, the thickness of the soft tissues varies considerably between a small- and large-breed dog. To get an accurate measurement of the amount of radioactivity originating from the canine kidney, it is necessary to correct the kidney counts for attenuation. Because of less or more consistent thickness of soft tissue dorsal to the kidney in the cat, attenuation correction is not as important. The percent attenuation caused by the overlying tissues is determined by the following equation:

$$\% \text{ Attenuation} = e^{-0.153 \times \text{kidney depth (cm)}}$$

The counts collected from the kidney ROI are now corrected for background and soft tissue attenuation and could be used to quantify renal function.

The estimation of GFR from dynamic renal scintigraphy can be performed by a variety of methods. The most commonly employed method used in veterinary medicine is a technique described by Gates (Gates 1982), and later modified by Twardock et al., for use in dogs and cats (Krawiec et al. 1986; Krawiec et al. 1988; Uribe et al. 1992). This technique estimates GFR from a regression correlation that was created from a plot of percent dose uptake of the radiopharmaceutical in the kidney to inulin clearance. The percent dose uptake of ^{99m}Tc-DTPA

Table 18.1 Slope (A) and intercept (B) values used in the regression equation for estimation of GFR in dogs and cats

Species	A (slope)	B (intercept)
Dog (attenuation and BKD corrected)	0.194	0.370
Cat (BKD corrected)	0.284	0.164

is determined by dividing the attenuation corrected net kidney counts by the injected dose.

$$\% \text{ dose uptake} = \frac{\text{Corrected kidney count (cpm)}}{\text{Pre} - \text{post syringe count (cpm)}}$$

Briefly, dynamic renal scintigraphy using ^{99m}Tc-DTPA was performed in normal dogs and cats before and after toxin-induced renal insufficiency. Inulin clearances (the gold standard for GFR) were performed within 72 hours to the ^{99m}Tc-DTPA scans over varying time intervals, such as 0–1 minutes, 0–3 minutes, 1–2 minutes, etc. Linear regression analysis was used to determine which time interval gave the best correlation of percent dose uptake of ^{99m}Tc-DTPA to GFR as determined by inulin clearance. This regression formula is used to predict GFR in mL/min/kg from a percent dose uptake measured from dynamic renal scintigraphy. As in people, the percent dose uptake of ^{99m}Tc-DTPA over the 1–3-minute period correlated very closely to the inulin clearance for the dog (r > 0.94) and cat (r > 0.81) (Krawiec et al. 1986; Krawiec et al. 1988; Uribe et al. 1992). Using the regression formula below, an estimation of GFR can be made from a calculation of the percent dose uptake in the kidney (Table 18.1). The formula is species-specific.

$$\text{GFR} \left(\frac{\frac{\text{mL}}{\text{min}}}{\text{kg}} \right) = \text{A } (\% \text{ dose uptake in the kidneys}) \times \text{B}$$

Another method to predict GFR from dynamic renal scintigraphy uses compartmental analysis (Kampa et al. 2007). The technique assumes a two-compartment model with unidirectional transfer of the ^{99m}Tc-DTPA from one compartment (plasma) to the other (kidney). The rate constant from the plasma to the kidney is the clearance rate. This clearance rate can be solved using a graphical analysis technique. The graphic is a Patlak–Rutland plot (Figure 18.1), which has as its y-axis as the function of kidney activity, $K(t)$, divided by plasma activity, $P(t)$: $K(t)/P(t)$, where $K(t)$ represents the attenuation corrected net kidney counts at time (t) and $P(t)$ represents plasma counts at time (t) (Peter 1994; Piepsz et al. 1996). The plasma activity is derived for an ROI drawn over the left ventricle (Kampa et al. 2006). The x-axis is a plot of integral of plasma activity $P(t)$ divided by $P(t)$: $\int P(t)dt/P(t)$. The points plotted are

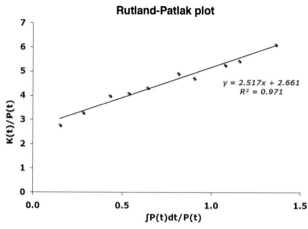

Figure 18.1 This is Patlak–Rutland plot. The y-axis is the function of kidney activity, $K(t)$, divided by plasma activity, $P(t)$. The x-axis is a plot of integral of plasma activity $P(t)$ divided by $P(t)$. The slope of this graph is equal or proportional to the clearance of the tracer from the blood to a tissue compartment.

reasonably straight except for the early points, which are influenced by extrarenal activity, and late points, which are influenced by passage of the radiopharmaceutical into the lower urinary tract (Piepsz et al. 1996). The slope of this graph is equal or proportional to the clearance of the tracer from the blood to a tissue compartment (Peter 1994).

A GFR value is expressed in terms of clearance per plasma volume (mL/min/L).

Dynamic renal scintigraphy is not an absolute measure of GFR (Finco 2005); however, there is strong correlation of GFR measurement derived from dynamic renal scintigraphy to inulin clearances (Krawiec et al 1986; Guyton and Hall 2006; Kowalsky 2006; Sykes et al 2006). Dynamic renal scintigraphy is less accurate than plasma clearance studies in determining GFR (Barthez et al. 1998). This is partially because of the fact that GFR measured from dynamic renal scintigraphy is based on a relatively short sampling of data (1–3 minutes postinjection for the Gates method, and 1–4 minutes for the Rutland–Patlak plot method) (Krawiec et al. 1986; Uribe et al. 1992; Kampa et al. 2007). Autoregulatory mechanisms alter the GFR to accommodate changes in RBF and pressure (Guyton and Hall 2006). Imaging GFR values may vary considerably in an animal (Kampa et al. 2003). This is especially true in animals with a normal or near-normal renal reserve capacity. GFR is also influenced by nonrenal factors, such as stress, hydration status, and dietary protein or sodium content (Greco et al. 1994; Finco and Cooper 2000; Singer 2003). Studies that measure GFR over a longer time interval, such as 24-hour inulin clearances or 3-hour plasma clearance studies, are more likely to give an accurate measurement of the animal's true GFR.

There is better accuracy in GFR measurement in animals with renal insufficiency because these animals have no reserve capacity and their kidneys are operating at or near maximum GFR.

The Gates method is based on an integral count of renal activity from 1–3 minutes. This technique assumes that the peak renal activity will occur between 3–4 minutes following injection. If the transit time of the ^{99m}Tc-DTPA molecule through the nephron is decreased, then the time to peak renal activity can be less than 3 minutes. If the total renal counts from 1–3 minutes is used in the calculation of the renal function and some of that activity has already left the kidney before 3 minutes, the measured GFR will be less. This was shown to be true in a study that was performed before and after saline diuresis. In this study, the renal mean transit time (MTT) was shortened with diuresis and the GFR was lower (Kunze et al. 2006).

There are other factors that influence the accuracy of GFR determination from image analysis (Kampa 2006). The gamma camera is a more complex instrument and factors such as field uniformly, linearity, and spatial resolution affect the image quantification. The patient must remain motionless during the imaging procedure. Movement decreases the ability to obtain accurate quantification of renal activity. In addition, ROI placement and depth attenuation can lead to errors in calculation of renal uptake (Kampa et al. 2002). Still, correlation of the imaging GFR values to inulin clearance values are good in animals, and the ease and speed that results can be obtained makes the imaging GFR technique useful.

The influence of hydration status or fluid loading can also influence GFR quantifications from imaging studies (Tabaru et al. 1993). Most imaging studies base their measurements of GFR during the first few minutes following injection of the radiopharmaceutical. A change in arterial pressure or RBF immediately before injection of the radiopharmaceutical influences the clearance rate and may not represent the true steady state GFR. To get the best estimate of the animal's true GFR, the animal should be well hydrated.

Interpretative principles

Interpretation of dynamic renal scintigraphy involves the analysis of serial images (Figure 18.2a), evaluation of a renogram curve created from time–activity data obtained from ROI analysis of both the kidneys (Figure 18.2b), and quantitative analysis of the data. In a normal animal, the aorta and kidney will be clearly seen, following the passage of the radiopharmaceutical through the heart and lungs.

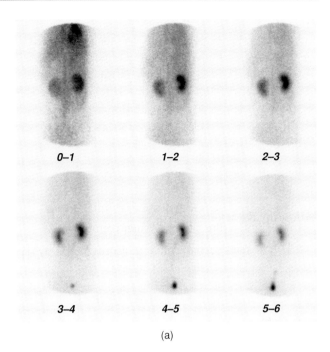

(a)

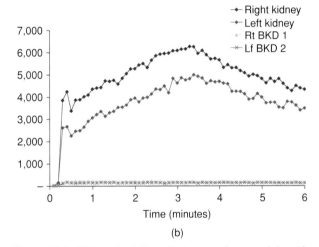

(b)

Figure 18.2 (a) Dorsal scintigraphic images of a normal dog. The animal's position with the head to the top and the animal's right is on the right side of the images. These are composite images created by summing all data into 1-minute intervals. The time is show below the images. Note the rapid increase in intensity of kidney uptake and the rapid clearance of the soft tissues. (b) Renogram curve created by plotting the activity within the left and right kidney over time. Note the initial arterial peak, then the gradual accumulation of the radiopharmaceutical within the kidneys. Peak renal activity was reached around 3 minutes following injection followed by renal clearance.

This initial renal activity is seen on the renogram curve as a rapidly rising slope that reaches an inflection point 15–30 seconds following injection. The kidney uptake decreases after the initial arterial blush. The decrease in kidney activity occurs because only 20% of the ^{99m}Tc-DTPA is extracted on each circulatory pass; therefore, some of the 99mTc-DTPA passes through the glomerulus and exits through the renal vein. In subsequent circulatory passes, the kidney gradually accumulates the radiopharmaceutical within the nephron through glomerular filtration. Peak renal radioactivity usually occurs between 2.5 and 3.5 minutes following injection. One study evaluating 8 normal dogs showed a range of 2–5.5 minutes (Barthez et al. 1999; Barthez et al. 2000). Time to peak renal radioactivity may be longer in poorly functioning kidneys or shorter if the animal is undergoing diuresis (Kunze et al. 2006). Renal radioactivity then decreases as the ^{99m}Tc-DTPA passes into the lower urinary tract. The rate of clearance from the kidney into the lower urinary tract can be used to assess outflow obstruction.

Global GFR values above 3 mL/min/kg are considered normal in a dog and global GFR values above 2.5 mL/min/kg are considered normal in a cat (Daniel et al. 1999; Twardock and Bahr 2006). Animals with subclinical renal insufficiency have global values between 1.2 and 2.5 mL/min/kg. Animals with global GFR values less than these levels (Figure 18.3) are often azotemic.

Global GFR values below 0.25 will have such poor renal uptake that quantitative renal scintigraphy with ^{99m}Tc-DTPA may be difficult to perform accurately.

Evaluation for obstructive uropathy

The renal (MTT) of the radiopharmaceutical can be calculated from the renal time–activity curve (Barthez et al. 1999). MTT can be calculated by various methods involving deconvolution of the renal time–activity curve with the vascular time–activity curve. Deconvolution of these curves allows creation of a renal time–activity curve that simulates a direct arterial injection of radiopharmaceutical into the renal artery. Various methods have been described in the human and veterinary literature. The most common method uses a matrix method for analysis. MTT can be used to detect ureteral obstruction. In one study, dogs were evaluated for 2–9 days after surgically induced partial ureteral obstruction (Barthez et al. 2000). There was a significant increase in renal transit times at 2 and 4 days following surgery. This was accompanied by decrease in renal uptake in some dogs. It was concluded that MTT may be useful in evaluation of upper urinary tract obstruction. A definitive value for obstruction has not been established in dogs.

Renal scintigraphy combined with injection of a diuretic is considered by many to be the method of choice to assess renal function and ureteral patency (Morton et al. 2007). The injection of the diuretic is necessary to differentiate between a dilated nonobstructed versus an obstructed ureter. Without the diuretic, both of these conditions can result in a lack of clearance from the kid-

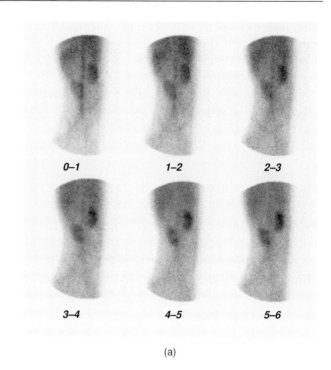

(a)

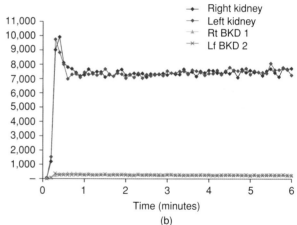

(b)

Figure 18.3 (a) Dorsal scintigraphic images of a dog in renal failure. Note the activity in the kidneys is less than the animal in Figure 18.2. Also note the persistence of activity in the extrarenal soft tissues and the lack of urinary bladder activity. (b) Renogram curve created by plotting the activity within the left and right kidney over time. Note the initial arterial peak indicating good renal blood flow; however, following the arterial blush of the kidneys, there is no accumulation of the radiopharmaceutical within the kidney. The flat renogram curve is characteristic of an animal with poor renal function.

ney. If the dynamic acquisition is terminated by 6 minutes following injection, the renogram curve will continue to increase to the end of the study in animals with a dilated renal pelvis and ureter. This ureteral dilation can occur secondary to obstruction, but can also be associated with nonobstructive disorders such as vesicoureteral reflux, trauma, infection, or congenital anomalies.

Table 18.2 Shape and diagnostic interpretation of the clearance phase of renogram curve

Type curve	Shape of clearance phase of renogram curve	Diagnosis
Type 1	Spontaneous clearance of activity from the kidney prior to lasix administration	Normal
	Clearance following lasix may appear flat if the collecting system has emptied prior to lasix	
Type 2	Progressive increase in renogram curve, even after lasix administration	High grade obstruction
Type 3a	Progressive increase in renogram curve until lasix is administered, then a rapid clearance from the kidney	Dilated, nonobstructed
Type 3b	Progressive increase in renogram curve until lasix is administered, then a slower than normal clearance from the kidney	Partial obstruction

Diuretic renography can be performed as a part of the routine renal scan using ^{99m}Tc-DTPA, only differing by the administration of 3.0 mg/kg furosemide IV at 4.5 minutes. The length of the dynamic acquisition is increased to 8 minutes. The shape of the renogram curve has been used to help in the diagnosis of obstructive uropathy (Table 18.2; Figure 18.4) (Morton et al. 2007).

The rate of renal excretion can be quantified from the downslope of the renogram curves. It is necessary to standardize the slope of the excretion phase to remove the effect of differing doses and plasma volumes. The standardized curve also helps in animals with poor renal function in which the peak renal activity will be less than a normal functioning kidney. The renogram curves are normalized so that the peak renal activity has a value of 10,000. A linear regression is used to fit the downslope of the renogram curve and measure the slope of the line. An excretion $T_{1/2}$ is derived from the slope of the fitted line. In normal dogs, the excretion $T_{1/2}$ median is 4.16 minutes with a range 3.62–5.90 minutes (Mitchell et al.

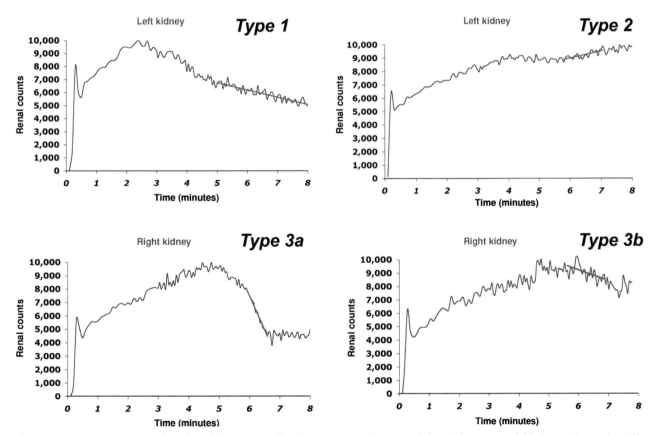

Figure 18.4 Renogram curves from four different animals. The type 1 curve is a normal dog with no ureteral dilation or obstruction. The type 2 curve is from a dog with ureteral calculi obstructing the left ureter. The type 3a curve is from a dog with renal pelvic calculi and mild ureteral dilation but no obstruction. The type 3b curve is a dog with a calculi in the right ureter causing partial obstruction.

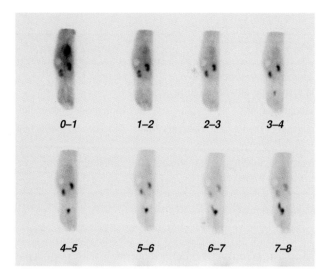

Figure 18.5 Dorsal scintigraphic images of a dog with bilateral nephroliths. The animal is positioned the same as the dog in Figures 18.2 and 18.3. The time is shown below the images. Lasix was injected intravenously at 4.5 minutes into the scan. Note the rapid decrease in renal activity after lasix injection indicating patency of the ureters.

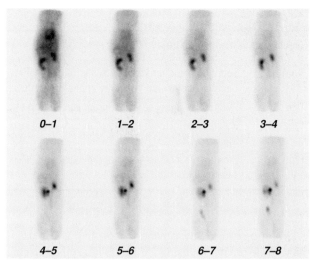

Figure 18.6 Dorsal scintigraphic images of a dog with bilateral nephroliths and right ureteral calculi. The animal is positioned the same as the dog in Figure 18.5. The time is shown below the images. Lasix was injected intravenously at 4.5 minutes into the scan. Note the left kidney is smaller than the right. There was a large photopenic void in the region of the right renal pelvis during the initial stages of the study consistent with renal pelvic. The radiopharmaceutical cleared from the left kidney. The activity in the right kidney passed from the renal pelvis into the proximal right ureter where it was retained. This dog had an obstructed proximal right ureter.

1998; Hecht et al. 2006a). Diuretic renal scintigraphy was performed in a series of 21 dogs with urolithiasis (Hecht et al. 2006b). In dogs with nonobstructed kidneys, renogram curves were type 1 or 3a (Figure 18.5).

The excretion phase of the renogram curve was similar to normal dogs and the excretion $T_{1/2}$ was not significantly difference. Obstructed kidneys showed a type 2 curve that continued to rise after lasix administration (Figure 18.6).

This study shows diuretic renography to be a useful tool to differentiate between obstructed and nonobstructed urolithiasis.

Plasma clearance studies

GFR can also be determined by clearance of ^{99m}Tc-DTPA from plasma (Cohen 1974). This method requires intravenous injection of ^{99m}Tc-DTPA followed by collection of blood samples at varying time intervals following injection (Heiene and Moe 1998). The in vitro counting technique is more laborious than imaging techniques (Figure 18.7); however, accuracy is improved since measurements are made over a longer time and are less susceptible to normal homoeostatic regulatory changes in renal function (Barthez et al. 1998).

In addition, the technique can be used in all the species using the same methods and formulas (Held and Daniel 1991; Matthews, Andrews et al. 1992). After a single intravenous injection of a radiopharmaceutical, disappearance of that substance from the plasma is related to

its distribution throughout the body and its excretion by the kidneys (Peter 2004). The plasma clearance curve of ^{99m}Tc-DTPA is described as biexponential for up to 4 hours (Figure 18.8).

The first exponential represents exchange of ^{99m}Tc-DTPA between plasma and the extracellular fluid space. In reality, there is another compartment that represents exchange of ^{99m}Tc-DTPA between subcompartments in the extracellular fluid space but it cannot be separated from the first compartment (Peter 2004). The second exponential is slower and represents the fractional rate at which ^{99m}Tc-DTPA is filtered at the glomerulus. The plasma clearance is equal to the administered amount of ^{99m}Tc-DTPA divided by the area under the plasma clearance curve (Cohen 1974; Daniel et al. 1999). The area under the plasma concentration curve can be defined by the sum of the area under these two compartments. The area is determined by a biexponential regression analysis of the decreasing plasma concentration data. Using commercial software, a least-squares approximation is used to determine the coefficients of the biexponential function using the following formula:

$$\text{GFR} = \frac{\text{Administered activity (dose)}}{^{A}/_{\alpha_a} + {^{B}/_{\alpha_b}}}$$

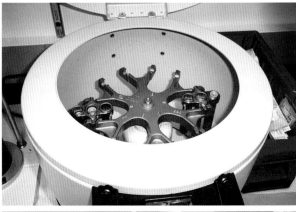
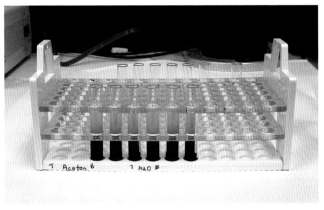
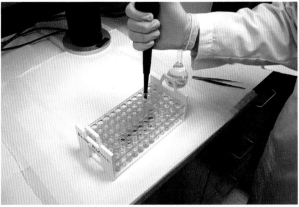
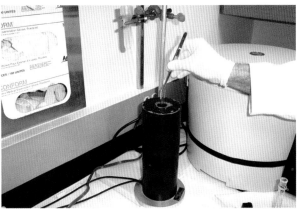

Figure 18.7 Step involved in a plasma clearance study. The plasma is separated by centrifugation. Aliquots of the plasma are removed and counted in a NaI well detector.

where A and B are the y-intercept of the fast and slow compartments, and α_a and α_b are the slopes of the clearance from the respective compartments.

The renal clearance formulas described above require that the dose be expressed in the same terms as the plasma activity. The radioactivity in the injected dose is recorded

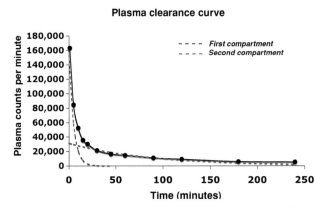

Figure 18.8 The activity within the plasma samples is plotted and fitted with by a biexponential function. The rapid drop in plasma activity represents redistribution in the plasma, that is, first compartment. The slower second compartment represents renal clearance.

in mCi or μCi, whereas the plasma activity is in counts per unit time. A standard is prepared to convert the expression of an injected dose in mCi or μCi to cpm. The standard is prepared by placing a measured quantity (approximately 80 μCi) (3 MBq) of the radiopharmaceutical into a 100-mL volumetric flask and expanding the volume to exactly 100 mL. An aliquot of the standard is removed and counted to determine the cpm per μCi of the standard, which is dependent on the efficiency of the well detector. The information from the standard is used to convert the injected dose from mCi to cpm detected using the well detector.

By using a radiopharmaceutical that is cleared exclusively by glomerular filtration, such as ^{99m}Tc-DTPA, this method can be used to determine GFR. Measurement of renal plasma flow is determined by clearance of a compound that is nearly completely extracted from the blood on its first passage through the kidney. Orthoiodohippuric Acid (OIH) is chemically similar to paraaminohippuric acid (PAH), which is the gold standard for measurement of renal plasma (Thrall and Ziessman 1995). OIH is the radiopharmaceutical of choice for evaluation of renal plasma flow because it has a high-first-pass extraction rate (95%). Tubular secretion accounts for

80% of OIH extraction from the blood with glomerular filtration accounting for the remaining 20%. OIH will equilibrate with the extracellular fluid space within minutes following intravenous injection. Disappearance of OIH is far more rapid than ^{99m}Tc-DTPA. OIH is commercially available in either an ^{123}I or ^{131}I form. ^{99m}Tc-Mercaptoacetyltriglycine(MAG$_3$) is an alternative to OIH and is now the radiopharmaceutical of choice for measuring ERPF (Itkin et al. 1994; Meyer et al. 1997). ^{99m}Tc-MAG$_3$ has biologic properties similar to OIH. Elimination of ^{99m}Tc-MAG$_3$ is primarily by tubular secretion (90%) with a small component by glomerular filtration (10%). ^{99m}Tc-MAG$_3$ has higher protein binding than OIH, which results in a lower plasma clearance, 70% of OIH. Since MAG$_3$ is a Tc-99 m agent, the radiopharmaceutical has better imaging properties than OIH.

Renal morphology scintigraphy with ^{99m}Tc-DMSA

^{99m}Tc-Dimercaptosuccinic acid (DMSA) is used as a renal cortical imaging agent (Thrall and Ziessman 1995). ^{99m}Tc-DMSA is partially bound in the proximal convoluted tubules and renal cortical uptake reaches maximum between 3 and 6 hours following radiopharmaceutical administration (Morton et al. 2007). ^{99m}Tc-DMSA is largely protein bound (90%) following injection and is therefore not available for glomerular filtration. The rate of extraction by the kidney tubules is slow with only 4–5% removed from the blood with each circulatory pass. Delayed imaging at 2–3 hours postinjection is recommended to allow adequate time for renal localization. By 4 hours postinjection, 51.7 ± 2.5% of the radiopharmaceutical will be bound to the kidney in normal dogs (Lora-Michiels et al. 2001). ^{99m}Tc-DMSA can be used to detect space occupying masses which displace renal tubular cells. These lesions will appear as a photopenic defects. Differential estimation of functioning tubular-renal mass can be made by determining the percent dose uptake of ^{99m}Tc-DMSA by the left and right kidneys (Morton et al. 2007). It is important to note that this provides an estimate of functioning tubular-renal mass and not renal function, as poor DMSA uptake in the presence of normal DTPA uptake has been seen in patients with tubulointerstitial renal disease. ^{99m}Tc-DMSA has also been used to detect acute pyelonephritis, and is considered superior to excretory urography for detection of renal scarring in children (Majd and Rushton 1992).

^{99m}Tc-DMSA is a static imaging agent. Unlike the other renal radiopharmacetical that are rapidly taken up and excreted by the kidneys, ^{99m}Tc-DMSA is taken up slowly and remains in the kidney. Instead of taking a series of

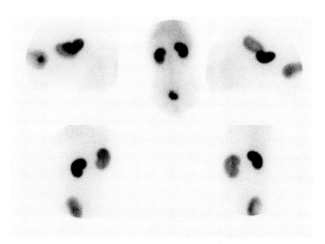

Figure 18.9 Images of a normal dog obtained 3 hours following injection of ^{99m}Tc-DMSA. The images on the top row are from left to right (right lateral, dorsal, and left lateral images). The images on the bottom row are from left to right (left dorsal oblique and right dorsal oblique). Note the majority of activity is located in the renal cortices. There is minimal extrarenal soft tissue or urinary bladder activity

images (dynamic acquisition), these studies are more similar to a bone scan in which individual images of the kidney are acquired 2–4 hours after injection. Images can be repeated if there is patient movement. Normally, ^{99m}Tc-DMSA uptake is uniformly distributed within the renal cortex (Figure 18.9) (Daniel et al. 1999).

Typically, dorsal, lateral, and oblique views are taken to free project as much of the renal cortex as possible. The kidneys are clearly visualized due to the high kidney

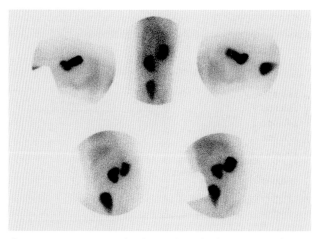

Figure 18.10 Images of a dog with multiple metastatic lesions to the kidney obtained 3 hours following injection of ^{99m}Tc-DMSA. The images on the top row are from left to right (right lateral, dorsal, and left lateral images. The images on the bottom row are from left to right (left dorsal oblique and right dorsal oblique). Note the multiple photopenic defects in both kidneys corresponding to the location of the metastatic lesions.

to background ratio. Space occupying masses devoid of normal tubules do not accumulate the radiopharmaceutical and appear as photopenic voids or "cold" lesions (Figure 18.10).

^{99m}Tc-DMSA has been used to diagnose acute pyelonephritis in people (Majd and Rushton 1992). Pyelonephritis results in multiple photopenic lesions due to a combination of focal tubular cell dysfunction and ischemia. ^{99m}Tc-DMSA can also be used to quantify relative (left versus right) functioning renal tubular mass (Lora-Michiels et al. 2001). In a study in dogs subjected to renal tubular damage by toxic doses of gentamicin, ^{99m}Tc-DMSA was able to detect disease earlier than either ^{99m}Tc-DTPA or ^{99m}Tc-MAG$_3$ (Lora-Michiels et al. 2001).

References

Barthez, P.Y., W.J. Hornof, et al. (1998). Comparison between the scintigraphic uptake and plasma clearance of Tc-99 m-diethylenetriaminepentacetic acid (DTPA) for the evaluation of the glomerular filtration rate in dogs. *Vet Radiol Ultrasound* **39** (5): 470–474.

Barthez, P.Y., D.D. Smeak, et al. (2000). Ureteral obstruction after ureteroneocystostomy in dogs assessed by technetium Tc 99 m diethylenetriamine pentaacetic acid (DTPA) scintigraphy. *Vet Surg* **29** (6): 499–506.

Barthez, P.Y., D.D. Smeak, et al. (1999). Effect of partial ureteral obstruction on results of renal scintigraphy in dogs. *Am J Vet Res* **60**(11): 1383–1389.

Barthez, P.Y., E.R. Wisner, et al. (1999). Renal transit time of Tc-99 m-diethylenetriaminepentacetic acid (DTPA) in normal dogs. *Vet Radiol Ultrasound* **40** (6): 649–656.

Berry, C.R. and G.B. Daniel (2006a). Radiation safety, personnel radiation monitoring and licensing issues. In: *Textbook of Veterinary Nuclear Medicine*, edited by G.B. Daniel and C.R. Berry. Harrisburg PA: American College of Veterinary Radiology, pp. 121–128.

Berry, C.R. and G.B. Daniel (2006b). Radiation Detectors. In: *Textbook of Veterinary Nuclear Medicine*, edited by G.B. Daniel and C.R. Berry. Harrisburg, PA: American College of Veterinary Radiology, pp. 25–38.

Cohen, M.L. (1974). Radionuclide Clearance Techniques. *Semin Nucl Med* **4** (1): 23.

Daniel, G.B. (2006). Quality control and image artifacts. In: *Textbook of Veterinary Nuclear Medicine*, edited by G.B. Daniel and C.R. Berry. Harrisburg, PA: American College of Veterinary Medicine, pp. 53–78.

Daniel, G.B., S.K. Mitchell, et al. (1999). Renal nuclear medicine: a review. *Vet Radiol Ultrasound* **40** (6): 572–587.

Evans, H.E. and G.C. Christensen (1993). The urogenital system. In: *Miller's Anatomy of the Dog*, edited by H.E. Evans and G.C. Christensen. Philadelphia, PA: WB Saunders, pp. 494–558.

Feeney, D.A. and G.A. Johnson (2007). The kidney and ureters. In: *Textbook of Veterinary Diagnostic Radiology*, edited by D.E. Thrall. St Louis, MO: Saunders Elsevier, pp. 693–707.

Finco, D.R. (2005). Measurement of glomerular filtration rate via urinary clearance of inulin and plasma clearance of technetium Tc 99 m pentetate and exogenous creatinine in dogs. *Am J Vet Res* **66** (6): 1046–1055.

Finco, D.R. and T.L. Cooper (2000). Soy protein increases glomerular filtration rate in dogs with normal or reduced renal function. *J Nutr* **130** (4): 745–748.

Gates, G.F. (1982). Glomerular filtration rate: estimation from fractional renal accumulation of 99mTc-DTPA (stannous). *AJR Am J Roentgenol* **138**: 565.

Greco, D.S., G.E. Lees, et al. (1994). Effect of dietary sodium intake on glomerular filtration rate in partially nephrectomized dogs. *Am J Vet Res* **55** (1): 152–159.

Greer, L.L., G.B. Daniel, et al. (2005). Evaluation of the use of technetium Tc 99 m diethylenetriamine pentaacetic acid and technetium Tc 99 m dimercaptosuccinic acid for scintigraphic imaging of the kidneys in green iguanas (*Iguana iguana*). *Am J Vet Res* **66** (1): 87–92.

Guyton, A.C. and J.E. Hall (2006). Urine formation by the kidneys: I. Glomerular filtration, renal blood flow and their control. In: *Textbook of Medical Physiology*, edited by A.C. Guyton and J.E. Hall. Philadelphia, PA: Elsevier, pp. 307–326.

Hecht, S., G.B. Daniel, et al. (2006a). Diuretic renal scintigraphy in normal dogs. *Vet Radiol Ultrasound* **47** (6): 602–608.

Hecht, S., G.B. Daniel, et al. (2006b). 99mTc-DTPA diuretic renography in dogs with urolithiasis. *14th Meeting of the International Veterinary Radiology Association*, Vancouver BC, IVRA-ACVR.

Heiene, R. and L. Moe (1998). Pharmacokinetic aspects of measurement of glomerular filtration rate in the dog: a review. *J Vet Intern Med* **12**: 401.

Held, J.P. and G.B. Daniel (1991). Use of nonimaging nuclear medicine techniques to assess the effect of flunixin meglumine on effective renal plasma flow and effective renal blood flow in healthy horses. *Am J Vet Res* **52** (10): 1619–1621.

Itkin, R.J., D.R. Krawiec, et al. (1994). Evaluation of the single-injection plasma disappearance of tc-99 m mercaptoacetyltriglycine method for determination of effective renal plasma-flow in dogs with normal or abnormal renal-function. *Am J Vet Res* **55** (12): 1652–1659.

Kampa, N. (2006). Renal scintigraphy in dogs. PhD Thesis, Department of Biomedical Sciences and Public Health, Uppsala Swedish University of Agricultural Sciences, Uppsala, Sweden.

Kampa, N., I. Bostrom, et al. (2003). Day-to-day variability in glomerular filtration rate in normal dogs by scintigraphic technique. *J Vet Med A Physiol Pathol Clin Med* **50** (1): 37–41.

Kampa, N., P. Lord, et al. (2007). Effects of measurement of plasma activity input on normalization of glomerular filtration rate to plasma volume in dogs. *Vet Radiol Ultrasound* **48** (6): 585–593.

Kampa, N., U. Wennstrom, et al. (2002). Effect of region of interest selection and uptake measurement on glomerular filtration rate measured by Tc-99 m-DTPA scintigraphy in dogs. *Vet Radiol Ultrasound* **43** (4): 383–391.

Kim, E.E., B.J. Barron, et al. (1996). Genitourinary nuclear medicine. In: *Diagnostic Nuclear Medicine*, edited by M.P. Sandlers, R.E. Coleman, F.J. Wacker, et al. Baltimore, MD: Williams & Wilkins, pp. 1191–1208.

Kowalsky, R.J. (2006). Radioactive decay, radioactivity, Tc-99 m generator and radiopharmaceuticals. In: *Textbook of Veterinary Nuclear Medicine*, G.B. Daniel and C.R. Berry. Harrisburg, PA: American College of Veterinary Radiology, pp. 1–24.

Krawiec, D.R., R.R. Badertscher, II, et al. (1986). Evaluation of 99mTc-diethylenetriaminepentaacetic acid nuclear imaging for quantitative determination of the glomerular filtration rate of dogs. *Am J Vet Res* **47** (10): 2175–2179.

Krawiec, D.R., A.R. Twardock, et al. (1988). Use of 99mTc diethylenetriaminepentaacetic acid for accessment of renal function in dogs with suspected renal disease. *J Am Vet Med Assoc* **192** (8): 1077–1080.

Kunze, C., A. Bahr, et al. (2006). Evaluation of Tc-99 m-diethylenetriaminepentaacetic acid renal scintigram curves in normal dogs after induction of diuresis. *Vet Radiol Ultrasound* **47** (1): 103–107.

Lora-Michiels, M., K. Anzola, et al. (2001). Quantitative and qualitative scintigraphic measurement of renal function in dogs exposed to toxic doses gentamicin. *Vet Radiol Ultrasound* **42** (6): 553–561.

Majd, M. and H.G. Rushton (1992). Renal cortical scintigraphy in the diagnosis of acute pyelonephtitis. *Semin Nucl Med* **22** (2): 98.

Matthews, H.K., F.M. Andrews, et al. (1992). Comparison of standard and radionuclide methods for measurement of glomerular-filtration rate and effective renal blood-flow in female horses. *Am J Vet Res* **53** (9): 1612–1616.

Mazze, R.I. (1986). Renal physiology and the effects of anesthesia. In: *Anesthesia*, edited by R.I. Mazze. NY: Chruchill Livingston, pp. 1223–1248.

Meyer, I., A. Westhoff, et al. (1997). Qualitative and quantitative renal function testing in the dog by means of MAG(3)-clearance measurement. *Berl Munch Tierarztl Wochenschr* **110** (5): 185–189.

Mitchell, S.K., G.B. Daniel, et al. (1998). Diuresis renography in normal dogs. *Annual Scientific Conference of the American College of Veterinary Radiology*. Chicago IL: American College of Veterinary Radiology *Veterinary Radiology & Ultrasound* **39**: 587.

Morton, K.A., P.B. Clarke, et al. (2007). Genitourinary. In: *Diagnostic Imaging: Nuclear Medicine*, edited by K.A. Morton and P.B. Clarke. Salt Lake City, UT: Amirsys, pp. 1–77.

Newell, S.M., J.C. Ko, et al. (1997). Effects of three sedative protocols on glomerular filtration rate in clinically normal dogs. *Am J Vet Res* **58** (5): 446–450.

Nilsson, K., E. Evander, et al. (1997). Pulmonary clearance of 99mTc-DTPA and 99mTc-Ablumin in smokers. *Clin Physiol* **14**: 183.

Nyland, T.G., J.S. Mattoon, et al. (2002). Small Animal Diagnostic Ultrasound 2nd ed. In: *Urinary Tract*, edited by T.G. Nyland and J.S. Mattoon. Philadelphia, PA: WB Saunders, pp. 158–195.

Peter, A.M. (1994). Editorial-Graphical analysis of dynamic data: the Patlak–Rutland plot. *Nucl Med Commun* **15**: 669.

Peter, A.M. (2004). The kinetic basis of glomerular filtration rate measurement and new concepts of indexation to body size. *Eur J Nucl Med* **31**: 137.

Piepsz, A., M. Kinthaert, et al. (1996). The robustness of the Patlak–Rutland slope for the determination of split renal function. *Nucl Med Commun* **17**: 817.

Singer, M.A. (2003). Dietary protein-induced changes in excretory function: a general animal design feature. *Comp Biochem Physiol B Biochem Mol Biol* **136B** (4): 785–801.

Sykes, J.M. IV, J. Schumacher, et al. (2006). Preliminary evaluation of ^{99m}technetium diethylenetriamine pentaacetic acid, ^{99m}technetium dimercaptosuccinic acid, and ^{99m}technetium mercaptoacetyltriglycine for renal scintigraphy in corn snakes (*Elaphe Guttata guttata*). *Vet Radiol Ultrasound* **47** (2): 222–227.

Tabaru, H., D.R. Finco, et al. (1993). Influence of hydration state on renal functions of dogs. *Am J Vet Res* **54** (10): 1758–1764.

Thrall, J.A. and H.A. Ziessman (1995). Genitourinary System. In: *Nuclear Medicine The Requisites*, edited by J.A. Thrall and H.A. Ziessman. St Louis, MO: Mosby, pp. 283–320.

Twardock, A.R. and A. Bahr (2006). Renal scintigraphy. In: *Textbook of Veterinary Nuclear Medicine*, edited by G.B. Daniel and C.R. Berry. Harrisburg, PA: American College of Veterinary Radiology, pp. 329–351.

Twardock, A.R., D.R. Krawiec, et al. (1991). Kidney scintigraphy. *Semin Vet Med Surg (Small Anim)* **6** (2): 164–169.

Uribe, D., D.R. Krawiec, et al. (1992). Quantitative renal scintigraphic determination of the glomerular-filtration rate in cats with normal and abnormal kidney-function, using tc-99 m-diethylenetriaminepentaacetic acid. *Am J Vet Res* **53** (7): 1101–1107.

Winter, M.D., K.G. Miles, et al. (2007). Effects of sedation protocol on glomerular filtration rate in cats as determined by quantitative renal scintigraphy. Annual Scientific Meeting of the American College of Veterinary Radiology, Chicago IL.

Young, K., G.B. Daniel, et al. (1997). Application of the pin-hole collimator in small animal nuclear scintigraphy: a review. *Vet Radiol Ultrasound* **38** (2): 83–93.

19

Diagnostic urologic endoscopy

Julie Byron and Dennis Chew

Introduction

Direct visualization of the lower urinary tract can be important for the diagnosis and treatment of many disease processes. Evaluation of the urinary bladder, ureters, and proximal urethra is possible via surgical exploration; however, uroendoscopy is a minimally invasive technique that allows assessment of the lower urinary and distal reproductive tract. In some situations, uroendoscopy may be valuable for the assessment of the upper urinary tract as in the case of unilateral renal hematuria. Uroendoscopy allows visual evaluation of the vaginal vestibule, vagina, entire urethra, urinary bladder, and ureteral openings. In some cases, the endoscope may be passed into the ureters for luminal evaluation as well. Diagnostic and therapeutic procedures may be performed via urinary endoscopy, including biopsy, urolith retrieval or lithotripsy, and laser surgical procedures. Uroendoscopy can be a valuable part of the diagnostic and therapeutic management of urinary tract diseases and can yield different information than that gained from other imaging modalities due to magnification of the luminal surfaces.

Indications

Many diseases of the urinary tract lend themselves to cystoscopic evaluation (Table 19.1). While it is often difficult to pass an endoscope into the ureters, it is possible to make some evaluation of the quality of the urine passing from one kidney or another by observing the pulsatile urine flow from the ureter openings. This is particularly relevant in cases of renal hematuria when only one kidney may be involved (Figure 19.1). Other indications for uroendoscopy include urinary incontinence, persistent hematuria, recurrent urinary tract infections, multiple types of dysuria, urinary tract obstruction, vulvar or penile discharge, and urethral or bladder masses. The potential for breakdown and retrieval of uroliths also makes uroendoscopy useful in these cases. In females, it is easy to confirm that all stones have been removed following voiding urohydropulsion (Messer et al. 2005).

Equipment

Rigid endoscope systems require a light source, camera, video monitor, and preferably an image capture system that allows for data storage onto CD or DVD. There are several manufacturers of these systems, and they are often purchased as part of a package with the endoscopes. Some incompatibilities exist between systems, so it is best to use components from the same manufacturer or verify their compatibility prior to purchase.

The best light sources for video uroendoscopy are xenon with automatic intensity adjustment. Halogen light sources can be used as well and are generally less costly, but have a lower intensity and produce lower image quality than xenon lights, especially when using smaller diameter cystoscopes. Although many rigid and flexible endoscopes have eyepieces, a camera and video system is essential for proper detailed viewing and documentation of uroendoscopic studies. Cameras are generally available in one- or three-chip models. The three-chip has higher image quality due to 3-color capture and processing and produces better images in low-light conditions, although one-chip models are adequate for most applications. Ideally, the camera has a focusing system and image capture controls mounted on the operating head,

Nephrology and Urology of Small Animals. Edited by Joe Bartges and David J. Polzin. © 2011 Blackwell Publishing Ltd.

Table 19.1 Indications for uroendoscopy of the dog and cat

Hematuria
Stranguria
Pollakiuria
Painful urination
Dysuria
Urinary incontinence
Attenuated urine stream
Urinary obstruction
Recurrent urinary tract infections
Urolithiasis
Urinary bladder masses
Vulvar discharge
Penile discharge

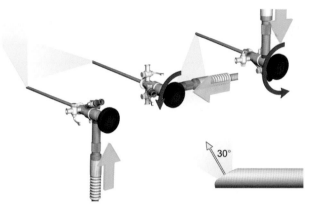

Figure 19.2 Artist's rendition of the path of view through the scope following rotation of the telescope while holding the camera in the same position. 30° viewing angle demonstrated from tip of telescope (Drawing by Tim Vojt).

although some have foot-pedal operation. A wide range of image capture systems are available from state-of-the-art high definition (HD) video to those that record only still images. Since dynamic imaging is desirable in uroendoscopy, a system that provides capture and recording of both still and video clip images is preferable.

Both rigid and flexible endoscopes may be used. Rigid cystoscopes consist of three parts, the telescope, sheath, and bridge. These may be separate components or integrated by the manufacturer. The glass fiber telescope provides an angled view of 0°, 12°, 30°, or 70° from the tip of the scope. The authors prefer 30°, which allows for visualization of all areas of the bladder with less manipulation as well as good visualization of the working field when using instruments (Figure 19.2). The sheath contains the irrigation and operating channels, and the bridge has

the light-source and camera connections as well as the instrument port (Figure 19.3). Rigid endoscope systems come in a variety of diameters and lengths. For small animal endoscopy, three sizes are generally recommended: 4.0 mm × 30 cm for medium to large female dogs, 2.7 mm × 18 cm for small and medium female dogs, and 1.9 mm × 18 cm for female cats and male cats with a perineal urethrostomy. Additionally, a flexible or semi-flexible 5 fr scope may be used to examine male cats. Male dogs with urethras that will accommodate an 8 fr diameter catheter can be examined using a flexible 7.5 fr × 45 cm human ureteroscope or other flexible endoscope of similar size.

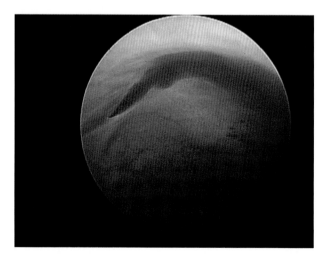

Figure 19.1 Renal hematuria can be detected by observing blood from either or both ureters. This dog had idiopathic renal hematuria coming from the right ureter/kidney.

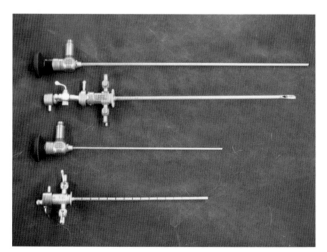

Figure 19.3 Two commonly used rigid telescopes and operating sheaths are the 4.0 mm × 30 cm telescope with a separate sheath and bridge (shown assembled here) and the 2.7 mm × 18 cm with an integrated sheath and bridge.

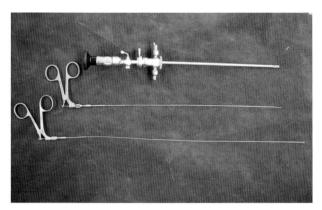

Figure 19.4 The assembled 4.0 mm × 30 cm rigid cystoscope with its operating sheath and compatible grasping and biopsy forceps are shown.

There is a large variety of accessories and instruments available for rigid endoscopes. At least one good quality biopsy forceps which fits through the operating channel is required for obtaining tissue samples. In addition, stone retrieval baskets, grasping forceps, and cautery tips are available (Figure 19.4).

Care of uroendoscopic equipment is similar to the care of other endoscopes. Rigid scopes are relatively durable; however, the small size of many of the instruments makes them especially fragile. Caution must be exercised to prevent overflexion of the instruments or excessive force in deploying and retracting them. The very small flexible and semiflexible endoscopes such as the 1 mm 6-inch Semi-Flexible Micro-Endoscope (MDS Inc., Brandon, FL) are also extremely fragile and need additional protection during cleaning and sterilization.

Patient preparation and procedure

Female dog and cat

Uroendoscopy can be performed with the patient in dorsal or lateral recumbency. The endoscopist is generally seated at the caudal end of the animal and the tail is secured out of the operating region. The external genitalia of the anesthetized patient is shaved and surgically prepared. The use of sterile technique is important to minimize iatrogenic contamination of the urinary tract. The endoscope is either gas or liquid sterilized and sterile gloves are worn during the procedure. Sterile 0.9% NaCl is passed through the irrigation channel to distend the anatomy and improve visualization. The endoscopist assembles the scope and its components and attaches the light and camera cables. The irrigation and efflux lines are attached and the scope is liberally coated with ster-

ile water-based lubricant. The scope is passed into the vaginal vestibule, and the vulvar folds are gently grasped around the scope to allow for fluid distension of the chamber.

Normal appearance during cystoscopy

The mucosa of the vestibule is light pink in color and smooth (Figures 19.5a–d). The vaginal opening, surrounded by a ridge of tissue, the cingulum, is seen at the craniodorsal aspect of the vestibule. Ventral to this is the smaller urethral opening. There may be a thin band of tissue crossing the opening dorsoventrally of the vagina, which has been called a hymenal membrane (Figures 19.6a,b). A thicker band referred to as the mesonephric remnant is often associated with abnormalities of development of the urethra and ureter. Most patients with ectopic ureter(s) have this thick band (Cannizzo et al. 2003). Either of these bands potentially may be a cause of breeding failure. The urethral opening is often covered by a dorsal fold of tissue in the intact female dog, is often exaggerated in size during heat, and should not be interpreted as a mass lesion (see Figures 19.5c,d). Lateral to the urethral opening are fossae, which may contain crypt-like areas. These can be normal findings and caution should be exercised to avoid mistaking these for ectopic ureter openings (Figure 19.7).

Next, the cystoscope is passed into the vagina, though this may be deferred to last in those with obvious discharge. The vaginal opening is encircled by a ring of fibrous tissue called the cingulum. Beyond the cingulum, the vaginal mucosa is pink with a prominent longitudinal fold running along the dorsal wall. The scope is passed cranially until the external uterine orifice at the caudal aspect of the cervix is reached. This has a folded appearance and passage of the scope beyond this point may be difficult and is rarely performed during routine urologic examinations (Figures 19.8a,b and 19.9).

The scope is redirected into the urethra and slowly passed cranially into the bladder. The urethra also has a dorsal fold and generally has smooth light pink mucosa (Figures 19.10a–c and 19.11). The length of the urethra may vary between normal dogs. Once the vesicourethral junction is reached, the bladder is drained of urine and debris and redistended with saline to provide a clear view. Urine is generally heavier than saline and pools in the dependent aspect of the bladder, obscuring structures in this area. Distension of the bladder is essential to get an adequate evaluation of the ureters and bladder wall; however, overdistension may lead to tearing of the urothelium and hemorrhage. To prevent this, the bladder should be manually palpated through the abdomen by an assistant

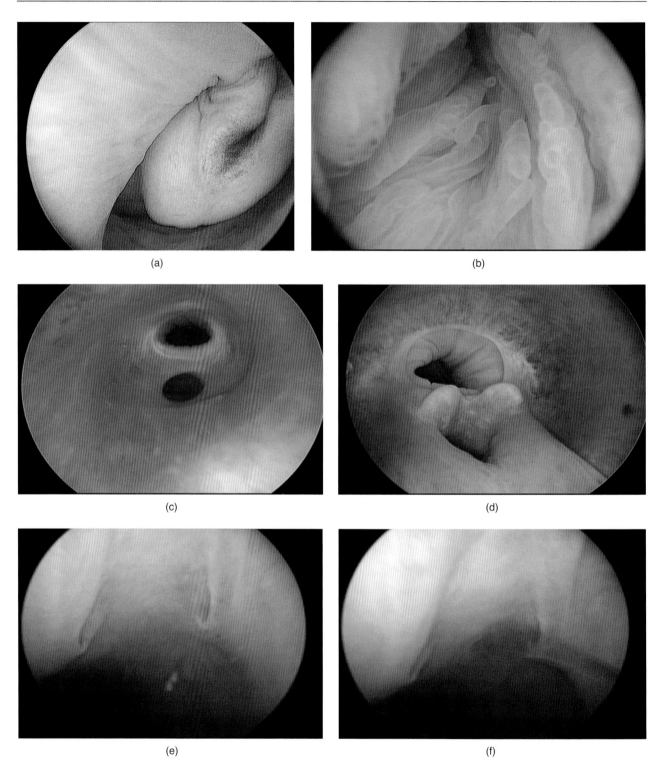

(a)

(b)

(c)

(d)

(e)

(f)

Figure 19.5 (a) and (b) The normal dog clitoris. Note the frond-like bands of tissue in the clitoral fossa. These are normal structures in the female dog. (c) and (d) The larger dorsal opening is the vagina with the thin band of tissue around its rim, the cingulum. The ventral opening is the external urethral meatus. The intact bitch has a flap of tissue dorsal to the external urethral meatus. The neutered female dog does not have this flap of tissue. (e) and (f) The ureters in the dog are normally placed slightly proximal to the vesicourethral junction and appear as two C-shaped openings facing each other. Normally, pulsatile urine flow can be seen from the ureters during cystoscopy.

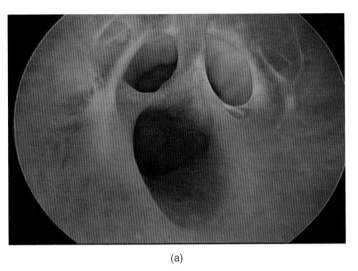

(a)

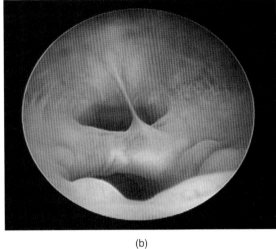

(b)

Figure 19.6 (a) A wide band of tissue, a mesonephric remnant, is often visualized across the vaginal opening in dogs with ectopic ureter. (b) A thin band across the vaginal opening is often referred to as a hymenal remnant and is common in dogs but is not associated with any lower urinary tract disease.

and distension ceased when it is slightly firm. If bleeding occurs, the bladder should be drained of fluid and chilled saline infused to induce vasoconstriction and reduce the impact on visibility. The infusion of cold fluid may cause the patient's body temperature to drop, and this should be closely monitored especially when multiple cycles of chilled fluid are infused and drained.

When the bladder is fully distended, the trigone is examined. The ureters are located dorsolateral to mid-

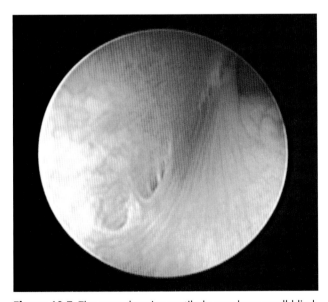

Figure 19.7 The normal canine vestibule may have small blind-end fenestrations on the lateral aspects of the urethral meatus. These are normal structures and should not be mistaken for ectopic ureters.

line as two crescent-shaped slits in the bladder wall. These two "C"-shaped structures should be facing each other as mirror images (Figures 19.5e,f and 19.10a). An inverted V- or Y-shaped ridge may run cranially from the openings and join at midline. Verification of their patency should be made by observing the pulsatile urine flow from each ureter. The cystoscope is then passed cranially to the apex of the bladder and the entire bladder wall is examined. The bladder mucosa is light pink with a fine vascular pattern (Figures 19.12a,b). Occasionally, the bladder wall will be semitransparent and abdominal organs may be faintly visualized from the lumen. It is important to examine all areas of the bladder interior in order not to miss small lesions or calculi, which may fall to its dependent aspect. Manual palpation and manipulation of the bladder through the abdomen can assist in a full evaluation. After completion of the examination, the efflux channel is opened and the fluid is drained from the bladder.

Male dog and cat

Uroendoscopy of the male is generally performed with a flexible endoscope. An assistant may be required to exteriorize the penis from the prepuce and atraumatic hemostats may be necessary to maintain retraction, particularly in the male cat. The endoscope is prepared and lubricated as with the female and is introduced directly into the external urethral orifice. Infusion of saline facilitates distension of the urethra ahead of the scope. It is important not to use the scope tip itself to dilate the urethra as this can cause injury to the delicate urothelium,

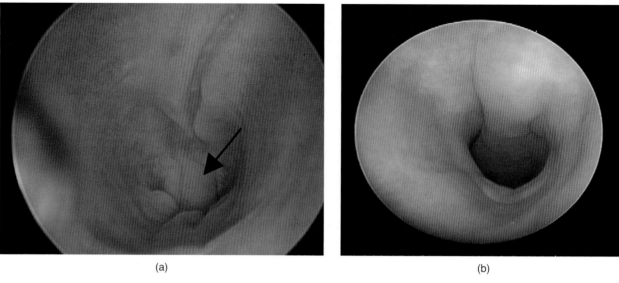

(a)   (b)

Figure 19.8 (a) The normal appearance of the vagina and cervix (arrow) in a neutered female dog. (b) The vaginal canal has a dorsal ridge of tissue that looks similar to that in the urethra.

which may be interpreted as lesions. As the scope is slowly passed from the perineal urethra into the prostatic urethra of the dog, tiny prostatic duct openings may be noted in the mucosa. These indentations are generally not seen in the male cat. Examination of the trigone, ureters, and bladder lumen are as with the female, but may be difficult due to the small size of the endoscope in relation to the size of the bladder lumen. Care must be taken to keep the tip of the scope close to the bladder wall to avoid missing lesions.

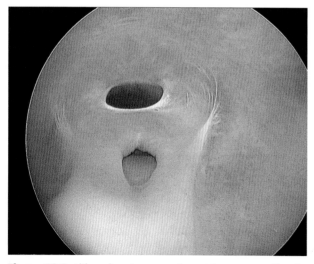

Figure 19.9 Although not necessarily a stricture, a smaller cingulum may be noted in some patients. The association of small cingulum size with incidence of lower urinary tract disease has been suggested but recently refuted to be of clinical relevance in most instances.

Abnormal appearance—uroendoscopic lesions

Several anatomic abnormalities can be observed using cystoscopy. The most widely recognized is the presence of ectopic ureters (see Chapter 58). Although several imaging modalities have been developed for the diagnosis and locating of ureteral ectopia, computed tomography (CT) (see Chapter 17) and uroendoscopy have been found to be the most reliable (Samii et al. 2004). Ectopic ureter openings may be seen at any point from the vesicourethral junction to the vestibule (Figures 19.13a–c). Many have large openings that can accommodate the diameter of a cystoscope. Care must be taken to differentiate the urethra from these large ureters. On the basis of embryology, ectopic ureter openings within the urethra are always dorsolateral and the path to the bladder ventral.

Within the vestibule, small white nodules may be noted, particularly in those patients with chronic or recurrent urinary tract infections (Figures 19.14a,b). These are often lymphoid in nature on histopathology and are likely secondary to the inflammatory process. Similar nodules are sometimes seen in the urethra and bladder. Presumptive abscesses may be noted in the wall of the bladder by their "fried egg" appearance, central pallor with a hyperemic rim around the nodule (Figure 19.15). These lesions may be biopsied and cultured to look for bacterial infection and occasionally have been read as lymphoplasmacytic infiltrates.

Mass lesions may be found within the vestibule, vagina, urethra, and bladder. Malignant neoplasia and benign or inflammatory polyps can look similar on gross

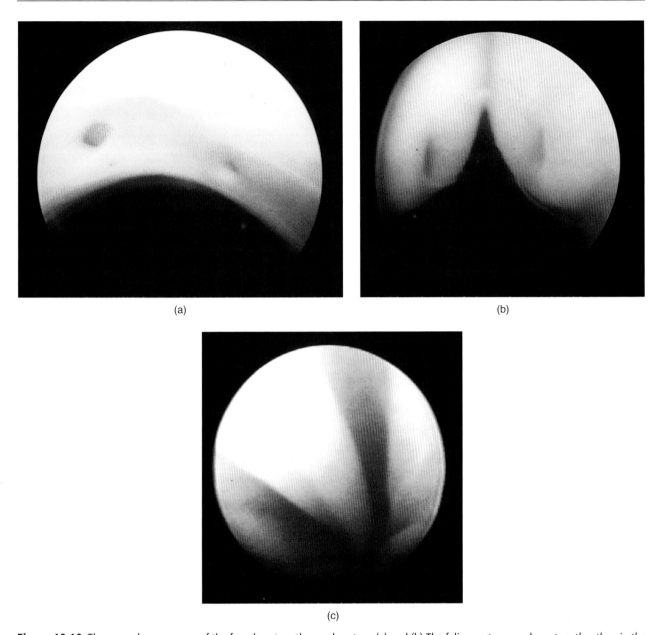

(a)

(b)

(c)

Figure 19.10 The normal appearance of the female cat urethra and ureters. (a) and (b) The feline ureters are closer together than in the dog and are more distal in the bladder neck, opening right at the vesicourethral junction. (c) The normal feline urethra in the female has a dorsal ridge that extends to the vesicourethral junction, especially prominent when the bladder is not fully distended.

examination, so it is important to sample all abnormal tissues (see Chapters 71 and 79). Proliferative urethritis (see Chapter 77) can resemble transitional cell carcinoma both in clinical presentation and cystoscopic appearance (Figure 19.16a,b) (Hostutler et al. 2004) though there are subtle cystoscopic differences (Figure 19.17a–c).

Small uroliths (see Chapter 69) are sometimes found on cystoscopic examination, despite the absence of ultrasonographic or radiologic evidence. Since most stones will fall to the dependent area of the bladder during

examination, it is important to thoroughly evaluate this area. Assessment of urolith size and feasibility of urohydropulsion can be made at this time (Figures 19.18–19.20a,b).

Additional abnormalities that may be encountered during cystoscopic examination include foreign material (Figures 19.21 and 19.22), ureteroceles, urachal diverticula (Figures 19.23a–c), and the glomerulations characteristic of idiopathic cystitis in cats (see Chapter 75) (Figure 19.24). Care must be taken to avoid interpretation

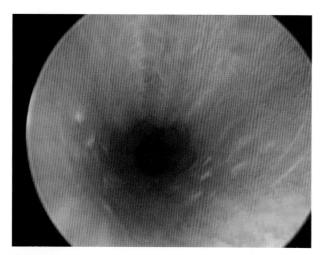

Figure 19.11 Normal appearance of the urethra in the dog.

of iatrogenic lesions from the uroendoscopy procedure (Figure 19.25).

Advanced diagnostic procedures and interventions

Additional procedures may be carried out during uroendoscopy. These should be performed after a thorough assessment of the urinary tract is completed due to the risk of secondary hemorrhage obscuring the view. Biopsy of lesions is the most common using a flexible biopsy instrument passed through the instrument port of the scope. Unfortunately, these samples are usually quite small, so several biopsies should be obtained for adequate analysis. An alternative is to identify a target area

for biopsy, remove the telescope from the sheath, and advance a larger biopsy instrument through the sheath to the desired area—in this case the biopsy is done without direct visualization. Another alternative is to pass the scope up to the mass lesion and use suction to obtain an aspiration biopsy through the operating port. The smallest flexible and semiflexible endoscopes do not have instrument ports, so biopsy may be necessary using ultrasound or fluoroscopic guidance in male cats and small male dogs.

If the ureter is dilated enough to allow passage of the scope into its lumen, a syringe may be attached to the instrument port and urine sterilely collected.

Several procedures may be performed to facilitate removal of uroliths. If the stones are small enough, they may be retrieved using a basket instrument or flushed from the bladder via urohydropulsion. Endoscopic evaluation of the urethra and bladder prior to urohydropulsion can facilitate passage of stones by lubricating and dilating the urethra. Single stones may be removed using grabbing instruments as well. Laser or electrohydraulic lithotripsy (see Chapter 34) may be performed to break the stones into smaller pieces, which may be safely flushed from the bladder (Figure 19.26) (Defarges 2006, 2008; Grant et al. 2007; Adams et al. 2008). A final evaluation should be made around the bladder lumen, particularly of the dependent areas, to determine if all uroliths have been removed before completing the procedure.

The use of injectable bulking agents to treat canine urinary incontinence has become more widely available in the last decade (see Chapters 38 and 76). The most common agent is bovine cross-linked collagen (Contigen®, C. R. Bard, Inc. Covington, GA), although other

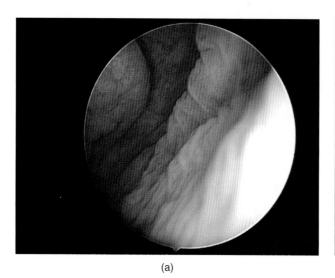

(a)

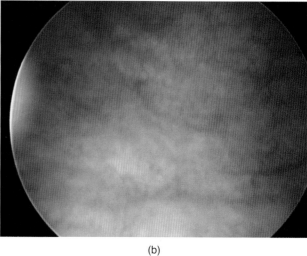

(b)

Figure 19.12 (a) The undistended bladder has a rough and undulating appearance, which flattens out when filled, (b).

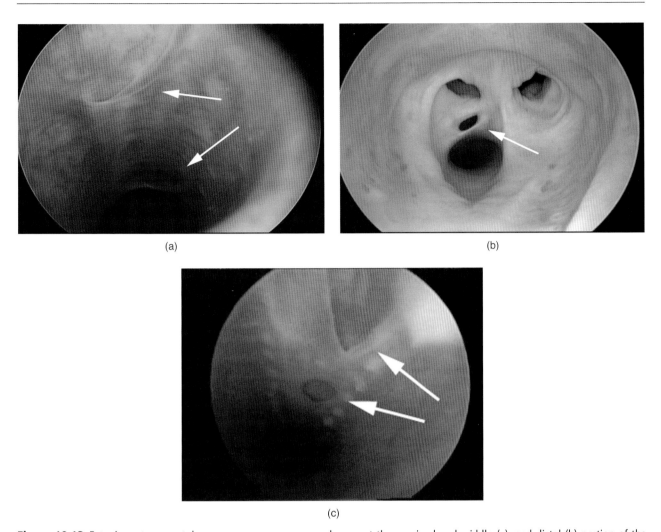

Figure 19.13 Ectopic ureters can take on many appearances and open at the proximal and middle (a), and distal (b) portion of the urethra (arrows). In (b), the patient also has a band of tissue bisecting the vaginal opening. (c) Ectopic ureters can also have fenestrations that lead to many openings along the urethra (arrows).

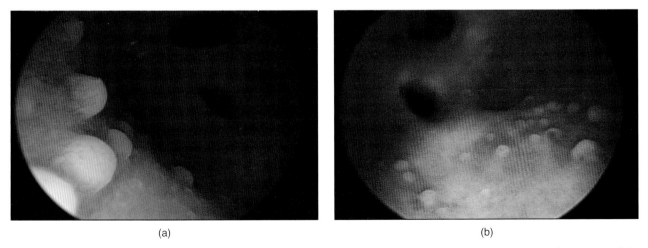

Figure 19.14 (a) and (b) Small nodular follicles may be seen in the vestibule or urethra of patients with chronic inflammation of the lower urinary tract.

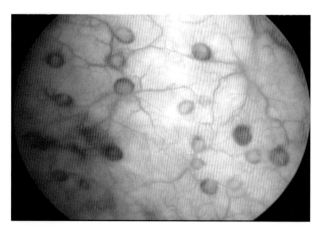

Figure 19.15 "Fried egg" appearance to the lesions on the bladder mucosa of a dog with chronic urinary tract infections. These lesions may be biopsied and cultured.

materials may be available such as Teflon paste. The material is injected through a needle passed through the instrument port of the cystoscope and embedded into the submucosa of the urethra near the vesicourethral junction. Visualization of the procedure using cystoscopy is essential for adequate placement and filling of the injection sites.

Urethral stricture can occur secondary to trauma, surgery, or the lodging of uroliths in the urethra. Strictures can be identified by uroendoscopy and those that are too proximal for surgical correction can be treated using balloon dilation. Follow-up evaluation of the affected area is important to assess the effectiveness of treatment.

Some surgical procedures have been described in dogs using cystoscopy. Electrocautery of bleeding vessels and

removal of masses has been performed (Elwick et al. 2003; Upton et al. 2006; Cerf et al. 2007). The ablation of the wall of ectopic ureters to a more cranial position using a neodymium or holmium: yttrium-aluminum-garnet (YAG) laser has also been performed in both male and female dogs (see Chapter 39) (McCarthy 2006; Berent et al. 2007, 2008). Use of a laser in cystoscopic procedures, including lithotripsy and tissue resection, requires cystoscopic experience and advanced training and is currently available at limited facilities around the United States.

Postoperative management and complications

Despite strict attention to sterility, the mild to moderate trauma to the urinary tract and the proximity of the anus may increase the likelihood of iatrogenic contamination during uroendoscopy. It is therefore recommended to place patients on 5–7 days of broad-spectrum antibiotics after the procedure. Alternatively, patients may have urine cultures evaluated 2–5 days after the procedure.

Both dogs and cats may experience a moderate amount of discomfort and pollakiuria after uroendoscopic procedures. Pain medication such as a nonsteroidal anti-inflammatory drug or mild opiate may be used for 2–3 days. In addition, mild hematuria may occur in patients after cystoscopy. This is generally short-lived and self-limiting but owners should be advised of its presence.

Several complications may arise during uroendoscopy. The most common complication is failure to be able to safely advance the cystoscope through the lumen of the urethra. Lodging of the endoscope in the urethra

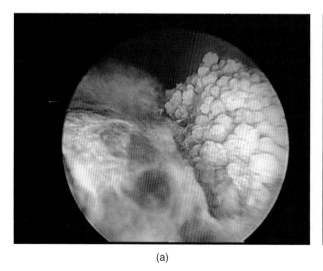
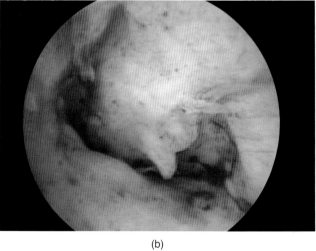

(a) (b)

Figure 19.16 (a) Polypoid cystitis, and (b) proliferative urethritis can grossly appear neoplastic. It is important to biopsy and perform histopathology on such lesions to differentiate them from carcinomas.

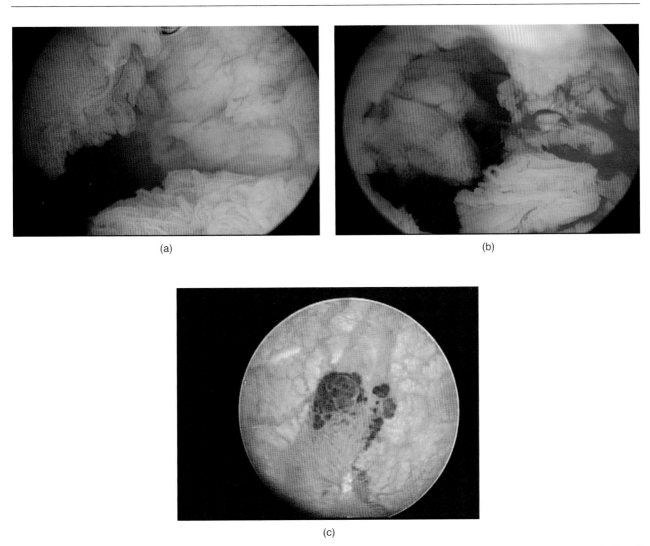

(a)

(b)

(c)

Figure 19.17 (a) and (b) Transitional cell carcinoma and other neoplasia can appear as a frondular mass on the bladder or urethral wall, or as a mass protruding from the urethra. (c) Small *in situ* carcinomas can develop at a site of incomplete resection of a neoplastic lesion.

can be avoided by proper selection of scope size for the patient and appropriate lubrication. The endoscope, whether flexible or rigid, should never be forced proximally through the urethra. This can lead to urethral damage or "hair-pinning" and lodging of a flexible scope in the urethra. Gentle pressure and, especially in the case of males, proper use of fluid to dilate the urethra ahead of the scope should be sufficient to allow for passage. If this is not successful, a smaller diameter scope should be used.

Perforation of the lower urinary tract is also a risk with uroendoscopy. This is particularly a risk in patients with a severely diseased urethral or bladder wall. The endoscopist must be attentive to the degree of fluid distention in the bladder and release any overfilling through the efflux channel. Depending on the size of the dam-

age, surgical repair may be necessary to correct a bladder tear. Rupture of the urethra can also occur, but may not require surgical intervention. Placing a urinary catheter for several days may be sufficient to allow for healing of the defect. The careful selection of an appropriately-sized scope and gentle technique will minimize these risks.

Summary

Urologic endoscopy is gaining widespread use in the diagnosis and treatment of lower urinary tract disorders in the dog and cat. The current trend toward minimally invasive interventions in veterinary medicine is leading to the development of numerous additional and therapeutic applications of this procedure.

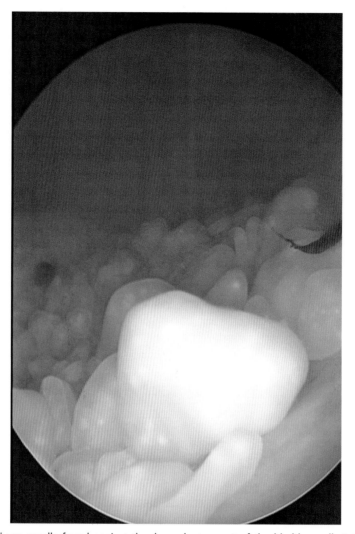

Figure 19.18 Bladder calculi are usually found against the dependent aspect of the bladder wall. A thorough examination of the dependent aspect is necessary during the cystoscopic procedure. These struvite stones were found in a female dog.

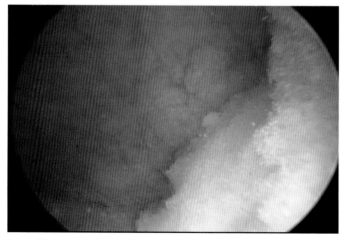

Figure 19.19 Large amounts of crystalline material may also be found on the dependent aspect of the bladder as shown in this female dog.

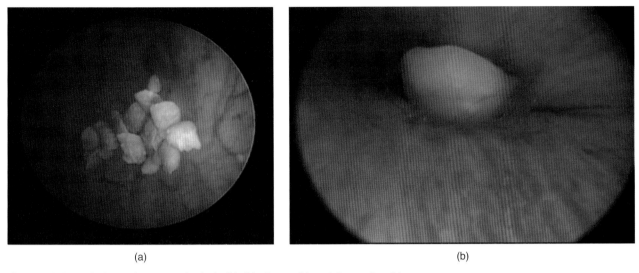

(a)   (b)

Figure 19.20 Calculi may be seen in both the bladder lumen (a) and the urethra (b).

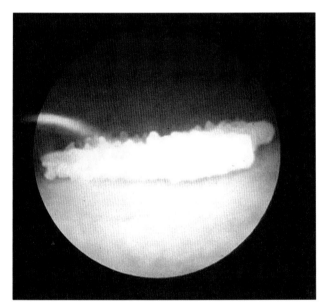

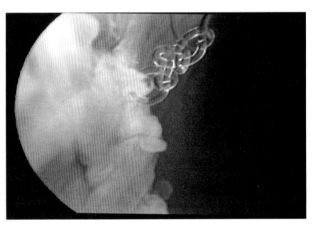

Figure 19.22 The presence of suture material can also predispose to recurrent lower urinary tract infections and local inflammation. This suture was a remnant from a ureteral transposition in a dog.

Figure 19.21 Calculi may form around a nidus of foreign material in the bladder lumen or wall. This calculus was formed by precipitation of struvite on suture material that was protruding into the bladder lumen from a previous cystotomy.

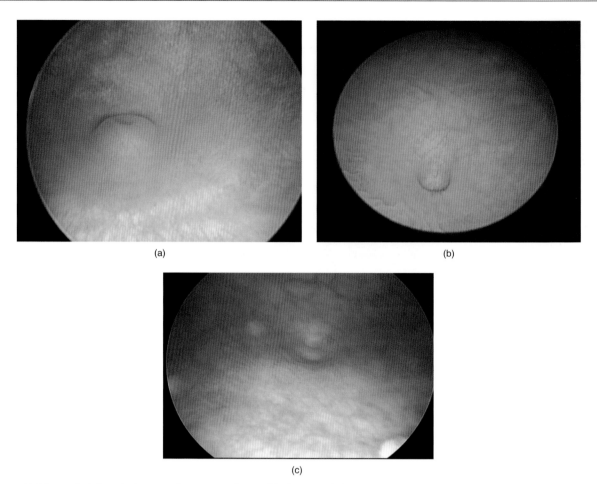

(a)   (b)

(c)

Figure 19.23 Urachal diverticula may take on many forms. (a) This ringed diverticulum appeared to be the cause of recurrent urinary tract infections in this female Maltese dog. Resection of the bladder apex led to resolution of clinical signs and infections. (b) This dog has a small but deep depression at the bladder apex. (c) This shallow depression contains two smaller depressions and may have been responsible for this dog's lower urinary tract signs.

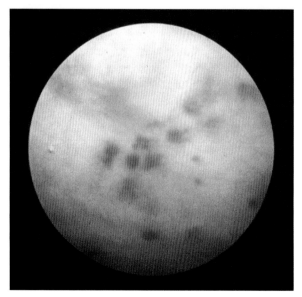

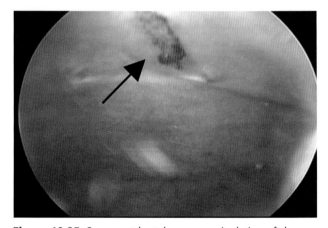

Figure 19.25 Care must be taken on manipulation of the cystoscope and observation of the urethral and bladder lumen. Operator-induced artifacts such as this mucosal damage (arrow) in the trigone can look like a lesion. A linear appearance suggests scope artifact.

Figure 19.24 Glomerulations on the bladder wall of a cat with feline idiopathic cystitis.

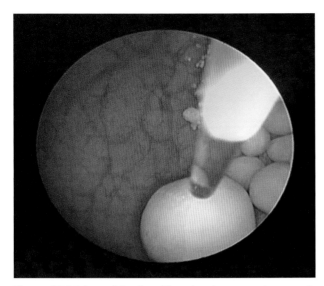

Figure 19.26 Laser lithotripsy fiber aimed at a struvite stone in the bladder of a dog.

References

Adams, L.G., A.C. Berent, et al. (2008). Use of laser lithotripsy for fragmentation of uroliths in dogs: 73 cases (2005–2006). *J Am Vet Med Assoc* **232**(11): 1680–1687.

Berent, A.C., P. Mayhew, et al. (2007). Cystoscopic-guided laser ablation of ectopic ureters in 12 dogs. *J Vet Intern Med* **21**(3): 600.

Berent, A.C., P.D. Mayhew, et al. (2008). Use of cystoscopic-guided laser ablation for treatment of intramural ureteral ectopia in male dogs: four cases (2006–2007). *J Am Vet Med Assoc* **232**(7): 1026–1034.

Cannizzo, K.L., M.A. McLoughlin, et al. (2003). Evaluation of transurethral cystoscopy and excretory urography for the diagnosis of ectopic ureters in female dogs: 25 cases (1992–2000). *J Am Vet Med Assoc* **223**(4): 475–481.

Cerf, D.J., E.C. Lindquist, et al. (2007). Ultrasound/endoscopy-guided diode laser ablation of nonresectable distal urinary transitional cell carcinoma in 19 female dogs. *J Vet Intern Med* **21**(3): 600.

Defarges, A. and M. Dunn (2006). Use of electrohydraulic shock-wave lithotripsy for the fragmentation of bladder calculi: a pilot study in dogs. *J Vet Intern Med* **20**(3): 737.

Defarges, A. and M. Dunn (2008). Treatment of urethral and bladder stones in 28 dogs with electrohydraulic lithotripsy. *J Vet Intern Med* **22**(3): 731–732.

Elwick K.E., L.D. Melendez, et al. (2003). Neodymium: Yttrium-aluminum-garnet (Nd: YAG) laser ablation of an obstructive urethral polyp in a dog. *J Am Anim Hosp Assoc* **39**(5): 506–508.

Grant, D.C., S.R. Were, et al. (2007). Holmium:YAG laser lithotripsy for urolithiasis in dogs. *J Vet Intern Med* **22**(3): 534–539.

Hostutler, R.A., D.J. Chew, et al. (2004). Cystoscopic appearance of proliferative urethritis in 2 dogs before and after treatment. *J Vet Intern Med* **18**(1): 113–116.

McCarthy, T.C. (2006). Peer-reviewed—transurethral cystoscopy and diode laser incision to correct an ectopic ureter. *Vet Med* **101**(9): 558–559.

Messer, J.S., D.J. Chew, et al. (2005). Cystoscopy: Techniques and clinical applications. *Clin Tech Small Anim Pract* **20**(1): 52–64.

Samii, V.F., M.A. McLoughlin, et al. (2004). Digital fluoroscopic excretory urography, digital fluoroscopic urethrography, helical computed tomography, and cystoscopy in 24 dogs with suspected ureteral ectopia. *J Vet Intern Med* **18**(3): 271–281.

Upton, M.L., C.H. Tangner, et al. (2006). Evaluation of carbon dioxide laser ablation combined with mitoxantrone and piroxicam treatment in dogs with transitional cell carcinoma. *J Am Vet Med Assoc* **228**(4): 549–552.

20

Vaginoscopy

Margaret Root Kustritz

Vaginoscopy is used to identify stage of the estrous cycle and to facilitate intrauterine insemination in bitches, to localize source of vulvar discharge, and as a component of a complete diagnostic work-up for persistent disease of the genitourinary tract. Use of vaginoscopy in breeding management will not be discussed.

Several different pieces of equipment can be used successfully to perform vaginoscopy in dogs. A vaginoscope head similar in size and length to a large otoscope cone and similarly attached to a handle that provides a light source is commercially available. Other sources describe use of a vaginal speculum. The author routinely uses a large otoscope cone attached to a handle with a light source for superficial vaginal examinations. The primary benefit of the use of these types of equipment is their ready availability in most veterinary clinics. However, only the caudal portion of the vagina and vestibule can be evaluated and concurrent dilation of the vaginal vault with fluid or air is not possible.

The vagina of the normal dog varies in length, with much of that variation associated with overall size of the dog (Wilson 2001; Wang et al. 2006). Total vaginal length in large breed dogs may be as much as 29 cm (Wilson 2001). If the entire vagina is to be examined, equipment of suitable length must be purchased. Rigid cystoscopes (Endoscopy Support Services, Inc., Brewster, NY, or Karl Storz Veterinary Endoscopy, Goleta, CA) varying in length from 18 to 36.5 cm are commercially available (see Chapter 19). If a single instrument is to be purchased for cystoscopy and vaginoscopy, the prudent choice may be an instrument of intermediate diameter and length, for example, a 4-mm diameter scope with 17 Fr sheath, which has a total length of 32 cm. The final consideration

is placement of the viewing lens on the tip of the scope. Scopes with no upward deflection permit good assessment of structures directly ahead of the scope only. A 30° upward deflection permits good assessment of structures in a wider range around the end of the scope. The operator may view the procedure through the eyepiece directly or may attach the eyepiece to an endoscopic camera. The latter is more comfortable for the operator and permits capture of images for the medical record.

If a rigid cystoscope is the instrument of choice, the dog should be placed under general anesthesia with appropriate preparation as for any anesthetic procedure. The perivulvar area should be cleaned and long hair clipped if necessary. Vaginoscopy is not a sterile procedure but care should be taken to minimize excessive contamination of the site. The recumbent dog can be placed in any orientation. Dorsal recumbency may be preferred as this minimizes fecal contamination of the site from the rectum and keeps the tail out of the way (Lulich 2006).

The scope is assembled and fluids attached to the irrigation port. The end of the scope should be lubricated with water-soluble lubricant. All instruments should be introduced into the dorsal commissure of the vulva and aimed toward the spine at a 45° angle. This prevents introduction of instruments into the blind-ended ventral clitoral fossa. Once the scope is in the vaginal vault, introduction of isotonic fluid distends the vaginal vault. To maintain distension, the vulvar lips should be occluded with the fingers of the free hand. Some leakage will occur so there should be fluid flowing into the vagina throughout the procedure and a catch basin for overflow should be placed beneath the dog.

Normal vulvar size and orientation varies tremendously in female dogs. In bitches, the most common variable altering vulvar size is stage of the estrous cycle, with significant increase in size and variation in tone of the

---

Nephrology and Urology of Small Animals. Edited by Joe Bartges and David J. Polzin. © 2011 Blackwell Publishing Ltd.

vulvar lips throughout proestrus and estrus (Nishiyama et al. 2000).

The ventral commissure of the vulva may be displaced excessively cranially or buried within perivulvar folds in some juvenile or spayed female dogs. This condition, commonly called recessed or juvenile vulva, has been associated with increased incidence of perivulvar dermatitis, especially in dogs with concurrent urinary incontinence (see Chapter 76) and with chronic urinary tract infection (see Chapter 71) (Hammel and Bjorling 2002). In one study comparing vulvar dimensions and orientation between dogs with and without lower urinary tract disease, recessed vulva was present in 68.4% of the affected dogs and 16.7% of the control dogs (Wang et al. 2006). Surgery (vulvoplasty) is the preferred corrective therapy. Allowing juvenile dogs to go through an estrous cycle will not effect permanent change in vulvar size or orientation.

The operator should avoid introduction of any instruments in the ventral clitoral fossa. However, if clitoral hypertrophy is present, the protruding clitoris may prevent ready introduction of equipment dorsally. Clitoral hypertrophy may occur secondary to irritation, including vulvar licking secondary to urinary incontinence or vaginitis. Male pseudohermaphroditism is reported to be associated with clitoral hypertrophy in 52% of cases, and true hermaphroditism in 100% of cases in dogs (Hare 1976). Hyperadrenocorticism is another reported pathologic cause of clitoral hypertrophy in dogs (Roberts 1986).

The vestibule contains the urethral papilla, which may or may not be visible as a distinct hillock of tissue. In a dog in dorsal recumbency, the urethral orifice is visible as a round opening dorsally. The vaginal os or junction of the vestibule and vagina (VV junction) is visible as an ovoid structure ventrally. The VV junction is a slight narrowing, commonly called the cingulum. Cranial to this by a variable length is a ventral tubercle that is the caudal end of dorsal median postcervical fold, which lies along the ceiling of the vaginal vault and restricts the vaginal vault in size by about 2/3, giving it a crescent shape. The size of the vaginal vault is greatly variable and is less well associated with overall size of the dog than is length of the vagina (Wilson 2001). The vaginal vault may be relatively small in maiden bitches and spayed dogs. Eventually, further passage of the scope cranially is stopped by the blind-ended fornix, ventral to which the cervix may be visible as a rosette of vaginal folds.

Normal vaginal mucosa is smooth, shiny, and pink, similar in appearance to oral mucous membranes. During estrus (standing heat), the vaginal epithelium is thickened and dehydrated, giving it a wrinkled and blanched appearance; this is normal. Inflammation is evidenced by diffuse or localized erythema of the mucosa. Be aware that the thin vaginal epithelium of spayed or nonestrous dogs is friable. In a small study evaluating use of vaginoscopy for diagnosis of vaginitis, significant erythema of the vaginal mucosa was present in 2 of 4 control dogs and 3 of 8 dogs in the study developed erythema quickly after other diagnostic testing (Schneider 2004).

Concurrent vaginitis and lower urinary tract disease may be present. Urinary incontinence (see Chapter 76) or chronic urinary tract infection (see Chapter 71) is reported to be present in 26–60% of cases of vaginitis (Johnson 1991; Parker 1998). Conversely, because the vagina is not sterile and urinary tract infections usually arise from bacteria in the distal urethra and surrounding area, it is not difficult to see how inflammation and overgrowth of vaginal flora may contribute to urinary tract disease (Olson and Mather 1978; Polzin and Jeraj 1979). One study evaluating risk factors for urinary tract infection identified both presence of vaginitis and performance of vaginoscopy as increasing risk for urinary tract infection in dogs (Freshman et al. 1989).

Vesicular lesions may be present in normal dogs or may be evidence of canine herpesvirus infection (Poste and King 1971; Hill and Mare 1974; Wang et al. 2006). Lymphoid follicles are nonspecific indicators of inflammation and may be present in asymptomatic dogs (Figure 20.1) (Wang et al. 2006).

Vaginal anatomic anomalies described in the dog include strictures and septae (see Chapter 80). These are readily demonstrated by vaginoscopy, with a reported diagnosis percentage of 95.8% (Figure 20.2) (Root et al. 1995; Kyles et al. 1996). Most commonly, these are found at the VV junction, where embryologically distinct tubular structures fuse during embryologic development. Significance of these structures as a component of urinary tract disease is equivocal. One study evaluating the ratio

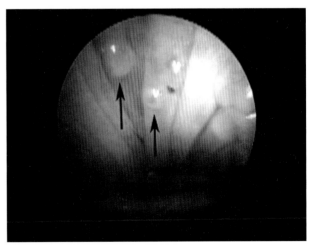

Figure 20.1 Lymphoid follicles on the vaginal mucosa of a bitch. Reprinted with permission: Lulich 2006.

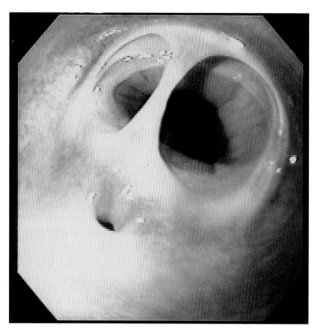

Figure 20.2 Vaginal septum in a standing bitch. Note urethral orifice ventrally. Reprinted with permission: Root Kustritz, M.V. (2005). *The Dog Breeder's Guide to Successful Breeding and Health Management*. St. Louis: Elsevier, p. 260.

of vaginal and vestibular sizes based on vaginography demonstrated a decreased response to treatment for urinary tract disease in dogs with a ratio of less than 0.2 and demonstrated that normal dogs had a ratio of greater than 0.35 (Crawford and Adams 2002). A subsequent study, which defined vestibular, vaginal, and vulvar measurements in clinically normal dogs, showed that normal dogs may have a ratio of less than 0.33 (Wang et al. 2006). Circumferential vaginal strictures most likely are significant when associated with urine pooling, evidenced as positional urinary incontinence. Vaginal septae also may be associated with urine pooling or other abnormalities, presumably due to alterations in drainage of fluids from the vagina as the septum pulls up on the vaginal floor. Several studies have documented an association between presence of vaginal anatomic anomalies and ectopic ureters (Cannizzo et al 2003; Samii et al. 2004).

Urine pooling may be difficult to assess in the presence of fluid distention of the vagina. If urine pooling is a concern, simple vaginoscopy as with a large otoscope cone on a lighted handle may be attempted on the unanesthetized, standing dog prior to endoscopic vaginoscopy (Davidson 2001). Oftentimes, urine pooling is best evidenced by a history of positional urinary incontinence.

Vulvar discharge may be mucoid, mucopurulent, or hemorrhagic. Mucoid discharge is a nonspecific indicator of inflammation. Mucopurulent discharge may be associated with urinary tract disease, vaginal disease, or uterine disease. Serosanguinous vulvar discharge is normal during proestrus and estrus; hemorrhagic discharge is associated with coagulopathy, blood parasites, or vaginal neoplasia (Johnston et al. 2001). Dogs with vaginal neoplasia usually present for a visible mass lesion but may present with stranguria or pollakiuria (Manothaiudom and Johnston 1991). The other mass lesion that may be present in the vagina is vaginal prolapse; this usually occurs in young dogs during proestrus and is very rarely associated with dysuria (Johnston et al. 2001).

References

Cannizzo, K.L., M.A. McLoughlin, et al. (2003). Evaluation of transurethral cystoscopy and excretory urography for diagnosis of ectopic ureters in female dogs: 25 cases (1992–2000). *J Am Vet Med Assoc* **223**: 475–481.

Crawford, J.T. and W.M. Adams (2002). Influence of vestibulovaginal stenosis, pelvic bladder, and recessed vulva on response to treatment for clinical signs of lower urinary tract disease in dogs: 38 cases (1990–1999). *J Am Vet Med Assoc* **221**: 995–999.

Davidson, A.P. (2001). Frustrating case presentations in canine theriogenology. *Vet Clin North Am Small Anim Pract* **31**: 411–420.

Freshman, J.L., J.S. Reif, et al. (1989). Risk factors associated with urinary tract infection in female dogs. *Prev Vet Med* **7**: 59–67.

Hammel, S.P. and D.E. Bjorling (2002). Results of vulvoplasty for treatment of recessed vulva in dogs. *J Am Anim Hosp Assoc* **38**: 79–83.

Hare, W.C.D. (1976). Intersexuality in the dog. *Can Vet J* **17**: 7–15.

Hill, H. and C.J. Mare (1974). Genital disease in dogs caused by canine herpesvirus. *Am J Vet Res* **35**: 669–672.

Johnson, C.A. (1991). Diagnosis and treatment of chronic vaginitis in the bitch. *Vet Clin North Am Small Anim Pract* **21**: 523–531.

Johnston, S.D., M.V. Root Kustritz, et al. (2001). Disorders of the canine vagina, vestibule, and vulva. In: *Canine and Feline theriogenology*. Philadelphia, PA: WB Saunders, pp. 225–242.

Kyles, A.E., S. Vaden, et al. (1996). Vestibulovaginal stenosis in dogs: 18 cases (1987–1995). *J Am Vet Med Assoc* **209**: 1889–1893.

Lulich, J.P. (2006). Endoscopic vaginoscopy in the dog. *Theriogenology* **66**: 588–591.

Manothaiudom, K. and S.D. Johnston (1991). Clinical approach to vaginal/vestibular masses in the bitch. *Vet Clin North Am Small Anim Pract* **21**: 509–521.

Nishiyama, T., K. Narita, et al. (2000). Shrinkage in the horizontal dimensions of the vulva (vulvar shrinkage) as an indicator of standing heat in the Beagle. *J Am Anim Hosp Assoc* **36**: 556–560.

Olson, P.N.S. and E.C. Mather (1978). Canine vaginal and uterine bacterial flora. *J Am Vet Med Assoc* **172**: 708–711.

Parker, N.A. (1998). Clinical approach to canine vaginitis: a review. *Proceedings, Society for Theriogenology*, Baltimore MD, pp. 112–115.

Polzin, D.J. and K. Jeraj (1979). Urethritis, cystitis and ureteritis. *Vet Clin North Am Small Anim Pract* **9**: 661–678.

Poste, G. and N. King (1971). Isolation of a herpesvirus from the canine genital tract: association with infertility, abortion, and stillbirths. *Vet Rec* **88**: 229–233.

Roberts, S.J. (1986). *Infertility and reproductive diseases in bitches and queens*. Woodstock, VT: SJ Roberts, pp. 709–751.

Root, M.V., S.D. Johnston, et al. (1995). Vaginal septa in dogs: 15 cases (1983–1992). *J Am Vet Med Assoc* **206**: 56–58.

Samii, V.F., M.A. McLoughlin, et al. (2004). Digital fluoroscopic excretory urography, digital fluoroscopic urethrography, helical computed tomography, and cystoscopy in 24 dogs with suspected ureteral ectopia. *J Vet Intern Med* **18**: 271–281.

Schneider, A.L. (2004). Plausible causes of vaginitis. Honors thesis, College of Agriculture, University of Minnesota.

Wang, K.Y., V.F. Samii, et al. (2006). Vestibular, vaginal, and urethral relations in spayed dogs with and without lower urinary tract signs. *J Vet Intern Med* **20**: 1065–1073.

Wilson, M.S. (2001). Transcervical insemination techniques in the bitch. *Vet Clin North Am Small Anim Pract* **31**: 291–304.

21

Urologic laparoscopy

Jacqueline Whittemore

Laparoscopy is the examination of the abdominal cavity using a rigid endoscope. It provides a way to thoroughly evaluate the abdomen without creating large incisions in the abdominal wall. Laparoscopy is divided into diagnostic procedures, involving visualization and tissue sampling, and interventional procedures.

Depending on the specific procedure, advantages of using a laparoscopic approach include direct visualization of organs, including surfaces that are difficult to visualize using other techniques; magnification of tissues so that subtle deviations from normal anatomy are visible; separation of organs from one another for closer examination; improved visualization in deep cavities; decreased pain and disruption of tissues, primarily due to decreased incision size; shorter procedure times, hospitalization stays, and decreased overall cost; decreased postoperative infection rates; and increased sample size, sample types, and sampling accuracy than can be obtained using other minimally invasive techniques.

Disadvantages of using a laparoscopic approach include the expense of laparoscopic-associated equipment, veterinary and technical training, and equipment maintenance; increased anesthesia time and procedural complications during the initial learning phase; difficulty in managing complications, particularly hemorrhage, because the abdomen is closed; and increased client cost compared to traditional surgery for some procedures.

Patient positioning

The approach utilized is dependent on the purpose of the laparoscopy. The right lateral approach is standard for exploratory laparoscopy. A left lateral approach may

be tried for visualization of the left kidney but is generally avoided, given the risk of splenic laceration. A ventral midline approach with the use of a rotating table is preferable for examination of this organ. The ventral midline approach is the preferred approach for surgical procedures, but the technique can be hindered by excessive falciform fat deposition. The operating table may be inclined 10–15° to move abdominal contents away from the particular organ of interest.

Laparoscopic equipment

The telescope acts as the surgeon's eyes. It is a glass and air column through which images are transmitted to a camera. Telescopes come in a variety of diameters and lengths. The most common telescope sizes for veterinary laparoscopy are 5 mm × 29 cm (standard) and 2.7 mm × 18 cm (often referred to as a pediatric scope). The tip of the telescope may be flat, usually 0–10° of deflection, or angled, 30–45 of deflection, for visualization around corners and objects (Figure 21.1). A high-intensity-light source cable is used to transmit light through the telescope to illuminate the abdomen, and a specialized camera is attached to the eyepiece of the telescope to capture images for processing and display on a monitor.

The abdomen can be entered by either a closed technique or an open approach (Leibl et al. 2001). The "closed" approach is used most commonly for procedures performed in lateral recumbency. A Veress needle is used to penetrate the abdominal wall and insufflate the abdomen with carbon dioxide before access ports are placed. This allows safe introduction of the access cannulae and facilitates separation of the organs for visualization and manipulation. The Veress needle has an inner blunt spring-loaded stylet that advances forward after puncture of the abdominal wall to prevent accidental organ impalement. An insufflator controls the flow of

Nephrology and Urology of Small Animals. Edited by Joe Bartges and David J. Polzin. © 2011 Blackwell Publishing Ltd.

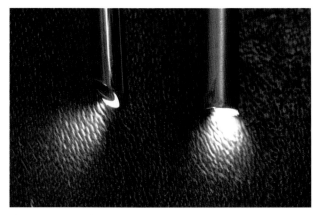

Figure 21.1 A photo of light being transmitted through 0° and 30° telescopes, demonstrating the difference in area of visualization created by deflection. Photo by Greg Hirshoren, © 2009 The University of Tennessee.

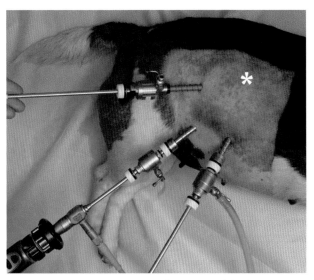

Figure 21.2 Access ports optimally positioned for laparoscopic-assisted percutaneous renal biopsy using a baseball diamond configuration: The right kidney is at home plate (denoted by the white asterisk), with the camera located in the center (the pitcher's mound) and instrument ports positioned on either side of the camera (first and third bases). Photo by Greg Hirshoren, © 2009 The University of Tennessee.

carbon dioxide into the abdomen and maintains appropriate intra-abdominal pressure, usually no more than 10 and 12 mmHg for cats and dogs, respectively. After insufflation of the abdomen is complete, trocar-cannulae are advanced through the abdominal wall to create access ports. The cannulae are equipped with one-way valves to prevent abdominal deflation once the trocars are removed, while allowing introduction and removal of equipment.

The Hasson technique is utilized for open approaches to the abdomen (Leibl et al. 2001), specifically procedures performed with the animal in dorsal recumbency. A mini-laparotomy is performed to place the first trocar, usually 2–3 cm caudal to the umbilicus and ideally the falciform fat. After incision of the linea alba, a hemostat or other blunt instrument is introduced and swept circularly to clear the insertion site of fat and confirm no tissues are adhered to the linea alba. A trocar is then placed to establish the first access port. An airtight seal is achieved by using either a positive-threaded cannula or placing a purse-string suture around the cannula opening. Once the access port is in place, the abdomen is insufflated as described above.

Access port placement is guided by the procedure to be performed. Once the first access port has been created, the laparoscope is introduced and used to observe additional trocars entering the abdomen to minimize the risk of iatrogenic damage. With exceptions as listed below, three access ports are typically utilized in what is often described as a baseball diamond configuration (Figure 21.2). In this configuration, the camera is placed at the "pitcher's mound" with the target organ located at "home base." By placing instruments at "first" and "third base," the operator is best able to manipulate organs without having the instruments interfere with one another or

the camera. A variety of instruments may be introduced through the access ports for abdominal exploration and tissue manipulations. Commonly utilized instruments include blunt palpation probes, cup and punch biopsy forceps, Babcock and dissecting forceps, retractors, and a variety of scissors.

Urologic procedures

Relevant organs accessible for examination during exploratory laparoscopy include the kidneys, portions of the ureters, urinary bladder, omentum, prostate, and regional lymph nodes. Urologic procedures for which laparoscopy may be indicated include renal biopsy, peritoneal dialysis catheter placement and omentectomy, cystotomy and bladder wall biopsy, cystostomy tube placement, cystopexy, prostate biopsy, and regional lymph node evaluation and biopsy. As veterinary laparoscopic technique improves, it is likely that pyelotomy and pyelolithotomy will also be performed laparoscopically.

Laparoscopic-assisted percutaneous renal biopsy

The use of laparoscopic assistance for percutaneous renal biopsies improves visualization of lesions, targeted biopsy of focal lesions, postprocedure hemorrhage surveillance,

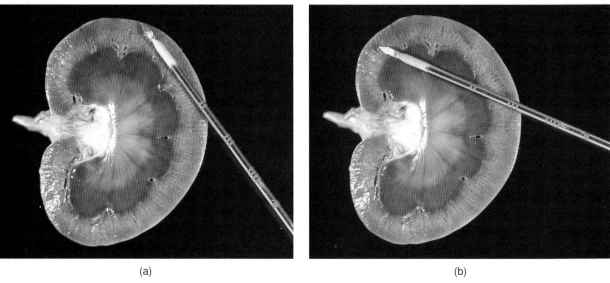

(a)   (b)

Figure 21.3 Left: Cross-section of a dog kidney illustrating optimal placement of the percutaneous biopsy instrument tangentially in the cortex. Right: Cross-section of a dog kidney illustrating suboptimal placement of the percutaneous biopsy instrument through the medulla and arcuate vessels. Photos by Robert Donnell, University of Tennessee College of Veterinary Medicine.

and diagnostic yield of biopsy samples (Grauer et al. 1983; Rawlings et al. 2003a). In one study, laparoscope-guided samples obtained with a 14-gauge Tru-cut style biopsy needle had better sample quality overall, less crush artifact, and 2.7 times as many glomeruli as samples from an 18-gauge needle (Rawlings et al. 2003a). Laparoscope-guided samples also had twice as many glomeruli, less crush artifact, and better sample quality, than ultrasound-guided samples obtained using the same-size biopsy needle. Although it has not been evaluated for renal biopsies specifically, the use of fully automatic biopsy needles is discouraged given the high rate of vagotonic complications associated with liver biopsy in cats (Proot and Rothuizen 2006).

Renal biopsy can be performed using either a midline or lateral approach. A lateral approach is generally preferred for diffuse disease processes because it allows better separation of the kidney from surrounding tissues, does not require repositioning of the patient during the procedure, and the right kidney is often less freely movable. For cases where biopsy of the left kidney—or both kidneys—is desired, a midline approach is utilized for initial insufflation and camera placement and then the patient is rotated into lateral recumbency. While monitoring the site through the laparoscope, the paralumbar area is palpated to determine the most appropriate location, caudal to the diaphragmatic reflection, for biopsy needle insertion. A small-skin incision is made and the percutaneous biopsy instrument is advanced through the abdominal wall. The kidney is isolated and stabilized using a blunt probe or fan retractor, before advancing the biopsy instrument to sample the affected area or,

in cases of glomerular disease, tangentially through the cortex, avoiding the arcuate vessels and medulla (Figure 21.3). The biopsy needle is deployed according to manufacturer's instructions (Figure 21.4). Pressure may be applied to the biopsy site with the palpation probe to control hemorrhage from the capsule after the biopsy needle is retracted.

Peritoneal dialysis catheter placement

Although increased availability of veterinary hemodialysis is decreasing the demand for peritoneal dialysis (see Chapter 30), it is still a regularly performed technique in

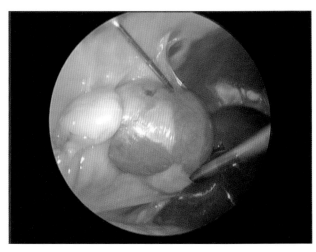

Figure 21.4 A blunt probe is utilized to stabilize and gently rotate the right kidney, optimizing placement of the percutaneous biopsy needle in the renal cortex.

both veterinary and human medicine. In addition to its usefulness for management of acute renal failure, peritoneal dialysis can be utilized for medical management of acute intoxication, electrolyte derangement, pancreatitis, and heatstroke cases (Dzyban et al. 2000). The benefits of peritoneal dialysis have historically been offset by the delay between catheter placement and safe initiation of dialysate exchanges. Streamlined-peritoneal dialysis catheters can be placed percutaneously using laparoscopy (Ash 2006; Seleem and Al-Hashemy 2007). Partial omentectomy, crucial to minimize catheter occlusion rates, may also be performed with relative ease. Finally, an abbreviated dialysate exchange may be administered through the access ports at the time of laparoscopy, prior to recovery from anesthesia. Since patients with anuric renal failure requiring peritoneal dialysis often are significantly volume overloaded, the ability to begin volume correction at time of surgery is a significant advantage. Because the exchange is performed through the laparoscopic cannula, there is little risk of dialysate dissection, with attendant cellulitis and infection, into subcutaneous tissues. Finally, the decrease in incision size allows for earlier use of the dialysis catheter for regular exchanges.

Laparoscopic-assisted cystotomy

There are a variety of advantages to using laparoscopic assistance for removal of cystic and urethral calculi. In addition to decreasing postoperative morbidity, the smaller size of incisions decreases potential abdominal contamination with urine (Rawlings et al. 2003b). For this procedure, the laparoscope is placed via the Hasson technique to guide bladder isolation and retrieval with Babcock forceps (Figure 21.5). It is important to carefully identify the apex of the bladder for retrieval. Malpositioning of the Babcock forceps will artificially compartmentalize the bladder, hindering thorough evaluation. Once the bladder has been isolated, exteriorized, and the cystotomy incision made, the laparoscope is advanced through the cystotomy site into the bladder to guide calculi retrieval (Figure 21.6). After all stones have been retrieved, the urethra and bladder can be carefully evaluated, decreasing the risk of overlooking an entrapped calculus and allowing targeted mucosal wall biopsy.

Laparoscopic-assisted incisional cystopexy

Cystopexy is performed most commonly for adjunctive management of urethral sphincter incontinence and to prevent urinary bladder entrapment in perianal hernias. Appropriate positioning of the bladder and cystopexy site is crucial to prevent postoperative micturition disorders, specifically urethral obstruction. A laparoscopic

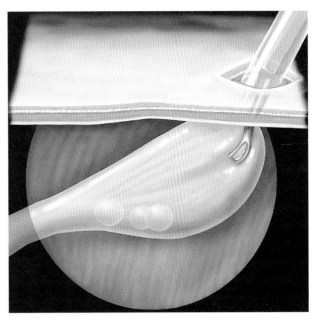

Figure 21.5 Illustration of bladder isolation and retrieval using Babcock forceps during laparoscopic-assisted cystotomy. Note the careful positioning of the forceps on the apex of the bladder. Image reproduced with permission from Rawlings, 2003b.

technique has been developed to decrease procedural complications (Rawlings et al. 2002). The most significant benefit of laparoscopic assistance is the ability to thoroughly evaluate the completed cystopexy to confirm appropriate alignment of the bladder and urethra and adequate cranial traction on the bladder before the animal is recovered from anesthesia (Figure 21.7). In severe cases of incontinence, this procedure may be coupled with cystoscopic urethral collagen injections (Barth et al. 2005). The same approach may be used for cystostomy tube placement.

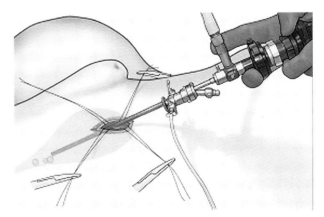

Figure 21.6 Illustration of laparoscope advancement into the bladder to guide cystolith removal during laparoscopic-assisted cystotomy. Image reproduced with permission from Rawlings, 2003b.

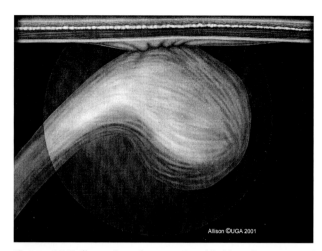

Figure 21.7 Illustration of appropriate bladder alignment and positioning during laparoscopic-assisted cystopexy. Image reproduced with permission from Rawlings, 2002.

Other procedures

Laparoscopy can also be used to guide prostatic biopsies, for prostatic omentalization, and for evaluation and biopsy of regional lymph nodes as part of cancer staging. Other procedures involving the reproductive tract for which laparoscopy may be quite useful include ovariectomy, ovariohysterectomy, and cryptorchidectomy.

References

Ash, S. (2006). Chronic peritoneal dialysis catheters: challenges and design solutions. *Int J Artif Organs* **29**(1): 85–94.

Barth, A., I. Reichler, et al. (2005). Evaluation of long-term effects of endoscopic injection of collagen into the urethral submucosa for treatment of urethral sphincter incompetence in female dogs: 40 cases (1993–2000). *J Am Vet Med Assoc* **226**(1): 73–76.

Dzyban, L., M.A. Labato, et al. (2000). Peritoneal dialysis: a tool in veterinary critical care. *J Vet Emerg Crit Care (San Antonio)* **10**(2): 91–102.

Grauer, G., D. Twedt, et al. (1983). Evaluation of laparoscopy for obtaining renal biopsy specimens from dogs and cats. *J Am Vet Med Assoc* **183**(6): 677–679.

Leibl, B.J., K. Kraft, et al. (2001). Access techniques for endoscopic surgery—types of trocards, ports and cannulae—an overview. *Minim Invasive Ther Allied Technol* **10**(1): 5–10.

Proot, S.J.M. and J. Rothuizen (2006). High complication rate of an automatic Tru-cut biopsy gun device for liver biopsy in cats. *J Vet Intern Med* **20**: 1327–1333.

Rawlings, C., E. Howerth, et al. (2002). Laparoscopic-assisted cystopexy in dogs. *Am J Vet Res* **63**(9): 1226–1231.

Rawlings, C., H. Diamond, et al. (2003a). Diagnostic quality of percutaneous kidney biopsy specimens obtained with laparoscopy versus ultrasound guidance in dogs. *J Am Vet Med Assoc* **223**(3): 317–321.

Rawlings, C., M. Mahaffey (2003b). Use of laparoscopic-assisted cystoscopy or removal of urinary calculi in dogs. *J Am Vet Med Assoc* **222**(6): 759–761.

Seleem, M. and A. Al-Hashemy (2007). Mini-laparoscopic placement of peritoneal dialysis catheter: New technique *Surgical Practice* **11**: 36–40.

22

Urodynamic studies

India F. Lane

Diagnosis of urinary dysfunction is usually made based on routine clinical data, including patient history, physical and neurological examination (see Chapter 4), urinalysis (see Chapter 7), and routine imaging (see Chapter 15). However, urodynamic studies may be indicated in select patients with urinary incontinence or urine retention, usually complex or refractory cases (Oliver 1987; Barsanti 1995). These studies require minimal technical skill but require appropriate investment in equipment and instrumentation, as well as frequent troubleshooting, quality control, and cautious interpretation of results. This chapter reviews indications, techniques, and interpretation of urodynamic procedures used commonly in dogs and cats (Table 22.1).

Instrumentation

Specially designed urinary catheters are available for urodynamic procedures. The most common catheters used in small animal practice include the urethral pressure profile catheter and double or triple lumen urodynamic catheters. The urethral pressure profile catheter is a small (6 Fr) polyvinylchloride (PVC) catheter with a single lumen but four opposing side holes placed around the circumference of the catheter (Figure 22.1). Multiple side holes provide a summation of urethral resistance from all quadrants of the urethra. Double and triple lumen urodynamic catheters also have multiple side holes, but the holes are spaced at different points along the length of the urethra (Figure 22.2). These urodynamic catheters are preferred for multichannel urodynamics; the separate lumens are used for infusion and pressure recording (double lumen) and for the simultaneous recording of

bladder and urethral pressure (triple lumen). Multilumen catheters are available in 6, 7, and 9 Fr diameters. The pediatric (6 Fr) size can be used even in small dogs and female cats. Microtip transducer (or microtransducer) recording catheters also have been applied for urodynamic testing; these catheters have one or two small sensor sites mounted on the exterior surface of the catheter (Figure 22.3). Most of these products are designed for single-use application, but can be resterilized by gas or cold sterilization methods.

Despite the value of the preferred catheter type, creative use of other urinary catheters also yields satisfactory results. Readily available Foley retention and polypropylene catheters were used for early studies in dogs (Rosin and Barsanti 1981; Richter and Ling 1985a; Barsanti 1995). Cystometric and uroflow studies using transabdominal catheters have also been reported (Moreau et al. 1983a). The author has used tom-cat catheters and infant feeding tubes to assess urethral function in male cats.

The only essential fixed equipment requirement for urodynamic studies is a pressure recording system. Physiographic recorders and analog recorders were the "workhorse" machines for years (Figure 22.4). Urodynamic machines purchased today are multichannel systems with automated software systems for recording, storage, and analysis of data (Figure 22.5). At least three channels are desired for quality studies. Automated catheter withdrawal devices also increase the precision and feasibility of urethral profiles (Figure 22.6). The most reliable and enduring manufacturer of urodynamic equipment in North America is Life-Tech International, based in Houston, Texas. Regular calibration and review of signal quality (sensitivity to movement and pressure change) is required with old or new equipment (Schafer et al. 2002).

Nephrology and Urology of Small Animals. Edited by Joe Bartges and David J. Polzin. © 2011 Blackwell Publishing Ltd.

Table 22.1 Overview of urodynamic studies adapted for small animals

Procedure	Primary application	Other indications	Limitations	Contraindications
Urethral pressure profile	Diagnosis or exclusion of USMI	Localization of urethral obstruction or spasm	Reflects urethral function during storage only, results affected by sedation, interindividual variability	Active UTI
Leak point pressure	Diagnosis of USMI with stress		Requires sedation or anesthesia	Active UTI; Bladder wall damage; Significant hematuria
Electromyography	Assessment of neurogenic disorders	Diagnosis of detrusor-striated muscle dyssynergia	Difficult to perform in small animals	
Cystometry	Diagnosis or exclusion of detrusor instability	Detrusor atony, evaluation of bladder compliance	Sedation and house-training can inhibit normal detrusor reflex	Active UTI; Bladder wall damage; Significant hematuria
Voiding studies	Diagnosis or exclusion of functional or dynamic urinary obstruction	Diagnosis of urine pooling	Nonphysiologic position, requires sedation or anesthesia	Contraindications to contrast media

General principles

Reporting for the International Continence Society, Schafer et al. (2002) outlined the elements of "good urodynamic practice," including (1) the selection of appropriate tests, (2) quality control for precise measurement, and (3) critical analysis of the results. He emphasized the formation of a clear "urodynamic question" for each patient, using all available data, prior to embarking on invasive testing. In small animals, the lack of subjective feedback from the patient makes identification of the core question even more important; objective uro-

dynamic data reviewed in a vacuum is likely to lead to misrepresentative diagnoses.

Urodynamic studies should be done in patients that are free from active urinary tract infection or inflammation. Diagnostic studies (see Chapter 9) ideally are performed prior to any trial pharmacologic treatments; if treatments have been initiated, they should be discontinued at least one week (preferably 2 weeks) prior to study. Posttreatment studies should be done at times of peak pharmacologic action as much as possible. Urodynamic procedures can be coordinated with other lower urinary tract procedures in order to best utilize sedation or anesthesia but should be performed first in sequence, because other procedures (cystoscopy, contrast studies)

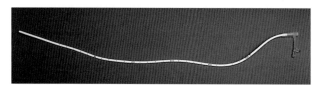

Figure 22.1 Urethral pressure profile catheter. Note the multiple small side holes for transmission of pressure from all sides of the urethra (UPP-8D, Life-Tech International, Stafford, TX).

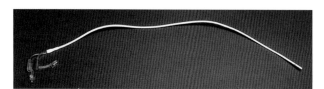

Figure 22.2 Double (or dual) lumen urodynamic catheter. One lumen can be used for fluid infusion and another for pressure recording (DLC-9D, Life-Tech International, Stafford, TX).

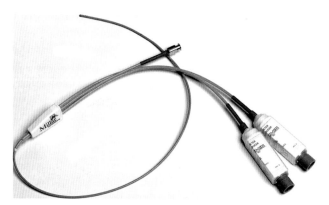

Figure 22.3 Microtransducer urodynamic catheter; pressures are recorded directly from transducers mounted on the catheter (Millar Mikro-Tip Catheter, Photo from Millar web catalog with permission).

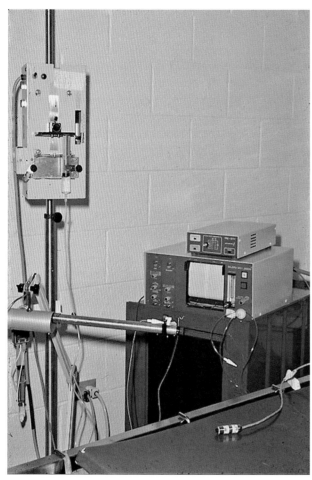

Figure 22.4 Analog pressure recording unit; this system includes a single channel pressure recorder, a catheter withdrawal arm and a syringe perfusion pump to accomplish most urodynamic studies.

are likely to affect results. Sedation and restraint are chosen as indicated in the best interests of the study and the patient. Most procedures are repeated two to three times during the study period to ensure reliability.

Urethral pressure studies

Indications

Urethral pressure profilometry (UPP) measures the pressures along the length of the urethra (Figure 22.7) (Rosin and Barsanti 1981). In some complicated incontinence or urine retention patients, the UPP may be useful for

- Evaluation of suspected USMI refractory to traditional medical therapies
- Evaluation of urethral function in patients with anatomic abnormalities (e.g., ectopic ureter)
- Perioperative evaluation of surgical treatment of USMI (e.g., urethral collagen injection, colposuspension)
- Confirmation/ localization of urethral spasm

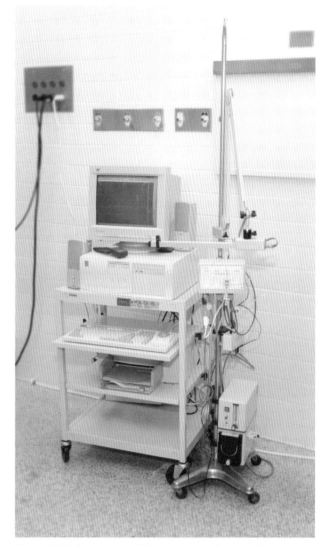

Figure 22.5 Desktop, multichannel system for recording and analyzing urodynamic studies (Janus System 4 is pictured, Life-tech International; current systems are Janus Urolab 6 available in desktop, notebook, or all in one mobile design packages).

- Assessment of outlet resistance in neurologic disorders
- Assessment of response to medical or surgical treatments
- Excluding urethral dysfunction in incontinent dogs (e.g., urine pooling, urge incontinence)

The urethral pressure profile is also applied extensively in prospective research, including assessment of pharmacologic treatments, surgical manipulation, and urethral devices.

Limitations

Although the urethral pressure profile has proven effective in documenting or excluding the diagnosis of USMI and has many applications in urologic research, the study

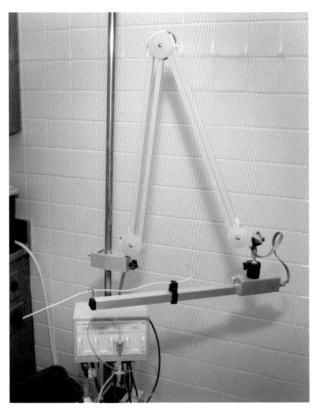

Figure 22.6 Withdrawal arm for recording urethral pressure studies. A UPP catheter (blue) is placed to illustrate how the catheter is attached and withdrawn during a urethral pressure profile.

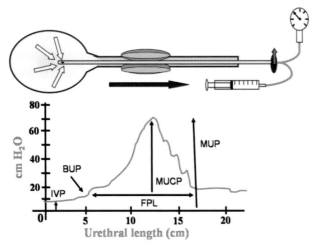

Figure 22.7 Schematic illustration of a female dog urethral pressure profile; fluid is infused via a syringe or other pump (blue arrow) while resistance to infusion is measured in cm H_2O (schematic recorder represents pressure transducer) at the catheter tip (multiple white arrows). IVP, intravesicular pressure; BUP, begin urethral pressure; MUP, maximum urethral pressure; MUCP, maximum urethral pressure; FPL, functional profile length. Illustration modified from Fischer, J.R. and I.F. Lane (2007). Incontinence and urine retention. In: *BSAVA Manual of Canine and Feline Nephrology and Urology*, edited by Elliott and Grauer. Gloucester: British Small Animal Veterinary Association, with permission.

is limited when more complex disorders are encountered. With the urethral pressure profile, the study is completed during a resting state, which is usually appropriate for storage disorders such as incontinence. The study is less likely to reflect urethral function during voiding, although inappropriate urethral contractions and high urethral resistance may be observed. The other major limitation of urethral studies is the inherent variability in results. Measurements can be affected by level of sedation or level of striated muscle activity and movement in awake dogs. Individual variation has been observed in dogs when studies are repeated over time, pressure, and length. Results are also affected by age, reproductive status (Salomon et al. 2006), and estrus cycle in intact females (Hamaide et al. 2005).

Sedation/restraint

Ideally, studies are conducted in awake patients. However, tracings from awake studies can be affected by movement artifact or active contraction of striated urethral or pelvic floor muscle. Transurethral catheterization may be difficult (and dangerous) in awake cats and small or anatomically abnormal dogs. The choice of approach depends on the patient, instrumentation used, and purpose of the study. For example, studies using urinary catheters with mounted microtip transducers must be completed under general anesthesia because the transducers are exquisitely sensitive to motion (Arnold et al. 1993). With the effects of sedation in mind, "apples" must be compared to "apples" and results must be interpreted by comparison to equivalent studies in normal animals. For most institutions, studies are done in a standardized fashion in order to feel most confident in results and to provide data suitable for research purposes. However, standardization across institutions is still lacking.

Urethral studies can usually be performed in awake, *nonsedated* male dogs and in female dogs whose size and conformation allow minimally traumatic transurethral catheterization. Light physical restraint is required to maintain the patient in relaxed lateral recumbency. Cats and small dogs require sedation or a light plane of general anesthesia. Unfortunately, virtually all sedatives or anesthetics depress urethral function. The variable absorption rate and duration of effect for injected sedatives also contributes to the variability of results. *Xylazine*, the preferred historical agent preferred for cystometry in veterinary patients, was also used for concurrent urethral pressure profiles out of convenience (Oliver and Young 1973b; Johnson et al. 1988). However, xylazine administration significantly depressed urethral pressure and functional length (Richter and Ling 1985). Intramuscular administration of medetomidine also depressed urethral pressure and was associated with increased variability of results in one group of healthy dogs (Rawlings et al. 2001). Currently, propofol or light inhalant anesthesia is recommended to facilitate catheterization and completion of urodynamic studies. A slow constant rate infusion of propofol had minimal effect on urethral pressure in two studies of healthy dogs (Combrisson et al. 1993; Byron et al. 2003). Some authors have advocated using propofol infusion for urinary catheterization, then allowing the patient to awaken to a degree that would have less impact the profile (Goldstein and Westropp 2005). However, the timing of the study (after withdrawal of sedation) could still complicate interpretation if this practice is followed.

Inhalant anesthetic agents may be preferred in cats and some challenging dogs, especially if propofol infusion is cost-prohibitive. Light anesthesia using isoflurane or sevoflurane (end tidal concentration 1.5–2.0%) is a reasonable choice for urethral studies (Byron et al. 2003), but often inhibits detrusor function for other urodynamic tests (Johnson et al. 1988; Cohen et al. 2009).

Procedure

Patients should be free of infection and active inflammation at the time of study. Recording equipment is prepared by accessing the study set-up program and zeroing transducers to atmospheric pressure (with open fluid columns placed at the level of the symphysis pubis). The patient is sedated if desired, and a transurethral urethral catheter is placed using aseptic technique. Ideally, a urethral pressure profile catheter is used. For a full urethral profile, the catheter is advanced so that the side holes are located in the neck of the bladder to begin the study. A preloaded fluid column (usually thin extension tubing) is attached to the recording transducer. Once the fluid column is attached to the external catheter port, low initial pressures (6–10 cm H_2O) are expected if the internal catheter port is free within the urinary bladder. If the initial pressure is significantly higher, adjustment of catheter placement or clearing the catheter with a little fluid may be required to ensure there is no interference. The UPP catheter port or one lumen of a multilumen catheter is connected to a pressure transducer. Some clinicians choose to zero transducers at this point in order to simplify calculation of closure pressure. Fluid is infused through a separate lumen of a multilumen catheter or using a stopcock (Figure 22.8) at a low infusion rate (2 mL/minute). Any resistance to fluid flow should be minimized. Pressures are recorded as the catheter is slowly withdrawn (usually at 0.5–1 mm/second). Alternately, a triple lumen catheter (Figure 22.9) can be used to record simultaneous bladder and urethral pressure dur-

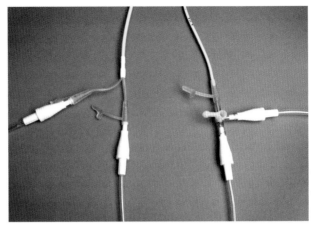

Figure 22.8 Method for recording urethral pressure (as resistance to flow) during slow fluid infusion. On the left, a double lumen catheter is used for single side-hole recording. Ideally, the side hole is oriented dorsally within the urethra. The infusion tubing is attached to one lumen (via the yellow port), whereas the fluid column for pressure recording is attached to the other. On the right, a single lumen, four-side-hole UPP catheter is attached to a stopcock and tubing that allows simultaneous infusion and pressure recording. In both cases, the tubing for fluid infusion is attached in direct line with the catheter so that there is minimal interference to flow. Note that air bubbles, kinks, or movements in the tubing will create artifacts.

ing withdrawal (Goldstein and Westropp 2005). Potential technical errors affect measurements, including variable or interrupted infusion flow (pump error), air bubbles, tubing kinks, inappropriate positioning of the catheter, or partial occlusion of the catheter. Analysis can be completed by urodynamic software system packages or manually (Figure 22.10). Automated software measurements are best utilized when the clinician selects key points on the tracing, instead of relying on selection parameters designed for human patients.

Interpretation

Maximal urethral pressure (MUP) is compared to resting urinary bladder pressure and to normal animals of the same species and sex (Figure 22.11). The key measure of urethral function is the maximal urethral closure pressure (MUCP), which is calculated by subtracting the resting bladder pressure from the maximum observed urethral pressure. The functional profile length (FPL or UFPL), the length over which urethral pressure exceeds bladder pressure, also reflects overall function. Some investigators report other parameters derived from the profiles, including area measures (area under the curve of the functional profile length). A visual assessment of the curve is important as well, the maximal pressure peak should be evident in the appropriate portion of the curve. Salomon et al.

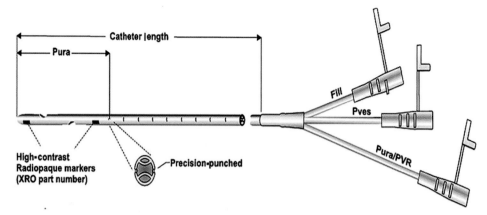

Figure 22.9 Schematic of a triple lumen catheter designed for simultaneous bladder and urethral pressure recording during urethral or bladder function studies. Pura, distance between catheter tip and side hole for urethral pressure measurement; Fill, port for fluid infusion lumen; Pves, port for lumen to remain in urinary bladder; Pura/PVR, port for lumen to record urethral pressures (Illustration reprinted from Life-Tech online catalog, with permission).

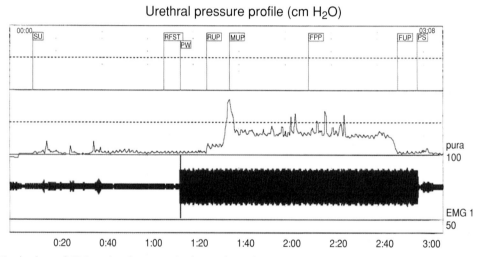

Figure 22.10 Single channel UPP tracing from a male dog with markings created using automated software (Life-Tech Janus System 4.03, Stafford, TX). Undulations reflect respiratory motion and movement during reset of catheter withdrawal. Note the blue activity reflected in the EMG channel; in this dog, EMG was not recorded, and the heavy activity recorded here is artifact.

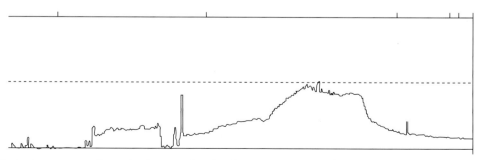

Figure 22.11 Urethral pressure profile tracing from a sedated male cat.

(2006) incorporated this point into their assessment of profiles from female dogs, reporting an area measurement for each of the cranial, middle, and caudal thirds of the functional profile length (in addition to a total integrated pressure).

The UPP has had considerable application in the evaluation of incontinence in small animals (see Chapter 76) and has been useful in the assessment of urethral responses to pharmacologic agents or surgical procedures (Rosin and Barsanti 1981; Gregory 1984; Richter and Ling 1985; Basinger et al. 1987; Holt 1988; Basinger et al. 1989; Mawby et al. 1990; Sackman et al. 1991; Frenier et al. 1992; Straeter-Knowlen et al. 1995; Marks et al. 1996; Fischer et al. 2003; Rawlings et al. 2001; Carofiglio et al. 2006; Byron et al. 2007). High urethral pressure zones are occasionally documented in dysfunctional voiding syndromes (Fillipich et al. 1989; Gookin and Bunch 1997; Lane et al. 2000). Multiple pressure spikes observed along the length of the membranous urethra have also been described in dogs with functional urinary obstruction (Lane et al. 2000). Additionally, finding a normal UPP in a dog with dysfunctional voiding and no evidence of obstruction has been considered supportive of a diagnosis of dyssynergia.

Leak point pressure

A "leak point pressure" can also be determined after moderate filling of the bladder for cystometric or other studies (Rawlings et al. 1999). In this test, the sphincter is challenged by pressure applied to the abdomen at the cranial level of the urinary bladder. Using a large blood pressure cuff around the caudal abdomen, and with progressively increasing infused volume (75–150 mL in mixed breed dogs >20 kg), the cuff is inflated until urine leakage is observed. Increased pressure can be applied by manual compression. In normal dogs, urine leakage was not observed until external pressure reached well over 100 cm H_2O in most dogs (Rawlings et al. 1999). Measurement of LPP is more commonly applied in the evaluation of incontinent women than it is in veterinary patients.

Complications

Complications from urethral pressure studies are rare and are usually related to instrumentation. Slight urethral and vaginal irritation is common and transient. Microscopic hematuria is common and not usually cause for concern. Careful aseptic technique must be followed during urethral catheterization and withdrawal in order to prevent iatrogenic urinary tract infection. Urethral catheters, infusion tubing, and transducers must also be sterilely prepared. Peri-procedural antimicrobials should be considered in animals with anatomical or functional compromise of urogenital host defenses (e.g., amoxicillin for 3 days). Since urodynamic studies are usually performed because of incontinence or urine retention, it can be argued that antimicrobials should be administered in all cases. Regardless of antimicrobial practice, a follow-up urine culture is recommended 5–7 days following the procedure to ensure the clearance of pathogens.

Electromyography

Electromyography (EMG) can be used to evaluate striated urethral musculature. Fine-wire recording electrodes are inserted percutaneously in or near periurethral muscle (Sackman and Sims 1991) or mounted on urinary catheters (Gregory 1984; Richter and Ling 1985; Basinger et al. 1987) used in urodynamic procedures. Addition of EMG to cystometric or urethral pressure studies provides some assessment of neurogenic innervation to the external urethral sphincter. In human patients, EMG activity is recorded throughout filling and voiding studies and is utilized primarily to assess synchrony of detrusor and striated urethral activity in neuropathic disease. EMG activity is expected to increase gradually during filling and to become silent during voiding. In veterinary medicine, EMG have predominantly been used to characterize urethral function at rest and following surgical procedures (Basinger et al. 1987, 1989; Sackman et al. 1999). However, EMG during voiding has been characterized in cats (Sackman and Sims 1990). In cases of urinary retention, EMG could be used to assess pudendal nerve innervation (helping to localize neurologic lesions) and recovery and in the assessment of dyssynergic voiding patterns (Lane 2000b).

Bladder function studies

Indications

Cystometrography (CMG) measures the pressure within the bladder as it is filled with fluid or gas (CO_2) (Figure 22.12). Most studies today are completed with fluid media. Bladder capacity and compliance may be estimated from calculations of infused volume and the pressure slope during filling. In some patients, detrusor contraction appears as a sharp steep pressure rise, accompanied by voiding. An atonic bladder, on the other hand, would be expected to have an expanded capacity and fill to large volumes at low pressure.

In small animal patients, the CMG is most useful for the diagnosis or exclusion of bladder overactivity, a rare cause of ("urge") incontinence in dogs and cats. A reduction in compliance can also contribute to urine storage disorders even if overt overactivity is not documented. CMG results can also be useful in raising suspicion of

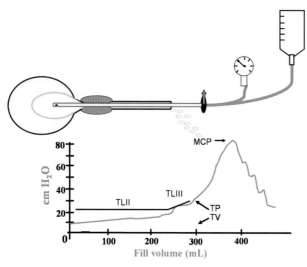

Figure 22.12 Schematic illustration of cystometric study. Intravesicular pressure is recorded while the urinary bladder is slowly filled by fluid infusion. TLII, slope of the filling phase; TLIII, slope change just before detrusor contraction (rarely observed in small animals); TP, threshold pressure; TV, threshold volume; MCP, maximum contraction pressure. Illustration modified from Fischer, J.R. and I.F. Lane (2007). Incontinence and urine retention. In: *BSAVA Manual of Canine and Feline Nephrology and Urology*, edited by Elliott and Grauer. Gloucester: British Small Animal Veterinary Association, with permission.

bladder dysfunction, so the procedure may be indicated in the following kinds of patients (see Chapter 76):

- Dogs with urinary incontinence refractory to traditional medical therapies
- Juvenile dogs with congenital functional or anatomical disorders
- Cats with urinary incontinence
- Dogs or cats with neurogenic disorders
- Dogs or cats with incomplete voiding
- Isolated cases of recurrent or chronic urinary tract infection
- To evaluate bladder function in animals with detrusor–urethral dyssynergia

Sedation/restraint

As for other urodynamic studies, cystometrographic results would be best obtained in nonsedated standing animals. However, most animals require sedation in order for this procedure to be performed to completion. Because the procedure involves potentially uncomfortable bladder distension, it may be inhumane to proceed without sedation. However, the author has completed studies in nonsedated dogs and has observed a few dogs that actually fall asleep during slow bladder filling. Goldstein and Westropp (2005) described experience with nonsedated cystometry in a small number of

cats, completed after cats were anesthetized for urinary catheterization and allowed to recover to consciousness.

Because sedation is usually required, a number of agents have been investigated. The optimal sedative for cystometry provides sufficient restraint and relaxation for both patient comfort and for obtaining quality tracings. Xylazine (with atropine) provided these benefits for years (Oliver and Young 1973a, 1973b; Barsanti et al. 1988; Johnson et al. 1988); medetomine (Rawlings et al. 2001) and oxymorphone (with acepromazine) were also considered reasonably acceptable.

However, xylazine significantly impacts urethral pressure and has numerous adverse effects, so smoother regimens have been sought. A tailored propofol infusion (0.82–1.38 mg/kg/minute) was effective for repeated studies of retrograde fill and diruesis cystometry in dogs (Hamaide et al. 2003). Low dose propofol at 0.2 mg/kg/minute was effective in providing adequate restraint and preserving the detrusor reflex in a small number of healthy cats undergoing infusion cystometry (Cohen et al. 2009). In this crossover study, a few cats were also studied using isoflurane at 1.75% and 2% for restraint. Lower threshold volume measures and fewer identifiable detrusor reflexes were observed (3 of 6).

Procedure

If possible, the animal is allowed to void normally prior to the study. Urinary catheterization is then routine, and the bladder is completely emptied. Residual volume can be measured and assessed in this fashion. Ideally, a balloon catheter is placed in the rectum in order to indirectly record abdominal pressure (Gregory et al. 1999; Goldstein and Westropp 2005). Once equipment and transducers are prepared, the ports of a double lumen catheter are connected to a pressure transducer line and fluid infusion line, respectively. Sterile water or saline is infused at 3–20 mL/minute depending on the size of the patient. Slower rates provide results more reflective of natural filling but are impractical in larger dogs (Barsanti 1995; Goldstein and Westropp 2005). Infusion rates of up to 100 mL/minute have been advocated for large dogs in order to speed the study, but rapid infusion has fallen out of favor. Filling rates of 5 and 10 mL/minute yielded more representative threshold pressure measurements and less evidence of bladder wall damage than did 20 mL/minute in female Beagle dogs. However, these dogs all weighed <20 kg (Hamaide et al. 2003). The pressure within the urinary bladder is recorded during filling, creating a graph of pressure versus volume infused. Filling is stopped when a detrusor contraction is observed or when intravesicular pressure reaches 30–40 cm H_2O in dogs. The urinary bladder in cats appears to tolerate higher pressure challenges; mean threshold pressure was 75 cm H_2O in one study (Cohen et al. 2009). Analysis of filling volume, compliance, threshold volume, and pressure can be completed either by urodynamic software system packages or manually.

Diuresis cystometry

The ability to assess bladder function during natural filling improves the validity of results. Of course, the time required for normal filling would increase study time to an impractical length. Diuresis cytometry incorporates the value of natural fill studies but speeds the process using fluid and diuretic administration (Nickel and Van Den Brom 1997). Bladder and urethral pressure are recorded as for retrograde fill cystometry; filling rate and threshold volume are determined by quantifying the urine volume at the time of micturition, either by interrupting micturition and withdrawing all the urine from the bladder (Hamaide et al. 2003) or by using tracer isotopes to calculate the volume of urine produced (Nickel and Van Den Brom 1997). These techniques, while adding to the cumbersome nature of the technique, have provided additional insight into the urinary bladder contribution to urinary incontinence. In a group of dogs with refractory urinary incontinence, 15/77 had urodynamic findings consistent with poor bladder storage function in addition to poor urethral function, and another 10 dogs had urodynamic abnormalities of bladder function alone (Nickel et al. 1999).

Interpretation

In normal animals, recorded intravesicular pressure is low in the empty bladder and remains low during most of the filling phase, because the urinary bladder muscle is highly compliant. In the CMG tracing, this phase is called tonus limb II (TLII) and is measured as the filling slope (end pressure—start pressure/end volume—start volume) (Figure 22.12). Sensation of pressure and the urge to urinate increase only when the bladder is stretched sufficiently to stimulate stretch receptors in the bladder wall. As a threshold volume is approached, the pressure rises more rapidly (tonus limb III, TLIII) and leads to urinary bladder contraction. A normal urinary bladder contraction should create a sustained high-pressure peak, sufficient to empty the bladder (Oliver and Young 1973).

As an isolated study, the cystometrogram best identifies failure of urinary bladder storage function, characterized by decreased capacity, decreased elasticity, and early involuntary detrusor contractions (Barsanti 1995). The study has been used to characterize bladder dysfunction in dogs with ectopic ureters (Lane et al. 1995) and assess the effects of anticholinergic agents in healthy

beagles (Lane 2000a). In a recent metanalysis, sensitivity (0.55–0.82) and specificity (0.66–0.92) of the single-channel cystometrogram were reasonable for the diagnosis of detrusor overactivity in women (Martin et al. 1996). In animals with urinary retention, the presence of an adequate detrusor contractile peak can be used to rule out detrusor atony, whereas large filling volumes, a prolonged flat filling slope, and a lack of a sustained detrusor contraction may support urinary bladder dysfunction of neurogenic or myogenic nature. However, many normal animals will inhibit detrusor contractions during the cystometrogram, a feature that may be overcome by repeated study (Johnson et al. 1988). The interpretation of an observed detrusor contraction also is limited by the fact that its magnitude may vary and is dependent on bladder volume at the time of contraction. Poor detrusor function confirmed by urodynamic studies may be neurogenic or myogenic in origin, and prognosis for recovery cannot be predicted on the basis of urodynamic measurements.

Contraindications and complications

As for other lower urinary tract manipulations, active urinary tract infection should be treated prior to cystometrography. Elimination of bacteriuria is especially important when bladder distension is anticipated. Retrograde infusion of fluid could lead to reflux of infected urine (or contaminated fluid) into the ureter and lead to ascending infection. Sterile fluid reflux can be damaging to the upper urinary tract as well. Juvenile animals may be most susceptible to fluid reflux, because the vesicoureteral junction is not completely functional until maturity.

Cystometry should be avoided in situations where the urinary bladder wall is compromised, for example by recent acute overdistension (obstruction) or cystotomy. Air cystometry should be avoided in patients with significant hematuria in order to avoid air embolism via compromised capillaries. Microscopic (and occasionally) gross hematuria are observed after cystometry in some dogs and can be prevented by avoiding rapid or excessive bladder distension (Hamaide et al. 2005). Hematuria was not observed in a small group of healthy cats undergoing fluid cystometry, even when high filling pressures were recorded (Cohen et al. 2009).

Voiding studies
Indications and procedures

Urodynamic studies that include parameters of urine flow, such as micturitional studies or uroflowmetry, are more likely to fully demonstrate the voiding phase of micturition. Cystometry combined with uroflowmetry is required for diagnosis of detrusor–urethral dyssynergia in people and is necessary for accurate interpretation of bladder and urethral components of voiding disorders. Methods of recording urine flow include weight recording, electromagnetic fields, air displacement, rotating trays, acoustic analysis, droplet dispersal analysis, and radionuclide techniques. The measurement of urine flow in small animals is difficult, however, owing to the difficulty of commanding urine flow, and of directing urine flow to an appropriate flowmeter. Urine flow measurements also are affected by position, bladder volume at voiding, age, and gender in people. A disadvantage of this technique is the requirement for transabdominal catheters. Micturition studies including intravesicular pressure and urine flow measurement have been described in dogs (Moreau et al. 1983a, 1983b). Fluid infusion and intravesicular pressure were recorded via percutaneously placed transabdominal catheters, and urine flow was diverted into an adapted electromagnetic flowmeter. The micturition study objectively identified outflow obstruction in one dog.

Functional obstructive syndromes in people are best diagnosed with micturitional urethral pressure profilometry or videourodynamic studies, procedures that allow objective or visual assessment of the bladder neck and urethra during voiding. Detrusor–urethral dyssynergia is documented by demonstration of poor urine flow or inappropriately high urethral pressures during sustained increased intravesicular pressure (Blaivas and Chancellor 1996; Steele et al. 1998). The micturitional urethral pressure profile is completed as a small multiport catheter is withdrawn during voiding. Detection of a pressure differential (drop off) along the urethra localizes outlet obstruction. Alternatively, a static transurethral catheter with multiple recording ports can be used to assess simultaneous bladder and multiple urethral pressures during filling and voiding (Yamanishi et al. 1997). Interpretation is enhanced when correlated with video recordings of bladder and urethral events. Uroflow studies are challenging in any species and rarely completed in small animal patients.

Imaging

Voiding videourography may demonstrate active outlet obstruction and may be a useful substitute for urine flow studies in veterinary patients. Postvoid images can be used to document residual urine volume although it must be stressed that voiding during imaging procedures may not be accurate due to contrived position, bladder volume, and nonphysiologic filling rates. Void-

ing cystourethrography with simultaneous urodynamic assessment should be feasible in small animal patients; however, the studies usually require general anaesthesia. Simultaneous contrast cystourethrography and cystometry was used to identify failure of urethral opening during induced voiding in one dog (Gookin and Bunch 1997).

Ultrasound examination of the urinary bladder prior to and following voiding can also be useful in determining residual volume. Crude estimates can be made by simple visualization; quantitative estimates have been validated (Atalan et al. 1998, 1999). Ultrasound examination of the urinary bladder wall and proximal urethral anatomy is a useful diagnostic tool in the evaluation of incontinence in women (Martin et al. 1996) but has not been investigated in dogs.

Conclusions

Urodynamic studies provide objective and repeatable measures of bladder and urethral function. Increased application of such studies would increase the evidence-based nature of urologic practice. However, the cumbersome nature of urodynamic procedures makes them impractical for routine veterinary practice. The many variable and technical details associated with urodynamic measurements emphasize the integration of multiple components of urodynamic information prior to conclusive diagnoses. Even with best practices, all urodynamic studies operate in an artificial situation that may or may not mimic the natural state. In veterinary practice, careful observation of voiding, with attention to initiation, apparent abdominal straining, quality and force of urine stream, and postvoid residual urine volume, usually suffices as "applied urodynamic testing" in veterinary patients. Further investigation of unusual or refractory cases should be undertaken by urologists familiar with the relative advantages and disadvantages of multiple lower urinary tract tests.

References

Arnold, S., D.J. Chew, et al. (1993). Reproducibility of urethral pressure profiles in clinically normal sexually intact female dogs by use of microtransducer catheters. *Am J Vet Res* **54**: 1347–1351.

Atalan, G., F.J. Barr, et al. (1998). Assessment of urinary bladder volume in dogs by use of linear ultrasonographic measurements. *Am J Vet Res* **59**(1): 10–15.

Atalan, G., F.J. Barr, et al. (1999). Comparison of ultrasonographic and radiographic measurements of bladder dimensions and volume determinations. *Res Vet Sci* **66**(3): 175–177.

Barsanti, J.A. (1995). Tests of lower urinary tract function. In: *Canine and Feline Nephrology and Urology*, edited by C.A. Osborne and D.R. Finco. Baltimore, MD: Williams and Wilkins, p. 316.

Barsanti, J.A., D.R. Finco, et al. (1988). Effect of atropine on cystometry and urethral pressure profilometry in the dog. *Am J Vet Res* **49**: 112–114.

Basinger, R.R., C.A. Rawlings, et al. (1987). Urodynamic alterations after prostatectomy in dogs without clinical prostatic disease. *Vet Surg* **16**: 405.

Basinger, R.R., C.A. Rawlings, et al. (1989). Urodynamic alterations associated with clinical prostatic diseases and prostatic surgery. *J Am Anim Hosp Assoc* **25**: 385.

Blaivas, J. and M. Chancellor (1996). Synchronous pressure/uroflow and video-urodynamics. In: *Atlas of Urodynamics*. Baltimore, MD: Williams and Wilkins, p. 88.

Byron, J.K., P.A. March, et al. (2003). Comparison of the effect of propofol and sevoflurane on the urethral pressure profile in healthy female dogs. *Am J Vet Res* **64**: 1288–1292.

Byron, J.K., P.A. March, et al. (2007). Effect of phenylpropanolamine and pseudoephedrine on the urethral pressure profile and continence scores of incontinent female dogs. *J Vet Intern Med* **21**: 47–53.

Carofiglio, F., A.J. Hamaide, et al. (2006) Evaluation of the urodynamic and hemodynamic effects of orally administered phenylpropanolamine and ephedrine in female dogs. *Am J Vet Res* **67**: 723–730.

Cohen, T.A., J.L. Westropp, et al. (2009). Evaluation of urodynamic procedures in female cats anesthetized with low and high doses of isoflurane and propofol. *Am J Vet Res* **70**: 290–296.

Combrisson, H., G. Robain, et al. (1993). Comparative effects of xylazine and propofol on the urethral pressure profile of healthy dogs. *Am J Vet Res* **54**: 1986–1989.

Fillippich, L.J., R.A. Read, et al. (1989). Functional urethral obstruction in a cat. *Aust Vet Pract* **19**: 202.

Fischer, J.R., I.F. Lane, et al. (2003). Urethral pressure profile and hemodynamic effects of phenoxybenzamine and prazosin in non-sedated male beagle dogs. *Can J Vet Res* **67**: 30.

Frenier, S.L., G.G. Knowlen, et al. (1992). Urethral pressure response to alpha-adrenergic agonist and antagonist drugs in anesthetized male cats. *Am J Vet Res* **53**: 1161.

Goldstein, R.E. and J.L. Westropp (2005). Urodynamic testing in the diagnosis of small animal micturition disorders. *Clin Tech Small Anim Pract* **20**: 65–72.

Gookin, J.L. and S.E. Bunch. (1997). Detrusor-striated sphincter dyssynergia in a dog. *J Vet Intern Med* **10**: 339.

Gregory, C.R. (1984). Electromyographic and urethral pressure profilometry: clinical application in male cats. *Vet Clin North Am (Sm Anim Pract)* **14**: 567.

Gregory, S.P., P.E. Holt, et al. (1999). Suitability of the cranial portion of the vagina as a site for measurement of intra-abdominal pressure variations in dogs. *Am J Vet Res* **60**: 1411–1414.

Johnson, C.A., J.M. Beemsterboer, et al. (1988). Effects of various sedatives on air cystometry in dogs. *Am J Vet Res* **49**: 1525.

Hamaide, A.J., J.G. Grand, et al. (2006). Urodynamic and morphologic changes in the lower portion of the urogenital tract after administration of estriol alone and in combination with phenylpropanolamine in sexually intact and spayed female dogs. *Am J Vet Res* **67**: 901–908.

Hamaide, A.J., J.P. Verstegen, et al. (2003). Validation and comparison of the use of diruesis cystometry and retrograde filling cystometry at various infusion rates in female Beagle dogs. *Am J Vet Res* **64**: 574–579.

Hamaide, A.J., J.P. Verstegen, et al. (2005). Influence of the estrous cycle on urodynamic and morphometric measurements of the lower portion of the urogenital tract in dogs. *Am J Vet Res* **66**: 1075–1083.

Holt, P.E. (1988). Simultaneous urethral pressure profilometry: comparisons between continent and incontinent bitches. *J Small Anim Pract* **22**: 98–104.

Lane, I.F. (2000a). Use of anticholinergic agents in lower urinary tract disease. In: *Kirk's Current Veterinary Therapy XIII*, edited by J.D. Bonagura. Philadelphia, PA: WB Saunders, pp. 899–902.

Lane, I.F. (2000b). Diagnosis and management of urine retention. *Vet Clin North Am* **30**: 25–57.

Lane, I.F., J.R. Fischer, et al. (2000). Functional urinary obstruction in three dogs: urethral pressure profile results and response to alpha adrenergic antagonists. *J Vet Intern Med* **14**: 43–49.

Lane, I.F., M.R. Lappin, et al. (1995). Evaluation of preoperative urodynamic measurements in nine dogs with ectopic ureters. *J Am Vet Med Assoc* **206**: 1348–1357.

Marks, S.L., I.M. Straeter-Knowlen, et al. (1996). Effects of acepromazine maleate and phenoxybenzamine on urethral pressure profiles of anesthetized, healthy, sexually intact male cats. *Am J Vet Res* **57**: 1497–1500.

Martin, J.L., K.S. Williams, et al. (2006). Systematic review and meta-analysis of methods of diagnostic assessment for urinary incontinence. *Neurourol Urodyn* **25**: 674–683.

Mawby, D.I., S.M. Meric, et al. (1990). Pharmacologic relaxation of the urethra in male cats: a study of the effects of phenoxybenzamine, diazepam, nifedipine, and xylazine. *Can J Vet Res* **55**: 28.

Moreau, P.M., G.E. Lees, et al. (1983a). Simultaneous cystometry and uroflowmetry (micturition study) for evaluation of the caudal part of the urinary tract in dogs: reference values for healthy animals sedated with xylazine. *Am J Vet Res* **44**: 1774.

Moreau, P.M., G.E. Lees, et al. (1983b). Simultaneous cystometry and uroflowmetry for evaluation of micturition in two dogs. *J Am Vet Med Assoc* **813**: 1084.

Nickel, R.F. and W. Van Den Brom (1997). Simultaneous diuresis cystourethrometry and multi-channel urethral pressure profilometry in female dogs with refractory urinary incontinence. *Am J Vet Res* **58**: 691–696.

Nickel, R.F., M.V. Vink-Noteboom, et al. (1999). Clinical and radiographic findings compared with urodynamic findings in neutered female dogs with refractory urinary incontinence. *Vet Rec* **145**: 11–15.

Oliver, J.E. and W.O.Young (1973a). Air cystometry in dogs under xylazine-induced restraint. *Am J Vet Res* **34**: 1433.

Oliver, J.E. and W.O. Young (1973b). Evaluation of pharmacologic agents for restraint in cystometry in the dog and cat. *Am J Vet Res* **34**: 665.

Oliver, J.E. Jr. (1987). Urodynamic assessment. In: *Veterinary Neurology*, edited by J.E. Oliver Jr., B.E. Hoerlein, and I.G. Mayhew. Philadelphia, PA: WB Saunders, p. 180.

Rawlings, C.A., J.A. Barsanti, et al. (2001a). Results of cystometry and urethral pressure profilometry in dogs sedated with medetomidine or xylazine. *Am J Vet Res* **62**: 167–170.

Rawlings, C., J.A. Barsanti, et al. (2001b). Evaluation of colposuspension for treatment of incontinence in spayed female dogs. *J Am Vet Med Assoc* **219**: 770–775.

Rawlings, C.A., J.R. Coates, et al. (1999). Stress leak point pressures and urethral pressure profile tests in clinically normal female dogs. *Am J Vet Res* **60**: 676–678.

Richter, K.P. and G.V. Ling (1985a). Clinical response and urethral pressure profile changes after phenylpropanolamine in dogs with primary sphincter incompetence. *J Am Vet Med Assoc* **187**: 605–611.

Richter, K.P. and G.V. Ling (1985b). Effects of xylazine on the urethral pressure profile of healthy dogs. *Am J Vet Res* **46**: 1881.

Rosin, A.E. and J.A. Barsanti (1981). Diagnosis of urinary incontinence in dogs: role of the urethral pressure profile. *J Am Vet Med Assoc* **178**: 814.

Sackman, J.E. and M.H. Sims (1990). Electromyographic evaluation of the external urethral sphincter during cystometry in male cats. *Am J Vet Res* **51**: 1237.

Sackman, J.E. and M.H. Sims (1991). Use of fine-wire electrodes for electromyographic evaluation of the external urethral sphincter during urethral pressure profilometry in male cats. *Am J Vet Res* **52**: 314.

Sackman, J.E., M.H. Sims, et al. (1991). Urodynamic evaluation of lower urinary tract function in cats after perineal urethrostomy with minimal and extensive dissection. *Vet Surg* **20**: 55.

Salomon, J.F., M. Gouriou, et al. (2006). Experimental study of urodynamic changes after ovariectomy in 10 dogs. *Vet Rec* **159**: 807–811.

Schafer, W., P. Abrams, et al. (2002). Good urodynamic practices: uroflowmetry, filling cystometry, and pressure-flow studies. *Neurourol Urodyn* **21**: 261–274.

Steele, G.S., M.P. Sullivan, et al. (1998). Urethral pressure profilometry: vesicourethral pressure measurements under resting and voiding conditions. In: *Practical Urodynamics*, edited by V.W. Nitti. Philadelphia, PA: WB Saunders, p. 108.

Straeter-Knowlen, I.M., S.I. Marks, et al. (1995). Urethral pressure response to smooth and skeletal muscle relaxants in anesthetized, adult male cats with naturally acquired urethral obstruction. *Am J Vet Res* **56**: 919.

Yamanishi, T., K. Yasuda, et al. (1997). The nature of detrusor bladder neck dyssynergia in non-neurogenic bladder dysfunction. *J Auton Nerv Sys* **66**: 163.

23

Renal biopsy

George E. Lees and Anne Bahr

The fundamental purpose of a renal biopsy usually is to obtain information that can help a clinician manage a patient's illness more astutely than might be possible without the biopsy and thus to obtain the best available outcome. This information can take the form of a diagnosis of a particular nephropathic illness for which specific therapeutic options can be defined or refined. Additionally, and usually independent of identifying a specific etiopathogenic diagnosis, renal biopsy typically yields information about the severity, activity, chronicity, and/or potential reversibility of pathologic changes that are present, which supports clinical decision-making about prognosis and treatment (Osborne et al. 1996; Vaden 2004; Vaden and Brown 2007).

In the past, renal biopsy has been utilized infrequently by veterinarians caring for animals with kidney diseases. This has been true for many reasons, but the most important contributing factors have been (1) initial detection of kidney disease only after it has reached an advanced stage, (2) infrequent use of the methods of pathologic examination of kidney that are required to make informative diagnoses, and (3) insufficient integration of pathologic findings with such clinical features of the illness as clinicopathologic findings, disease course, and response to treatment. In these circumstances, renal biopsy has been unable to aid the care of many patients with kidney disease; clinicians generally have been able to make appropriate clinical decisions without information derived from a renal biopsy.

Going forward, renal biopsy can be expected to have a more useful and prominent role in the management of kidney diseases in animals. This is partly because renal diseases are more often being detected in their earlier stages by screening tests used to monitor health status. Benefits arise from this because it is in such earlier stages that the pathologic changes associated with specific renal diseases are most distinctive and treatment is more likely to be effective. Additionally, a growing number of veterinarians have the expertise required to manage complex disorders affecting the kidneys, and the number and scope (from administration of medications to renal replacement therapies) of effective treatments that are available for patients with renal diseases are increasing.

Indications for renal biopsy

Clinical settings in which renal biopsy may be considered include acute renal failure (see Chapter 49), glomerular disease manifested by proteinuria (i.e., protein-losing nephropathies) (see Chapter 53), and chronic renal failure (see Chapter 48). Our preference is to subdivide and approach each of these categories as follows.

Acute renal failure

Episodes of acute renal failure generally can be subdivided as acute nephritis or acute nephrosis, with the nephritis category being marked by clinical evidence of an inflammatory process either at the systemic level (e.g., fever and hematologic changes) or within the urinary tract (e.g., urinalysis findings). In acute nephritis, there often are sufficient grounds for presumptive diagnosis of some disorder (e.g., leptospirosis) that can be managed appropriately without a biopsy. However, when there is recent active and ongoing renal injury due to an uncertain cause, a renal biopsy should be strongly considered. The goals of biopsy in this setting are to clarify etiopathogenesis, refine the therapeutic plan, and assess severity and prognosis.

A second category of acute renal failure is nephrosis, which usually is due to some toxic and/or ischemic cause. Among all possible causes of acute nephrosis, only a few

Nephrology and Urology of Small Animals. Edited by Joe Bartges and David J. Polzin. © 2011 Blackwell Publishing Ltd.

(e.g., ethylene glycol, other crystal-associated forms of tubular injury) can be identified on the basis of biopsy findings. Moreover, even when a cause is identified, the finding rarely has direct therapeutic implications (i.e., for administration of specific therapy, as opposed to continuing nonspecific and/or supportive therapy). In this setting, the goals of biopsy can be partly to exclude other possibilities when the etiopathogenic diagnosis is in doubt, but usually are mainly to assess the severity and potential reversibility of the changes that are present. This prognostic information can have a large impact on clinical decisions about whether or not to continue ongoing care that often is a difficult burden (financially and otherwise) for everyone concerned (patient, clinician, and owners).

Biopsy of animals with chronic kidney disease (CKD) in IRIS stage IV or late stage III usually is unrewarding and should be avoided. Nonetheless, one potential indication for biopsy in animals known to have CKD is detection of an abrupt increment in magnitude of azotemia that might be due to superimposition of a process of an acute (i.e., potentially treatable) injury on the chronic disease. In such circumstances, the lower (milder) the azotemia initially (i.e., before the recent increment), the more likely the biopsy is to be informative. The more advanced CKD becomes, the more difficult it is to discern signs of acute injury among the chronic changes. Additionally, although CKD often exhibits a slow and steady pattern of progression, some animals with CKD show an erratic pattern of progression characterized by periods of stability that are interrupted from time to time by abrupt decrements of function that do not have any specific cause that can be identified even with a biopsy.

Protein-losing nephropathies

Animals with protein-losing glomerular disease also may be subdivided on clinical grounds into several categories, namely, nephritic or nephrotic glomerulopathies and glomerular disease characterized by persistent subclinical renal proteinuria.

Nephritic glomerulopathies are characterized by proteinuria that can have a wide range of magnitude but often is in the nephrotic range (arbitrarily defined as UPC > 3.5), with or without accompanying hypoalbuminemia that usually is of mild to moderate severity when it is present, and urinalysis findings that include signs of inflammation in the urinary tract (e.g., microscopic hematuria, mild pyuria). Most animals with nephritic glomerulopathies exhibit some degree of azotemia (the magnitude of which can range from mild to severe) that typically also shows a rising trend in cases of acute nephritic glomerular disease. Additionally, hypertension that often is severe and difficult to control medically is frequently present; however, edema or ascites is uncommon.

The nephritic clinical picture most often is associated with glomerular diseases having a substantial component of endocapillary inflammation, the most common example of which is membranoproliferative glomerulonephritis, type I, particularly during the earlier phases of the process of injury. The goals of biopsy in animals with nephritic glomerulopathies are to obtain an accurate diagnosis, to refine the therapeutic plan, and to assess prognosis (i.e., severity and activity of the changes that are present). In animals with acute, rapidly worsening nephritic glomerular diseases, very aggressive therapeutic interventions may be justified, provided that the diagnosis is well established in part by biopsy findings.

Animals with nephrotic glomerulopathies exhibit nephrotic range proteinuria that is associated with hypoalbuminemia that can be severe but may or may not be associated with clinically evident edema or third-space accumulation of transudates (e.g., ascites, pleural effusion). Animals with nephrotic glomerulopathies usually have totally inactive urine sediments and often do not have azotemia, especially early in the course of the nephropathy. Hypertension is a variable feature of nephrotic glomerulopathies.

The nephrotic clinical presentation most often is associated with glomerular diseases that disrupt visceral epithelial cell (podocyte) function without generating inflammation in the endocapillary compartment. The prototypical condition that does this is membranous glomerulopathy. Minimal change disease is another condition that might be considered, but this diagnosis has been very uncommon in dogs and cats that have been evaluated to date. Additionally, amyloidosis often produces marked proteinuria that is not accompanied by glomerular inflammation.

Goals of biopsy in animals with nephrotic glomerulopathies are to obtain an accurate diagnosis as a basis for planning therapy, and to assess indicators of disease severity and/or activity that might correlate with prognosis or anticipated response to treatment. Animals with nephrotic glomerulopathies exhibit a wide range of stages of disease, and it is likely that biopsy-derived information about the stage of disease can help to predict clinical course and outcome.

Animals with persistent subclinical renal proteinuria (i.e., proteinuria that is not of prerenal or postrenal origin and has been repeatedly documented over a period of a month or more in an animal that exhibits no related clinical signs) may have proteinuria of any magnitude, but it usually is of mild to moderate severity and associated with normal or only mildly decreased circulating albumin concentrations. These animals may or may not be azotemic. Indeed, this category overlaps with CKD, especially in IRIS stages I and II, and early in stage III (see aforementioned text). These animals are among the most challenging ones in which to decide whether or not a biopsy will be useful. It is fair to say that the higher the UPC and the lower (more normal or near normal) the serum creatinine concentration, the more a recommendation to biopsy can be supported; however, each case should be considered individually (i.e., rather than by applying any specific UPC or serum creatinine cutoffs). Nonetheless, in border-line cases, it makes sense to be swayed toward biopsy by finding a lack of response to or worsening trends during nonspecific interventions (i.e., feeding an appropriate diet and administering drugs to block portions of the renin–angiotensin–aldosterone system).

Whether or not the animal might benefit from administration of immunosuppressive therapy often is a key question that the clinician is hoping to address when performing renal biopsy in animals with subclinical renal proteinuria. Criteria that can be used to answer this question, particularly regarding when it can or will be beneficial, have not been developed. However, there are two situations that occur fairly frequently in which biopsy findings helpfully show that immunosuppressive therapy is not appropriate. One is when there is no evidence of glomerular deposition of immune complexes shown by either ultrastructural evaluation or immunostaining. The second is when despite the presence of some immune complex deposits, the predominant glomerular changes are those of chronic scarring (i.e., glomerulosclerosis) rather than of any active, ongoing process of injury that might be mitigated by immunosuppressive therapy.

Miscellaneous circumstances

There are a few other circumstances in which renal biopsy deserves consideration. One of these is when an animal exhibits a juvenile-onset nephropathy. In some cases, definitive diagnosis of the type of changes present (or their likelihood to be attributable to an inherited defect) is sufficiently important to justify biopsy. Although the pathologic findings rarely have a direct impact on therapy (i.e., because the more frequent types of congenital or inherited renal disease do not have specific treatments that are effective), biopsy-derived information can influence breeding decisions for related animals and contribute to a more informed prognosis than might otherwise be available. Yet another special circumstance occurs when owners of dialysis-dependent animals are faced with difficult choices that hinge on the likelihood that adequate renal function will be regained if treatment is continued.

Contraindications for renal biopsy

Regardless of the indications for a renal biopsy, it should not be performed (or it should at least be delayed until the patient's condition is stabilized) if it cannot be performed safely. The main renal biopsy complication of clinical concern is life-threatening hemorrhage (Bigge et al. 2001; Vaden et al. 2005). Factors that are associated with increased risk of this complication are small patient size (i.e., small size of the biopsy target relative to adjacent large vessels), especially animals that weigh less than 5 kg, as well as the presence of disordered hemostasis (thrombocytopenia, prolonged bleeding time, etc.) or uncontrolled hypertension. Other relative or absolute contraindications to renal biopsy include infection, especially abscesses or localized infections that might be pierced or disseminated by the biopsy procedure, large renal cysts, inadequate control of patient pain or motion (including breathing), and inadequate operator competence.

Timing of renal biopsy

Animals with acute nephritis or nephrosis, as well as those with acute nephritic glomerular disease, generally should be biopsied as soon as they are sufficiently well stabilized to permit performing the procedure safely. Animals with nephrotic glomerular diseases usually do not need to be biopsied as urgently as animals with nephritic conditions, and they sometimes need reduction of their fluid accumulations, especially ascites, before the biopsy is performed. For animals with subclinical renal proteinuria, the timing of renal biopsy is an issue that requires clinical judgment. One should be guided first by verifying that the proteinuria is persistent and then by the magnitudes and rates of change of the proteinuria and any associated azotemia. In animals with juvenile-onset nephropathies, a renal biopsy sometimes can be obtained in concert with anesthetic episodes or surgery performed for other reasons (e.g., elective castration or ovariohysterectomy). Similarly, renal biopsy may be indicated during exploratory laparotomy or laparoscopy procedures.

Renal biopsy methods

Performing a renal biopsy requires selection of a suitable method of approaching or locating the target kidney and choice of a device or method for retrieving the tissue. Ultrasound-guided needle biopsy techniques are commonly employed and generally are quite satisfactory when the expected changes are likely to be diffusely distributed in the renal cortex (as is the case in most glomerular disorders and instances of acute renal failure).

A variety of automated biopsy devices that procure satisfactory specimens when they are used properly are available commercially. The size of needle used, both in terms of its diameter and depth of penetration (i.e., length of throw), should be appropriate for the size of the target, which can be assessed directly when using sonographic guidance. When the cortex is thin either because the animal is small or because of effects of disease, use of a short-throw needle (e.g., 11-mm throw; 7-mm specimen notch) is recommended to aid in keeping the biopsy tracts entirely within the cortex even if it is necessary to take a few more samples in order to obtain sufficient tissue for all intended evaluations (Groman et al. 2004). If the samples are intact (i.e., not fragmented) and are handled carefully, the cores of tissue provided by 18-gauge needle biopsy devices generally are quite satisfactory for most purposes. Nonetheless, all other things being equal, larger diameter needles (e.g., 16 ga, rather than 18 ga) often yield more informative samples and are preferable when they can be used safely.

Ultrasound-guided needle biopsy of kidney generally should be performed under general anesthesia so as to have sufficient control over patient discomfort and motion, including breathing, during the procedure. There are several different combinations of patient positions, scanning angles, needle directions, and aspects of the kidney to be the biopsy target(s) that can be used successfully depending on operator preferences. Some prefer to biopsy the right kidney because it typically is less mobile (i.e., it holds still better) than the left kidney; however, others prefer the left kidney due to its more caudal location. Some operators prefer to use a biopsy guide attached to the scanning probe to direct the needle biopsy device, but others prefer a "free hand" technique in which the probe and biopsy device are not connected to one another and can be manipulated independently until the operator is certain that the needle is positioned optimally. Although a scan plane that includes both cortex and medulla often makes the kidney easy to recognize, a scan plane that includes only cortex (within which the biopsy tract will be confined) is recommended for renal biopsy. After identifying the kidney, the operator should rotate or shift the scan plane so that only cortex remains in the plane in which the biopsy needle will be placed. When the scan plane and direction of needle placement have been identified, a small stab incision is made through the skin at the entry point to minimize dulling of the biopsy needle before it is advanced through the body wall to the kidney.

Needle biopsy devices also can be used in combination with other aiming methods, including manual palpation (e.g., in cats), laparoscopy, and a keyhole or fully open celiotomy (Grauer et al. 1983; Osborne et al. 1996; Vaden 2004; Vaden and Brown 2007). However, one observation is that when surgeons use biopsy needles to obtain specimens of kidney during a laparotomy, they often direct the devices too deeply. This problem is avoided when a wedge biopsy is obtained at surgery. Additionally, this type of biopsy is better for evaluation of renal changes that are not uniformly distributed in cortex, as often is the case in animals with juvenile-onset nephropathies.

Adequate planning for a renal biopsy also requires prior procurement of the materials needed to process and submit tissue samples that will be suitable for the examinations required to perform an appropriate evaluation. For glomerular disorders and some other conditions, light microscopic examination alone is not sufficient (Walker et al. 2004). Moreover, the specimens required for electron microscopic examination or immunostaining must be appropriately processed and placed into the proper fixatives and preservatives when the tissue specimens are first obtained. The centers that perform these evaluations provide renal biopsy kits containing the materials and instructions needed to obtain, process, and submit satisfactory specimens to their laboratories.

The cortex of the kidney is the proper target for all renal biopsy procedures for two important reasons, the first of which is safety (Figure 23.1). Biopsy needle tracts that cross the corticomedullary junction are associated with risk of damaging the large vessels (e.g., arcuate arteries) that are located there and thus causing both excess hemorrhage and greater damage to the renal parenchyma as a

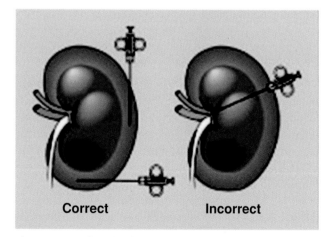

Correct   **Incorrect**

Figure 23.1 Schematic illustrations of correct and incorrect methods of directing a needle biopsy device for renal biopsy. Note that the needle should be directed such that the entire biopsy tract is within the renal cortex. The needle should not cross the corticomedullary junction or enter either the renal medulla or pelvis. Reprinted by permission from Elsevier: Vaden, S.L. (2004). Renal biopsy: methods and interpretation. *Vet Clin North Amer: Sm Anim Pract* **34**: 887–908, copyright 2004.

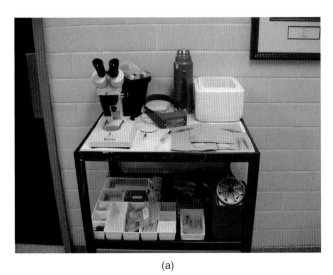

(a)

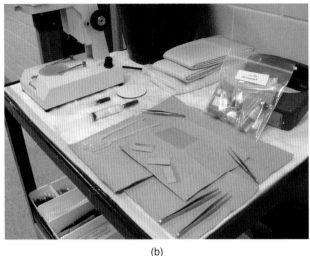

(b)

Figure 23.2 Mobile cart used at Texas A&M University to aid the processing of renal biopsy specimens. The cart is readily taken to whatever site in the hospital (e.g., surgery or ultrasound suite, etc.) where specimen collection is planned. (a) View of the cart as prepared for processing a biopsy on-site. Note the dissecting microscope and magnifying loupe, either of which can be used to assess specimen content. There also is an ice bucket to keep the fixative for electron microscopy chilled, as well as a thermos containing liquid nitrogen used to snap freeze samples for immunofluorescence microscopy after a shallow puddle of the liquid nitrogen is poured into the styrofoam freezing box. (b) View of the cart as prepared for processing specimens off-site utilizing the materials provided in renal biopsy kits that are available from centers that perform comprehensive pathologic evaluations. The reclosable plastic bag contains appropriate fixatives [10% formalin (green-top vial) for light microscopy; 3% glutaraldehyde (vial with red label) for electron microscopy] and a preservative [Michel's transport medium (vial with blue label) for immunofluorescence microscopy]. Tissue samples are placed on the glass slides for examination and kept moist with the saline solution in the syringe. The forceps have no teeth and are suitable for delicate manipulation of the samples. There are a sufficient number of forceps and single-edge razor blades used to separate instruments for specimens intended for each type of fixative or preservative to prevent cross-contamination. The pipettes are used to transfer fluids from the sample containers to the surface of the glass slides and then to wash the samples off the glass slides into their respective specimen containers.

result of ischemia or infarction of the region(s) served by the damaged vessel(s). Secondly, renal cortex is the primary tissue of interest for almost all purposes for which biopsies of kidney are obtained. Indeed, all glomeruli are in the cortex, and a renal biopsy for evaluation of glomerular disease is wholly inadequate if it does not contain an adequate sample of cortical tissue.

Visual assessment of the composition of the tissue cores obtained to verify that they contain glomeruli (i.e., that the samples to be submitted for evaluation are cortical tissue) is an important step in performing a renal biopsy that often is overlooked (Figure 23.2). This task is best accomplished with a low level of magnification (10–40×), such as can be achieved with a dissecting microscope, an ocular loupe, or a hand held lens, and good illumination. With such magnification, several aspects of the appearance of core biopsy specimens aid differentiation of cortex from medulla (Figure 23.3). One is that glomeruli often can be seen in cortical tissue as small spherical structures (or merely as spherical disruptions in the surrounding pattern of tubules). However, even when individual glomeruli are not recognized, the cortex usually can be distinguished from medulla based

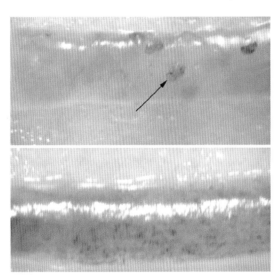

Figure 23.3 Renal biopsy specimen as seen with a dissecting microscope. (a) Renal cortex, not the glomeruli, recognized as round red areas (wet preparation ×10). (b) Renal medulla, reddish vasculature is present by no glomeruli seen (wet preparation ×10, photographs contributed by Alexis Harris, MD). Reprinted by permission from Macmillan Publishers, Ltd: Walker, P.D., et al. (2004). Practice guidelines for the renal biopsy. *Mod Pathol* **17**(12): 1555–1563, copyright 2004.

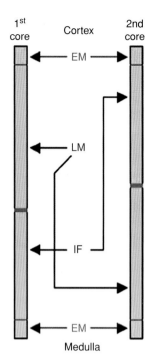

1st core   Cortex   2nd core

EM

LM

IF

EM

Medulla

Figure 23.4 Diagram to illustrate division of renal biopsy cores in the absence of a dissecting microscope for laboratories using immunofluorescence. The ends from all cores are taken for electron microscopy with the remainder divided for light microscopy and immunofluorescence. Reprinted by permission from Macmillan Publishers, Ltd: Walker, P.D., et al. (2004). Practice guidelines for the renal biopsy. *Mod Pathol* **17**(12): 1555–1563, copyright 2004.

on the general architecture of the tissue because tubules in cortical tissue are convoluted (i.e., they appear jumbled in an irregular pattern), whereas those in medulla are straight and arrayed in parallel with one another. Additionally, the specimens should be kept moist (i.e., never placed on dry sponges) with physiologic saline solution and manipulated with great care (i.e., very gently and without grasping them with forceps) as they are collected, assessed, processed, and placed in appropriate fixatives or preservatives.

In general, it is best to collect at least two cortical cores if each is >10 mm long. When the cores are shorter than 10 mm each, 3 cores usually are required. Needle biopsy cores do not need to be cut into smaller pieces except as needed to subdivide them appropriately separate evaluations (Figure 23.4); however, a portion of a wedge biopsy specimen must be carefully cut into pieces that are no greater than 1–2 mm in any dimension before placement in the fixative (e.g., 3% glutaraldehyde in phosphate buffer) for electron microscopy.

References

Bigge, L.A., D.J. Brown, et al. (2001). Correlation between coagulation profile findings and bleeding complications after ultrasound-guided biopsies: 434 cases (193–1996). *J Am Anim Hosp Assoc* **37**: 228–233.

Grauer, G.F., D.C. Twedt, et al. (1983). Evaluation of laparoscopy for obtaining renal biopsy specimens from dogs and cats. *J Am Vet Med Assoc* **183**: 677–679.

Groman, R.P., A. Bahr, et al. (2004). Effects of serial ultrasound-guided renal biopsies on kidneys of healthy adolescent dogs. *Vet Radiol Ultrasound* **45**: 62–69.

Osborne, C.A., J.W. Bartges, et al. (1996). Percutaneous needle biopsy of the kidney; indications, applications, technique, and complications. *Vet Clin North Am Small Anim Pract* **26**: 1461–1504.

Vaden, S.L. (2004). Renal biopsy: methods and interpretation. *Vet Clin North Am Small Anim Pract* **34**: 887–908.

Vaden, S.L., and C.A. Brown (2007). Renal biopsy. In: *BSAVA Manual of Canine and Feline Nephrology and Urology*, edited by J.A. Elliott and G.F. Grauer, 2nd Edition. Quedgeley, Gloucester, UK: British Small Animal Veterinary Association, pp. 167–177.

Vaden, S.L., J.F. Levine, et al. (2005). Renal biopsy: a retrospective study of methods and complications in 283 dogs and 65 cats. *J Vet Intern Med* **19**: 794–801.

Walker, P.D., T. Cavallo, et al. (2004). Practice guidelines for the renal biopsy. *Mod Pathol* **17**: 1555–1563.

24

Renal pathology

Cathy Brown

Introduction

Evaluation of the morphologic changes occurring in the diseased kidney requires an appreciation of normal renal structure and function and an understanding of how the kidney may respond to injury. The lesions present in renal biopsies represent a spectrum between primary injury (acute or chronic) with minimal secondary changes to chronic disease in which the secondary changes may obscure the etiology of the initial insult. The goal of pathologic evaluation and characterization of both primary and secondary disease processes occurring in a renal biopsy is to provide the veterinary clinical nephrologist with accurate information important for treatment and prognosis. Renal biopsies are most often obtained from animals with either clinically acute renal disease or protein-losing nephropathy. As the renal lesions causing these clinical diseases are occurring in the cortical tubulointerstitium or glomeruli, the biopsy should be composed entirely or predominantly of cortical tissue. While acute pyelonephritis or acute papillary necrosis are potential causes of acute renal disease that cannot be diagnosed based on examination of cortical renal tissue alone, diagnostic methods other than renal biopsy are more appropriate for these diseases.

Initial approach to renal biopsy evaluation

The normal renal cortex contains numerous tubules and scattered glomeruli within a scant interstitium. The distribution of proximal tubules versus distal tubule/collecting ducts can be readily appreciated with immunohistochemical staining for cytokeratin, which intensely stains the distal tubules and collecting ducts (Figure 24.1).

The proximal tubule is approximately twice as long as the distal segment, so more tubular cross-sections in the cortex are proximal. Proximal tubules are also distinguished from distal tubules by their prominent brush border (Figure 24.2). While most toxins and ischemic insults affect proximal tubules, some toxins (most notably melamine/cyanuric acid) affect distal tubules. Lesions present within glomeruli may be focal (less than 50% of glomeruli involved) or generalized (all or almost all glomeruli involved). Within an affected glomerulus, the lesion may be segmental (only part of the capillary tuft affected) or global (the entire tuft involved). As most primary glomerular diseases in dogs and cats are generalized, it is possible that a diagnosis could be made based on the appearance of a single glomerulus. However, as there may be variability both in the severity of the primary glomerular lesion and the secondary glomerular changes, a minimum of five glomeruli should be present in the submitted biopsy. The number of glomeruli present in the biopsy should be stated in the biopsy report as an indication of the adequacy of the biopsy.

Glomeruli, tubules, the interstitium, and blood vessels (arteries and arterioles) are initially evaluated in slides stained with hematoxylin and eosin (H&E) in order to determine lesion distribution, severity, and the primary site of renal disease. The primary site of injury within the nephron may be suspected prior to biopsy based on clinical data, and it is important to convey this information to the nephropathologist. Animals with severe proteinuria that are not azotemic will be more likely to have lesions confined to the glomerulus, while those with increasing severity of azotemia are more likely to have secondary interstitial and glomerular changes. It may be impossible to determine the primary site of injury (glomerular versus tubulointerstitial) in animals

Nephrology and Urology of Small Animals. Edited by Joe Bartges and David J. Polzin. © 2011 Blackwell Publishing Ltd.

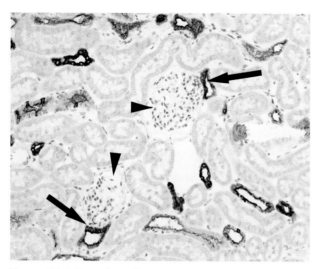

Figure 24.1 Normal renal cortex containing glomeruli (arrowheads) and numerous tubular profiles, dog. Distal tubular profiles (arrows, darkly staining with cytokeratin) are fewer in number than proximal tubules, reflecting the longer length of the proximal segment. Immunohistochemistry, pancytokeratin, original magnification 200×.

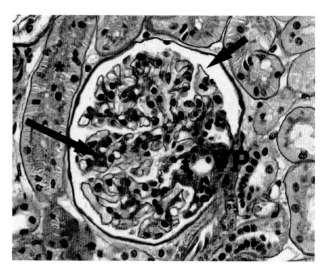

Figure 24.2 Normal renal glomerulus stained with PASH, dog. Note the dark pink staining of the tubular basement membranes, Bowman's capsule, the glomerular basement membrane (short arrow), mesangial matrix (long arrow), and the proximal tubular brush border (asterisk). The vascular pole (VP) and adjacent macula densa are also evident. PASH, original magnification 400×.

with more chronic renal disease with moderate azotemia and mild to moderate proteinuria. In addition to H&E stains, a battery of other stains is routinely used for evaluation of the renal biopsy. As thicker sections will appear more cellular, have more mesangial matrix, and have thicker glomerular capillary loops, renal biopsies should be routinely sectioned and evaluated at 2–3 um. Thin sections are stained with periodic acid-Schiff hematoxylin (PASH) and Masson's trichrome. As listed in Table 24.1, PASH stains all basement membranes (BM) and the mesangial matrix dark pink (Figure 24.2).

In the absence of significant interstitial pathology, the BM of tubules will be touching each other; subtle tubular separation is readily appreciated with this stain. PASH also demonstrates wrinkling of the tubular BM, indicative of tubular atrophy, and thickening of the tubu-

lar BM, which may occur as a nonspecific response to ischemia. This stain is also used to evaluate the quantity of mesangial matrix; mesangial matrix expansion or glomerulosclerosis is indicative of mesangial cell activation and may be a primary or secondary response to injury. The mesangium acts as scaffolding for the capillary tuft, and is normally present as fine anastomosing branches confined to the central portions of the capillary tuft (Figure 24.2). PASH is also used to evaluate changes in the glomerular capillary wall in suspected cases of glomerulonephritis (BM spikes or reduplication). Alternatively, methanamine silver stains with various counterstains may also be used to effectively demonstrate GBM changes. Masson's trichrome stain accentuates interstitial fibrosis by staining collagen blue. Fibrosis is indicative of chronic disease, and the severity of fibrosis is positively

Table 24.1 Special stains used in evaluation of renal biopsies

Stain	Features	Use
PASH	Dark pink staining of BMs of glomerular capillaries, Bowman's capsule, and tubules; mesangial matrix; and proximal tubule brush border	Initial evaluation of GBM thickness, GBM spikes, GBM splitting, mesangial matrix expansion, highlights any tubular separation or tubular atrophy, tubular injury with loss of brush border
Masson's trichrome	Dark blue staining of interstitial collagen, lighter blue staining of BMs and mesangial matrix, magenta staining of glomerular immune deposits	Assessment of amount of interstitial fibrosis, demonstration of immune deposits in glomerulonephritis
Congo red	Amyloid deposits in glomeruli, vessels, tubular BMs, or interstitium stain red-orange; confirmed by apple-green birefringence of stained material under polarized light	Identification of eosinophilic deposits as amyloid

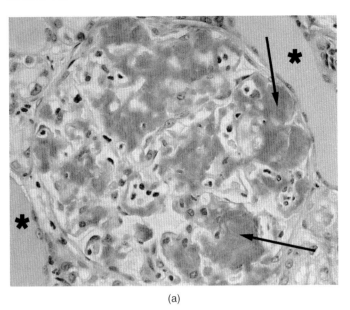 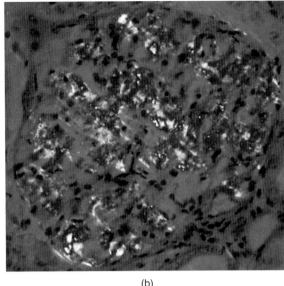

(a)   (b)

Figure 24.3 Glomerular amyloidosis, dog. (a) Nodular accumulations of red-orange homogeneous material (arrows) expand the glomerulus, separating resident cells. Hyaline casts (asterisk), indicative of proteinuria, are present within distal tubules. Congo red. (b) When view under polarized light, Congo red-stained deposits exhibit apple-green birefringence. Original magnification 600×.

correlated with the degree of renal dysfunction. Interstitial fibrosis is a poor prognostic indicator, as it is associated with irreversible renal injury and nephron loss. Masson's trichrome may also be used to detect immune deposits in the glomerular capillary, which stain magenta with this stain. Biopsies with glomerular deposits suggestive of amyloid should be cut at 5–8 um, stained with Congo red or Standard Toluidine Blue, and viewed with polarized light to confirm this diagnosis (Figure 24.3). Thick sections are required for sufficient binding of the dye for visualization of birefringence under polarized light.

Lesions of acute intrinsic renal disease

Renal biopsy may be indicated in animals with acute renal failure, as the lesions may suggest a cause with a specific treatment and may facilitate prognostication (Vaden and Brown, 2007) The lesions of acute renal failure typically involve the tubulointerstitium and can be evaluated with light microscopy alone. Acute intrinsic renal failure in dogs and cats is most often toxic in etiology, resulting in acute tubular necrosis (ATN) (Worway, 2008; Behrend, 1996). In contrast, ATN causing acute renal failure in people is more often ischemia in nature and is due to decreased renal blood flow associated with hypotension/shock, blood loss, hypovolemia, or sepsis. Although ischemia may play a contributing role in some cases of ATN in dogs and cats, particularly when there is evidence of underlying chronic renal disease, it appears as though the canine and feline kidney are relatively resis-

tant to renal failure during conditions that cause ischemic ATN in people.

The proximal tubule is the segment of the nephron most susceptible to toxic (and ischemic) injury. This susceptibility of the proximal tubule is a reflection of their large microvillous surface area, their normal high absorptive and excretory function (may excrete toxins into this segment), and their high oxygen requirements. As not all cortical tubules are proximal and because the proximal tubule may be segmentally affected, the tubular necrosis will appear patchy in distribution, with affected tubules being adjacent to relatively normal tubules. This "patchy" distribution of ATN will be present similarly throughout the cortex, so the lesion should be present in any cortical biopsy. The histologic severity of toxic ATN may vary from mild (often described as "nephrosis") with sloughing of small numbers of necrotic of epithelial cells and brush border loss ("tubular simplification") to frank epithelial cell necrosis affecting most cells in the affected tubular segment (lily toxicosis). Depending on the disease process, there may be severe functional abnormalities despite relatively minor morphologic changes. For example, young dogs with **acute septicemic leptospirosis** may have severe azotemia and extra-renal lesions of uremia (uremic gastritis and pneumonitis, vascular fibrinoid necrosis) but only mild, potentially unrecognized lesions of renal tubular dilation due to brush border loss and mild ATN. The cause of the mild ATN in these dogs is thought to be due to toxic factors released by the spirochetes (Davila de Arriga et al., 1982). Due to the acute nature of the infection, these dogs will typically not yet have

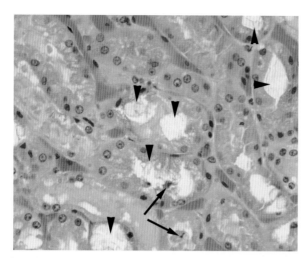

Figure 24.4 Acute tubular nephrosis, ethylene glycol toxicosis, dog. Large numbers of pale green oxalate crystals are present within tubules (arrowheads). There is mild associated renal tubular necrosis characterized by individual cell pyknosis and hypereosinophilia; these necrotic cells often slough into the tubular lumen (arrows). H&E, original magnification 400×.

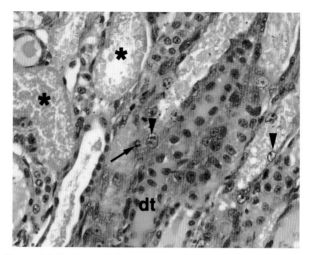

Figure 24.5 Acute tubular necrosis, lily toxicosis, cat. Some segments of the proximal tubule exhibit massive necrosis (asterisks), while others are lined by fewer attenuated viable epithelial cells. There is evidence of epithelial regeneration with large nuclei (arrowheads) and mitotic figures (arrow) present. Note relative sparing of distal tubule (DT). H&E, original magnification 400×.

positive serologic leptospira titers, and renal inflammation is minimal or not present. **Ethylene glycol toxicosis** results in the deposition of large numbers of calcium oxalate crystals in both proximal and distal tubules (Figure 24.4).

Microscopically, there are only small numbers of necrotic tubular epithelial cells, and this necrosis is often confined to cells in direct contact with the crystals. The renal diagnosis "severe oxalate nephrosis" reflects the large numbers of crystals present and the minimal histologic evidence of necrosis. Calcium oxalate crystals may result in tubular obstruction and cause direct tubular damage by altering membrane structure and function, increasing reactive oxygen species, and interfering with epithelial cell oxidative phosphorylation (McMartin, 2009). The presence of large numbers of oxalate crystals in tubules is virtually diagnostic of ethylene glycol toxicosis. However, small numbers of oxalates (secondary oxalosis) may be observed in tubules in animals with any renal tubular dysfunction.

In contrast to the minimal histologic tubular changes seen with ethylene glycol toxicosis, other toxins may cause acute severe ATN of the proximal tubules as observed in cats with **lily nephrotoxicosis**. Severe ATN affecting segments of the proximal tubule is observed in cats ingesting flowers (most toxic) or leaves of Easter lilies, Tiger or lilies, and Asiatic hybrid lilies (Figure 24.5). Affected cats exhibit acute renal failure with azotemia, vomiting, and depression with evidence of proximal tubular dysfunction (glucosuria, tubular proteinuria) (Rumbeiba et al., 2004). Initial degenerative changes include nuclear pyknosis, swelling and granularity of the cytoplasm, and

indistinct cell borders. As the cell damage progresses, this is nuclear fragmentation or lysis, and cells slough into the lumen. In more severely affected cats and in cats dying of lily nephrotoxicosis, the lining epithelium may be completely absent in some proximal tubular cross-sections and the lumen filled with a granular hypereosinophilic coagulum (Figure 24.5).

Other tubules are lined by attenuated cells as the tubular epithelium spreads to cover areas of denuded BM. The ultrastructural finding of enlarged "megamitochrondria" in proximal tubular epithelial cells suggests that the mitochondria are the cellular target in lily toxicosis.

Aminoglycoside nephrotoxicity may manifest as proximal tubule brush border loss, although in higher doses or in conjunction with preexisting renal disease tubular cell necrosis may occur (Maxie et al., 2007).

Some toxins, most notably melamine/cyanuric acid, affect the distal rather than the proximal tubules in affected dogs and cats. A large outbreak of **melamine/cyanuric-acid associated renal failure (MARF)** occurred in the United States in 2007, a similar outbreak in Asia in 2004 was retrospectively determined to be of the same cause (Brown et al, 2007). While both MARF and ethylene glycol toxicosis are characterized by polarizable intratubular crystals, there are distinct differences between these two crystal types. Crystals are typically more numerous in ethylene glycol toxicosis than in MARF. Oxalate crystals are predominantly in proximal tubules, lighter green with a glassy appearance, often oblong in shape, and more difficult to appreciate without polarization (Figure 24.4). In contrast, melamine/cyanuric acid crystals are predominantly within distal

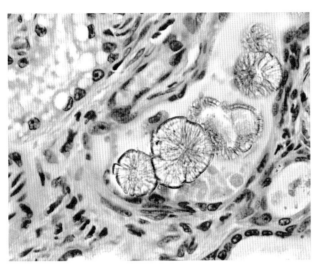

Figure 24.6 Acute distal tubular necrosis with intratubular crystals, melamine/cyanuric acid toxicosis, cat. Characteristic round striated crystals within distal tubule. Note attenuation of the tubular epithelium and small numbers of sloughed necrotic cells. H&E, original magnification 400×.

tubular segments, green to blue in appearance, often exhibit striations, and are easily visualized histologically without polarization (Figure 24.6).

Animals with MARF will often have small numbers of oxalate crystals (secondary oxalosis) in proximal tubules.

Acute MARF is characterized by distal nephron segments (distal tubules and collecting ducts) dilation both in the presence and absence of associated crystals. Dilated distal tubules contain fewer epithelial nuclei, epithelial cells are attenuated, and small numbers of necrotic cells are observed in tubular lumina. Mild anisokaryosis with occasional mitotic figures, indicative of tubular epithelial regeneration, is often present. In some animals, there may be an associated acute tubulitis, typically within the medulla, with intratubular and peritubular neutrophils. Focal proliferation of tubular epithelial cells over the intraluminal crystals is occasionally observed. Renal lesions seen in animals that have been ingesting melamine/cyanuric acid for longer periods of time include distal tubular necrosis with characteristic intratubular crystals, mild to moderate renal interstitial fibrosis, and lymphoplasmacytic inflammation. The inflammation surrounding crystal-containing tubules is more prominent than in acute MARF and consists of moderate numbers of lymphocytes, plasma cells, and macrophages, with only rare neutrophils. Larger crystals are more common in the medulla in cases of chronic MARF, and crystal-containing tubules may rupture. Liberated interstitial crystals are surrounded by macrophages, multinucleated giant cells, and fibrous connective tissue. Large aggregates of crystals may be present in the papilla, and grossly visible renoliths may be observed in some animals.

Acute renal injury is potentially reversible and is dependent on cessation of the original pathologic process and, in ATN, requires a sufficient epithelial pool to regenerate and sufficient maintenance of function to allow time for regeneration to occur. Tubular epithelial changes such as anisokaryosis, increased cytoplasmic basophilia (indicative of increased protein synthesis), and increased numbers of mitotic figures are indicative of regeneration following ATN, which is a favorable prognostic sign (Figure 24.5). In diseases associated with frank ATN such as lily, grape, or aminoglycoside nephrotoxicosis, the severity of the ATN may have prognostic significance. Secondary changes may occur following ATN and these changes may also affect prognosis. Interstitial fibrosis is associated with nephron loss and, as nephron loss is permanent, is indicative of some degree of permanent renal dysfunction. Tubulitis may occur in ethylene glycol toxicosis and MARF and may exacerbate tubular injury, which may or may not be reversible. Animals with more chronic forms of MARF may have tubular rupture; these released crystals are surrounded by granulomatous inflammation and fibrous connective tissue. These crystals would also be expected to persist longer than intratubular crystals following withdrawal of contaminated pet food.

Some **infectious diseases** may cause acute intrinsic renal failure by causing acute severe tubulointerstitial nephritis. **Subacute or classic leptospirosis** is characterized by severe neutrophilic to lymphoplasmacytic tubulointerstitial nephritis and serologic evidence of leptospirosis. **Embolic suppurative nephritis** occurs when bacteria localize in the kidney of bacteremic animals. Bacteria lodge in glomeruli and peritubular capillaries and result in multiple areas of abscessation. Finally, **feline infectious peritonitis** is fairly commonly associated with pyogranulomatous interstitial nephritis and vasculitis. However, methods other than renal biopsy (serology or bacterial culture) are typically used to diagnose these diseases. Fulminant glomerular diseases, such as **glomerular thrombosis, hemolytic uremic syndrome**, and **rapidly progressive glomerulonephritis** (typically with crescents) may also result in acute renal failure. Because of the severe and often irreversible nature of these diseases, diagnosis is more often made on necropsy rather than biopsy specimens.

Protein-losing nephropathy – normal glomerular structure and function

Renal biopsy is perhaps most commonly performed on animals with evidence of protein-losing nephropathy. Accurate histologic evaluation of the glomerulus is dependent upon an appreciation of the normal morphology of the glomerulus, both at the light and electron

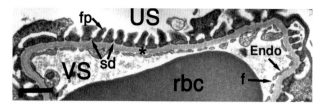

Figure 24.7 Normal glomerular filtration apparatus, dog. The capillary vascular space, containing a red blood cell (RBC), is lined by a layer of fenestrated endothelial cells. The GBM is between the endothelial cell and the podocyte (present in the urinary space; US). The slit diaphragm (sd) is the central size-selective component of the filtration apparatus. Bar = 1 μm.

microscopic level, as well as the relation of structure to function. The glomerulus is a tuft of highly branched capillaries that invaginate into an extension of the proximal tubule. The afferent arteriole enters the glomerulus and arborizes to form the glomerular capillary tuft, which reforms and exits as the efferent arteriole; these arterioles enter and exit at the vascular pole (Figure 24.2). The capillary loops are supported by scaffolding made up of mesangial cells and their surrounding extracellular mesangial matrix. The capillary tuft is draped by glomerular BM and is covered by a layer of interdigitating visceral epithelial cells (podocytes).

The function of the glomerulus is to form an ultrafiltrate of plasma; a small portion of this filtrate will eventually be voided as urine. Fenestrated endothelial cells line the glomerular capillaries and restrict the passage of blood cells (Figure 24.7). Macromolecules with a molecular weight similar to albumin are small enough to fit through these fenestrate or pores. However, the negatively charged sialoproteins that coat the endothelial cells normally repel negatively charged macromolecules such as albumin. The glomerular BM is between the endothelial cells and podocytes within capillary loops, and between mesangial cells and podocytes in other areas. It is important to note that the mesangial cell is not separated from the vascular space by GBM, but is in direct communication with the endothelium and subendothelial space. The GBM is composed primarily of nonfibrillar type IV collagen, laminin, and heparin sulfate containing proteoglycans. Type IV collagen forms a "chicken wire"-like structure made up of heavily cross-linked triple helixes of $\alpha3:\alpha4:\alpha5$ collagen chains. This form of collagen contains more intermolecular disulfide crosslinks than the type IV collagen present in other vascular BM, which are thought to provide more structural strength to the GBM. This is particularly important as the glomerular capillary walls do not have the supportive fibrillar type III collagen of other blood vessels and they are subject to high pressures and fluid shifts not present in other capillaries. The "holes" in the chicken wire allow macromolecules below

a certain size to pass through, acting as an important size selective barrier to the passage of large uncharged plasma macromolecules. Attached to the collagen "wire" are negatively charged heparin sulfate containing proteoglycans and laminin that contribute to the charge selective filtration barrier of the GBM. The filtration of smaller molecular weight molecules is inhibited by slit pores or filtration slits, which are present between the foot processes of the visceral epithelial cells. The slit diaphragm is now thought to be the central size-selective component of the filtration barrier. Nephrin has been recently identified as a key structural component of the slit diaphragm. Congenital defects in nephrin in people result in Congenital Nephrotic Syndrome with massive proteinuria; congenital nephrin defects have not been documented in animals. However, nephrin synthesis may be altered in acquired glomerular diseases with proteinuria.

Proteinuria results when there is disruption of the filtration barrier, which may be caused by the deposition of immune complexes, complement, or amyloid; by an increase or change (either acquired or congenital) in the composition of the glomerular BM; or by injury to the endothelial cells or podocytes. Glomerular injury may also affect mesangial cells, resulting in mesangial cell proliferation and/or increased production of mesangial matrix. Diseases primarily affecting mesangial cells are associated with proteinuria of lesser magnitude than diseases affecting the filtration apparatus.

The goal of renal biopsy in glomerular diseases is to accurately identify the specific changes occurring in the glomerulus in order to determine the prognosis and potential treatment options for the identified glomerular disease. Glomeruli should be evaluated for cellularity, matrix increase, amyloid deposition, hyalinization, necrosis, fibrin thrombosis, crescents, protein deposits, adhesions, and glomerular BM changes. PASH and Masson's trichrome stains, in addition to hematoxylin and eosin, should be used when evaluating glomerular morphology in diseases other than amyloidosis. In the normal glomerulus stained with PASH, the thickness of the capillary walls should be assessed in peripheral capillary loops, and when cut at a right angle, the normal loops will be thin, uniform, and crisp. The mesangial matrix can be seen as disconnected branches containing mesangial cells (Figure 24.2). Matrix typically surrounds one or two mesangial cell nuclei; mesangial matrix expansion is present if matrix extends to encircle more cells. More than three mesangial cell nuclei in close proximity are indicative of mesangial hyperplasia.

Glomerular diseases are a leading cause of renal disease in dogs but are reported less commonly in cats. In human beings, specific glomerular diseases are characterized by their light microscopic, immunopathologic, and electron

Table 24.2 Classification of glomerular lesions[a]

Morphologic classification	LM findings	EM findings	Immuno-pathology	Current status in dogs and cats
Amyloidosis	Nodular hyalinosis of capillary wall, positive Congo red staining	Mesangial and subendothelial fibrils	Immune deposits absent	Most often diagnosed in advanced stage of disease, early stages poorly recognized
Membranous GN (MGN), stage I–IV	Diffuse capillary wall thickening, normal cellularity, magenta deposits with trichrome, PASH spikes	Subepithelial immune deposits	Primarily IgG	Early cases not detected with LM alone
Membranoproliferative glomerulonephritis (MPGN) type I/III	Increased glomerular cellularity and capillary wall thickness, magenta deposits with trichrome, tram-track GBM with PASH	Deposits subendothelial, +/− mesangial and sub-epithelial deposits, mesangial interposition	Primarily IgG, C3, and other Ig may be present	Requires EM for accurate dx, specific Ig classes or type of MPGN, described in dogs and rarely in cats
MPGN type II	As MPGN type I	Intramembranous linear dense deposits	Deposits composed of C3	Described in dogs with inherited complement abnormalities
Mesangioproliferative GN/IgA nephropathy	Typically, increased mesangial cellularity, other lesions possible	Mesangial deposits	IgA	Difficult to dx with LM, requires FA; not documented in dogs or cats
Focal segmental glomerulosclerosis (FSGS)	Segmental hypercellularity and solidification of capillary tuft affecting some glomeruli	Deposits not present	Not typically present	May be primary (suspected in dogs) or secondary to decreased renal mass (common)
Minimal change disease	Normal histology	Foot process effacement	Not present	Rarely described in dogs
Glomerular vasculopathy (DIC, HUS)	Fibrin thrombosis, endothelial swelling, vasculitis	Fibrin, endothelial swelling/necrosis	Fibrin	Described in greyhounds, occasionally suspected in other dogs
Hereditary nephritis	Nonspecific and varied changes	Thin or focally/diffusely split GBM	Not expected	Described in several breeds, suspected in others

[a]Modification of preliminary classification system developed by the WSAVA Renal Standardization Group.

microscopic features that are correlated with the clinical and clinicopathologic findings. While veterinary pathologists have attempted to characterize glomerular diseases in dogs using a classification system similar to that used in human nephropathology, they have based their diagnoses primarily on light microscopic findings. Relying on light microscopy alone often results in misdiagnoses, leading to errors in treatment and prognosis and loss of clinician confidence in the utility of the renal biopsy. Adaptation of the diagnostic approach to glomerular disease routinely used in human nephropathology (electron microscopy and immunopathology in addition to light microscopy)

to veterinary nephropathology will result in the accurate classification of canine glomerular disease (Table 24.2). Correlation of different glomerular diseases/lesions with efficacy of different treatment modalities and patient outcome should establish the importance of the renal biopsy for optimal patient management.[1]

Lesions of protein-losing nephropathy

Amyloidosis is one of the most common glomerular diseases in dogs, accounting for approximately one-fourth of dogs with glomerular disease; cats less commonly develop glomerular amyloidosis (Cook et al., 1996; Vaden and Brown, 2009). While glomerular amyloidosis in later stages can be diagnosed with light microscopy alone, early stages may require ultrastructural evaluation. With the exception of the Chinese Shar Pei, amyloid is deposited primarily in the glomeruli of affected dogs. Amyloid is first deposited in mesangial areas, with eventual subendothelial deposition. Because proteinuria associated with glomerular amyloidosis may be massive, many dogs will present with nephrotic syndrome or pulmonary thromboembolism (due to loss of antithrombin III). Chinese Shar Pei dogs and Abyssinian cats have a familial form of reactive amyloidosis that is characterized by glomerular and medullary amyloid deposition, with medullary deposits typically predominating. Affected Shar Pei dogs and Abyssinian cats are more likely to present clinically with azotemia rather than proteinuria, as medullary interstitial amyloid deposition leads to ischemia, chronic interstitial fibrosis, papillary necrosis, and nephron loss.

In H&E stained slides, glomerular amyloid appears as eosinophilic nodular deposits that expand the mesangium and glomerular capillary walls. Interstitial amyloid may be present as perivascular and peritubular deposits primarily within the medulla. Dogs with amyloid only in the glomerulus will typically not have interstitial fibrosis, even when azotemia is present. If interstitial fibrosis is observed in dogs with glomerular amyloid, medullary deposits of amyloid causing ischemia and nephron loss are also likely present. When stained with Congo red and evaluated by conventional light microscopy, amyloid deposits take on various shades of orange-red, depending upon the amount of amyloid and the thickness of the section (Figure 24.3a). Deposits stained with Congo red and evaluated by polarizing microscopy are birefringent and have an apple green color (Figure 24.3b).

Early stages of renal amyloidosis may have some degree of proteinuria, but the amyloid deposits may not be detectable histologically. In these cases, electron microscopy is required for diagnosis. Amyloid deposits occur between the capillary endothelial cells and the GBM and within mesangial areas (Figure 24.8).

If not previously verified by Congo red positivity, the fibrils are identified as amyloid based on their morphology (nonbranching fibrils of variable length) and size (7–15 nm in diameter).

Rarely, fibrillary deposits that do not polarize with Congo red staining are observed in glomeruli in people and have also been rarely reported in dogs and cats (Cavana et al., 2008). The Congo red-negative fibrillary deposits are composed of organized immunoglobulin or extracellular matrix protein and are typically larger in diameter than amyloid fibrils.

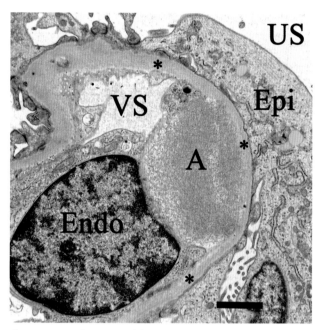

Figure 24.8 Ultrastuctural features of glomerular amyloid, dog. There is a nodular accumulation of amyloid fibrils (a) beneath the endothelium (Endo) lining the vascular space (VS) of the glomerular capillary. There is diffuse podocyte (epithelial cell, Epi) foot process effacement, and the glomerular basement membrane (asterisks) is normal. Bar = 2 μm. Electron micrograph courtesy of Ralph Nichols, Texas Heart Institute.

Glomerulonephritis is an immune mediated disease typically associated with deposition of immune complexes within the glomerulus. Intact antigen–antibody complexes may be circulating and passively trapped within the mesangium or subendothelial space during normal glomerular filtration. As the kidney receives 25% of the cardiac output, circulating immune complexes pass through glomeruli at a high rate. Intraglomerular capillary pressures are higher than in other capillary beds, and these capillaries provide a large, highly permeable negatively charged surface area that facilitates the nonspecific trapping of positively charged macromolecules. These circulating preformed immune complexes are too large to pass through the GBM, although in some cases they may dissociate, cross the GBM, and reform in situ in the subepithelial space. Alternatively, immune complexes may form "in situ" when circulating antibody binds to normal glomerular antigens or to soluble antigens trapped within subendothelial, subepithelial, or mesangial areas. The associated immunologic and glomerular responses to the immune deposits within these different glomerular sites results in the different forms of glomerulonephritis.

While light microscopy may be highly suggestive of glomerulonephritis, electron microscopy is required to verify the presence of deposits, to detect small deposits not evident by light microscopy, and to identify the location (subendothelial, subepithelial, intramembranous, and/or mesangial) of the deposits in the glomerulus. Immunofluorescence, to determine the specific nature of the immune deposits (IgG, IgA, IgM, and/or complement), further defines the disease process.

Membranous glomerulonephritis/membranous nephropathy (MGN/MN) is the most common cause of the nephrotic syndrome in adult people, occurs in 10–45% of reported cases of GN in dogs, and is the most common type of GN described in cats (Vaden and Brown, 2009; Jaenke et al.). MGN results from the in situ deposition of immune complexes, most often containing IgG and largely unidentified antigens, on the subepithelial aspect of the glomerular BM. In uncomplicated cases of MGN, glomeruli are of normal cellularity, and there may be diffuse uniform thickening of the capillary loops. PASH stain may demonstrate either spikes or holes in the thickened GBM (Figure 24.9).

The changes that may be seen with light microscopy are better appreciated by understanding the response of the glomerulus to the presence of these subepithelial immune complexes. The subepithelial immune deposits cause local complement activation with C5b-9-mediated podocyte injury. Sublethal C5b-9 attack of podocytes causes the injured epithelial cells to produce oxygen radicals and proteases and causes dissociation of nephrin from the actin cytoskeleton. Proteinuria in MN is the result of oxidative and protease-mediated damage to the GBM and podocyte cytoskeletal changes disrupting the normal filtration slit diaphragm (Nangaku and Couser, 2005). This injury is reflected ultrastructurally

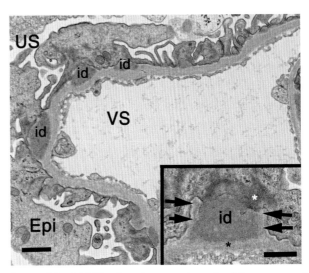

Figure 24.10 MGN, dog. Immune deposits (id) are present between the visceral epithelial cell (Epi) and the GBM. There is diffuse epithelial cell foot process effacement, but minimal change in the GBM. Inset: Later stage MGN, dog. The GBM extends as "spikes" (arrows) around an immune deposit. These spikes may be appreciated with PASH as in figure 9. Bar = 1 μm. Electron micrograph courtesy of Ralph Nichols, Texas Heart Institute.

by diffuse foot process effacement and reorganization of actin filaments (Figure 24.10).

Podocytes have limited proliferative capability, so increased glomerular cellularity due to podocyte proliferation is not a feature of MGN. In some cases of MGN, increased cellularity associated with focal segmental glomerulosclerosis may occur; this secondary scarring is likely irreversible and is considered a negative prognostic indicator. Very early cases of MGN will have subepithelial deposits and foot process effacement but minimal changes in the GBM (stage I MGN, Figure 24.10). After a period of time, new GBM is deposited next to the immune deposits, resulting in the spikes that may be visualized with PASH staining (stage II MGN, Figure 24.10, inset). PASH stains the original and new GBM dark pink without staining the immune deposits. With more chronic disease, additional GBM may expand these spikes to encircle the immune deposits (stage III MGN) and this change may be seen as "holes" in the thickened GBM with PASH (Figure 24.9). In some chronic cases of MGN, there may be loss of immune deposits with empty holes present in the GBM ultrastructurally. These four stages of MGN are well characterized in people and have been described in dogs (Jaenke and Allen, 1986). More advanced stages in cats and dogs have been shown to correlate with more severe azotemia, whereas animals with milder disease are more likely to have nephrotic syndrome. Staging of MGN will likely have prognostic significance, as earlier stages may be more amenable to therapy.

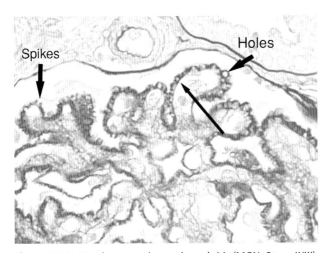

Figure 24.9 Membranous glomerulonephritis (MGN, Stage II/III), cat. The GBM has well-defined spikes and holes, caused by increased production of GBM between (spikes) and around (holes) the immune deposits. The glomerulus is not hypercellular and the endothelial aspect of the capillary wall is smooth (arrow). PAS, original magnification 1,000X.

There is no inflammatory cell participation in MGN, as the immune deposits are sequestered on the urinary aspect of the GBM where they are separated from circulating inflammatory cells and platelets. For this reason, MGN is often referred to as membranous nephropathy (MN) to reflect the lack of cellular inflammation within the glomerulus. Depending on the duration of the disease and resultant changes in the GBM, changes may or may not be appreciated in PASH-stained sections so confirmation of a diagnosis of MGN is dependent on ultrastructural demonstration of immune deposits in a subepithelial position. Immunofluorescent staining of glomeruli is used to verify the presence or absence of immune deposits and to further characterize the deposits in terms of their composition and distribution in the glomerulus. Secondary changes of focal glomerulosclerosis and/or glomerular adhesions to Bowman's capsule may be present in some cases of MN; this irreversible glomerular scarring may be associated with a less favorable prognosis.

Membranoproliferative   glomerulonephritis (MPGN) is probably the most common form of glomerulonephritis in dogs, accounting for 20–60% of cases in various studies, and is rarely reported in cats (Vaden and Brown, 2009; Inoue et al., 2001). The term MPGN refers to the light microscopic findings of thickening of the peripheral capillary wall with increased glomerular cellularity and is caused by the presence of immune complexes on the subendothelial aspect of the GBM (type I MPGN), with additional deposits within the mesangium or on the subepithelial aspect of the GBM (type III MPGN). Type II MPGN, also called dense deposit disease, is characterized by the deposition of complement as a homogeneous dense band in the GBM and has only been described in dogs and pigs with genetic deficiencies in the complement system (Jansen et al., 1998). Type III MPGN appears to be the most common type of MPGN in dogs and cats.

Immune deposits in the subendothelial space are not separated from the vascular space by GBM. In this location they activate complement and are readily accessible to circulating neutrophils, macrophages, and platelets. These cells produce inflammatory mediators, such as cytokines, growth factors, and proteases, and activate the coagulant cascade resulting in severe capillary wall damage, inflammatory cell infiltration, and mesangioal proliferation (Nangaku and Couser, 2005). MPGN is characterized histologically by increased cellularity of the glomerular capillary tuft with diffuse irregular thickening of glomerular capillary walls. The increased glomerular cellularitiy is due primarily to mesangial proliferation; endothelial proliferation and intravascular inflammatory cells may also be present (Figure 24.11).

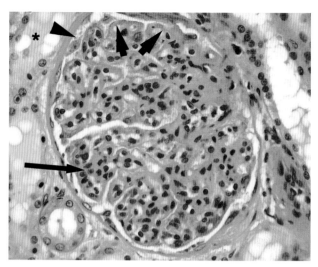

Figure 24.11 Membranoproliferative glomerulonephritis (MP-GN), dog. The glomerulus is globally hypercellular (long arrow) and the capillary walls, evaluated in peripheral loops, are thickened (short arrows). A parietal epithelial cell is hypertrophied and contains protein droplets indicative of proteinuria. H&E, original magnification 400×.

There is mesangial matrix expansion, which along with the increase in cellularity may lead to an accentuated lobular appearance of the glomerular tuft. With a PASH stain, splitting and reduplication of the thickened GBM evident. This GBM change is also referred to as having a "double contour" or "tram-track" appearance. This GBM change is due to movement/extension of mesangial cells from the mesangial area to the subendothelial area of the capillary loops and is referred to as mesangial interposition. The deposition of new GBM between the interposed mesangial cell and the overlying endothelium results in the double contour of the GBM. Larger immune deposits may stain magenta with trichrome stain (Figure 24.12). Confirmation of the diagnosis of MPGN is dependent on demonstration of subendothelial deposits (immune complexes) via electron microscopy (Figure 24.13). Subendothelial immune deposits are readily accessible to circulating inflammatory cells (particularly neutrophils) and platelets and are associated with more severe capillary wall injury and greater activation of resident glomerular cells. Mesangial deposits injure and activate mesangial cells, causing mesangial cell proliferation and increased production of mesangial matrix.

Crescents may be observed in some cases of MPGN and are indicative of more severe glomerular injury causing breaks or gaps in the damaged GBM that allow the passage of fibrinogen, and later macrophages, into the urinary space (Figure 24.14). Fibrin and macrophages induce parietal epithelial cell and fibroblast proliferation, and glomerular crescents form. Glomerular diseases with

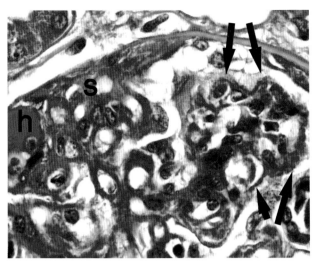

Figure 24.12 MPGN, dog. Globular magenta-staining immune deposits are evident within capillary loops (arrows). There is an adhesion (synechia, s) between the capillary tuft and Bowman's capsule with hyalinosis (h). Masson's trichrome, original magnification 1,000×.

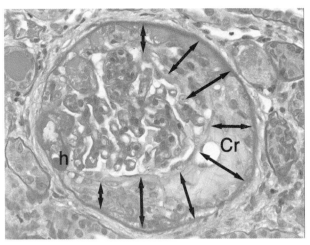

Figure 24.14 MPGN with serocellular crescent, dog. There is a crescent-shaped proliferation of cells (Cr, arrows) within Bowman's capsule and outside the glomerular capillary tuft. H&E, original magnification 400×.

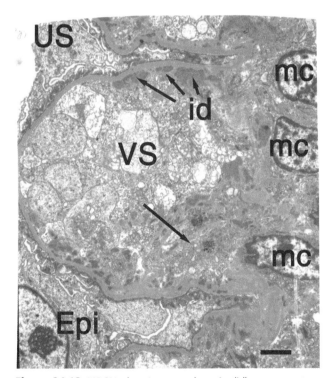

Figure 24.13 MPGN, dog. Immune deposits (id) are present on the subendothelial aspect of the GBM. There is mesangial cell interposition (long single arrow) and mesangial cell hyperplasia (n, nuclei of 3 mesangial cells). The capillary lumen (vascular space, VS) is filled with swollen cell cytoplasm. Diffuse epithelial (Epi) foot process effacement is present. Urinary space, US. Bar = 2 μm. Electron micrograph courtesy of Ralph Nichols, Texas Heart Institute.

significant crescent formation are typically more severe and have a rapidly progressive clinical course. Crescents are commonly seen in dogs with Lyme nephritis.

MPGN may be of unknown cause, or secondary to a variety of underlying systemic and infectious diseases. In some cases of MPGN, glomeruli may be infiltrated with monocytes or neutrophils; this inflammatory infiltrate is characteristic of exudative or postinfectious GN. Postinfectious glomerulonephritis of people most commonly occurs following a streptococcal infection but has also been identified with other infections (e.g., staphylococcal infection). It is of interest to note that this pattern of disease is usually caused by infections of limited duration that have often resolved prior to clinical signs of glomerular disease.

Mesangioproliferative glomerulonephritis (GN) accounted for only 2–16% of glomerular lesions in dogs of two studies (Vaden and Brown, 2009). Proteinuria and renal failure (mild to moderate, acute or chronic) are the expected presenting signs in affected dogs. Like MPGN and MGN, mesangioproliferative GN is an immune-complex-mediated disease caused by deposition of immune complexes within the mesangial area. Mesangial deposits injure and activate resident mesangial cells, causing mesangial cell proliferation and increased production of transforming growth factor (TGF)-B and platelet derived growth factor (PDGF), cytokines, and extracellular matrix (Nangaku and Couser, 2005).

Mesangioproliferative GN is characterized histologically by mesangial cell hyperplasia, defined as more than three cells per mesangial area, which is accompanied by an increase in mesangial matrix. As these changes are also common in animals with chronic renal disease (glomerulosclerosis), this disease must be verified with electron microscopy and immunofluorescence. On electron microscopy, immune complexes are present primarily within the mesangium and are mainly of the IgA class (IgA nephropathy).

Minimal change nephropathy (MCN) or minimal change disease derives its name from the lack of significant histologic renal abnormalities on light microscopy. MCN accounts for 15–20% of the cases of idiopathic nephrotic syndrome in adults and is the most common cause of the nephrotic syndrome in children. This disease has been described rarely in the dog, which may be due to its low prevalence and/or failure of detection if tissues are only evaluated at the light microscopic level.

MCN is due to injury to podocytes, a cell type with limited potential for repair or replacement. The mechanism of this injury is poorly understood, but a soluble T-cell factor is suspected to be involved in most cases. People with MCN tend to be highly responsive to corticosteroids, with an expected response rate of 80–90%. Rarely, MCN is precipitated by a drug and will resolve once the offending drug is withdrawn. Drug-induced MCN has also been observed in dogs, with rapid resolution of proteinuria after drug withdrawal (Sum et al., 2010).

While glomeruli are typically entirely normal on light microscopy, there are characteristic ultrastructural lesions. Changes are confined to the glomerular epithelial cells, which exhibit diffuse foot process effacement or flattening in the absence of electron-dense immune deposits (Figure 24.15).

Villous transformation, a nonspecific change associated with proteinuria, is commonly observed. These changes are reversible, and complete resolution of pro-

teinuria is expected if the cause (immunologic or drug) of the podocyte injury can be eliminated.

Alport syndrome (hereditary nephritis) is a glomerular disease characterized by inherited glomerular BM structural abnormalities. In people, Alport syndrome is characterized by hematuria, progressive nephritis with proteinuria, declining renal function, and, in some people, hearing and ocular abnormalities. Alport-like syndromes have been described in young Samoyeds, Doberman Pinschers, English Cocker Spaniels, Bull Terriers, Dalmatian dogs, and mixed breed dogs (Wakamatsu et al., 2007). These dogs have proteinuria and progressive renal disease, without hematuria, hearing, or visual abnormalities. Alport syndrome is the result of congenital defect in the molecular structure of type IV collagen, which is the major structural component of the GBM. Type IV collagen in the mature GBM is present predominantly as extensively crosslinked trimers of $\alpha3$, $\alpha4$, and $\alpha5$ type IV isoforms. Mutations of the COL4A3, COL4A4, or COL4A5 genes result in a structurally and functionally abnormal and weakened GBM, which becomes progressively thickened and split with the eventual development of glomerulosclerosis.

Histologic renal findings in people and dogs include mild mesangial hypercellularity, global to segmental glomerulosclerosis, immature glomeruli, tubular atrophy, and interstitial fibrosis, with eventual evolution to end-stage renal disease. Although the light microscopic findings in this disease are nonspecific, the ultrastructural changes are diagnostic. The GBM is less electron dense and of variable thickness because of a complex interwoven "basket-weave" replication of the lamina densa. There may be podocyte foot process effacement, and the epithelial aspect of the capillary wall is typically irregular.

The glomerular changes of increased glomerular cellularity and irregular thickening of the capillary loops were initially misinterpreted as MPGN in some dog breeds with Alport syndrome. Although MPGN is also characterized by increased glomerular cellularity and thickened capillary loops, MPGN is a consequence of immune complex or complement deposition in the glomerular capillary wall. A diagnosis of MPGN is dependent on the demonstration of these immune deposits by electron microscopy and, for optimal characterization, immunofluorescent techniques. Immune deposits are not a feature of Alport syndrome. Although there is variability in the light microscopic renal lesions among breeds of dogs and people with Alport syndrome, the GBM ultrastructural changes of lamellation are pathognomonic for this disease. Therefore, a diagnosis of this disease is absolutely dependent on ultrastructural examination of the kidney.

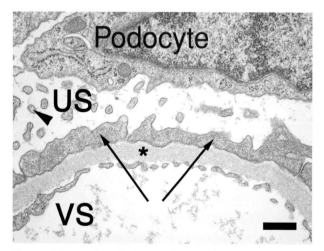

Figure 24.15 Minimal change disease, dog. There is diffuse podocyte foot process effacement (arrows) with mild podocyte villous transformation (arrowheads). The GBM (asterisk) is normal and no deposits are present. VS, vascular space. Bar = 1 μm.

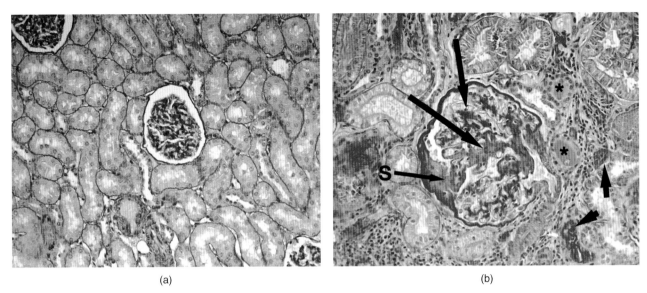

Figure 24.16 Glomerular hypertrophy and glomerulosclerosis, remnant kidney, dog. (a) Normal renal biopsy from a dog prior to partial loss of renal mass. PASH, original magnification 200×. (b) Same dog following renal mass reduction. Note the marked glomerular hypertrophy and glomerulosclerosis characterized by increased mesangial matrix and mesangial proliferation (arrows) with a synechia (s). There is also evidence of proteinuria (hyaline casts, asterisk), tubular atrophy with wrinkling of the tubular basement membranes (short arrows), and lymphoplasmacytic interstitial inflammation. PASH, original magnification 200×.

Focal segmental glomerulosclerosis (FSGS) is a glomerular lesion that, like MCN, is thought to be due to podocyte injury (Mathieson, 2007). It differs significantly from MCN in that the lesions in FSGS are irreversible. Focal segmental glomerulosclerosis (FSGS) occurs as a primary glomerular disease in people and is the most common cause of the nephrotic syndrome in adults. Like MCN, FSGS associated with the nephrotic syndrome is also thought to be immunologically mediated and immunosuppressive therapy may be effective in its treatment. It has been proposed that MCN and FSGS may represent opposite ends of a single spectrum of disease: reversible podocyte injury in MCN and irreversible focal podocyte loss resulting in focal sclerosis in FSGS. Because the podocyte injury in MCN is reversible, progressive loss of renal function is rare. As podocyte injury is more severe in FSGS and potentially irreversible, progressive loss of renal function may be more likely.

While FSGS associated with the nephrotic syndrome is seldom recognized in nephrotic dogs and cats, secondary FSGS is an expected finding in chronic kidney disease and a common finding secondary to underlying primary glomerular disease. Chronic kidney disease is characterized by the gradual loss of nephrons with hyperfunction of the remaining nephrons. The normal adaptive responses of the glomerulus to decreased numbers of functioning nephrons include an increase in single nephron filtration rate (glomerular hyperfiltration) associated with an increase in capillary pressure (glomerular hypertension) due to preferential afferent arteriole

dilation and an increase in glomerular size (glomerular hypertrophy). These responses increase GFR, an obviously beneficial effect, but may also lead to further glomerular injury, resulting in glomerulosclerosis and, in some animals, progression of chronic renal disease (Brown et al., 1997).

The glomerulosclerosis seen in animals with chronic renal disease is also seen in normal dogs and cats following experimental reduction of renal mass by 75% or more. Following significant experimental or natural nephron loss, remaining glomeruli are markedly hypertrophied and glomerulosclerosis occurs (Figure 24.16).

The sclerotic segments of the affected glomeruli exhibit mesangial hypercellularity and mesangial expansion that eventually causes solidification of peripheral capillary loops. Although mesangial cells and endothelial cells proliferate during glomerular hypertrophy, podocyte numbers remain the same, resulting in a decrease in podocyte density. If podocytes are unable to cover the increased glomerular surface area or if there is podocyte detachment or death, portions of the GBM become exposed and synechiae may form. Synechia or adhesions occur between sclerotic portions of the capillary tuft and Bowman's capsule, and secondary hyalinosis is common. With a PASH stain, hyalinosis appears as glassy eosinophilic material in the capillary wall; this material is serum lipoproteins, which have leaked across the adhered portion of the glomerular BM. In animals without an underlying primary glomerular disease, the degree of proteinuria will be mild in FSGS occurring as a consequence of decreased functioning renal mass and there will be other evidence of renal disease.

Secondary FSGS is a common glomerular lesion seen in necropsy tissues, as chronic or end stage kidney disease is a relatively common renal abnormality. On light microscopy, there will typically be other nonspecific lesions associated with chronic renal disease, such as lymphoplasmacytic interstitial inflammation, interstitial fibrosis, BM mineralization, glomerular obsolescence, tubular dilation and atrophy, and collecting duct hyperplasia.

Correlation of morphologic type of acute glomerular injury with clinical presentation

Patients with primary glomerular disease may present clinically with either the nephrotic or the nephritic syndrome, with the different morphologic types of glomerular disease more likely to present with primarily one or the other syndrome (Madaio et al., 2001). The nephrotic syndrome is characterized by marked proteinuria with hypoalbuminemia, hyperlipidemia, and edema (more commonly seen in people); these animals may or may not be azotemic. Diseases expected to be associated with the nephrotic syndrome include amyloidosis, membranous nephropathy, primary focal segmental glomerulosclerosis and minimal change disease. These diseases cause disruption of the normal filtration barrier but are not associated with active inflammatory cell participation and more severe glomerular injury. The nephritic syndrome is characterized by moderate proteinuria, active urine sediment (red cells or casts), azotemia, and hypertension. Diseases with more severe glomerular injury or inflammation, such as membranoproliferative glomerulonephritis or hemolytic uremic syndrome, are more likely to be associated with the nephritic syndrome.

While some animals with primary glomerular disease may have features of both clinical syndromes and so may not be easily classified, where possible distinction between the nephrotic and nephritic syndrome is helpful in establishing initial differential diagnoses prior to biopsy. Using light, electron, and immunofluorescent microscopy, the specific type and severity of the glomerular disease can be determined, with the ultimate goal of identifying and instituting optimal treatment strategies.

Endnote

1. WSAVA Renal Standardization Group, supported by Hills Pet Nutrition and Bayer Animal Health)

References

Behrend, E.N., G.F. Grauer, et al. (1996). Hospital-acquired acute renal failure in dogs: 29 cases (1983–1992). *J Am Vet Med Assoc* **208**(4): 537–541.

Brown, S.A., W.A. Crowell, et al (1997). Pathophysiology and management of progressive renal disease. *Vet J* **154**: 93–109.

Brown, C.A., K-S. Jeong K-S, et al. (2007). Outbreaks of melamine and cyanuric acid associated renal failure (MARF) in dogs and cats in 2004 and 2007. *J Vet Diag Invest* **19**: 525–531.

Cavana, P., M.T. Capucchio, et al. (2008). Noncongophilic fibrillary glomerulonephritis in a cat. *Vet Pathol* **45**: 347–351.

Cook, A.K. and L.D. Cowgill (1996). Clinical and pathological features of protein-losing glomerular disease in the dog: a review of 137 cases (1985–1992). *J Am Anim Hosp Assoc* **32**(4): 313–322.

Davila de Arriaga, A.J., Rocha, A.S. et al. (1982). Morpho-functional patterns of kidney injury in experimental leptospirosis of the guinea pig (*L. icterohaemorrhagiae*). *J of Pathol* **138**(2): 145–161.

Inoue, K., J. Kami-Ie, et al. (2001). Atypical membranoproliferative glomerulonephritis in a cat. *Vet Pathol* **38**: 468–470.

Jaenke, R.S. and T.A. Allen (1986). Membranous nephropathy in the dog. *Vet Pathol* **23**: 718–733.

Jansen, J.H. Hogasen, K., et al. (1998). In situ complement activation in porcine membranoproliferative glomerulonephritis type II. *Kidney Int* **53**(2): 331–349.

Madaio, M.P. and J.T. Harrington (2001) The diagnosis of glomerular diseases: acute glomerulonephritis and the nephrotic syndrome. *Arch Intern Med* **161**: 25–34.

Mathieson, P.W. (2007). Minimal change nephropathy and focal segmental glomerulosclerosis. *Semin Immunopathol* **29**: 415–426.

Maxie, M.G. and S.J. Newman (2007). Urinary system. In: *Jubb, Kennedy, and Palmer's Pathology of Domestic Animals*, edited by M.G. Maxie, Vol. 2, 5th edition. Philadelphia, PA: Elsevier, pp. 425–500.

McMartin, K. (2009). Are calcium oxalate crystals involved in the mechanism of acute renal failure in ethylene glycol poisoning? *Clin Toxicol* **47**(9): 859–869.

Nangaku, M. and W.G. Couser (2005). Mechanisms of immune-deposit formation and the mediation of immune renal injury. *Clin Exp Nephrol* **9**: 183–191.

Rumbeiha, W.K., et al. (2004). A comprehensive study of Easter lily poisoning in cats. *J Vet Diagn Invest* **16**: 527–541.

Sum, S.O., Hansel, P., et al. (2010). Drug-induced minimal change nephropathy in a dog. *J Vet Intern Med* **24**: 431–435.

Vaden, S.L. and C.A. Brown (2007). Renal biopsy. In: *Manual of Canine and Feline Nephrology and Urology*, edited by J. Elliot and G. Grauer, Chapter 12, 2nd edition. Birmingham, UK: British Small Animal Veterinary Association, pp. 167–177.

Vaden, S.L. and C.A. Brown (2009) Glomerular disease.In: Kirk's Current Veterinary Therapy XIV, edited by J. Bonagura and D. Twedt, Chapter 188, 14th edition. Saunders Elsevier Publishers, pp. 863–868.

Wakamatsu, N., K. Surdyk, et al. (2007). Histologic and ultrastructural studies of juvenile onset renal disease in four Rottweiler dogs. *Vet Pathol* **44**: 96–100.

Worwag, S. and C.E. Langston (2008). Acute intrinsic renal failure in cats: 32 cases (1997–2004). *J Am Vet Med Assoc* **232**(5): 728–732.

25

Biopsy of the lower urinary tract

Jody Lulich and Carl Osborne

Differentiation of potentially reversible disease from progressive irreversible disease is the single most important factor in the management of persistent or recurrent lower urinary tract signs. Biopsy of the urinary bladder and urethra is helpful to make this distinction in the living patient. Many options are available to obtain tissue for microscopic evaluation (Table 25.1). If structures to be biopsied can be palpated, they are usually accessible for aspiration with a needle and syringe. If larger samples are desired, minimally invasive techniques, such as transurethral catheter biopsy, have been commonly recommended (Osborne and Lulich 1995). A practical alternative to catheterization biopsy is use of flexible endoscopy forceps to retrieve tissue samples from the lower urinary tract (Lulich et al. 2000). Obtaining samples using endoscopy forceps has the advantage of procuring samples with minimal architectural disruption. Likewise, the procedure is as convenient as urinary catheterization.

Materials needed for biopsy

Flexible endoscopy biopsy forceps can be obtained from a variety of vendors in a variety of sizes and lengths. We have had the best results using forceps with a fenestrated oval or elongated cup (Figure 25.1). The fenestrated cup minimizes tissue crushing. Although some prefer biopsy forceps with a central spear to help anchor the biopsy cup to the biopsy site, in our experience the spear becomes dull after several uses. Once damaged, the spear no longer anchors tissue, but inadvertently pushes the target tissue away from the grasping cup. For this reason, we no longer use biopsy forceps with a central spear.

Depending on the location and size of the lesion, additional equipment can be used to guide the biopsy forceps and visualize the procedure. For example, biopsy forceps inserted through the biopsy channel of a cystoscope greatly facilitates procurement of samples from the lateral walls of the urinary bladder. If operators are not familiar with cystoscopy, ultrasound can be used to guide the biopsy forceps (Figure 25.2).

Performing forceps biopsy

Obtaining tissue samples using the endoscopy forceps is similar to methods used to obtain gastrointestinal mucosal with an endoscope. Since the endoscope is not inserted into the urethra, other methods, such as palpation, cystoscopy, or medical imaging, are needed to localize the lesion and direct the biopsy forceps.

1. Allow the patient to void urine prior to biopsy. If micturition is difficult due to partial or complete obstruction, urine can be removed by transurethral catheterization or decompressive cystocentesis. An empty bladder will facilitate patient comfort and cooperation.
2. Sedate or anesthetize the patient. To biopsy urethral masses, general anesthesia may not be needed. However, mild tranquilization will facilitate urethral catheterization, will permit palpation of the urethra and bladder, and will minimize patient discomfort and anxiety. In lieu of generalized sedation, local anesthesia can be achieved by applying water soluble lubricants containing lidocaine or other topical anesthetics to the vaginal/prepucial mucosa and/or urethra.[1] To anesthetize urethral mucosa, the same lubricant can be diluted and injected into the urethral lumen through a catheter and applied to the biopsy forceps prior to urethral insertion. It has been

Nephrology and Urology of Small Animals. Edited by Joe Bartges and David J. Polzin. © 2011 Blackwell Publishing Ltd.

Table 25.1 Methods for biopsying the lower urinary tract

Method	Principal indication	Relative limitations	Reliability	Potential complications	Procedures to guide biopsy
Exfoliative wrine cytology	Inexpensive screening	Small sample Size Loss of cellular and tissue architecture Cellular autolysis Some tissues exfoliate poorly	Poor to variable high false-negative rate	Tumor seeding via collection by cystocentesis (Nyland et al. 2002; Vignoli et al. 2007)	NA
Fine needle aspirate	Extramural masses	Small sample Size Loss of tissue architecture Some tissues exfoliate poorly	Poor to moderate depending on exfoliative tendency	Tumor seeding (Nyland et al. 2002; Vignoli et al. 2007)	Palpation, ultrasonography. A Franzen biopsy guide facilitates transrectal acquisition of proximal urethral masses (Lulich et al. 2000)
Transurethral catheter aspirate	Urethral masses	Small sample size Loss of architecture Some tissues exfoliate poorly Difficulty obtaining samples from lateral walls urinary bladder Subepithelial lesions may be inaccessible	Poor to moderate	Urinary tract infection Urinary tract perforation	Palpation, ultrasonography (Lamb et al. 1996). Fluoroscopy-consider catheters with radiographic markers
Transurethral forceps pinch	Urethral and bladder vertex masses	Small sample size Some subepithelial lesions may be inaccessible	Moderate to good	Urinary tract infection Urinary tract perforation	Palpation, ultrasonography, fluoroscopy, cystoscopy
Grasping loops	Benign peduculated masses	Usually requires cystoscopy	Moderate to good	Striping the urothelium as the mass is pulled from its attachment	Cystoscopy
Surgical	Deep intramural lesions and small masses that can be completely excised	Proximal urethral tumors may be inaccessible	Good	Tumor seeding	NA

our experience that most cats require general sedation to manipulate and catheterize their urethra.

3. Identify the site for biopsy by palpation, catheterization, cystoscopy, and/or medical imaging.

4. With the grasping unit at the end of the forceps closed, insert the flexible endoscopy forceps (not the endoscope) into the urethra.

5. Advance the forceps until the grasping unit is near the area to be biopsied. The tip of the grasping unit can be positioned by abdominal palpation, transrectal urethral palpation, radiography, ultrasonography, or cystoscopy. For most urethral lesions, the biopsy site is easily determined during insertion and advancement of the forceps through the urethral

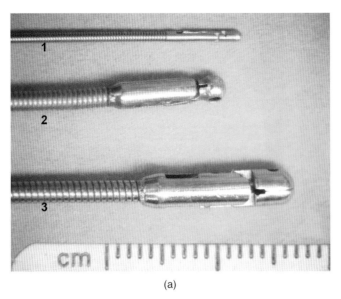
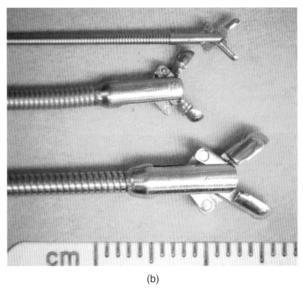

(a)   (b)

Figure 25.1 Biopsy forceps vary in their length and diameter (a; 1 = 1 mm diameter and 120 cm long, 2 = 2.8 mm diameter and 155 cm length, 3 = 3 mm and 40 cm length). Obtaining samples with large biopsy cups (b) improve diagnostic potential by obtaining samples deeper below the urothelium.

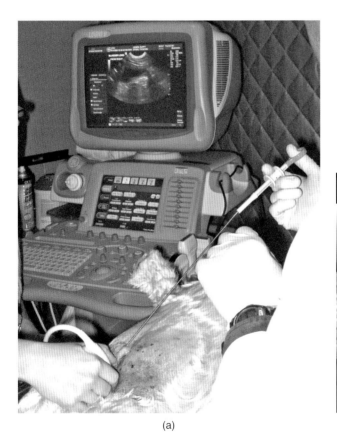
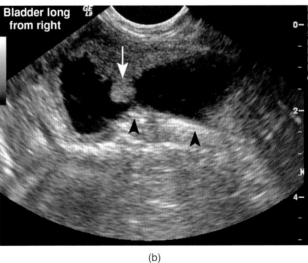

(a)   (b)

Figure 25.2 Abdominal ultrasonography of a14-year-old, male-neutered, West Highland white terrier revealed an intraluminal bladder mass attached to the right wall. To biopsy the mass, the dog was sedated and positioned in dorsal recumbency (a). Biopsy forceps was inserted into the external urethral orifice and advanced to the bladder. Ultrasonography was used to guide the grasping end of the biopsy forceps (arrow heads) to obtain a sample of the mass (arrow) for evaluation (b).

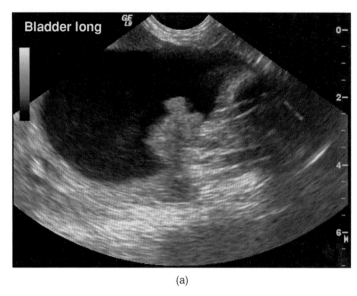
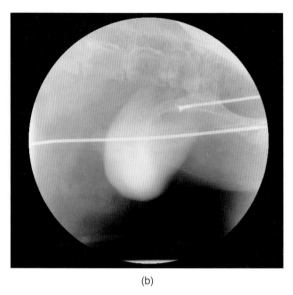

(a)   (b)

Figure 25.3 Ultrasonography of the urinary bladder of a 10-year-old, male-neutered cocker spaniel revealed a 1.1 cm intraluminal filling defect originating from the dorsal bladder wall (a). Following contrast urethrocystography, the tip of the biopsy forceps was inserted into the external urethral orifice and advanced to the bladder. Fluoroscopy was used to guide the biopsy forceps and obtain a sample of the mass for evaluation (b).

lumen; increased friction and force is often required to advance the forceps at the biopsy site. The distance of the biopsy site within the urethra can also be measured by using previous radiograms to determine how far the forceps must be inserted into the urethral lumen to reach the lesion. Diffuse urothelial lesions at the vertex (i.e., dome) of the bladder can be sampled by advancing the forceps to the most cranial portion of the bladder. Positioning the forceps fluoroscopically, immediately following contrast urethrocystography is also an effective method of positioning the biopsy instrument adjacent to the lesion (Figure 25.3). When using cystoscopy, we usually insert the biopsy forceps alongside of the cystoscopy. Narrow biopsy forceps can also be inserted through the biopsy channel of the cystoscope; however, the samples obtained with narrow forceps are small. In some cases, the samples may be nondiagnostic. Therefore, when using the smaller biopsy forceps (1 mm diameter), we took twice as many samples (10–15 samples compared to 3–5 with larger forceps) to improve our diagnostic ability.

6. After the biopsy forceps is properly positioned, open the grasping unit and slightly advance the forceps against the lesion.

7. Close the grasping unit. With the grasping unit closed, the forceps and tissue sample are retracted from the urinary tract.

8. The biopsy sample can be removed from the forceps by lifting the sample from the cup of the grasping unit with a 22 or 25 gauge needle. The sample should then be transferred to formalin for histologic processing.

9. Impression smears for immediate cytologic evaluation can be made prior to placing the sample in formalin. Tissue samples are first lightly blotted on filter paper or dry gauze pads to remove surface blood. Then, impressions can be made on glass slides and stained prior to microscopic evaluation.

10. Several samples (3–5) should be retrieved to ensure complete representation of the area in question.

Patient care following biopsy

Following bladder biopsy, hematuria and dysuria may be more pronounced. In most cases, bleeding quickly stabilizes (hours to a day) without treatment. Administration of antibiotics is indicated because the integrity of the mucosal surface of the lower urinary tract is disrupted by this procedure, further altering normal host defenses. If possible, infections diagnosed during initial evaluation should be eradicated prior to biopsy. Eliminating infection prior to biopsy will minimize hematuria and dysuria associated with sampling of inflamed tissues and also the potential of extending the infection into the biopsy site and adjacent tissues. In the absence of prior infection, we routinely administer antibiotics orally for the next 3–5 days. The need for medication to minimize pain and inflammation should be determined on the basis of the underlying disease and the degree of tissue disruption during procurement of the sample and the type and dose of preanesthetic agents used.

Limitations of forceps biopsy

Standard flexible biopsy forceps are approximately the diameter of an 8 Fr catheter (2.7 mm). As a general rule, one should be able to insert the biopsy forceps into the urethral lumen of most male dogs greater than 4 kilograms and into the urethral lumen of most, if not all, female cats and dogs. The lumen of the penile urethra of male cats is usually too narrow to accommodate insertion of standard flexible biopsy forceps used for endoscopy. For male cats, consider using forceps with a shaft diameter less that 1–1.67 mm in diameter (i.e., less than 3.5–5 Fr). Most cystoscopes cannot be inserted in the urethra of male cats, and those scopes that fit into the urethra generally do not have a biopsy channel. Therefore, consider transurethral palpation or medical imaging to direct the biopsy procedure.

It is possible that a thin or weakened bladder wall could be perforated by this procedure. For this reason we do not recommend biopsy of the lower urinary tract at sites proximal to sites of partial or complete obstruction because increases in intravesicular pressure may result in extravasation of urine into the abdominal cavity or retroperitoneal space. If a tissue sample proximal to a urinary obstruction is desired, constant bladder evacuation by indwelling urethral catheterization or antepubic percutaneous catheterization (Stone 1992) of the urinary bladder should be considered. Minimizing intravesicular pressure should allow small perforations of the bladder wall to spontaneously heal.

Endnote

1. Anestacon, Polymedica Indeustries, Divison of Alcon Labs Inc., Woburn, MA 01801.

References

Lamb, C.R., N.D. Trower, et al. (1996). Ultrasound-guided catheter biopsy of the lower urinary tract: technique and results in 12 dogs. *J Small Anim Pract* **37**: 413–416.

Lulich, J.P., C.A. Osborne, et al. (2000). Caniine lower urinary tract disorders. In: *Textbook of Veterinary Internal Medicine*, edited by S.J. Ettomger and E.C. Fledman, 5th edition. Philadelphia, PA: WB Saunders Company, pp. 1749–1750.

Nyland, T.G., S.T. Wallack, et al. (2002). Needle-tract implanatation following US-guided fine needle aspiration of transitional cell carcinomal of the bladder, urethra, and prostate. *et Radiol Ultrasound* **43**: 50–53.

Osborne, C.A. and J.P. Lulich (1995). Catheter and forceps biopsy of the urethra, urinary bladder, and prostate. In: *Canine and Feline Nephrology and Urology*, edited by C.A. Osborne and D.R. Finco. Baltimore, MD: Williams and Wilkins, pp. 329–332.

Vignoli, M., F. Rossi, et al. (2007). Needle tract implantation after fine needle aspiration biopsy of transitional cell carcinoma of the urinary bladder and adenocarcinoma of the lung. *Schweiz Arch Tierheilkd* **149**(7): 314–318.

26

Cytology of the urinary tract and prostate

Michael M. Fry

The aim of this chapter is to provide a concise overview of cytology of the urinary tract and prostate in dogs and cats, including indications, advantages and disadvantages of cytology compared to histology, sample preparation, and cytologic findings typical of common lesions. Techniques for obtaining cytologic specimens and recommended therapies are covered elsewhere in this text (see Chapters 16, 20, 21, 23, 25, and 78). Other sources with good information about urinary tract cytology in small animals are also available (Baker and Lumsden 2000; Baker and Lumsden 2000; Borjesson 2001; Henson 2001; Ewing et al. 2008; Zinkl 2008).

Indications, advantages, and disadvantages

The main indications for cytologic examination of urinary tract specimens are detection of a mass or masses, organomegaly, or infiltrative lesions. Advantages of cytology compared to histology include lower cost, faster turnaround time, better morphologic detail, a less invasive sample collection procedure, and, depending on the practioner's level of expertise, the option of interpreting samples in-house. Disadvantages of cytology compared to histology are the greater risk of obtaining a sample that is not representative of the lesion and, especially, the lack of tissue architecture. In general, cytology is a good means of diagnosing inflammatory lesions and neoplastic lesions that exfoliate easily (especially round cell and epithelial tumors), and a less reliable means of diagnosing lesions that tend to exfoliate less readily (such as fibrotic lesions and sarcomas).

Limitations of urine as a cytologic sample

Microscopic examination of the urine sediment is an essential component of routine urinalysis (see Chapter 7) and is a good way of detecting some types of urinary system pathology. However, urine samples submitted for cytologic evaluation because of a suspicion of neoplasia are often nondiagnostic because the neoplastic cells have not exfoliated into the urine in sufficient numbers or because the cellular morphology has deteriorated. Occasionally, urinary tract neoplasia may be diagnosed from examination of urine, but in general it is more productive to sample a suspected neoplastic lesion directly.

Sample acquisition and slide preparation

Whether interpreting cytologic specimens in-house or sending them to a diagnostic laboratory, it is to a practitioner's advantage to become proficient at obtaining samples and evaluating their adequacy for diagnosis. Adequacy of a cytologic specimen depends on quantity (cellularity or the number of cells) and quality (preservation of cell structure and appropriate monolayer distribution of the cells on the slide). The best cytologic specimens are typically of high cellularity and have mostly intact, rather than disrupted, cells. Detailed sample collection methods are discussed elsewhere in this text, but common ways of obtaining samples from the urogenital tract include fine-needle aspiration, traumatic catheterization, prostatic wash, and surgical biopsy. Regardless of the collection method and cellularity of the sample, the keys to making good quality cytologic preparations are minimizing trauma to cells during sampling, gently creating a cell monolayer on a glass slide, rapidly air drying the smear after it is made, proper staining, and avoiding exposure of the sample to formalin or formalin fumes at any point.

Nephrology and Urology of Small Animals. Edited by Joe Bartges and David J. Polzin. © 2011 Blackwell Publishing Ltd.

To create slides from aspirates, detach the aspiration needle from the syringe, draw a few milliliters of air into the syringe, and reattach the needle. Next, position the needle bevel down and gently express the contents onto the slide. *Slide preparation should be done with minimal trauma to the cells, and air-dried as quickly as possible.* If the sample has a fluid consistency, smears can be made in the same fashion as a blood smear—that is, with the edge of a spreader slide, without applying any downward pressure. For samples that do not spread easily in this manner, an alternative is to place a clean slide face down on the one with the sample, and then draw the slides apart horizontally without applying any downward pressure. For samples that are too thick or chunky even to use this method, one may compress ("squash") the slides before drawing them apart; however, this method may crush enough cells to render the sample uninterpretable. Of course, other factors may also render a cytologic sample nondiagnostic—for example, if the tissue of interest was missed or did not exfoliate readily.

To create slides from impression smears, the freshly cut tissue should be blotted gently to remove excess tissue fluid. The impression smear is made by gently touching the tissue to the glass slide or by touching the cutaneous lesion with the glass slide. If the lesion is poorly exfoliative, a scalpel blade can be repeatedly scraped across the tissue and the accumulated cells along the edge of the blade can then be transferred to a glass slide for squash prep.

Once a cytology smear has been prepared, it should be air dried as quickly as possible and then stained. Unlike biopsy samples for histologic evaluation, no chemical fixation is necessary for cytology specimens. In fact, *it is critical that the sample not be exposed to formalin fumes*, which interfere with normal cytologic staining and almost always make the sample uninterpretable. Staining is usually done with a rapid stain (e.g., Camco Stain Pak, Cambridge Diagnostic Products, Ft. Lauderdale, FL) in the practice setting and Wright's or Wright's-Giemsa stain in the reference laboratory setting.

Cytologic findings

This section describes cytologic findings typical of normal tissue and common neoplastic and non-neoplastic lesions of the urinary tract and prostate.

Normal tissue

Although the intent in collecting samples for cytologic examination from the urinary tract or prostate is usually to obtain cells representative of a pathologic lesion, normal cells may also be present. Aspirates of renal lesions occasionally contain normal tubular epithelial cells (Figure 26.1) or glomeruli (Figure 26.2). Epithelial cells may be present individually or in clusters that retain tubular characteristics. Normal renal tubular cells have round nuclei and moderate amounts of finely granular medium-blue cytoplasm. Feline renal tubular cells often contain low numbers of small punctate clear vacuoles. Except for the distal urethra, which is lined by squamous epithelium, the lower urinary tract is lined by transitional epithelium (also known as urothelium). Normal transitional epithelial cells may be present in samples from the lower urinary tract, singly or in clusters. These cells have fairly uniform morphology, round to polygonal in shape, with round nuclei and medium-blue cytoplasm. Normal prostatic epithelial cells usually exfoliate in sheets or clusters of uniform cells with round nuclei and lightly basophilic cytoplasm.

Neoplastic lesions

The most common neoplasms of the upper urinary tract diagnosed cytologically in dogs and cats are lymphoma (especially renal lymphoma in cats) and renal carcinoma (see Chapter 57). Renal lymphoma typically occurs bilaterally. The neoplastic cells are usually large round cells with large round nuclei and small amounts of deep blue cytoplasm that in cats often contains low numbers of small punctate clear vacuoles (Figure 26.3). As with lymphoma in other anatomic locations, there are frequently many lysed cells and cytoplasmic fragments in addition to intact neoplastic cells. Carcinomas tend to produce cells in cohesive clusters, in addition to individual cells, and the malignant cells typically have multiple features of malignancy (Figures 26.4 and 26.5). Carcinomas of extrarenal origin may metastasize to the kidney(s). Renal sarcomas are uncommon. In general, aspirates of sarcomas tend to yield samples of relatively low cellularity, in which the neoplastic cells are present individually or in loose aggregates. The neoplastic cells often have tapering cytoplasmic projections and are often associated with pink extracellular matrix (Figure 26.6).

The most common neoplasm of the lower urinary tract is transitional cell carcinoma (also known as urothelial carcinoma), especially in dogs (see Chapter 79). The neoplastic cells typically exfoliate in cohesive clusters and have prominent features of malignancy (Figure 26.7). Sarcomas of the lower urinary tract are uncommon but are likely to have cytologic characteristics of sarcomas from other anatomic locations (Figure 26.8).

Non-neoplastic lesions

Cytology may help to characterize non-neoplastic lesions specific to the urinary tract, such as hyperplasia,

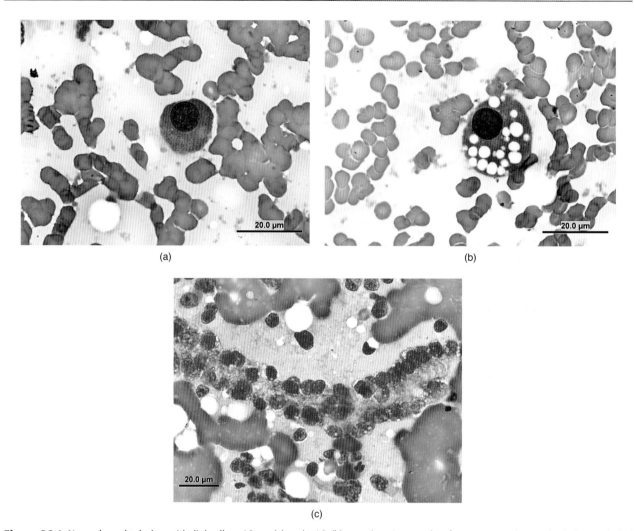

(a)

(b)

(c)

Figure 26.1 Normal renal tubular epithelial cells, without (a) and with (b) cytoplasmic vacuoles, from a cat, and a renal tubular epithelial structure (c) from a dog.

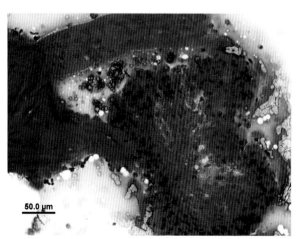

Figure 26.2 Glomerulus (bottom) and associated tubular structure (top) from a cat.

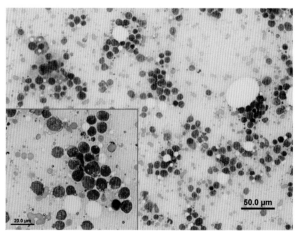

Figure 26.3 Aspirate from a cat with renal lymphoma. The neoplastic cells are large round cells with large round nuclei. There are also many basophilic cytoplasmic fragments (sometimes called "lymphoglandular bodies"), a common feature of aspirates of both lymphoma lesions and non-neoplastic lymphoid tissue.

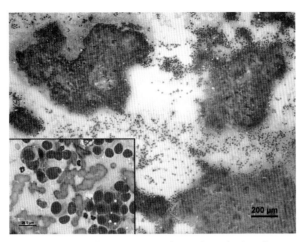

Figure 26.4 Renal carcinoma in a dog. The low magnification image shows the cohesive clusters typical of epithelial tumors. The inset more clearly shows the features of malignancy, including increased variability in cell and nuclear size, increased nuclear:cytoplasmic ratios, and irregularly condensed chromatin.

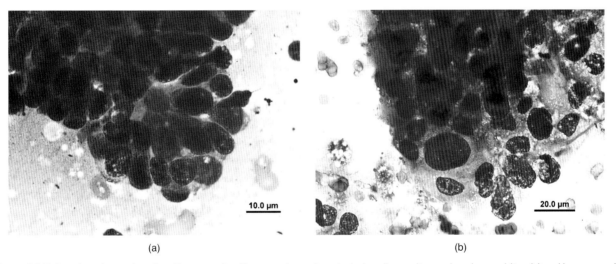

(a)   (b)

Figure 26.5 Renal carcinoma in a dog. Features of malignancy shown here include cell crowding and nuclear molding (a) and karyomegaly (b). The amorphous blue material (b) is necrotic debris.

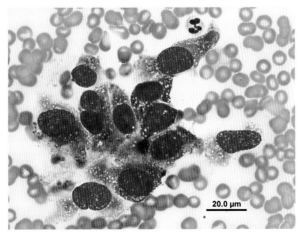

Figure 26.6 Renal sarcoma in a cat. The specific cell type in this case was not determined. These cells have the fusiform shape, indistinct cell margins, tapering cytoplasmic processes, loosely aggregated arrangement, and pink extracellular material that are characteristic of mesenchymal cells. Features of malignancy shown here include anisocytosis, anisokaroysis, and loose chromatin with 1 or 2 prominent nucleoli.

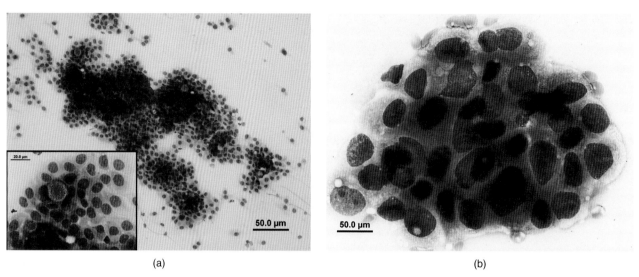

(a)   (b)

Figure 26.7 Transitional cell carcinoma from the urethra (a) and urinary bladder (b) in two dogs. The low magnification image shows the high cellularity and cohesive clustering typical of epithelial tumors. The high magnification images more clearly show features of malignancy, including anisocytosis and anisokaryosis, high N:C ratios, and irregularly condensed chromatin. Variably sized round granular pink cytoplasmic inclusions are often present in these tumors, but may also be a feature of prostatic adenocarcinomas (LeBlanc et al, 2004).

dysplasia, or metaplasia of epithelial cells. Hyperplasia/dysplasia of epithelial cells (such as urothelium or prostatic epithelium) often occurs in response to inflammation, and it is common to see atypical epithelial cells in samples from patients with cystitis or prostatitis (see Chapters 71 and 78). The morphologic changes that occur in response to inflammation are similar to those that occur with malignant transformation—for example, increased anisocytosis, nuclear:cytoplasmic ratios, and cytoplasmic basophilia—so it is advisable to be conservative in interpreting these findings. Usually, the most prudent approach is to repeat cytologic examination after the

inflammation is resolved. Hyperplastic prostatic epithelium has a characteristic uniform "honeycomb" arrangement of polygonal cells with round nuclei and moderate amounts of lightly basophilic cytoplasm (Figure 26.9). Squamous metaplasia of the prostate (Figure 26.10) is a recognized complication of estrogen excess in dogs with Sertoli cell tumors or that have been treated with exogenous estrogens (Merk et al. 1986; MacLachlan and Kennedy 2002).

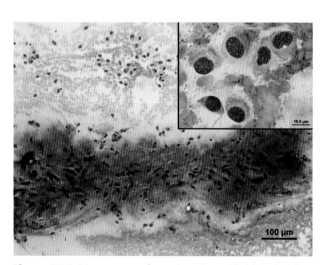

Figure 26.8 Myxosarcoma from the urinary bladder of a dog. Note the abundant magenta extracellular matrix.

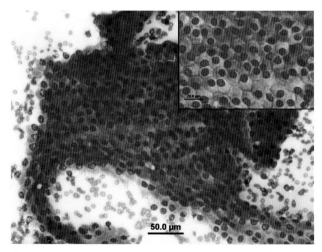

Figure 26.9 Benign prostatic hyperplasia in a dog. The low magnification image shows a sheet of cells of uniform morphology. The inset more clearly shows the "honeycomb" arrangement of the cells.

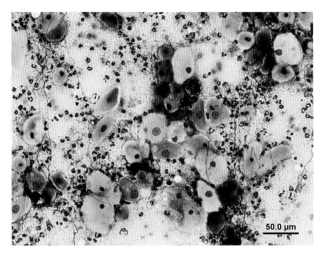

Figure 26.10 Squamous metaplasia and neutrophilic inflammation in the prostate of a dog with a Sertoli cell tumor. The angular shapes and turquoise cytoplasm are characteristic of squamous cells.

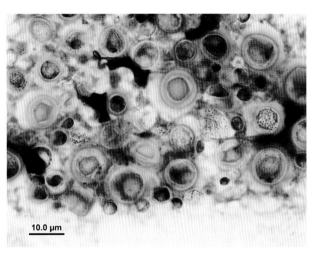

Figure 26.12 Renal cryptococcosis in a cat. The thick clear capsule and occasional narrow-based budding are characteristic of *C. neoformans* yeast forms. Slide courtesy of Dr. David F. Edwards.

Cytology may also be useful to characterize non-neoplastic lesions that are not unique to the urinary tract and may be cytologically indistinguishable from similar lesions from other anatomic locations, such as infections, inflammation, cysts, or hemorrhage. Infectious agents that may be detectable cytologically include, but are not limited to, bacteria (Figure 26.11) and fungi (Figure 26.12). Suppurative inflammation (predominantly neutrophilic) (Figures 26.10 and 26.11) suggests the possibility of a bacterial infection, even if organisms are not detected. Pyogranulomatous inflammation (characterized by an infiltrate of neutrophils and macrophages)

is consistent with feline infectious peritonitis in cats, or with fungal infection, actinomycosis/nocardiosis, or foreign body reactions in any species. Cystic fluid often contains cholesterol crystals (Figure 26.13), which form as a result of breakdown of cellular lipids. Virtually all cytologic specimens contain some degree of sampling-induced blood contamination. Prior "true" hemorrhage can be distinguished from sampling-related iatrogenic hemorrhage if there is evidence of erythrophagocytosis or the erythrocyte breakdown products hemosiderin or hematoidin (Figure 26.14).

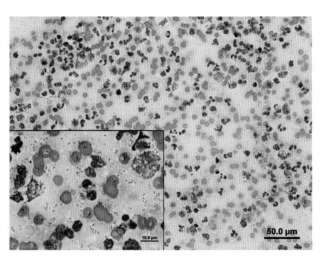

Figure 26.11 Marked septic suppurative inflammation in the prostate of a dog. Bacterial rods are present extracellularly and phagocytosed within neutrophils.

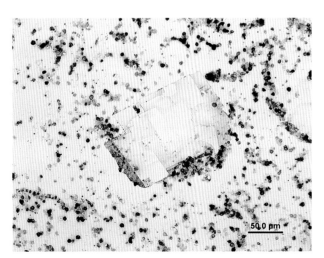

Figure 26.13 Fluid from a renal cyst in a dog. This image shows overlapping cholesterol crystals (clear rectangular forms that often have a notch in one corner) in the center, surrounded by amorphous to granular (possibly mineralized) debris.

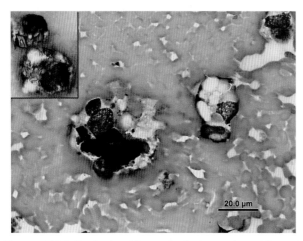

20.0 μm

Figure 26.14 Cytologic evidence of prior hemorrhage. The main image shows two erythrophagocytic macrophages; the one on the left also contains coarse granular dark green pigment consistent with hemosiderin. The inset shows macrophages and hematoidin crystals. Inset image courtesy of Dr. Bente Flatland.

References

Baker, R. and J.H. Lumsden (2000). The reproductive tract—vagina, uterus, prostate, and testicle. In: *Color Atlas of Cytology of the Dog and Cat*, edited by R. Baker and J.H. Lumsden. St. Louis, MO: Mosby, pp. 235–252.

Baker, R. and J.H. Lumsden (2000). The urinary tract—kidney, bladder, and urethra. In: *Color Atlas of Cytology of the Dog and Cat*, edited by R. Baker and J.H. Lumsden. St. Louis, MO: Mosby, pp. 223–234.

Borjesson, D.L. (2001). Cytologic examination of the urinary tract. In: *Atlas of Canine and Feline Cytology*, edited by R.E. Raskin and D.J. Meyer. Philadelphia, PA: WB Saunders, pp. 253–260.

Ewing, P.H., J.H. Meinkoth, et al. (2008). The kidneys. In: *Diagnostic Cytology and Hematology of the Dog and Cat*, edited by R.L. Cowell, R.D. Tyler, J.H. Meinkoth, and D.B. DeNicola, 3rd edition. St. Louis, MO: Mosby Elsevier, pp. 339–349.

Henson, K.L. (2001). Reproductive system. In: *Atlas of Canine and Feline Cytology*, edited by R.E. Raskin and D.J. Meyer. Philadelphia, PA: WB Saunders, pp. 277–312.

LeBlanc, C.J., C.S. Roberts, et al. (2004). Firm rib mass aspirate from a dog. *Vet Clin Pathol* **33**(4): 253–256.

MacLachlan, N.J. and P.C. Kennedy (2002). Tumors of the genital systems. In: *Tumors in Domestic Animals*, edited by D.J. Meuten, 4th edition. Ames: Iowa State Press, pp. 547–573.

Merk, F.B., M.J. Warhol, et al. (1986). Multiple phenotypes of prostatic glandular cells in castrated dogs after individual or combined treatment with androgen and estrogen. Morphometric, ultrastructural, and cytochemical distinctions. *Lab Invest* **54**(4): 442–456.

Zinkl, J.G. (2008). The male reproductive tract: prostate, testes, and semen. In: *Diagnostic Cytology and Hematology of the Dog and Cat*, edited by R.L. Cowell, R.D. Tyler, J.H. Meinkoth, and D.B. DeNicola, 3rd edition. St. Louis, MO: Mosby Elsevier, pp. 369–377.

27

Diagnosis of infectious diseases of the urinary tract

Meryl P. Littman

Introduction

Infectious pathogens may gain access and colonize organs of the urinary tract by ascending from the distal urogenital tract, hematogenously, via direct trauma or by descending from the kidneys to the lower urinary tract. Commonly, localized bacterial infection within the tract may damage the kidneys (pyelonephritis), ureters (ureteritis), bladder (cystitis), prostate gland (prostatitis), and/or urethra (urethritis) (see Chapter 71). Less commonly, infections with fungal, protozoal, viral, or parasitic organisms affect these organs, possibly more likely in immunocompromised individuals (see Chapters 72, 73, and 74).

Infectious agents may cause multiorgan involvement hematogenously and may target the kidneys for colonization, for example, bacterial septicemia, Leptospirosis, Toxoplasmosis, Brucellosis, Cryptococcosis, Aspergillosis, etc. (see Chapters 49, 52, 71, 72, 73, and 74). Some agents cause vasculitis, which may affect the kidney, for example, infectious canine hepatitis (Adenovirus I), Rocky Mountain spotted fever (*Rickettsia rickettsii*), and feline infectious peritonitis (FIP coronavirus). Also, infectious agents may cause renal damage indirectly by immune-mediated mechanisms, via antigenic stimulation that may cause pathology not so much by the presence of intact organisms in the kidney but by deposition of immune (antigen–antibody) complexes, especially in the glomeruli of the kidneys (see Chapter 53) (Sykes 2003). Examples implicated include chronic active infections (e.g., endocarditis, pyoderma, dental

disease) and diseases that cause carrier states (so-called "stealth pathogens") with antigenic variation, ongoing immune stimulation, and circulating immune complexes (CIC) that may deposit in glomeruli (e.g., Anaplasmosis, Babesiosis, Bartonellosis, Borreliosis (Lyme disease), Dirofilariasis, Ehrlichiosis, Hepatozoonosis, Leishmaniasis, Mycoplasmosis, Trypanosomiasis). Immune-mediated glomerulonephritis (IMGN) causes protein-losing nephropathy (PLN), and proteinuria may then further damage the rest of the nephron.

In order to diagnose infectious causes of damage to the kidneys or urinary tract, integrate information from history and physical examination (see Chapter 4), imaging (see Chapters 15, 16, and 17), blood and urine tests (see Chapters 7, 8, and 9), and sometimes aspirates or biopsies (see Chapters 23, 24, 25, and 26). Depending on clinical signs, clinicopathologic findings, and localization of disease, prioritize infectious agent suspects and determine which confirmatory test(s) will be most helpful to identify the agent. Sometimes, a search for antigen is done, for example, by direct visualization of cytologic preparations of urine sediment, blood, fine needle aspirate, or biopsy and by culture, ELISA agar-gel immunodiffusion, or PCR technology to find specific DNA of the agent. A search for antigen in blood, urine, or tissue is best done during the acute phase, before treatment is begun. Sometimes, a search for serum antibodies directed against the agent is most helpful, by IFA, ELISA, IgM/IgG, immunoassay, Western blot, agglutination test, etc. For some diseases, animals may present during an acute phase, before seroconversion takes place, in which case paired (acute and convalescent) titers including a titer taken 2 weeks into the illness may be necessary to make the diagnosis. Treatment will depend on which agent is found as well as where the infection is localized. For diseases with carrier

Nephrology and Urology of Small Animals. Edited by Joe Bartges and David J. Polzin. © 2011 Blackwell Publishing Ltd.

states, if quantitative titers are available, they should be repeated 6 months post treatment to check for decline and to get a new baseline.

Suspicion for urinary tract infection

Bacterial infections affecting the kidneys and urinary tract are very common in small animals (see Chapter 71); 14% of dogs have urinary tract infection (UTI) sometime in their lifetime and *E. coli* is the most common culprit (Barsanti 2006). Urinalysis and urine aerobic culture and sensitivity are recommended (preferably by cystocentesis) for animals with signs of lower urinary tract disease (e.g., pollakiuria, stranguria, dysuria, hematuria, urinary incontinence, "sawhorse" stance, prostatic pain, or abnormal vaginal/preputial discharges; prostatitis cases may also need a prostatic wash done (see Chapter 78)); renal disease (e.g., polyuria/polydipsia (PU/PD), anorexia, vomiting, abnormal renal size or architecture, painful kidneys, or azotemia); vague or nonspecific signs (e.g., anorexia, lethargy, fever, weight loss, heart murmur, leukocytosis, or left shift), or with diseases or medications that predispose for UTI (e.g., uroliths; neoplasia; neurologic (see below), musculoskeletal, or anatomic abnormalities associated with urine stasis, obstruction, or incontinence; immunosuppressive conditions such as steroid treatment (Ihrke et al. 1985), hyperadrenocorticism, or Diabetes mellitus (>40% of dogs with hyperadrenocorticism and/or Diabetes mellitus have UTIs (Forrester et al. 1999)), cancer, or chemotherapy; systemic infections such as endocarditis, dental disease, pyometra, lymphadenopathy, diskospondylitis; or previous instrumentation, catheterization, or surgery (e.g., perineal urethrostomy).

Spayed female dogs were found to be most at risk for UTI, probably due to their short urethra, followed by neutered males, intact females, and lastly, intact males (Barsanti 2006). Dogs having surgery for type I thoracolumbar intervertebral disc extrusion often had UTI (27% of 92 dogs had positive bacterial cultures), especially females and dogs unable to walk or voluntarily urinate. The UTI was found before surgery (15% of dogs) or after surgery (12% had UTI at 2–3 days, 16% at 4–5 days, and 20% at 7 days) (Stiffler et al. 2006). Decreased prevalence of UTI in this population was found in dogs that had received perioperative cefazolin and in dogs whose body temperature stayed above 35°C during anesthesia.

Occult UTI was often found in dogs receiving long-term corticosteroids for chronic skin diseases (Ihrke et al. 1985). Despite inactive microscopic sediment, 39% of 71 dogs had positive bacterial cultures, most often growing *E. coli* (59%). Mixed infections (in 28% of the dogs) and recurrent infections (in 38%) were seen. Females and

neutered males had higher risk of UTI; no association was found in relation to steroid dose, duration of treatment, or daily versus alternate day therapy.

Cats with lower urinary tract signs that have not been catheterized or have a urethrostomy generally have sterile cystitis (see Chapter 75). Feline calicivirus may localize in the upper and lower urinary tract in cats, possibly causing clinical signs (see Chapter 73) (Kruger et al. 2007; Larson et al. 2007). Bacterial UTI in cats is more commonly seen in older cats, affecting the kidneys. Urine cultures were positive for bacterial growth in roughly 15% of cats sick with a variety of illnesses, including hyperthyroidism (24% had positive cultures), neurologic disease (24%), neoplasia (20%), renal failure (18%), Diabetes mellitus (13%), lower urinary tract disease (10%), respiratory disease (9%), and gastrointestinal disease (4%) (Bailiff et al. 2004). In another study, positive cultures were found in cats with uncontrolled hyperthyroidism (21.7%), chronic kidney disease (16.9%), Diabetes mellitus (13.2%), and only 4.9% of cats with lower urinary tract signs (Bailiff et al. 2007). *E. coli* was the most common organism isolated and was found in 67% of diabetic cats with UTI (Bailiff et al. 2006) and 51% of nondiabetic cats (Bailiff et al. 2004) but was not isolated in cats with only lower urinary tract signs (Bailiff et al. 2007). Dilute urine specific gravity, contrary to presumption, was not associated with positive culture results in these cats (Bailiff et al. 2004, 2007). Increased risk for UTI was related to the Persian breed, female sex, increasing age, and decreasing body weight (Bailiff et al. 2007).

History can give clues to determine if a bacterial urinary tract infection is likely acute, with recent onset of signs, or chronic, with signs for more than 2 or 3 weeks; simple or complicated; intermittent (sporadic), relapsing, or rarely, a superinfection. Simple UTIs are defined as occurring relatively rarely in the individual, for instance, no more than one or two UTIs per year in an individual. Complicated or relapsing infections require further diagnostic work-up to find and treat underlying predisposing factors. Localization of the site of damage within the urinary system is important when making treatment decisions concerning medications, type of antibiotic that can penetrate the affected organ(s), length of treatment, and prognosis. For example, chronic prostatitis requires lengthy treatment with an antibiotic that can breach the prostate–blood barrier (see Chapter 78). Localization of UTI (upper versus lower urinary tract and acute versus chronic prostatitis) is reviewed elsewhere (Bartges 2005).

Urinalysis (see Chapter 7) including cytologic examination of sediment and urine cultures/sensitivity (see Chapter 9) are most helpful to confirm UTI. The leukesterase dipstick square frequently (20%) shows false-negative results, so urinary sediment examination should always be done. Urinalysis findings of bacteriuria and/or pyuria suggest UTI, but bacteria and cells from vagina or prepuce may contaminate voided samples (and the absence of inflammatory cells does not rule out occult UTI). Among 50 normal dogs with sterile cystocentesis samples, 26% of catheterized samples and 85% of voided samples grew bacteria on culture (Comer and Ling 1981), so if not contraindicated, sampling by cystocentesis is most preferred. Allowable numbers of WBC in the microscopic sediment and bacteria in the quantitative culture vary depending on how the specimen was collected. Host defenses from ascending urogenital flora (see Chapters 9 and 71) normally keep bacterial numbers low in the bladder. Contamination may allow growth of 10^4 (dog) or 10^3 (cat) colony forming units (CFU) per mL of urine in a mid-stream voided or manually expressed sample, 10^3 (dog) or 10^2 (cat) CFU/mL in a catheterized sample, and 10^2 (dog or cat) in cystocentesis samples (Osborne 1995). Normal numbers of WBC in the urine are 0–8 WBC/HPF ($\times 450$) in catheterized or mid-stream voided, and 0–3 WBC/HPF in a cystocentesis sample (Osborne 1995). A catalase test for early detection of UTI (Uriscreen, Savyon Diagnostic Ltd, Israel) needs more study in veterinary medicine. One study showed 92% sensitivity, 77% specificity, 55% positive predictive value, and 97% negative predictive value; it may be helpful in deciding which urine samples need cultures done (Bellino et al. 2002).

Occult UTI is fairly common in small animals. Among 85 asymptomatic intact male dogs, 9% had UTI; clinical signs of UTI were absent in 95% of dogs with hyperadrenocorticism and/or Diabetes mellitus, which had UTI (Barsanti 2006). Lack of pyuria may occur because of decreased margination of WBC to the site of inflammation due to hyperadrenocorticism, iatrogenic steroid administration, diabetes, or immunosuppressive states, and requires that urine aerobic cultures be done even when the urinary sediment is inactive. Anaerobic cultures are generally not necessary unless emphysematous cystitis is seen. False-negative urine cultures may occur if samples contain antibiotics, bacteriostatic radiocontrast dye, alcohol, or cleansing agents. Bacteriuria from pyelonephritis may be intermittent, and cultures of bladder urine may be negative when the few bacteria are phagocytized by WBC; therefore, pyelocentesis may be necessary (see Chapter 6). Urine cultures may be falsely positive if contaminated by bacteria from the skin, colon, prepuce, or vagina. Quantitation of bacterial colonies, interpreted in light of how the sample was obtained, helps rule out contamination and false-positives (see aforementioned text). Brownian motion of dust particles may be mistaken for bacteriuria. If rods were noted in sediment, there was a 92% likelihood that rods would be cultured, but if cocci were noted, only 80% of the time was there a positive culture (Barsanti et al. 2006a). No bacteria were seen in microscopic sediment in 8% (rods) and 12% (cocci) positive cultures (Barsanti et al. 2006a).

Finding proteinuria and/or glucosuria warrants doing urine cultures. Dogs with UTI showed significant proteinuria 77% of the time while 61% had <10 WBC/HPF (Barsanti et al. 2006a). Diabetics with glucosuria are of course prone to UTI, and glucosuria in nondiabetics suggests a tubular reabsorptive problem that may be associated with pyelonephritis.

When UTI is suspected, based on clinical signs, urinalysis, or the existence of predisposing factors, urine culture is recommended to identify the type and number of bacteria present. Urine is plated on agar plates and grown in vitro. Antibiotic sensitivity testing can then be done by using Kirby-Bauer disc diffusion methodology with the viewing of inhibition zones or by automated MIC (mean inhibitory concentration) testing to find which antibiotics are best to use for treatment (see Chapter 35).

Rarely, nonbacterial infectious agents colonize the urinary tract and can be visualized in sediment, or cultured from urine or tissue specimens (see Chapters 72 and 74). Clinical signs of organ involvement may suggest a search for such agents (Table 27.1).

Suspicion for infection as a trigger for glomerulonephritis

Immune-mediated damage to the urinary tract targets the renal glomeruli, causing proteinuria. Proteinuria may be occult and may only be recognized in healthy appearing animals during annual health screening tests including testing for proteinuria by urinalysis and sulfosalicylic acid (SSA), microalbuminuria (MA) by E.R.D. test (HESKA), quantitative MA (Antech), or a urine protein/creatinine ratio evaluation (see Chapter 8).

Whenever noted, consistent and significant proteinuria without gross hematuria or an active urinary sediment suggests PLN, which may present with signs of hypertension (e.g., blindness due to retinal hemorrhage or detachment, neurologic signs due to cerebrovascular accident; see Chapter 68), thromboembolic events (e.g., hindleg paresis due to saddle thrombus, dyspnea due to pulmonary embolism, pancreatitis due to portal venous thrombosis), or ascites, effusion/edema (see Chapter 44), even before signs of renal failure (e.g., PU/PD, vomiting) are seen. Blood tests may show hypoalbuminemia and hypercholesterolemia with or without azotemia. Signs suggestive of infectious agents that may cause PLN include other signs of immune-mediated or systemic disease, for example, fever, cytopenias (anemia, leucopenia,

Table 27.1 Diagnostic clues for infectious diseases associated with renal proteinuria and/or renal azotemia. Additional references beyond text: Houser et al. 2006, Littman 2008

Infectious agent	Site of renal injury	Infected cell/organ	Other signs of illness					Diagnostic tests	
			Lameness	Oculo-neural	↓RBC Anemia	↓WBC	↓Platelets	Search for antigen	Search for antibody
Bacterial diseases									
Bacteria (Many spp.)	G, T	Many	Possibly, if sepsis, endocarditis, etc.					C, micro, PCR	
Bartonella	I, G?	V, M, epi-rbc	x	x	x		x	C, PCR	FA, WB
Brucella	G, T	Many	x	x	x			C, micro, PCR	AGID, RSAT, TAT, FA, ELISA
Mycoplasma/ureaplasma	T	Uro-genital	?					C, PCR	
Rickettsial diseases									
Anaplasma	G	WBC	x	x	x	x	x	PCR, micro	ELISA, FA
Ehrlichia	G	WBC	x	x	x	x	x	PCR, micro	ELISA, FA
RMSF	G	V	x	x	x	x	x	PCR, FA	FA, LA
Spirochetes									
Leptospira spp.	T	EC, V, T		x	x		x	PCR, micro, C, FA	MAT, LA, ELISA, WB
Borrelia burgdorferi (Lyme)	G	EC, fibroblasts	x	Rare			x	PCR, micro, C, IHC, FA	C6, ELISA, WB, FA, Elution
Parasitic and other diseases									
Balamuthia (amoebae)	I	Kidney, neuro		x				Micro, IHC, PCR	
Capillaria		Bladder						Micro	
Dioctophyma renale	I	Kidney, abdomen						Micro, gross	
Dirofilaria (Heartworm)	G	Heart, V			x			ELISA, micro	IA (for feline heartworm)
Prototheca (algae)	I			x				Micro, C	
Protozoal diseases									
Babesia spp.	G, T	RBC		x	x		x	Micro, PCR	FA, CF
Hepatozoon	G	Muscle	x		x			PCR, micro	
Leishmania	G	EC, M	x	x	x	x	x	PCR, micro	ELISA, FA, WB
Toxoplasma	I	Many	Rare	x	x			PCR, micro	IgM/IgG, ELISA, FA, CF, LA, HA
Trypanosoma	G	Many	x					PCR, micro, C	FA, radioimmuno-precipitin

Viral diseases

Adenovirus I	G	Liver		x	x	x	PCR, micro, VI, FA, IHC	ELISA, FA, SN, CF, HAI
Calicivirus	I	URI, bladder	Rare				VI, IHC, PCR	VN
FeLV	G or whole	Many		x	x	x	FA, ELISA, C VI, PCR, IHC	VN (rarely done)
FIV		Many	See secondary infections				PCR	ELISA, FA, WB
FIP	I	V, many		x		x	x	x

Fungal diseases

Aspergillus	I	Nasal, many	x	x	x		Micro, C, ELISA	AGID, ELISA, CF
Blastomyces	I	Bone, lung, many	x		x		C, micro, ELISA, EIA	CF, AGID
Candida	I	Various					C, micro, PCR	
Coccidioides	I	Lung, many	x		x		C, micro, PCR	ELISA, AGID, CF, FA, IgM/IgG
Cryptococcus	I	Nasal, many			x		C, micro, FA ELISA, LA	

AGID, agar gel antibody immunodiffusion test; C, culture; CF, complement fixation; EC, extracellular; EIA, enzyme immunoassay; ELISA, enzyme-linked immunosorbent assay; FA, fluorescent antibody test; G, glomerular; HAI, hemagglutination inhibition; I, infiltrative; IA, immunoassay; IHC, immunohistochemistry; LA, latex agglutination; M, macrophages; MAT, microagglutination test; Micro, cytology, histopathology; PCR, polymerase chain reaction test; RMSF, Rocky Mountain spotted fever (Rickettsia rickettsii); RSAT, rapid slide agglutination test; SN, serum neutralization; T, tubular;TAT, tube agglutination test; URI, upper respiratory infection; V, vasculature; VI, virus isolation; VN, virus neutralizing antibody.

and/or thrombocytopenia), epistaxis, petechiation, ecchymoses, icterus, polyarthropathy, vasculitis, uveitis, chorioretinitis, meningitis, and lymphadenopathy. A screening test for proteinuria should always be done on animals (whether asymptomatic or not) that have positive test results for diseases that can cause carrier states, such as heartworm, Lyme, *Ehrlichia*, *Anaplasma*, *Bartonella*, *Babesia*, *Brucella*, *Leishmania* spp., etc.

Infectious disease examples (Table 27.1)

Adenovirus I

See "Infectious canine hepatitis" later.

Anaplasmosis

See "Ehrlichiosis" later.

Aspergillosis

This fungal infection generally causes nasal disease in dogs with possible extension through the cribriform plate leading to CNS signs. However, dissemination may occur, especially in middle-aged female German Shepherds (Schultz et al. 2008), to kidneys, bones, etc. Histopathology or cytology/culture of tissue may show fungal elements; serum antibody tests are not always positive.

Babesiosis

Canine Babesiosis may be due to several species of *Babesia*, including large (*B. canis* and a novel unnamed *Babesia* species (Birkenheuer et al. 2004; Sikorski et al. 2008)) and small (*B. gibsoni* and a *B. microti*-like/*Theileria annae* species). In the United States, dogs at risk include Greyhounds (*B. canis*), Pit Bull Terriers or dogs that have fought with them (*B. gibsoni*), and splenectomized dogs (novel large *Babesia* sp.). Common signs include immune-mediated hemolytic anemia, but less commonly seen are acute renal failure and thrombocytopenia syndromes, as described in Spain with a *B. microti*-like agent (Camacho et al. 2001, 2004). Pigmenturia is mostly due to hemoglobinuria (due to intravascular hemolysis) and bilirubinuria. Organisms may be missed in RBCs; blood smears of the buffy coat or ear sticks may be helpful. Since antibodies to different *Babesia* spp. may not cross-react with IFA tests for *B. canis* or *B. gibsoni* antibodies, *Babesia* PCR using primers that can pick up all types of *Babesia* and/or *Theileria*-like organisms should be used.

Balamuthia mandrillaris

This amoeba caused granulomatous nephritis and meningoencephalitis in a dog. Antigenic tests include microscopic identification of trophozoite and cystic forms, IHC, or PCR on affected tissues (Foreman et al. 2004).

Bartonellosis

Various *Bartonella* spp. may cause carrier states in dogs and cats, and as such may cause chronic immune stimulation as "stealth" pathogens. Organisms may be associated with RBCs and endothelial cells. Lymphadenopathy, endocarditis, hepatitis, vasculitis, uveitis, polyarthropathy, granulomatous disease, neurologic, and other syndromes have been described (Breitschwerdt et al. 2004). The clinical importance of Bartonellosis in dogs and cats is still controversial; proving causation of illness may be difficult even when evidence of exposure or carrier status is found. One study found 10.1% and 27.2% seroprevalence in healthy versus sick dogs, respectively (Goodman et al. 2005). Diagnostic tests include searching for antigen by PCR or 5–6 week culture of blood or tissue samples in special media for this gram-negative fastidious bacterium and searching for antibody by IFA or Western blot.

Blastomycosis

This dimorphic fungal disease may invade skin, lung, bone, eyes, kidneys, etc. Chronic antigenic stimulation may cause IMGN. Testing for antigen in urine or serum was found to be more sensitive than testing for serum antibodies (Spector et al. 2008).

Borreliosis

See "Lyme nephropathy" later.

Brucellosis

Brucella canis may cause diskospondylitis, epidydimitis, orchitis, reproductive failure, and sometimes uveitis, meningoencephalitis, lymphadenitis, etc. in dogs. Organisms persist in the prostate and are shed in the urine for months to years. Renal involvement may occur by extension, or chronic immune stimulation may lead to IMGN in some carrier dogs. The gram-negative rods may be cultured from blood, semen, urine, aborted fetuses, or disk material, but diagnosis is usually by serum antibodies identified by the rapid slide agglutination test (RSAT) or tube agglutination test (TAT), which may be confirmed with the more specific agar gel immunodiffusion test (AGID). Seroconversion is slow and may take 1–3 months (Scheftel 2003).

Calicivirus

This viral infection usually causes upper respiratory signs, but is implicated in some cases of feline cystitis (see Chapter 73) (Kruger et al. 2007; Larson et al. 2007).

Candidiasis

This yeast may invade urinary organs, usually in immunosuppressed animals by extension from lower urogenitalia (Pressler et al. 2003, 2004). Diagnosis is by visualization or culture of organisms in urine, bladder, or rarely, renal samples (see Chapter 72).

Capillariasis

Lower urinary tract signs may be seen in cats and dogs with double operculated ova in urinary sediment. Rule out fecal contamination with *Trichuris* spp. Ova (see Chapter 74).

Coccidioidomycosis

Also known as San Joaquin Valley Fever, the fungus may disseminate to many organs, including kidneys, and/or may cause IMGN. Detection of the agent, antigen, or antibodies has been recently reviewed (Taboada 2008).

Coronavirus

See "Feline infectious peritonitis" later.

Cryptococcosis

Usually causing nasal and/or CNS disease in cats, this fungal infection sometimes colonizes the kidneys, causing renomegaly and renal failure. Organisms may be cultured (takes 2–42 days) or directly visualized in urine or renal tissue specimens with methylene blue, India ink, or gram stains. They appear similar to fat droplets but are all the same size and focus at the level of the sediment (fat droplets vary in size and float under the coverslip). Histopathology specimens may use Mayer's mucicarmine stain, which colors the agent's capsule rose-red as compared to the blue background. Antigens may be captured by latex agglutination or ELISA with monoclonal antibodies (Larsson 2002).

Dioctophyma renale

The giant kidney worm of dogs and cats comes from eating raw fresh water fish or frogs. Hematuria, ureteral obstruction, or, if bilateral, azotemia, may result. Ova may be seen in urine or abdominal fluid; adult worms may be seen on ultrasound or grossly in the kidney or peritoneal cavity (see Chapter 74).

Dirofilariasis

Heartworm disease may cause IMGN, possibly involving antigens from the endosymbiont rickettsial *Wolbachia* spp., which live in the heartworms, assisting their fertility. Heartworm disease may cause no signs, cough or hemoptysis (dogs), emesis (cats), signs of heart failure, coughing, pulmonary thromboembolic events, etc. Heartworm infestation may be diagnosed by finding microfilaria on blood smears or by finding circulating heartworm antigens by immunoassay with in-house tests such as the SNAP-3Dx, SNAP-4Dx (IDEXX), or Solo Step CH (HESKA) in dogs. Since the antigens tested for are from gravid female worms, animals (especially cats) with small burdens may have negative results; the Solo Step FH (HESKA) feline heartworm test is used to detect antibodies.

Ehrlichiosis/anaplasmosis

These rickettsial organisms may cause chronic carrier states with no signs of illness, or they may cause polyarthropathy, uveitis, meningitis, IMGN with PLN, vasculitis, cytopenias (especially thrombocytopenia), gammopathy mimicking multiple myeloma, lymphadenopathy, etc. Cytologic examination of buffy coat or blood smears' feathered edge, bone marrow aspirates, or joint taps may reveal white blood cells with intracytoplasmic morulae in granulocytes (e.g., *E. ewingii* and *A. phagocytophilum* organisms) or mononuclear cells (e.g., *E. canis* and *E. chaffeensis* organisms). The in-house SNAP-4Dx (IDEXX) test qualitatively tests for antibodies directed against *E. canis* (cross-reaction detects antibodies to *E. chaffeensis*) and *A. phagocytophilum* (cross-reaction detects antibodies to *A. platys*, a platelet rickettsial infection). Whole cell ELISA and IFA tests are available to quantitate height of titers for *E. canis* and *A. phagocytophilum* (the latter used to be called *E. equi*). Since animals may present during an acute phase of illness before seroconversion has occurred, paired testing (acute and convalescent) may be needed, or one titer 10–14 days into the illness. The SNAP tests are likely to remain positive for years after treatment, because of immune memory. Pre- and 6-month post-treatment quantitative titers for *Ehrlichia* or *Anaplasma* may be helpful to check for a decline, indicating possible clearance or decreased burden, and to get a new baseline to compare with future quantitative titers should signs recur or worsen. Older IFA tests for *E. canis* antibodies inconsistently cross-reacted with antibodies directed against other *Ehrlichia* or *Anaplasma* spp.

PCR testing on whole blood using primers to identify any species of *Ehrlichia* or *Anaplasma* is available, and is best done before doxycycline treatment is started, lest the result be negative. The SNAP test does not pick up antibodies to *E. ewingii*, and since organisms may be missed cytologically, the PCR test would help find evidence of *E. ewingii* DNA and is best done before treatment is started. During and after treatment, PCR testing became negative in dogs that had *A. phagocytophilum* infection (Alleman et al. 2006). But with steroid challenge, PCR testing was positive again, proving lack of clearance with a 2-week course of doxycycline.

FeLV/FIV

Immunosuppression due to feline leukemia virus and/or feline immunodeficiency virus may predispose cats to secondary urinary tract infections. Risk also occurs for IMGN due to CIC associated with FeLV or FIV carrier status, secondary infections, or antigens from FeLV-associated neoplasia or myelodysplasia. Diagnostic tests for FeLV find soluble virus (ELISA) or cell-associated virus (FA) on blood or bone marrow smears and PCR or IHC on tumor or bone marrow specimens. Culture of bone marrow may reveal latent infections. Antibody testing for FeLV is rarely done. Diagnosis of renal lymphoma usually requires renal FNA or biopsy, since affected cats are often FeLV-negative. ELISA for FIV antibodies is standard even though it cross-reacts with FIV vaccinal antibodies. The SNAP Feline Triple Test (IDEXX) is an in-house test for FeLV and heartworm antigens and FIV antibodies.

Feline infectious peritonitis (FIP coronavirus)

The immune-mediated vasculitis of FIP may affect kidneys, with granulomatous infiltration and renomegaly. Other organ involvement (liver, eye, CNS) may occur; blood tests may show hyperglobulinemia, icterus, azotemia, etc. Renal biopsy is the main way to diagnose renal FIP when it occurs in the "dry form" of FIP. In the "wet form" of FIP, PCR may be done on effusions. Since FIP is caused by a mutant coronavirus and antibodies cross-react with those against the common enteric coronavirus, which many cats have, titers may not be as helpful.

Hepatozoonosis

Carriers of *Hepatozoon americanum* or *H. canis* in southeast United States (Allen et al. 2008) may develop IMGN. *H. americanum* causes severe wasting myositis. Long bone periosteal proliferation may be seen radiographically. Diagnosis is confirmed by muscle biopsy (PCR and visualization of schizonts).

Infectious canine hepatitis (Adenovirus I)

This virus may cause vasculitis, cytopenias, renal and hepatic failure, but not usually icterus. Disease is now rare because vaccination is very effective. If suspected, virus isolation, PCR, etc. are done.

Leishmaniasis

In the United States, this protozoal systemic infection is primarily seen in Foxhounds and may cause IMGN. Besides signs due to nephrotic syndrome/hypertension/renal failure, signs may include epistaxis, dermal, ocular, musculoskeletal signs, and/or lymphadenopathy. Labwork may show proteinuria, cytopenias, hypoalbuminemia, hyperglobulinemia, and/or azotemia. Promastigotes may be seen in macrophages by aspirating lymph node, bone marrow, spleen, etc. Many tests for antigen and antibody detection exist. A new rapid in-house ELISA test is available for serum antibodies, the SNAP *Leishmania* Test (IDEXX) (Ferroglio et al. 2007).

Leptospirosis

This systemic spirochetal infection usually enters the body via mucous membranes or damaged skin, and targets the kidneys hematogenously. The organisms localize in renal tubular cells and are shed in the urine intermittently for months to years by carriers. Many pathogenic species exist and can cause clinical signs in dogs, farm animals, and humans, but interestingly, cats are relatively resistant even though they are exposed to urine of small rodents that can carry *Leptospira* spp. organisms. *Leptospira* spp. shed in urine can survive in a wet environment, for example, on organic material or on biofilms of rocks in neutral or alkaline waterways. In the past, serovars *L. canicola* and *L. icterohemorrhagica* were predominant in sick dogs; now illness is likely due to *L. pomona*, *L. grippotyphosa*, *L. bratislava*, or *L. autumnalis*. Signs of Leptospirosis are variable and range from occult infection to acute or chronic signs, which may include renal, hepatic, gastrointestinal, myalgia/arthralgia, and/or uveitis signs. Clinicopathologic abnormalities may include cytopenias, leukocytosis, azotemia, liver enzyme elevations (especially cholestatic), isosthenuria, glycosuria, bilirubinuria, and active sediment with negative bacterial urine cultures.

With the exception of PCR (Harkin et al. 2003), diagnostic tests to look for *Leptospira* spp. antigens are generally not helpful. The spirochetes are difficult to isolate (require special media) or visualize (require dark-field microscopy, Giemsa or silver stains, FA, or PCR). Testing for antibodies is currently the main way to look for exposure, but cross-reactive antibodies makes interpretation difficult. Differentiating between vaccinal and natural exposure antibodies may be available in the future with Western blot or immunoblotting (Goldstein 2008). Cross-reaction also exists between members of serogroups. Contrary to previous thought, the highest titer may not be the infecting serovar; convalescent titers show less serogroup cross-reaction over time, allowing for better prediction of the offending serovar (Lunn 2008). The microagglutination test (MAT) is the current "gold standard" but ELISA, IgG/IgM, and macroagglutination tests are also available. Since acute illness may occur before seroconversion, paired titers (acute and convalescent) are needed, if the dog presents during the first 10–14 days of illness, to see seroconversion or a fourthfold rise in titer. Standardization is difficult; interlaboratory results do not always agree, and the cut-off for significance is arbitrary. For instance, some would accept a titer of 1:200 for a non-vaccinal serovar as a positive titer; others use 1:800 as a cut-off. For vaccinal serovars, some use 1:3200 while others use 1:800 as a cut-off for natural exposure antibodies >10 weeks postvaccine. As higher titers are used as a cut-off, specificity is gained but sensitivity is lost. Most agree that chronic urinary shedders can be serologically negative, and since shedding may be intermittent, urine PCR may be negative as well.

Lyme nephropathy

The diagnosis of disease caused by Lyme (*Borrelia burgdorferi*) is difficult because seropositivity is so common in Lyme endemic areas, and the vast majority of seropositive dogs remain asymptomatic, without illness or proteinuria, even though most remain chronic carriers (Littman et al. 2006). In some Lyme endemic areas, 50–90% of normal dogs are seropositive. So when sick dogs are seropositive, it is difficult to know whether Lyme disease is causing their illness. Less than 5% of exposed Lyme + dogs show a "classic Lyme arthritis" syndrome including anorexia, fever, and oligoarthritis, which is self-limiting over a few days in experimental models and is quickly responsive to antibiotics such as doxycycline or amoxicillin in cases seen in the field. Response to doxycycline does not prove cause, since many other infectious diseases that mimic Lyme disease are doxycycline-responsive and since doxycycline has anti-inflammatory and antiarthritic properties in addition to its antimicrobial ones. Some Lyme + dogs may have immune-mediated polyarthropathy (IMPA, often with swollen

painful hocks and carpi), which may be due to Lyme-triggered immune-mediated synovitis (or coinfections with Anaplasmosis) and responds to doxycycline with corticosteroids. At Penn, 57% of dogs with IMPA were Lyme + when compared with 37% of the rest of the hospital population (Rondeau et al. 2005).

An unknown but small number of Lyme + dogs become sick with an immune-mediated nephropathy caused by Lyme antigen–antibody complex deposition in glomeruli (Chou et al. 2006; Goldstein 2007 and personal communication presented during that ACVIM 2007 talk). The disease is not due to colonization of the kidneys with spirochetes and few if any organisms are actually present in the kidneys (different than Leptospirosis) (Chou et al. 2006; Hutton et al. 2008). Glomerular deposits (immune complexes) in dogs with Lyme nephropathy were found to include Lyme-specific antibodies, for example, directed against Lyme antigens p31 (ospA), p34 (ospB), and p83 (Chou et al. 2006; Goldstein 2007). Dogs with Lyme nephropathy may or may not have had a history of lameness or past exposure to Lyme vaccinations (Littman 2008). The use of Lyme vaccine is controversial, since increased levels of circulating Lyme-specific immune complexes (Lyme-CIC) are associated with Lyme nephropathy and can be found in dogs after vaccination, circulating for many months (longer with bacterin than with subunit ospA vaccine, and longer in dogs that were seropositive before vaccination) (Goldstein and Atwater 2006; Goldstein 2007); theoretically dogs may have increased immune-complex deposition or sensitization if they are genetically so inclined. Asymptomatic as well as sick dogs were found to have Lyme-specific CIC, but sick dogs had higher CIC than asymptomatic dogs (Goldstein 2006).

Any breed can be affected; however, Labrador and Golden Retrievers were found to be at high risk for Lyme nephropathy (Dambach et al. 1997). At Penn, 85% of Retrievers with PLN were Lyme + when compared with 24% of healthy Retrievers (there was no association found in German Shepherds) (Littman et al. 2006a). But even among Lyme + Labrador Retrievers, the incidence of Lyme nephropathy is very low (Goldstein et al. 2007), and currently, there is no way to predict which seropositive dogs will be at risk. Height of antibody titer does not appear to predict illness, and many asymptomatic dogs have high titers (Littman et al. 2006; Levy et al. 2008). In Europe, although a high percentage of Bernese Mountain Dogs are Lyme +, there was no association between proteinuria and seropositive status (Gerber et al. 2005).

All Lyme + dogs should be monitored for proteinuria whether they are sick with Lyme disease or not. Sick dogs with Lyme nephropathy may present due to signs of PLN, including nephrotic syndrome, hypertension, thromboembolic events, and/or renal failure. The diagnosis of Lyme nephropathy is supported by a history of exposure to *Ixodes* ticks in a Lyme endemic area (95% of cases are in just 12 states, including PA, NY, NJ, MA, CT, RI, WI, MD, MN, DE, VA, and NH) and evidence of antibodies directed against the organism. Transmitted after 2–4 days of tick attachment, the spirochetes migrate through the tissues and do not circulate via the bloodstream. The organisms are associated with collagen and fibroblasts, and are difficult to find cytologically or culture from blood, joint taps, biopsy, etc. Therefore, proof of exposure is generally shown by finding antibodies directed against the antigens that would be present in the dog due to natural exposure (as opposed to vaccination). Since vaccinal antibodies include those directed against antigens expressed by *B. burgdorferi* as found in the tick or in vitro, certain tests can be done on vaccinated dogs, which can differentiate for natural exposure antibodies. The most sensitive and specific test for natural exposure antibodies is the C6 peptide test, which is included on the SNAP-3Dx and SNAP-4Dx tests (IDEXX). These in-house tests give a qualitative positive or negative. For quantitation of level (height) of antibodies, C6 Quant (IDEXX) can be done by the reference laboratory. The in-house SNAP tests are very sensitive and may show a positive result even when the C6 Quant is <30, which is the level below which clinical illness would not be expected to be associated with Lyme disease. Since normal dogs may have C6 Quant even higher than 600, the height of the C6 Quant does not prove causation.

The old tests of IFA and whole cell ELISA are not specific for natural exposure to *B. burgdorferi*. They may become positive due to exposure to other *Borrelia* spp. or to Lyme vaccination. They would need to be followed up with a Western blot test to look for specific banding pattern usually seen with natural infection/exposure to *B. burgdorferi*, or preferably a C6 peptide test (SNAP or C6 Quant). Doing paired (acute and convalescent) titers are not necessary, and IgG and IgM testing is not helpful for Lyme disease, since illness would not be expected during early infection (with IgM+/IgG– status) based on the experimental finding that dogs did not show any illness until 2–5 months after exposure. Having IgM+/IgG+ status does not prove recent exposure, since antigenic variation during the chronic carrier phase can cause novel antigen exposures and new IgM antibodies to rise.

There is no experimental model for Lyme nephropathy, and since renal biopsies are not usually done on mildly affected dogs, histopathologic changes during the early stages of Lyme nephropathy is not yet characterized. Histopathologic changes on pet dogs sick with moderate to severe Lyme nephropathy showed a combination of IMGN, tubular necrosis/regeneration, and interstitial nephritis (Dambach et al. 1997). Urinalysis shows proteinuria, casts, sometimes bilirubinuria, and possibly evidence of tubular disease (glucosuria, decreased concentration).

Sophisticated elution studies showing Lyme-specific antigens or antibodies in the glomerular immune deposits are used in research but are not readily available for the clinician to help diagnose whether PLN is actually due to Lyme disease or not. Imaging (radiographs, ultrasound) are not helpful in differentiating Lyme nephropathy from other forms of PLN. Response to treatment is fair to poor. Doxycycline, angiotensin-converting enzyme inhibitors, antithrombotic low dose of aspirin, omega-3 fatty acids, and modified protein/phosphorus diet are generally used. Antihypertensives, antiemetics/protectants, colloid therapy, etc. are added as needed. Studies with immunosuppressives and plasmapheresis therapy to remove CIC need to be critically evaluated.

Prototothecosis

This systemic algal disease may be seen in immuno-compromised animals. Dissemination to kidneys may cause renal failure. Other signs may include diarrhea/hematochezia, lymphadenopathy, anterior uveitis, dermal ulcers, and neurologic signs. Organisms may be seen in urine sediment, aerobic urine cultures, or renal histopathology (Pressler et al. 2005).

Rocky Mountain spotted fever (RMSF)

Dogs exposed to *Rickettsii rickettsia* may have no signs of illness or variable signs including fever, vasculitis, bleeding, vomiting/diarrhea, acute renal failure, vestibular or other neurologic signs, lameness, and pancreatitis. Anemia and thrombocytopenia are common; pancytopenia may occur. Vasculitis affecting the kidney may cause proteinuria and renal failure. Organisms invade vascular endothelial cells and are not found in the blood. Dogs present acutely, often before seroconversion; therefore, paired titers (acute and convalescent) are often necessary. Contrary to other rickettsial infections, there is no known carrier state.

Toxoplasmosis

Toxoplasma gondii protozoal organisms may infiltrate the kidneys and cause renomegaly and renal failure. Other organs may be affected, including the eye, CNS, lung, liver, muscle, etc. Cats are the definitive hosts and may shed oocysts in the feces but sick cats do not necessarily shed oocysts when they are ill. PCR or cytologic examination of renal aspirates or biopsies may show organisms (tachyzoites). Antibody titers (paired) can check for both IgM and IgG, to show active or recent infection (IgM) versus chronic carrier status (IgG).

Trypanosomiasis

This protozoal infection may mimic Leishmaniasis in clinical presentation, cytologically, and by serology and immunohistochemistry, due to cross-reactive antibodies. PCR analysis may be helpful (Nabity et al. 2006). Chagas disease in S. America (*T. cruzi*) causes myositis, heart disease, and IMGN; a new rapid dipstick test is used on canine sera (Cardinal et al. 2006).

Ureaplasma/mycoplasma spp

Ureaplasma spp. are in the Mycoplasma family and are too small to be seen in the urinary sediment. They are associated with urogenital/reproductive problems and possibly lower urinary tract signs due to colonization. Tests include PCR or culture on special media. Infection with *Ureaplasma* spp. may be suspected in animals with lower urinary tract signs, active sediment (WBC), and negative bacterial cultures.

References

Allen, K.E., Y. Li, et al. (2008). Diversity of *Hepatozoon* species in naturally infected dogs in the southern United States. *Vet Parasitol* **154**(3/4): 220–225.

Alleman, A., R. Chandrashekar, et al. (2006). Experimental inoculation of dogs with a human isolate (NY18) of *Anaplasma phagocytophilum* and demonstration of persistent infection following doxycycline therapy. *J Vet Intern Med* **20**(3): 763.

Bailiff, N., J. Westropp, et al. (2007). Comparison of urinary tract infections in cats presenting with lower urinary tract signs and cats with chronic kidney disease, hyperthyroidism, and Diabetes mellitus. *J Vet Intern Med* **21**(3): 649.

Bailiff, N.L., R.W. Nelson, et al. (2006). Frequency and risk factors for urinary tract infection in cats with Diabetes mellitus. *J Vet Intern Med* **20**(4): 850–855.

Bailiff, N., R. Nelson, et al. (2004). Prevalence of urinary tract infections in diabetic cats. *J Vet Intern Med* **18**(3): 442–443.

Barsanti, J.A. (2006). Genitourinary infections. In: *Infectious Diseases of the Dog and Cat*, edited by C.E. Greene, 3rd edition. St. Louis, MO: W.B. Saunders Company, Elsevier, Inc, pp. 935–961.

Barsanti, J.A., S. Sanchez, et al. (2006a). Accuracy of urinalysis in predicting the type of infecting bacteria in urinary tract infection. *J Vet Intern Med* **20**(3): 738.

Bartges, J.W. (2005). Urinary tract infections. In: *Textbook of Veterinary Internal Medicine*, edited by S.J. Ettinger and E.C. Feldman, 6th Edition. Philadelphia, PA: WB Saunders, Elsevier, pp. 1800–1808.

Bellino, C., A.M. Farca, et al. (2002). The validity of a catalase test for early detection of urinary tract infection (UTI) in dogs and cats. *12th ECVIM-CA/ESVIM Congress.* Available at: http://www.vin.com/Members/Proceedings/Proceedings.plx?CID=ecvim2002&PID=pr02291&O=VIN (accessed October 15, 2010).

Birkenheuer, A.J., J. Neel, et al. (2004). Detection and molecular characterization of a novel large *Babesia* species in a dog. *Vet Parasitol* **124**(3/4): 151–160.

Breitschwerdt, E.B., K.R. Blann, et al. (2004). Clinicopathological abnormalities and treatment response in 24 dogs seroreactive to *Bartonella vinsonii (berkhoffii)* antigens. *J Am Anim Hosp Assoc* **40**(2): 92–101.

Camacho, A.T., E. Pallas, et al. (2001). Infection of dogs in northwest Spain with a *Babesia microti*-like agent. *Vet Rec* **149**(18): 552–555.

Camacho, A.T., E.J. Guitian, et al. (2004). Azotemia and mortality among *Babesia microti*-like infected dogs. *J Vet Intern Med* **18**(2): 141–146.

Cardinal, M.V., R. Reithinger, et al. (2006). Use of an immunochromatographic dipstick test for rapid detection of *Trypanosoma cruzi* in sera from animal reservoir hosts. *J Clin Microbiol* **44**(8): 3005–3007.

Chou, J., A. Wunschmann, et al. (2006). Detection of *Borrelia burdorferi* DNA in tissues from dogs with presumptive Lyme borreliosis. *J Am Vet Med Assoc* **229**(8): 1260–1265.

Comer, K.M. and G.V. Ling (1981). Results of urinalysis and bacterial culture of canine urine obtained by antepubic cystocentesis, catheterization, and the midstream voided methods. *J Am Vet Med Assoc* **179**(9): 891–895.

Dambach, D.M., C.A. Smith, et al. (1997). Morphologic, immunohistochemical, and ultrastructural characteristics of a distinctive renal lesion in dogs putatively associated with *Borrelia burgdorferi* infection: 49 cases (1987–1992). *Vet Pathol* **34**(2): 85–96.

Ferroglio, E., E. Centaro et al. (2007). Evaluation of an ELISA rapid device for the serological diagnosis of *Leishmania infantum* infection in dog as compared with immunofluorescence assay and Western blot. *Vet Parasitol* **144**(1–2): 162–166.

Foreman, O., J. Sykes, et al. (2004). Disseminated infection with *Balamuthia mandrillaris* in a dog. *Vet Pathol* **41**(5): 506–510.

Forrester, S.D., G.C. Troy, et al. (1999). Retrospective evaluation of urinary tract infection in 42 dogs with hyperadrenocorticism or Diabetes mellitus or both. *J Vet Intern Med* **13**(6): 557–560.

Gerber, B., S. Eichenberger, et al. (2005). Urine protein excretion of healthy Bernese Mountain Dogs and other dogs with and without antibodies against *Borrelia burgdorferi*. *J Vet Intern Med* **19**(3): 431.

Goldstein, R.E. and D.Z. Atwater (2006). Evaluation of serology and circulating immune complexes in dogs naturally infected with *Borrelia burgdorferi*. *J Vet Intern Med* **20**(3): 713.

Goldstein, R.E. (2007). Current understanding of Lyme nephropathy. *Proc 25th ACVIM Forum*, Seattle, WA. pp. 672–673.

Goldstein, R.E., A.P. Cordner, et al. (2007). Microalbuminuria and comparison of serologic testing for exposure to *Borrelia burgdorferi* in nonclinical Labrador and Golden Retrievers. *J Vet Diagn Invest* **19**(3): 294–297.

Goldstein, R.E. (2008). Advances in the diagnosis of Leptospirosis. *Proc 26th ACVIM Forum*, San Antonio, TX. pp. 622–623.

Goodman, R.A. and E.B. Breitschwerdt (2005). Clinicopathologic findings in dogs seroreactive to *Bartonella henselae* antigens. *Am J Vet Res* **66**(12): 2060–2064.

Harkin, K.R., Y.M. Roshto, et al. (2003). Clinical application of a polymerase chain reaction assay for diagnosis of leptospirosis in dogs. *J Am Vet Med Assoc* **222**(9): 1224–1229.

Houser G., A. Ayoob, et al. (2006). Laboratory testing for infectious diseases of dogs and cats. In: *Infectious Diseases of the Dog and Cat*, edited by C.E. Greene, 3rd edition. St. Louis, MO: WB Saunders, Elsevier, pp. 1139–1168.

Hutton, T.A., R.E. Goldstein, et al. (2008). Search for *Borrelia burgdorferi* in kidneys of dogs with suspected "Lyme nephritis." *J Vet Intern Med* **22**(4): 860–865.

Ihrke, P.J., A.L. Norton, et al. (1985). Urinary tract infection associated with long-term corticosteroid administration in dogs with chronic skin diseases. *J Am Vet Med Assoc* **186**(1): 43–46.

Kruger, J.M., C.P. Pfent, et al. (2007). Feline calicivirus-associated urinary tract disease in specific-pathogen-free cats. *J Vet Intern Med* **21**(3): 648–649.

Larson, J., J.M. Kruger, et al. (2007). Epidemiology of feline calicivirus urinary tract infection in cats with idiopathic cystitis. *J Vet Intern Med* **2**(3): 648.

Larsson, C.E. (2002). Cryptococcosis. *Proc WSAVA Congress.* Available at: http://www.vin.com/Members/Proceedings/Proceedings.plx?CID=wsava2002&PID=pr02548&O=VIN (accessed October 15, 2010).

Levy, S.A., T.P. O'Connor, et al. (2008). Quantitative measurement of C6 antibody following antibiotic treatment of *Borrelia burgdorferi* antibody-positive nonclinical dogs. *Clin Vaccine Immunol* **15**(1): 115–119.

Littman, M.P. (2008). Polyarthropathy, cytopenias, and proteinuria. *Proc 22nd NAVC Conference*, Orlando, FL. **22**: 701–703.

Littman, M.P., R.E. Goldstein, et al. (2006). ACVIM small animal consensus on Lyme disease in dogs: diagnosis, treatment, and prevention. *J Vet Intern Med* **20**(2): 422–434.

Littman, M.P., U. Giger, et al. (2006a). Seroprevalence of *Borrelia burgdorferi* antibodies in dogs at a veterinary teaching hospital in a Lyme endemic area. *J Vet Intern Med* **20**(3): 761–762.

Lunn K.F. (2008). Limitations of MAT for the serodiagnosis of canine Leptospirosis. *Proc 26th ACVIM Forum*, San Antonio, TX. pp. 615–616.

Nabity, M.B., K. Barnhart, et al. (2006). An atypical case of *Trypanosoma cruzi* infection in a young English Mastiff. *Vet Parasitol* **140**(3–4): 356–361.

Osborne, C.A. (1995). Three steps to effective management of bacterial urinary tract infections: diagnosis, diagnosis, and diagnosis. *Compend Cont Educ* **17**(10): 1233–1248.

Pressler, B.M. (2004). Fungal urinary tract infections. *Proc 22nd ACVIM Forum.* Available at: http://www.vin.com/Members/Proceedings/Proceedings.plx?CID=acvim2004&PID=pr06067&O=VIN (accessed October 15, 2010).

Pressler, B.M., J.L. Gookin, et al. (2005). Urinary tract manifestations of Protothecosis in dogs. *J Vet Intern Med* **19**(1): 115–119.

Pressler, B.M., S.L. Vaden, et al. (2003). *Candida* spp. urinary tract infections in 13 dogs and seven cats: predisposing factors, treatment, and outcome. *J Am Anim Hosp Assoc* **39**(3): 263–270.

Rondeau, M.P., R.M. Walton, et al. (2005). Suppurative, nonseptic polyarthropathy in dogs. *J Vet Intern Med* **19**(5): 654–662.

Scheftel, J. (2003). *Brucella canis*: Potential for zoonotic transmission. *Compend Cont Educ* **25**(11): 846–852.

Schultz, R.M., E.G. Johnson, et al. (2008). Clinicopathologic and diagnostic imaging characteristics of systemic aspergillosis in 30 dogs. *J Vet Intern Med* **22**(4): 851–859.

Sikorski L.E., A.J. Birkenheuer, et al. (2008). Clinical and molecular characterization of a novel canine *Babesia* species. *J Vet Intern Med* **22**(3): 780.

Spector, D., A.M. Legendre, et al. (2008). Antigen and antibody testing for the diagnosis of Blastomycosis in dogs. *J Vet Intern Med* **22**(4): 839–843.

Stiffler, K.S., M.A. Stevenson, et al. (2006). Prevalence and characterization of urinary tract infections in dogs with surgically treated type 1 thoracolumbar intervertebral disc extrusion. *Vet Surg* **35**(4): 330–336.

Sykes, J. (2003). Mechanisms of renal injury by infectious agents. *Proc 21st ACVIM Forum.* Available at: http://www.vin.com/Members/Proceedings/Proceedings.plx?CID=acvim2003&PID=pr04349&O=VIN (accessed October 15, 2010).

Taboada, J. (2008). Systemic mycoses. In: *Handbook of Small Animal Practice*, edited by R.V. Morgan, 5th edition. St. Louis, MO: WB Saunders, Elsevier, pp. 1073–1086.

Section 3

Therapeutic techniques

28

Hemodialysis

Cathy Langston

Terminology

Renal replacement therapies include dialysis and transplantation. Dialytic therapies include peritoneal dialysis (Chapter 30), an intracorporeal technique, and extracorporeal renal replacement therapies (ERRT), which include intermittent and continuous hemodialysis (Chapter 29). The principles of intermittent and continuous therapies are the same, but there are practical differences between the techniques, and the reader is referred to the chapter on continuous renal replacement therapy for further information.

The basic premise of ERRT involves withdrawing blood from the patient, circulating it through a dialyzer composed of a semi-permeable membrane to allow removal of uremic toxins, and returning the cleansed blood to the patient. By creating a continuous loop of blood circulation, although only a portion of the blood volume is out of the patient at any given time, the entire blood volume is circulated through the dialyzer many times over during the course of the treatment. At the conclusion of the treatment, the blood in the circuit is generally returned to the patient. Dialysate may be circulated through the dialyzer to allow diffusive clearance (hemodialysis), or fluid may be removed from the patient to allow convective clearance (hemofiltration), or both techniques may be used simultaneously (hemodiafiltration). Intermittent hemodialysis relies on diffusive clearance, but may include hemofiltration. Continuous therapies may be diffusive, convective, or both.

In this chapter, the term dialysis is used to indicate peritoneal dialysis (PD), intermittent hemodialysis (IHD), and continuous renal replacement therapy (CRRT), and the term extracorporeal renal replacement therapy (ERRT) is used to include intermittent and continuous hemodialysis therapies.

Epidemiology

Who to dialyze and when

In veterinary medicine, dialysis is used most commonly for acute kidney injury (Chapter 49). Dialysis is indicated for patients with anuria or oliguria, life-threatening fluid overload (i.e., pulmonary edema), or hyperkalemia (Chapter 62), if attempts to induce urine production are unsuccessful. In human pediatric patients, fluid overload (>10%) is associated with a worse outcome (Gillespie et al. 2004; Goldstein et al. 2005). Uremic symptoms, progressive azotemia, or azotemia that does not improve with standard medical therapy are indications for dialysis, even if urine output is adequate or increased. In one human study, nonoliguric patients were referred for dialysis later during hospitalization compared to oliguric patients, and they suffered a worse outcome (Liangos et al. 2005). Whether initiating dialysis early in the course of AKI improves outcome compared to later initiation is unresolved. Some studies have shown an advantage to early initiation, although others have not (Gettings et al. 1999; Bouman et al. 2002; Liu et al. 2006). However, these studies are all confounded by differences in defining early versus late, only one was randomized, and cohort size was generally small. In many situations, AKI is reversible, and because there are no studies that clearly predict which patients will need dialysis, it is possible that results of studies on early versus late initiation will be biased toward early initiation because of inclusion of patients in the early group that did not need dialysis (Waikar and Bonventre 2006). Despite the lack of an adequate study to answer this question, waiting until uremic symptoms are severe and patient condition has deteriorated may be disadvantageous, but the risk of early initiation in a patient

Nephrology and Urology of Small Animals. Edited by Joe Bartges and David J. Polzin. © 2011 Blackwell Publishing Ltd.

that may not need dialysis must be weighed against the potential risks and cost of ERRT.

Dialysis is reserved until standard medical management has been attempted. Standard medical management includes adequate volume expansion. Because dehydration of less than 5% cannot be clinically detected, patients that appear normally hydrated but not overhydrated should receive a dose of IV fluid equal to 5% of body weight. The systemic blood pressure should be adequate to perfuse the kidneys (>80–100 mmHg systolic or >60–80 mmHg mean arterial pressure). The use of diuretics is widespread in both human and veterinary medicine despite lack of conclusive evidence of a positive impact on outcome (Bagshaw et al. 2008). Loop diuretics, specifically furosemide, are most commonly used. If loop diuretics, osmotic diuretics (i.e., mannitol), or other diuretics fail to induce adequate urine production within hours, early referral for dialysis is appropriate.

In people, hemodialysis is used primarily to treat end-stage renal disease (Stage V chronic kidney disease; Chapter 48). People may be maintained on chronic hemodialysis for years while waiting for a renal transplant (Chapter 31) or for decades if transplantation is not possible. Transplantation is generally preferred over chronic hemodialysis, as it more completely replaces renal function, but transplantation is not readily available for dogs. Chronic hemodialysis is an alternative in those cases and in cats in which there are clear contraindications to transplantation. The goal of chronic hemodialysis is to maintain a satisfactory quality of life, which should take precedence over longevity. Chronic hemodialysis should be recommended when the signs of uremia are no longer controlled by medical management (Chapter 41). The serum creatinine concentration is generally over 5 mg/dL. In some patients, the main sign of uremia is anorexia. If few other uremic signs are present or can be controlled, placement of a feeding tube prior to initiating dialysis may be prudent. Although patients may decompensate acutely and unpredictably, the decision to initiate chronic dialysis ideally should be planned in advance, allowing scheduling of surgical placement of a permanent hemodialysis catheter in conjunction with feeding tube placement. Although return of a normal appetite is expected with adequate dialysis, anorexia can be expected during prolonged interdialysis intervals, when catheter function is temporarily inadequate, or when concurrent illness is present, and use of a feeding tube during those times allows better over all patient care.

Outcome

Overall survival of dogs and cats treated with hemodialysis for AKI is 41–52%, but survival is dependent on

Table 28.1 Survival rates with intermittent hemodialysis for various etiologies of renal failure

Category	Survival rate
Obstructive (cats)	70–75%
Infectious	58–86%
Metabolic/hemodynamic	56–72%
Other	29–56%
Toxic	18–35%

etiology, with infectious and ischemic causes faring better than toxic causes, in general (Table 28.1) (Langston et al. 1997; Adin and Cowgill 2000; Francey and Cowgill 2002; Fischer et al. 2004b; Pantaleo et al. 2004; Francey 2006a). Of the nonsurviving patients, about half of those die or are euthanatized due to extra-renal conditions (e.g., pancreatitis, respiratory complications). About a third of nonsurvivors are euthanized due to failure of recovery of renal function. On going uremic signs, dialysis complications, and unknown causes account for the remaining patient deaths. Of the surviving patients, approximately half regain normal renal function (defined by normal serum creatinine concentration) and half have persistent chronic kidney disease.

A clinical scoring system for outcome prediction of dogs with AKI receiving hemodialysis has been developed (Chapter 49). The model uses data that is commonly available prior to instituting dialysis, although knowledge of the specific etiology, which is frequently not known initially, improves the accuracy of the outcome prediction. Although this scoring system has not yet been independently validated and should not be used in the decision-making process for an individual patient, use of scoring systems will hopefully help in determining appropriate candidates for dialysis (Segev et al. 2008).

Equipment

Vascular access

Catheter design

An adequately functioning dialysis catheter allows smooth and efficient treatment and patient management; a poorly functioning catheter frustrates the technician, doctor, and patient. In veterinary medicine, catheters are the predominant form of vascular access. Much thought and care should go into choosing the appropriate catheter, placing it, and maintaining it.

A variety of materials can be used to make a catheter that is minimally thrombogenic, flexible, and nonirritating to the vessel wall. Polyurethane, polyethylene, polytetrafluoroethylene (PTFE), silicone, and carbothane are suitable choices. Polyethylene is stiff and kinks when bent. It can be used for temporary catheters but is not appropriate for long-term use (Ash 2007). Polyurethane has some rigidity at room temperature, which assists in placement, but it becomes softer and more flexible at body temperature. Alcohol containing antibiotic ointments will weaken the material (Ash 2007).

To allow simultaneous removal and return of blood, a dialysis catheter has two lumens. Although catheters are placed in a central vein, the lumen that provides blood egress from the body is generally referred to as the "arterial" port, and the lumen that provides blood return to the body is termed the "venous" port. The arterial lumen is usually shorter than the venous return lumen, to avoid uptake of blood returning from the dialyzer (access recirculation), which would decrease the efficiency of treatment (Figure 28.1). In some situations, two single lumen catheters are placed to provide blood egress and return, either in separate vessels or in the same vessel. In lumens with a single opening (either at the tip or a side port), partial occlusion from thrombosis or a fibrin sheath can decrease catheter function to the point of being unable to provide adequate dialysis. The risk of complete occlusion is lessened by having multiple ports (Figure 28.2). If the ports are positioned circumferentially around the catheter, even if the vessel wall is sucked against the ports on one side of the catheter, blood flow can continue on the opposite side. If the side ports are small, blood will preferentially flow through the tip, making the side ports superfluous. If the side ports are large, they weaken the catheter and increase the amount of heparin that diffuses out of the catheter between dialysis treatments (Depner 2001).

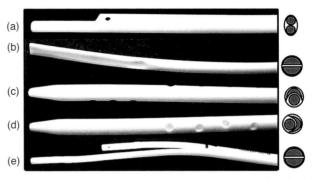

Figure 28.2 Common ERRT catheter configurations. (a) and (b) are tunneled cuffed catheters. (c) is a nontunneled noncuffed catheter ("temporary"). (d) shows catheter C rotated 90° to demonstrate placement of multiple openings. (e) is a split tip catheter. Cross-section of lumen configurations on right.

A double D configuration provides the highest lumen volume with lowest surface contacting the blood to diminish shear stress, while maintaining a modest outer circumference (Ash 2007). Other configurations are commonly used, however, including round or C-shaped lumens (Figure 28.2) (Wentling 2004). Temporary catheters are generally designed with a tapering tip to facilitate percutaneous placement. Permanent catheters may have the tips separated, such that the intravenous portion acts like two separate catheters placed in the same vein, whereas the external portions are bound together. By having separated tips, side ports can be placed circumferentially, and the increased flexibility of the tips and their movement with each cardiac cycle may help decrease fibrin sheath formation (Depner 2001). An arteriovenous fistula or graft is the preferred access in people receiving chronic hemodialysis. An artery is surgically anastomosed to a vein with a section of autologous vein or synthetic graft (typically, PFTE). Within approximately a month, endothelial cells line the graft, and the endothelial cells of the autologous vein segment take on characteristics of arterial endothelium instead of venous. The access can be then used by percutaneous puncture of the arterial and venous segments with large gauge needles at each dialysis treatment. Between treatments, no anticoagulant is needed because blood is continually flowing through the graft/fistula. Because it is completely enclosed under the skin, the infection rate is extremely low in comparison to catheters. A model of AV fistula has been developed for canine hemodialysis, and a brachial-cephalic access could be considered for dogs receiving chronic dialysis (Adin et al. 2002).

Catheter placement and care

Temporary, nontunneled catheters can be placed in an operating room, but are frequently placed in a clean

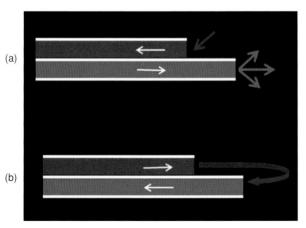

Figure 28.1 Configuration of arterial and venous lumen catheter tips. The tip of the "arterial" port, or intake port, is shorter than the "venous" port, or blood return port (1A). If the connections are reversed (1B), there is a greater percentage of returned blood that is immediately recirculated through the catheter.

Table 28.2 Common ERRT catheter specifications and approximate blood flow rates[a]

Manufacturer	Type	Lumens	Fr size	Length (cm)	Max blood flow (mL/min)
Quinton PermCath	Cuffed	2	15	45	370
Quinton PermCath	Cuffed	2	15	40	400
Quinton PermCath	Cuffed	2	15	36	410
MedComp Pediatric	Cuffed	2	8	18	120
Hohn	Cuffed	2	7	36	30
MedComp Temporary	Noncuffed	2	11.5	24	360[b]
Arrow[c]	Noncuffed	2	7	20	100
Arrow, 20 ga lumen[c]	Noncuffed	3	5.5	13	40
Arrow, 22 ga lumen[c]	Noncuffed	3	5.5	13	20
Arrow, 20 ga lumen[c]	Noncuffed	3	5.5	8	50
Arrow, 22 ga lumen[c]	Noncuffed	3	5.5	8	30
Intracath through the needle[c]	Noncuffed	1	19 ga	30.5	20

[a]Maximum blood flows determined in vitro using canine packed red blood cell solution (29% packed cell volume). Arterial chamber pressure maintained at −250 mmHg or higher. Maximum blood flow rates in vivo may be lower.
[b]Maximum blood flow determined in vivo.
[c] Not designed for dialysis.

procedure room. Caps, masks, gowns, gloves, and a large sterile drape should be used to maintain sterility during placement. Sedation and/or a local anesthetic may be necessary depending on the patient's clinical status and demeanor. These catheters are usually placed percutaneously (or through a small skin incision) with a guidewire using the Seldinger technique. Temporary hemodialysis catheters are intended for acute dialysis of less than a few weeks duration.

So-called permanent hemodialysis catheters have an external cuff, generally made of Dacron. The catheter is placed with a portion in a subcutaneous pocket, which separates the site where the catheter exits the skin from the site where the catheter enters the vessel by several centimeters. The Dacron cuff is positioned in this subcutaneous pocket and allows fibroblasts to adhere, thus securing the catheter in place and decreasing bacterial migration to the vessel. These catheters are intended for use for up to two years.

Cuffed, tunneled hemodialysis catheters should be placed in an operating room with full sterile technique. Although they can be placed with sedation and a local anesthetic in humans, general anesthesia is generally used when placing permanent catheters in veterinary patients. A skin incision is made over the vessel, and the jugular vein is cleared of all fascia. A separate small incision just large enough to allow placement of the catheter is made through the skin at the exit site. The tip of the catheter is placed through this incision and tunneled under the skin to exit at the skin incision over the vessel. A small venotomy incision is made and the catheter introduced into the vessel and advanced. Alter-

nately, the catheter can be tunneled under the skin and exit a small incision near the vessel. Instead of dissecting to the vessel for a venotomy, a guidewire can be placed into the vessel, followed by placement of a dilator inside a sheath. The dilator is removed and replaced with the catheter, and the sheath peels away, leaving the catheter in place. An esophagostomy or gastrostomy feeding tube is frequently placed at the same time as catheter placement.

The largest catheter that can be placed is preferred. Flow is proportional to the catheter diameter and inversely proportionally to catheter length. Minor changes in catheter diameter have very large changes in flow, based on Poiseuille equation: $Q_b = k \cdot P \cdot D^4/(L \cdot V)$, where Q_b is blood flow, k is a proportionality constant, P is the change in pressure, D is the luminal diameter, L is catheter length, and V is blood viscosity. A 19% increase in diameter doubles the blood flow; a 50% increase in the diameter of the catheter increases the flow five-fold (Depner 2001). Approximate blood flow rates for various catheters are presented in Table 28.2. For intermittent treatment, the catheter should ideally provide over 15 mL/kg/min blood flow. Flow rates of 3–5 mL/kg/min are adequate for CRRT.

With any method of placement, flow through both lumens of the catheter should be brisk when aspirated with a large syringe. Fluoroscopic guidance is helpful to ensure that the tip of the catheter is appropriately placed at the junction of the cranial vena cava and right atrium. If fluoroscopy is not used during placement, a postprocedure radiograph to confirm accurate placement should be performed.

The ERRT catheter should be used only for ERRT procedures and should be handled only by ERRT personnel. At each ERRT treatment, the exit site should be inspected and cleaned with antiseptic solution. When the ERRT catheter is accessed at the beginning and end of each ERRT treatment, or at any other time, the catheter ports should receive an aseptic scrub for 3–5 minutes. The ERRT technician should wear examination gloves and a mask when opening or closing the catheter. When not in use, the catheter is bandaged in place.

Between ERRT treatments, each lumen of the catheter is filled with an anticoagulant solution. Unfractionated heparin is currently used most commonly. A concentration of 500–1,000 unit/mL is generally used for cats, and 1,000–5,000 u/mL for dogs. A portion (15–20%) of the instilled heparin will diffuse out of the tip of the catheter (Sungur et al. 2007). An alternative locking solution is sodium citrate. A 4% trisodium citrate solution has similar rates of catheter thrombosis, dysfunction, and infection compared to 5000 u/mL heparin locking solution, with fewer episodes of major systemic bleeding (Grudzinski et al. 2007; MacRae et al. 2008). Higher citrate concentrations (>30%) are also antimicrobial (Weijmer et al. 2002; Weijmer et al. 2005). Any locking solution should be removed prior to the next use of the catheter, but with catheter malfunction, it is sometimes not possible to aspirate the locking solution. Injection of a highly concentrated (46.7%) citrate solution may cause symptomatic hypocalcemia and sudden death. Aspirin is routinely used in veterinary patients as an antiplatelet agent (0.5–2 mg/kg PO q 24 h in dogs, q 48 h in cats) to decrease catheter-associated thrombosis. Catheter function can decrease over time if thrombosis or stenosis occurs gradually, or it can decline abruptly. A simple way of monitoring function at each dialysis treatment is recording the blood speed when the pressure in the arterial chamber (pre-pump) is −200 mmHg. A gradual decline in the blood speed at a standardized pressure predicts catheter malfunction. The arterial pressure should be maintained above −200 to −250 mmHg, because at more negative values, the pump speed indicated on the machine is likely higher than the actual blood flow (Depner 2001).

Access recirculation decreases the efficiency of treatment by "diluting" the blood being withdrawn with blood that has just returned from the dialyzer and has a low concentration of uremic solutes. With the extracorporeal circuit blood lines attached in the normal configuration, recirculation is usually less than 5%, but reversing the connections such that blood is withdrawn from the distal port ("venous") increases recirculation to 13–24% (Carson et al. 2005). If the blood flow rate that can be achieved in this reversed configuration is much greater than the blood flow rate in the normal configuration, the increase in flow more than offsets the decrease in efficiency (Carson et al. 2005). During initial IHD treatments when efficiency is purposefully limited to decrease complications, the blood lines may be reversed to create recirculation.

Access recirculation can be measured by a variety of techniques, all of which seek to alter the venous line blood in some fashion and then detect the presence of altered blood in the arterial line blood. Some alterations include dilution with saline (detected by ultrasound or light transmission), change in temperature (cooling) or conductivity (added hypertonic saline), and hemoconcentration (via ultrafiltration) (Sherman and Kapoian 2008). The indicator dilution method is the most accurate method of determining access recirculation (Transonic Systems, Inc., Ithaca, NY). Injection of a bolus of saline in the venous line will dilute the blood, which will be detected by an ultrasonic sensor placed on the venous blood line. If there is recirculation, the blood entering the arterial line will also be diluted, to a smaller degree, which is measured by an arterial line ultrasonic sensor. The percent of blood recirculation is then calculated by the machine. Hemoglobin monitors (i.e., Critline III TQA, Hemametrics) can detect access recirculation by injection of saline first in the venous line, followed by saline injection in the arterial line, but are not accurate measures of recirculation compared to ultrasonic dilution technique (Lopot et al. 2003). Some dialysis machines have incorporated technology to automate measurement, utilizing changes in dialysate in lieu of injection of a substance directly into the blood line, and include use of temperature or conductivity changes. These measurements can be made repeatedly throughout the dialysis treatment.

Catheter complications

Despite the use of the least thrombogenic materials possible, hemodialysis catheters have a high rate of thrombosis. Thrombosis may be intraluminal or extraluminal. Both ports of the catheter should be flushed with saline or heparinized saline after every use (approximately 10–12 cc for a large catheter, 3–6 cc for smaller gauge catheters) to prevent intraluminal thrombosis. Each port is then filled with the locking solution (heparin, citrate, or other). Systemic anticoagulation has not been shown to decrease intraluminal thrombosis (Beathard 2001). Treatment of thrombosis should be initiated as soon as detected. Delays in treatment may decrease the adequacy of dialysis and may allow the thrombus to enlarge. Signs of intraluminal thrombosis include inadequate blood flow during dialysis, or an inability to aspirate the catheter. A first step to attempt is forceful flushing of the catheter with saline.

Dislodgement of the thrombus does not appear to cause clinically relevant pulmonary thromboembolic disease (Beathard 2001). If a saline flush does not restore catheter flow, tissue plasminogen activator (tPA) can be instilled in the occluded lumen (Alteplase, CathFlow, Genentech). The lumen is aspirated after a 10 minute dwell time, and if the thrombus is not aspirated, the dwell time is prolonged to 1–2 hours, with intermittent aspiration. If the catheter can be cleared sufficiently to perform a dialysis treatment, but flow remains suboptimal, tPA can be instilled in the catheter lumen for up to 48 hours and removed at the start of the next dialysis treatment (Lok et al. 2006). In our experience, tPA dwell protocols are successful in allowing sufficient blood flow to perform a dialysis treatment, but the effects are short-lived, with re-treatment or catheter replacement being necessary within a week.

Other methods of improving function of an occluded or partially occluded catheter include mechanical disruption. A guidewire can be placed in the catheter to dislodge a thrombus at the tip of the catheter, but is less effective at dislodging thrombi that have formed at side ports.

Extraluminal thrombi include thrombi that form around the tip of the catheter and may be attached to the vessel wall, and thrombi in the right atrium. These thrombi may act as a ball valve, allowing infusion but occluding the catheter and preventing aspiration. Thrombi in the right atrium and in the cranial vena cava near the heart may be imaged with echocardiography (Figure 28.3). Risk factors for thrombosis include venous stasis (from volume depletion, hypotension, immobilization, CHF), enhanced coagulability, and vessel wall trauma (Liangos et al. 2006). In our experience, over 50% of patients with a catheter in place for over 3 weeks

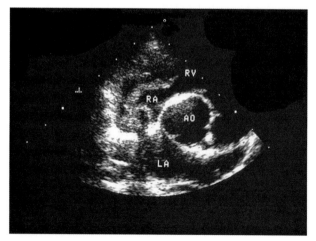

Figure 28.3 Echocardiogram of thrombus on tip of dialysis catheter. Thrombus is visible in the right atrium (RA), trailing into the right ventricle (RV). AO, aorta; LV, left ventricle.

have thrombus formation, based on routine surveillance. Thrombi can be detected echocardiographically in about 20% of our patients within 1 week of catheter placement, although catheter flow problems become apparent around 2 weeks after catheter placement.

Prophylactic administration of aspirin or warfarin decreases catheter thrombosis when compared with no treatment. Bleeding complications were more common with warfarin, and its routine use is not recommended for thrombus prevention (Willms and Vercaigne 2008).

If a small mural or right atrial thrombus is detected, the recommendation for people is 6 months of systemic anticoagulation. If the thrombus is large, the catheter should be removed and systemic anticoagulation started with unfractionated or low-molecular weight heparin for 5–7 days and warfarin for at least 1 month. If the thrombus is large and infected, surgical thrombectomy is recommended (Liangos et al. 2006). In veterinary patients, a long-standing thrombus may become covered with endothelium or fibrous tissue. Surgical removal has not been attempted in veterinary patients.

A sheath of fibrin may form around the catheter within 24 hours of placement, and this form of obstruction accounts for 38–50% of catheter malfunctions in people (Figure 28.4) (Liangos et al. 2006). In people, tPA infusion should likely be specified here. Infusion through the dialysis catheter over 2–3 hours during or after a dialysis treatment may be effective in disrupting a fibrin sheath (Lok et al. 2006).

Thrombolytic infusion to dissolve extraluminal thrombi or a fibrin sheath has been used with variable results in veterinary patients. A technique of fibrin sheath stripping involves placement of a femoral catheter advanced to cranial vena cava. A snare is used to encircle the fibrin sheath around the dialysis catheter and gently remove the sheath. This technique has not been attempted in veterinary medicine.

Replacement of the catheter over a guidewire is a simple and effective method of treating intraluminal thrombosis or fibrin sheath formation. A guidewire is placed in the dysfunctional catheter. If angiography is desired, the catheter is partially removed, leaving the tip within the vessel, and contrast agent is injected through the catheter. If a fibrin sheath is detected, the old catheter is removed and a balloon catheter inserted over the guidewire. The balloon is inflated to disrupt the fibrin sheath. A new catheter is placed over the guidewire, through the same exit site and subcutaneous tunnel (if present). Disrupting the fibrin sheath with catheter replacement has better results than catheter replacement alone in people (Oliver et al. 2007).

Careful attention to asepsis is necessary during the entire procedure. If angiography is not performed,

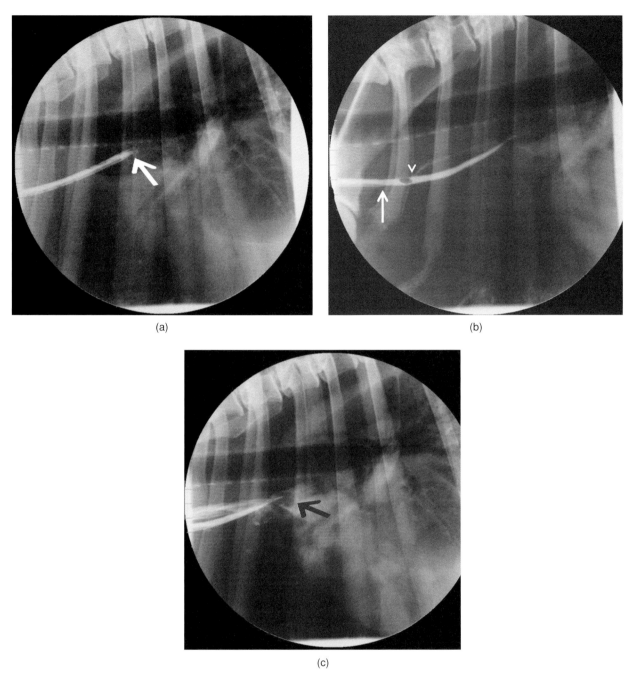

(a)

(b)

(c)

Figure 28.4 Nonselective angiogram of fibrin sheath. (a) Dialysis catheter is visible in cranial vena cava. The distal tip of the catheter is indicated by white arrow. (b) Catheter was partially retracted (distal tip indicated by white arrow) and contrast was injected through the catheter. A very narrow stream of contrast is visible within the fibrin sheath, with a breach in the fibrin sheath (arrowhead) allowing contrast to stream out of the sheath and into the surrounding cranial vena cava. (c) Contrast in and around the fibrin sheath demonstrates partial filling of the cranial vena cava. A filling defect (black arrow) indicates a thrombus that was at the tip of the dialysis catheter.

catheter replacement over a guidewire can be performed in the dialysis unit if needed.

Central venous stenosis occurs in 27–38% of human patients but is frequently asymptomatic (Liangos et al. 2006). The incidence and significance of this condition in veterinary patients is unknown, but facial edema, which can be a sign of cranial vena caval stenosis or obstruction, is a common finding in dogs receiving hemodialysis and stenosis may cause a marked decrease in dialysis treatment efficiency.

Infections are the most frequent serious complication of catheter use in people and are discussed more thoroughly in "Patient Management" section later (Himmelfarb et al. 2005). Inadvertent catheter dislodgement is an infrequent complication. During each dialysis treatment, the extracorporeal tubing is securely taped to a harness placed on dogs or directly to the forelimb in cats so that exuberant motion of the patient does not unduly stress the sutures anchoring the catheter in place.

Dialyzer

Almost all dialyzers used today are configured with the semi-permeable membrane arranged in hollow fibers. Blood flows through the center of the fibers, and the fibers are bathed in dialysate. This configuration provides a large surface area for diffusive clearance while minimizing the volume of blood used to fill the dialyzer. The fibers are held in place by potting material (termed header or footer, depending on position), and careful design helps allow blood to completely fill every fiber equally. Blood enters at the top of the dialyzer and exits at the bottom. Dialysate generally enters at the bottom and exits at the top, in order to maintain a countercurrent flow pattern that maximizes the concentration gradient across the length of the dialyzer.

The most common methods of dialyzer sterilization are ethylene oxide gas, heat, or gamma-irradiation, although some membranes cannot withstand heat sterilization (Hoenich and Ronco 2008a). All dialyzers need to be rinsed prior to use to remove any sterilant byproducts and microorganisms killed by the sterilization process (Hoenich and Ronco 2008a). In veterinary medicine, dialyzers are used for one dialysis treatment and then discarded. For people receiving chronic hemodialysis, a dialyzer may be rinsed, disinfected, and reused for up to 30 treatments in the same individual. Advantages of dialyzer reuse include cost savings (although the cost of disinfecting offsets replacement cost) and decrease in bioincompatibility reactions (see below). Disadvantages include increased time and equipment for the disinfection process, risk of infection, and risk of exposure of the patient to the disinfectant.

Semi-permeable membranes can be categorized as cellulosic, modified cellulosic, or synthetic. Cuprophane is an example of a cellulosic membrane. Modified cellulosic membranes, such as hemophan, have substituted hydroxyl groups with a substance less likely to activate the patient's complement system (Hoenich and Ronco 2008a). Although hemophan was the most commonly used dialyzer membrane in early years in veterinary dialysis, synthetic membranes are used almost exclusively now. Synthetic membranes have larger pores and allow better middle molecule clearance. They are also less reactive, thus decreasing bioincompatibility reactions. Examples of synthetic membranes include polysulfone, polymethylmethacrylate (PMMA), polycar-

bonate, polyamide, polyacrylonitrile and methallyl sulfonate (AN-69), and polyacrylonitrile polyacrylonitrile (PAN).

The ideal pore size in a dialyzer would allow easy passage of small- to middle-sized uremic toxins while restricting loss of albumin. Cellulosic and modified cellulosic membranes have smaller pores than synthetic membranes, which limits clearance of middle molecules. Synthetic membranes are thicker than cellulose-based membranes (20–55 μm versus 5–11 μm). The synthetic membranes have an asymmetric structure, with a dense blood contact surface and more open supporting structure (Hoenich and Ronco 2008a). Most dialyzer membranes have limited adsorptive capacity.

During the course of dialysis, blood is exposed to the dialysis catheter, blood lines, potting material of the dialyzer, the dialyzer membrane, and any contaminants in the water or dialysate. Any of these could potentially cause an adverse reaction. However, the dialysis membrane has the largest surface area and is the most likely component to induce the strongest biologic reaction. Cellulosic materials generally induce the strongest reaction, although clinically significant reactions may occur with the more biocompatible synthetic membranes.

Exposure of blood to the dialysis membrane activates the complement cascade, which activates the coagulation cascade. In addition to causing inflammation and thrombosis, contact proteins activated by exposure to the dialysis membrane convert high molecular weight kininogen to kinin. The kinins, including bradykinin, increase vascular permeability, diminish arterial resistance, and mediate inflammatory responses.

Within 15 minutes of starting dialysis, neutrophil and platelet counts decrease as these cells become sequestered in the pulmonary capillaries. The effect of a bioincompatibility reaction on lymphocytes is fairly minimal. Macrophages/monocytes play a more prominent role in this phenomenon. Monocytes become activated and increase production of cytokines such as interleukin-1β, tumor necrosis factor α, and interleukin-6. Within 3 to 4 hours, neutrophil and platelet counts return to pretreatment values. Neutrophil and platelet aggregation in the pulmonary capillaries impairs oxygen transport. Additionally, complement components induce airway and vessel constriction and increase edema in the lungs due to an increase in permeability, further decreasing oxygen transport. Other clinical signs of a dialyzer reaction include hypertension, hypotension, dyspnea, cough, sneezing, wheezing, choking, rhinorrhea, conjunctival injection, headache, muscle cramps, back pain, abdominal pain, chest pain, nausea, vomiting, fever, chills, flushing, urticaria, pruritis, and death (Jaber and Pereira 2005; Hoenich and Ronco 2008b).

Complement activation can be decreased by cooling the blood, which can be achieved by setting the dialysate temperature slightly lower than body temperature. Adhesion of proteins such as albumin to the dialyzer membrane decreases the bioincompability reaction, and subsequent reuse of dialyzers reduces the reaction. Since synthetic membranes are much less likely to induce significant first use reactions, reuse is becoming less common in human hemodialysis.

Clearance of a dialyzer is the volume of blood completely cleared of a certain solute during a single pass through the device and is identical to the concept of clearance in the kidney. Dialyzer clearance is calculated by measuring the concentration of the substance at the inlet and outflow of the dialyzer, at standardized blood flow (usually 200, 300, and 400 mL/min), dialysate flow (500 mL/min), and ultrafiltration (0) rates. Clearance of urea, creatinine, phosphorus, vitamin B12, and inulin are commonly reported, as substances of interest, or markers of other solute clearance (i.e., vitamin B12 (MW 1355 Da) and inulin (MW 5200 Da) as markers of middle molecule clearance). Clearance is reported in mL/min and abbreviated $K_{d[solute]}$. Dialyzer specification data is derived from in vitro measurements, and actual performance is generally slightly lower.

The coefficient of ultrafiltration (K_{UF}) is a measure of the hydraulic permeability of the membrane, or the water flux. It is the number of milliliters of water that can be removed per hour for each 1 mmHg transmembrane pressure (the difference in hydraulic pressure between the blood compartment and the dialysate compartment). Dialyzers with a higher K_{UF} can remove larger volumes of fluid from the patient in a given time with a lower transmembrane pressure. In the average veterinary dialysis patient, even dialyzers with a low K_{UF} can remove adequate volumes of fluid to normalize patient hydration. Because of the decrease in hydrostatic pressure from the top to the bottom of the blood fibers, and because of the increase in oncotic pressure at the bottom of the dialyzer due to ultrafiltration and the resultant hemoconcentration, it is possible to get back-filtration at the bottom of the dialyzer. Back-filtration allows endotoxins or other contaminants from the dialysate to enter the blood compartment. Back-filtration is more likely to occur when a dialyzer with a high K_{UF} is used without ultrafiltration. In order to prevent this from occurring when a dialyzer with a high K_{UF} is being used, a nominal rate of ultrafiltration should always be applied, with intravenous fluid replacement if the patient does not need fluid removal.

High-flux dialyzers are characterized by a membrane with larger pore size, which possess high ultrafiltration coefficients and permits clearance of middle molecules (Jaber and Pereira 2005; Yeun and Depner 2005). High-efficiency dialyzers have high urea clearance by virtue of the large surface area, but they also have a larger priming volume (Table 28.3).

Extracorporeal circuit

Extracorporeal circuit is the tubing that carries the blood from the catheter to the machine and dialyzer and returns it to the patient. It should be made from a nonthrombogenic material. The pressure in the extracorporeal circuit before and after the dialyzer is routinely monitored by the dialysis machine, to detect any unsafe conditions, such as a line disconnection or occlusion. Any air–blood interface creates a potential site for thrombosis. The dialysis machine detects any air bubbles in the venous return segment, which triggers automatic clamping of the blood line until the situation is corrected. The volume of blood contained in the extracorporeal circuit depends on the specific tubing used and should be selected based on the patient's size.

Dialysate

Dialysate is the solution that bathes the blood-filled hollow fibers in the dialyzer. It is physiologically similar to the aqueous portion of plasma. A typical IHD treatment uses 150 L of water for dialysate. Contaminants in the water can diffuse into the bloodstream, and as discussed above, some small volume of dialysate may enter the blood compartment via back-filtration. Multiple steps are involved in purifying water used for dialysate.

Water quality

The appropriate design of a water treatment system depends on the quality of source water and may include all or most of the following components. A filter, such as a mixed bed multimedia filter, removes particulate matter in the water. An ion exchanger absorbs cations and anions and releases sodium and chloride in exchange. The predominant ions removed in this fashion are calcium and magnesium. Carbon filtration adsorbs organic toxins, including chlorine and chloramines. A small filter is placed after the carbon tanks to catch small particles of carbon that became dislodged. Reverse osmosis is usually the final step in water purification. Pressure applied to the water forces it through a semi-permeable membrane that excludes contaminants. Deionization can be used instead of reverse osmosis. With deionization, cations are bound to the resin, releasing H^+, and anions are bound, releasing OH^-. All of the pipes and materials the water contacts should be PVC, stainless steel, or glass to avoid leeching of potentially toxic components (such as copper or zinc). There should be no dead-end loops in the system because

Table 28.3 Common dialyzers used in veterinary ERRT

Manufacturer/ machine	Dialyzer	Membrane	Surface area (m^2)	Priming volume — dialyzer (mL)	Priming volume — dialyzer and tubing (mL)	Kd$_{urea}$ (mL/min)	Kd$_{creat}$ (mL/min)	Kd$_{phos}$ (mL/min)	Kd$_{B12}$ (mL/min)	K$_{UF}$ (mL/h/mmHg)
Conventional										
Gambro	100HG[bcd]	Hemophan	0.22	18		102	82	69	25	2.0
Fresenius	F3	Polysulfone	0.4	28		125	95	50	20	1.7
Fresenius	F4	Polysulfone	0.7	42		155	128	78	32	2.8
Fresenius	F5	Polysulfone	1.0	63		170	149	103	45	4.0
High-efficiency										
Gambro	500HG[c]	Hemophan	1.1	58		184	171	144	66	7.6
Fresenius	F8	Polysulfone	1.8	110		186	172	138	76	7.5
Medium-flux										
Fresenius	F40	Polysulfone	0.7	42		165	140	138	75	20
Fresenius	F80 M	Polysulfone	1.8	110		190	177	170	110	27
High-flux										
Fresenius	F160 NR	Polysulfone	1.5	84		194	181	178	128	45
Fresenius	F200 NR	Polysulfone	2	112		195	191	183	148	56
Gambro	Polyflux 140 H	Polyamix™	1.4	94		193	181	174	128	60
Gambro	Polyflux 170 H	Polyamix™	1.7	115		196	186	180	137	70
Prisma CRRT sets										
Gambro Prisma	M10[g]	AN-69	0.042	3.5	45	9.7	8.1		3.6	
Gambro Prisma	M60[a,e]	AN-69	0.6	48	90	37	30	29	25	15
Gambro Prisma	M100[b,e,f]	AN-69	0.9	65	107	43	33	32	35	22

Measurements performed in vitro at Qb = 200 mL/min, Qd = 500 mL/min, UF = 0, except where otherwise noted.
[a] Q_b = 100 mL/min, UF = 5 mL/min
[b] Q_b = 150 mL/min
[c] UF = 13 mL/min
[d] Discontinued
[e] Q_d = 2 L/h (33 mL/min)
[f] UF = 10 mL/min
[g] Q_b = 20 ml/min, Q_d = 1 L/h, UF = 1 ml/min
Polyamix™ = Polyarylethersulfone, polyvinylpyrrolidone, and polyamide
With some dialysis machines, various tubing configurations are available, allowing flexibility with tubing volume. The Gambro CentrySystem 3 and Phoenix machines have specific tubing sets. The tubing volume for the neonatal set is 40 mL, and the volume for the pediatric set is 75 mL. The volume of the dialyzer is added to this volume to determine the total extracorporeal circuit volume. With the Gambro Prisma, the tubing and dialyzer are one integrated set.

they increase the risk of bacterial growth. Hot and cold water entering the system are usually blended to enhance function because excessively hot or cold water decreases the efficiency of the reverse osmosis machine. Routine maintenance of the system is performed to maintain adequate function and to disinfect the system. In most new models of dialysis machines, an additional filtration step is provided by the dialysis machine, using a device similar to a dialyzer. Using the same principles of ultrafiltration, dialysate entering the device is ultrafiltered, and the ultrafiltrate is passed to the patient dialyzer, leaving behind any

bacterial contaminants or endotoxins, producing what is termed ultrapure dialysate.

Water treatment systems can be sized to produce adequate water for one or many dialysis machines. Self-contained water treatment systems with the capacity to produce only enough water for one dialysis machine are available and are designed to attach to the back of the dialysis machine.

Water and dialysate should routinely be tested for chemical and bacterial contamination. Culture media should be restricted in nutrients (i.e., tryptic soy agar) and a pour plate method is preferable to a calibrated loop method. The Association for the Advancement of Medical Instrumentation (AAMI) has established standards for dialysis water quality. Standard dialysis water should have a bacterial count of less than 200 CFU/mL, and prepared dialysate should have a count less than 2,000 CFU/mL. Endotoxin levels are commonly measured using the limulus ameobocyte lysate assay and should be less than 0.25 endotoxin units/mL. Ultrapure dialysate should have fewer than 0.1 CFU/mL bacterial count and <0.03 endotoxin units/mL. Continuous renal replacement therapies generally use prepackaged sterile dialysate, thus avoiding the necessity for a water treatment system and associated monitoring. In addition to bacterial contaminants, AAMI has established guidelines for acceptable levels of chemical components of water (Table 28.4).

Production of cytokines in dialysis patients is related to the endotoxin load in the dialysate and the permeability of the dialysis membrane to endotoxin. Whether use of ultrapure dialysate will decrease chronic inflammatory conditions associated with dialysis has not clearly been established yet (Bommer and Jaber 2006).

Table 28.4 AAMI guidelines for dialysate water

Contaminant	Allowable range (mg/L = ppm)
Sodium	0–70
Potassium	0–8
Alminum	0–0.01
Calcium	0–2
Copper	0–0.1
Magnesium	0–4
Selenium	0–0.09
Zinc	0–0.1
Chromium	0–0.014
Lead	0–0.005
Arsenic	0–0.005
Mercury	0–0.0002
Cadmium	0–0.001
Beryllium	0–0.0004
Antimony	0–0.006
Thallium	0–0.002
Silver	0–0.005
Barium	0–0.1
Fluoride	0–0.2
Nitrate	0–2
Sulfate	0–100

Bacteriological:
• Maximum 200 CFU (colony forming unit) for RO water
• Maximum 2,000 CFU for dialysate
Endotoxin: 2 EU (endotoxin units)

Clinical toxicity may occur with inadequately treated water. Municipal water treatment facilities add aluminum sulfate or alum to water to clear flocculent debris, and this aluminum must be completely removed before use in dialysate. Signs of aluminum toxicity in people include neurologic signs, including personality change, decreased short-term memory, speech disturbance, myoclonic muscle spasm, hallucinations, seizures, and dementia; bone disease (such as osteomalacia, osteodystrophy); and microcytic hypochromic anemia. Chloramines are added to water as bactericidal agents. Toxic effects of chloramines are primarily hematologic, including hemolysis, heinz body anemia, and methemoglobinemia. Fluoride is added to prevent dental disease, but overexposure to fluoride can cause osteomalacia and osteoporosis. Copper can leech from copper pipes in the water system. Signs of copper toxicosis include chills, nausea, headaches, liver damage, and hemolysis. Zinc can also leech from pipes or galvanized containers and causes nausea, vomiting, fever, and anemia. Nitrates are not added to water via the treatment process, but may appear due to bacterial contamination or run-off from fertilizers used in the area of the source water. Nitrates cause methemoglobinemia, cyanosis, hypotension, nausea, and potentially hemolysis. Sulphates may cause nausea, vomiting, or metabolic acidosis. Although calcium and magnesium are normally found in the body, extremely high levels, as may occur with malfunction of the water-softening process, can cause nausea, vomiting, muscular weakness, skin flushing, hypertension, or hypotension. An extremely high sodium level could occur if the ion exchanger goes through a regeneration cycle during the dialysis treatment (D'Haese and De Broe 1996; Langston 2004).

Dialysate production

Purified water is combined with the electrolyte and buffer solutions to create the final dialysate. With IHD, the dialysis delivery machine performs this procedure, creating dialysate at a rate of 300–800 mL/min. A highly concentrated salt solution, containing sodium, chloride, glucose, and other components as desired (potassium, calcium, magnesium) is diluted with the purified water to the desired sodium concentration, based on measurement of conductivity. The concentration of other components will be proportional to the sodium concentration and cannot be individually adjusted by the dialysis machine. However, different salt solutions can be used, such as potassium-free or calcium-free solutions. Bicarbonate is provided individually, and the concentration can be adjusted independent of the sodium concentration. An alternate method of producing dialysate involves mixing the salt and buffer solutions with water in a large bulk tank, where it is stored until being piped to the individual dialysis machines in the unit. Every patient in the unit would use the same dialysate composition. With continuous therapies (CRRT), dialysate is prepackaged in sterile bags, similar to intravenous fluids. This has the advantage of sterility and ease of use, but the disadvantages of large storage requirements and higher cost. Dialysate flow rates are much lower in CRRT (0–2.5 L/hour) compared to IHD ($\approx$30 L/hour).

Dialysis machine

There are several basic types of dialysis machines, also called the dialysis delivery system. In general, machines are designed to be used either for intermittent or for continuous therapy. IHD machines can be used to provide sustained low-efficiency dialysis (SLED) treatments in addition to highly efficient intermittent treatments. CRRT machines are usually smaller and more mobile because they do not need to produce dialysate. In the past several years, "hybrid" machines have become available, which are intended to perform both intermittent and continuous therapies. Some machines (e.g., Fresenius 2008 K) are adaptations of intermittent machines. The NxStage machine is intended to be a portable home hemodialysis machine for intermittent treatment, using prepackaged dialysate in bags. Many machines approved for use in Europe have the capability of on-line hemodialfiltration, which means they can provide large volumes of solutions to infuse into the patient as replacement fluid, in addition to producing large volumes of dialysate.

In the United States most veterinary units performing IHD use either Gambro (Centrysystem 3 or Phoenix models) or Fresenius machines. The Gambro machines have a cartridge system for the extracorporeal circuit that includes all the necessary tubing in one piece. The dialyzer is separate. The snap-in cartridge simplifies machine set-up, but limits tubing choices. In the Fresenius machine, several tubing components are incorporated separately during machine set-up. This provides more flexibility with tubing sizing and volumes, as well as multiple choices for independent manufacturers, but lacks the simplicity of the Gambro machines. Most US units performing CRRT use the Gambro Prisma (now discontinued) machine. The Prisma utilizes a combined dialyzer and extracorporeal circuit. This allows almost automated machine set-up, but limits selection to three available options (plus a plasmapheresis cartridge option).

The ERRT machine has many built-in sensors and alarms to ensure patient safety. In addition to pressure sensors and air bubble detectors mentioned above, the dialysis machine monitors the waste dialysate for evidence of blood leak. Dialysate composition and tempera-

ture are constantly monitored. If any unsafe or potentially unsafe conditions are detected in the dialysate, dialysate flow is diverted from the dialyzer. If blood path conditions are potentially compromised, the blood pump stops and the blood lines are automatically clamped. On-screen instructions notify the operator of the specific alarm, which must be remedied in order to restart the treatment. Despite the myriad, and in many cases, duplicate, monitors installed in the machine, operator error can still occur. Only personnel specifically trained to use and troubleshoot the specific machine should be performing ERRT treatments.

Prescription

Methods of clearance

Diffusion is defined as the movement of particles from an area of higher concentration to an area of lower concentration. Particles in solution have kinetic energy causing movement, and smaller particles tend to have more movement than larger particles. If two identical solutions are separated by a membrane that is permeable to a substance, individual particles may cross the membrane in either direction, and although the individual particle on either side of the membrane may change, there is no net change in the concentration of particles. If, however, the concentration on one side is lower, there will be net diffusion from the higher concentration to the lower concentration. Over time, the two solutions will equilibrate to the same concentration on both sides. The higher the concentration gradient between the two sides, the faster the rate of diffusion. With dialytic therapies (including extracorporeal and peritoneal), the solution on one side of the membrane is the blood, and dialysate is the solution on the other side of the membrane. By constant replenishment of the dialysate, a large concentration gradient is maintained and equilibrium is never reached, so diffusive clearance continues. Extracorporeal therapies have a constant dialysate flow, although the rate of dialysate flow generally varies dramatically between intermittent and continuous therapies. Extremely fast dialysate flow rates maximize diffusive clearance, and flow rates of 300–800 mL/min are typical with IHD (usually 500 mL/min). Continuous therapies in a diffusive clearance mode typically use lower dialysate flow rates (up to 40 mL/min). PD involves instillation of a discrete volume of dialysate that is periodically removed and replaced with fresh dialysate. During the dwell time, diffusion occurs.

Although we are composed of approximately 60% water and could not live without it, water can be considered a "uremic toxin" that needs to be removed in the oliguric renal failure patient. Diuretics may be ineffective in this patient population, leaving ultrafiltration (UF) as the only effective means of removing fluid. As opposed to diffusion, in which a concentration gradient causes solute movement, UF involves a hydrostatic pressure gradient to cause water movement. By creating negative pressure on the side opposite the blood compartment, water is "pulled" out of the blood. The water removed in this fashion is termed ultrafiltrate. With machines used today, the transmembrane pressure is automatically controlled by the dialysis machine to achieve the desired fluid removal in the time specified.

Convective clearance removes solutes by removing the water in which they are dissolved, a process that is also called solute drag. Middle molecules (compounds with a molecular weight of 500 to 5,000 Da) are more efficiently cleared with convection compared to diffusion, whereas diffusion is a very efficient method of removing small molecules (e.g., urea, creatinine, sodium). The term hemofiltration indicates using convective clearance for uremic toxin removal. When UF is used for net fluid removal, convective clearance will occur. If a larger degree of convective clearance is desired, the UF rate can be increased dramatically (up to 35 mL/kg/h or higher), with administration of intravenous fluids to avoid volume depletion.

Certain substances, like cytokines, will bind to the dialyzer membrane and thus can be removed from the circulation. The adsorptive capacity of the dialysis membrane is limited, and some studies show saturation after about 30 minutes, making this an ineffective method of removal (Lonneman et al. 2001). Charcoal and other hemoperfusion techniques are better suited for significant adsorption.

Prescription components

Although the overall goal of hemodialysis is to control uremic symptoms, the specific goals of an individual treatment vary based on the situation. The components of a dialysis prescription include modality (i.e., intermittent versus continuous), schedule (i.e., daily versus alternate day), intensity (i.e., amount of blood processed, convective clearance rate, and diaysate flow rate), dialyzer type and size, dialysate composition, and UF rate.

Prescribing the dialysis dose requires an ability to predict the adequacy of treatment. The most commonly used measure of clearance in veterinary hemodialysis is the urea reduction ratio (URR), which can be calculated by the formula: (pre-treatment BUN—post-treatment BUN)/pre-treatment BUN. The most commonly used measure of dialysis dose in humans is Kt/V, a dimensionless unit of measurement that incorporates the dialyzer clearance, time on dialysis, and volume of distribution. The adequacy of dialysis is discussed more fully below.

Mode and schedule

The mode and schedule recommended differs for acute and chronic disease. With acute kidney injury, the two major initial considerations are the rate of clearance and the intensity of treatment. When azotemia is severe, rapid clearance may induce dialysis disequilibrium syndrome. One method of limiting clearance during the initial few dialysis treatments is a short dialysis treatment time, coupled with a moderately slow blood flow rate. The target URR of 0.25–0.5 can be reached in 1.5 hours at a blood flow rate of 3–5 mL/kg/min. Despite the low overall clearance, this rate can induce complications, particularly in severely uremic patients (BUN > 200 mg/dL) or small patients. An alternative approach would be sustained low efficiency dialysis (SLED) or CRRT. SLED is performed with an IHD machine and involves a very slow blood flow rate (1–3 mL/kg/min) for 6–24 hours. CRRT also uses a similar slow blood flow rate, markedly slower dialysate flow rate (0–40 mL/min for CRRT versus 300–500 mL/min for IHD), and frequently relies on more convective clearance than most IHD prescriptions. Despite these differences, SLED and CRRT appear to have similar outcomes (Berbece and Richardson 2006; Ghahramani et al. 2008).

The hemodynamic stability of the patient is another factor that is generally included in the decision of dialysis modality. CRRT and SLED are generally preferred in the hemodynamically unstable patient. Rapid fluid removal in IHD treatments can cause hypotension, which is thought to induce on going renal damage (Conger 1990). Slow or continuous fluid removal in SLED or CRRT intuitively is less likely to cause intermittent hypotension. Although clinical impressions support this, there is no evidence of superior hemodynamic stability in SLED or CRRT compared to IHD in randomized trials (John et al. 2001; Gasparovic et al. 2003; Uchino 2008).

Treatment intensity for acute kidney injury is an area of on going research. Although CRRT does not improve survival rates compared to IHD, early studies suggested that renal recovery was more complete with CRRT, with more patients becoming dialysis independent (Mehta et al. 2001; Bell et al. 2007; Uchino et al. 2007). In a recently published meta-analysis, modality did not affect survival or renal recovery outcomes, although a subsequent study did find a lower rate of dialysis dependence with CRRT compared to IHD (Bell et al. 2007; Ghahramani et al. 2008). However, intermittent IHD is less resource-intensive. Daily 6–8 hour treatments (6–7 days a week) can be performed by day staff. Although some studies have shown a survival advantage with a higher dialysis dose, results have been inconsistent, and a recently published randomized trial showed no advantage to intensive therapy (daily IHD/daily SLED with a

Kt/V of 1.2 per treatment or CRRT with a total effluent of 35 mL/kg/h) compared to less intensive therapy (alternate day IHD/SLED with a Kt/V of 1.2 per treatment or CRRT with a total effluent of 20 mL/kg/h) (Ronco et al. 2000; Bouman et al. 2002; Schiffl et al. 2002; Saudan et al. 2006; Network 2008; Tolwani et al. 2008). During the recovery phase of acute kidney injury, a less intensive schedule (4–5 hour treatments three times a week, decreasing to twice weekly as function improves) may be adequate.

The typical human patient on hemodialysis for chronic kidney disease has traditionally been treated 3–4 hours three days a week. In veterinary medicine, treatment times have been longer (4 hours for cats, 5 hours for dogs) to provide better clearance. Occasionally, patients with significant residual renal clearance may be maintained on twice weekly treatments, although this likely represents the minimal recommendation that will be beneficial to the patient (Cowgill 2008).

Alternative schedules for chronic hemodialysis are being used more frequently for human patients. Daily dialysis with 1.5–2.5 hour treatments 6–7 days a week provides more complete control of uremia (Kjellstrand et al. 2008). Nocturnal dialysis involves 7–10 hour treatments while the patient sleeps and allows people on chronic dialysis to maintain a more normal daytime schedule, but this schedule is not advantageous in veterinary dialysis. Home hemodialysis for chronic kidney disease is possible for people, with remote monitoring and ready access to support staff via telephone (for both daytime and nocturnal dialysis treatments), but is unlikely to be feasible in veterinary dialysis because most patients currently have acute rather than chronic disease, and the support network is not established.

Guidelines for treatment intensity for veterinary patients have been established through clinical experience (Table 28.5). After determining the desired URR, the number of liters of blood to be processed to achieve the goal are based on weight of the patient and can be estimated from Figures 28.5 and 28.6. In early treatments, a slow rate of reduction decreases complications, so a longer treatment duration is selected, whereas in later treatments, a rapid blood flow rate can achieve the treatment goals faster (or achieve greater clearance in a set time interval). Once the desired amount of blood to be processed and the duration of treatment are selected, the average blood flow rate to achieve these goals can easily be calculated.

Limiting factors for blood flow rate are the catheter and the patient. Larger diameter catheters can provide much faster blood flow rates than smaller catheters (Table 28.2). Minor hemolysis may occur if the pressure in the "arterial" limb of the extracorporeal circuit before the

Table 28.5 Treatment intensity prescription guidelines (adapted from Cowgill 2008)

1st treatment	
BUN <200 mg/dL	URR < 0.5 @ no greater than 0.1 URR per hour
200–300 mg/dL	URR 0.3–0.5 @ no greater than 0.1 URR per hour
>300 mg/dL	URR ≤ 0.3 @ no greater than 0.05–0.07 URR per hour
2nd treatment	
BUN < 200 mg/dL	URR 0.6–0.7 @ 0.01–0.15 URR per hour
200–300 mg/dL	URR 0.4–0.6 @ 0.10–0.12 URR per hour
>300 mg/dL	URR ≤ 0.4 URR @ no greater than 0.05–0.1 URR per hour
3rd and subsequent treatments	
BUN < 150 mg/dL	URR > 0.8 @ > 0.15 URR per hour
150–300 mg/dL	URR 0.5–0.6 @ 0.10–0.15 URR per hour
>300 mg/dL	URR 0.5–0.6 @ < 0.1 URR per hour

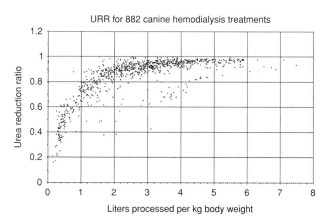

Figure 28.5 Treatment intensity (urea reduction ratio) as a function of amount of blood processed in dogs. Treatments with over 8 L/kg of processed blood were excluded.

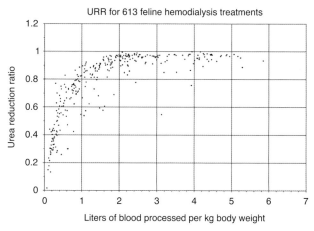

Figure 28.6 Treatment intensity (urea reduction ratio) as a function of amount of blood processed in cats.

Table 28.6 Recommended extracorporeal volumes for ERRT in dogs and cats (adapted from Cowgill 2008)

Species	Body weight	Dialyzer volume	Total extracorporeal volume (mL)	% Blood volume
Cats, dogs	<6 kg	<20 mL	<60 mL	13–40%
Cats	>6 kg	<30 mL	<70 mL	<23%
Dogs	6–12 kg	<45 mL	<90 mL	9–19%
Dogs	12–20 kg	<80 mL	100–160 mL	6–17%
Dogs	20–30 kg	<120 mL	150–200 mL	6–13%
Dogs	≥30 kg	>80 mL	150–250 mL	6–10%

blood pump is more negative than -350 mmHg (Twardowski 2000). Of more clinical significance, prepump pressures more negative than -200 mmHg will cause the pump to deliver less blood flow than is indicated, causing an overestimation of the amount of dialysis delivered (Daugirdas 1994). If the blood flow rate is less than desired due to catheter flow problems, the treatment time may need to be prolonged to achieve the desired clearance.

Dialyzer and extracorporeal circuit selection

Various dialyzers are available. Differences in the membrane type were discussed above. The choice of dialyzer size depends on desired clearance and patient size. Although pediatric hemodialysis recommendations include limiting the total volume of the extracorporeal circuit and dialyzer to less than 10% of the infant's blood volume, this guideline may be impractical in veterinary dialysis (Table 28.6) (Ellis 2008). In a standard treatment, the largest feasible dialyzer is generally preferred, but for the first 1–3 treatments, when slower clearance is desired, a slightly smaller dialyzer is generally recommended.

When preparing for the dialysis treatment, the dialyzer is flushed with saline to remove any particulate matter or residual disinfectant or materials from production. This solution is discarded and refreshed with saline that will be infused into the patient as the blood is being withdrawn, and this volume of saline helps maintain the patient's blood pressure. In small animals, if the total extracorporeal circuit volume represents >20% blood volume, a colloid solution is used instead of saline. Dextran 70 6% can be diluted with an equal volume of saline, to provide colloid support without risking excessive volume overload, or other colloid solutions such as Hetastarch can be used. In rare situations, diluted oxyglobin can be used as a priming solution. Priming with banked blood is commonly performed with human pediatric patients. At the end of the treatment, the patient's blood is not returned, to avoid volume overload. A blood prime is not commonly used in veterinary medicine for IHD for

various practical reasons, including limited availability of blood for daily treatments and concern about transfusion reaction due to the rapid infusion rate. With CRRT, theoretically the same circuit can be used for 3 days, potentially reducing some of the mentioned concerns.

Dialysate composition

The composition of dialysate is similar to the composition of plasma water. The sodium concentration can be readily adjusted to avoid large or rapid changes in the patient. Sodium profiling is a feature of most machines that allows the dialysate sodium concentration to automatically adjust throughout the treatment to a match a preset pattern. The dialysate sodium may be set slightly higher than the patient's at the start of the treatment and gradually decreased to normal over the course of the treatment. This profile enhances diffusion of sodium into the patient early in the course of treatment when urea removal is most rapid, and helps maintain a stable patient osmolality, thus decreasing the risk of dialysis disequilibrium syndrome. The sodium concentration is lowered by the end of the treatment to avoid loading the patient with sodium, which can enhance thirst and water retention in the interdialysis interval (Stiller et al. 2001). Sodium profiling is not possible with CRRT because dialysate is supplied in premixed sterile bags, but sodium profiling is not necessary given the slow and continual nature of CRRT.

Because the dialysis machine proportions the dialysate concentrate based on the sodium concentration, individual adjustments of other dialysate components are not possible, but can be made by using different concentrates. Dialysate typically contains approximately 3 mEq/L of potassium, but potassium-free dialysate is used for hyperkalemic patients. Several concentrations of dialysate calcium are available, including calcium-free dialysate, used with some citrate anticoagulation protocols (see below). Various magnesium concentrations are also available. Bicarbonate is incorporated separately and can be adjusted independently from sodium concentration. To combat metabolic acidosis that is commonly present, the dialysate bicarbonate concentration is usually higher than the patient's, allowing diffusion of bicarbonate from the dialysate into the patient. The typical dialysate bicarbonate concentration used in people (35 mEq/L) leads to panting in dogs; a slightly lower concentration (30 mEq/L) is typically used in veterinary hemodialysis. If acidosis is severe, a high dialysate bicarbonate concentration may cause paradoxic CNS acidosis and dialysis disequilibrium syndrome.

Although most intermittent dialysis treatments use a dialysate flow rate of 500 mL/min, the dialysate flow rate is adjustable. With IHD, clearance depends more on blood flow rate than on dialysate flow rate. At a slow blood flow rate and rapid dialysate flow rate, blood leaving the dialyzer may be completely cleared of a solute. With a fast blood flow rate and the same dialysate flow rate, the blood spends less time in the dialyzer and a lower percentage of the solute is extracted. For example, at a blood flow rate of 20 mL/min, blood entering the dialyzer with a urea concentration of 100 mg/dL may have a 0 mg/dL concentration when leaving the dialyzer. At a blood flow rate of 200 mL/min, blood entering the dialyzer with a urea concentration of 100 mg/dL may have a 30 mg/dL concentration when leaving. In the first example, 20 mL/min of blood are completely cleared of urea, whereas in the second example, 140 mL/min of blood are completely cleared. Thus, despite the decrease in efficiency from 100% to 70% clearance in one pass, there is an overall greater clearance with a higher blood flow rate. Increasing the dialysate flow rate from 500 mL/min to 800 mL/min will increase the clearance by 5–10%, if the blood flow rate is already at very high rate (>350 mL/min). A lower dialysate flow rate (i.e., 300 mL/min) will modestly decrease clearance. Dialysate flow rates in CRRT are generally between 0 and 40 mL/min. With CRRT, dialysate is saturated with one pass through the dialyzer, and faster dialysate flow rates have a substantial effect on clearance (Clark and Ronco 2001).

In most treatments, dialysate flows from the bottom of the dialyzer to the top, while blood flows in the opposite direction, to maximize the concentration gradient across the length of the dialyzer. By reversing the dialysate connectors, dialysate can flow in a concurrent direction instead of countercurrent, thus decreasing efficiency by about 10%, which may be indicated in the first 1–3 treatments (Yeun and Depner 2005).

Blood leaving the dialyzer is in thermic equilibrium with the dialysate. Higher patient temperatures promote vasodilation of the skin and periphery, which may cause cardiovascular instability and intradialytic hypotension. A dialysate temperature slightly (2°C) below body temperature promotes mild patient cooling and vasocon-

striction to the periphery and decreases the risk of intradialytic hypotension (Selby and McIntyre 2006). Because basal temperatures of dogs and cats are higher than that for humans, dialysate temperature settings available with currently used machines are typically slightly below normal for veterinary patients.

When dialysis is used for nonrenal indications, such as removal of a toxin, hypophosphatemia can develop as a result of rapid clearance of phosphorus. Although phosphorous concentration may rebound shortly after the dialysis treatment, there is a risk of hemolysis with severe hypophosphatemia (serum phosphorus <1.0 mg/dL). Addition of phosphate to the dialysate may prevent this from occurring. Addition of 16 mL of a neutral sodium phosphate (Fleet Enema, Fleet Brand Pharmaceuticals, C.B. Fleet Company, Inc., Lynchbrg, VA) per liter of dialysate concentrate produces a dialysate concentration of approximately 2 mg/dL (Cowgill 2008).

Ethylene glycol intoxication is efficiently treated with hemodialysis. Fomepizole (Antizole-Vet, Jazz Pharmaceuticals, Palo Alto, CA) or ethanol should be administered intravenously as soon as possible to delay metabolism of ethylene glycol while the patient is being prepared for dialysis. Because ethanol is also readily dialyzable, addition of ethanol to the dialysate can maintain a steady state in the patient. Enough ethanol is added to create a 0.1% ethanol concentration in the dialysate (Cowgill 2008).

Ultrafiltration

The desired volume of UF depends on the patient's hydration status. Some patients may be 10–25% overhydrated, in the most severe cases. In severe cases, the excess fluid cannot generally be removed in a single short dialysis treatment because the rate of fluid removal should not exceed 20 mL/kg/h, to avoid intradialytic hypotension. Some newer machines can be set to remove fluid at variable rates during the dialysis treatment. An effective profile involves a faster rate of fluid removal at the beginning of the treatment, when the extra fluid is readily accessible in the bloodstream, and a slower rate toward the end, to account for a slower transfer from the interstitium to bloodstream and thus to dialyzer as the patient nears the optimal fluid status (Stiller et al. 2001). In IHD, with its high dialysate flow rate, the addition of UF for convective clearance contributes relatively little to the overall solute clearance (Yeun and Depner 2005).

Single needle dialysis

If only one vascular access lumen is available, either because a single lumen catheter was placed or because one lumen of a double lumen catheter is nonfunctional, dialysis can be performed in what is termed single-needle mode. A Y-connector is attached to the single lumen so that both the "arterial" and "venous" extracorporeal tubing segments can be attached. The venous side is automatically clamped while the blood pump draws blood from the arterial side into the dialyzer. Blood already in the dialyzer is displaced into a reservoir placed in the extracorporeal circuit on the venous return side (after the dialyzer but before the clamp). The arterial side is then clamped and the venous side is unclamped, allowing the dialyzed blood to be returned to the patient, and the cycle is repeated. Single-needle dialysis is far less efficient than double needle, as less than half of the dialysis time is spent withdrawing blood. There is also a decrease in efficiency due to recirculation of the returned blood in the catheter that is withdrawn on the next cycle. By maintaining a fast blood flow rate and a higher stroke volume (amount of blood removed in each cycle), the effect of recirculation is decreased, but in many situations, a fast blood flow rate is limited by the type and condition of the functional lumen of the catheter.

Anticoagulation

Exposure of blood to the extracorporeal circuit and dialyzer membrane induces coagulation, and some method of eliminating or decreasing this effect is necessary. The most common method of anticoagulation of the extracorporeal circuit in IHD is unfractionated heparin. An intravenous bolus of heparin (20–50 units/kg) is given at the start of the dialysis treatment, followed by a constant infusion during the treatment. The infusion rate is adjusted during treatment to maintain the clotting time at about 1.6–2 times normal. Most dialysis machines can be programmed to discontinue the heparin infusion prior to the end of treatment (generally 30–60 minutes), allowing the clotting times to start decreasing toward normal. The half-life of heparin is 40–120 minutes (Ward 2005).

The coagulation cascade is heavily dependent on calcium as a cofactor at several steps. Because citrate binds calcium, it is an effective anticoagulant. Regional citrate anticoagulation involves infusing citrate into the extracorporeal circuit as the blood is being withdrawn from the patient, anticoagulating only the blood in the extracorporeal circuit. In order to avoid hypocalcemia in the patient, calcium is infused into the patient, preferably through a catheter separate from the extracorporeal circuit and dialysis access. If no other venous access is available, calcium can be infused into the extracorporeal circuit at the point where the blood is returned to the patient. This increases the risk of thrombosis in the catheter, however. Regional citrate anticoagulation has the advantage of not causing systemic anticoagulation,

which is desirable, especially in patients at high risk for bleeding (i.e., patients with GI ulceration or bleeding diathesis or after surgery). Disadvantages include an increase in complexity of treatment, because the citrate infusion rate is adjusted based on both the blood flow rate and the ionized calcium concentration of the extracorporeal circuit, and the calcium infusion rate is adjusted based on the citrate infusion rate and the patient's ionized calcium concentration. The dialysate should not contain calcium. Although protocols have been investigated using calcium-containing dialysate to avoid the need for intravenous calcium administration, thrombosis in the circuit occurs more frequently (Buturovic-Ponikvar et al. 2008). Because citrate is metabolized by the liver, regional citrate anticoagulation is contraindicated in patients with hepatic dysfunction. Metabolic alkalosis may occur since citrate is metabolized to bicarbonate; use of a lower dialysate bicarbonate concentration may be advisable.

In high-risk patients, dialysis can sometimes be performed without anticoagulation. The extracorporeal circuit is flushed with saline (50–150 mL) every 15–30 minutes to flush any fibrin strands that are starting to form. The extra volume infused is removed by UF to avoid volume overload in the patient. Rapid blood flow rates are necessary to decrease clotting. An increase in transmembrane pressure may predict clotting; careful attention to this parameter and narrow alarm settings are recommended if performing dialysis without anticoagulation. It has been the author's clinical experience that even with aggressive saline flushing, dialyzer and circuit clotting limit treatment to less than 1.5 hours without anticoagulation in many patients.

Protamine counteracts the effects of heparin and can be administered to the patient as a constant IV infusion to reverse the heparin anticoagulation in the patient while heparin maintains anticoagulation in the extracorporeal circuit. This technique of regional heparinization is rarely used. Low-molecular weight heparin can be used instead of unfractionated heparin in patients at high risk of bleeding, but is not commonly used in routine patients, due to the additional expense and inability to monitor in real time. Other anticoagulants have been investigated, including prostacyclin, recombinant hirudin (lepirudin), danaparoid (a heparinoid), and argatroban (direct thrombin inhibitor) (Pun and Kovalik 2008).

Complications of anticoagulation include excessive bleeding or thrombosis in the patient (discussed below) or thrombosis in the catheter or extracorporeal circuit. Thrombosis is most likely to occur in the dialyzer, which decreases the surface area available for diffusive clearance and decreases the efficiency of treatment. Thrombosis may also occur at the air–blood interface in the arterial or venous drip chamber. Catastrophic coagulation of the entire extracorporeal circuit can occur, necessitating discontinuation of the treatment and preventing return of the blood to the patient, but this complication is uncommon if rapid blood flow is maintained without excessive periods of stopped flow due to catheter malfunction.

Intradialysis patient monitoring

Blood pressure disorders are common in the dialysis patient population during and between dialysis treatments. Numerous factors contribute to hypotension during dialysis. The volume of blood in the extracorporeal circuit compared to the blood volume is a major contributor in smaller patients. The smallest extracorporeal circuit currently available for IHD is about 70 mL (including the dialyzer volume). Removal of this volume of blood, which may be 15–40% of the total blood volume of a cat or small dog, consistently causes a decrease in blood pressure. In stable patients, the magnitude of decrease may only be 20–30 mmHg, and most patients have compensatory mechanisms that increase the blood pressure within 30 minutes of starting the treatment. Some patients seem to be unable to autoregulate, however. UF removes fluid from the intravascular compartment, which is then refilled from the interstitial and intracellular compartments. Rapid UF can induce hypotension that generally responds rapidly to a temporary discontinuation of UF or small boluses of crystalloid fluid. Exposure of the blood to the dialysis membrane can activate the complement cascade, leading to hypotension. The AN69 membrane is particularly capable of activating bradykinin, especially in an acidic environment. Blood pressure should be monitored carefully throughout the entire dialysis treatment. In stable patients, monitoring every 30 minutes is generally adequate.

The intravascular blood volume can be monitored during dialysis using a continuous hemoglobin monitor (Figure 28.7). The hemoglobin content can be measured optically with a sensor placed on the blood tubing. Presuming the patient is neither gaining hemoglobin (transfusion) nor losing hemoglobin (bleeding), changes in the hemoglobin concentration reflect changes in plasma volume from UF or fluid infusion. Monitoring the rate of decline in the intravascular volume can allow prediction of hypotension from rapid UF before it occurs. A general guideline is that if the blood volume decreases by more than 10% per hour, the rate of UF should be decreased.

Some method of monitoring anticoagulation is necessary during hemodialysis. Activated clotting time (ACT) is the most commonly used method. ACT evaluates the intrinsic and common pathways of coagulation, and reliable automated measurement is available at the bedside.

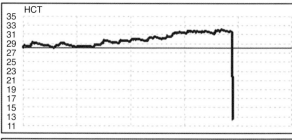
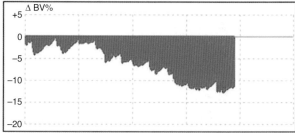

Figure 28.7 Change in blood volume as predicted by CritLine Monitor. Two liters were removed via ultrafiltration during a 3.5 hour dialysis treatment.

Heparin affects the intrinsic pathway, and the effects of heparin can be monitored by ACT or by partial thromboplastin time (PTT). ACT is generally measured before treatment, 30 minutes after starting or any dose adjustment, and then hourly once a stable dose has been reached.

Extracorporeal circuit ionized calcium can be measured in lieu of ACT in patients receiving citrate anticoagulation. An ionized calcium concentration of less than 0.25–0.40 mmol/L will provide sufficient anticoagulation.

Dialysis adequacy

There are many ways to gauge the adequacy of dialysis treatment. The patient's quality of life is a crude (but important) measure, but there are many other factors that impact on quality of life beyond the dialysis treatment, including the nature of the kidney injury, amount of residual renal function and comorbid conditions.

Uremia (Chapter 41) involves a number of metabolic disturbances resulting from the accumulation of a variety of substances, in addition to hormonal imbalances and inflammation. Commonly measured markers of renal function include urea, creatinine, phosphorus, and potassium, but these represent only a small subset of the uremic toxins. In fact, urea is not highly toxic unless present at extremely high concentrations. Despite that, urea concentrations are correlated to outcome, because urea is a suitable marker for other small molecular weight molecules (<500 Da) that diffuse readily. Urea clearance is not a suitable marker for middle molecular weight uremic toxins (500–15,000 Da) or high molecular weight (>15,000 Da) toxins.

Routine measurement of solutes (urea, creatinine, phosphorus, electrolytes) prior to and immediately following a dialysis treatment provides a simple measure of dialysis adequacy. However, these values are affected by factors beyond the adequacy of dialysis treatment. For example, the predialysis urea concentration may be low due to adequate dialysis or protein malnutrition. Conversely, a high predialysis urea concentration may reflect inadequate dialysis, high protein intake, dehydration, or increased catabolism. Because of vacillations in the predialysis BUN over the week, the time-averaged urea concentration (TAC) has been used to provide a measure of the average urea exposure over the week. It is calculated as the area under the urea measurement curve divided by time of the measurement interval (Leypoldt 2005; Francey 2006b).

Accurate and consistent timing of the postdialysis blood sampling is necessary to avoid introducing error, due to the potential for significant postdialysis rebound of urea. With rapid blood and dialysate flow rates in a short dialysis treatment, the blood compartment is readily cleared of urea, but the intracellular compartment lags behind in clearance. After the end of the dialysis treatment, the intracellular and blood compartments equilibrate, and the blood concentration rapidly (30–60 minutes) increases compared to the immediately postdialysis measurement.

The URR is another simple marker of ERRT adequacy. It is calculated from blood urea measurements taken before and immediately after dialysis. It is calculated from the formula: $URR = (BUN_{pre} - BUN_{post})/BUN_{pre}$. In IHD, URR can be predicted by the volume of blood processed through the dialyzer, presuming standard dialysate flow and no convective clearance. If the actual URR is lower than predicted, there may be substantial clotting of fibers of the dialyzer or substantial catheter recirculation.

The most common measure of dialysis dose in human ERRT is Kt/V, in which K is the clearance of the dialyzer, t is time on dialysis, and V is volume of distribution. Various equations are based on different presumptions about the urea pool and the kinetics of urea movement. The simplest is single pool, in which urea is presumed to diffuse freely and rapidly throughout the entire volume of distribution. The double pool kinetic model presumes differential rates of urea clearance from certain regions (i.e., intracellular space).

The dialyzer clearance can be measured or estimated. Urea is measured in blood entering and leaving the dialyzer, and the clearance is calculated from the formula: $K_d = Q_b \times ((BUN_{in} - BUN_{out})/BUN_{in})$. Note that the

blood flow rate readings from the dialysis machine may vary from the actual blood flow rate. Some newer dialysis machines incorporate ionic dialysance measurement. Dialysance is a measure of solute mass transfer from blood to dialysate when the solute is present in both the blood and dialysate. The collective dialysance of small molecular weight ions (such as sodium) is considered equivalent to the dialysance of urea. For conventional single pass hemodialysis circuits, urea dialysance becomes equal to urea clearance. By programmed alterations in dialysate conductivity (by changes in sodium concentration) and measurement of conductivity at the dialysate inlet and outlet, the dialysis machine can calculate the dialyzer ionic dialysance and thus the dialyzer urea clearance. Repeated measurements are made throughout the treatment, allowing calculation of Kt for each dialysis treatment.

The urea volume of distribution is considered to be the same as the total body water and is generally estimated as 58% of body weight. Alterations in water balance and in lean body mass are common in patients with renal failure. Measurement of body water can be performed with dilution techniques or bioimpedance.

More thorough discussions of dialysis adequacy have previously been published for human and veterinary ERRT (Leypoldt 2005; Yeun and Depner 2005; Francey 2006b).

Patient management

Patients with AKI or CKD severe enough to require ERRT are prone to a variety of concurrent conditions induced by the inciting cause of the renal failure, derangement due to the renal failure itself or its treatment, or preexisting comorbid conditions in some. ERRT is able to maintain patients with more severe renal failure for longer periods of time than medical management, which allows development of some late-stage complications that are not commonly encountered in the nondialysis renal failure population. The following discussion will focus on complications unique to the ERRT population or uncommon manifestations that are more likely to be encountered in the ERRT population. The reader is referred to chapters on AKI (Chapter 49) and CKD (Chapter 48) for a general discussion of common manifestations of uremia and appropriate treatment.

Neurologic system

There are a number of potential disturbances of the neurologic system in the dialysis patients. Correctly differentiating the cause of the signs may allow more targeted therapy.

Dialysis Disequilibrium Syndrome (DDS) is characterized by a variety of neurologic signs, including restlessness, nausea, vomiting, muscle twitching, disorientation, tremor, hypertension, obtundation, seizure, coma, and death (Liangos et al. 2005). DDS is more likely to occur in the first few dialysis treatments in patients that are severely azotemic. Risk factors seem to include severe azotemia, small patient size, preexisting neurologic disease, rapid dialysis, and low dialysate sodium relative to the patient. The exact cause of DDS is not clearly defined, but interstitial cerebral edema is a feature (Chen et al. 2007). One theory holds that slower diffusion of urea from cells of the CNS in relationship to removal of urea from the blood compartment during dialysis leads to a relative intracellular hyperosmolality. A decrease in urea transporters and an increase in aquaporins in the brain of uremic rats support this theory (Trinh-Trang-Tan et al. 2005). However, the urea gradient between brain and blood is quantitatively insufficient to cause cerebral edema (Patel et al. 2008). An alternative theory involves paradoxic CNS acidosis from rapid correction of systemic metabolic acidosis during dialysis. The presence of idiogenic osmoles in the brain has been postulated as a contributor to DDS, but concentrations of specific brain organic osmolytes (glutamine, glutamate, taurine, and myoinositol) do not increase with rapid dialysis (Patel et al. 2008). Gradual correction of uremia, as with CRRT or SLED, decreases the risk of DDS. A higher dialysate sodium concentration during periods of rapid urea removal may help decrease the incidence of DDS. In high-risk patients, prophylactic administration of mannitol (0.5 g/kg) about 30–60 minutes after the start of dialysis is recommended. Signs may occur during dialysis or up to 48 hours afterwards and can be treated with mannitol and supportive care. Some patients will recover completely, but this complication can be fatal.

Hypertension can cause neurologic signs that include lethargy, ataxia, blindness, stupor, and seizures (Brown et al. 2005). This condition is called posterior reversible encephalopathy syndrome in people and is characterized by MRI findings suggestive of cerebral edema (Servillo et al. 2007). Hypertensive encephalopathy is not caused by dialysis, but many patients requiring dialysis are hypertensive.

Uremic encephalopathy in people is characterized by diminished concentration, slowed and inefficient cognitive functioning, restlessness, and lowered arousal level or drowsiness (Brown 2008). There are only a few reports of uremic encephalopathy in the veterinary literature. The author has seen a small number of patients that exhibited behavior changes (predominantly agitation and aggression) that resolve immediately after dialysis and return prior to the next dialysis treatment.

Aluminum toxicity can occur acutely from contaminated dialysate source water or chronically from oral aluminum-containing phosphate binders. In addition to hematologic toxicity, aluminum toxicity can cause encephalopathy and neuromuscular disorders (Segev et al. 2008).

Human hemodialysis patients are more likely to suffer from subdural hematoma than the general population, but this complication has not been noted in veterinary dialysis patients (Sood et al. 2007). Other causes of acute localizing neurologic symptoms include intracerebral hemorrhage or ischemic stroke (Murakami et al. 2004).

Uremic polyneuropathy is a common complication of chronic kidney disease in people. Sensory symptoms such as paresthesia, pain, and a burning sensation usually precede motor symptoms, which include muscle weakness and atrophy, myoclonus, and areflexia (Avram and Mittman 2008). Adequate dialysis will usually stabilize the signs, but improvement is rare.

Blood pressure

Hypertension commonly occurs with acute or chronic kidney disease (Chapter 68). Correction of overhydration over the first several days of treatment may decrease the blood pressure, although many patients will need antihypertensive medications. Patients receiving long-term dialysis who are prone to intradialytic hypotension should not receive the antihypertensive medications on the morning of dialysis treatment. Intradialytic hypotension has many potential causes (see Intradialytic Patient Monitoring). Interdialytic hypotension may occur due to sepsis, systemic inflammatory response syndrome, electrolyte and acid–base disturbances, and hypoxia (Waddell 2005).

Hemostasis

Anticoagulation during dialysis (or between treatments) and uremic bleeding tendencies contribute to the risk of hemorrhage in the dialysis patient. Clinical signs may include obvious bleeding, such as bleeding from the catheter exit site or melena, or may be more insidious. A decreasing hemoglobin concentration may not be apparent on continuous monitors because of the concurrent UF. Hypotension that rapidly responds to small bolus of crystalloid fluid but rapidly recurs may be an indication of ongoing bleeding. An acute onset of dyspnea may denote pulmonary hemorrhage.

The three issues to be addressed in a patient that is actively hemorrhaging is (1) decrease ongoing loss, (2) correct anemia, and (3) support affected organs. Immediate cessation of anticoagulant administration is intuitive. Protamine can be given to reverse the effects of heparin, at a dose of 1 mg protamine for each 100 units of heparin to be reversed, although an overdose of protamine can cause a coagulopathy. If bleeding is due to systemic diseases associated with coagulation factor deficiency, plasma transfusion may be helpful. A major component of uremic bleeding is thrombocytopathy; platelet transfusion is unlikely to be helpful. Dialysis partially corrects the platelet dysfunction (Kaw and Malhotra 2006). Other treatments to prevent or treat uremic bleeding in people include erythropoietin, desmopressin, cryoprecipitate, and conjugated estrogen (Hedges et al. 2006; Kaw and Malhotra 2006).

Blood transfusion is usually indicated for moderate to severe hemorrhage associated with clinical signs. Although erythropoiesis stimulating agents are commonly necessary in most chronic hemodialysis patients, a significant increase in hematocrit generally takes several weeks to effect. Hemorrhage into critical areas such as the lungs or CNS may cause damage that slowly resolves, but this is frequently a catastrophic fatal event.

Thrombosis

Right atrial thrombosis occurs in 22% of human hemodialysis patients who have a catheter for vascular access (Bolz et al. 1995). The presence of right atrial thrombosis is associated with a 68% chance of concurrent infection and 27% mortality (Negulescu et al. 2003). Right atrial thrombosis detected primarily by echocardiography is common in veterinary patients and can routinely be seen within 2 weeks of catheter placement. Catheter thrombosis is discussed in catheter complications section.

Electrolyte and acid–base disorders

Hyperkalemia (Chapter 62) is usually associated with anuria or severe oliguria. In the chronic dialysis patient, however, hyperkalemia can occur in the nonoliguric patient, but usually only when the GFR is less than 10% of normal (Allon 2005). Patients with acute kidney injury are more likely to develop hyperkalemia than those with chronic disease, because the kidney can compensate by increasing the efficiency of potassium excretion. Factors that contribute to hyperkalemia, in addition to the limited ability of the kidney to excrete potassium, include certain drugs [ACE inhibitors, potassium-sparing diuretics (spironolactone, amiloride, triamterene), prostaglandin inhibitors, heparin, nonspecific beta-blockers (propranolol), high doses of potassium penicillin], aldosterone deficiency, inorganic acidosis, and high dietary intake. Commonly used renal diets are supplemented with potassium.

Potassium is a small molecule that is rapidly removed by dialysis. Use of a potassium-free dialysate will normalize serum potassium. In acute dialysis, using a prescription of short treatments with slow blood flow for the first few treatments, the potassium level will generally normalize by the end of each treatment, but the total body excess of potassium has probably not been removed. After cessation of that dialysis treatment, serum potassium levels will increase. Usually after the second or third dialysis treatment, the potassium rebound is less exaggerated. SLED or CRRT may be used for more sustained potassium control in the first day. EKG abnormalities start to improve within the first 15 minutes of dialysis, even though the potassium concentration has not yet been corrected. It has been the author's clinical experience that treatment of hyperkalemia with agents that translocate potassium intracellularly (i.e., insulin, dextrose, bicarbonate) within the hour or two prior to the dialysis treatment limit the total body removal of potassium in a short initial dialysis treatment. Conceptually, potassium is less available in the bloodstream for diffusive clearance during a short treatment, but starts translocating out of the cells after several hours (after the end of the treatment), potentially leading to symptomatic hyperkalemia in the interdialysis interval. In those settings, SLED or CRRT should be considered.

In patients with chronic hyperkalemia between dialysis treatments, sodium polystyrene resin (Kayexalate, Sanofi-Aventis, Bridgewater, NJ) can be administered orally (or by enema). Sodium is released when potassium binds the resin and potassium is trapped for removal via the GI tract. Side effects include anorexia, nausea, vomiting, constipation, hypokalemia, hypocalcemia, and hypernatremia. Drugs that will transiently decrease potassium concentrations include insulin, dextrose, bicarbonate, and beta agonists (e.g., albuterol) (Allon 2005; Kogika and de Morais 2008).

Life-threatening ventricular arrhythmia is the most serious complication of hyperkalemia. EKG abnormalities are usually not seen at potassium concentration of less than 6.5 mEq/L. The earliest EKG changes include peaked T wave. Above 6.5 mEq/L, PR interval prolongation and widened QRS complex may be seen. Above 8–9 mEq/L, a sinoventricular rhythm may occur and P waves are not apparent. Above 10 mEq/L, the classic sine-wave EKG pattern appears, and ventricular fibrillation and asystole are imminent (Parham et al. 2006). In the author's clinical experience, acute elevations in potassium are more likely to induce symptomatic EKG changes, whereas patients with chronic renal disease and chronic hyperkalemia may sustain higher potassium concentrations without obvious signs.

Sodium disorders are commonly encountered and include both hyponatremia and hypernatremia. Sodium is readily diffusible, and the sodium dialysate composition can be used to normalize patient sodium concentration.

Metabolic acidosis (Chapter 66) occurs due to a failure of the kidney to excrete an adequate amount of acid and to reabsorb bicarbonate. Dialysis corrects acidosis by two methods. First, it removes organic and inorganic acid solutes. Second, bicarbonate in the dialysate diffuses into the blood to buffer retained acids. Standard dialysate bicarbonate concentration in veterinary medicine is 30 mEq/L, which loads the patient with bicarbonate during dialysis, to delay the reoccurrence of metabolic acidosis in the interdialysis interval.

Magnesium (Chapter 63) is a divalent cation that is excreted by the kidney. Hypermagnesemia may occur with renal failure, but is corrected by dialysis.

Anemia

Anemia is almost a universal problem in patients on dialysis, even those with acute kidney injury. There are several sources of blood loss, including gastrointestinal bleeding, diagnostic blood sampling, and blood loss in the dialyzer. About 5–10 mL of blood remains in the dialyzer after even the most complete blood rinseback at the end of the treatment, and substantially more blood can be lost if there is any dialyzer clotting. In addition, anticoagulation necessary for dialysis can increase the risk of hemorrhage. Red cell survival times are shortened with uremia. Hemolysis is unlikely to occur in the blood pump segment with the gentle roller pumps employed currently, but can be a problem if excessive negative pressure (from inadequate access flow) occurs. ERRT patients are unable to produce sufficient replacement red blood cells primarily due to lack of erythropoietin production. Additionally, uremic toxins and inflammation inhibit erythropoiesis. Iron, vitamin B, and other nutritional deficiencies may contribute. Myelofibrosis from renal osteodystrophy related to renal secondary hyperparathyroidism has been reported in humans. Aluminum toxicity, which can occur chronically from aluminum-containing phosphate binders and inadequate dialysate water treatment, or acutely from dialysate water contamination, can cause anemia.

Treatment of anemia in dialysis patients in the acute setting generally involves blood transfusion. Oxyglobin can be used in emergency settings. Most patients receiving dialysis for more than a few weeks will benefit from administration of an erythropoiesis stimulating agent such as darbepoetin, although there is a risk of pure red cell aplasia from antibody formation. Iron supplementation is of paramount importance in obtaining an adequate response, as iron losses in the dialysis patient are 3–6 times higher than in the normal patient (Schmidt and Besarab 2008).

Bone and mineral

Approximately 60% of ingested phosphorus is absorbed from the GI tract normally, and up to 80% is absorbed in the presence of active vitamin D. The bulk of the body's phosphorus (85%) is located in bones and teeth. Approximately 14% is located in the soft tissues, 0.5% in interstitial fluid, and 0.02% is in the plasma compartment. Phosphorus (Chapter 65) that is removed during dialysis comes from the intracellular pool. The main determinant of phosphate removal during the first 60–90 minutes of dialysis is the serum phosphate concentration. After the phosphate gradient between blood and the dialysate is decreased, the slow diffusion rate of phosphate out of cells determines the rate of phosphate removal during dialysis. There is a large rebound effect after dialysis, with phosphate values returning to 80% of predialysis values. The kinetics of phosphate removal with hemodialysis make thrice weekly hemodialysis relatively ineffective at controlling hyperphosphatemia. Phosphate removal during short daily dialysis treatments (1.5–3 hours for 6 days a week) is dependent on predialysis phosphate concentration. Nocturnal dialysis (6–10 hours six nights a week) removes twice as much phosphate weekly as conventional thrice weekly hemodialysis. Patients on short daily or nocturnal dialysis have better control of phosphate despite higher phosphate intake and lower phosphate binder doses (Kooienga 2007).

Parathyroid hormone (PTH) is considered a uremic toxin. Concentrations of PTH are elevated in patients with renal disease because of variety of factors, including hyperphosphatemia, inadequate calcitriol formation, and alterations in parathyroid gland sensitivity. PTH is considered a middle molecule, and removal is limited during conventional dialysis. Use of a high-flux dialyzer and convective clearance help remove this substance.

Ionized calcium concentration (Chapter 64) must be regulated within a narrow range to preserve appropriate neurologic and muscular function. The ionized fraction of calcium is available for diffusive transfer; complexed or protein-bound calcium does not diffuse with dialysis. Acute hypocalcemia is suspected as a contributor to intradialytic hypotension, because of an inability of the vasculature to constrict in the absence of calcium. Various dialysate calcium concentrations are available to suit the individual patient's needs.

Water balance

Maintaining water balance can be a significant challenge in patients who require dialysis. Volume overload is common, as the kidneys are not able to excrete water appropriately, and even modest fluid administration rates may cause fluid accumulation in patients with anuria, oliguria, or relative oliguria. Additionally, many patients with acute kidney injury are hypoalbuminemic or have a vasculitis, leading to interstitial fluid accumulation, which complicates assessment of hydration status by physical examination. The traditional veterinary end-stage chronic kidney disease patient is polyuric with a tendency to develop dehydration. Most of these patients die or are euthanized due to uremia prior to (or at the time of) development of oliguria, unless maintained with dialysis. Volume overload, frequently exacerbated by nutritional support via an enteral feeding tube, is common in this group. These patients may need some degree of UF at each dialysis treatment.

Nutrition

Malnutrition is a significant concern in the dialysis patient. Both enteral and parenteral feeding involves an obligate water load, which many patients cannot excrete. The administered water can be removed via UF, with either intermittent or continuous therapies. Acute kidney injury is a highly catabolic disease. Provision of adequate protein can ameliorate (although not eliminate) the negative nitrogen balance that occurs with AKI, and protein restriction, a standard recommendation for patients with chronic kidney disease, may not be appropriate for patients with AKI (Druml 2001).

Standard diets for chronic kidney disease may not be appropriate for chronic dialysis patients. With each dialysis treatment, amino acids are lost into the dialysate, and the protein restriction of renal diets may be insufficient to replenish these losses. Most renal diets are potassium rich, because hypokalemia may occur in the pre-dialysis CKD patient, but these diets induce hyperkalemia in the dialysis patient that has extremely limited renal potassium excretory capability. Supplementation with carnitine and taurine, amino acids that may be lost in the dialysate, is recommended for patients on dialysis for over a month (Fischer 2006).

Infection

Infection is the second most common cause of mortality in human dialysis patients, accounting for 14% of deaths (Evers 1995; Tokars et al. 2005; Katneni and Hedayati 2007). In one study, bacterial infection is responsible for more than 30% of all causes of morbidity and mortality in human patients, with vascular access infection being the culprit in 73% of all bacteremias (Ponce et al. 2007). Bacteremia occurs in human hemodialysis outpatients at a rate of 0.6–1.7% of patients per month, and vascular access infections occur in 1.3–7.2% of patients per month (Tokars et al. 2005). Data is not available in animals, but appears to be similar or higher. Most infections in human dialysis patients are catheter related (28–33% in one study) (Tokars et al. 2005).

Catheter-related infections include exit site infections, catheter infections, and bacteremia. Catheter exit site infections are characterized by erythema, warmth, induration, swelling, tenderness, breakdown of skin, loculated fluid, or purulent exudates (Tokars et al. 2005).

The catheter itself can become infected. Bacteria can produce a biofilm that adheres to the walls of the catheter and protect the bacteria. Blood cultures obtained through the catheter may be positive even if bacteremia is not present. To document bacteriemia, blood for culture must be obtained from a separate venipuncture site.

Signs of catheter-related bacteremia include fever, chills, nausea, headache, hypotension, or elevated white blood cell count. The frequency of catheter-associated bacteremia in humans is 2–4 episodes per 1,000 patient days (0.7–1.5 bacteremias per catheter year) (Himmelfarb et al. 2005). With catheter-related bacteremia, 3 weeks of an appropriate antibiotic and exchange over a guidewire, if minimal signs are present, results in cure in 88% of patients, whereas immediate catheter removal with replacement after defervesence is required in patients with severe septic symptoms (Beathard 1999). One study showed that 51% of catheters could be salvaged without exchange with an antibiotic lock and 3 weeks of systemic antibiotics (Krishnasami et al. 2002). Mupirocin or bacitracin to the catheter exit site may decrease catheter-related bacteremia (Sesso et al. 1998; Johnson et al. 2002; Lok et al. 2003). Thrombosis is correlated with an increased rate of infection (Shah et al. 2004).

The most common bacteria isolated from catheter infections and associated bacteremia in humans is *Staphylococcus aureus* and coagulase negative Staphylococci (Tokars et al. 2005; Katneni and Hedayati 2007). In veterinary patients, half of positive catheter-related cultures (including cultures of blood and/or heparin lock obtained through the catheter and the tip of the catheter) are Staphylococcus spp., and gram-negative organisms comprise 32% of positive catheter-related cultures (unpublished data, Langston 2008).

Although catheter-related infections account for the majority of infections in dialysis patients, other common sites in humans include lung (25%), urinary tract (23%), skin and soft tissue (9%), and other or unknown sites (15%) (Tokars et al. 2005). Gram-negative organisms, predominantly Klebsiella and *E. coli*, account for the majority (77%) of positive urine cultures in veterinary dialysis patients (personal observation).

Respiratory system

Respiratory dysfunction can be caused by a variety of mechanisms. Exposure of blood to the dialysis membrane can activate complement, leading to temporary sludging of activated neutrophils and platelets in pulmonary capillaries, impairing oxygen diffusion. Oxygen pressure can decrease by 5–30 mmHg (Liangos et al. 2005). This effect is most profound within 30–60 minutes of starting the treatment, and resolves within hours. Cellulose and substituted cellulose membranes elicit a stronger reaction; more biocompatible synthetic membranes activate compliment to a lesser degree. Other causes of respiratory impairment can be seen in the dialysis patient. Pulmonary hemorrhage has been noted in dogs with leptospirosis and is a potential complication of excessive anticoagulation (Greenlee et al. 2004). Pulmonary edema can occur as a result of volume overload in the face of oliguria or anuria. Uremia increases pulmonary vascular permeability, similar to that observed in acute respiratory distress syndrome (Rabb et al. 2003). Pulmonary thromboembolic disease is a potential complication of an indwelling catheter.

Gastrointestinal system

Gastrointestinal signs, including vomiting, diarrhea, and anorexia, are pervasive in the dialysis population. With adequate dialysis, these signs may resolve. Aggressive therapy with antiemetic drugs is frequently necessary, but rarely completely resolves vomiting and nausea (Ljutic et al. 2002).

Drug dosing

Drugs that are primarily excreted by the kidneys require dose adjustment with advanced renal failure (Chapter 40). In general, the loading dose does not need to be adjusted unless the volume of distribution is significantly altered, as with patients with large changes in body water. Extending the dosing interval is useful for drugs with a long half-life. Dose reduction while maintaining the interval between doses generally leads to more constant serum levels. A variety of factors affect removal of drugs by dialysis. Drugs with a molecular weight >500 Da are poorly cleared by conventional dialysis, although clearance may be enhanced with synthetic membranes commonly used in veterinary ERRT. Drugs that are highly protein or tissue bound or are highly lipid soluble are not dialyzed to a significant degree due to the high volume of distribution. Drugs that are significantly cleared by dialysis may require supplemental dosing after the dialysis treatment to maintain therapeutic levels. Drug level monitoring is available for some drugs, but may be impractical in many situations. Tables of recommended dose adjustments in dialysis patients are available (Aronoff 2005; Johnson 2008; Olyaei and Bennett 2008). With continuous therapies utilizing convective clearance, molecular size and volume of distribution become less limiting than with IHD, but limited pharmacokinetic data is available (Bugge 2001). Although using specific pharmacokinetic data to adjust dosing is preferred, some suggested guidelines for humans in the absence of necessary data are to presume CRRT is equivalent to a GFR of 10–50 mL/min (normal GFR for humans is >90 mL/min/1.73 m^2) or to increase the dose of nontoxic drugs by 30% over the drug dose estimated for the degree of renal failure (Bugge 2001).

Nonrenal uses

Certain toxins can be removed by hemodialysis or a related technique, hemoperfusion. Characteristics of substances that might be removed by dialysis are small molecular weight, minimal protein binding, and a small volume of distribution. Hemoperfusion involves placing a charcoal-filled cartridge in the extracorporal circuit. As blood passes through the cartridge, activated charcoal adsorbs the toxin. Charcoal perfusion can remove substantial amounts of substances that are protein bound. A list of substances that can be removed can be found in Table 28.7 (Fischer et al. 2004a).

Dialytic therapy can be used for other nonrenal indications. Isolated UF can be used for diuretic resistant congestive heart failure. Dialysis removes cytokines and other inflammatory mediators (both proinflammatory and anti-inflammatory) from septic patients, but there is insufficient evidence to support dialysis (specifically, CRRT) as a treatment for sepsis in the absence of acute renal failure. Two separate systems (Molecular Adsorbants Recirculating System and Prometheus) have been developed to treat liver failure with an extracorporeal clearance system. Commonly used dialysis machines (intermittent and continuous) can be used for therapeutic plasmapheresis.

Table 28.7 Substances that can be removed by extracorporeal purification (adapted from Fisher et al. 2004; Cowgill 2008)

Substance	Conventional dialysis	High-flux	Hemoperfusion
Alcohols			
Ethanol	X		
Ethylene glycol	X		
Methanol	X		
Analgesics/anti-inflammatory			
Acetaminophen	X		
Aspirin	X		
Mesalamine (5-ASA)	X		
Morphine		X	
NSAIDs			X
Salicylates	X		X
Pentazocine	X		
Antibacterials			
Amikacin	X		
Amoxicillin (most penicillins)	X		
Cephalexin (most 1st generation cephalosporins)	X		
Cefotetan (many 2nd generation cephalosporins)	X		
Cefoxitin	X		
Ceftriaxone (many 3rd generation cephalosporins)	X		
Chloramphenicol	X		
Enrofloxacin			X
Gentamicin	X		
Imipenem/cilastin	X		
Kanamycin	X		
Linezolid	X		
Nitrofurantoin	X		
Ofloxacin	X		
Metronidazole	X		
Sulbactam	X		
Sulfamethoxazole	X		
Sulfisoxazole	X		
Trimethoprim	X		
Vancomycin		X	
Anticonvulsants			
Gabapentin	X		
Phenobarbital	X		
Phenytoin		X	
Primidone	X		
Antifungals			
Dapsone	X		
Fluconazole	X		
Flucytosine	X		
Antineoplastics			
Busulfan	X		
Carboplatin	X		
Cytarabine		X	
Cyclophosphamide	X		
Fluorouracil (5-FU)	X		
Ifosfamide	X		
Methotrexate	X		
Mercaptopurine	X		
Vincristine			X

(Continued)

Table 28.7 (*Continued*)

Substance	Conventional dialysis	High-flux	Hemoperfusion
Antivirals			
Acycylovir	x		
Famciclovir	x		
Valvcyclovir	x		
Zidovudine	x		
Cardiac/vasoactive medications			
Atenolol	x		
Bretylium	x		
Captopril	x		
Enalapril	x		
Esmolol	x		
Lisinopril	x		
Metoprolol	x		
Mexiletine	x		
Nitroprusside	x		
Procainamide	x		
Sotalol	x		
Tocainide	x		
Chelating agents			
Deferoxamine	x		
Ethylendiamine tetraacetic acid (EDTA)	x		
Penicillamine	x		
Immunosuppressive agents			
Azathioprine	x		
Methyl prednisone	x		
Miscellaneous medications			
Allopurinol	x		
Amatoxins			x
Amitriptyline	x		x
Ascorbic acid	x		
Barbiturates			x
Caffeine	x		
Carisoprodol	x		
Chloral hydrate	x		
Chlorpheniramine	x		
Diazoxide	x		
Foscarnet	x		
Iohexol	x		
Iopamidol	x		
Lithium	x		
Mannitol	x		
Metformin	x		
Minoxidil	x		
Octreotide	x		
Ranitidine	x		
Theophylline	x		x

Appendix: Extracorporeal Renal Replacement Therapy Units

United States
Animal Medical Center
510 E. 62nd Street
New York, NY 10065
(212)838-8100 (phone)
(212)329-8618 (hemodialysis unit)
(212)752-2592 (fax)
Dr. Cathy Langston, cathy.langston@amcny.org
hemodialysis@amcny.org
www.amcny.org
IRRT

Advanced Critical Care
City of Angels Veterinary Specialty Center
9599 Jefferson Blvd
Culver City, CA 90232
(310)558-6100 (phone)
(310)558-6199 (fax)
Dr. Richard Mills
Dr. Jon Perlis
www.cityofangelsvets.com
CRRT

Center for Specialized Veterinary Care
609-5 Cantiague Rock Road
Westbury, NY 11590
(516)420-0000 (phone)
(516)420-0122 (fax)
www.vetspecialist.com
CRRT

Companion Animal Hemodialysis Unit
Veterinary Medical Teaching Hospital
University of California-Davis
Davis, CA 95616
(530)752-1393 (phone)
(530)752-8662 (fax)
Dr. Larry Cowgill, ldcowgill@ucdavis.edu
www.vetmed.ucdavis.edu
IRRT

Louisiana State University
Veterinary Medical Teaching Hospital
Baton Rouge, LA 70803
(225)578-9600 (phone)
(225)578-9559 (fax)
Dr. Mark Acierno
www.vetmed.lsu.edu
CRRT

Advanced Critical Care and Internal Medicine
2965 Edinger Avenue
Tustin, CA 92708
(949)654-8950 (phone)
(949)936-0079 (fax)
Dr. Ravi Seshardri
accimvet@aol.com
www.accim.net
CRRT

California Animal Referral And Emergency Hospital
301 Haley St.
Santa Barbara, CA 93101
(805)899-2273 (phone)
(805)965-0070 (fax)
Dr. Andrea Wells
www.carehospital.org
CRRT

Chicago Veterinary Kidney Center
1515 Bush Parkway
Buffalo Grove, IL 60089
(847)459-7535 (phone)
(847)459-3576 (fax)
Dr. Jerry Thornhill, jthornhill@vetspecialty.com
www.vetspecialty.com
CRRT

Companion Animal Hemodialysis Unit
University of California Veterinary Medical Center
10435 Sorrento Valley Road, Suite 101
San Diego, CA 92121
(858)875-7505 (phone) or (858)875-7505 (HD unit)
(858)875-7584 (fax)
Dr. Larry Cowgill
Dr. Sherri Ross
sdhemodialysis@vmth.ucdavis.edu
IRRT

Tufts University Foster Hospital for Small Animals
School of Veterinary Medicine
200 Westboro Road
North Grafton, MA 01536
(508)839-5395 or (508)839-5302 (phone)
(508)839-7951 (fax)
Dr. Mary Anna Labato, mary.labato@tufts.edu
Dr. Linda Ross, linda.ross@tufts.edu
Vet.tufts.edu
IRRT

(Continued)

Appendix: (*Continued*)

University of Florida
Veterinary Medical Center
2015 SW 16th Ave
Gainesville, FL 32608
(352)392-2235
Dr. Carsten Bandt
www.vetmed.ufl.edu
IRRT

Worldwide
Anubi Companion Animal Hospital
Strada Genova 299/A
10024 Moncalieri
Italy
+39 011 6813033 (phone)
+39 011 6813047 (fax)
Dr. Claudio Brovida
info@anubi.it
www.anubi.it
IRRT

Hospital Veterinario Montenegro
Rua Pereira Reis – 191
4200-477 Porto
Portugal
+351 225 089989 or 225 089639 (phone)
+351 966 291916 (fax)
Dr. Luis Montenegro
www.hospvetmontenegro.com
IRRT

Renal Vet Rio de Janeiro
Rua Tereza Buimaraes
42 Botafogo
Rio de Janerio – RJ
CEP 22280-050
Brazil
+55 21 2275 2391 or 3902 7158 (phone)
renalvet@veterinariaonline.com.br
www.veterinariaonline.com
IRRT

Vetsuisse Faculty University of Berne
Small Animal Clinic
Laenggass-Strasse 128, PO Box 8466
CH-3001 Berne
Switzerland
+41 0 31 6312943 (phone)
+41 0 31 6312275 (fax)
Dr. Thierry Francey, Thierry.francey@kkh.unibe.ch
www.vetdialyse.unibe.ch
IRRT

Veterinary Specialists of South Florida
9410 Stirling Road
Cooper City, FL 33024
(954)432-561 (phone)
(954)437-7207 (fax)
Dr. Brian Roberts
info@amccc.com
www.amccc.com
CRRT

Centro Nefrologico Veterinario
Clinica Veterinaria Citta di Catania
V.le V. Veneto 313
Catania
Italy
+39 095 503924 (phone)
+39 095 441542 (fax)
Dr. Angelo Basile, angel.basile@tiscali.it
www.nefrovet.com
IRRT

Manhattan Animal Hospital
1 Fl NO 77, Sec 4, Civic Blvd
Taipei
Taiwan
+886 229815203 (phone)
+866 227735118 (fax)
Dr. David Tan
IRRT

Renal Vet Sao Paulo
Rua Heitor Penteado
99 Sumare
Sao Paulo – SP
Brazil
+55 11 3875 2666 (phone)
renalvet@veterinariaonline.com.br
www.veterinariaonline.com
IRRT

Tierärztliche Klinik für Kleintiere Kabels
Stieg 41 D-22850
Norderstedt
Germany
(040) 52 98 94-0 (phone)
(040) 52 98 94-55 (fax)
info@tierklinik-norderstedt.de
www.tierklinik-norderstedt.de/page1.aspx?pageid=50
IRRT

IRRT = Intermittent Renal Replacement Therapy (Intermittent Hemodialysis)
CRRT = Continuous Renal Replacement Therapy
Other web-based resources:
www.vetcrrt.net – Home page of the Veterinary CRRT Society
www.queenofthenephron.com – listing of units performing extracorporeal renal replacement therapies and/or renal transplantation

References

Adin, C.A. and L.D. Cowgill (2000). Treatment and outcome of dogs with leptospirosis: 36 cases (1990–1998). *J Am Vet Med Assoc* **216**(3): 371–375.

Adin, C.A., C.R. Gregory, et al. (2002). Evaluation of three peripheral arteriovenous fistulas for hemodialysis access in dogs. *Vet Surg* **31**(5): 405–411.

Allon, M. (2005). Disorders of potassium metabolism. In: *Primer on Kidney Diseases*, edited by A. Greenberg. Philadelphia, PA: WB Saunders, pp. 110–119.

Aronoff, G.R. (2005). Drug dosing in chronic kidney disease. In: *Chronic Kidney Disease, Dialysis and Transplantation*, edited by B.J.G. Pereira, M.H. Sayegh, and P. Blake. Philadelphia, PA: Elsevier Saunders, pp. 853–869.

Ash, S.R. (2007). Fluid mechanics and clinical sussess of central venous catheters for dialysis—answers to simple but persisting problems. *Semin Dial* **20**(3): 237–256.

Avram, M.M. and N. Mittman (2008). Management of uremic peripheral neuropathy. In: *Handbook of Dialysis Therapy*, edited by A.R. Nissenson and R.N. Fine. Philadelphia, PA: Saunders Elsevier, pp. 943–950.

Bagshaw, S.M., et al. (2008). Oliguria, volume overload, and loop diuretics. *Crit Care Med* **36**(4 Suppl.): S172–S178.

Beathard, G. (1999). Management of bacteremia associated with tunnelled hemodialysis catheters. *J Am Soc Nephrol* **10**(5): 1045–1049.

Beathard, G. (2001). Catheter thrombosis. *Semin Dial* **14**(6): 441–445.

Swing, B.M., F. Granath, et al. (2007). Continuous renal replacement therapy is associated with less chronic renal failure than intermittent haemodialysis after acute renal failure. *Intensive Care Med* **33**: 773–780.

Berbece, A.N. and R.M.A. Richardson (2006). Sustained low-efficiency dialysis in the ICU: cost, anticoagulation, and solute removal. *Kidney Int* **70**: 963–968.

Bolz, K.D., G. Fjermeros, et al. (1995). Catheter malfunction and thrombus formation on double-lumen hemodialysis catheters: an intravascular ultrasonographic study. *Am J Kid Dis* **25**(4): 597–602.

Bommer, J. and B.L. Jaber (2006). Ultrapure dialysate: facts and myths. *Semin Dial* **19**(2): 115–119.

Bouman, C., H.M. Oudemans-van Straaten, et al. (2002). Effects of early high-volume continuous venovenous hemofiltration on survival and recovery of renal functions in intenstive care patients with acute renal failure: a prospective, randomized trial. *Crit Care Med* **30**(10): 2205–2211.

Brown, C.A., J.S. Munday, et al. (2005). Hypertensive encephalopathy in cats with reduced renal function. *Vet Pathol* **42**: 642–649.

Brown, W.S. (2008). Electroencephalography in the evaluation of neurologic function. In: *Handbook of Dialysis Therapy*, edited by A.R. Nissenson and R.N. Fine. Philadelphia, PA: Saunders Elsevier, pp. 951–957.

Bugge, J.F. (2001). Pharmacokinetics and drug dosing adjustments during continuous venovenous hemofiltration or hemodiafiltration in critically ill patients. *Acta Anaesthesiol Scand* **45**: 929–934.

Buturovic-Ponikvar, J., S. Cerne, et al. (2008). Regional citrate anticoagulation for hemodialysis: calcium-free vs. calcium containing dialysate—a randomized trial. *Int J Artif Organs* **31**(5): 418–424.

Carson, R.C., M. Kiaii, et al. (2005). Urea clearance in dysfunctional catheters is improved by reversing the line position despite increased access recirculation. *Am J Kid Dis* **45**: 883–890.

Chen, C.L., P.H. Lai, et al. (2007). A preliminary report of brain edema in patients with uremia at first hemodialysis: evaluation by diffusion-weighted MR imaging. *Am J Neuroradiol* **28**(1): 68–71.

Clark, W.R. and C. Ronco (2001). Factors influencing therapy delivery in acute dialysis. *Contrib Nephrol* **132**: 304–312.

Conger, J.D. (1990). Does hemodialysis delay recovery from acute renal failure? *Semin Dial* **3**(3): 146–148.

Cowgill, L.D. (2008). *Hemodialysis Prescriptions*. New York: Advanced Renal Therapies Symposium 2008.

D'Haese, P.C. and M.E. De Broe (1996). Adequacy of dialysis: trace elements in dialysis fluids. *Nephrol Dial Transplant* **11**(Suppl 2): 92–97.

Daugirdas, J.T. (1994). Chronic hemodialysis prescription: a urea kinetic approach. In: *Handbook of Dialysis*, edited by J.T. Daugirdas and T.S. Ing. Boston, MA: Little, Brown and Company, pp. 92–120.

Depner, T.A. (2001). Catheter performance. *Semin Dial* **14**(6): 425–431.

Druml, W. (2001). Nutritional support in patients with acute renal failure. In: *Acute Renal Failure: A Companion to Brenner and Rector's The Kidney*, edited by B.A. Molitoris and W.F. Finn. Philadelphia, PA: WB Saunders, pp. 465–489.

Ellis, E.N. (2008). Infant hemodialysis. In: *Handbook of Dialysis Therapy*, edited by A.R. Nissenson and R.N. Fine. Philadelphia, PA: Saunders Elsevier, pp. 1262–1270.

Evers, J. (1995). Approach to fever in dialysis patients. *Nephron* **69**(1): 110.

Fischer, J.R. (2006). *Chronic Hemodialysis and its Complications*. New York: Advanced Renal Therapies Symposium 2006.

Fischer, J.R., V. Pantaleo, et al. (2004a). Clinical and clinicopathological features of cats with acute ureteral obstruction managed with hemodialysis between 1993 and 2004: a review of 50 cases (abstract). *J Vet Intern Med* **18**(3): 418.

Fischer, J.R., V. Pantaleo, et al. (2004b). Veterinary hemodialysis: advances in management and technology. *Vet Clin North Am Small Animal Pract* **34**(4): 935–967.

Francey, T. (2006a). *Outcomes of Hemodialysis*. New York: Advanced Renal Therapies Symposium.

Francey, T. (2006b). *Dialysis Quantification and Adequacy*. New York: Advanced Renal Therapies Symposium 2006.

Francey, T. and L.D. Cowgill (2002). Use of hemodialysis for the management of ARF in the dog: 124 casese (1990–2001) (abstract). *J Vet Intern Med* **16**(3): 352.

Gasparovic, V., I. Filipovic-Grcic, et al. (2003). Continuous renal replacement therapy (CRRT) or intermittent hemodialysis (IHD)—what is the procedure of choice in critically ill patients? *Renal Failure* **25**(5): 855–862.

Gettings, L., H.N. Reynolds, et al. (1999). Outcome in post-traumatic acute renal failure when continuous renal replacement therapy is applied early vs. late. *Intensive Care Med* **25**(8): 805–813.

Ghahramani, N., S. Shadrou, et al. (2008). A systematic review of continuous renal replacement therapy and intermittent hemodialysis in management of patients with acute renal failure. *Nephrology* **13**(7): 570–578.

Gillespie, R.S., K. Seidel, et al. (2004). Effect of fluid overload and dose of replacement fluid on survival in hemofiltration. *Pediatr Nephrol* **19**: 1394–1399.

Goldstein, S.L., M.J. Somers, et al. (2005). Pediatric patients with multiorgan dysfunction syndrome reciving continuous renal replacement therapy. *Kidney Int* **67**(2): 653–658.

Greenlee, J.J., C.A. Bolin, et al. (2004). Clinical and pathologic comparison of acute leptospirosis in dogs caused by two strains of *Leptospira kirschneri* serovar grippotyphosa. *Am J Vet Res* **65**(8): 1100–1107.

Grudzinski, L., P. Quinan, et al. (2007). Sodium citrate 4% locking solution for central venous dialysis catheters—an effective, more cost-efficient alternative to heparin. *Nephrol Dial Transplant* **22**: 471–476.

Hedges, S.J., S.B. Dehoney, et al. (2006). Evidence-based treatment recommendations for uremic bleeding. *Nat Clin Pract Nephrol* **3**(3): 138–153.

Himmelfarb, J., L.M. Dember, et al. (2005). Vascular access. In: *Chronic Kidney Disease, Dialysis, and Transplantation*, edited by B.J.G. Pereira, M.H. Sayegh, and P. Blake. Philadelphia, PA: Elsevier Saunders, pp. 341–362.

Hoenich, N.A. and C. Ronco (2008a). Selecting a dialyzer: technical and clinical considerations. In: *Handbook of Dialysis Therapy*, edited by A.R. Nissenson and R.N. Fine. Philadelphia, PA: Saunders Elsevier, pp. 263–278.

Hoenich, N.A. and C. Ronco (2008b). Biocompatibility of dialysis membranes. In: *Handbook of Dialysis Therapy*, edited by A.R. Nissenson and R.N. Fine. Philadelphia, PA: Saunders Elsevier, pp. 279–294.

Jaber, B.L. and B.J.G. Pereira (2005). Biocompatibility of hemodialysis membranes. In: *Chronic Kidney Disease, Dialysis, and Transplantation*, edited by B.J.G. Pereira, M.H. Sayegh, and P. Blake. Philadelphia, PA: Elsevier Saunders, pp. 363–387.

John, S., D. Griesbach, et al. (2001). Effects of continuous haemofiltration vs. intermittent haemodialysis on systemic haemodynamics and splanchnic regional perfusion in septic shock patients: a prospective, randomized clinical trial. *Nephrol Dial Transplant* **16**: 320–327.

Johnson, C.A. (2008). *Dialysis of Drugs*. Verona, Wisconsin: CKD Insights.

Johnson, D.W., R. MacGinley, et al. (2002). A randomized controlled trial of topical exit site mupirocin application in patients with tunnelled, cuffed haemodialysis catheters. *Nephrol Dial Transplant* **17**(10): 1802–1807.

Katneni, R. and S.S. Hedayati (2007). Central venous catheter-related bacteremia in chronic hemodialysis patients: epidemiology and evidence-based management. *Nat Clin Pract Nephrol* **3**: 256–266.

Kaw, D. and D. Malhotra (2006). Platelet dysfunction and end-stage renal disease. *Semin Dial* **19**(4): 317–322.

Kjellstrand, C.M., U. Bunocristiani, et al. (2008). Short daily haemodialysis: survival in 415 patients treated for 1006 patient-years. *Nephrol Dial Transplant* **23**: 3283–3289.

Kogika, M.M. and H.A. de Morais (2008). Hyperkalemia: a quick reference. *Vet Clin North Am Small Animal Pract* **38**(3): 477–480.

Kooienga, L. (2007). Phosphorus balance with daily dialysis. *Semin Dial* **20**(4): 342–345.

Krishnasami, Z., D. Carlton, et al. (2002). Management of hemodialysis catheter-related bacteremia with an adjunctive antibiotic lock solution. *Kidney Int* **61**: 1136–1142.

Langston, C.E. (2004). *Water Treatment for Dialysis*. New York: Advanced Renal Therapies Symposium 2004.

Langston, C.E., L.D. Cowgill, et al. (1997). Applications and outcome of hemodialysis in cats: a review of 29 cases. *J Vet Intern Med* **11**(6): 348–355.

Leypoldt, J.K. (2005). Hemodialysis adequacy. In: *Chronic Kidney Disease, Dialysis, and Transplantation*, edited by B.J.G. Pereira, M.H. Sayegh, and P. Blake. Philadelphia, PA: Elsevier Saunders, pp. 405–428.

Liangos, O., A. Gul, et al. (2006). Long-term management of the tunneled venous catheter. *Semin Dial* **19**(2): 158–164.

Liangos, O., B.J.G. Pereira, et al. (2005). Acute complications associated with hemodialysis. In: *Chronic Kidney Disease, Dialysis, and Transplantation*, edited by B.J.G. Pereira, M.H. Sayegh, and P. Blake. Philadelphia, PA: Elsevier Saunders, pp. 451–471.

Liangos, O., M. Rao, et al. (2005). Relationship of urine output to dialysis initiation and mortality in acute renal failure. *Nephron Clin Pract* **99**(2): c56–c60.

Liu, K.D., J. Himmelfarb, et al. (2006). Timing of initiation of dialysis in critically ill patients with acute kidney injury. *Clin J Am Soc Nephrol* **1**(5): 915–919.

Ljutic, D., D. Perkovic, et al. (2002). Comparison of ondansetron with metoclopramide in the symptomatic relief of uremia-induced nausea and vomiting. *Kidney Blood Press Res* **25**(1): 61–64.

Lok, C.E., K.E. Stanley, et al. (2003). Hemodialysis infection prevention with polysporin ointment. *J Am Soc Nephrol* **13**(1): 169–179.

Lok, C.E., A. Thomas, et al. (2006). A patient-focused approach to thrombolytic use in the management of catheter malfunction. *Semin Dial* **19**(5): 381–390.

Lonneman, G., L. Sereni, et al. (2001). Pyrogen retention by highly permeable synthetic membranes during in vitro dialysis. *Artif Organs* **25**(12): 951–960.

Lopot, F., B. Nejedly, et al. (2003). Comparison of different techniques of hemodialysis vascular access flow evaluation. *Int J Artif Organs* **26**(12): 1056–1063.

MacRae, J.M., I. Dojcinovic, et al. (2008). Citrate 4% versus heparin and the reduction of thrombosis study (CHARTS). *Clin J Am Soc Nephrol* **3**(2): 369–374.

Mehta, R.L., B.R. McDonald, et al. (2001). A randomized clinical trial of continuous versus intermittent dialysis for acute renal failure. *Kidney Int* **60**: 1154–1163.

Murakami, M., T. Hamasaki, et al. (2004). Clinical features and management of intracranial hemorrhage in patients undergoing maintenance dialysis therapy. *Neurol Med Chir (Tokyo)* **44**: 225–233.

Negulescu, O., M. Coco, et al. (2003). Large atrial thrombus formation associated with tunneled cuffed hemodialysis catheters. *Clin Nephrol* **59**(1): 40–46.

Network, V.N.A.R.F.T. (2008). Intensity of renal support in critically ill patients with acute kidney injury. *N Engl J Med* **359**(1): 7–20.

Oliver, M.J., D.C. Mendelssohn, et al. (2007). Catheter patency and function after catheter sheath disruption: a pilot study. *Clin J Am Soc Nephrol* **2**(6): 1201–1206.

Olyaei, A.J. and W.M. Bennett (2008). Principles of drug usage in dialysis patients. In: *Handbook of Dialysis Therapy*, edited by A.R. Nissenson and R.N. Fine. Philadelphia, PA: Saunders Elsevier, pp. 1089–1195.

Pantaleo, V., T. Francey, et al. (2004). Application of hemodialysis for the management of acute uremia in cats: 119 cases (1993–2003) (abstract). *J Vet Intern Med* **18**(3): 418.

Parham, W.A., A.A. Mehdirad, et al. (2006). Hyperkalemia revisited. *Tex Heart Inst J* **33**: 40–47.

Patel, N., P. Dalal, et al. (2008). Dialysis disequilibrium syndrome: a narrative review. *Semin Dial* **21**(5): 493–498.

Ponce, P., J. Cruz, et al. (2007). A prospective study on incidence of bacterial infections in Portuguese dialysis units. *Nephron Clin Pract* **107**(4): c133–C138.

Pun, P.H. and E.C. Kovalik (2008). Methods of hemodialysis anticoagulation. In: *Handbook of Dialysis Therapy*, edited by A.R. Nissenson and R.N. Fine. Philadelphia, PA: Saunders Elsevier, pp. 224–238.

Rabb, H., Z. Wang, et al. (2003). Acute renal failure leads to dysregulation of lung salt and water channels. *Kidney Int* **63**(2): 600–606.

Ronco, C., R. Bellomo, et al. (2000). Effects of different doses in continuous veno-venous haemofiltration on outcomes of acute renal failure: a prospective randomised trial. *Lancet* **356**(9223): 26–30.

Saudan, P., M. Niederberger, et al. (2006). Adding a dialysis dose to continuous hemofiltration increases survival in patients with acute renal failure. *Kidney Int* **70**(7): 1312–1317.

Schiffl, H., S.M. Lang, et al. (2002). Daily hemodialysis and the outcome of acute renal failure. *N Engl J Med* **346**(5): 305–310.

Schmidt, R.J. and A. Besarab (2008). Anemia in patients with end-stage renal disease. In: *Handbook of Dialysis Therapy*, edited by A.R. Nissenson and R.N. Fine. Philadelphia, PA: Saunders Elsevier, pp. 761–770.

Segev, G., C. Bandt, et al. (2008). Aluminum toxicity following administration of aluminum-based phosphate binders in two dogs with renal failure. *J Vet Intern Med* **22**(6): 1432–1435.

Segev, G., P.H. Kass, et al. (2008). A novel clinical scoring system for outcome prediction in dogs with acute kidney injury managed by hemodialysis. *J Vet Intern Med* **22**(2): 301–308.

Selby, N.M. and C.W. McIntyre (2006). A systematic review of the clinical effects of reducing dialysate fluid temperature. *Nephrol Dial Transplant* **21**: 1883–1898.

Servillo, G., F. Bifulco, et al. (2007). Posterior reversible encephalopathy syndrome in intensive care medicine. *Intensive Care Med* **33**: 230–236.

Sesso, R., D. Barbosa, et al. (1998). *Staphylococcus aureus* prophylaxis in hemodialysis patients using central venous catheter: effect of mupirocin ointment. *J Am Soc Nephrol* **9**(6): 1085–1092.

Shah, A., M. Murray, et al. (2004). Right atrial thrombi complicating use of central venous catheters in hemodialysis. *Int J Artif Organs* **27**(9): 772–778.

Sherman, R.A. and T. Kapoian (2008). Dialysis access recirculation. In: *Handbook of Dialysis Therapy*, edited by A.R. Nissenson and R.N. Fine. Philadelphia, PA: Saunders Elsevier, pp. 102–108.

Sood, P., G.P. Sinson, et al. (2007). Subdural hematomas in chronic dialysis patients: significant and increasing. *Clin J Am Soc Nephrol* **2**(5): 956–959.

Stiller, S., E. Bonnie-Schorn, et al. (2001). A critical review of sodium profiling for hemodialysis. *Semin Dial* **14**(5): 337–347.

Sungur, M., E. Eryuksel, et al. (2007). Exit of catheter lock solutions from double lumen acute haemodialysis catheters—an in vitro study. *Nephrol Dial Transplant* **22**(12): 3533–3537.

Tokars, J., M.J. Alter, et al. (2005). Nosocomial infections in hemodialysis units. In: *Chronic Kidney Disease, Dialysis and Transplantation*, edited by B.J.G. Pereira, M.H. Sayegh, and P. Blake. Philadelphia, PA: Elsevier Saunders, pp. 429–450.

Tolwani, A.J., R.C. Campbell, et al. (2008). Standard versus high-dose CVVHDF for ICU-related acute renal failure. *J Am Soc Nephrol* **19**(6): 1233–1238.

Trinh-Trang-Tan, M.-M., J.-P. Cartron, et al. (2005). Molecular basis for the disequilibrium syndrome: altered aquaporin and urea transporter expression in the brain. *Nephrol Dial Transplant* **20**: 1984–1988.

Twardowski, Z.J. (2000). Safety of high venous and arterial line pressures during hemodialysis. *Semin Dial* **13**(5): 336–337.

Uchino, S. (2008). Choice of therapy and renal recovery. *Crit Care Med* **36**(Suppl): S238–S242.

Uchino, S., R. Bellomo, et al. (2007). Patient and kidney survival by dialysis modality in critically ill patients with acute kidney injury. *Int J Artif Organs* **30**(4): 281–292.

Waddell, L.S. (2005). Hypotension. In: *Textbook of Veterinary Internal Medicine*, edited by S.J. Ettinger and E.C. Feldman, Vol **1**. St. Louis, MO: Elsevier Saunders, pp. 480–483.

Waikar, S.S. and J.V. Bonventre (2006). Can we rely on blood urea nitrogen as a bomarker to determine when to initiate dialysis? (Editorial). *Clin J Am Soc Nephrol* **1**(5): 903–904.

Ward, D.M. (2005). Anticoagulation in patients on hemodialysis. In: *Clinical Dialysis*, edited by A.R. Nissenson and R.N. Fine. New York: McGraw-Hill, pp. 127–152.

Weijmer, M.C., Y.J. Debets-Ossenkopp, et al. (2002). Superior antimicrobial activity of trisodium citrate over heparin for catheter locking. *Nephrol Dial Transplant* **17**: 2189–2195.

Weijmer, M.C., M.A. Van Den Dorpel, et al. (2005). Randomized, clinical trial comparison of trisodium citrate 30% and heparin as catheter-locking solution in hemodialysis patients. *J Am Soc Nephrol* **16**(9): 2769–2777.

Wentling, A.G. (2004). Hemodialysis catheters: materials, design and manufacturing. *Contrib Nephrol* **142**: 112–127.

Willms, L. and L. Vercaigne (2008). Does warfarin safely prevent clotting of hemodialysis catheters? *Semin Dial* **21**(1): 71–77.

Yeun, J.Y. and T.A. Depner (2005). Principles of hemodialysis. In: *Chronic Kidney Disease, Dialysis, and Transplantation*, edited by B.J.G. Pereira, M.H. Sayegh, and P. Blake. Philadelphia, PA: Elsevier Saunders, pp. 307–340.

29

Continuous renal replacement therapy

Mark J Acierno

Continuous renal replacement therapy (CRRT) is a new blood purification technique that is quickly gaining acceptance for treatment patients with acute kidney injury (see Chapter 49). As its name implies, CRRT relies on gradual and continuous operation to remove uremic toxins, establish electrolyte/acid–base balance and regulate fluids. CRRT, like traditional intermittent hemodialysis (ID) (see Chapter 28), utilizes semipermeable membranes contained within a dialyzer to replace normal kidney function. However, unlike ID, which primarily employs diffusion to modify blood composition, CRRT employs both diffusion and convection.

CRRT has several potential advantages over ID. Its continuous nature and ability to remove larger molecules allows CRRT to more closely approximate normal kidney function (Clark et al. 1994). In addition, studies have demonstrated that CRRT is superior to ID for controlling acid–base and electrolyte balance (Bellomo et al. 1995). Since ID relies primarily on diffusion for blood purification, large amounts of sterile dialysate must be produced onsite. This requires specialized water treatment facilities, which adds significantly to the complexity and expense of operating and maintaining the dialysis equipment (Langston 2002). CRRT units utilize prepackaged fluids, which significantly reduces maintenance and cost and allows the system to be used cage-side. Studies in human patients have shown that CRRT can be safely used in patients weighing as little 2.3 kg (Symons et al. 2003).

Indications

Treatment of acute kidney injury is the most common application for CRRT. CRRT removes uremic toxins while

correcting electrolyte, acid–base, and fluid imbalances. In addition, CRRT can also be used to expedite the removal of drugs and toxins. The ability to remove a substance by CRRT is dependent on the size of the molecule, its volume of distribution, as well as its degree of protein binding (Johnson and Simons 2006). A small toxin with a minimal volume of distribution and low protein binding would be most amenable to filtering. The extent to which many drugs and toxins can be dialyzed has been published (Johnson 2007). CRRT has also been used to treat humans with congestive heart failure (Clark and Ronco 2004).

Blood purification

The purification of blood using a semipermeable membrane relies on two distinct mechanisms: diffusion and convection. Diffusion is the tendency for molecules in solution to move from an area where they are in a high concentration to an area where they are in a lower concentration (Clark and Ronco 2004). Changing the composition of canine blood using diffusion across a semipermeable membrane was first demonstrated in 1914 (Abel et al. 1914). In this classic experiment, blood was diverted from dog and into a glass cylinder where the blood was divided into tube-like semipermeable membranes bathed in solution. The blood was then returned to the patient. By changing the composition of the fluid bathing the semipermeable membranes, substances could be made to diffuse in or out of the blood. This remains the basis of all hemodialysis.

Convection also takes place in the semipermeable membranes of the dialyzer. In this process, blood is perfused through the dialyzer at a pressure exceeding that on the opposite side of the dialyzer membrane, thereby producing a positive transmembrane pressure that pushes

Nephrology and Urology of Small Animals. Edited by Joe Bartges and David J. Polzin. © 2011 Blackwell Publishing Ltd.

SCUF

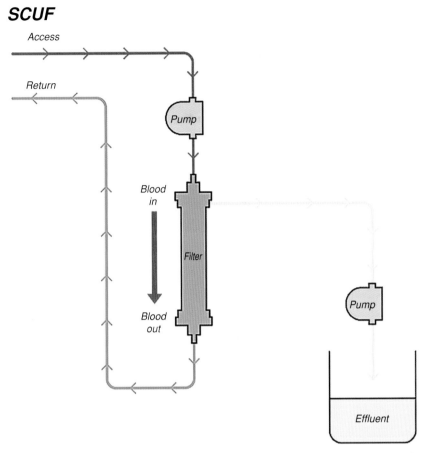

Figure 29.1 Slow continuous ultrafiltration (SCUF)—a purely convective modality generates large amounts of ultrafiltrate, which is not replaced (Used with permission, Veterinary Learning Systems).

fluid (called ultrafiltrate) across the membrane (Golpher 2002). Toxins, electrolytes, and other small molecules are then carried out of the blood with the ultrafiltrate, which is then disposed of as "effluent." Convection is more challenging than diffusion as it removes large amounts of water and electrolytes from the blood that must be replaced with great accuracy. The benefit is that it is more effective than diffusion in clearing larger molecules such as beta-macroglobulin from the bloodstream (Ronco et al. 2001).

Modes of operation

CRRT units utilize the principles of diffusion and convection to produce four different filtration modalities. Slow continuous ultrafiltration (SCUF) (Figure 29.1) is a purely convective modality in which ultrafiltrate is removed from the blood and not replaced (Bellomo and Ronco 2002a). This modality has been used in human medicine to treat congestive heart failure (Clark and Ronco 2004).

Continuous veno-venous hemofiltration (CVVH) (Figure 29.2) is similar to SCUF in that it is a purely convective modality; however, in CVVH, the ultrafiltrate is replaced with a sterile balanced electrolyte solution (Bellomo and Ronco 2002a). This replacement fluid can be added before or after the blood passes through the dialyzer. Adding fluid after the dialyzer is an extremely efficient way to remove uremic toxins; however, as the blood travels through the dialyzer, it becomes hemoconcentrated, thereby increasing the risk of clotting (Henderson 1979). Adding the replacement fluid prior to the dialysis cartridge avoids the problems of hemoconcentration but is significantly less efficient (Parakininkas and Greenbaum 2004). Since approximately 25% of the plasma volume (filtration fraction) can be safely removed and replaced after the dialyzer, we have most commonly employed postfilter fluid replacement. Until recently, there were no FDA-approved replacement solutions, and CRRT dialysate solution was used (Davenport 2004a). Although several approved solutions now exist, off-label use of dialysis solution as a replacement fluid is still commonly employed.

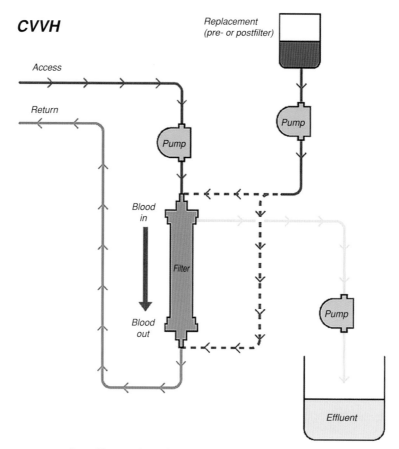

Figure 29.2 Continuous veno-venous hemofiltration (CVVH) is a convective modality that generates large amounts of ultrafiltrate. In CVVH, the ultrafiltrate is replaced with a sterile balanced electrolyte solution. This replacement fluid is added before or after the dialyzer (Used with permission, Veterinary Learning Systems).

Continuous veno-venous hemodialysis (CVVHD) is a diffusive therapy similar to ID (Figure 29.3) (Bellomo and Ronco 2002b). Unlike ID, CVVHD relies on prepackaged dialysate that is made possible due to relatively slow dialysate flow rates (Davenport 2004b).

Continuous veno-venous hemodiafiltration (CVVHDF) combines the diffusive aspects of CVVHD and convective aspects of CVVH (Figure 29.4) (Bellomo and Ronco 2002b). Blood flowing through the dialyzer's semipermeable membranes are bathed in dialysis solution and exposed to elevated transmembrane pressure so that both diffusion and ultrafiltration guides the movement of solutes. This modality offers the greatest treatment flexibility (Clark and Ronco 2004).

At this time, it is not clear which CRRT modality provides the most effective blood purification. Although CVVH and CVVHDF provide a significant advantage in the removal of middle-sized molecules, the role of these substances in uremic toxicity remains unresolved. Nevertheless, in most cases, we currently utilize HVVD or CVVHDF.

Blood access

To provide adequate blood flow, a dual lumen temporary dialysis catheter is placed in the jugular vein using the Seldinger technique. A 11.5 Fr. catheter is placed in very large dogs while a 8 Fr. catheter is typically used in smaller dogs and cats. In the smallest patients, two single lumen 5 Fr. catheters can be placed in the jugulars.

Anticoagulation

Despite the highly biocompatible nature of dialysis catheters, tubing, and dialyzers, appropriate anticoagulation is essential. Clotting of the CRRT setup necessitates the costly replacement of dialyzer and tubing, leads to a significant loss of patient blood, and delays access to treatment. There are two drugs commonly used for anticoagulation: citrate and heparin.

Historically, constant rate infusion of heparin has been the most widely employed method of anticoagulation (Davenport 2004a). Heparin increases the activity of

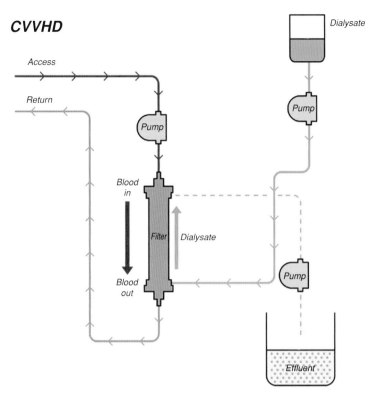

Figure 29.3 Continuous veno-venous hemodialysis (CVVHD) is a diffusive therapy in which the movement of small molecules is guided by their relative concentration in the blood and dialysate (Used with permission, Veterinary Learning Systems).

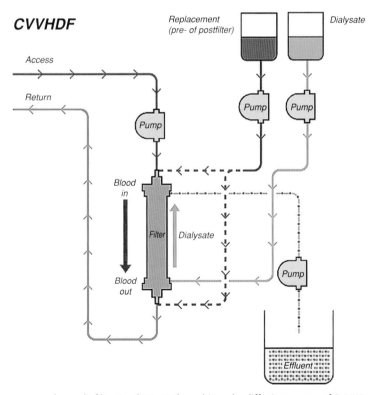

Figure 29.4 Continuous veno-venous hemodiafiltration (CVVHDF) combines the diffusive aspects of CVVHD with the convective properties of CVVH. Diffusion guides the movement of some uremic toxins and electrolytes while a difference in the transmembrane pressure causes lead to the creation ultrafiltrate and removal of solutes (Used with permission, Veterinary Learning Systems).

Table 29.1 LSU heparin work sheet

Start of therapy
  Check ACT
  In the absence of coagulopathy (ACT > 150) give 25 unit/kg heparin bolus
  Record total units given ____
  Recheck ACT. If <180, repeat bolus (maximum 3 TOTAL bolus)
  Record number of boluses given ____
  ACT at start of therapy ____
During hemofiltration
  Start heparin infusion 20 units/kg/hour
  If ACT <180 increase heparin by 1 unit/kg/hour
  If ACT >220 decrease heparin by 1 unit/kg/hour
  If ACT <170 bolus 10 unit/kg heparin & increase CRI
  If ACT <160 bolus 15 unit/kg heparin & increase CRI
Monitor ACT q30 minutes after any change
  Monitor ACT q2 hours once stable

antithrombin, a circulating protease inhibitor (Ganong 2001). Since the patient is systemically anticoagulated, there is a risk of hemorrhagic complications (Davenport 2004a). This risk can be minimized by periodically monitoring the activated clotting time (ACT) (Davenport 2004a) and adjusting the heparin dosage to maintain the ACT between 180 and 220 seconds (Table 29.1)

Calcium is an important cofactor throughout the clotting cascade and blood is unable to clot in its absence (Gibney 2005). As blood enters the CRRT circuit, citrate can be infused to chelate serum calcium. As the blood leaves the system, calcium chloride is then infused to restore serum calcium to physiologic levels (Davenport 2004). Citrate therapy has the advantage of providing only local anticoagulation. Nevertheless, there are significant risks of systemic hypocalcemia and metabolic alkalosis necessitating frequent calcium and acid/base monitoring (Bellomo and Ronco 2002c; Gibney 2005). Because of the ease of monitoring, lower cost, and personal experience, our preference is to use heparin as an anticoagulant.

Treatment adequacy

Although the exact toxins responsible for uremia are not known, blood urea nitrogen (BUN) is easily measured and used as a surrogate for all low molecular weight substances removed by CRRT (Ricci et al. 2005). A commonly used measure of CRRT treatment adequacy is Kt/V where K is a measurement of instantaneous urea clearance (removal rate/concentration) (Ricci et al. 2005). Total solute removal per period of time is then defined as the product of instantaneous clearance (K mL/minute) and time (t minutes) receiving CRRT per day. This product is then normalized for volume of distribution (V mL). Urea is approximately equally distributed in all body water compartments, and therefore, in CRRT, V is equal to total body water, which is estimated as 60% of body weight in kilograms.

Although relevant veterinary studies are lacking, evidence from the human literature suggest that Kt/V values greater than 1.4 are associated with decreased morbidity and mortality (Ronco et al. 2000; Ricci et al. 2005). Values for K can be estimated before treatment starts (K_{calc}) and then actual K calculated (K_{del}) (Table 29.2). For example, a 32 kg Labrador retriever suffering from AKI secondary to heat stroke is to be started on CVVH. Blood rate (Q_b) will be set at 100 mL/minute and ultrafiltration rate 20%. From experience, we know that the patient will receive 1320 minutes (22 hours) of therapy per day. From Table 29.1, we see that in CVVH K = ultrafiltrate rate or 20 mL/ minute. Therefore Kt/V_{calc} = (20 mL/minute * 1,320 minutes)/19,200 mL or 1.37. Since this is less than our goal, we can increase the blood flow rate, the ultrafiltration rate, or both.

Complications

In our experience, problems associated with anticoagulation are perhaps the most challenging. Despite regular monitoring of the activated clotting time, the CRRT circuit eventually becomes obstructed by a clot. Conversely, some patients develop bleeding at the catheter site. Hypotension is another potential complication that is thought to be the result of the large amount of blood needed to fill and maintain the CRRT circuit (50 – 84 mL). In an attempt to address this problem in smaller patients, neonatal dialyzers can be used, and the blood

Table 29.2 *Kt/V* formulae

K_{calc} = calculated (estimated) urea clearance
K_{DEL} = actual delivered urea clearance

CVVH – Post-dialyzer replacement fluid
K_{calc} = Ultrafiltration rate (mL/minute)
K_{DEL} = Ultrafiltrate urea concentration (mg/dL) *Ultrafiltration rate (mL/minute)/Predialyzer urea concentration (mg/dL)

CVVH – Pre-dialyzer replacement fluid
K_{calc} = Ultrafiltration rate (mL/minute)/[1+(Fluid replacement (mL/minute)/blood flow rate (mL/minute)]
K_{DEL} = Ultrafiltrate urea concentration (mg/dL) *Ultrafiltration rate (mL/minute)/Predialyzer urea concentration (mg/dL)

CVVHD
K_{calc} = dialysate rate (mL/minute)
K_{DEL} = Postdialyzer dialysate urea concentration (mg/dL) *dialysate rate (mL/minute)/prefilter blood urea level (mg/dL)

CVVHDF – Post-dialyzer replacement fluid
K_{calc} = Ultrafiltration rate (mL/minute) + dialysate rate (mL/minute)
K_{DEL} = Ultrafiltrate urea concentration (mg/dL) *(Ultrafiltration rate (mL/minute) + dialysate rate (mL/minute))/Predialyzer blood urea level (mg/dL)

pathway can be primed with blood or other colloids. It is important to note that stored blood products can become acidic. When blood with a low pH interacts with AN69 dialyzer membranes, bradykinins are activated (Brophy et al. 2001). This can lead to a catastrophic cardiovascular event. Therefore, if blood priming is used, the blood should be allowed to undergo diffusion or convection in the CRRT circuit to allow the pH to become physiologic and bradykinins cleared (Brophy et al. 2001). We have successfully used this strategy to treat patients weighing only 2.5 kg. Dialysis disequilibrium, a concern in ID, has not been reported in CRRT (Bagshaw et al. 2004).

Patient care

Planning for adequate patient care is probably the most overlooked aspect in providing CRRT. Once a patient is started on CRRT, there is an obligation to provide trained, competent 24 hour a day care for extended periods of time. This can be extremely taxing. In addition, an advanced knowledge of renal physiology and the mechanics of the CRRT unit are essential for hourly treatment decisions.

Conclusion

CRRT comprises four different modalities for the treatment of acute kidney injury, toxin exposure, and fluid overload. Its slow continuous nature and self-contained design offers several advantages over traditional ID. Nevertheless, the need for constant expert supervision and a skilled nursing staff should not be underestimated. Therefore, application of CRRT is likely to be most suc-

cessful when utilized in specialized referral intuitions with appropriately trained staff.

References

Abel, J., L. Rowntree, et al. (1914). On the removal of diffusible substances from the circulating blood of living animals by dialysis. *J Pharmacol Exp Ther* **5**: 275–316.

Bagshaw, S.M., A.D. Peets, et al. (2004). Dialysis disequilibrium syndrome: brain death following hemodialysis for metabolic acidosis and acute renal failure—a case report. *BMC Nephrol* **5**: 9.

Bellomo, R., M. Farmer, et al. (1995). Severe acute renal failure: a comparison of acute continuous hemodiafiltration and conventional dialytic therapy. *Nephron* **71**: 59–64.

Bellomo, R. and C. Ronco (2002a). An introduction to continuous renal replacement therapy. In: *Atlas of Hemofiltration*, edited by R. Bellomo, I. Baldwin, C. Ronco, et al. London: WB Saunders, pp. 1–9.

Bellomo, R. and C. Ronco (2002b). Nomenclature for continuous renal replacement therapy. In: *Atlas of Hemofiltration*, edited by R. Bellomo, I. Baldwin, C. Ronco, et al. London: WB Saunders, pp. 11–14.

Bellomo, R. and C. Ronco (2002c). Anticoagulation during CRRT. In: *Atlas of Hemofiltration*, edited by R Bellomo, I. Baldwin, C. Ronco, et al. London: WB Saunders, pp. 63–68.

Brophy, P.D., T.A. Mottes, et al. (2001). AN-69 membrane reactions are pH-dependent and preventable. *Am J Kidney Dis* **38**: 173–178.

Clark, W.R., B.A. Mueller, et al. (1994). A comparison of metabolic control by continuous and intermittent therapies in acute renal failure. *J Am Soc Nephrol* **4**: 1413–1420.

Clark, W.R. and C. Ronco (2004). Continuous renal replacement techniques. *Contrib Nephrol* **144**: 264–277.

Davenport, A. (2004a). Anticoagulation for continuous renal replacement therapy. *Contrib Nephrol* **144**: 228–238.

Davenport, A. (2004b). Replacement and dialysate fluids for patients with acute renal failure treated by continuous veno-venous haemofiltration and/or haemodiafiltration. *Contrib Nephrol* **144**: 317–328.

Ganong, W. (2001). Circulating body fluids. In: *Review of Medical Physiology*. New York: Lange Medical Books, pp. 499–527.

Gibney, N. (2005). Anticoagulation 2: special techniques citrate. *Proc 11th Annual International Conference on Continuous Renal Replacement Therapies*, San Diego, CA, pp. B30–B31.

Golpher, T. (2002). Solute transport in CRRT. In: *Atlas of Hemofiltration*, edited by R. Bellomo, I. Baldwin, C. Ronco, et al. London: WB Saunders, pp. 15–18.

Henderson, L.W. (1979). Pre vs. post dilution hemofiltration. *Clin Nephrol* 11: 120–124.

Johnson, C. and W. Simmons (2006). *Dialysis of Drugs*. Verona, WI: Nephrology Pharmacy Associates.

Johnson, C. (2007). *Dialysis of Drugs*. Verona, WI: Nephrology Pharmacy Associates.

Langston, C. (2002). Hemodialysis in dogs and cats. *Compendium* 24: 540–549.

Parakininkas, D. and L.A. Greenbaum (2004). Comparison of solute clearance in three modes of continuous renal replacement therapy. *Pediatr Crit Care Med* 5: 269–274.

Ricci, Z., G. Salvatori, et al. (2005). In vivo validation of the adequacy calculator for continuous renal replacement therapies. *Crit Care* 9: R266–R273.

Ronco, C., R. Bellomo, et al. (2000). Effects of different doses in continuous veno-venous haemofiltration on outcomes of acute renal failure: a prospective randomised trial. *Lancet* 356: 26–30.

Ronco, C., R. Bellomo, et al. (2001). Continuous renal replacement therapy in critically ill patients. *Nephrol Dial Transplant* 16(Suppl 5): 67–72.

Symons, J.M., P.D. Brophy, et al. (2003). Continuous renal replacement therapy in children up to 10 kg. *Am J Kidney Dis* 41: 984–989.

30

Peritoneal dialysis

Mary Anna Labato

Dialysis is the process by which water and solutes move between two compartments that are separated by a semi-permeable membrane. In peritoneal dialysis (PD), the two compartments consist of blood in the peritoneal capillaries and fluid (dialysate) instilled into the peritoneal cavity. The peritoneum serves as the semi-permeable membrane. The primary indication for PD in animals is in kidney failure to correct the resulting water, solute, and acid–base imbalances and to remove uremic toxins. Experimental abdominal lavage was performed as early as the late nineteenth century; however, Putnam in 1923 was the first to characterize the peritoneum as a dialyzing membrane in dogs (Lameire et al. 1998).

PD has been used to treat acute kidney failure in humans since 1923 when Georg Ganter used PD to treat a patient with kidney disease. PD temporarily replaces the kidney's excretory function by using the peritoneum as the semi-permeable membrane across which unwanted solutes are eliminated. Currently, in human medicine, PD is used to treat both acute and chronic kidney failure (Chapters 48 and 49) as well as to remove dialyzable toxins such as ethylene glycol, ethanol, and barbiturates. It is one of the most common forms of therapy for acute kidney injury in children (Posen and Luisello 1980; Mendoza et al. 1993; Wong et al. 1996; Passadakis and Oreopoulos 2007). PD is also used as a treatment for uroabdomen (Chapter 11), hyperthermia, hypothermia, pancreatitis, fluid volume overload secondary to congestive heart failure, and to reduce life-threatening metabolic disturbances and peritonitis (Henrich and Paganini 1992). In veterinary medicine, the most common indication for PD has been acute kidney injury.

Pathophysiology

The peritoneal membrane is a thin translucent porous layer of tissue with numerous blood vessels. It consists of two layers, the parietal layer that lines the inner surface of the abdominal wall and the visceral layer that covers the abdominal organs (Kelly 2004). The visceral peritoneum accounts for about 80% of the total peritoneal surface area (Blake and Daugirdas 2001). The space between the parietal and visceral peritoneum is called the peritoneal cavity. It normally contains less than 10 mL of fluid but can accommodate several hundred milliliters to several liters of fluid without patient discomfort (Khanna et al. 1993; Kelly 2004). This membrane is semi-permeable and acts as a dialyzer, permitting waste to cross (filter through) the membrane from the blood to the dialysis solution in the peritoneal cavity (Figure 30.1)

The most important function of the peritoneal membrane is to provide a protective lubricating surface for the abdominal organs. Mesothelial cells secrete glycosaminoglycans including hyaluronic acid, proteoglycans such as decorin and biglycan, and phosphatidylcholine-containing lamellar bodies (Nagy and Jackman 2000). Recent studies have shown that mesothelial cells play a role in a number of other processes, including antigen presentation, control of inflammation, tissue repair, coagulation, and fibrinolysis (Chegini 2002; Jorres 2003). Some studies suggest that mesothelial cells can play an active role in fluid transport. Plasmalemmal vesicles may mediate transport across the mesothelial cells. Mesothelial cells may also affect blood flow through peritoneal capillaries by secretion of various vasoactive substances, including nitric oxide and endothelin (Nagy and Jackman 2000). It is generally felt that the mesothelial cells do not represent a significant barrier to water transport.

The anatomic structures that appear to play the most important role in fluid and solute transport are the walls of the capillaries and the extracellular matrix

Nephrology and Urology of Small Animals. Edited by Joe Bartges and David J. Polzin. © 2011 Blackwell Publishing Ltd.

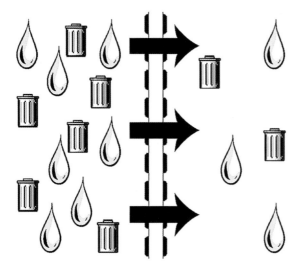

Figure 30.1 This figure illustrates the process of diffusion across the semi-permeable peritoneal membrane. Reprinted from Nephrology Nursing Journal, 2004, Volume 31, Number 5, p. 448. Reprinted with permission of the publisher, the American Nephrology Nurses' Association (ANNA); East Holly Avenue, Box 56, Pitman, NJ 08071–0056; (856) 256–2300; FAX (856) 589–7463; E-mail: ana@ajj.com; web site: www.annanurse.org.

located in the submesothelial cell connective tissue (Stelin and Rippe 1990; Flessner 1991; Flessner et al. 2003). Peritoneal capillaries are composed primarily of non-fenestrated endothelial cells supported by a basement membrane. Endothelial cells contain aquaporins, which are responsible for water transport. Intercellular clefts between endothelial cells also play a role in solute transport (Khanna 2000). When the peritoneum is thought of as a dialyzer, it should be considered as six resistances in series consisting of a stagnant capillary fluid film overlying the endothelium of the peritoneal capillaries, the capillary endothelium, the endothelial basement membrane, the interstitium, the mesothelium, and a stagnant fluid film overlying the peritoneal membrane.

The dynamics of fluid and solute exchange across a semi-permeable membrane is the foundation of PD. Large molecules such as proteins pass very slowly or not at all through the membrane. Smaller molecules such as urea, glucose, and ions (sodium and potassium) move easily across the membrane down a concentration gradient until equilibration is reached on both sides of the membrane. Water moves across the membrane from the solution of lower osmolality to that of higher osmolality until equilibration is reached. Normal plasma osmolality has been measured from 285 to 310 mOsm/L. Uremic animals may have an osmolality of about 350–400 mOsm/L (Labato 2000). Various solutes and water can be added to or removed from plasma by altering the electrolyte composition and osmolality of the dialysate fluid.

The peritoneal transfer of solutes reflects two simultaneous and interrelated transport mechanisms: diffusion and convection. Diffusion refers to the movement of solute across a semi-permeable membrane in response to differing concentrations of that solute on either side of the membrane. The solute moves from the side with higher to the side with lower concentration, down an electrochemical gradient and in accordance with basic thermodynamic principles. Convection refers to the movement of solutes swept across the membrane within the flux of fluid that arises as a consequence of ultrafiltration. Convective transport is determined by the ultrafiltration rate. Studies of peritoneal membrane function have classically characterized membrane transport properties in terms of effective membrane surface area and solute permeability, fluid transfer (ultrafiltration), and peritoneal lymphatic absorption (Alexander et al. 1999). Ultrafiltration refers to the movement of water across a semi-permeable membrane as a result of favorable osmotic or hydrostatic gradients. Effective ultrafiltration can occur during PD only by manipulating the osmotic gradient by changing the tonicity of the dialysate solution. Ultrafiltration is frequently desired when performing PD in animals because they are often over-hydrated as a result of fluid therapy.

Kinetics of PD

Dialysis occurs during the dwell time through the process of diffusion. Diffusion allows solutes to cross the peritoneal membrane from an area of higher to lower concentration. Uremic solutes and potassium diffuse from the capillary blood vessels across the membrane into the dialysis solution. Glucose and lactate diffuse in the opposite direction.

Peritoneal diffusion depends on the following factors:

1. The concentration gradient: urea is maximal in the blood at the start of the dwell when the concentration in the dialysis fluid is zero. It gradually decreases during the course of the dwell as it is removed from the blood.
2. The effective peritoneal surface area: depends on the total peritoneal surface area and the degree of vascularity.
3. The fill volume: where diffusion can also be increased by using larger fill volumes.
4. The molecular weight of solutes: solutes with lower molecular weight such as urea (MW 60) are more easily transported than those with higher molecular weights such as creatinine (MW113) (Kelly 2004).

Convection occurs when solutes are carried along with the bulk flow of water during ultrafiltration. This movement can occur even when the concentrations of solute on either side of the semi-permeable membrane would not promote diffusion of the solute. This effect does not play an important role in PD (Ross and Labato 2006).

A variety of mathematical models have been proposed over the years to account for movement of water and solutes across the peritoneum. The three-pore model appears to best describe peritoneal transport (Stelin and Rippe 1990; Flessner 1997; Anglani et al. 2001). Large pores greater than 150 A in diameter allow the transport of macromolecules. They are present in only small numbers, accounting for 5–7% of the total pore surface area. Small pores 20–25 A in diameter allow the passage of low molecular weight substances such as urea, creatinine, and glucose. It is believed that the clefts between capillary endothelial cells function as small pores and are present in large numbers representing more than 90% of the pore surface area. Ultra-small pores 3–5 A in diameter allow water only to pass. These ultra-small pores are believed to be aquaporins (molecular water channels). Aquaporins are a family of transport membrane polypeptides that permit water transport across the cellular membrane in response to an osmotic gradient. Aquaporin 1 appears to be the channel that is involved in water transport across the peritoneum. The location and number of Aquaporin 1 molecules are not yet well understood. Aquaporin 1 molecules have been identified in both peritoneal endothelium as well as peritoneal mesothelial cells.

Indications for PD

The primary indication for PD in animals is for the treatment of acute kidney injury (Chapter 49). This includes oliguric or anuric kidney failure, acute polyuric kidney failure with severe uremia that is not responsive to fluid therapy, and postrenal uremia resulting from ureteral obstruction or a rupture in the urinary collecting system (Chapters 58, 59, 70, 77, and 82). PD is a less efficient treatment modality than hemodialysis (Chapters 28 and 29) in correcting uremia and water and solute abnormalities; however, it still has a number of therapeutic advantages. The decreased efficiency may actually be beneficial in treating cats and small dogs in which rapid fluid and electrolyte shifts can result in serious clinical consequences. The equipment and supplies used for PD are easily obtained, and the technique for performing PD, although labor-intensive, is not difficult (Table 30.1). This actually makes PD a useful therapeutic modality for private practices especially those located in areas distant from intermittent or continuous dialysis facilities.

There are many other indications for the use of PD (Table 30.2). PD can be used for the treatment of toxicities in which the offending toxin can be removed by

Table 30.1 Comparison of peritoneal dialysis and hemodialysis

Peritoneal dialysis	Hemodialysis
Labor-intensive	Requires high level of technological expertise
Technologically simple	Requires expensive equipment and supplies
More efficacious in removing uremic middle molecules	More efficacious in altering water and solute balance

diffusion across the peritoneal membrane. These toxins include ethylene glycol, ethanol, and barbiturates. In addition to toxicities, severe metabolic disturbances such as hyperkalemia, resistant metabolic acidosis, hypercalcemia, and hepatic encephalopathy can be corrected with PD (Dyzban et al. 2000a, 2000b; Garcia-Lacaze et al. 2002; Ross and Labato 2006). PD with hypertonic dialysate can be used to remove excess water in animals with life-threatening fluid overload that may be seen with congestive heart failure. There are other disorders in which peritoneal lavage using solutions and techniques very similar to PD may be therapeutic. These include hypothermia, hyperthermia, and pancreatitis (Dyzban et al. 2000a, 2000b; Ross and Labato 2006).

Published reports of the clinical use of PD in small animals with kidney disease are few (Kirk 1957; Jackson 1964; Avellini et al. 1973; Thornhill et al. 1984; Fox et al. 1987; Crimp et al. 1989; Beckel et al. 2005; Wojick

Table 30.2 Indications for acute peritoneal dialysis

Oliguric or anuric acute kidney injury
Chronic kidney disease associated with nonresponsive
  uremia
Postrenal failure
  Ureteral obstruction
  Rupture in urine collecting system
Removal of dialyzable toxins
  Ethylene glycol
  Ethanol
  Barbiturates
Metabolic disorders
  Hepatic encephalopathy
  Hyperkalemia
  Hypercalcemia
  Severe metabolic acidosis
Fluid overload
Hyperthermia caused by heatstroke
Hypothermia
Pancreatitis

et al. 2008; Cooper and Labato in press). Although most described improvements in renal function during dialysis overall survival remained poor. In an early study involving 27 dogs and cats, 24% improved and were discharged from the hospital (Crimp et al. 1989). This study included 2 cats, and neither one survived. Eleven of twenty-one of these animals with acute kidney injury suffered from ethylene glycol intoxication, which is known to result in a mortality rate approaching 100% (Vaden et al. 1997; Forrester et al. 2002). A recent study of dogs with leptospirosis-induced kidney injury reported a survival rate of 80% (Beckel et al. 2005). The survival rate of dogs with leptospirosis treated with a standard approach of intravenous fluids and antibiotics has been reported to be 59–85% (Harkin and Gartrell 1996; Rentko et al. 1992; Adin and Cowgill 2000). The success of PD must be compared with the overall survival rate of animals with acute kidney injury treated with other means because animals undergoing dialysis traditionally have been those with the most severe kidney failure. In a study of 99 dogs with acute kidney injury, 43% were discharged from the hospital (Vaden et al. 1997). Of these, 24% were left with residual kidney dysfunction and only 19% had return to normal kidney function. In another report of 80 dogs with acute kidney injury of which 44% had ethylene glycol intoxication, only 20% survived to discharge (Forrester et al. 2002). In a recent review of 22 cats, the most common indication for PD was acute and chronic kidney injury (7/22, 32%). Urolithiasis accounted for 23% (5/22) of cases; 18% (4/22) of cats as presented with acute kidney injury due to toxicity, three of which were lily intoxication and one was an unknown toxin. Acute kidney injury was attributed to spay complications in 14% (3/22) of cats (bilateral ureteral ligation in two animals and unknown in one animal). Three cats were presented with acute kidney injury for unknown reasons (Cooper and Labato in press). Ten of twenty-two cats (45.5%) were discharged from the hospital after PD. The average number of days from initiation of PD to discharge for these cats was 9.4 (median 7.5, range 5–19). The average number of days on PD in this group was 3.5 (median 2.5, range 0–10). One animal was discharged from the hospital with the PD catheter intact and came back daily for PD catheter flushes for 10 days in the event that PD would be necessary again. The PD catheter in this cat was removed 10 days after discharge from the hospital after renal profiles showed that azotemia was being controlled with subcutaneous fluid administration (Cooper and Labato in press).

Indications for the use of PD in human medicine are acute kidney injury in children and chronic kidney disease in adults. In countries where hemodialysis is not readily available, PD is also used for acute kidney injury in adults. There are a number of studies comparing PD to continuous renal replacement therapies such as continuous venovenous hemofiltration, and there is still much debate as to which modality is superior (Phu et al. 2002; Passadakis and Oreopoulos 2007).

PD could theoretically be used for the long-term management of chronic kidney disease in dogs and cats. Technical problems with catheter flow and complications with infection make chronic PD challenging and definitely require a committed owner only a few cases have been reported (Simmons et al. 1980; Rubin et al. 1983; Thornhill et al. 1984; Carter et al. 1989; Crimp et al. 1989; Cooper and Labato in press).

Contraindications to PD

There are few situations in which PD is absolutely contraindicated. In humans, these include peritoneal adhesions that prevent fluid distribution throughout the peritoneal cavity and pleuroperitoneal leaks that would result in pleural effusion and respiratory compromise. Adhesions are not often seen in dogs and cats. Diaphragmatic or pericardiodiaphragmatic hernias are seen in animals and could result in respiratory or cardiac dysfunction. However, there was an early report of the use of pleural dialysis in two dogs with acute kidney injury (Shahar and Holmberg 1985). PD is contraindicated in severe catabolic states in which marked hypoalbuminemia exists because large amounts of protein can be lost through the peritoneum during dialysis exchanges. Marked ascites, obesity, recent abdominal surgery, bowel distention, or abdominal masses may interfere with catheter placement or adequate volume exchanges and are relative contraindications for PD (Labato 2000)

Protocol for PD

Catheter types and placement

The key to successful PD is the catheter and its placement. An ideal catheter allows efficient inflow and outflow. It is biocompatible and resists infection of both the peritoneum and the subcutaneous tunnel (Labato 2000; Bersinas 2006; Ross and Labato 2006). There are many catheter designs available and most are modifications of a fenestrated silicone tube with Dacron (INVISTA, Wichita, KS) cuffs positioned to promote fibrous adhesions at the peritoneal and cutaneous exit sites (Table 30.3)

Simple tube catheters with stylets can be placed percutaneously in conscious animals using local anesthetics in an emergency situation (Dyzban et al. 2000; Bersinas 2006; Ross and Labato 2006). A percutaneous cystotomy

Table 30.3 Suppliers of peritoneal dialysis catheters

Covidien/Kendall/Tyco Healthcare
15 Hampshire St.
Mansfield, MA 02048
800-962-9888
www.Kendallhq.com/healthcarecatalog.asp
www.covidien.com

A variety of peritoneal dialysis catheters
Medigroup Inc.
(division of Janin Group Inc)
505 Weston Ridge Drive
800-323-5389
www.medigroupinc.com
Ash Advantage Fluted-T Catheter
Flex-neck PD catheters

Medcomp
1499 Delp Drive
Harleyville, PA 19438
215-256-4201
www.medcompnet.com
Straight and curled, one and two cuff peritoneal dialysis
  catheters

Cook Medical Inc.
PO Box 4195
Bloomington, IN 47402–4195
www.cookmedical.com
Stamey and other suprapublic PD catheters

Smiths Medical PM, Inc.
N7W22025 Johnson Drive
Waukeshsa, WI 53186
888-745-6562
www.surgivet.com
acute peritoneal dialysis catheter

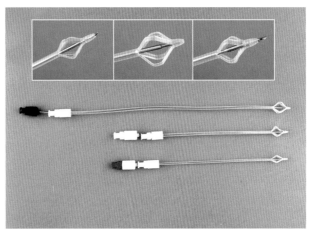

Figure 30.2 The Stamey percutaneous suprapubic catheter set (Cook Medical, Bloomington, IN) has been used successfully for acute short-term PD.

timeters, then insert through the abdominal muscles in the abdomen. The catheter is advanced over the trocar until it is fully in the abdomen. Ideally, the subcutaneous tunnel should create a snug fit. Use a purse string suture pattern to secure the catheter.

There are a variety of straight and curled catheters with straight and flexed necks for placement for long-term use (Figures 30.3 and 30.4).

The two catheters that have been most successful in veterinary medicine for long-term use are the fluted-T catheter and the Missouri catheter (Ash 1993; Ross and Labato 2006; Yerram 2007). The pediatric lengths are best used in cats and ferrets. When it is believed PD will be performed for longer than 24 hours, a surgically placed catheter should be utilized. Although some catheters such as the Fluted-T and the Missouri Swan

tube catheter (Stamey percutaneous suprapubic catheter set, Cook Medical, Bloomington, IN) has been used successfully for acute short-term PD (Figure 30.2)

The Tenckhoff catheter, developed in 1968, is a straight soft silastic tube fenestrated at the distal end and furnished with two Dacron velour cuffs that can be placed with a trocar or a laparascope (Thornhill et al. 1980; Gokal et al. 1998; Chada 2000; Harvey 2001). Because of the high rate of omental entrapment, surgical omentectomies are advocated when using this catheter in animals in which more than 3 days of dialysis is anticipated. PD for acute kidney failure should be performed for a minimum of 48–72 hours, the duration of treatment is predicated by the animal's condition. The patient should have the abdomen shaved and aseptically cleaned as for a surgical procedure. A stab incision should be made 3–5 cm lateral to the umbilicus. Insert the trocar toward the pelvis and inguinal canal. Tunnel subcutaneously for several cen-

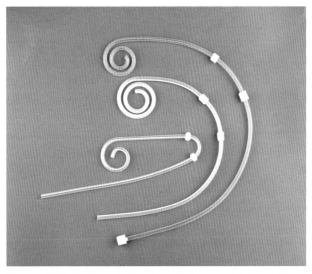

Figure 30.3 Peritoneal dialysis catheters: straight and flexed Swan neck curl catheters.

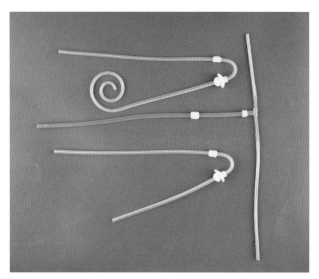

Figure 30.4 Peritoneal dialysis catheters: Missouri straight and flexed Swan neck curl catheters and fluted-T catheter.

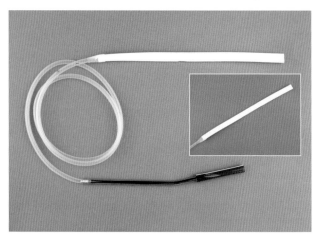

Figure 30.5 The Blake surgical drain (Johnson and Johnson, Arlington, TX) functions in a manner similar to the fluted-T catheter and has been utilized for PD in human infants.

Neck curled catheter have been designed to be placed either via laparoscope or blind trocarization in human medicine, it is preferable to place these catheters surgically in dogs and cats. Omentectomy is necessary to provide adequate exchanges for long durations. The curled tip should be positioned in the inguinal area. The fluted aspect of the fluted-T catheter is placed against the parietal peritoneum and oriented in a cranial to caudal plane. It is placed in a paramedian location with the long aspect directed toward the inguinal ring. The subcutaneous tunnel should be such that there is a gentle bend in the catheter that does not kink and that exits caudally and off midline by 3–5 cm. When a cuffed catheter is used, the cuffs should be soaked in sterile saline before placement to remove air and facilitate fibroblast cuff invasion. The inner cuff is placed in the rectus muscle, and the other cuff is placed in the subcutaneous tunnel. A tight subcutaneous tunnel with fibrous ingrowth into the cuff decreases the incidence of dialysate leak (Labato 2000; Langston 2003). Although not specifically designed for PD, the Blake surgical drain (Johnson and Johnson, Arlington, TX) functions in a manner similar to the fluted-T catheter and has been utilized for PD in human infants (Dyzban et al. 2000) [Figure 30.5].

Initially, large volumes of dialysate should be avoided to minimize excess intra-abdominal pressure, which can promote leaks and retard healing of exit sites (Lane et al. 1992; Goldraich and Mariano 1993; Cowgill 1995). It is recommended that one-quarter to one-half of the calculated prescription volume for the first 24 hours be infused at the start of dialysis exchanges. This author has found that the smaller volume leads to less fluid leakage into the subcutaneous tissue. If it is possible to wait for

12–24 hours postsurgical catheter placement that is ideal; unfortunately, in most cases in veterinary medicine, we do not have that luxury and exchanges need to begin immediately.

The catheter should be attached to a sterile closed exchange system and carefully bandaged into position with dry sterile dressings. The use of topical antibiotic ointments is not recommended because of the potential to cause maceration of the exit site tissues and fibroblast inhibition. Minimizing catheter movement during the invasion of fibroblasts into the cuffs is crucial for minimizing exit leaks and infections. After placement of the dialysis catheter, the tail of the catheter tubing is connected to a transfer tubing set, which previously has been attached to and primed with a pre-warmed bag of dialysate. Strict sterile technique should be maintained throughout all manipulations. Connections should be protected with povidone-iodine connection shields or chlorhexidine-soaked sponges.

Delivery technique and the exchange procedure

Aseptic technique during delivery of dialysate is essential to minimize the risk of peritonitis. Hands should be thoroughly washed with soap or cleaned with a hand sanitizer and sterile gloves used while changing the dialysate bag or lines, because the most common cause of peritonitis is contamination of the bag spike (Carter et al. 1989; Ross and Labato 2006). Routine use of a face mask while doing bag exchanges and catheter maintenance has been shown to be unnecessary as long as proper hand care is maintained (Figueiredo et al. 2000). Every line connection should be covered with a povidone-iodine connection shield or chlorhexidine-soaked dressings covered with sterile gauze. All injection ports should be scrubbed with chlorhexidine and alcohol before injections, and the use of multiple-dose vials (e.g., heparin or potassium chloride) for dialysate supplements should be avoided to decrease the risk of introducing microorganisms.

Although dialysis can be performed with a straight-line transfer set, use of a closed, flush system has been associated with lower infection rates (Maiorca and Cancarini 1990; Maiorca et al. 1991; Rippe 2007). The closed "Y" system allows the lines to be flushed free of possible bacterial contamination before each dialysate infusion without opening the system to outside air (the drain, flush, instill method).

For the first 24–48 hours after catheter placement, the exchange volumes should be one-quarter the calculated ideal volume to assess the degree of abdominal distention, the effect on respiratory function, and the potential for dialysate leakage. After the first 48 hours, the dialysate can be infused at a dosage of 20–40 mL/kg during a 10-minute period (Christie and Bjorling 1993; Labato 2000). The dialysate is allowed to remain in the peritoneal cavity for 30–40 minute dwell time and then is drained into a collection bag by gravity during a 20–30 minute period. A 90–100% recovery of dialysate is expected. This process is repeated continually and the dialysate formula and dwell times are adjusted every 12–24 hours according to the animal's needs. This form of continuous exchanges or cycling is referred to as continuous PD (Alarabi et al. 1994).

A Y-set tubing with a fresh dialysate bag and a drainage container attached to either segment is connected to the catheter tubing or transfer set. First, a small amount of fresh dialysate is flushed into the drainage bag, and then the peritoneal cavity is drained so that any contaminants introduced during the connection procedures are flushed into the drainage bag and not into the peritoneal cavity (Figure 30.6).

After drainage, the fresh dialysate is infused. This "drain first—infuse later" principle has markedly decreased the incidence of peritonitis in humans on PD as compared with the "infuse first–drain later" principle used in the straight single-spiked system (Ash et al. 1995).

The exchange procedure for severe azotemia should follow the described protocol. The dialysate should remain in the abdomen for 30–40 minutes. Dialysis cycles should be repeated every 1–2 hours until the animal is clinically improved, blood urea nitrogen (BUN), and serum creatinine concentrations have decreased and volume overload has been corrected. This initial intensive dialysis typically continues for 24–48 hours. Do not attempt to bring the BUN and creatinine concentrations into the normal range. A reasonable goal is a BUN concentration of 60–100 mg/dL and a serum creatinine con-

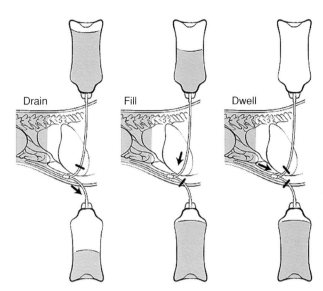

Figure 30.6 The drain, fill, and dwell protocol. Peritonitis is decreased by employing the Y-set and flushing of catheter line prior to each fill.

centration of 4.0–6.0 mg/dL. The animal can then be switched to a chronic dialysis schedule. A chronic dialysis schedule involves allowing the dialysate solution to remain in the abdomen for 3–6 hours. Three to four exchanges per day are performed. The dialysate should remain in the abdomen during these extended exchange periods. The rate of infusion can be rapid in most cases without problems. If the animal shows signs of discomfort during infusion, check that the solution temperature is not too hot or too cold. Also, slow the rate of infusion.

The frequency of the exchanges and the dwell time duration are adjusted for each animal's individual needs. The goal of PD for an animal with renal failure is to remove enough urea to maintain the BUN concentration at ≤ 70 mg/dL (Ross and Labato 2006). The amount of solute transferred across the peritoneal membrane is determined by the concentration gradient for each solute. If there is a need to increase removal of large molecules such as creatinine, the dwell time for each exchange is extended.

Dialysis should be continued until kidney function has normalized or is adequate to maintain the patient without dialysis as determined by urine output and the stabilization of blood values and clinical signs. Gradual reduction of the number of exchanges and having exchange free periods are recommended. This intermittent PD should be done during a 3–4 day period with continual reevaluation of the patient's clinical state. If the animal receiving aggressive, well-managed continual PD has not improved according to biochemical parameters or uremic signs after several days, chronic PD, chronic hemodialysis, renal transplantation, or euthanasia should be considered.

Dialysate solutions

The biocompatibility of a PD solution can be defined as the ability of a solution formulation to permit long-term dialysis without any clinically relevant changes in the functional characteristics of the peritoneum and is of paramount importance not only in maintaining the health of the membrane but also in permitting PD to be a successful long-term therapy. Solution components can affect leukocyte, mesothelial cell, endothelial cell, and fibroblast function, resulting in alterations in cytokine, chemokine, and growth factor networks, up-regulation of pro-inflammatory and pro-fibrotic pathways, impaired peritoneal host defense, and the induction of carbonyl and oxidative stress (Cooker et al. 2002). Such perturbations of normal physiology have been proposed as causative factors contributing to changes in peritoneal structure, such as peritoneal fibrosis, sclerosis, and vasculopathy, and changes in peritoneal function including increased solute permeability and ultrafiltration failure (Cooker et al. 2002; Crawford-Bonadio and Diaz-Buxo 2004; terWee and van Ittersum 2007). The majority of PD fluids used today have the composition of a lactate-buffered, balanced salt solution devoid of potassium, with glucose as the osmotic agent. Lactate is used as a buffer instead of bicarbonate because bicarbonate and calcium may precipitate (to form calcium carbonate) during storage. However, with the advent of newer multi-chambered PD delivery systems, it is currently possible to replace lactate with bicarbonate and to make a number of other solution modifications that previously were not feasible. However, the high cost of a number of the newer, more physiologic fluid formulations should be kept in mind (Rippe 2007). Very few of these newer solutions will be utilized during the relatively short durations PD is utilized in veterinary medicine.

The ideal solution for PD should not be unduly hypertonic, should not impair host defenses, and should not damage the peritoneal membrane. It should be sterilized in a manner that does not promote generation of glucose degradation products (GDPs). Most existing glucose-based solutions are lactate-based, have low pH and high tonicity, contain GDPs, and glycosylate the peritoneal membrane.

Commercially prepared dialysate solutions containing various concentrations of dextrose are available. Dialysis for removal of solutes is generally performed using 1.5% dextrose. Dialysates containing 2.5% and 4.25% dextrose are used in moderate to severely over-hydrated patients. Dialysate solutions are buffered, slightly hyper-osmolar crystalloid solutions designed to pull fluid, creatinine, urea, electrolytes, and phosphates from the plasma into the dialysate while providing diffusible buffer and other needed compounds such as magnesium and calcium (Lane and Carter 1997).

Hyperosmolar dextrose-containing dialysate solutions are effective for minimizing edema in over-hydrated patients and for enhancing ultrafiltration (removal of water) in all patients. Hyperosmolar dextrose appears to favor capillary vasodilation and promotes solute drag. A 1.5% dextrose dialysate is used in dehydrated or normovolemic patients. The 2.5% and 4.25% dialysates should be used in mildly to severely over-hydrated patients. Intermittent use of a 4.25% dialysate solution may increase the efficiency of dialysis in all patients (Ross and Labato 2006). Heparin (250–1,000 U/L) should be added to the dialysate for the first few days after catheter placement to help prevent occlusion of the catheter by fibrin deposition. This heparin is minimally absorbed by the patient's circulation and is unlikely to prolong clotting times (Lane et al. 1992; Cowgill 1995; Dzyban et al. 2000b; Sjoland et al. 2004; Ross and Labato 2006). The dialysate should be warmed to 38°C to improve permeability of the peritoneum. The dialysate line should be placed in a fluid warmer to help maintain this temperature.

In an emergency situation where there is no commercially prepared dialysate solution available, a suitable dialysate solution can be made by adding dextrose to lactated Ringer's solution. Osmolality should closely approximate that of the patient and the dextrose concentration should be at least 1.5%. Adding 30 mL of 50% glucose to 1 L of lactated Ringer's solution will result in a 1.5% dextrose solution.

Glucose is harmful to the peritoneum. The glucose concentration of dialysate solution is high. The tissues of the peritoneal membrane are continuously exposed to glucose concentrations that are clearly in the diabetic range. These concentrations of glucose are toxic to the mesothelium. Glucose activates the polyol pathway and the secretion of transforming growth factor-beta1 (TGF-B1), monocyte chemoattractant protein-1 (MCP-1), and fibronectin. There are studies suggesting that glucose is involved in the development of peritoneal fibrosis (Van Biesen et al. 1998; Vardhan et al. 2003). Glucose is likely to be involved in the development of peritoneal neoangiogenesis. The clinical importance of this finding is that it leads to enlargement of the peritoneal vascular surface area, resulting in loss of the osmotic gradient that impairs ultrafiltration. A third mechanism by which glucose can damage the peritoneal tissue is by inducing nonenzymatic glycosylation of tissue proteins that leads to the formation of advanced glycoslyation end products (AGEs). The deposition of AGEs in the vascular wall leads to ultrafiltration failure (Dasgupta, 1989; Vardhan et al. 2003).

GDPs are formed during the heat stabilization process of dialysate solutions. GDPs consist of aldehydes such as formaldehyde and dicarbonyl products such as glyoxal and methylglyoxal. GDPs may affect the peritoneal membrane by three mechanisms. They are toxic to fibroblasts. Methylgloxal enhances the production of vascular endothelial growth factor (VEGF). And the final mechanism is the GDPs trigger of the formation of AGEs at a much faster rate than glucose (Vardhan et al. 2003). However, for short-term use in veterinary medicine, no adverse effects have been recognized.

Ideally, the osmotic agent used in PD fluids should be biocompatible, effective in inducing ultrafiltration, nonabsorbable, easy to manufacture, and inexpensive. At present, glucose, polyglucose, and amino acids are being used in commercial PD fluids. Amino acid solutions are not available in the US market. Polyglucose (icodextrin, Extrarenal, Baxter Healthcare Corporation, Deerfield, IL) is available. Icodextrin (7.5% polyglucose) is a mixture of high molecular weight, water-soluble glucose polymers isolated by fractionation of hydroloyzed cornstarch. Icodextrin is a glucose polymer of molecular weight 16,8000 and osmolality of 285 mOsm. No diffusion into the blood occurs and the colloid osmotic gradient and ultrafiltration are maintained as the dwell proceeds. Ultrafiltration occurs by colloid osmosis via small pores. Minimal ultrafiltration occurs via ultrapores through which glucose mainly acts, and consequently there is no sodium sieving. Iso-osmolar polyglucose solutions achieve peritoneal ultrafiltration by colloid osmosis, allowing net ultrafiltration during long dwell exchanges due to its slow absorption. The ultrafiltration achieved with polyglucose after 12 hours is superior to 4.25% glucose, particularly in patients with high peritoneal transport (Admad 2008). Icodextrin is absorbed via lymphatics and metabolized to maltose (Vardham 2003; Crawford-Bonadio and Diaz-Buxo 2004). No toxicity has been identified. There are a number of adverse effects that have been noted with Icodextrin, which include sterile peritonitis, peritoneal mononucleosis, and antibody formation. In humans undergoing CAPD, Icodextrin is utilized during the long dwell times (Moberly 2003; Martin et al. 2003). At this time, the future role of Icodextrin in veterinary medicine remains to be seen.

Bicarbonate-based solutions are being developed to increase solution biocompatibility and thus protect the peritoneal membrane. Their formulation also reduces infusion pain associated with the low acidity of most conventional commercial preparations. These solutions require use of a double chamber bag to separate bicarbonate from calcium (Crawford-Bonadio and Diaz-Buxo

2004; Ross and Labato 2006). A 1.1% amino acid solution is now available in many countries to supplement protein intake and treat or prevent malnutrition. One exchange of the 1.1% amino acid solution per day has been shown to improve nitrogen balance and biochemical markers for nutrition in malnourished CAPD patients (Kopple et al. 1995; McIntyre 2007; Tjiong et al. 2007).

Complications

Complications with PD are common but manageable if recognized early. The most common complications include catheter flow problems, exit site leaks, hypoalbuminemia, peritonitis, pleural effusion, dyspnea caused by increased abdominal pressure, changes in hydration status, and electrolyte abnormalities (Table 30.4) (Labato 2000; Maaz 2004; Ross and Labato 2006).

Catheter flow obstruction by fibrin or omentum leading to dialysis retention is common (Christie and Bjorling 1993; Ash 1999). In one study, 30% of dogs undergoing PD developed such obstructions (Crimp et al. 1989). In a review of cats treated with PD, 77% had dialysis retention with 3/22 or 13.6% having a clogged catheter. Fifty-eight percent of cats with surgically placed catheters experienced dialysate retention while 100% of those cats with percutaneously placed catheters had retention problems. Careful catheter placement and management are important preventative steps. Heparinized saline flushes of the catheter for the first few days may decrease the occurrence of omentum wrapping around the catheter (Dzyban et al. 2000). If a clot in the catheter is suspected, a high pressure saline flush or the addition of 15,000 U of urokinase to the catheter for 3 hours may dislodge clots (Ash et al. 1995). Decreasing volumes of dialysate during outflow or abdominal pain on dialysate inflow are evidence of omental entrapment. If omental entrapment occurs, catheters can be repositioned or replaced to correct this

Table 30.4 Potential complications of peritoneal dialysis

Catheter related
Catheter obstruction
Exit site and tunnel infection
Dialysate leakage
Hypoalbuminemia
Electrolyte disorders
Peritonitis
Diagnosis based on presence of at least 2 of 3 criteria
Cloudy dialysate effluent
Detection of >100 inflammatory cells/uL, or organisms in gram stain or cultures
Clinical signs of peritonitis
Acute pleural effusion

problem. For this reason, it is strongly recommended that catheters be surgically placed and an omentectomy performed if use of the PD catheter is anticipated for longer than 48 hours.

The most frequent complication at the author's institution is dialysate leakage into the subcutaneous tissue. Sixty-two percent of cats with percutaneously placed catheters experienced subcutaneous leakage and 50% of cats with surgically placed catheters had subcutaneous leakage. This complication is managed by having the surgeon closely appose the abdominal incision (simple interrupted suture pattern only), starting the initial exchange volumes at one-quarter of the calculated infusion amount, and if leakage does occur, intermittently wrapping the limbs to promote mobilization of the edema. If at all possible, it is beneficial to wait a minimum of 12 hours after surgical placement to begin the exchanges; unfortunately, because the indication for PD is typically associated with an acute process, this opportunity to wait is typically not an option. Additionally, if subcutaneous leakage occurs, the dialysate solution should be changed to the lowest possible osmolality formulation available.

Acute pleural effusion is an uncommon complication and usually occurs early in the course of treatment. A common PD complication is overhydration of the patient. If the patient is gaining weight, the central venous pressure is increasing, or the effluent recovered is not at least 90% of the dialysate infused, the prescription should be changed to ultrafiltration with more concentrated dextrose (2.5 or 4.25%) solutions.

Protein losses can be clinically important with PD (Young et al. 1987). Losses may increase dramatically (50–100%) when peritonitis is present. Hypoalbuminemia was the most common complication in a review of PD cases in dogs and cats, and 41% of the animals were affected (Crimp et al. 1989). In another study, 16% of cats developed hypoalbuminemia (Cooper and Labato in press). Hypoalbuminemia may be the result of low dietary protein intake, gastrointestinal or renal protein loss, loss in the dialysate itself, uremic catabolism, and concurrent diseases. Usually, the animal can maintain normal serum albumin levels if nutritional intake is adequate. Adequate enteral nutrition may be difficult to maintain, given the anorexia and vomiting common in uremic patients. Supportive measures to maintain positive nitrogen balance often must be utilized. Nutritional support includes feeding tubes, partial or total parenteral nutrition, and the technique of PD utilizing 1.1% amino acid solutions (Kopple et al. 1995; Jones et al. 1998; Dzyban et al. 2000a; terWee and van Ittersum 2007; Tjiong et al. 2007). Gastrostomy and jejunosotomy tubes are contraindicated during PD because of increased risk of infection and abdominal wall exit site dialysate leaks.

The prevalence of peritonitis in veterinary patients on PD had previously been reported as being higher than that reported for humans 22% versus 15% (Crimp et al. 1989; Tzandoukas 1996). Additionally, exit site infection is a troublesome problem in humans (Peng et al. 1998). In recent studies, at the author's institution, peritonitis was not identified in any of the PD cases in dogs reviewed during a 4-year period and was reported in only one of 22 cats (2.5%) over a 5 year period (Beckel et al. 2005; Cooper and Labato in press). The most common source of peritonitis is contamination of the bag spike or tubing by the handler, but intestinal, hematogenous, and exit site sources of infection do occur. It is important to recognize peri-catheter leaks to minimize exit site sources on infection (Dzyban et al. 2000a). Peritonitis is diagnosed when two of the following three criteria are recognized: (1) cloudy dialysate effluent, (2) greater than 100 inflammatory cells/uL of effluent or positive culture results and, (3) clinical signs of peritonitis. The incidence of peritonitis has dramatically decreased with the use of the closed Y-system and drain first protocol. Because *Staphylococcus* spp. is the most common organism cultured, cephalosporins administered systemically and intra-peritoneally are empirically recommended. The author commonly will administer one dose of cefazolin in one dialysate exchange daily and also administer the antibiotic intravenously as well.

Dialysis disequilibrium is a rare complication characterized by dementia, seizures, or death. Dysequilibrium may occur during early exchanges especially in patients with extreme azotemia, acidosis, hypernatremia, or hyperglycemia. Rapid removal of urea and other small solutes apparently causes influx of water into brain cells and neurological dysfunction (Ross and Labato 2006) The reverse urea effect results from more efficient removal of urea from plasma as compared with the brain, with development of a reverse osmotic gradient. This intracellular accumulation of solutes such as urea favors movement of water to the intracellular space, leading to cerebral edema and an increase in intracranial pressure. Other compounds such as idiogenic osmoles are thought to play a role as well as paradoxical intracellular acidosis (Ali and Pirzada 2004). If evidence of disequilibrium occurs, the dialysate prescription should be adjusted to remove urea and small solutes at a slower rate (i.e., fewer exchanges or longer dwell times).

Monitoring

Monitoring of the PD patient should include carefully recording the volume of the dialysate infused and recovered during each exchange period as well as the volume

Date	Dialysate	#	Please note AM or PM. Also note date on each sheet inflow time	Dwell time	Outflow time	Dialysate volume in	Dialysate volume out	Current exchange net balance of dialysate only (volume out − volume in = balance)	Running total of balance of dialysate only	IV fluids in	Urine out	Total fluids in	Total fluid out	Current exchangeFluid difference (total fluid in − total fluids out = fluid diff)	Running total of Fluid difference	Exchange	Comments
		1						0	0			0	0	0	0	1	
		2						0	0			0	0	0	0	2	
		3						0	0			0	0	0	0	3	
		4						0	0			0	0	0	0	4	
		5						0	0			0	0	0	0	5	
		6						0	0			0	0	0	0	6	
		7						0	0			0	0	0	0	7	
		8						0	0			0	0	0	0	8	
		9						0	0			0	0	0	0	9	
		10						0	0			0	0	0	0	10	

Figure 30.7 Peritoneal dialysis flow sheet. Flow sheet used for monitoring dialysate and fluid volumes.

of urine produced and any additional fluids administered (Figure 30.7).

If the patient is volume overloaded and a high osmolality fluid is utilized, the fluid recovered from the abdomen may be greater than that delivered for the first few exchanges. As dialysis proceeds, outflow should approximate or exceed inflow if the patient is adequately hydrated. If less fluid is recovered with subsequent exchanges, the patient should be evaluated for dialysate leakage into subcutaneous fluids or for dialysate retention. At that point, the catheter should be checked for evidence of obstruction to outflow.

In the acute setting, body weight and hydration status should be monitored frequently, with body weight recorded consistently on the same scale and either with or without dialysate in the abdomen. Measurement of central venous pressure (CVP) through a jugular catheter is a relatively sensitive method for detecting overhydration or hypovolemia and should be performed every 4 hours. Determination of packed cell volume (PCV) and total protein should be performed at least twice daily. Serum electrolyte concentrations and other blood chemistries such as BUN, creatinine, albumin, and acid–base should be assessed initially every 8–12 hours and then daily (Table 30.5).

A number of metabolic aberrations may occur in patients on PD, including alterations in serum sodium, potassium, magnesium, and glucose concentrations as well as changes in acid–base status. Frequent monitoring and adjustment in dialysate and supplemental parenteral fluid composition may be necessary (Burkart 2004; Ross and Labato 2006).

Conclusion

In cases of acute kidney failure, the objectives of PD are to reduce azotemia, resolve the clinical signs of ure-

mia, and to help correct fluid, electrolyte, and acid–base imbalances until the animal's kidney function can recover sufficiently. Conversion of the anuric or oliguric state to a polyuric state and stabilization or improvement of azotemia are the primary indications for discontinuation of PD.

PD is a realistic option for veterinary patients with acute nonresponsive kidney failure or dialyzable toxin exposure. The protocol requires careful intraperitoneal catheter placement and care, aggressive exchange prescriptions, and careful monitoring for complications. Veterinarians should recognize that PD is an extremely effective tool in human medicine and should consider it as a treatment modality in an acute critical care setting.

The future role of PD in veterinary medicine may be as alternative management therapy for end-stage kidney failure when hemodialysis and transplantation are not options. As advanced renal replacement therapy becomes

Table 30.5 Monitoring parameters for patients receiving peritoneal dialysis

1. Weigh the animal twice daily before dialysate infusion
2. Check central venous pressure (CVP) every 4–6 hours
3. Check systemic arterial blood pressure every 6–8 hours
4. Record heart rate and respiratory rate every 2 hours. Note if there is respiratory difficulty with dialysateo infusion
5. Monitor body temperature every 6–8 hours
6. Perform adequate peritoneal catheter exit site care and evaluate for exit site infection daily
7. Record or weigh the amount of dialysate infused and recovered with each exchange
8. Evaluate packed cell volume (PCV), total protein, serum urea nitrogen (BUN), creatinine, electrolytes, albumin, and venous blood gas analysis once to twice daily depending on severity of azotemia

a more common treatment modality, we may find chronic ambulatory PD is the next area to emerge. In some patients, chronic hemodialysis is not a viable option because of poor vascular access, other underlying diseases, size of the animal, or unavailability of a hemodialysis center. Continuous ambulatory PD (CAPD) may serve as a treatment option for these patients. Cats that are not transplant candidates and are too small for hemodialysis are ideal candidates for CAPD. The active lifestyles of most dogs traditionally have made PD challenging for them. However, with a dedicated owner, CAPD may serve a role in renal replacement therapy. Typically, the patient is maintained in the hospital while the dialysis prescription is formulated, the incision heals, and the animal becomes accustomed to the dialysis process. Long-term care at home with outpatient visits is a goal for the future. Success will necessitate active cooperation among the owner, veterinarian, and technical staff. The challenge of maintaining a CAPD catheter will require developing and establishing excellent aseptic technique, daily bandage changes, and early recognition of any signs of infection. Investigational use of intradialytic amino acid solution and alternatives to traditional dialysate solutions will become areas of investigation in veterinary PD as more chronic dialysis is performed (Ross and Labato 2006).

References

Adin, C.A. and L.D. Cowgill (2000). Treatment and outcome of dogs with leptospirosis: 36 cases (1990–1998). *J Am Vet Med Assoc* **216**: 371–375.

Admad, M., T. Jeloka, et al. (2008). Icodextrin produces higher ultrafiltration in diabetic than in non-diabetic patients on continuous cyclic peritoneal dialysis. *Int Urol Nephrol* **40**: 219–223.

Alarabi, A.A., T. Petersson, et al. (1994). Continuous peritoneal dialysis in children with acute renal failure. *Adv Perit Dial* **10**: 289–293.

Alexander, S.R., W.E. Harmon, et al. (1999). Chronic dialysis in children. In: *Principles and Practice of Dialysis*, edited by W.L. Henrich, 2nd edition. Baltimore, MD: Lippincott, Williams and Wilkins, p. 511.

Ali, I.I. and N.A. Pirzada (2004). Neurologic complications associated with dialysis and chronic renal insufficiency. In: *Principles and Practice of Dialysis*, edited by W.L. Henrich, 3rd edition. Philadelphia, PA: Lippincott, Williams & Wilkins, pp. 502–512.

Anglani, F., M. Forino, et al. (2001). Molecular biology of the peritoneal membrane: in between morphology and function. *Contrib Nephrol* **131**: 61–73.

Ash, S.R. (1999). Acute peritoneal dialysis in the treatment of ARF. *ASN 32nd Annual Meeting*. Miami, FL, pp. 452–475.

Ash, S.R., D.J. Carr, et al. (1995). Peritoneal access devices: hydraulic function and biocompatibility. In: *Clinical Dialysis*, edited by A. Nissenson. Stanford: Appleton and Long, pp. 212–236.

Ash, S.R., E.M. Janles. (1993). T-fluted peritoneal dialysis catheter. *Adv Perit Dial* **9**: 223–226.

Avellini, G., G. Fruganti, et al. (1973). Peritoneal dialysis in the treatment of canine leptospirosis. *Atti della Società Italiana Delle Scienze Veterinairie* **27**: 377.

Beckel, N., T. O'Toole, et al. (2005). Peritoneal dialysis in the management of acute renal failure in five dogs with leptospirosis. *J Vet Emerg Crit Care (San Antonio)* **15**(3): 201–205.

Bersinas, A. (2006). Peritoneal Dialysis. *Proceedings of Advanced Renal Therapies Symposium*. New York, pp. 1–7.

Blake, P.G. and J.T. Daugirdas (2001). Physiology of peritoneal dialysis. In: *Handbook of Dialysis*, edited by J.T. Daugirdas, P.G. Blake, and T.S. Ing. Philadelphia, PA: Lippincott, Williams and Wilkins, pp. 281–296.

Burkart, J. (2004). Metabolic consequences of peritoneal dialysis. *Semin Dial* **17**(6): 498–504.

Carter, L.J., W.E. Wingfield, et al. (1989). Clinical experience with peritoneal dialysis in small animals. *Compend Cont Educ Pract Vet* **11**: 1335–1343.

Chada, V., B.A. Warady, et al. (2000). Tenckhoff catheters prove superior to cook catheters in pediatric acute peritoneal dialysis. *Am J Kidney Dis* **35**(6): 1111–1116.

Chegini, N. (2002). Peritoneal molecular environment, adhesion formation and clinical implication. *Front Biosci* **7**: 91–115.

Christie, B.A. and D.E. Bjorling (1993). Kidneys. In: *Textbook of Small Animal Surgery*, edited by D. Slatter, 2nd edition. Philadelphia, PA: WB Saunders, pp. 1439–1440.

Cooker, L.A., C.J. Holmes, et al. (2002). Biocompatibility of icodextrin. *Kidney Int* **62**: S34–S45.

Cooper, R.L. and M.A. Labato (in press). Peritoneal dialysis in cats with acute kidney injury: 22 cases (2001–2006). JVIM, Jan-Feb, 2011.

Cowgill, L.D. (1995). Application of peritoneal dialysis and hemodialysis in the management of renal failure. In: *Canine and Feline Nephrology and Urology*, edited by C.A. Osborne. Baltimore MD: Lea and Febiger, pp. 573.

Crawford-Bonadio, T.L. and J.A. Diaz-Buxo (2004). Comparison of peritoneal dialysis solutions. *Nephrol Nurs J* **31**(5): 500–509.

Crimp, M.S., D.J. Chew, et al. (1989). Peritoneal dialysis in dogs and cats: 27 cases (1976–1987). *J Am Vet Med Assoc* **195**: 1262–1266.

Dasgupta, M.K. (1998). Glycosylated end-products and peritoneal membrane damage. *Dial Transplant* **27**(2): 79–86.

Dzyban, L.A., M.A. Labato, et al. (2000a). CVT update: peritoneal dialysis. In: *Kirk's Current Veterinary Therapy XIII*, edited by J.D. Bonagura. Philadelphia, PA: WB Saunders, pp. 859–861.

Dzyban, L.A., M.A. Labato, et al. (2000b). Peritoneal dialysis: a tool in veterinary critical care. *J Vet Emerg Crit Care* **10**: 91–102.

Figueiredo, A.E., C.E. de Figueiredo, et al. (2000). Peritonitis prevention in CAPD: to mask or not? *Perit Dial Int* **20**: 354–358.

Flessner, M.F. (1991). Peritoneal transport physiology: insights from basic research. *J Am Soc Nephrol* **2**: 122–135.

Flessner, M.F. (1997). The peritoneal dialysis system: importance of each component. *Perit Dial Int* **17**: S91–S97.

Flessner, M., J. Heneoar, et al. (2003). Is the peritoneum a significant transport barrier in peritoneal dialysis? *Perit Dial Int* **23**: 542–549.

Forrester, S.D., N.S. McMillan, et al. (2002). Retrospective evaluation of acute renal failure in dogs (abstract). *J Vet Intern Med* **16**: 354.

Fox, L.E., G.F. Grauer, et al. (1987). Reversal of ethylene glycol-induced nephotoxicosis in a dog. *J Am Vet Med Assoc* **191**: 1433–1435.

Garcia-Lacaze, M., et al. (2002). Peritoneal dialysis: not just for renal failure. *Compend Cont Educ Pract Vet* **24**(10): 758–771.

Gokal, R., S. Alexander, et al. (1998). Peritoneal catheters and exit-site practices toward optimum peritoneal access: 1998 update. *Perit Dial Int* **18**: 11–33.

Goldraich, I. and M. Mariano (1993). One-step peritoneal catheter replacement in children. *Adv Perit Dial* **9**: 325–328.

Harkin, K.R. and C.L. Gartrell (1996). Canine leptospirosis in New Jersey and Michigan: 17 cases (1990–1995). *J Am Anim Hosp Assoc* **32**: 495–501.

Harvey, E.A. (2001). Peritoneal access in children. *Perit Dial Int* **21**(3): 5218–5222.

Henrich, W.L. and E.P. Paganini (1992). Dialytic support in ICU nephrology. ASN short courses in the clinical practice of nephrology, Baltimore, p. 43.

Jackson, R.F. (1964). The use of peritoneal dialysis in the treatment of uremia in dogs. *Vet Rec* **76**: 1481.

Jones, M., T. Hagen, et al. (1998). Treatment of malnutrition with 1.1% amino acid peritoneal dialysis solution: results of a multicenter outpatient study. *Am J Kidney Dis* **32**: 761–769.

Jorres, A. (2003). PD: a biological membrane and a non-biological fluid. *Contrib Nephrol* **140**: 1–9.

Kelly, K.T. (2004). How peritoneal dialysis works. *Nephrol Nurs J* **31**(5): 481–491.

Khanna, R., K.D. Nolph, et al. (1993). *The Essentials of Peritoneal Dialysis*. Norwell, MA: Kluwer Academic Publishers, p. **4**.

Khanna R. (2000) Peritoneal transport: Clinical implications. In Dialysis and Transplantation, Philadelphia, PA: WB Suanders, pp. 129–143.

Kirk, R.W. (1957). Peritoneal lavage in uremia in dogs. *J Am Vet Med Assoc* **131**: 101–103.

Kopple, J.D., D. Bernard, et al. (1995). Treatment of malnourished CAPD patients with an amino acid based dialysate. *Kidney Int* **47**: 1216–1224.

Labato, M.A. (2000). Peritoneal dialysis in emergency and critical care medicine. *Clin Tech Small Anim Pract* **15**(3): 126–135.

Lameire, N., W. Van Biesen, et al. (1998). Experimental models in peritoneal dialysis: a European experience. *Kidney Int* **54**: 2194–2206.

Lane, I.F. and L.J. Carter (1997). Peritoneal dialysis and hemodialysis. In: *Veterinary Emergency Medicine Secrets*, edited by W. Wingfield. Philadelphia, PA: Hanley and Belfus, pp. 350–354.

Lane, I.F., L.J. Carter, et al. (1992). Peritoneal dialysis: an update on methods and usefulness. In: *Kirk's Current Veterinary Therapy XI*, edited by J.D. Bonagura. Philadelphia, PA: WB Saunders, pp. 865–870.

Langston, C. (2003). Advanced renal therapies: options when standard treatments are not enough. *Vet Mod* **98**: 999–1008.

Maaz, D.E. (2004). Troubleshooting non-infectious peritoneal dialysis issues. *Nephrol Nurs J* **31**(5): 521–533.

Maiorca, R., E.F. Vonesh, et al. (1991). A multicenter, selection-adjusted comparison of patient and technique survivals on CAPD and hemodialysis. *Perit Dial Int* **11**: 118–127.

Maiorca, R. and G. Cancarini (1990). Experiences with the Y-system. *Contemp Issue Nephrol Perit Dial* **22**: 167–190.

Martin, J., G. Sansone, et al. (2003). Severe peritoneal mononucleosis associated with icodextrin use in continuous ambulatory peritoneal dialysis. *Adv Perit Dial* **19**: 191–194.

McIntyre, C.W. (2007). Update on peritoneal dialysis solutions. *Kidney Int* **71**: 486–290.

Mendoza, S.A., W.R. Griswold, et al. (1993). Acute peritoneal dialysis in critically ill infants and children. *Dial Transplant* **22**: 129–132.

Moberly, J.B., S. Mujais, et al. (2003). Pharmacokinetis of icodextrin in peritoneal dialysis patients. *Kidney Int* **62**: S23–S33.

Nagy, J.A. and R.W. Jackman (2000). Peritoneal membrane biology. In: *Dialysis and Transplantation*. Philadelphia, PA: WB Saunders, pp. 109–128.

Passadakis, P.S. and D.G. Oreopoulos (2007). Peritoneal dialysis in patients with acute renal failure. *Adv Perit Dial* **23**: 7–16.

Peng, S.J., C.S. Yang, et al. (1998). The clinical experience and natural course of peritoneal catheter exit site infection among continuous ambulatory peritoneal dialysis patients. *Dial Transplant* **27**(2): 71–78.

Phu, N.H., T.T. Hien, et al. (2002). Hemofiltration and peritoneal dialysis in infection-associated acute renal failure in Vietnam. *N Engl J Med* **347**(121): 895–902.

Posen, G.A. and J. Luisello (1980). Continuous equilibration peritoneal dialysis in the treatment of acute renal failure. *Perit Dial Bull* **1**: 6–8.

Rentko, V.T., N. Clark, et al. (1992). Canine leptospirosis: a retrospective study of 17 cases. *J Vet Intern Med* **6**: 235–244.

Rippe, B. (2007). Peritoneal dialysis: principles, techniques and adequacy. In: *Comprehensive Clinical Nephrology*, edited by J. Feehally, J. Floege, and R.J. Johnson, 3rd edition. Philadelphia, PA: Elsevier, pp. 979–990.

Ross, L.A. and M.A. Labato (2006). "Peritoneal dialysis." In: *Fluid Electrolyte and Acid-Base Disorders in Small Animal Practice*, edited by S.P. DiBartola, 3rd edition. Philadelphia, PA: WB Saunders, pp. 635–649.

Rubin, J., Q. Jones, et al. (1983). A model of long-term peritoneal dialysis in the dog. *Nephron* **35**: 259–263.

Shahar, R. and D.L. Holmberg (1985). Pleural dialysis in the management of acute renal failure in two dogs. *J Am Vet Med Assoc* **187**: 952–954.

Simmons, E.E., A.S. Lockard, et al. (1980). Experience with continuous ambulatory peritoneal dialysis and maintenance of a surgically anephric dog. *Southwest Vet* **33**: 129–135.

Sjoland, J.A., R.S. Pedersen, et al. (2004). Intraperitoneal heparin reduces peritoneal permeability and increases ultrafiltration in peritoneal dialysis patients. *Nephrol Dial Transplant* **10**: 1264–1268.

Stelin, G. and B. Rippe (1990). A phenomenological interpretation of the variation in dialysate volume with dwell time in CAPD. *Kidney Int* **38**(3): 465–472.

terWee, P.M. and F.J. van Ittersum (2007). The new peritoneal dialysis solutions: friends only, or foes in part? *Nat Clin Pract Nephrol* **3**(11): 604–612.

Tjiong, H.L., T. Rietveld, et al. (2007). Peritoneal dialysis with solutions containing amino acids plus glucose promotes protein synthesis during oral feeding. *Clin J Am Soc Nephrol* **2**: 74–80.

Thornhill, J.A., J. Hartman, et al. (1984). Support of an anephric dog for 54 days with ambulatory peritoneal dialysis and a newly designed peritoneal catheter. *Am J Vet Res* **45**(6): 1156–1161.

Thornhill, J.A., S.R. Ash, et al. (1980). Peritoneal dialysis with the Purdue column disc catheter. *Minn Vet* **20**: 27–33.

Tzandoukas, A.H. (1996). Peritonitis in peritoneal dialysis patients: an overview. *Adv Ren Replace Ther* **3**(3): 232–236.

Vaden, S.L., J. Levine, et al. (1997). A retrospective case control of acute renal failure in 99 dogs. *J Vet Intern Med* **11**: 58–64.

Van Biesen, W., R. Vanholder, et al. (1998). Recent developments in osmotic agents for peritoneal dialysis. *Adv Ren Replace Ther* **5**(3): 218–231.

Vardhan, A., M.M. Zweers, et al. (2003). A solutions portfolio approach in peritoneal dialysis. *Kidney Int* **64**: S114–S123.

Wong, W., E. McCall, et al. (1996). Acute renal failure in the paediatric intensive care unit. *N Z Med J* **109**: 459–461.

Wojick, K., D. Berube, et al. (2008). Clinical technique: peritoneal dialysis and percutaneous peritoneal dialysis catheter placement in small mammals. *J Exotic Pet Med* **17**(3): 181–188.

Yerram, P., A. Gill, et al. (2007). A 9-year survival analysis of the presternal Missouri swan-neck catheter. *Adv Perit Dial* **23**: 90–93.

Young, G.A., A.M. Brownjohn, et al. (1987). Protein losses in patients receiving continuous ambulatory peritoneal dialysis. *Nephron* **45**: 196–201.

31

Renal transplantation

Christopher A. Adin

History of renal transplantation

Vascular surgery techniques and suture materials that enabled surgeons to perform canine and feline renal transplantation were described in experimental models as early as 1902 (Ullman 2002). Unfortunately, it would be another 70 years before modern immunosuppressive medications would allow this experimental technique to become a viable treatment for end-stage renal disease in any species (Borel et al. 1994). Since that time, renal allograft transplantation has been the undisputed treatment of choice in human beings with end-stage renal disease (ESRD). Renal transplantation in animals has shown similar benefits, although cost, availability, and lower success rates in companion animals have caused organ transplantation to be more slowly adopted. Recent decreases in the cost of chronic drug therapy, opening of new transplant centers, and constant advances in immunosuppression have continued to improve the environment for clinical application of renal transplantation in cats and dogs with ESRD. Nonetheless, the majority of data related to clinical renal transplantation has been obtained in human beings and this information will be included throughout the chapter as a background for the current status of veterinary renal transplantation.

Transplantation immunology

The major histocompatibility complex

Our current concepts of transplantation immunology hinged upon the characterization of the major histocompatibility complex (MHC), a genetically-determined, cell-surface protein that is involved in the recognition of foreign protein fragments or antigens derived from the donor tissue. This work, for which George Snell and Baruj Banacerraf shared the Nobel Prize for Physiology or Medicine in 1980, was performed using simple genetic studies in mice. Later studies showed that the mouse MHC complex (termed H-2) was analogous to the MHC region in other vertebrates. The MHC has now been characterized in several species and given specific names: the human leukocyte antigen (HLA), dog leukocyte antigen (DLA), and feline leukocyte antigen (FLA). In each species, the MHC locus one of the largest and most variable (polymorphic) regions of the genome, with up to 40 histocompatibility alleles identified for each gene (Abbas et al. 1991). Inheritance of the MHC phenotype follows Mendelian genetic patterns, and alleles from both parents are expressed codominantly in the MHC phenotype of the offspring. Despite the extreme polymorphism noted in the MHC, breeding studies showed that after 20 generations of sibling matings, mice became syngeneic, with identical genes occurring even at the variable MHC loci (Abbas et al. 1991). Transplanted tissue from these genetically identical individuals is termed an isograft and typically results in no rejection episodes. In contrast, tissue that is transplanted from one outbred strain to another is termed an allograft and will nearly always stimulate a vigorous immune response. Later studies have described the structure of the MHC complex, a peptide chain with cytoplasmic, transmembrane, and cell surface regions. There are two distinct classes of MHC (class I and class II MHC) and the majority of the extracellular portion of these molecules is nonvariable. The extreme polymorphism of the MHC is reflected primarily in the composition of a small peptide binding region. This region binds to protein fragments that range from 8–20 amino acids in length (Dallman 2001). A variety of nucleated cell types will express the MHC I and II proteins on the cell surface, either constitutively or when stimulated by cytokines.

Nephrology and Urology of Small Animals. Edited by Joe Bartges and David J. Polzin. © 2011 Blackwell Publishing Ltd.

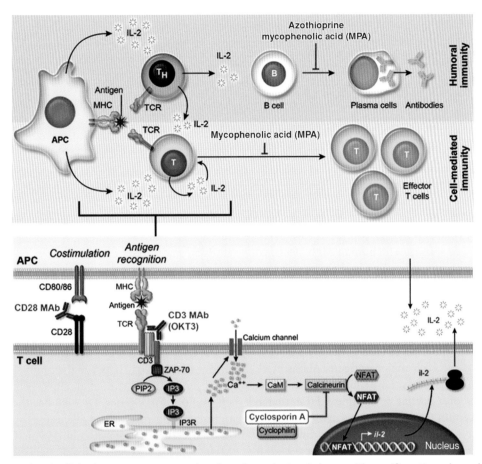

Figure 31.1 Humoral and cellular immune response to the allograft are depicted above, with specific antigen dependent and antigen-independent (costimulation) activation of the T-cell is depicted below. Specific drug and monoclonal antibody targets are indicated in red. Abbreviations: APC, antigen-presenting cell; T, T-cell; T$_H$, T-helper cell; IL-2, interleukin-2; IL-2, interleukin-2 messenger RNA; MHC, major histocompatibility complex; TCR, T-cell receptor; CaM, calmodulin; NFAT, nuclear factor of activated T-cells; PIP3, phosphatidylinositol triphosphate; PIP2, phosphatidylinositol diphosphate; MAb, monoclonal antibody.

These MHC proteins combine with protein fragments from the cell itself to form a complex that is bound by specific T-cell subtypes, depending upon the MHC class involved (see Figure 31.1). MHC I-antigen complexes are bound by CD8+ T-cells, while MHC II-antigen complexes are bound by CD-4+ T-cells (Welsh and Bunce 2001). It is important to note that T-cells are not activated by free or soluble antigens, only antigen that is bound to the MHC protein will stimulate an immune response. Studies using knockout mice with selective deletion of either MHC I or MHC II have shown that incompatibility involving either one of these proteins is sufficient to produce the rejection response (Dallman 2001). The immune response to the transplanted organ is actually aided by a group of professional antigen-presenting cells (also known as dendritic cells) that arise from the donor organ and rapidly migrate into the recipient's lymphoid tissue where they present foreign antigen to host T-cells. MHC is also expressed by a variety of other cells,

including dendritic cells from the recipient, as well as on the vascular endothelium of the graft itself. CD4+ and CD8+ T-cells are activated by this interaction with the antigen-presenting cell, MHC complex and antigen, initiating a variety of intracellular signaling pathways, causing cytokine production, expression of new cell-surface proteins, and alteration in gene expression that mark the beginning of graft rejection (Figure 31.1). In addition to the antigen-dependent activation provided by the T-cell receptor signal, complete activation of CD4+ T-cells appears to be dependent on a nonantigen-dependent interaction between the cell-surface proteins on the T-cell (CD28, CTLA4) and those on the antigen-presenting cell (CD80, CD86) as seen in Figure 18.1. Without this process, termed "co-stimulation," the CD4+ T-cell can enter a state of anergy or inactivity, halting the immune response of this cell line (Welsh and Bunce 2001). Each aspect of T-cell activation has been very carefully studied, with interest in discovering specific targets for pharmacologic intervention that would prevent T-cell activation and allograft rejection, while preserving the function of other aspects of the immune system. Immunosuppressive strategies using T-cell receptor antibodies, costimulation blockade, inhibitors of intracellular signaling, or cytokine production have provided effective means of prolonging allograft survival in various models of transplantation (see Figure 31.1), although no one area of intervention can provide complete protection at this time.

MHC typing

There is great variability in the complexity of MHC genetics in different species. The human MHC (termed the human lymphocyte antigen) has three major alleles: HLA-A, HLA-B, and HLA-DR, which are encoded on chromosome 6. Each individual has one copy from each parent, producing a total of 6 alleles (Dallman 2001). Within the human population, there is incredible polymorphism within these HLA genes, with 50–100 different variants for each major antigen (Abbas et al. 1991). Since family members share similar genetic material, the chances of a partial or complete HLA match are high. However, on the basis of the polymorphism at each allele, there is a very low chance of finding a perfect match in the general population. As expected, graft survival is directly proportional to the number of compatible antigens obtained when matching a donor and recipient pair, with the greatest graft retention occurring in donor recipient matches for all 6 HLA (Cecka 1998). It is interesting to note that occasional transplants performed between identical twins have demonstrated that histocompatibility is even more complex than described herein, including additional proteins termed minor histocompatibility antigens. While minor histocompatibility antigens may prove to be of some significance in fine tuning of immunosuppression in the future, current concepts in clinical transplantation are focused on the more powerful response to MHC reactions as described above.

The cat MHC (also known as the FLA) has not been well characterized, since this species is rarely used as an experimental model for human diseases. However, it has long been known that transplant immunosuppression is relatively simple to achieve in the cat, and there was some suspicion that there was minimal polymorphism at the MHC loci in this species. Surprisingly, DNA restriction analysis actually showed that there was significant polymorphism in the cat MHC, with 24 alleles detected amongst 12 family groups of cats (Winkler et al. 1989). However, cDNA isolated from a cat T-cell lymphoma line revealed that there is only a single heterogenous MHC I locus in the cat, a finding that may explain the ease of

transplant immunosuppression that has been noted in this species, as well as the susceptibility to viral infection (Yuhki et al. 1989). On the basis of the clinical success of renal allograft transplantation between nontissue matched pairs, donor screening is typically limited to blood typing and crossmatch evaluation. Cats are typically blood typed, then cross-matched to three potential donors. Because of the prevalence of blood type A in the domestic short-haired cats in the United States, identification of a compatible donor has proved to be simple unless an exotic or imported feline recipient is being considered.

The dog MHC has been comparatively well-studied, due to the fact that the dog is considered an excellent translational model for solid organ transplant studies. The use of dogs as an animal model is based on the fact that the complexity of the MHC in the dog is similar to that of the human being, making the dog a very stringent model for evaluation of new immunosuppressive regimes. Four discrete DLA genes have been identified in the dog (DLA-12, -88, -79, and -64) with a significant degree of homology between the canine DLA and human HLA genes (Graumann et al. 1998; Wagner et al. 1999). Of the four DLA genes, DLA-88 has the greatest degree of polymorphism, with 44 alleles for this gene identified in 63 breeds (Graumann et al. 1998). The other class I MHC loci are less polymorphic, with less than 12 alleles each (Wagner et al. 1999). However, each dog has a total of eight genes (four from each parent), making the total level of genetic diversity quite high. As in the human transplant recipient, tissue matching is required to achieve maximal success in the dog. Genes are inherited in a Mendelian pattern and are expressed codominantly, so a genetically related donor is preferred. Because of genetic selection that has occurred in pure-bred dogs, a donor and recipient combination that arose from the same breed would also be more likely to achieve some degree of tissue matching. Since it is not common to identify a related dog that is both suitable and available for organ donation, most of the efforts at transplantation in dogs with naturally occurring renal disease have been focused on achieving successful immunosuppression in nontissue-matched renal transplant recipients. Despite the challenges in finding a tissue-matched donor, it is still recommended that clinicians perform tissue cross-matching between canine transplant candidates and any potential donors. Using this information will allow the transplant team to make a more individualized plan for immunosuppressive regime and will allow the collection of data on the prognostic significance of tissue matching in canine transplant recipients. Both canine and feline histocompatibility testing is available through the Immunohematology and Serology Laboratory at Michigan State University (*msuhla.chm.msu.edu*).

Immunosuppression

The science of immunosuppression has blossomed over the past 40 years with constant refinement in protocols that have the ultimate goal of preventing allograft rejection and with minimal effect on the recipients' response to infectious agents or neoplasia. Experience has demonstrated that single-agent drug protocols are less successful in preventing rejection and produce more side-effects when compared to combined immunosuppressive protocols using multiple drug classes. The classic combination of drugs that has been applied in human beings over the past three decades is termed "triple drug therapy" and includes a glucocorticoid, a calcineurin inhibitor and an antimetabolite. Various other nonpharmacologic means have been added in more recent years, including monoclonal antibody therapies and nonmyeloablative irradiation. Immunosuppressive protocols that have been reported in clinical or experimental studies in nonmatched cats and dogs have paralleled efforts in human beings, with selected protocols summarized in Table 31.1. Specific drugs and immunosuppressive techniques are described in more detail later.

Glucocorticoids

Corticosteroids, in combination with azathioprine, constituted the first effective immunosuppressive protocol that fueled efforts in renal allograft transplantation from the 1960s until the addition of cyclosporine in the 1980s. Steroids act through a variety of complex mechanisms to aid in preservation of allograft function. Corticosteroids are absorbed into the cytoplasm where they bind with intracytoplasmic receptors before entering the nucleus.

After entering the nucleus, the corticosteroid receptor complexes stimulate synthesis of IκB-α, a protein that inhibits the transcription NF-κB, essentially halting this important early step in the generation of cytokines that stimulate several aspects of the inflammatory response (Tizard 2004). As such, corticosteroid have both anti-inflammatory and immunomodulatory effects. Anti-inflammatory effects of corticosteroids are mediated through inhibition of arachidonic acid metabolism by phospholipase A. Immunomodulatory effects are broad and have not been completely elucidated, though they include inhibition of both cell-mediated and humoral immunity. Specific mechanisms include suppression of IL-2, IL-6, and interferon-γ, inhibition of lymphocyte proliferation, and inhibition of monocyte migration to areas of inflammation (Ray and Sehgal 1992; Paliogianni and Boumpas 1995; Calandra and Bucala 1997). Increased rate of rejection episodes occurred in a small trial involving substitution of a cyclooxygenase inhibitor (ibuprofen) for glucocorticoids, suggesting that it is the immunosuppressive rather than the anti-inflammatory properties of these drugs that are most important in maintenance antirejection therapy (Kreis et al. 1984). However, the anti-inflammatory effects of glucocorticoids are believed to be of value in the treatment of acute rejection (Abrahamian and Cosimi 2001).

A variety of forms of glucocorticoids are available for oral or parenteral administration. Traditionally, high-dose injectable methylprednisolone is used human renal transplant recipients during the immediate perioperative period. Patients are then switched to low-dose (20 mg/day) prednisone or prednisolone for oral maintenance therapy. Glucocorticoid therapy causes a

Table 31.1 Selected immunosuppressive protocols and survival times using nonmatched kidney donors

Species	Immunosuppressive protocol	Study type	Median survival	Complications	Reference
Cat	Prednisolone Cyclosporine	Clinical Nonmatched	22 months	Opportunistic infection, neoplasia	Mathews 1996
Dog	Glucocorticoid Cyclosporine Azathioprine	Clinical Nonmatched	<2 months	Thromboembolism, opportunistic infection	Gregory 2006
Dog	RADTS Glucocorticoid Cyclosporine Azathioprine	Clinical	8 months	Opportunistic infection	Mathews 2000
Dog	Myeloablative radiation Donor bone marrow transplant Glucocorticoid Mycofenolate Cyclosporine	Experimental	>200 days	Mild chronic rejection, GI toxicity	Broaddus 2004

Abbreviations: RADTS, Rabbit anti-dog thymocyte serum; GI, gastrointestinal.

variety of serious side effects in human beings, ranging from avascular necrosis of bone to gastric ulcers, diabetes, obesity, cataracts, and pancreatitis (Shun-Shin et al. 1990; Isoniemi et al. 1993; Slakey et al. 1997; Morris 2001). Because of the severity and frequency of complications associated with steroid therapy, steroid-sparing or steroid-free protocols have been the major focus in transplantation immunology for the last 20 years (Rajab et al. 2006; Aoun et al. 2007; Matas 2009).

Fortunately, cats have proven to be far more tolerant of chronic glucocorticoid therapy. Dosage and tapering schedule in cats has been purely empirical, with an initial twice-daily dose of oral prednisolone (2.5–5 mg every 12 hours) tapering to once daily treatment after 1–3 months. Long-term therapy with 2.5–5 mg/day is often continued for the remainder of the post-transplant period, unless evidence of hyperglycemia and diabetes occurs. In cats that develop diabetes following renal transplantation, steroid administration is either decreased or discontinued and insulin therapy is used, as needed, to control the hyperglycemic state (Case et al. 2007). Dogs are far less tolerant of chronic high dose steroid therapy and are known to manifest many of the side effects seen in human transplant recipients. As such, steroid sparing protocols are typically pursued, with initial doses of 10 mg/kg methylprednisolone at the time of surgery, followed by oral prednisolone 1 mg/kg per day (Mathews et al. 2000; Gregory et al. 2006). Steroid dosage is halved monthly, then discontinued after 3 months (Gregory et al. 2006).

Azathioprine

Azathioprine, a purine synthesis inhibitor, is an antimetabolite that is relatively specific for T-cell and B-cell proliferation. The concept of applying a purine synthesis inhibitor as a selective immunosuppressive agent was based on the observation that certain people with congenital defects in purine biosynthesis suffered from severe T- and B-cell deficiencies and immunosuppression (Allison et al. 1975). Unlike other cell lines, T- and, to a lesser extent, B-cells rely on de-novo synthesis of purines for DNA and RNA synthesis (Allison et al. 1977). Azathioprine was produced in 1960 as a derivative of the antiproliferative agent 6-mercaptopurine in an effort to achieve antiproliferative effects without the toxicity noted after 6-MP administration (Elion et al. 1960a, 1960b). Azathioprine (Figure 31.1) was shown in experimental models to have efficacy in preventing organ rejection through inhibiting T-cell proliferation and decreasing production of interleukin-2 (Morris 2001; Bach 1975), but had improved safety profile when compared to previous antimetabolites. Nonetheless, azathioprine continues to carry risks of gastrointestinal toxicity, bone marrow

suppression, and occasional hepatotoxicity. Antimetabolites were found to be sufficient to produce long-term acceptance of allografts and are now included as part of a combination therapy that would include a corticosteroid component and a calcineurin inhibitor, such as cyclosporine. Although other more potent antiproliferative agents are now available, the low cost of azathioprine will likely encourage the continued use of this drug for many years to come (Morris 2001).

Azathioprine is metabolized in the liver to form 6-mercaptopurine and other inactive metabolites, which are excreted in the urine. Xanthine oxidase is one of the major enzymes involved in azathioprine metabolism, and co-administration of azathioprine with allopurinol greatly reduces the dose requirement for azathioprine. Azathioprine is myelotoxic in cats and must be used with great caution. Because of this risk and the relative success of simple two-drug immunosuppression using corticosteroids and cyclosporine, azathioprine is not typically used in feline renal transplant recipients. Nonetheless, azathioprine has been used at a dose of 0.3 mg/kg once every 3 days, to supplement standard cyclosporine and prednisolone therapy in cats with high risk or organ rejection due to inflammatory bowel disease (Gregory 2009). Unlike the cat, prednisolone and cyclosporine alone do not provide long-term survival of renal allografts in the dog. Accordingly, azathioprine has been used as part of a three-drug protocol in dogs receiving unmatched renal allografts (Gregory et al. 2006). In this study, rejection was effectively prevented in all dogs, although mortality due to thromboembolism and excessive immunosuppression were extremely high.

Cyclosporine

Cyclosporine was arguably the first example of a selective immunosuppressive agent, with the primary effects of this drug being conveyed on the T-helper cell, a necessary component in the organ rejection response. The cyclosporine polypeptide is derived from the natural fungus *Tolypocladium inflatum* and has a unique lipophilic molecular structure with two distinct protein binding surfaces (Tizard 2004). In the cytoplasm, this structure allows cyclosporine to simultaneously bind cytophilin, an intracellular receptor, and calcineurin, a serine-threonine phosphatase that is involved in the intracellular, calcium-dependent signaling cascade (Figure 31.1). Through this action, cyclosporine effectively prevents transcription of the cytokines IL-2 and IFN-γ by T-helper cells, suppressing an essential step in the activation of the cytotoxic T-cell response (Figure 31.1).

Cyclosporine is available in several preparations, including oral liquid, oral capsules, and intravenous forms. Use of the original oil-based formulation

(Sandimmune®, Novartis AG) has been largely replaced by use of a microemulsified version of the drug (Neoral®, Novartis AG), which has been shown to have improved bioavailability and more predictable absorption after oral administration (Pollard et al. 2003; Acott et al. 2006). Generic forms of the drug are also available, but clinicians must be careful to specify the microemulsified or "modified" form of cyclosporine when prescribing from an outside pharmacy, as dosing is not equivalent between the various formulations. In addition, some physicians question whether generic drugs, which have been confirmed as "bioequivalent" to Neoral® by single dose studies in healthy volunteers, will have identical pharmacokinetics in transplant recipients (Pollard et al. 2003). While several sizes of preloaded of cyclosporin gelatin capsules are now available for use in animals and humans, the oral liquid preparation (100 mg/mL) allows the most precise adjustments in dosing and can be applied in both dogs and cats. Many animals will consider this drug to be unpalatable, and it is recommended that the liquid is placed in an empty gelatin capsule before oral administration (Gregory 2009).

Because of variability in pharmacokinetics between individual animals and variability over time within individual animals, drug monitoring is performed throughout the course of cyclosporine therapy. Ideally, transplant recipients would be admitted to the hospital for multiple blood samples over a several hour period, allowing determination of an "area under the curve" or AUC for cyclosporine that provides a more accurate representation of total exposure to the drug. However, the cost and inconvenience associated with the AUC method has led to the measurement of a single cyclosporine whole blood concentration at the 12-hour trough period (Gregory 2009). Measurement of whole blood concentrations (rather than plasma concentrations) using the HPLC technique provides the most consistent results. Samples should be obtained in an EDTA tube and shipped according to instructions provided by the laboratory.

Dosing in cats is typically begun at 3–4 mg/kg every 12 hours and is then modified based on 12-hour trough cyclosporine blood levels. Target range for cyclosporine whole blood levels in cats range from 300–500 ng/mL in the initial perioperative period and are decreased to 250–400 ng/mL after 4–6 months. In dogs, cyclosporine dose varies from 5–10 mg/kg every 12 hours and target drug levels are based on the desired level of immunosuppression. Whole blood cyclosporine levels of 500–600 ng/mL are required for initial post-transplantation immunosuppression in the dog, while lower levels may be sufficient for management of immune-mediated diseases such as perianal fistulas (Mathews et al. 2000). Serious side effects of cyclosporine administration are rare in both species, although excessively high drug levels (>1000 ng/mL) will cause acute vomiting, lethargy, and azotemia. Long-term side effects from cyclosporine administration include gingival hyperplasia, hypertrichosis (especially around the paws), diabetes, and chronic allograft nephropathy.

Cyclosporine is metabolized by hepatic glucuronidation and is therefore subject to drug interactions with medications that alter the rate of hepatic glucuronidation. Co-administration of cimetidine, ketoconazole, imipenem, and metoclopramide may increase whole blood levels of the drug, while phenobarbital or trimethoprim sulfa may cause decreased drug levels by upregulating hepatic glucuronidation (Davidson and Plumb 2003). These interactions have been manipulated in attempts to decrease drug costs in patients receiving cyclosporine, with ketoconazole being the most frequently reported substance (McAnulty and Lensmeyer 1999). Ketoconazole provides not only a cost benefit by decreasing dosage requirements for cyclosporine, but may also have immunomodulatory and antifungal properties that are desirable in the transplant recipient population and allows conversion to a once a day dosing regimen in some cats (McAnulty and Lensmeyer 1999). Administration of ketoconazole at a dose of 10 mg/kg once daily increased the whole blood concentrations of cyclosporine 1.8 fold at 12 hours and increased terminal phase elimination half life from 10.7 to 22.2 hours in normal cats (McAnulty and Lensmeyer 1999). A similar study in normal dogs showed that administration of a low therapeutic dose of ketoconazole (13.6 mg/kg per day) allowed for a 75% reduction in cyclosporine dose levels and an estimated 57.8% cost savings compared to cyclosporine alone (Dahlinger et al. 1998).

Tacrolimus

Tacrolimus (also known as FK-506) is a calcineurin inhibitor that prevents T-cell activation by interrupting calcium-dependent signaling, similar to the actions of cyclosporine. However, Tacrolimus is 50–100 times more potent than cyclosporine in T-cell inhibition, when evaluated in vitro (Bierer et al. 1993; Kulkarni et al. 2001). On the basis of the increased potency of this drug, tacrolimus has been applied in human beings both as a primary immunosuppressive agent for high risk recipients and as a "rescue" agent during periods of solid organ rejection. In fact, Tacrolimus has replaced cyclosporine as the primary immunosuppressive agent in human liver transplantation and is used in approximately 1/3 of all renal allograft recipients (Kulkarni et al. 2001). Unfortunately, clinical experience with application of tacrolimus in veterinary medicine is limited and experimental studies suggest that anorexia, intestinal intussusceptions, and a potentially fatal vasculitis will limit the applications of this drug in dogs (Gregory 2009).

Mycofenolate mofetil

Mycofenolate mofetil (Cellcept®, Roche) is a prodrug for mycofenolic acid, a powerful immunosuppressive agent produced by several *Penicillum* species (Smak Gregoor et al. 2000). This drug was actually discovered as early as 1896, but was not applied clinically for transplant immunosuppression until it was rediscovered in the early 1980s by researches searching for novel purine biosynthesis inhibitors (Mathew 2001). Mycofenolate mofetil or MMF is a potent inhibitor of inosine monophosphate dehydrogenase (IMPDH), a rate-limiting enzyme in the process of de-novo purine synthesis, leading to T- and B-cell-specific immunosuppression (Figure 31.1). Interestingly, the immunosuppressive effects of MMF are reversible by supplementing the patient with guanosine, the product of IMPDH (Mathew 2001).

Mycofenolate is available in oral capsules (250 or 500 mg), oral suspension, or injectable solution. In human beings, mycofenolate is nearly completely absorbed after oral ingestion and is converted to the active metabolite, mycophenolic acid, or MPA. MPA is metabolized by glucuronidation into MPAG, an inactive metabolite, which is then excreted in the bile and urine. However, considerable enterohepatic circulation occurs, with conversion of MPAG back into the active metabolite MPA. Mean half life is 17.9 hours after oral ingestion, and the drug is typically administered twice daily in human transplant recipients. Mycofenolate mofetil is not considered potent enough to be used as a single agent for transplant immunosuppression. The most common application of MMF is as a substitute for azathioprine in triple drug regimens that include a corticosteroid and calcineurin inhibitor (Mathew 2001). In very rigorous studies of drug efficacy, MMF has been shown to reduce the risk of graft rejection by 60% compared to similar protocols using azathioprine (Halloran et al. 1997). Toxic effects are similar to those of azathioprine, affecting the gastrointestinal system or causing leukopenia through its actions on T- and B-cells.

Clinical experience with mycofenolate in animals is limited, although Broaddus and other reported the successful use of MMF (10 mg/kg, every 12 hours) in combination with total body irradiation, cyclosporine, and corticosteroids in an experimental transplantation model using healthy dogs (Table 31.1). Experience in this model did suggest that MMF has the potential for significant gastrointestinal toxicity, causing death in two dogs when administered at full dosage immediately following total body irradiation. The authors subsequently decreased initial dosage to 5 mg/kh every 12 hours and eliminated further mortality (Broaddus et al. 2006).

Antilymphocyte serum

Initial efforts at drug-free immunotherapy involved the development clinical protocols for preparation of anti-lymphocyte serum (ALS) for use in dogs and human beings (Starzl et al. 1967). The protocols began simply, culturing human lymphoblasts and injecting them into horses or rabbits to produce a serum that contained a polyclonal mixture of antiglobulins, many of which arose from the previous immune activity of the animal rather than being specific to the human lymphocyte antigens. Because of the importance of the T-cell in allograft rejection, more specific antithymocyte serum (ATS) preparations were performed, using cadaveric human thymus or thymic tissue obtained during cardiac surgery on live donors. Even after fractionation of the IgG components, only a small portion of the product is considered to be specifically reactive with target human lymphocytes (Greco et al. 1983) with the remainder being undesired components. Initial proof of efficacy for ATS was obtained in humans that were experiencing acute rejection episodes. ATS has subsequently been incorporated into the induction protocol of many institutions and is still applied today, despite the disadvantages of a polyclonal preparation. Commercial products are available for use in human beings, while a few institutions prepare their own ATS (Abrahamian and Cosimi 2001). Approximately 20% of human transplant recipients experience a cutaneous hypersensitivity reaction and chills, termed a "first dose reaction," which lessens during subsequent doses. This reaction, which can also manifest as a more severe anaphylactic reaction, is caused by increases in IL-2, IL-3, IL-6, tumor necrosis factor, and complement activation (Ferran et al. 1990).

Rabbit anti-dog thymocyte serum (RADTS) has been applied in clinical dog transplants for a number of years with some success (Mathews et al. 2000). RADTS is prepared according to a protocol that was developed by Dr. Karol Mathews at Guelph (Mathews et al. 1993) and is not commercially available at this time. A median survival of 18 months was obtained in 15 dogs, using a standard triple-drug therapy (cyclosporine, prednisone, and azathioprine) supplemented with intramuscular RADTS. To date, this study represents the most successful survival data generated in dogs with naturally occurring disease (Table 31.1).

Monoclonal antibodies

As technologies improved, monoclonal antibodies to T-cell antigens have been developed, allowing specific targeting of T-cell subsets without the nonspecific immunoglobulins contained in polyclonal preparations (Figure 31.1). The first successful product, termed OKT3, was directed against the CD3 protein, an essential component of T-cell receptor signaling. OKT3 causes nearly total elimination of circulating T-cells by opsonization and complement-mediated lysis or by reticuloendothelial uptake within minutes of IV administration (Abrahamian and Cosimi 2001). Clinical trials of OKT3 have shown it to be as effective as ATS and OKT3 is now the treatment of choice in steroid-resistant acute rejection episodes. Despite the high success rate in treating refractory rejection with OKT3, a relatively large number of recipients (10–15%) will experience a repeated rejection episode 4–6 weeks after OKT3 therapy. Repeat treatment with OKT3 is associated with a risk of sepsis due to excessive suppression of cell-mediated immunity, increased risk of viral disease, and lymphoproliferative disorders. Other potential risks of therapy include a first-dose effect similar to that described for ATS, including chills, fever, diarrhea, and respiratory difficulty (Thistlethwaite et al. 1988; Abrahamian and Cosimi 2001). With the explosion in discovery of T-cell associated proteins, a wide array of other monoclonal antibodies are being developed for clinical use. Two drugs that are already approved and in clinical use are basiliximab and daclizumab, monoclonal antibodies against the IL-2 receptor that were prepared by forming chimeric antibodies based on a "humanized" mouse antibody (Abrahamian and Cosimi 2001). Since IL2 is an essential step in activation of cytotoxic T-cells, induction therapy with these medications have proven to be very effective in rejection prophylaxis, decreasing 1-year rejection rate by 28% in controlled studies (Kahan et al. 1999). Because of their mechanism of action, IL2Ra are not typically used only in prophylaxis rather than in treatment of active rejection. Clinical application of monoclonal antibody therapy has not been described in the dog or cat, and there is some question as to whether the humanized antibody will be reactive to canine or feline T-cells without some modification (Sandusky et al. 1986). Success of applying these techniques in veterinary medicine will hinge on availability of canine and feline monoclonal reagents that equate to those already commercially produced for experiments in mice and clinical application in humans.

Irradiation

Nonmyeloablative irradiation has been applied in a variety of forms, including total lymphoid irradiation (TLI) or total body irradiation (TBI). Original application of TLI was performed as an adjunct therapy for Hodgkin's disease in human beings and included two ports: the "mantle" port that included the cervical and mediastinal lymph nodes and an "inverted Y" port that covered the aortic iliac and pelvic lymph nodes (Kaplan 1980). Over time, researchers noted that TLI was associated with a decrease in number of circulating T-cells, suppression of mixed lymphocyte reactivity testing in vitro, and induction of suppressor T-cells, but these individuals did not experience a greatly increased risk of opportunistic infections (Goffinet et al. 1972; Waer et al. 1984). Subsequent application of TLI with concurrent donor bone marrow transplantation was found to induce hematopoietic chimerism and tolerance in mouse models of organ transplantation (Strober et al. 1979). This exciting work has been somewhat tempered by results in human clinical renal transplantation, in which only a small fraction of the transplant recipients go on to develop tolerance (Waer 2001). Widespread application of TLI and donor bone marrow transplantation has also been slowed by the risks of graft versus host disease, a rare but life-threatening complication of bone marrow transplantation.

Experimental application of TBI and donor bone marrow transplantation has been performed in association with renal allograft transplantation in non-matched dogs (Broaddus et al. 2006). Although this technique was highly successful in preventing rejection when combined with immunosuppressive drug therapy, it failed to induce organ-specific tolerance in this species.

Selection of appropriate candidates

Timing

Because of the fear of applying an expensive, invasive procedure in client-owned animals, veterinarians will often reserve consideration of renal transplantation until an animal has reached a life-threatening crisis. Unfortunately, veterinary transplant centers require several weeks to identify a compatible donor, to perform thorough screening of the transplant candidate and to assemble a team to perform the procedure. In both human and animal transplant recipients, there is mounting evidence that early intervention will minimize the risk of perioperative complications and will prolong survival (Katz et al. 1991; Anonymous 1993; Obrador and Pereira 1998; Abecassis et al. 2008). Pet owners must also be given adequate time to consider the responsibilities of caring for a transplant recipient prior to making a decision to perform this procedure. As a result, it is recommended that veterinarians offer referral to a transplant center early in the course of treatment; as soon as the animal begins to show the signs of weight loss, poor appetite, or anemia that indicate the onset of end-stage disease. In humans with chronic renal disease, it is recommended that a patient is referred to a nephrologist for management when serum creatinine concentrations exceed 1.5 mg/dL for a woman or 2.0 mg/dL for a man (Anonymous 1993). Early referral to a nephrologist has been to shown to improve management of hypertension and metabolic derangements. While it has been clearly shown that pre-emptive transplantation (transplantation as an initial therapy) improves patient survival and decreases morbidity, organ availability and delayed referral has limited the number of patients that receive pre-emptive transplant to only 2.5% of those with chronic kidney disease (Abecassis et al. 2008). Unfortunately, there have been no comparable objective criteria for referral of dogs or cats with CKD. Rather, authors have focused on levels of azotemia that would preclude transplantation due to severe uremia, indicating that animals with blood urea nitrogen concentrations (BUN) in excess of 100 mg/dL or serum creatinine concentrations exceeding 10 mg/dL despite adequate fluid diuresis may require hemodialysis prior to transplantation. Ideally, transplantation would be performed in an animal with stable chronic renal disease that has just begun to decompensate despite appropriate medical therapy. Objective guidelines for timing of surgical intervention will require outcome analysis in a large number of cats in order to determine the appropriate time for referral.

Screening of candidates

Identification and screening of candidates for renal transplantation is typically carried out by the primary care provider. Renal transplantation and associated immunosuppression can pose great risk in a patient with an underlying cardiovascular, neoplastic, or infectious disease. In addition, the involvement of a live donor in veterinary transplantation necessitates that only the most viable candidates are selected for transplantation. Thus, thorough systemic diagnostic evaluations are performed to identify any comorbid diseases prior to referral. A list of diagnostic evaluations for the recipient and donor are summarized in Tables 31.2 and 31.3, with more specific information on each area of interest to follow.

Primary disease

Renal allograft transplantation may be used to treat nearly all forms of chronic renal disease (Chapter 48), presuming that the chances of recurrent primary disease are low and that the process of immunosuppression will not increase the risk of further complications. In human beings, renal transplantation is performed to treat a wide variety of congenital and acquired conditions, with glomerulomephritis (26%), reflux nephropathy/interstitial nephritis (16%), polycystic kidney disease

Table 31.2 Diagnostic screening of renal transplant candidates

Laboratory tests	Complete blood count
	Serum biochemistry panel
Cardiovascular	Thoracic radiographs
	Electrocardiography
	Echocardiography
	Indirect blood pressure
Infectious	FeLV/FIV test (cat)
	Heartworm antigen test (dog)
	Toxoplasma IgG and IgM
Urinary	Urinalysis
	Urine culture (cystocentesis)
	Abdominal ultrasound
	Urine protein:creatinine
Immune	Blood typing
	Major/minor blood crossmatch to donor
	Tissue histocompatibility testing (dog)
Endocrine	Thyroid evaluation

Abbreviations: FeLV, feline leukemia virus; FIV, feline immunodeficiency.

(14%), and diabetes mellitus (11%) being the most common (Briggs 2001).

In cats, the vast majority of transplant candidates are diagnosed with chronic tubulo-interstitial nephritis, with no known primary injury (Adin et al. 2001b). Several animals with ethylene glycol toxicity have been treated using renal allograft transplantation, although the acute, oliguric nature of this syndrome can make medical support during the pre-transplant evaluation very challenging. Initially, clinicians questioned the wisdom of renal allograft transplantation in cats suffering from calcium oxalate urolithiasis, due to fears of stone formation in the allograft (Aronson et al. 2006). Although allograft urolithiasis did occur in 26% of 19 cats in one retrospective study, survival in this group of cats (median

Table 31.3 Diagnostic evaluation of renal transplant donors

Laboratory tests	Complete blood count
	Serum biochemistry panel
Infectious	FeLV/FIV test (cat)
	Heartworm antigen test (dog)
	Toxoplasma IgG and IgM
Urinary	Urinalysis
	Urine culture
	Abdominal ultrasound, IVP, or CTA
Immune	Blood typing
	Major and minor crossmatch to donor
	Tissue histocompatibility testing (dog)

Abbreviations: FeLV, Feline leukemia virus; FIV, Feline immunodeficiency virus; Ig, immunoglobulin; IVP, intravenous pyelogram; CTA, computerized tomography with angiography.

602 days) appears to parallel that of the general transplant-population (Aronson and Drobatz 2000). While the 5 year recurrence rate of glomerulonephritis is only 2% in human transplant recipients (Raine et al. 1992; Briggs 2001), there is no data available regarding the use of renal allograft transplantation in dogs or cats with protein losing nephropathies (Chapter 53). Typically, PLN in dogs and cats are the result of systemic immune disease or hereditary conditions, and renal failure is only a secondary, end-stage complication. As such, renal allograft transplantation is not commonly practiced in the treatment of animals with glomerulonephritis or amyloidosis. Historical or current bacterial urinary tract infections are common in animals that are being evaluated for renal allograft transplantation and are typically treated as a relative contraindication for transplantation. Most transplant centers will require that bacterial culture is performed immediately before referral for transplantation. Animals with an active infection are treated with antimicrobials based on culture and sensitivity testing. After confirmation of a negative bacterial culture, animals are subjected to a cyclosporine challenge consisting of a 2-week period of immunosuppression using microemulsified cyclosporine orally at a dose of 4 mg/kg, twice daily. Urine samples are obtained by cystocentesis and re-cultured at the completion of this period to verify that infection does not recur during immunosuppressive drug therapy.

Cardiovascular disease

Cardiovascular disease is the number one cause of death in human renal allograft recipients. Initially, human transplant candidates with evidence of left ventricular failure were declined due to expectations of a poor outcome after renal transplantation. Further study has confirmed that chronic renal failure is a risk factor for cardiac events in patients with atherosclerosis and coronary heart disease. However, physicians are becoming increasingly aware that many cardiac events in human beings with ESRD are not related to coronary heart disease, but rather are the result of left ventricular dysfunction produced by chronic uremia and hypertension. Interestingly, left ventricular failure secondary to uremic cardiomyopathy can actually be reversed by successful renal transplantation (Zolty et al. 2008).

A study performed in feline renal transplant candidates at the University of California, Davis, revealed similar findings. Cardiac murmurs and abnormal echocardiographic findings associated with the left ventricle and septum were common in cats with chronic renal disease, but were not associated with an increased risk of congestive heart failure after renal transplantation (Adin et al. 2001a). Currently, cats and dogs that are candidates for renal transplantation are screened with thoracic radiographs and echocardiography. In animals with overt evidence of congestive heart failure, or subjective evidence of primary hypertrophic cardiomyopathy, transplantation is not recommended. However, focal areas of hypertrophy or mild left ventricular hypertrophy are not considered contraindications for renal transplantation. It is hoped that more specific genetic tests for feline and canine hypertrophic or dilated cardiomyopathies will be available in the future, allowing clinicians to distinguish between primary cardiac disease and uremic cardiomyopathy that may be ameliorated by renal transplantation.

Hypertension

Post-transplant hypertension (Chapter 68) is a common problem in human renal transplant recipients and is often the result of multiple factors, including activation of the renin–angiotensin system by the retained native kidneys, renal artery stenosis in the allograft, or drug-related factors (Curtis 1993). Other investigators have shown that increased activation of the sympathetic nervous system continues after renal transplantation, despite resolution of uremia (Hausberg et al. 2002). Unlike primary or essential hypertension, transplant-related hypertension is often treatable using simple interventions, such as angiotensin-converting enzyme inhibitors or interventional radiologic techniques, to treat native kidney hypertension or vascular stenoses, respectively. On the basis of the potential for cardiovascular complications and end organ damage, identification and medical management of preoperative hypertension is indicated prior to scheduling transplantation surgery (Briggs 2001).

In veterinary transplantation, severe acute hypertension in the immediate postoperative period has proven to be one of the most frustrating and common complications, with a significant effect on perioperative neurologic complications and mortality. One study documented that 18% of cats presenting for renal transplantation had preoperative hypertension, but 62% experienced acute postoperative hypertension (Kyles et al. 1999). Occurrence of postoperative hypertension was associated with an increased risk of neurologic complications after surgery. Interestingly, preoperative administration of propranolol did not appear to prevent the occurrence of this complication (Kyles et al. 1999). Preoperative hypertension does not appear to be a good predictor for the occurrence of postoperative complications in cats, and we do not have any strong data to support specific therapy aside from standard antihypertensive medications. Typically, animals are screened using indirect arterial blood pressure measurements obtained in a controlled environment. Animals with preoperative hypertension are treated with amlodipine at a dose of 0.05 mg/kg (0.025 mg/lb) orally every 12–24 hours, until the desired effect is achieved.

Neoplasia

Neoplasia is the number 2 cause of death in human transplant recipients, second only to cardiovascular events (Wong and Chapman 2008). A number of studies have documented that human renal transplant recipients experience a 3–5-fold increase in incidence of neoplasia when compared to an age-matched population (Wong and Chapman 2008). Neoplasms may be de-novo, recurrent, or transferred via the transplanted organ and pathophysiology is widely believed to be the related to chronic immunosuppression. Recently, a more specific analysis of the data has suggested that it may only be viral-related tumors that occur with increased incidence in transplant recipients, while epithelial neoplasms occur at a similar frequency to that seen in a control population (Grulich et al. 2007), adding more evidence to the argument that immunosuppression is the key factor in the pathophysiology of this complication. Screening of human candidates for renal transplantation is largely extrapolated from screening procedures used in the general population, including sigmoidoscopy to evaluate for colorectal cancer, cytologic screening for cervical cancer, total body skin evaluation by a dermatologist, mammography, prostate specific antigen tests, and imaging to evaluate for intracavitary neoplasia (Wong and Chapman 2008). On the basis of the relationship between viral disease and post-transplant neoplasia, viral testing is considered essential in screening human renal transplant recipients. Prognosis for human transplant recipients with malignant cancer is very poor as definitive chemotherapy is often precluded by comorbidities that increase the risk of cardiac toxicity, renal toxicity, or other drug interactions (Wong and Chapman 2008). As a result, human beings with active malignant neoplasia are not considered candidates for renal transplantation.

Although limited information is available for veterinary transplant recipients, a single retrospective study does suggest that cats experience an increased risk of de-novo neoplasia, with an incidence of 9.5% in a population of 95 cats (Wooldridge et al. 2002). Lymphoma is the most frequently identified type of neoplasia in feline transplant recipients, and it is interesting to hypothesize whether this may be related to latent viral infection as in the human population. Although FeLV and FIV status at the time of diagnosis was not reported in these cats (Wooldridge et al. 2002), a previous report did document the development of lymphoma in association with

FeLV virus infection following renal transplantation in a cat (Gregory et al. 1991). Screening for neoplasia in the dog and cat population is not nearly as detailed as the previously described protocols used in aged human beings. Rather, veterinarians perform standard imaging including 3-view thoracic radiographs and abdominal ultrasonography, while using the history and physical examination to guide any further specific testing. In animals with active or historical malignancy, medical management of renal disease is typically recommended, as the risks of transplant related immunosuppression may outweigh the benefits of improved renal function.

Infectious disease

Because of the requirement for life-long immunosuppression following renal allograft transplantation, infectious diseases are one of the most common and serious sequelae in transplant recipients. In particular, transplant candidates with preexisting viral, bacterial, fungal, or parasitic diseases have an extremely high rate of morbidity and mortality after transplant immunosuppression is initiated (Chapters 27, 71–74). On the basis of the data available in human transplant recipients, patients are routinely screened for urinary tract infections, respiratory infections including tuberculosis, cytomegalovirus, human immunodeficiency virus, and hepatitis B and C (Browne and Kahan 1994). Sporadic case reports in the veterinary literature demonstrated that disseminated toxoplasmosis or mycobacterial infection could also develop in companion animals after initiating immunosuppressive therapy, with uniformly fatal consequences (Bernsteen et al. 1999; Griffin et al. 2003; Nordquist and Aronson 2008). A large retrospective study has recently confirmed suspicions that infectious diseases are more common than the individual case reports would suggest, with 47 infections being documented in 43 of 169 cats (Kadar et al. 2005). Infections included bacterial (25/47), viral (13/47), fungal (6/47), and protozoal (3/47) etiologies; overall, infection was the second most common cause of death in this series, comprising 14% of deaths (Kadar et al. 2005). Similar problems have occurred in canine renal transplants. After overcoming problems with acute rejection, recent studies have shown an opposite trend, with excessive immunosuppression leading to opportunistic infections in nearly all patients and causing significant mortality in canine transplant recipients that survive the perioperative period (Mathews et al. 1994; Gregory et al. 2006).

Donor selection and screening

Although renal allograft transplantation is the treatment of choice for most human beings with ESRD, a severe shortage of donor organs exists, leaving a large number of candidates to receive chronic hemodialysis therapy while awaiting a suitable donor organ. Previously, only a small portion of human renal transplant recipients received organs from living donors (typically, a spouse or primary relative), while the majority received organs from cadaveric donors through a matching system termed the United Organ Sharing Network. Despite ongoing recruitment, the number of cadaveric donor organs has stabilized while the number of candidates waiting for donated organs increases with each year. To compensate for this increasing shortfall, recruitment of living donors has increased, and in the year 2001, the use of living donors surpassed the use of cadaveric organs for the first time. Living donors undergo both medical and psychological screening before surgery. Patients are carefully screened for evidence of familial renal disease, hypertension, or other factors that may increase their risk of undergoing unilateral nephrectomy. In addition, donors are screened for infectious diseases, pyelonephritis and neoplasia, in an effort to prevent the spread of disease to the recipient.

In veterinary medicine, transplant centers lack the financial resources to support a cadaveric organ sharing network. Thus, all reported clinical organ transplants in dogs and cats have been performed using living donors. Because of the simplicity of the feline MHC gene and the relative ease of preventing allograft rejection in cats, veterinary transplant centers have focused on the use of unrelated donor cats that are obtained from research colonies. Owners of the recipient are required to sign an agreement that the donor cat will be provided with a good home for the remainder of their life, regardless of the outcome for the recipient. It would seem that the use of cats from animal shelters would be even more desirable, but policies at many humane societies prevent the adoption of animals for the purpose of organ donation, even if the cat is destined for euthanasia. The use of cats from animal shelters also carries significant risk of transferring infectious diseases to the immunosuppressed recipient. After any potential donors are identified, blood typing and crossmatching with the recipient are performed to confirm compatibility. In dogs, initial inquiries are made as to the availability of any related donors, to improve the chances of histocompatibility. If no related donors are available, then identification of an unrelated donor is pursued as described for cats, attempting to identify an animal that is in need of adoption and would benefit from the provision of an excellent home. The potential donor is then screened using physical examination, laboratory testing and imaging, to ensure that there is no evidence of renal disease, anatomic anomalies, or infectious diseases that would preclude safe performance of unilateral nephrectomy (Table 31.3). Particular concern

is now given to screening for species-specific infectious diseases, as significant mortality has been documented in donors following transmission of infectious diseases to the immunosuppressed organ recipient, either directly or via the transplanted tissue (Bernsteen et al. 1999; Kadar et al. 2005). In addition to standard screening, some centers have adopted the use of CT angiography to specifically identify anomalies in renal vasculature that may aid in surgical planning or exclusion of some donors, based on duplication of renal arteries or veins (Bouma et al. 2003).

Renal transplantation

Preoperative care of the recipient

The recipient is admitted to the transplant center 2–3 days prior to the planned surgery. A preoperative checklist is often helpful in assuring that all aspects of patient care are achieved. Re-evaluation of complete blood count, serum biochemistry panel, and any remaining screening tests that were unable to be performed prior to referral are completed at this time. Blood crossmatch to the donor is repeated, to ensure that incompatibility has not developed as a result of previous transfusion therapy. The donor is also crossmatched to three additional units of whole or packed red blood cells, to allow for rapid therapy in the perioperative period. The transplant team may choose to place a multilumen jugular catheter prior to surgery, in order to allow for repeated blood sampling in the perioperative period.

Preoperative fluid therapy is planned based on the results of the most recent laboratory evaluations. Most animals will have chronic, polyuric renal failure and are diuresed using crystalloids at a rate of 5–6 mL/kg/h until the time of surgery. Because of the frequency of electrolyte disorders in renal transplant candidates, careful consideration is given to choice of a magnesium-containing fluid and intravenous fluids are supplemented with potassium chloride, as indicated (Wooldridge and Gregory 1999). Whole blood transfusions are administered to achieve a packed cell volume of 30% prior to surgery (Gregory et al. 1992), with up to 73% of cats requiring transfusion therapy to achieve this goal (Valverde et al. 2002). Careful monitoring of hydration status and daily evaluation of body weight should be performed in an effort to avoid volume overload. Animals with advanced renal disease have little ability to increase urine output to compensate for large volumes of fluid administration and concurrent administration of blood products with large volumes of crystalloids may produce volume overload. Indirect arterial blood pressure is evaluated after acclimatization to the hospital environment. Antihypertensive therapy with propranolol is prescribed for cats with evidence of preoperative systemic hypertension (systolic BP >170 mmHg) to prevent end organ damage associated with chronic severe hypertension. Unfortunately, prophylactic treatment of feline renal transplant recipients with propranolol did not prevent episodes of malignant hypertension in the postoperative period and prophylactic therapy does not appear to be indicated at this time (Kyles et al. 1999). If cyclosporine is initiated prior to the procedure, 12-hour trough whole blood levels are measured after 2–4 doses, to allow adjustment in the perioperative period (Gregory et al. 1992).

Anesthesia

Recipient

Debilitated candidates for renal transplantation are affected by a number of metabolic, fluid-balance, and nutritional abnormalities, leading to a variety of challenges in anesthetic management. Despite these challenges, severe intraoperative anesthetic complications are rare, with 0% mortality in nearly all reported case series (Valverde et al. 2002). Typically, cats are premedicated with a combination of an anticholinergic (atropine 0.02 mg/kg or glycopyrrolate 0.005 mg/kg) and an opioid (oxymorphone 0.05 mg/kg) (Valverde et al. 2002). In the published studies describing anesthetic management of veterinary transplant recipients, the vast majority of animals were induced using isoflurane and oxygen administered via a face mask, rather than with an injectable product (Gregory et al. 1992; Mathews and Gregory 1997; McAnulty 1998; Valverde et al. 2002). Cephazolin, 22 mg/kg, IV, is administered to the recipient within 20 minutes of induction for antimicrobial prophylaxis. Anesthetic maintenance is achieved using isoflurane and oxygen, with supplemental crystalloids (5–10 mL/kg/h) and dopamine infusion (2.5–7ug/kg/minute) titrated to maintain systolic blood pressure >80 mmHg (Valverde et al. 2002). Controlled ventilation was performed in 87% of cats, with supplemental atracurium (0.25 mg/kg loading dose followed by 0.1 mg/kg IV) used in a small number of animals for intraoperative paralysis (Valverde et al. 2002). Patient warming is performed at all times after induction using a circulating warm water blanket over the operating table and a forced air warming device surrounding the torso. Monitoring during anesthesia should include ECG, indirect blood pressure, core body temperature, blood gas analysis, pH, and electrolytes, including sodium, potassium, and ionized calcium. Intraoperative administration of sodium bicarbonate (base deficit × 0.3 × body weight in kg) and 10% calcium chloride (0.2 mL/kg, IV over 20 minutes) are performed to correct acidosis and hypocalcemia, respectively (Valverde

et al. 2002). Mannitol (0.5–1 g/kg, IV) is administered immediately after the release of the vascular clamps to induce diuresis after reperfusion. Perioperative anticoagulant therapy with standard heparin or enoxaparin have been described in dogs, based on the high rate of thromboembolic complications in a recent study (Gregory et al. 2006). Interestingly, perioperative use of anticoagulants does not appear to be necessary in cats, as thromboembolism has been exceedingly rare in this species.

Donor

Anesthesia for the donor is performed as described above for the recipient. Pre-medication and induction are performed approximately 30 minutes prior to the recipient to minimize total anesthetic time in the recipient if concurrent harvest and organ implantation are planned (Gregory et al. 1992; Mathews and Gregory 1997). When cold storage techniques are used, the donor harvest and recipient organ implantation may be separated by 3.5–7 hours, allowing staged procedures (McAnulty 1998). Mannitol is administered to the donor cat approximately 20–30 minutes prior to harvest of the organ, to induce diuresis and aid in free radical scavenging during ischemia (Gregory et al. 1992; Mathews and Gregory 1997).

Donor nephrectomy

In human renal allograft transplantation, many centers are now offering laparoscopic or laparoscopic-assisted donor nephrectomy to minimize patient morbidity. In veterinary patients, donor nephrectomy is still performed through a standard ventral midline approach, with an incision extending from the xyphoid to pubis to allow for retrieval of the entire length of ureter during kidney harvest. Preferably, the left kidney is harvested, as this kidney has the longest renal vein segment. The abdominal cavity is explored to confirm normal anatomy and then the vascular pedicle to the left kidney is bluntly dissected. Intermittent topical application of lidocaine (20%) is performed to prevent vasospasm. If exposure of the vascular pedicle reveals duplication of the renal artery or a major arborization within 5 mm of the renal pelvis, the contralateral kidney is examined and harvested. If bilateral renal vascular anomalies exist, surgical techniques are available to address the anomalies (Aguilo et al. 1991; Singh et al. 2008), although application of these techniques has not been described in reports of renal transplantation in dogs or cats. After confirmation of suitable vascular anatomy, the kidney is dissected free from its retroperitoneal attachments, and the ureter is isolated down to the level of the bladder, carefully preserving the ureteral blood supply. When dissection is complete, the renal artery and vein are ligated with suture or using hemostatic clips placed close to the aorta and vena cava. The vessels are then transected distal to the ligations. The renal artery is flushed immediately with either chilled heparinized saline (Gregory et al. 1992) or with preservation solution if cold storage is planned (McAnulty 1998). The renal artery is dilated with forceps and the adventitia is trimmed from the distal 1 mm of the vessel. The kidney is then immersed in chilled heparized saline or preservation solution and is transferred to the recipient for implantation.

Allograft implantation

Although a number of refinements have been made to the procedure of renal allograft implantation in cats and dogs, the initial concept remains unchanged. The allograft is implanted in a heterotopic location, typically in the caudal abdomen. This location allows easy access to a vascular supply from the aorta or its terminal branches and is in close proximity to the urinary bladder for implantation of the ureter without excessive tension. As in human renal transplantation, most veterinary transplant surgeons have adopted the policy of maintaining the native kidneys to provide a mechanism of fluid elimination in the case of delayed graft function or during later episodes of acute rejection. One group has described prophylactic bilateral native nephrectomy to prevent the development of refractory hypertension in

dogs (Mathews et al. 2000). Native nephrectomy may also be indicated in isolated cases when expansile polycystic disease has become advanced enough to hinder exposure during surgery.

Vascular anastomosis

Feline renal transplantation requires a moderate level of microsurgical skill and is typically carried out using an operating microscope, due to the small vessel and ureteral lumen diameters in this species. Originally, feline renal transplantation was carried out using simple interrupted sutures to perform an end-to-end arterial anastomosis of the recipient external iliac artery to the donor renal artery (Gregory et al. 1992). The renal vein was then anastomosed in an end-to-side fashion with the common iliac vein. This technique led to acceptable results in the majority of recipients, although a small number of cats suffered from ischemic injury to the left pelvic limb, with neuropraxia occurring in 12% of cats and severe ischemic necrosis requiring pelvic limb amputation in one cat (Mathews and Gregory 1997). End-to-end arterial and venous anastomoses may also be performed using a microanastomotic device as depicted in Figure 31.2 (Newell et al. 1999). This technique has the great advantage of speed and technical simplicity when compared to hand suturing, but retains the possibility for serious ischemic complications in the left pelvic limb. The end-to-end anastomosis also creates some technical

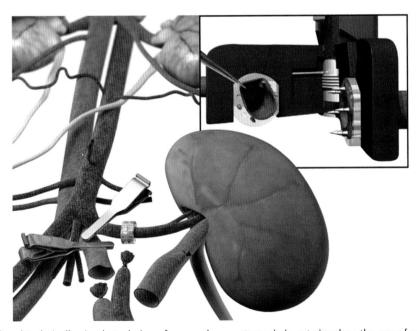

Figure 31.2 An rapid and technically simple technique for vascular anastomosis in cats involves the use of an anastomotic coupling device. Because of the configuration of the device, an end-to-end technique using the external iliac artery and common iliac vein is required. The vessel ends are pulled through the anastomostic rings, and the vessel is pulled over the sharp pegs, everting the endothelium at the level of the anastomosis. The device is then engaged, compressing the anastomotic rings into apposition.

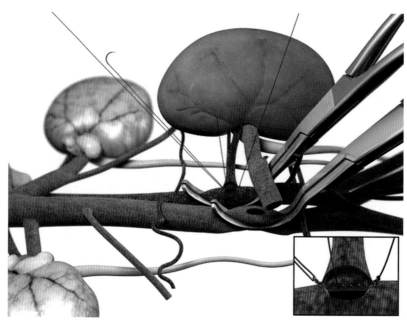

Figure 31.3 An aorto-caval side-to-side vascular anastomotic technique is used for renal allograft implantation in cats and small dogs. The caudal abdominal aorta and vena cava are exposed, and partial occlusion clamps are placed between the gonadal vessels and the caudal mesenteric artery. Separate continuous suture patterns are run for the front and back wall (inset). Note that the native kidneys are retained in most recipients.

difficulties when there is a disparity in the donor and recipient vessel diameter. A later modification of the technique was proposed to address these concerns (Figure 31.3), using an end-to-side anastomosis technique, in which the donor artery and vein were anastomosed directly to the caudal abdominal aorta and vena cava, respectively (Bernsteen et al. 1999). Aortocaval anastomosis preserves the circulation to the pelvic limbs, without ligation of any terminal arterial branches, and ischemic times are similar to previously described hand-sutured anastomotic techniques.

In large dogs, collateral circulation to the pelvic limb has prevented any serious complications associated with ligation of the iliac vessels and a standard iliac artery to donor renal vein anastomosis is typically performed with an end-to-end technique. The renal vein is sutured end-to-side with the recipient common iliac vein (Figure 31.4). In dogs less than 10 kg, one group has described the application of the modified caudal aortic and caval anastomosis technique that is used in cats (Gregory et al. 2006). Because of the larger vessel diameter in most dogs, vascular anastomosis can be carried out using magnifying loupes (3.5×) rather than with an operating microscope.

Ureteral implantation

The small luminal diameter of the feline ureter has made ureteral implantation one of the more challenging aspects of renal transplantation, with neoureterocys-

tostomy causing partial to complete ureteral obstruction for a period of 3–7 days in most animals (Mehl et al. 2005). Initial attempts at renal transplantation in the cat were performed using a "drop-in" technique that was described in human beings. This technically simple technique involves tunneling the ureter through the bladder wall, then tacking the ureteral mucosa to the bladder mucosa with two sutures, making no efforts to achieve perfect mucosal apposition (Kochin et al. 1993). Unfortunately, clinical application of this technique led to a 34% incidence of postoperative ureteral obstruction due to granulation tissue formation, requiring surgical revision of the ureteral implantation site in 12 of 37 ureters (Mathews and Gregory 1997). On the basis of this experience, the ureteral implantation technique was modified (Figure 31.5), performing mucosal apposition of the implanted ureter and bladder using an interrupted technique with 8–0 Nylon (Gregory et al. 1996). After switching to the mucosal apposition technique, no further ureteral revision surgeries were required (Mathews and Gregory 1997). Since this time, two alternative techniques have been presented for neoureterocystostomy in cats: an extravesicular implantation technique (Mehl et al. 2005) and a ureteral papilla implantation technique (Hardie et al. 2005). Both of these techniques (Figure 31.5) may be performed without creating a large cystotomy, reducing both operative morbidity and time.

Ureteral implantation in dogs can be performed using any of the aforementioned mucosal apposition

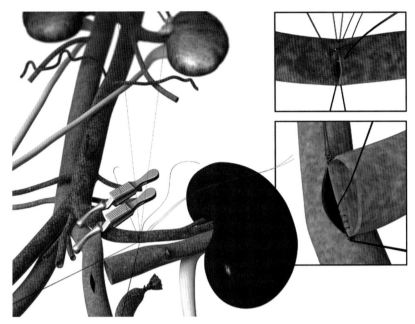

Figure 31.4 An end-to-end anastomosis is performed in larger dogs, using the recipient external iliac artery. The anastomosis is triangulated using three interrupted sutures placed at 120 degree intervals around the vessels, then the vessels are apposed using an interrupted pattern. A continuous end-to-side technique is used to anastomose the renal vein and the common iliac vein, due to disparity in vessel diameters.

techniques. Although the larger luminal diameter of the canine ureter has not been reported to cause clinical problems in canine renal transplantation, neoureterostomy appears to produce temporary ureteral obstruction in this species as well (Barthez et al. 2000).

Nephropexy

After implantation in the caudal abdomen, the renal allograft is attached only at the vascular pedicle and ureteral implantation sites, allowing the kidney to torse on this attachment point and cause vascular occlusion

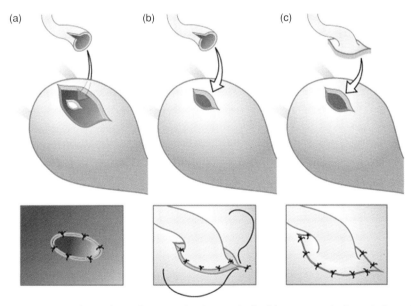

Figure 31.5 Ureteral implantation may be performed using either intravesicular (a) or extravesicular techniques (b) and (c). Intravesicular neoureterocystostomy (a) requires that a large cystotomy incision is made to allow direct visualization of mucosal apposition. In extravesicular neoureterocystostomy, the ureter is spatulated and sutured to the bladder mucosa from the exterior. A seromuscular tunnel is then created by closing the incision in the bladder wall (b). Implantation of the ureter may also be simplified by resecting a patch of bladder wall during harvest of the donor kidney (c).

and thrombosis. Clinical reports of kidney torsion and vascular avulsion in several cats (Mathews and Gregory 1997) have led to the empirical application of a variety of nephropexy techniques. Nephropexy can be performed by simply affixing the kidney directly to the adjacent transversus muscle and peritoneum using interrupted, nonabsorbable sutures (Mathews and Gregory 1997). Alternatively, a ventrally based musculoperitoneal flap may be elevated and sutured to the renal capsule (Bernsteen et al. 1999).

Enteropexy

Multiple reports have confirmed that intussusception is a frequent complication following renal allograft transplantation in the dog (Libro and Proto 1964; Kelly et al. 1971; Du Toit et al. 1981; Finco et al. 1985; McAnulty et al. 1989; Klinger et al. 1990; Kyles et al. 2003a). Postoperative intussusception is an exceedingly rare complication in this species, and the etiology for the increased incidence seen in transplant recipients is not known, although the administration of opioid analgesics appears to significantly decrease the incidence of this complication (McAnulty et al. 1989; Klinger et al. 1990). Prophylactic enteroplication has also been recommended following renal transplantation in the dog (Kyles et al. 2003a). Postoperative intussusception has never been reported in feline renal transplant recipients; as a result, enteroplication is not currently performed in the cat.

Feeding device

Renal transplant recipients are commonly affected by chronic nutritional deficiencies that will continue throughout the perioperative period. Placement of a percutaneous feeding tube (esophagostomy or gastrostomy tube) is typically performed at the time of surgery, if not already present at the time of admission. Presence of a feeding tube facilitates maintaining caloric intake after surgery and simultaneously provides a reliable route for drug administration. The feeding tube is typically removed in 1–2 months after surgery, when oral food intake has returned to normal. After conferring with the pet owners, some clinicians may elect to place a low-profile silicone gastrostomy tube that will be maintained to improve compliance with long-term immunosuppressive drug administration.

Postoperative care

For the first 24–48 hours after surgery, the recipient is recovered in an intensive care unit facility with 24-hour observation. Staff are carefully instructed about precautions with regard to transfer of infectious diseases to the immunosuppressed recipient and are warned against any aggressive restraint of a fractious patient following surgery, which has caused avulsion of the vascular pedicle in a small number of animals. Latex gloves are worn when treating the patient and a high level of aseptic technique is maintained with use of the intravenous catheter and cleaning of the surgical sites. Analgesia is provided with opioids as a continuous rate infusion or by intermittent bolus injections for 24–48 hours. Intravenous crystalloid therapy is initiated at a rate of 4–6 mL/kg/h and is adjusted based on assessment of hydration. Urine output may be estimated by weighing absorbent pads that are placed in the litter box and cage, although urinary catheterization is avoided to minimize the risk of introducing a urinary tract infection. Bladder expression is strictly forbidden, to prevent avulsion of the vascular pedicle or ureteral implantation site. If oliguria or anuria is suspected, bladder size may be investigated using ultrasound of the abdomen with gentle restraint. Postoperative antibiotic therapy is performed using cefazolin (22 mg/kg IV, every 6–8 hours) until oral medications are tolerated. Amoxicillin-clavulanic acid is continued orally for 1–2 weeks after surgery. Famotidine is administered intravenously (0.5 mg/kg IV, every 12 hours) to prevent gastric ulceration and uremic gastritis. Feeding is initiated via the gastrostomy tube at 24 hours after surgery. Caloric intake is limited to 33% of daily maintenance requirements and then increased by 33% per day until full maintenance requirements are being met. Daily intake is divided into four or more feedings using a liquefied diet. Initially, a renal diet is often required, but may be transitioned to a high caloric density recovery diet after azotemia has resolved.

Indirect arterial blood pressure is monitored hourly during the first 48 hours after surgery, with instructions to administer hydralazine (2.5 mg) subcutaneously if the systolic blood pressure exceeds 170 mmHg. Recipients are also serially examined for evidence of neurologic abnormalities such as anisocoria, blindness, ataxia, obtundation, and seizures (Kyles et al. 1999). Detection of neurologic abnormalities should prompt evaluation of venous blood gas, electrolytes, osmolality, and blood glucose concentrations (Gregory et al. 1997). If no metabolic cause for the signs is detected, mannitol may be administered (1–2 g/kg) IV, over 20 minutes.

Blood samples are obtained via the multilumen catheter at 12–24 hours after surgery to allow analysis of blood urea nitrogen and serum creatinine concentrations, packed cell volume, blood glucose and serum electrolytes. Immunosuppressive therapy is performed according to the protocol developed for the individual (Table 31.1) and a 12-hour trough sample for cyclosporine analysis is obtained 24 hours after surgery and repeated every 48 hours until 12-hour trough levels are between 350–500 ng/mL for cats or 500–600 ng/mL for dogs (Mathews et al. 1993; Mathews and Gregory 1997).

Care of the donor is standard for an animal undergoing nephrectomy. Analgesia is provided using opioid analgesics, as for the recipient. Crystalloid therapy is typically performed at a rate of 4–6 mL/kg/h for 24 hours after surgery and then discontinued when oral intake of food and water is documented. Discharge of the donor may be performed at 48 hours after surgery, allowing acclimatization of the donor to the home environment before the recipient is released.

Home care

Transplant recipients are discharged when azotemia has resolved and cyclosporine levels have been adequately regulated to the desired therapeutic range. Total hospitalization time ranges from 7 to 14 days, depending upon the clinical condition of the recipient. Before discharge is considered, the owners of the recipient are also instructed to identify and contact a veterinary center that provides 24-hour care that is located in their local area. At the time of discharge, clients are instructed on the measurement and administration of cyclosporine. The client is observed while administering the medications to reaffirm compliance with medication administration after discharge. Clients are also instructed on daily cleaning of the feeding tube entry site and on the preparation and administration of food. Animals that experience delayed graft function are supported as indicated by the level of ongoing azotemia.

Precautions

Immunosuppressive regimes used in renal transplantation carry a number of potential hazards, including susceptibility to infectious diseases and specific drug interactions. In general, owners are recommended to avoid boarding of transplant recipients in a kennel or animal hospital environment as upper respiratory pathogens such as *Bordetella* and Herpesvirus 1 have proven to be serious or fatal complications in a number of dogs and cats (Mathews et al. 1994; Kadar et al. 2005). Cats must be maintained indoors to avoid bite wounds, exposure to feline leukemia or feline immunodeficiency virus, and to ensure availability for consistent administration of immunosuppressive drugs. Animals undergoing prophylactic dental cleanings should receive fluid diuresis and broad spectrum intravenous antibiotic therapy during the anesthetic period. There is some question as to whether immunization is effective in patients receiving transplant immunosuppression. Veterinarians are also cautioned to avoid administration of any live virus vaccines.

Clients and veterinarians must be aware of medications that would interact with immunosuppressive drug administration. In particular, drugs such as phenobarbital will affect hepatic metabolism of cyclosporine via the cytochrome P-450 pathway and may lower drug levels (Campana et al. 1996). On the contrary, diltiazem or ketoconazole may inhibit hepatic metabolism of cyclosporine and will increase drug levels in recipient (Wagner et al. 1988; Campana et al. 1996). Nephrotoxic potential of aminoglycosides or trimethoprim sulfa may be increased by co-administration of cyclosporine and concurrent use of these drugs is contraindicated (Bennett 1986). In general, it is prudent for the referring veterinarian to contact the transplant coordinator before administering any medication or vaccine that is outside of the specified immunosuppressive regime.

Follow-up visits

Because of the long distances that owners travel to reach veterinary transplant centers, the majority of follow-up is typically performed by the local primary care veterinarian. As a result, it is crucial this veterinarian becomes a well-educated and communicative member of the transplant team. In particular, any problems must be recognized early and pursued aggressively to allow rapid intervention if needed. Follow-up visits for complete physical examination (including body temperature) and laboratory evaluations occur weekly until drug levels and allograft function are stabilized, then the interval between visits is slowly increased to a maximum of 3 months. Visits should be scheduled at a time that is 12 hours after the administration of cyclosporine and owners must be reminded not to administer the medication until after the sample is obtained. Blood tests to be evaluated at each visit will include a complete blood count, 12-hour trough cyclosporine level, and serum biochemistry panel. All results should be forwarded to the transplant center for evaluation to allow constant communication between team members. Particular concern should be taken to check the gastrostomy tube site for any evidence of opportunistic infection; this is a frequent complication following surgery that can become life-threatening if not addressed.

Therapy for acute rejection

Acute rejection can be difficult to recognize and must be differentiated from other causes of azotemia or anorexia. Common differentials include ureteral obstruction, cyclosporine toxicity, or sepsis. Acute rejection occurs most frequently during the first 3 months following transplantation and is suspected when acute azotemia occurs in coordination with sub-therapeutic levels of cyclosporine therapy. Clinical signs can be vague and include inappetance, lethargy, and elevations in body temperature (Mathews and Gregory 1997; Halling et al. 2004). The gold standard for confirmation of allograft rejection is percutaneous needle biopsy. Unfortunately, waiting for results of cyclosporine blood levels or biopsy reports will incur an unacceptable delay in most cases, and recipients are frequently treated for rejection while diagnostic results are pending. Diagnostic ultrasound can be helpful in supporting a clinical diagnosis of acute rejection in ruling out an obstructive etiology. However, serial examinations of crosssectional area were the only reliable indicator of rejection in cats (Halling et al. 2003). Serologic markers of oxidative stress were not useful as indicators of acute rejection in cats (Halling et al. 2004). Initial therapy for suspected rejection episodes involves intravenous administration of prednisolone sodium succinate, 10 mg/kg (4.5 mg/lb) every 12 hours. Clients are also provided with an emergency dose of intravenous cyclosporine and instructions for the referring veterinarian on administration of the drug in the event of acute rejection: 6.6 mg/kg (3 mg/lb) diluted in 20–100 mL 0.9% NaCl and given over 4–6 hours, once daily until azotemia resolves. Between 85–90% of human transplant rejection episodes are steroid responsive (Morris 2001), while the reported response rate in cats is only 58% (Mathews and Gregory 1997).

Prognosis

To date, survival and quality of life after renal transplantation has been highly variable between species. Human renal allograft transplantation centers frequently report a 1-year patient and kidney graft survival rate of 100% (Aoun et al. 2007). These success rates are certainly a tribute not only to the great skills of the nephrologists and surgeons that are involved in leading transplant centers, but also to their vast experience, with many performing 200–300 renal transplants per year. Human transplant centers also pool data, allowing critical comparison of medical versus surgical therapy in the treatment of human ESRD. These analyses have clearly indicated that human renal transplant recipients have improved survival, better quality of life, and decreased medical costs in comparison to equivalent patients managed with medical therapy (Abecassis et al. 2008).

Unfortunately, available data for analysis of success in veterinary transplantation are limited. Most of the published information pertains to cats and has been derived from a single renal transplant center (Gregory et al. 1992;

Mathews and Gregory 1997; Adin et al. 2001b). Data indicate that outcomes are less successful in cats than in human beings, with approximately 60% of cats surviving to 6 months (Adin et al. 2001b). Highest mortality occurs in the perioperative period, and cats that survive past 1 year can experience long-term survival, with 42% survival being maintained at 3 years after surgery (Adin et al. 2001b). Delay in treatment may be a major contributor to the decreased success seen in veterinary transplant recipients. Transplantation is typically performed as an alternative to euthanasia, with cats having a mean serum creatinine concentration of nearly 8 mg/dL at the time of transplantation (Adin et al. 2001b). Data are not available to indicate whether earlier intervention would improve outcome in cats. Causes of death included graft failure, infectious complications secondary to immunosuppression, and neoplasia. Of all factors analyzed, only recipient age was predictive of outcome, with increasing recipient age having a significant negative effect on postoperative survival.

The dog has been found to present the most rigorous challenges in clinical renal transplantation. As noted previously, the canine MHC shows much greater diversity when compared to that of the domestic cat, greatly increasing the likelihood of allograft rejection when using non-related organ donors. After initial battles with achieving adequate immunosuppression, successful long-term survival (>100 days) has now been achieved in DLA mismatched research dogs using a variety of experimental protocols (Kyles et al. 2001; Kyles et al. 2002; Bernsteen et al. 2003; Kyles et al. 2003b; Broaddus et al. 2006). Long-term survival has also been achieved in recipients with naturally occurring disease using DLA-matched related donors. Unfortunately, sibling donors are rare and these clinical successes have not been reproduced using nonmatched dogs. Median survival in a recent clinical study using triple-drug immunosuppression (azathioprine, cyclosporine and prednisolone) was 18 days, with only 50% of dogs surviving past 2 months (Gregory et al. 2006). Survival data from a second center using RADTS in addition to similar triple drug immunosuppressive regime was notably better, with a median survival of 8 months (Mathews et al. 2000). In both reports, dogs that did survive long-term suffered from frequent opportunistic infections, suggesting that these protocols lead to excessive immunosuppression.

Ethics

Ethical considerations regarding renal transplantation hinge upon the health and rights of the living kidney donor. In human beings, similar concerns have led to extensive investigations of the health risks associated with kidney donation. Long-term follow-up studies have shown that unilateral nephrectomy has no significant effect on life expectancy in human beings (Narkun-Burgess et al. 1993); lifetime risk of renal failure is extremely small in kidney donors (0.1%) and occurs at an incidence that is similar to the general population (Hou 2000). There is only one report of donor follow-up pertaining to veterinary transplantation. This retrospective study reported normal BUN and serum creatinine concentrations in 15 donor cats at 2–5 years after unilateral nephrectomy, and showed no evidence of mortality or morbidity associated with kidney donation.

A separate consideration is that performing an elective surgery on a patient that is not a medical necessity may be interpreted to contradict the Hippocratic and veterinary oaths. In human beings, any risks associated with kidney donation are explained to the prospective donors and the "voluntary" aspect of the process can be used to argue against the ethical and legal considerations above. However, it has been debated that when a spouse, relative, or friend with appropriate histocompatibility matching is identified, the pressures on that individual will likely create a situation in which the prospective donor cannot comfortably withdraw from the process. In canine and feline transplantation, donors are typically obtained from research colonies or shelters and, after organ donation, are provided with an excellent home. In most cases, these animals are being rescued from euthanasia. Nonetheless, the animal organ donor does not have an ability to participate in the decision-making process, raising the ethical concerns of some veterinarians. Much of the debate on the ethics of donor nephrectomy has occurred in the United Kingdom, where veterinary law prohibits surgical procedures that do not provide a demonstrable health benefit to the individual.

Organization of an organ-harvesting network using nonliving donors is unlikely to be feasible in veterinary health care. However, the application of autogenous or cell-based therapies, artificial organs, and other aspects of regenerative medicine would bypass many of these ethical considerations.

References

Abbas, A.K., A.H. Lichtman, et al. (1991). *Cellular and Molecular Immunology*. Philadelphia, PA: WB Saunders.

Abecassis, M., S.T. Bartlett, et al. (2008). Kidney transplantation as primary therapy for end-stage renal disease: a national kidney foundation/kidney disease outcomes quality initiative (NKF/KDOQITM) conference. *Clin J Am Soc Nephrol* 3(2): 471–480.

Abrahamian, G.A. and A.B. Cosimi (2001). Antilymphocyte globulin and monoclonal antibodies. In: *Kidney Transplantation :Principles and Practice*, edited by P.J. Morris, 5th edition. Philadelphia, PA: WB Saunders, pp. 289–309.

Acott, P.D., J.F. Crocker, et al. (2006). Evaluation of performance factors affecting two formulations of cyclosporine in pediatric renal transplant patients. *Transplant Proc* 38(9): 2835–2841.

Adin, D., W.P. Thomas, et al. (2001a). Echocardiographic evaluation of cats with chronic renal failure (abstract). *J Vet Intern Med* 13(3): 337A.

Adin, C.A., C.R. Gregory, et al. (2001b). Diagnostic predictors of complications and survival after renal transplantation in cats. *Vet Surg* 30(6): 515–521.

Aguilo, J., O. Rodriguez, et al. (1991). Vascular anastomosis techniques in renal transplants. *Int Angiol* 10(1): 39–43.

Allison, A.C., T. Hovi, et al. (1975). Immunological observations on patients with lesch-nyhan syndrome, and on the role of de-novo purine synthesis in lymphocyte transformation. *Lancet* 2(7946): 1179–1183.

Allison, A.C., T. Hovi, et al. (1977). The role of de novo purine synthesis in lymphocyte transformation. *Ciba Found Symp* (48): 207–224.

Anonymous. (1993). NIH consensus statement, morbidity and mortality of dialysis. *NIH Consens Statement* 11(2): 1–33.

Aoun, M., P. Eschewege, et al. (2007). Very early steroid withdrawal in simultaneous pancreas-kidney transplants. *Nephrol Dial Transplant* 22(3): 899–905.

Aronson, L.R. and K. Drobatz (2000). Hypercalcemia following renal transplantation in a cat. *J Am Vet Med Assoc* 217(7): 1034–1037.

Aronson, L.R., A.E. Kyles, et al. (2006). Renal transplantation in cats with calcium oxalate urolithiasis: 19 cases (1997–2004). *J Am Vet Med Assoc* 228(5): 743–749.

Bach, J.F. (1975). The mode of action of immunosuppressive agents. *Front Biol* 41: 1–374.

Barthez, P.Y., D.D. Smeak, et al. (2000). Ureteral obstruction after ureteroneocystostomy in dogs assessed by technetium TC 99 m diethylenetriamine pentaacetic acid (DTPA) scintigraphy. *Vet Surg* 29(6): 499–506.

Bennett, W.M. (1986). Comparison of cyclosporine nephrotoxicity with aminoglycoside nephrotoxicity. *Clin Nephrol* 25(Suppl 1): S126–S129.

Bernsteen, L., C.R. Gregory, et al. (1999). Acute toxoplasmosis following renal transplantation in three cats and a dog. *J Am Vet Med Assoc* 215(8): 1123–1126.

Bernsteen, L., C.R. Gregory, et al. (2003). Microemulsified cyclosporine-based immunosuppression for the prevention of acute renal allograft rejection in unrelated dogs: preliminary experimental study. *Vet Surg* 32(3): 213–219.

Bernsteen, L., C.R. Gregory, et al. (1999). Comparison of two surgical techniques for renal transplantation in cats. *Vet Surg* 28(6): 417–420.

Bierer, B.E., G. Hollander, et al. (1993). Cyclosporin A and FK506: molecular mechanisms of immunosuppression and probes for transplantation biology. *Curr Opin Immunol* 5(5): 763–773.

Borel, J.F., C. Feurer, et al. (1994). Biological effects of cyclosporin A: a new antilymphocytic agent. 1976. *Agents Actions* 43(3–4): 179–186.

Bouma, J.L., L.R. Aronson, et al. (2003). Use of computed tomography renal angiography for screening feline renal transplant donors. *Vet Radiol Ultrasound* 44(6): 636–641.

Briggs, J.D. (2001). The recipient of a renal transplant. In: *Kidney Transplantation: Principles and Practice*, edited by P.J. Morris, 5th edition. Philadelphia, PA: WB Saunders, pp. 45–59.

Broaddus, K.D., D.M. Tillson, et al. (2006). Renal allograft histopathology in dog leukocyte antigen mismatched dogs after renal transplantation. *Vet Surg* 35(2): 125–135.

Browne, B.J. and B.D. Kahan (1994). Renal transplantation. *Surg Clin North Am* 74(5): 1097–1116.

Calandra, T. and R. Bucala (1997). Macrophage migration inhibitory factor (MIF): a glucocorticoid counter-regulator within the immune system. *Crit Rev Immunol* **17**(1): 77–88.

Campana, C., M.B. Regazzi, et al. (1996). Clinically significant drug interactions with cyclosporin: an update. *Clin Pharmacokinet* **30**(2): 141–179.

Case, J.B., A.E. Kyles, et al. (2007). Incidence of and risk factors for diabetes mellitus in cats that have undergone renal transplantation: 187 cases (1986–2005). *J Am Vet Med Assoc* **230**(6): 880–884.

Cecka, M. (1998). Clinical outcome of renal transplantation: factors influencing patient and graft survival. *Surg Clin North Am* **78**(1): 133–148.

Curtis, J.J. (1993). Management of hypertension after transplantation. *Kidney Int Suppl* **43**: S45–S49.

Dahlinger, J., C. Gregory, et al. (1998). Effect of ketoconazole on cyclosporine dose in healthy dogs. *Vet Surg* **27**(1): 64–68.

Dallman, M.J. (2001). Immunology of graft rejection. In: *Kidney Transplantation: Principles and Practice*, edited by P.J. Morris, 5th edition. Philadelphia, PA: WB Saunders, pp. 9–31.

Davidson, G. and D.C. Plumb (2003). *Veterinary Drug Handbook*, Client information edition. Ames, Iowa: Distributed by Iowa State Press.

Du Toit, D.F., W.P. Homan, et al. (1981). Canine intestinal intussusception following renal and pancreatic transplantation. *Vet Rec* **108**(2): 34–35.

Elion, G.B., S. Bieber, et al. (1960a). A summary of investigations with 2-amino-6-[(1-methyl-4-nitro-5-imidazolyl)thio]purine (B.W. 57–323) in animals. *Cancer Chemother Rep* **8**: 36–43.

Elion, G.B., S.W. Callahan, et al. (1960b). The metabolism of 2-amino-6-[(1-methyl-4-nitro-5-imidazolyl)thio]purine (B.W. 57–323) in man. *Cancer Chemother Rep* **8**: 47–52.

Ferran, C., M. Dy, et al. (1990). Reduction of morbidity and cytokine release in anti-CD3 MoAb-treated mice by corticosteroids. *Transplantation* **50**(4): 642–648.

Finco, D.R., C.A. Rawlings, et al. (1985). Kidney graft survival in transfused and nontransfused sibling beagle dogs. *Am J Vet Res* **46**(11): 2327–2331.

Goffinet, D.R., E.J. Glatstein, et al. (1972). Herpes zoster-varicella infections and lymphoma. *Ann Intern Med* **76**(2): 235–240.

Graumann, M.B., S.A. DeRose, et al. (1998). Polymorphism analysis of four canine MHC class I genes. *Tissue Antigens* **51**(4 Pt 1): 374–381.

Greco, B., L. Bielory, et al. (1983). Antithymocyte globulin reacts with many normal human cell types. *Blood* **62**(5): 1047–1054.

Gregory, C.R. (2009). Immunosuppressive agents. In: *Kirk's Current Veterinary Therapy*, edited by J.D. Bonagura and D.C. Twedt, 14th edition. Philadelphia, PA; London: Elsevier Saunders, pp. 254–259.

Gregory, C.R., I.M. Gourley, et al. (1992). Renal transplantation for treatment of end-stage renal failure in cats. *J Am Vet Med Assoc* **201**(2): 285–291.

Gregory, C.R., A.E. Kyles, et al. (2006). Results of clinical renal transplantation in 15 dogs using triple drug immunosuppressive therapy. *Vet Surg* **35**(2): 105–112.

Gregory, C.R., R.A. Lirtzman, et al. (1996). A mucosal apposition technique for ureteroneocystostomy after renal transplantation in cats. *Vet Surg* **25**(1): 13–17.

Gregory, C.R., B.R. Madewell, et al. (1991). Feline leukemia virus-associated lymphosarcoma following renal transplantation in a cat. *Transplantation* **52**(6): 1097–1099.

Gregory, C.R., K.G. Mathews, et al. (1997). Central nervous system disorders after renal transplantation in cats. *Vet Surg* **26**(5): 386–392.

Griffin, A., A.L. Newton, et al. (2003). Disseminated mycobacterium avium complex infection following renal transplantation in a cat. *J Am Vet Med Assoc* **222**(8): 1097,1101, 1077–1078.

Grulich, A.E., M.T. van Leeuwen, et al. (2007). Incidence of cancers in people with HIV/AIDS compared with immunosuppressed transplant recipients: a meta-analysis. *Lancet* **370**(9581): 59–67.

Halling, K.B., G.W. Ellison, et al. (2004). Evaluation of oxidative stress markers for the early diagnosis of allograft rejection in feline renal allotransplant recipients with normal renal function. *Can J Vet Res* **45**(10): 831–837.

Halling, K.B., J.P. Graham, et al. (2003). Sonographic and scintigraphic evaluation of acute renal allograft rejection in cats. *Vet Radiol Ultrasound* **44**(6): 707–713.

Halloran, P., T. Mathew, et al. (1997). Mycophenolate mofetil in renal allograft recipients: a pooled efficacy analysis of three randomized, double-blind, clinical studies in prevention of rejection. The international mycophenolate mofetil renal transplant study groups. *Transplantation* **63**(1): 39–47.

Hardie, R.J., C. Schmiedt, et al. (2005). Ureteral papilla implantation as a technique for neoureterocystostomy in cats. *Vet Surg* **34**(4): 393–398.

Hausberg, M., M. Kosch, et al. (2002). Sympathetic nerve activity in end-stage renal disease. *Circulation* **106**(15): 1974–1979.

Hou, S. (2000). Expanding the kidney donor pool: ethical and medical considerations. *Kidney Int* **58**(4): 1820–1836.

Isoniemi, H.M., J. Ahonen, et al. (1993). Long-term consequences of different immunosuppressive regimens for renal allografts. *Transplantation* **55**(3): 494–499.

Kadar, E., J.E. Sykes, et al. (2005). Evaluation of the prevalence of infections in cats after renal transplantation: 169 cases (1987–2003). *J Am Vet Med Assoc* **227**(6): 948–953.

Kahan, B.D., P.R. Rajagopalan, et al. (1999). Reduction of the occurrence of acute cellular rejection among renal allograft recipients treated with basiliximab, a chimeric anti-interleukin-2-receptor monoclonal antibody. United states simulect renal study group. *Transplantation* **67**(2): 276–284.

Kaplan, H.S. (1980). Hodgkin's disease: unfolding concepts concerning its nature, management and prognosis. *Cancer* **45**(10): 2439–2474.

Katz, S.M., R.H. Kerman, et al. (1991). Preemptive transplantation—an analysis of benefits and hazards in 85 cases. *Transplantation* **51**(2): 351–355.

Kelly, G.E., J.M. Drummond, et al. (1971). Intussusception in dogs following renal homograft transplantation. *Aust Vet J* **47**(12): 597–600.

Klinger, M., J. Cooper, et al. (1990). The use of butorphanol tartrate for the prevention of canine intussusception following renal transplantation. *J Invest Surg* **3**(3): 229–233.

Kochin, E.J., C.R. Gregory, et al. (1993). Evaluation of a method of ureteroneocystostomy in cats. *J Am Vet Med Assoc* **202**(2): 257–260.

Kreis, H., N. Chkoff, et al. (1984). Nonsteroid antiinflammatory agents as a substitute treatment for steroids in ATGAM-treated cadaver kidney recipients. *Transplantation* **37**(2): 139–145.

Kulkarni, S., A. Kopelan, et al. (2001). Tacrolimus therapy in renal transplantation. In: *Kidney Transplantation: Principles and Practice*, edited by P.J. Morris, 5th edition. Philadelphia, PA: WB Saunders, pp. 251–262.

Kyles, A.E., C.R. Gregory, et al. (2001). Leflunomide analog, MNA-715, plus cyclosporine reduces renal allograft rejection in mismatched dogs. *Transplant Proc* **33**(1–2): 368–369.

Kyles, A.E., C.R. Gregory, et al. (2003a). Modified noble plication for the prevention of intestinal intussusception after renal transplantation in dogs. *J Invest Surg* **16**(3): 161–166.

Kyles, A.E., C.R. Gregory, et al. (2003b). Immunosuppression with a combination of the leflunomide analog, FK778, and microemulsified cyclosporine for renal transplantation in mongrel dogs. *Transplantation* **75**(8): 1128–1133.

Kyles, A.E., C.R. Gregory, et al. (2002). An evaluation of combined immunosuppression with MNA 715 and microemulsified cyclosporine on renal allograft rejection in mismatched mongrel dogs. *Vet Surg* **31**(4): 358–366.

Kyles, A.E., C.R. Gregory, et al. (1999). Management of hypertension controls postoperative neurologic disorders after renal transplantation in cats. *Vet Surg* **28**(6): 436–441.

Libro, V. and M. Proto (1964). Observations on some cases of intestinal invagination in dogs operated for homoplastic transplant of the kidneys. *Osp Maggiore* **59**: 809–815.

Matas, A.J. (2009). Minimization of steroids in kidney transplantation. *Transpl Int***22**: 38–48.

Mathew, T.H. (2001). Mycofenolate mofetil. In: *Kidney Transplantation: Principles and Practice*, edited by P.J. Morris, 5th edition. Philadelphia, PA: WB Saunders, pp. 263–278.

Mathews, K.A., G.J. Gallivan, et al. (1993). Clinical, biochemical, and hematologic evaluation of normal dogs after administration of rabbit anti-dog thymocyte serum. *Vet Surg* **22**(3): 213–220.

Mathews, K.A., D.L. Holmberg, et al. (1994). Renal allograft survival in outbred mongrel dogs using rabbit anti-dog thymocyte serum in combination with immunosuppressive drug therapy with or without donor bone marrow. *Vet Surg* **23**(5): 347–357.

Mathews, K.A., D.L. Holmberg, et al. (2000). Kidney transplantation in dogs with naturally occurring end-stage renal disease. *J Am Anim Hosp Assoc* **36**(4): 294–301.

Mathews, K.G. and C.R. Gregory (1997). Renal transplants in cats: 66 cases (1987–1996). *J Am Vet Med Assoc* **211**(11): 1432–1436.

McAnulty, J.F. and G.L. Lensmeyer (1999). The effects of ketoconazole on the pharmacokinetics of cyclosporine A in cats. *Vet Surg* **28**(6): 448–455.

McAnulty, J.F. (1998). Hypothermic storage of feline kidneys for transplantation: successful ex vivo storage up to 7 hours. *Vet Surg* **27**(4): 312–320.

McAnulty, J.F. and G.L. Lensmeyer (1999). The effects of ketoconazole on the pharmacokinetics of cyclosporine A in cats. *Vet Surg* **28**(6): 448–455.

McAnulty, J.F., J.H. Southard, et al. (1989). Prevention of postoperative intestinal intussusception by prophylactic morphine administration in dogs used for organ transplantation research. *Surgery* **105**(4): 494–495.

Mehl, M.L., A.E. Kyles, et al. (2005). Comparison of 3 techniques for ureteroneocystostomy in cats. *Vet Surg* **34**(2): 114–119.

Morris, P.J. (2001). Azathioprine and steroids. In: *Kidney Transplantation: Principles and Practice*, edited by P.J. Morris, 5th edition. Philadelphia, PA: WB Saunders, pp. 217–226.

Narkun-Burgess, D.M., C.R. Nolan, et al. (1993). Forty-five year follow-up after uninephrectomy. *Kidney Int* **43**(5): 1110–1115.

Newell, S.M., G.W. Ellison, et al. (1999). Scintigraphic, sonographic, and histologic evaluation of renal autotransplantation in cats. *Am J Vet Res* **60**(6): 775–779.

Nordquist, B.C. and L.R. Aronson (2008). Pyogranulomatous cystitis associated with toxoplasma gondii infection in a cat after renal transplantation. *J Am Vet Med Assoc* **232**(7): 1010–1012.

Obrador, G.T. and B.J. Pereira (1998). Early referral to the nephrologist and timely initiation of renal replacement therapy: a paradigm shift in the management of patients with chronic renal failure. *Am J Kidney Dis* **31**(3): 398–417.

Paliogianni, F. and D.T. Boumpas (1995). Glucocorticoids regulate calcineurin-dependent trans-activating pathways for interleukin-2 gene transcription in human T lymphocytes. *Transplantation* **59**(9): 1333–1339.

Pollard, S., B. Nashan, et al. and CONSENT: Consensus on Substitution in European Transplantation. (2003). A pharmacokinetic and clinical review of the potential clinical impact of using different formulations of cyclosporin A. *Clin Ther* **25**(6): 1654–1669.

Raine, A.E., R. Margreiter, et al. (1992). Report on management of renal failure in europe, XXII, 1991. *Nephrol Dial Transplant* **7**(Suppl. 2): 7–35.

Rajab, A., R.P. Pelletier, et al. (2006). Excellent clinical outcomes in primary kidney transplant recipients treated with steroid-free maintenance immunosuppression. *Clin Transplant* **20**(5): 537–546.

Ray, A. and P.B. Sehgal (1992). Cytokines and their receptors: molecular mechanism of interleukin-6 gene repression by glucocorticoids. *J Am Soc Nephrol* **2**(12 Suppl): S214–S221.

Sandusky, G.E., P.J. Horton, et al. (1986). Use of monoclonal antibodies to human lymphocytes to identify lymphocyte subsets in lymph nodes of the rhesus monkey and the dog. *J Med Primatol* **15**(6): 441–451.

Shun-Shin, G.A., P. Ratcliffe, et al. (1990). The lens after renal transplantation. *Br J Ophthalmol* **74**(5): 267–271.

Singh, P.B., N.K. Goyal, et al. (2008). Renal transplantation using live donors with vascular anomalies: a salvageable surgical challenge. *Saudi J Kidney Dis Transpl* **19**(4): 554–558.

Slakey, D.P., C.P. Johnson, et al. (1997). Management of severe pancreatitis in renal transplant recipients. *Ann Surg* **225**(2): 217–222.

Smak Gregoor, P.J., T. van Gelder, et al. (2000). Mycophenolate mofetil, cellcept, a new immunosuppressive drug with great potential in internal medicine. *Neth J Med* **57**(6): 233–246.

Starzl, T.E., T.L. Marchioro, et al. (1967). The clinical use of antilymphocyte globulin in renal homotransplantation. *Transplantation* **5**(4):Suppl: 1100–1105.

Strober, S., S. Slavin, et al. (1979). Allograft tolerance after total lymphoid irradiation (TLI). *Immunol Rev* **46**: 87–112.

Thistlethwaite, J.R. Jr., J.K. Stuart, et al. (1988). Complications and monitoring of OKT3 therapy. *Am J Kidney Dis* **11**(2): 112–119.

Tizard, I.R. (2004). *Veterinary Immunology: An Introduction*, 7th edition. Philadelphia, PA: WB Saunders.

Ullman, E. (2002). Experimental kidney transplantation. 1902. *Wiener Klinische Wochenschrift* **114**(4): 126–127.

Valverde, C.R., C.R. Gregory, et al. (2002). Anesthetic management in feline renal transplantation. *Vet Anaesth Analg* **29**(3): 117–125.

Waer, M. (2001). Total lymphoid irradiation. In: *Kidney Transplantation: Principles and Practice*, edited by P.J. Morris, 5th edition. Philadelphia, PA: WB Saunders, pp. 320–325.

Waer, M., K.K. Ang, et al. (1984). Influence of radiation field and fractionation schedule of total lymphoid irradiation (TLI) on the induction of suppressor cells and stable chimerism after bone marrow transplantation in mice. *J Immunol* **132**(2): 985–990.

Wagner, J.L., R.C. Burnett, et al. (1999). Organization of the canine major histocompatibility complex: current perspectives. *J Hered* **90**(1): 35–38.

Wagner, K., M. Henkel, et al. (1988). Interaction of calcium blockers and cyclosporine. *Transplant Proc* **20**(2 Suppl. 2): 561–568.

Welsh, K.I. and M. Bunce (2001). HLA typing, matching and crossmatching in renal transplantation. In: *Kidney Transplantation: Principles and Practice*, edited by P.J. Morris, 5th edition. Philadelphia, PA: WB Saunders, pp. 135–157.

Winkler, C., A. Schultz, et al. (1989). Genetic characterization of FLA, the cat major histocompatibility complex. *Proc Natl Acad Sci USA* **86**(3): 943–947.

Wong, G. and J.R. Chapman (2008). Cancers after renal transplantation. *Transplant Rev* **22**(2): 141–149.

Wooldridge, J.D. and C.R. Gregory (1999). Ionized and total serum magnesium concentrations in feline renal transplant recipients. *Vet Surg* **28**(1): 31–37.

Wooldridge, J.D., C.R. Gregory, et al. (2002). The prevalence of malignant neoplasia in feline renal-transplant recipients. *Vet Surg* **31**(1): 94–97.

Yuhki, N., G.F. Heidecker, et al. (1989). Characterization of MHC cDNA clones in the domestic cat: diversity and evolution of class I genes. *J Immunol* **142**(10): 3676–3682.

Zolty, R., P.J. Hynes, et al. (2008). Severe left ventricular systolic dysfunction may reverse with renal transplantation: uremic cardiomyopathy and cardiorenal syndrome. *Am J Transplant* **8**(11): 2219–2224.

32

Indwelling urinary catheters and stents

Allyson Berent

Urinary catheters and stents can be used for various purposes to divert urine throughout the entire urinary collection system. Catheters are defined as flexible or rigid hollow tubes employed to drain fluids from body cavities. Most "catheters" in the urinary system are used for temporary drainage of the renal pelvis, ureter, or urinary bladder. Urinary catheters are classically soft, comfortable, polyurethane type tubes that have an open lumen, permitting temporary drainage. Stents are defined as small tubes, often expandable, inserted across a blocked lumen to restore patency. Urinary "stents" are typically used for permanent or long-term diversion in the kidney, ureter, bladder, or urethra. Stents are most often completely indwelling tubes that can be placed for various purposes, most commonly to bypass a malignant obstruction, stricture, or embedded stone (i.e., ureterolithiasis). Stents come in different materials (metal, polyurethrane, plastic, rubber, etc.), shapes, and sizes (Weisse, 2009). This chapter will discuss various types of catheters and stents that are currently being used in the urinary tract of veterinary patients for various purposes. An anatomic organization will be used to discuss different applications in the kidney, ureter, bladder, and urethra.

Kidney

The most common reason for stent or catheter placement in the kidney is for drainage of the renal pelvis due to hydronephrosis. This is called a *nephrostomy tube*. Ureteral obstructions secondary to ureterolithiasis, malignancy, strictures, or trauma can result in severe hydronephrosis and/or life-threatening azotemia, par-

ticularly when presenting bilaterally or in animals with concurrent preexisting renal insufficiency/failure. Some patients can be managed medically with supportive care until a ureterolith passes, others may require surgery to avoid permanent damage and/or hemodialysis for stabilization prior to a prolonged anesthesia for ureteral surgery. Ureterotomies can be relatively prolonged and complicated surgeries in these debilitated patients with an unclear outcome of residual renal function (Kyles 2005, 2005; Snyder 2005). One possibility is to place a nephrostomy tube percutaneously (via a modified Seldinger Technique) to quickly relieve the obstruction, minimize morbidity, and determine whether adequate renal function remains prior to a prolonged anesthesia for ureteral surgery or a ureteral stent placement. Hydronephrosis is most commonly due to ureteral obstructions from either ureterolithiasis, trigonal neoplasia obstructing the ureterovesicular junction (UVJ), ureteral strictures, accidental ureteral ligation, ureteral trauma, ureteral edema after ureteral surgery, pyelonephritis, etc. Nephrostomy tubes are also helpful postintervention while a surgical site is healing (postureterotomy) or in a patient awaiting future intervention that is not possible at the time of the initial presentation (i.e., ureteral resection anastomosis, ureteral stent placement, or renal transplantation). These tubes allow the clinician to follow ureteral patency serially with contrast pyeloureterography and are relatively well tolerated by patients. Nephrostomy tubes can be placed either percutaneously using ultrasound and/or fluoroscopic guidance, or surgically. The ideal catheter for this procedure is a locking-loop pigtail catheter (Figure 32.1). Foley urinary catheters and red rubber catheters have also been used historically, but have a tendency to back out after placement with an absent locking mechanism. In humans, nephrostomy tubes are commonly placed for temporary urinary diversion for hydronephrosis

Nephrology and Urology of Small Animals. Edited by Joe Bartges and David J. Polzin. © 2011 Blackwell Publishing Ltd.

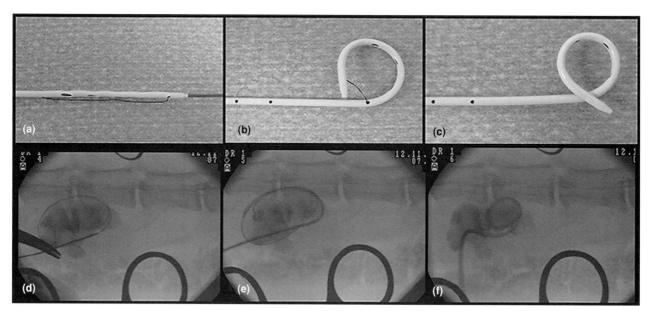

Figure 32.1 Placement of a percutaneous nephrostomy tube using a locking loop pigtail catheter in a cat. (a) 6 Fr locking loop pigtail catheter straightened over a 0.035-inch guidewire. Notice the loose string connecting the distal hole to the most proximal hole. (b) Once the stylette and trocar are removed from the catheter, the pigtail loop can form as the string is tightened. (c) The pigtail is locked in place by the string being completely taught. (d) Fluoroscopy image of an 18-guage needle in the renal pelvis after contrast was infused for a pyelogram. A 0.018-inch guidewire was advanced through the needle and coiled inside the renal pelvis. (e) The needle is removed over the wire and the locking loop pigtail catheter is being advanced over the guidewire so that a coil is made inside the renal pelvis. (f) Once the string is pulled, the loop is tightly formed in the renal pelvis to prevent inadvertent removal.

secondary to severe pyelonephritis, ureterolithiasis, or urinary malignancies. These tubes can be easily left in place in humans without the concern of tube contamination, accidental removal, or excessive tube maintenance. This is a little different in our veterinary patients, making complete indwelling tubes more desirable (see Ureteral stenting).

Percutaneous nephrostomy tube placement

This is usually suggested for renal pelvis dilation greater than 1 cm in diameter so that the locking loop can easily form in the pelvis and prevent the tube from backing out. Ultrasound is best used to perform a pyelocentesis using an over-the-needle venous catheter to aid in a modified Seldinger technique for serial wire and catheter exchanges (Figure 32.1d; dog—18 guage, cat—22 guage). Once the tip of the catheter is in the renal pelvis, about 3 mL of urine is drained (pyelocentesis) and an equal amount of contrast (Iohexol[1]) material is infused into the renal pelvis (pyelogram). This allows the renal pelvis to be seen clearly with fluoroscopy. Then the stylette is gently removed from the catheter and an angle tipped hydrophilic guidewire (Figure 32.1e Weasel wire[2]—for dog, 0.035-inch wire fits through the 18 gauge catheter; for cat, the 0.018-inch wire fits through the 22 gauge catheter) is advanced through the over-the-needle

catheter and monitored with fluoroscopy to document it coiling in the dilated renal pelvis. We aim to get 2–3 loops in the pelvis if possible to be sure the stiff shaft of the guidewire is inside the kidney. Then the catheter is removed over the wire and a locking loop pigtail catheter (5 Fr[3] or 6 Fr[4]) is advanced, over the appropriate sized wire (6 Fr over 0.035-inch; 5 Fr over 0.018-inch wire), through the renal parenchyma and into the renal pelvis (Figure 32.1f). For this process, the stylette is initially left in place to keep the catheter rigid during renal penetration, but the trocar is removed so it can be advanced easily over the guidewire. Once the tip of the catheter is in the renal pelvis, as seen via fluoroscopy (Figure 32.1d,e), the stylette is gently removed as the catheter is simultaneously advanced over the guidewire to form its loop (Figure 32.1e,f). Once the loop of the pigtail is completely within the renal pelvis, the loop of the catheter is locked in place by pulling on the string, as seen in Figure 32.1b,c,f. The catheter is then secured to the body wall using a purse-string and Chinese-finger-trap suture pattern, and a urine collection system is attached to the catheter for gravity drainage (Figure 32.5b).

Surgical nephrostomy tube placement

This technique described above can also be performed surgically by an approach to the greater curvature of the kidney. Ideally, this is done with fluoroscopy as well, but can be done with digital palpation. As described above, an over-the-needle catheter can be directed through the greater curvature of the kidney into the renal pelvis using the modified Seldinger technique. Once urine is visualized to drain, the guidewire can be advanced and curled into the kidney and the catheter can be removed over the wire. Next, the locking loop catheter can be advanced over the wire as described above. Another approach is via digital palpation without fluoroscopy or ultrasound. The locking loop catheter, with the trocar left in place through the stylette, can be directly advanced through the body wall, punctured through the greater curvature of the kidney, and into the renal pelvis. Then the trocar is removed and urine is drained through the stylette to assure proper location. The loop is then advanced over the stylette and into the pelvis, and the loop is locked into place. Then the kidney should be secured to the body wall with a purse string around the tube at its insertion site and secured to the skin as described above. Other tubes that can be

used in a similar manner is a 5 or 8 Fr Foley catheter or red rubber catheter in a similar manner, though these do not have a locking mechanism and have a tendency to back out after placement. The safest way to place these tubes is over a guidewire as described above, which would require the very tip of the catheter to be carefully cut to have an open-ended catheter to advance over the wire.

For catheters placed percutaneously, a seal must form to the body wall, and this can take 2–4 weeks. If the patient is taken to surgery or the obstruction is relieved by other interventional techniques before a seal is formed (i.e., ureteral stenting, shockwave lithotripsy, etc), the tube can either be removed with the site surgically repaired or the tube can be capped and wrapped so the pet can go home without the need for gravitational drainage, and the tube can be left in place for 2–4 weeks prior to being removed (Figure 32.2). Removal of the nephrostomy tube is recommended to be done under fluoroscopic guidance. A sterile hypdrophilic guidewire is advanced down the

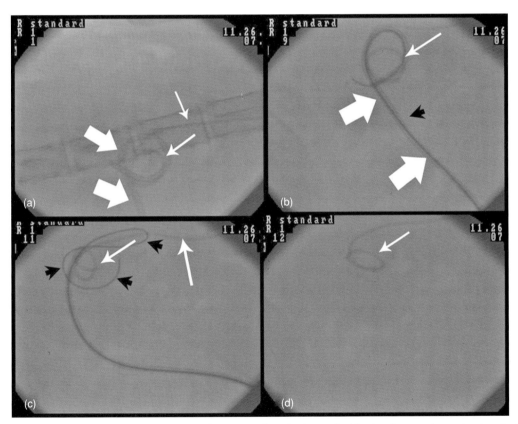

Figure 32.2 Removal of a locking loop nephrostomy tube in a cat that also has a double pigtail ureteral stent in place (red arrows). (a) The locking loop pigtail catheter (6 Fr) is locked in place in the renal pelvis (large white arrows). (b) A guidewire (0.035-inch black arrow) is advanced through the pigtail catheter (large white arrows) and the string is cut proximally to release the locking mechanism. (c) The guidewire (back arrows) is advanced into the renal pelvis to straighten out the locking loop pigtail. Care is taken to not manipulate the indwelling ureteral stent (small white arrows). (d) The nephrostomy tube is retracted over the guidewire until it is completely exteriorized and the double pigtail ureteral stent (small white arrow) remains in place with one loop in the renal pelvis and the shaft going down the ureter.

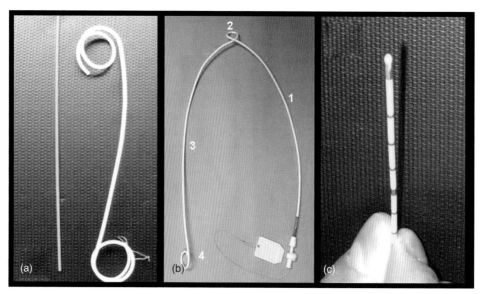

Figure 32.3 Three different types of ureteral stents/catheters. All are made of polyurethrane material. (a) A 3 Fr variable length (8–12 cm) double pigtail ureteral stent that remains indwelling. The proximal loop remains in the renal pelvis and the distal loop in the urinary bladder. The tubing (asterisk) is a pushing catheter that is used to push the ureteral stent over the guidewire when it is straightened out endoscopically so that it can remain indwelling. (b) An 8 Fr nephroureteral stent. This stent (1) exits the body wall from the nephrostomy side and transverses the renal parenchyma until it reaches the renal pelvis at the proximal loop (2). The shaft of the stent sits in the ureter (3) and the distal loop (4) remains in the urinary bladder for complete collection system drainage. (c) This catheter is an open-ended ureteral catheter (5 Fr). It has 1 cm marks along its entire length for endoscopic size guidance. This is classically used for retrograde ureteropyelography done endoscopically.

tube and curled into the renal pelvis. The string is cut and loosened. The tube is then withdrawn over the wire with gentle traction until it is out of the animal's body, and the wire is subsequently removed. The site can be wrapped for a few hours thereafter. A seal should form over the opening in a few hours, and the wrap can be removed.

Ureter

Ureteral stenting has been performed for a variety of disorders in both dogs and cats. The goal of ureteral stenting is four fold: (1) to divert urine from the renal pelvis into the urinary bladder to bypass a ureteral obstruction, (2) to encourage passive ureteral dilation (for ureteral stenosis/strictures or future ureteroscopy), (3) to decrease surgical tension on the ureter after/during surgery (i.e., resection and anastomosis) and prevent post-operative leakage and edema, or (4) to aid in extracorporeal shockwave lithotripsy for large obstructive ureteroliths or nephroliths that could result in serial ureteral obstructions if the stones do not completely pass down the ureter, a term called Steinstrasse (Al-Awadi 1999). There are three main types of ureteral stents/catheters: (1) an indwelling double pigtail ureteral stent,[5] which is the most common type used in veterinary and human

medicine, (2) a nephroureteral stent,[6] and (3) an open-ended ureteral catheter[7] (Figure 32.3). The double pigtail stent is completely intracorporeal and can remain in place for numerous months if necessary (recommended for <3–6 months but has been left in place for over 2 years without a problem in some cats).

The first report of ureteral stent placement was in 1967 in a human for malignant obstruction (Zimskind 1967). Since that time, nonresectable trigonal or ureteral tumors are treated similarly, with an indwelling double pigtail ureteral stent used to bypass the obstruction. These tumors have been shown to be more easily accessed though a antegrade percutaneous approach, in order to gain access down the ureter, which is exactly what we have appreciated in veterinary patients. In humans, there is a 96–98% success in stent placement with this antegrade approach (Uthappa 2005; Yossepowitch 2001). It was not until 1977 that a report of ureteral stenting for benign disease was published, and this was for a ureteral stricture (Goldin 1977). Then, in 2005, a report in pediatics came out showing the use of ureteral stenting for passive ureteral dilation prior to ureteroscopy for ureterolithiasis (Hubert 2005). Very few reports in dogs exist, one study done in dogs, as a model for human disease, was performed in 1997 and showed that canine ureters did have associated passive ureteral dilation after a stent was in place (Lennon 1997), but there have been few veterinary studies (Berent et al. 2007) or clinical cases reported in either dogs or cats with ureteral stenting to this point. At the author's institution, over 25 dog or cat ureters have been stented for various clinical purposes.

Ureteral stents are classically used to bypass obstructions from ureterolithiasis, malignant obstructive neoplasia, trauma, and ureteral stenosis/strictures. After interventional procedures (ureteroscopy, ureteral balloon dilation, retrograde ureteral lithotripsy, or percutaneous nephroureterolithotomy-PCNL), a ureteral stent can be placed to prevent temporary obstructions from ureteral edema or spasm. Following surgical ureterotomy, ureteral resection and anastomosis, or ureteral tears, a ureteral stent may allow for tension relief and healing, prevent postoperative ureteral leaking, and prevent ureteral stricture formation while the surgical site heals. Ureteral stenting is also ideal in patients with large (>5 mm) nephroliths or ureteroliths that are undergoing extracorporeal shockwave lithotripsy (ESWL) to aid in ureteral stone localization and stone fragment passage following the ESWL treatment (Block 1996; Lennon 1997; Adams 1999; Mustafa 2007). Ureteral stenting has been shown to allow passive ureteral dilation in children over 2–4 weeks to permit the passage of a ureteroscope or spontaneous stone passage of obstructive ureteroliths (Lennon 2005). This theory is still under investigation

in our veterinary patients, but initial experience would support a similar finding.

Ureteral stents are most often placed cystoscopically in a retrograde manner through the ureteral orifice at the UVJ. They can also be placed antegrade, through the renal pelvis percutaneously or surgically during a cystotomy or ureterotomy. Under general anesthesia, the *retrograde technique* uses cystoscopy and concurrent fluoroscopy. An angle-tipped hydrophilic guidewire is advanced into the distal ureter from the UVJ. The wire is advanced up the length of the ureter and curled into the renal pelvis. Care is taken to bypass the obstruction carefully without perforating the ureter (Figure 32.4). An open-ended ureteral catheter[6] (Figures 32.3c and 32.4b) is then advanced over the wire under fluoroscopic guidance, and the guidewire is removed. A retrograde contrast ureteropeylogram is performed to help identify any lesions, stones, or filling defects in the ureter or renal pelvis (Figure 32.4c). The wire is re-advanced through the catheter into the renal pelvis and the catheter is withdrawn. An indwelling double pigtail ureteral stent,[4] is placed over the guidewire under fluoroscopic guidance with one curl remaining in the renal pelvis in front of the obstruction and the other in the urinary bladder (Figure 32.4d). The *antegrade technique* requires percutaneous renal access with a renal access needle[8] or over-the-needle catheter, as described above. This can be done with either

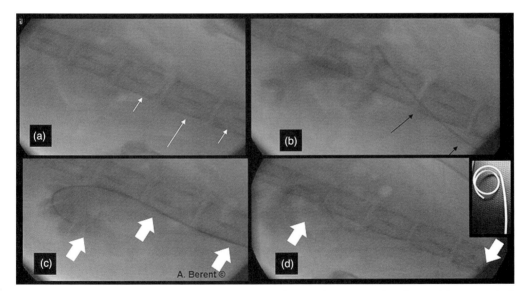

Figure 32.4 Fluoroscopic images of a placement of a double pigtail ureteral stent in a female cat. (a) A 0.018-inch angle tipped hydrophilic guidewire (small white arrows) is advanced up the right ureter to the level of the obstruction under endoscopic and fluoroscopic guidance. (b) A 3 Fr open-ended ureteral catheter (black arrows) is advanced over the guidewire, and the wire is removed for a retrograde ureteropyelogram to be performed using contrast material. This helps document the obstructed area of the ureter and guide the catheter and stent into the renal pelvis. (c) The guidewire is re-advanced into the renal pelvis to create a curl and the stent (large white arrow) is pushed over the guidewire so the proximal end forms a pigtail inside the pelvis. (d) The wire is then removed and the pigtail forms in the proximal end inside the renal pelvis (large white arrow) and the distal end inside the urinary bladder. The picture is the upper right corner of (d) is one of the loops of the double pigtail ureteral stent prior to placement.

ultrasound or fluoroscopy. The guidewire is passed down the ureter, into the urinary bladder, and out the urethra to have through-and-through access ("flossed"). This is the typical approach for a trigonal-induced malignant ureteral obstruction when the ureteral orifice cannot be identified cystoscopically or for small male dogs and male cats where cystoscopy for retrograde ureteral access is not possible. The stent is then placed in a retrograde fashion over the wire, as described above to keep the hole in the kidney as small as possible. These procedures can also be done intraoperatively when surgical success is in question, leakage is a concern, or obstructive neoplasia is found. Indwelling drainage is an ideal, long-term, and safe option.

The nephroureteral (NU) stent[5] is classically used for a combination of maintaining a tract into the renal pelvis, down the ureter, and into the bladder after percutaneous nephrolithotomy (PCNL) procedures. This stent is partially indwelling and partially external. It protects the ureter after lithotripsy from a PCNL, allowing any ureteral edema to subside and residual stone fragments to pass (Figure 32.5). In order for a seal to form from the kidney to the body wall after a larger sheath was placed in the renal pelvis, the catheter must exit the body wall from the renal pelvis and maintain a tight seal. The catheter forms a loop in the renal pelvis with multiple fenestrations for drainage and then passes down the ureter and

into the urinary bladder. This maintains a draining tract from the renal pelvis to the bladder, bypassing the ureter temporarily, as well as allowing a seal to form to the body wall from the kidney. It usually remains in place for 2–4 weeks after PCNL.

Retrograde ureterpyelography allows for the infusion of contrast in a retrograde manner up the ureter, under fluoroscopic guidance, in order to image ureteral patency, space occupying lesions, stone disease, tortuosities of the ureter, and ureter diameter/length for stent placement (Figure 32.4c). This is seemingly more accurate than intravenous pyelography (IVP) since ureteral distension is not possible without mild pressure irrigation in the ureter. This procedure is also less invasive than antegrade pyelography, eliminating the need for renal needle access and the risk of subsequent urinary leakage through the renal parenchyma if a ureteral obstructive lesion persists. As described above, the guidewire is advanced up the ureteral orifice via cystoscopic and fluoroscopic guidance, and an open-ended ureteral catheter (Figure 32.3c) is advanced over the wire and the wire is subsequently removed. Then contrast is injected through the catheter for ureteral visualization. This allows subtle lesions and filling defects to be evaluated with repetition if needed without extravasation of contrast into the retroperitoneal space (i.e., antegrade pyeloureterography) and under mild to moderate pressure allowing

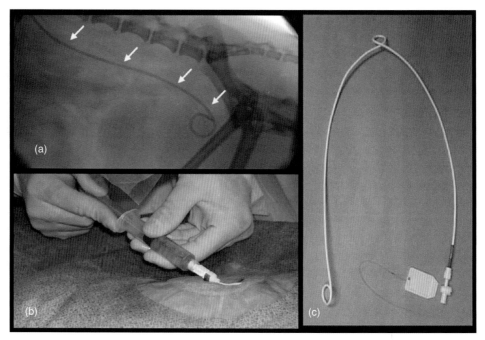

Figure 32.5 A nephroureteral stent in a 3.6 kg female spayed Yorkshire terrier placed after a percutaneous nephrolithotomy (PCNL) procedure. (a) Fluoroscopic image of the catheter down the ureter (white arrows) and the pigtail is curled in the urinary bladder. (b) The external drainage of the catheter from the body wall, through the skin, and into the renal pelvis with urine being drained out of the catheter. (c) The nephroureteral stent (see Figure 32.3b).

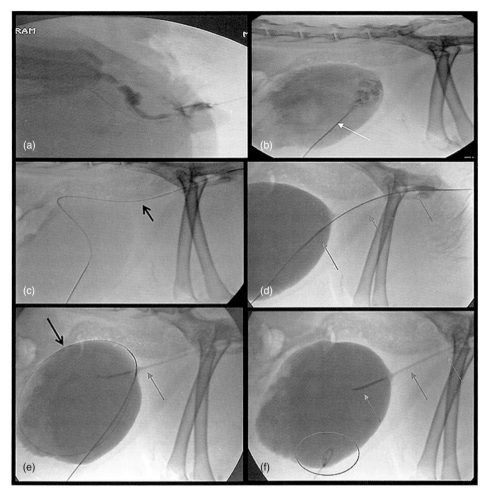

Figure 32.6 A male neutered cat with a urethral tear that occurred during catheterization. (a) Contrast urethrogram from the distal end of the penis showing extravasation of contrast into the subcutaneous space around the urethra at the level of the tear. (b) An 18 guage over-the-needle catheter is used to perform a cystocentesis (small white arrow), and contrast is injected through the needle to highlight the bladder during fluoroscopy. (c) A guidewire (0.035-inch) (black arrow) is aimed through the catheter, into the bladder, and out through the urethra in an antegrade manner gaining through-and-through access. (d) An open-ended urethral catheter (5 Fr red rubber catheter) is advanced over the guidewire through the urethral lumen (grey arrows) into the urinary bladder and sutured in place at the prepuce. (e) The guidewire (black arrow) is then removed from the urethral catheter (grey arrow) and curled into the bladder and a locking loop pigtail catheter is advanced over the guidewire through the body wall for the placement of a percutaneous cystostomy tube. (f) The wire is removed and the lock is formed (grey oval) on the locking loop pigtail catheter to secure it inside the bladder for a percutaneous cystostomy tube.

ureteral distension. It also prevents any risk of contrast-induced nephropathy, since the contrast agent remains in the renal collection system and is not injected intravascularly.

Bladder

Cystostomy tubes are often placed to bypass a urethral obstruction or "buy time" while a urethral/trigonal lesion is healing. This can be secondary to malignant neoplasia (trigonal, urethral, prostatic tumors), proliferative/granulomatous urethritis, urethral strictures, urethral tears, or urethral stones that are difficult to remove

surgically. With the advent of urethral stents (see below), the use of cystostomy tubes has declined. Cystostomy tubes can either be placed percutaneously or surgically. With the locking loop pigtail catheter (Figure 32.1), percutaneous cystostomy tube placement has become a relatively fast and easy technique when necessary (Figure 32.6). As described above for nephrostomy tubes, an 18-guage over-the-needle catheter is advanced into the urinary bladder like a cystocentesis (paramedian), until urine is draining. The stylette is removed and the hydrophilic guidewire is advanced though the catheter and into the urinary bladder. The wire is curled around the bladder 2–3 times. This can also be done under fluoroscopic guidance, but this is not always necessary. Then the locking loop catheter is advanced over the wire with the stylette still in place (and the trocar removed). Once the entire loop of the catheter is well within the urinary bladder, the stylette is removed and the loop is locked. The bladder can then be easily drained and the catheter is secured tightly to the body wall as described above. This tube would need to remain in place, since it is not surgically pexied, for at least 2–4 weeks prior to removal. Other tubes, such as latex mushroom-tipped catheters, Foley catheters, or Low Profile tubes, can be placed with either an open or laparoscopic-assisted surgical technique (Smith 1995; Stiffler 2003). This allows for a cystopexy to be performed at the same time. These tubes should remain in place for approximately 2 weeks after placement. Cystostomy tubes are commonly associated with secondary infections (at least 86% in one study) due to the external nature of the tube and complications with the tubes have been reported in as high as 49% of patients, involving inadvertent tube removal, eating of the tube by the patients, fistulous tract formation, and mushroom-tip breakage during removal (Beck 2007). This is not ideal in circumstances where chemotherapy (for malignant obstructions) or immunosuppressive therapy (for immune-mediated disease-proliferative urethritis) is being used.

Urethra

Urethral catheterization is typically a fairly simple and routinely performed procedure in veterinary patients primarily used to monitor urine output, establish urine drainage in patients that are recumbent, have mechanical/functional urethral obstructions, urethral tears, or to provide urethral patency following urethral or urinary bladder surgery. The most common urethral catheters used are either Foley catheters that have a balloon tip to prevent the catheter from backing out into the urethra or a red rubber catheter that is more rigid, but do not have a safety mechanism for inadvertent removal like a Foley. In male dogs, catheters are easily advanced in a retrograde manner, up the penile urethra and into the urinary bladder. All catheters in the urinary system should be placed with sterile technique. In female dogs and cats, this is a little more difficult, requiring digital palpation of the urethral papilla for catheter advancement, and sometimes the use of a speculum or cystoscope/vaginoscope to aid papilla cannulization. There are various types of catheters developed for male cats, and it is most important to use an atraumatic type of catheter. Rigid catheters, like a TomCat, can result in urethral tears and are not recommended by the author. More hydrophilic soft catheters, like a Slippery Sam, or small 3.5 or 5 Fr frozen red rubber catheters are stiff enough, but also less traumatic. Urethral tears are most commonly seen in male cats and occurs most often while trying to unblock the patient or from vehicular trauma. The management of urethral trauma has recently been reported by the use of urethral catheterization alone (Meige 2008), and this is the author's recommended treatment of choice if the urethra can be cannulated with a catheter (see Antegrade catheterization).

Antegrade catheterization

For animals that are either very difficult or too small to easily catheterize (small female dogs, cats; or have a urethral tear or malignant obstruction), antegrade access can be attempted (Figure 32.6). Under general anesthesia or heavy sedation, this can be accomplished. The patient can be placed in lateral recumbency and an area in the caudal lateral abdomen just over the bladder should be clipped and aseptically prepared. A cystocentesis should be performed with an 18-gauge over-the-needle catheter directed toward the trigone of the bladder, as described for the cystostomy tube above. Then 5–15 mL of urine is drained from the bladder and replaced with an equal amount of contrast material. Once the stylette is removed, a hydrophilic guidewire is advanced into the bladder and aimed toward the bladder trigone under fluoroscopic guidance. This can then be aimed down the urethra and out of the body, gaining through-and-through access from the bladder, though the urethra, and out the urethral orifice. Once the wire is outside the urethra, a urinary catheter (open-ended; Foley, red rubber, Locking Loop catheter, etc.) is advanced over the wire in a retrograde manner, through the urethra and into the urinary bladder. This is ideal for male cats with urethral tears, because the tear is usually longitudinal and made in a retrograde manner. Longitudinal urethral tears will usually heal within 5–10 days without surgical intervention, and the catheter should be maintained for that length of time (Meige 2008).

Urethral stents

Urethral stents are most commonly used for the relief of malignant urothelial obstructions in the urethra. They have also been placed for benign diseases like proliferative/granulomatous urethritis, urethral strictures, and reflex dyssynergia, when standard medical intervention has failed or surgery is either declined or not indicated. Extraluminal urethral compressions secondary to neoplasia have also been successfully stented. Urethral stents are compressed metallic tubes that are typically of two types: self-expanding metallic stents (SEMS)[9] made of laser-cut nitinol metal and Balloon-Expanding Metallic

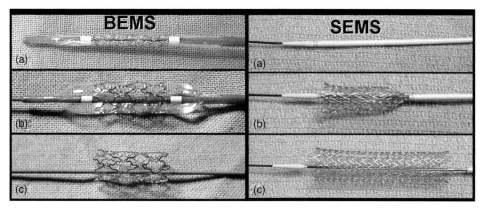

Figure 32.7 Metallic stents used for urethral obstructions. BEMS, balloon expandable metallic stent: (a) A BEMS is preloaded on a percutaneous transluminal angioplasty (PTA) balloon that is guided over a guidewire before it is deployed. (b) The PTA balloon is inflated using an insufflation device to the predetermined pressure, and the stent is then expanded to its predetermined diameter. (c) Once the PTA balloon is deflated and removed, the stent remains in place, over the guidewire in the desired location. SEMS, self-expanding metallic stent: (a) This stent is compressed onto a stylette and covered with a sheath to prevent premature deployment. It is advanced over a guidewire and situated in the desired location. The sheath is then deployed off the stylette and the stent opens up to its predetermined diameter and length. (c) Once the stent is fully deployed, the stylette is removed over the wire and the stent remains in place.

Stents (BEMS)[10] made of either stainless steel or nitinol metal (Figure 32.7). They are placed transurethrally under fluoroscopic guidance, in a minimally invasive manner, without necessitating surgical intervention. Malignant obstructions of the urethra can cause severe discomfort, dysuria, and life-threatening azotemia. Greater than 80% of animals with transitional cell carcinoma (TCC) of the urethra and/or prostatic carcinoma experience dysuria and approximately 10% developing complete urinary tract obstruction (Norris 1992; Knapp 2000). Chemotherapy and radiation therapy have been successful in slowing tumor growth but complete cure is uncommon. When signs of obstruction occur, more aggressive therapy is indicated. Placement of cystostomy tubes, transurethral resections, and surgical diversionary procedures have been described, but are invasive and potentially associated with an undesirable outcome due to manual urine drainage, associated morbidity, frequent urination, and infection (Norris 1992; Stiffler 2003; Liptak 2004). Placement of metallic stents using fluoroscopic guidance through a transurethral approach can be a fast, reliable, and safe method to establish urethral patency in both male and female dogs (and potentially cats) with an 85–90% good to excellent palliative outcome in over 60 canine cases currently performed at the author's institution (Weisse 2006).

A contrast cystourethrogram is performed and transurethral retrograde, or antegrade, guidewire access across the narrowing is obtained, as described above. Measurements of the normal urethral diameter and the length of obstruction are obtained (Figure 32.8) during a powerful cystourethrogram for maximal urethral distension. A marker catheter, which is typically placed in the colon to adjust for magnification, is used for determining the appropriate stent size. A SEMS is chosen (approximately 10–15% greater than the normal urethral diameter and 1 cm longer than the obstruction on both the cranial and caudal ends). The stent is deployed under fluoroscopic guidance and a repeat contrast cystourethrogram is performed to document restored urethral patency. Self-expanding metallic stents come in various sizes from 6–12 mm diameters and 40–80 mm lengths. Because of the longer size of these stents, which is needed for tumor coverage, a BEMS is more commonly used when stenting obstruction due to strictures or very narrow obstructions. The reason for this is that strictures are often very short in nature, and a BEMS is usually under 30 mm length (15–30 mm). They also come in variable diameters ranging from 3–10 mm. It is very important to only stent the length that is necessary in order to decrease the risk of urinary incontinence (5–10 mm beyond the visible obstruction).

Metallic stents remain in place once they are deployed and are very difficult to remove. It is rare for a tumor to grow through the interstices of the stent, but we have seen a rare number of cases where the tumor grew behind or in front of the stent and an additional stent was added.

There are many uses for various urinary catheters and stents in the urinary tract of dogs and cats, all of which can be placed in a minimally invasive fashion. Fluoroscopy is recommended for the placement of most stents, though surgical placement has been successful for ureteral stents and nephrostomy tubes without the benefit of fluoroscopy. There are some people who use ultrasound alone to place locking loop pigtail catheters in the renal pelvis

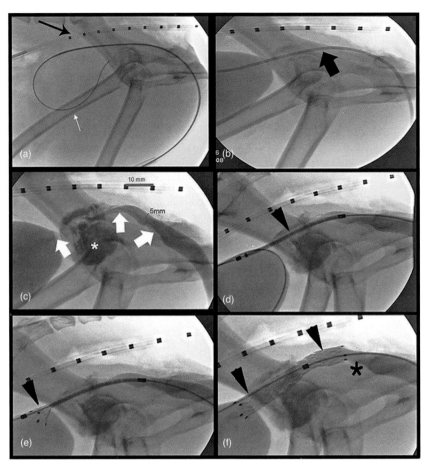

Figure 32.8 Urethral stent placement in an 8-year-old mixed breed dog with prostatic carcinoma and a urethral obstruction. (a) A marker catheter (small black arrow) is placed in the colon in order to adjust for magnification and measure the maximal urethral diameter and obstructive length for appropriate stent size selection. A guidewire (small white arrow) is advanced up the urethra and into the urinary bladder. (b) A catheter is advanced over the guidewire (large black arrow) and once the guidewire is removed, a cystourethrogram is performed. It is important that the bladder be maximally distended prior to the urethrogram to fully appreciate the location of the bladder trigone. (c) The urethral lumen is maximally distended behind the tumor and contrast is seen extravisating into the prostatic carcinoma (white asterisk). The urethral obstruction is appreciated by the very narrow lumen (large white arrows) in front of and behind the prostate. The marker catheter is used to get a maximal urethral diameter measurement (5 mm) and a stent size is chosen. It is ideal to oversize the diameter by 10–15%. (d) The SEMS (self-expanding metallic stent) is advanced over the guidewire into the urethra (black arrowhead) and the length of the stent is predetermined to cover approximately 5–10 mm cranial and caudal to the urethral obstruction. (e) The stent is initially deployed from the cranial aspect until the mesh is seeded into the urethra at the bladder trigone, and the remainder is then en-sheathed to cover the length of the obstruction. (f) The stent is fully deployed (black arrowheads). There is a small amount of nonobstructive tumor behind the caudal end of the stent appreciated by the filling defect (black asterisk). Since this area of the urethra is not obstructed and is fully patent, it was elected not to stent this region to decrease the risk of urinary incontinence.

and bladder, and if fluoroscopy is not available, this too can be considered. The introduction to advanced urinary catheters and stents in veterinary medicine in the past 5 years has truly given our patients alternatives they never had before. Avoiding invasive surgeries with excessive morbidity in animals with non-resectable malignant cancer for ureteral or urethral obstructions is the basis for how many of these techniques were first discovered in human medicine, and the same principles apply to our patients.

Endnotes

1. Iohexol, 240 mg/mL, Omnipaque, GE Healthcare Inc, Princeton, NJ
2. Weasel Wire (0.035-, 0.025-, 0.018-inch) hydrophilic angle-tipped guidewire, Infiniti Medical LLC, West Hollywood, CA.
3. Dawson-Meuller Drainage Catheter, 5 Fr., Cook Medical, Bloomington, IN.
4. Infiniti 6 Fr. Locking loop drainage catheter, Infiniti Medical LLC, West Hollywood, CA.
5. Vet Stent, Double pigtail Ureteral stent, Infiniti Medical LLC, West Hollywood, CA.

6. Nephroureteral catheter, Cook Medical, Bloomington, IN.
7. Open ended ureteral catheter, Cook Medical, Bloomington, IN.
8. Disposable Trocar Needle, 18 g × 15 cm, Cook Medical, Bloomington, IN.
9. Vet Stent-Urethra, Infiniti Medical, West Hollywood, CA.
10. Balloon Expandable Metallic Stent, Infiniti Medical, West Hollywood, CA.

References

Adams, L.G. (1999). Electrohydraulic and extracorporeal shock-wave lithotripsy. *Vet Clin North Am Small Anim Pract* **29**: 293–302.

Al-Awadi, K.A. (1999). Steinstrasse: a comparison of incidence with and without J stenting and the effect of J stenting on subsequent management. *BJU Int* **84**: 618.

Beck, A.L. (2007). Outcome of and complications associated with tube cystostomy in dogs and cats: 76 cases (1995–2006). *J Am Vet Med Assoc* **230**: 1184–1189.

Berent, A., C. Weisse, et al. (2007). Ureteral stenting for benign and malignant disease in dogs and cats. *Abstract presented at American College of Veterinary Surgery*, 17–21 October, Chicago, IL.

Block, G. (1996). Use of extracorporeal shock wave lithotripsy for treatment of nephrolithiasis and ureterolithiasis in five dogs. *J Am Vet Med Assoc* **208**(4): 531–536.

Goldin, A.R. (1977). Percutaneous ureteral splinting. *Urology* **10**(2): 165–168.

Hubert, K.C. (2005). Passive dilation by ureteral stenting before yeteroscopy: eliminating the need for active dilation. *J Urol* **174**(3): 1079–1080.

Knapp, D.W. (2000). Naturally occurring canine transitional cell carcinoma of the urinary bladder. A relevant model of human invasive bladder cancer. *Urol Oncol* **5**: 47.

Kyles, A. (2005). Management and outcome of cats with ureteral calculi: 153 cases (1984–2002). *J Am Vet Med Assoc* **226**(6): 937–944.

Kyles, A. (2005). Clinical, clinicopathologic, radiographic, and ultrasonographic abnormalities in cats with ureteral calculi: 163 cases (1984–2002). *J Am Vet Med Assoc* **226**(6): 932–936.

Lennon, G.M. (1997). Double pigtail ureteric stent versus versus percutaneous nephrostomy: effects on stone transit and ureteric motility. *Eur Urol* **31**(1): 24–29.

Liptak, J.M. (2004). Transurethral resection in the management of urethral and prostatic neoplasia in 6 dogs. *Vet Surg* **33**: 505.

Meige, F. (2008). Management of traumatic urethral reupture in 11 cats using primary alignment with a urethral catheter. *Vet Comp Orthop Traumatol* **21**: 76–84.

Mustafa, M. (2007). The role of stenting in relieving loin pain following ureteroscopic stone therapy for persisting renal colic with hydronephrosis. *Int Urol Nephrol* **39**(1): 91–94.

Norris, A.M. (1992). Canine bladder and urethral tumors: a retrospective study of 115 cases (1980–1985). *J Vet Intern Med* **16**: 145.

Smith, J.D. (1995). Placement of a permanent cystostomy catheter to relieve urine outflow obstruction in dogs with transitional cell carcinoma. *J Am Vet Med Assoc* **206**: 496–499.

Stiffler, K.S. (2003). Clinical use of low-profile cystostomy tubes in four dogs and a cat. *J Am Vet Med Assoc* **223**(3): 325–329.

Stone, E.A. (1988). Ureterocolonic anastomosis in ten dogs with transitional cell carcinoma. *Vet Surg* **17**: 147.

Snyder, D. (2005). Diagnosis and surgical management of ureteral calculi in dogs: 16 (1990–2003). *New Zealand Vet Journal* **53**(1): 19–25.

Uthappa, M.C. (2005). Retrograde or antegrade double-pigtail stent placement for malignant ureteric obstruction? *Clin Radiol* **60**: 608–612.

Weisse, C. and A. Berent (2009). Interventional radiology and endosurgery of the urinary system. *Current Veterinary Therapy, XIV*.

Weisse, C. (2006). Evaluation of palliative stenting for management of malignant urethral obstructions in dogs. *J Am Vet Med Assoc* **229**(2): 226–234.

Yossepowitch, O. (2001). Predicting the success of retrograde stenting for managing ureteral obstruction. *J Urol* **166**: 1746–1749.

Zimskind, P.D. (1967). Clinical use of long-term indwelling silicone rubber ureteral splints inserted cystoscopically. *J Urol* **97**: 840–844.

33

Extracorporeal shock wave lithotripsy

Larry G. Adams and Corinne K. Goldman

Lithotripsy is crushing or fragmenting uroliths by high-energy shock waves or by laser energy. Types of lithotripsy include extracorporeal shock wave lithotripsy (ESWL), electrohydraulic lithotripsy, and laser lithotripsy (Chapter 34). ESWL utilizes repeated shock-waves generated outside the body to fragment the uroliths into smaller fragments that can pass spontaneously through the excretory system.

In 1980, ESWL was first used to successfully fragment nephroliths in a human patient in Germany (Chaussy et al. 1982b). In 1984, the initial clinical trial of ESWL in the United States showed excellent results for treatment of nephroliths (Lingeman et al. 1986). The widespread use of ESWL and the subsequent development of laser lithotripsy have changed the treatment approach to uroliths in humans such that minimally invasive techniques are utilized for approximately 99% of upper tract uroliths versus less than 1% treated by open surgical methods (Lingeman et al. 2002).

In humans, the relative roles of ESWL, laser lithotripsy and percutaneous nephrolithotomy have been established through prospective clinical trials (Lingeman et al. 1987; Lingeman 1989; Lam et al. 1992; Albala et al. 2001). In humans, ESWL is usually the first choice for treatment of nephroliths and proximal ureteroliths because of its high success rate and non-invasive nature (Segura et al. 1997; Lingeman et al. 2002). Ureteroscopy with laser lithotripsy is successful for removal of ureteroliths in over 90% of human patients and this approach is considered the first choice for impacted distal ureteroliths (Segura et al. 1997; Grasso et al. 1998; Denstedt et al. 2001; Bagley 2002). For large staghorn nephroliths in humans, percutaneous nephrolithotomy with or without shock wave lithotripsy is the preferred technique (Kahnoski et al. 1986; Segura et al. 1994). Percutaneous nephrolithotomy involves fragmentation and removal of nephroliths with a nephroscope via a percutaneous approach into the renal pelvis. For large staghorn nephroliths, ESWL is not recommended because of the risk of ureteral obstruction during passage of large amounts of nephrolith fragments.

The relative roles of ESWL, laser lithotripsy, and percutaneous nephrolithotomy have not yet been fully determined in dogs and cats. Although percutaneous nephrolithotomy has been performed in large breed research dogs, (Donner et al. 1987) the technique has only recently been performed in dogs with spontaneously occurring nephroliths (Weisse et al. 2008). Laser lithotripsy may be utilized for fragmentation and removal of lower urinary tract uroliths in dogs and cats that can be visualized using a rigid or flexible cystoscope or ureteroscope (see Chapter 34) (Adams et al. 2008; Grant et al. 2008). Although electrohydraulic lithotripsy can also be performed in dogs, (Defarges and Dunn 2008), this technique has been largely replaced by laser lithotripsy because of greater efficiency and efficacy of laser lithotripsy compared to electrohydraulic lithotripsy (Adams et al. 2008; Defarges and Dunn 2008; Grant et al. 2008). In veterinary medicine, ESWL is used primarily for fragmentation of nephroliths or ureteroliths in dogs and for ureteroliths in cats. The remainder of this chapter will be limited to discussion of ESWL in dogs and cats.

Overview of extracorporeal shock wave lithotripsy

ESWL treatment of nephroliths and ureteroliths results in comminution of uroliths into smaller fragments which are able to pass down the ureter and subsequently be voided with the urine (Figure 33.1). We originally reported the safety and efficacy of ESWL for the treatment

Nephrology and Urology of Small Animals. Edited by Joe Bartges and David J. Polzin. © 2011 Blackwell Publishing Ltd.

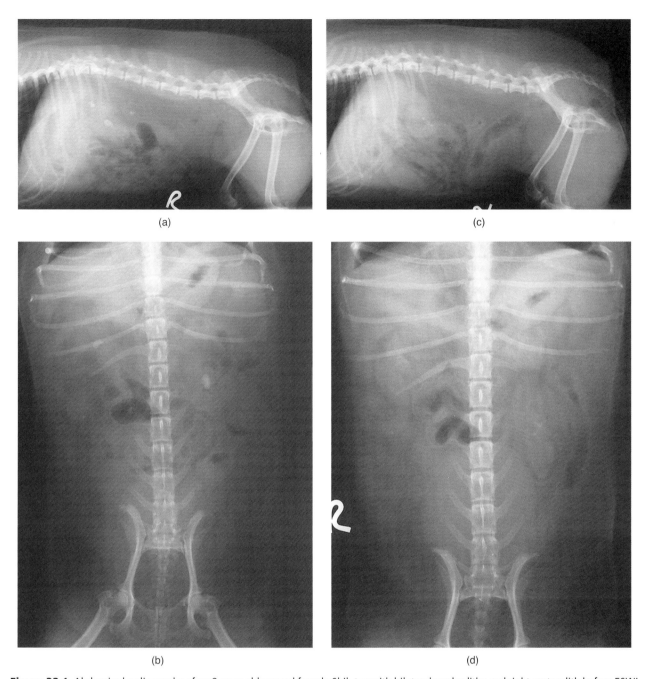

(a)

(c)

(b)

(d)

Figure 33.1 Abdominal radiographs of an 8-year-old spayed female Shih tzu with bilateral nephroliths and right ureterolith before ESWL (a) and (b). Abdominal radiographs after ESWL (c) and (d) showing fragmentation of the nephroliths and right ureterolith. All urolith fragments passed and were voided within one month.

of canine nephrolithiasis and ureterolithiasis from our first five cases (Block et al. 1996). Currently, we have treated over 150 dogs with ESWL using an unmodified Dornier HM3 lithotriptor. In ESWL, shock waves are generated outside the body and then reflected to converge on a focal point which is a defined distance from the shock wave generator. The patient is positioned such that the urolith is placed within the focal point. The

shock wave is directed at the urolith by an integrated targeting system using either fluoroscopy or ultrasonography. Shock waves are high-amplitude sound waves generated by electrohydraulic, electromagnetic or piezoelectrical energy sources. Like ultrasound waves, shock waves travel through media of fluid or soft tissue density until reaching a tissue interface at the "hard" acoustic surface of the urolith.

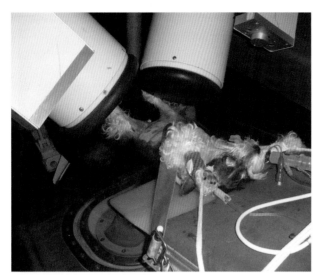

Figure 33.2 A 7-year-old spayed female Miniature Schnauzer positioned in the Dornier HM-3 lithotriptor for ESWL treatment of bilateral nephroliths. Note the water level on the side of the water bath and the biplanar fluoroscopy used for targeting the uroliths.

The initial lithotriptor used for human clinical use, the Dornier HM3 (Dornier, Marietta, GA), relied upon transmission of shock waves through a water bath medium, requiring the patient to be partially submerged during treatment. This lithotriptor is still used by the authors for treatment of uroliths in dogs (Figure 33.2). In the Dornier HM-3, shock waves are generated by an underwater spark created by an electrohydraulic electrode. Newer lithotriptors utilize other types of shock wave generators and "dry" methods, in which shock waves are transmitted to the patient through a fluid filled cushion while the patient lies on a dry treatment table (Figure 33.3). While dry lithotriptors are easier to use and more widely available, the efficacy of dry lithotriptors is lower than that of the Dornier HM-3, because of smaller focal zones and in some cases, lower peak pressure (Lingeman et al. 2002). This narrow focal zone limits shock wave damage to surrounding tissues, but requires precision in targeting uroliths. For either type of lithotriptor, the hair overlying the entry point of the shock waves should be clipped to prevent trapping of air bubbles under the hair that could attenuate the shock wave at the skin surface. With dry lithotriptors, the treatment head of the lithotriptor must be carefully coupled to the body wall with copious amounts of ultrasonic coupling gel to assure transmission of the shock waves into the body.

Prior to initiation of ESWL, the urolith must be accurately identified by fluoroscopy, ultrasonography or both. The patient is positioned such that the urolith is placed within the focal spot of the lithotriptor utilizing the inte-

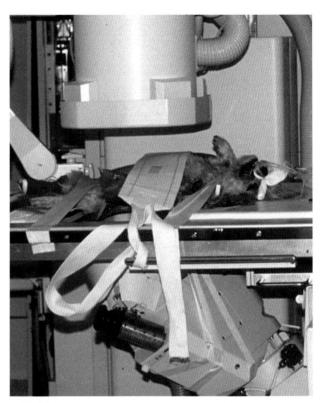

Figure 33.3 A 12-year-old spayed female Lhasa apso positioned on a dry lithotriptor for ESWL. Note the fluid-filled cushion used for coupling the shock wave generator to the patient below and fluoroscopy unit above the patient.

grated targeting system of the lithotriptor. Accurate targeting is essential to fragment uroliths and prevent damage to other organs. This is particularly important with dry lithotriptors with small intense focal spots. The lung field should be shielded from the shock wave to prevent pulmonary contusion since lung parenchyma has different acoustical impedance than soft tissues. Once ESWL therapy is initiated, the targeted urolith should be periodically monitored to confirm that fragmentation is occurring and that positioning is accurate. For larger uroliths, several different areas of the urolith should be targeted during ESWL. Uroliths or urolith fragments may migrate within dilated ureters or within the urinary bladder lumen, thus the patient may need to be re-positioned during ESWL to assure complete fragmentation of all uroliths.

Mechanisms of urolith fragmentation by shock wave lithotripsy

Fragmentation of uroliths during ESWL occurs by mechanical stresses on the urolith produced by the shock wave itself or by collapse of cavitation bubbles on the surface of the urolith (Chaussy et al. 1982a, 1982b; Lingeman et al. 2002; McAteer et al. 2005). The major proposed mechanisms of urolith comminution include (1) compressive fracture, (2) spallation, and (3) cavitation (Lingeman et al. 2002).

As the shock wave enters the front edge of a urolith, positive pressure waves generate compression-induced cracks or fractures that often occur along preexisting defects in the urolith. Reflection of a compressive wave at the far surface of the urolith at the urolith–urine interface results in a reflected wave that is inverted in phase referred to as a tensile (negative) wave. If the tensile wave exceeds the tensile strength of the urolith, microcracks within the urolith occur, and then coalesce to fragment the urolith near the posterior surface of the urolith. This process is called spallation.

Cavitation is the process of rapid formation and collapse of air bubbles in the fluid medium on the surface of uroliths. During the collapse of these air bubbles, a liquid jet or microjet occurs and accelerates to extremely high speeds which impact on the surface of the urolith resulting in surface pitting (Crum 1988; Pishchalnikov et al. 2003; Chitnis and Cleveland 2006). Cavitation is thought to be a particularly important mechanism for comminution of uroliths smaller than 2–3 mm. The inability of cavitation bubbles to form and collapse from lack of fluid-urolith interface around impacted ureteroliths may contribute to the observed lower success rates for fragmentation of impacted ureteroliths compared to nephroliths (Lingeman et al. 2002).

Principles of extracorporeal shock wave lithotripsy treatment of uroliths

In dogs and cats, ESWL treatments are performed under general anesthesia to provide analgesia during the procedure and to facilitate accurate targeting of the uroliths. Treatment of nephroliths by ESWL may cause injury to the kidney, therefore the total dose delivered to the kidney and/or proximal ureter must be below the threshold for inducing clinically relevant renal injury (Webb and Fitzpatrick 1985; Newman et al. 1987; Jaeger et al. 1995). Shock wave-induced renal injury occurs primarily by formation and collapse of microscopic air bubbles within the kidney tissues, especially within the blood vessels (Williams et al. 1999; Evan et al. 2002; Sapozhnikov et al. 2002; Pishchalnikov et al. 2003). Severity of the renal injury is influenced by the rate of shock wave administration such that slower rates (60/minutes) are less damaging to renal parenchyma than more rapid rates (120/minutes) (Sapozhnikov et al. 2002). Furthermore, the efficacy of urolith fragmentation is improved by slower rates of shock wave administration compared to faster rates (Paterson et al. 2002; Pace et al. 2005). Given

this information, ESWL treatment strategies for dogs and cats with upper tract uroliths should include using slower treatment rates and maintaining total shock wave dose delivered to an individual kidney below approximately 1,500 shock waves depending on the lithotriptor utilized.

Voltage stepping is the term used to describe ESWL protocols that begin with low voltage settings per shock wave and progressively increase the voltage during treatment as compared to the conventional approach of setting the lithotriptor at a constant voltage for the entire duration of shock wave therapy. Voltage stepping (e.g., increasing voltage from 16 to 18 kV) results in the improved fragmentation of upper uroliths compared to using the same voltage (18 kV) for all shock waves administered (Zhou et al. 2004; Maloney et al. 2006; Demirci et al. 2007). Patient tolerance of ESWL therapy is also improved with voltage stepping allowing for lighter planes of anesthesia during ESWL (Lingeman et al. 2002). Therefore, ESWL protocols for dogs and cats should include voltage stepping by increasing the shock wave voltage from a lower initial setting up to a maximum safe dose during ESWL.

Based on available research and our clinical experience, we have the developed treatment recommendations for ESWL protocols for treatment of nephroliths, ureteroliths and urocystoliths using the Dornier HM3 lithotriptor. The approach when using other lithotriptors should be adjusted based on relative power and safety profile of the lithotriptor compared to the HM3 (Lingeman et al. 2002).

Treatment of nephroliths and ureteroliths in dogs using shock wave lithotripsy

Dogs with nephroliths should be treated with a full therapeutic dose of 1,400–1,500 shocks per kidney at energy levels that are gradually increased from 13 to 16 kV. The rate of shock wave administration should be 60–90 shock waves per minute. The Dornier HM-3 is designed to trigger shock waves based on the patient's ECG (termed ECG gating) to avoid shock wave-induced arrhythmias. The Dornier HM-3 can be programmed to trigger a shock wave with every heart beat or every other heart beat allowing the rate of shock wave administration to be adjusted to within the target range. As ECG gating of ESWL therapy is not required for dry lithotriptors, they can be triggered at preset rates of 60–120 shock waves per minute or faster for some models. Following the principle that slower rates result in less renal injury and greater urolith fragmentation, we recommend slower rates of 60–90 shock waves per minute.

Treatment with sub-therapeutic shock wave doses may result in lower fragmentation rates or higher re-treatment rates, thus full therapeutic doses are recommended. In most dogs with bilateral nephroliths, both kidneys can be safely treated during the same anesthetic episode. For larger bilateral nephroliths, pre-placement of double pig-tailed ureteral stents, minimizes the risk of ureteral obstruction during passage of nephrolith fragments through the ureters (Figure 33.4). In female dogs,

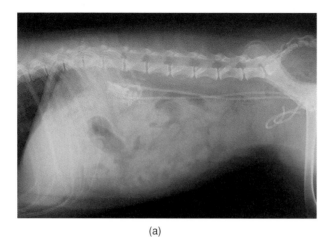

(a)

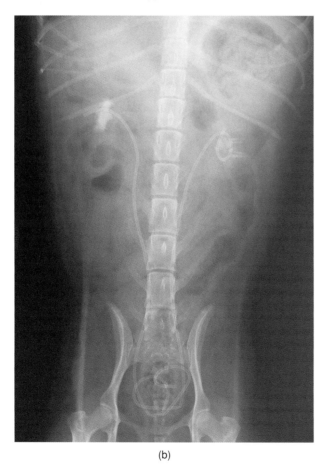

(b)

Figure 33.4 Abdominal radiographs of a 7-year-old spayed female miniature poodle with bilateral ureteral stents prior to ESWL treatment of bilateral nephroliths.

ureteral stents may be placed retrograde up the ureter over a urologic guide wire via cystoscopy. Once the ureteral stent is no longer needed, the stent can be easily extracted via cystoscopy by grasping the distal end of the ureteral stent and providing gentle traction to withdraw the stent through the urethra. In dogs with large bilateral nephroliths treated without ureteral stents, ESWL treatment of the kidneys may be intentionally staggered with treatments administered ≥ 4 weeks apart to minimize the risk of bilateral ureteral obstruction during passage of ureteral fragments.

For dogs with ureteroliths in the mid to distal ureter, aggressive ESWL treatment protocols are more likely to result in successful fragmentation. Ureteroliths are more difficult to fragment by ESWL compared to nephroliths (Pace et al. 2000; Paterson et al. 2005). This difficulty appears to be due to the inability of cavitation bubbles to form and collapse on the surface of the ureterolith (Pishchalnikov et al. 2003; Chitnis and Cleveland 2006). ESWL treatment of the ureteroliths in the proximal ureteral may result in the caudal pole of the kidney being included within the treatment focal spot while targeting the ureterolith. If the kidney is included in the treatment focal spot, the total dose targeting the nephrolith and ureterolith should not exceed 2,000 shock waves. For mid to distal ureteroliths in dogs, ESWL treatment should be aggressive with doses of 2,000–3,000 shock waves at progressively increasing voltages from 15 to 18 kV. These higher ESWL doses can be used as long as the kidney is not included within the treatment focal spot while targeting the most proximal ureterolith. The maximum number of shock waves we have safely administered to target multiple distal ureteroliths was 4,400 shock waves at 18–19 kV. When targeting multiple ureteroliths, it is recommended to treat the most distal ureterolith first and move proximally up the ureter towards the kidney.

Placement of ureteral stents is not essential for treatment of ureteroliths, but there are advantages of ureteral stents that facilitate ESWL and patient management. Ureteral stents allow urine to bypass ureteral obstruction at the site of the ureterolith and prevent additional renal damage from obstructive uropathy. Because ureteral stents are radiopaque, they facilitate accurate targeting of ureteroliths during SWL (Figure 33.4). When treating ureteroliths using fluoroscopy without ureteral stents, administration of intravenous contrast iodinated agent such as iohexol may be required to delineate the ureter and to accurately target smaller ureteroliths. Fluid diuresis during ESWL treatment may hinder opacification of the ureter during the excretory phase following intravenous iohexol administration. Ureteral stents also induce passive ureteral dilation thus increasing the diameter of the ureter lumen by approximately threefold

(Culkin et al. 1992). This has the theoretical advantage of allowing for greater urolith-fluid interface for cavitation bubble formation and collapse to increase the efficiency of urolith fragmentation. Passive dilation of the ureter should also facilitate passage of nephrolith and ureterolith fragments following ureteral stent removal.

Nephroliths are successfully fragmented and removed by ESWL in approximately 85% of dogs. Approximately 30% of dogs require more than one ESWL treatment for complete fragmentation of nephroliths. Re-treatment rates in humans vary by type of lithotriptor and are generally higher with dry lithotriptors (Lingeman et al. 2002). For dogs with obstructed ureteroliths, nearly 80% of ureteroliths can be resolved by ESWL, although roughly 50% require two or more ESWL treatments which is a higher re-treatment rate than for dogs with nephroliths. This is similar to observations in humans and in research models that confirm impacted ureteroliths are more difficult to fragment compared with nephroliths (Pace et al. 2000; Lingeman et al. 2002; Paterson et al. 2005). Since the development of smaller flexible ureteroscopes and laser lithotripsy, humans with ureteroliths that fail ESWL are usually treated by ureteroscopy and laser lithotripsy rather than having repeated ESWL (Lingeman et al. 2002; Pace et al. 2000). Ureteroscopy with laser lithotripsy of ureteroliths has not been reported in dogs due to the smaller ureteral diameter compared to available flexible ureteroscopes. Dr. India Lane has reported successful ESWL treatment of ureteroliths in dogs and cats using large numbers of shock waves per treatment which has subsequently modified our approach to treatment of ureteroliths (Lane 2003; Lane et al. 2005).

Extracorporeal shock wave lithotripsy of urocystoliths in dogs

Although ESWL is better suited for fragmentation of uroliths fixed in one location such as nephroliths or ureteroliths, the authors have successfully fragmented urocystoliths using ESWL. As the urocystoliths tend to move out of the focal spot of the lithotriptor, uniform fragmentation does not occur consistently. Recently, we have changed our ESWL protocol urocystoliths to administer 2,000 shocks at 18–19 kV using the Dornier HM-3, which is higher than the typical ESWL dose for nephroliths (Goldman et al. 2008). The dogs are also positioned in lateral recumbency for targeting of urocystoliths (Figure 33.5).

In our experience, urocystoliths can be fragmented by ESWL into fragments small enough to pass through the urethra in 85% of the dogs (Goldman et al. 2008). Results of ESWL treatment of urocystoliths using newer dry lithotriptors may be significantly lower because of the

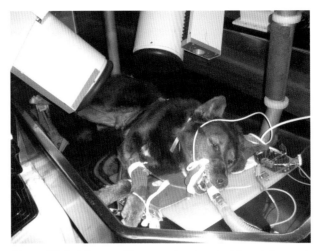

Figure 33.5 A 9-year-old neutered male mixed breed dog positioned in the Dornier HM-3 lithotriptor for ESWL treatment of urocystoliths.

much smaller treatment focal spots of most dry lithotriptors. When using these machines, use of higher shock wave doses and frequent monitoring of fragment size and location within the bladder via fluoroscopy may improve efficacy of this approach. If the fragments are too large to be removed through the urethra following an initial ESWL session, ESWL may be repeated or a secondary procedure such as laser lithotripsy may be required to remove larger urocystolith fragments. For male dogs that are too small for transurethral laser lithotripsy, ESWL followed by voiding urohydropropulsion provides an attractive alternative for non-invasive urolith removal.

Treatment of nephroliths and ureteroliths in cats using shock wave lithotripsy

Preliminary research with ESWL in cats revealed that the shock wave dose must be reduced in cats compared to dogs to prevent shock wave induced injury to the kidney. Using the Dornier HM3, shock wave doses greater than 750 shock waves at an energy level of 13 kilovolts result in renal parenchyma injury and reduction in renal function. We have treated six cats with spontaneously occurring calcium oxalate ureteroliths and chronic renal failure with ESWL. Five of these cats also had concurrent nephroliths. We were only successful in ESWL treatment of one of these six cats (complete resolution of the ureterolith). We were unsuccessful in the other five cats. Partial fragmentation of the nephroliths occurred in two of five cats. Ineffective ESWL fragmentation of ureteroliths in cats may be due to intrinsic factors in feline uroliths that make them less susceptible to fragmentation by shock waves (Adams et al. 2005). Another possible explanation is that impacted ureteroliths are less susceptible to fragmentation by ESWL compared to nephroliths (Paterson et al. 2005). This resistance to fragmentation of ureteroliths may be due to the lack of urine around the impacted ureterolith preventing cavitation which is thought to be important for fragmentation of smaller uroliths (Crum 1988; Pishchalnikov et al. 2003). Because of these poor initial results, we discontinued ESWL treatment of cats using the Dornier HM3.

Recent reports indicate that dry lithotriptors with small focal spots can be safely used to treat cats without compromising renal function. Shock wave treatment of normal cats with the Dornier MFL-5000 did not cause significant renal injury or renal functional problems (Labato 2001; Gonzalez et al. 2002). Cats with ureteroliths have been successfully treated by ESWL with dry lithotriptors using large numbers of shock waves per ESWL session (Labato 2001; Lane 2003; Lane et al. 2005). Therefore, dry lithotriptors may be used to attempt ESWL therapy of ureteroliths in cats. Berent et al. have recently reported successful retrograde ureteral stent placement in cats with ureteroliths (Berent et al. 2007; Weisse et al. 2008). Ureteral stent placement prior to ESWL may improve efficacy of fragmentation of ureteroliths as discussed above.

We previously demonstrated in vitro that feline calcium oxalate uroliths are significantly more difficult to fragment using ESWL than were paired canine calcium oxalate uroliths (Adams et al. 2005). Shock wave lithotripsy is unlikely to be as effective for treatment of nephroliths in cats as in dogs because the small diameter of the feline ureter requires that all fragments be fine sand. Even with sand-like fragments, ureteral obstruction is likely to occur in some cats unless ureteral stents are placed before ESWL. Therefore, the authors believe that ESWL treatment of uroliths in cats should be limited to fragmentation and removal of ureteroliths by dry lithotriptors only and that nephroliths in cats should not be treated by ESWL until more research is available to determine safe and effective protocols.

Complications of ESWL

We have observed several complications from ESWL treatment. The most common complication has been the development of transient ureteroliths that partially obstructed the ureter in approximately 10% of dogs treated for nephroliths. Unlike humans, clinical signs of acute abdominal pain attributable to ureteral "colic" are uncommon in dogs during passage of ureteral fragments. Acute bilateral ureteral obstruction from nephrolith fragments may require surgery or placement of ureteral stents to relieve the obstruction. In dogs with large bilateral nephroliths undergoing staggered ESWL treatment of

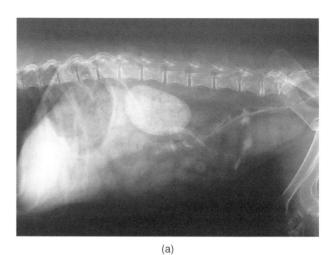

(a)

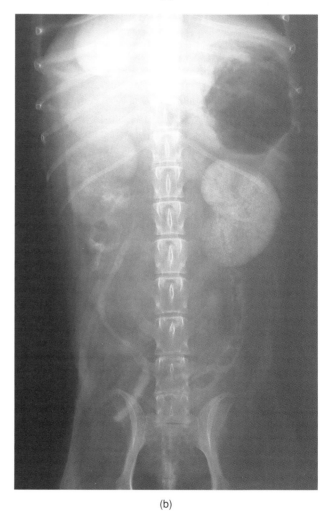

(b)

Figure 33.6 Abdominal radiographs of an 8-year-old spayed female Bichon friese showing contrast accumulation in both kidneys (more severe in left kidney) consistent with contrast nephropathy. These radiographs were obtained approximately 24 hours after intravenous iohexol administration for targeting of a proximal ureterolith during ESWL. Note that some of the iohexol was excreted via the biliary system resulting in opacification of the gall bladder, small intestines, and colon.

nephroliths, any ureteral fragments that occur from treatment of the first kidney can be treated by ESWL during the second ESWL session along with treatment of the second kidney.

Treatment of the right kidney in small dogs by ESWL often results in mild asymptomatic increases in amylase and lipase, suggestive of pancreatic injury. The pancreas is probably included in the shock wave focal spot during the treatment of the right kidney because of these dogs' small size (<5 kg), the large focal spot of the HM-3, and the proximity of the pancreas to the right kidney. Only 3% of dogs treated by ESWL with the HM-3 have developed clinical acute pancreatitis following ESWL treatment of the right kidney (Daugherty et al. 2004).

One dog developed a fatal ventricular arrhythmia during ESWL treatment. The origin of the arrhythmia was not definitively determined. This dog had mitral regurgitation and left ventricular hypertrophy which may have contributed to the arrhythmia. Although heart and lungs are shielded from the primary shock wave to prevent pulmonary contusions, the heart might have been affected by secondary shock waves from reflection of the primary shock wave off the inside of the water bath and gantry. Alternatively, the arrhythmia might have been anesthetic associated and unrelated to ESWL. We utilize the ECG gating feature of the Dornier HM-3 to minimize the risk of shock wave-induced arrhythmias.

One dog developed contrast nephropathy from iohexol given during ESWL to facilitate targeting of ureteroliths (Figure 33.6). Radiographic contrast was administered to assist targeting of ureteroliths or radiolucent nephroliths in 42 other dogs without any adverse effects. In normal dogs, iohexol administration had no adverse effects when administered multiple times before, during and after ESWL (Karlsen et al. 1993).

Follow-up serum chemistry profiles and urinalyses did not reveal decreased renal function compared to pretreatment evaluation in most dogs. Mean serum creatinine concentration was not significantly different before, one day after and one month after ESWL. In four dogs with preexisting renal failure, there was a transient increase in serum creatinine concentration which returned to pre-treatment levels within 48 hours after ESWL. In cats treated by ESWL using the Dornier HM-3, serum creatinine concentrations were transient increased after ESWL treatment in two of six cats. One additional cat had marked decline in renal function after ESWL for greater than one month.

Conclusions

ESWL treatment is an efficacious and safe minimally invasive approach to treatment of uroliths in dogs. ESWL also has been successful for removal of ureteroliths in a limited number of cats. Careful patient selection and attention to detail during ESWL are important factors for determining success of ESWL therapy.

References

Adams, L.G., et al. (2005). In vitro evaluation of canine and feline urolith fragility by shock wave lithotripsy. *Am J Vet Res* **66**: 1651–1654.

Adams, L.G., et al. (2008). Use of laser lithotripsy for fragmentation of uroliths in dogs: 73 cases (2005–2006). *J Am Vet Med Assoc* **232**: 1680–1687.

Albala, D.M., et al. (2001). Lower pole I: a prospective randomized trial of extracorporeal shock wave lithotripsy and percutaneous nephrostolithotomy for lower pole nephrolithiasis-initial results. *J Urol* **166**: 2072–2080.

Bagley, D.H. (2002). Expanding role of ureteroscopy and laser lithotripsy for treatment of proximal ureteral and intrarenal calculi. *Curr Opin Urol* **12**: 277–280.

Berent, A.C., et al. (2007). Ureteral stenting for benign and malignant disease in dogs and cats (Abstract). *Vet Surg* **36**: E3.

Block, G., et al. (1996). Use of extracorporeal shock wave lithotripsy for treatment of spontaneous nephrolithiasis and ureterolithiasis in dogs. *J Am Vet Med Assoc* **208**: 531–536.

Chaussy, C., et al. (1982a). *Extracorporeal Shock Wave Lithotripsy: New Aspects in the Treatment of Kidney Stone Disease.* Munich: Krager, pp. 1–109.

Chaussy, C., et al. (1982b). First clinical experience with extracorporeally induced destruction of kidney stones by shock waves. *J Urol* **127**: 417–420.

Chitnis, P.V. and R.O. Cleveland (2006). Quantitative measurements of acoustic emissions from cavitation at the surface of a stone in response to a lithotripter shock wave. *J Acoust Soc Am* **119**: 1929–1932.

Crum, L.A. (1988). Cavitation microjets as a contributory mechanism for renal calculi disintegration in ESWL. *J Urol* **140**: 1587–1590.

Culkin, D.J., et al. (1992). Anatomic, functional, and pathologic changes from internal ureteral stent placement. *Urology* **40**: 385–390.

Daugherty, M.A., et al. (2004). Acute pancreatitis in two dogs associated with shock wave lithotripsy (Abstract). *J Vet Intern Med* **18**: 441.

Defarges, A. and M. Dunn (2008). Use of electrohydraulic lithotripsy in 28 dogs with bladder and urethral calculi. *J Vet Intern Med* **22**: 1267–1273.

Demirci, D., et al. (2007). Comparison of conventional and step-wise shockwave lithotripsy in management of urinary calculi. *J Endourol* **21**: 1407–1410.

Denstedt, J.D., et al. (2001). A prospective randomized controlled trial comparing nonstented versus stented ureteroscopic lithotripsy. *J Urol* **165**: 1419–1422.

Donner, G.S., et al. (1987). Percutaneous nephrolithotomy in the dog: an experimental study. *Vet Surg* **16**: 411–417.

Evan, A.P., et al. (2002). Kidney damage and renal functional changes are minimized by waveform control that suppresses cavitation in shock wave lithotripsy. *J Urol* **168**: 1556–1562.

Goldman, C.K., et al. (2008). Extracorporeal shock-wave lithotripsy for the treatment of urocystoliths in dogs (Abstract). *Urol Res* **36**: 179.

Gonzalez, A., et al. (2002). Evaluation of the safety of extracorporeal shock-wave lithotripsy in cats (Abstract). *J Vet Intern Med* **16**: 376.

Grant, D.C., et al. (2008). Holmium: YAG laser lithotripsy for urolithiasis in dogs. *J Vet Intern Med* **22**: 534–539.

Grasso, M., et al. (1998). Retrograde ureteropyeloscopic treatment of 2 cm. or greater upper urinary tract and minor Staghorn calculi. *J Urol* **160**: 346–351.

Jaeger, P., et al. (1995). Morphological and functional changes in canine kidneys following extracorporeal shock-wave treatment. *Urol Int* **54**: 48–58.

Kahnoski, R.J., et al. (1986). Combined percutaneous and extracorporeal shock wave lithotripsy for staghorn calculi: an alternative to anatrophic nephrolithotomy. *J Urol* **135**: 679–681.

Karlsen, S.J., et al. (1993). Does the administration of systemic radiographic contrast media influence the acute changes in renal physiology following exposure to extracorporeal shock waves in dogs? *J Urol* **150**: 219–222.

Labato, M.A. (2001). Managing urolithiasis in cats. *Vet Med* **96**: 708–718.

Lam, H.S., et al. (1992). Staghorn calculi: analysis of treatment results between initial percutaneous nephrostolithotomy and extracorporeal shock wave lithotripsy monotherapy with reference to surface area. *J Urol* **147**: 1219–1225.

Lane, I.F. (2003). Dry extracorporeal lithotripsy in small animals. *Proceedings 21st Annual ACVIM Forum*, pp. 13–14.

Lane, I.F., et al. (2005). Lithotripsy. In: *Consultations in Feline Internal Medicine*, edited by J.R. August. St. Louis, MO: Elsevier Saunders, pp. 407–414.

Lingeman, J.E. (1989). Relative roles of extracorporeal shock wave lithotripsy and percutaneous nephrostolithotomy. In: *Shock Wave Lithotripsy 2*, edited by J.E. Lingeman and D.M. Newman. New York: Plenum Press, pp. 303–308.

Lingeman, J.E., et al. (1986). Extracorporeal shock wave lithotripsy: the Methodist Hospital of Indiana experience. *J Urol* **135**: 1134–1137.

Lingeman, J.E., et al. (1987). Comparison of results and morbidity of percutaneous nephrostolithotomy and extracorporeal shock wave lithotripsy. *J Urol* **138**: 485–490.

Lingeman, J.E., et al. (2002). Surgical management of urinary lithiasis. In: *Campbell's Urology*, edited by A.B. Retik, E.D. Vaughan Jr., and A.J. Wein. Philadelphia, PA: WB Saunders, pp. 3361–3451.

Maloney, M.E., et al. (2006). Progressive increase of lithotripter output produces better in-vivo stone comminution. *J Endourol* **20**: 603–606.

McAteer, J.A., et al. (2005). Ultracal-30 gypsum artificial stones for research on the mechanisms of stone breakage in shock wave lithotripsy. *Urol Res* **33**: 429–434.

Newman, R., et al. (1987). Pathologic effects of ESWL on canine renal tissue. *Urology* **29**: 194–200.

Pace, K.T., et al. (2000). Low success rate of repeat shock wave lithotripsy for ureteral stones after failed initial treatment. *J Urol* **164**: 1905–1907.

Pace, K.T., et al. University of Toronto Lithotripsy Associates. (2005). Shock wave lithotripsy at 60 or 120 shocks per minute: a randomized, double-blind trial. *J Urol* **174**: 595–599.

Paterson, R.F., et al. (2002). Stone fragmentation during shock wave lithotripsy is improved by slowing the shock wave rate: studies with a new animal model. *J Urol* **168**: 2211–2215.

Paterson, R.F., et al. (2005). Shock wave lithotripsy of stones implanted in the proximal ureter of the pig. *J Urol* **173**: 1391–1394.

Pishchalnikov, Y.A., et al. (2003). Cavitation bubble cluster activity in the breakage of kidney stones by lithotripter shockwaves. *J Endourol* **17**: 435–446.

Sapozhnikov, O.A., et al. (2002). Effect of overpressure and pulse repetition frequency on cavitation in shock wave lithotripsy. *J Acoust Soc Am* **112**: 1183–1195.

Segura, J.W., et al. (1994). Nephrolithiasis Clinical Guidelines Panel summary report on the management of staghorn calculi. The American Urological Association Nephrolithiasis Clinical Guidelines Panel. *J Urol* **151**: 1648–1651.

Segura, J.W., et al. (1997). Ureteral Stones Clinical Guidelines Panel summary report on the management of ureteral calculi. *The American Urological Association*. J Urol **158**: 1915–1921.

Webb, D.R. and J.M. Fitzpatrick (1985). Percutaneous nephrolithotripsy: a functional and morphological study. *J Urol* **134**: 587–591.

Weisse, C.W., et al. (2008). Potential applications of interventional radiology in veterinary medicine. *J Am Vet Med Assoc* **233**: 1564–1574.

Williams, J.C. Jr., et al. (1999). Effect of macroscopic air bubbles on cell lysis by shock wave lithotripsy in vitro. *Ultrasound Med Biol* **25**: 473–479.

Zhou, Y., et al. (2004). The effect of treatment strategy on stone comminution efficiency in shock wave lithotripsy. *J Urol* **172**: 349–354.

34

Intracorporeal laser lithotripsy

Jody P. Lulich, Carl A. Osborne, and Hasan Albasan

The term "laser" is an acronym for "Light Amplification by Stimulated Emission of Radiation". A laser is a device which transmits light of various frequencies into an extremely intense, small, and nearly non-divergent beam of monochromatic radiation with all the waves in phase. Lasers are capable of mobilizing immense heat and power when focused in close range.

Use of laser energy for intracorporeal lithotripsy is a relatively new concept. In 1968, investigators first reported in vitro fragmentation of uroliths with a ruby laser. (Mulvaney and Beck 1968) However, because fragmentation of stones was associated with generation of sufficient heat that would likely damage adjacent tissues, it could not be used to treat patients. Likewise, use of carbon dioxide laser energy was considered unsuitable for clinical use because it could neither be delivered through nontoxic fibers nor through a liquid medium. However, in 1986, using a 504 nm pulsed dye laser, researchers successfully and safely treated human patients with ureteroliths (Dretler et al. 1987). The Holmium: YAG laser is one of the newest and safest lasers available for clinical lithotripsy (Razvi et al. 1996; Pierre and Preminger 2007).

Holmium (Ho) is a rare earth element named in honor of the Swedish chemist who discovered it (the Greek word "holmia" means Sweden). A Holmium:YAG laser is a laser whose active medium is a crystal of yttrium, aluminum, and garnet (YAG) doped with holmium (chromium and thulium), and whose beam falls in the near infrared portion of the electromagnetic spectrum (2,100 nm). Several commercial models of Holmium:YAG lasers for lithotripsy are available, and the pulse duration ranges from 250 to 750 microseconds, the pulse energy ranges

from 0.2 to 4.0 J/pulse, the frequency ranges from 5 to 45 Hz, and the power output ranges from 3.0 to 100 Watts (W). The power that one chooses is based on the desired application. The Holmium: YAG laser that we use has a maximum power output of 20 W with a 350-microsecond pulse width.

The mechanism of stone fragmentation with the Holmium:YAG laser is mainly photothermal, and involves a thermal drilling process rather than a shockwave effect (Adams et al. 2008). Laser energy is transmitted from the energized crystal to the urolith via a flexible quartz fiber. With each pulse, water at the tip of the laser fiber is vaporized creating a vapor bubble that when transmitted to the urolith causes thermal decomposition. Rapid expansion and collapse of vaporization bubbles shear the stone into fragments. To achieve optimum results, the tip of the laser fiber should be in direct contact with the surface of the urolith during laser activation. If the tip of the laser fiber is not close to the stone (<0.5–1 mm), the surrounding fluid absorbs the energy and the stone remains unaltered.

Performing intracorporeal laser lithotripsy

Laser lithotripsy is performed via cystoscopy in anesthetized patients. Although patient positioning may be chosen according to operator preference, we usually place female dogs and cats in dorsal recumbency (Figure 34.1), and male dogs in lateral recumbency. Once uroliths are visualized with the aid of the cystoscope, the laser fiber is passed through the operating channel of the cystoscope (Figures 34.2–34.5). The tip of the fiber is placed in direct contact and in a perpendicular orientation to the surface of the urolith. In our experience, the initial energy setting to fragment stones is approximately 0.6–0.8 Joules at 6–8 Hertz. Energy settings can be increased as desired, but levels greater than 1 Joule and 12 hertz are rarely needed

Nephrology and Urology of Small Animals. Edited by Joe Bartges and David J. Polzin. © 2011 Blackwell Publishing Ltd.

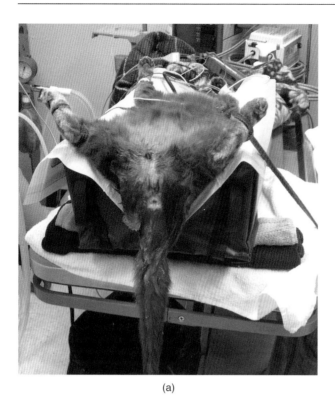

(a)

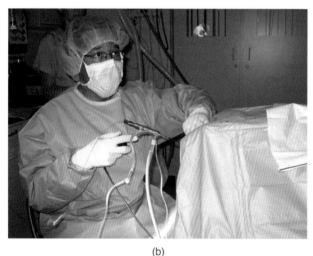

(b)

Figure 34.1 To perform laser lithotripsy, female patients are placed in dorsal recumbency. (a) An anesthetized 4-year-old cat with urate uroliths. The patient is draped so that only the vulva is exposed to allow entry of the cystoscope (b).

to efficiently fragment uroliths. During lithotripsy, sterile saline is continuously flushed through the working channel of the cystoscope to wash debris from the visual field and absorb stray laser energy.

Once uroliths have been sufficiently fragmented such that they are small enough to pass through the urethra, fragments can be removed by a variety of methods. Initially, we use a stone basket to remove the largest urolith fragments. This permits visual verification that uroliths

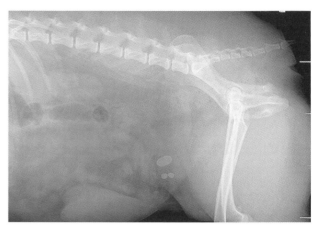

Figure 34.2 Survey lateral radiograph of a 5-year-old female spayed, Miniature Schnauzer with three urocystoliths. The radiograph appearance of these stones is unique in that their outer layer is denser than their inner core. These findings are consistent with the diagnosis of a compound urolith.

have been reduced to pieces that will easily traverse the urethral lumen. Voiding urohydropropulsion (Figure 34.6) is an efficient and rapid process to remove the remaining fragments; however, in cases with large stone burdens, we continue to remove the larger fragments via basket retrieval to insure a successful urohydropropulsion at the end of the procedure. In our experience, the urethral becomes impacted when voiding a large number of irregular fragments even though individual fragments would have passed easily. We adopted this approach to minimize the number of times a clean cystoscopy field needs to be re-established to retrieve retained urolith fragments with the stone basket or to repeat laser applications for fragments that fail to be expelled during voiding

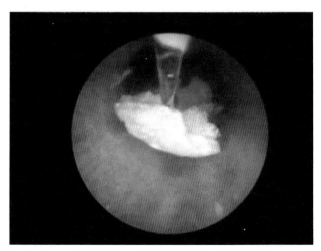

Figure 34.3 Cystoscopic view of a urocystolith in the female Miniature Schnauzer described in Figure 34.2. Holmium: YAG laser energy transmitted through a 520 μm quartz fiber fractures the urocystolith.

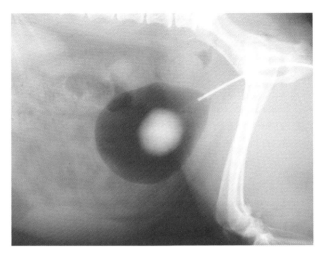

Figure 34.4 Lateral double-contrast cystogram of the female Miniature Schnauzer described in Figure 34.2. The radiograph was obtained following lithotripsy to fragment uroliths and voiding urohydropropulsion to flush urolith fragments out of the urinary bladder. The lack of radiolucent filling defects in the central puddle of contrast agent confirms the effectiveness of these procedures to remove stones.

urohydropropulsion. Table 34.1 lists additional strategies to improve efficiency of urolith removal during laser lithotripsy.

In some patients with substantial inflammation of the lower urinary tract, transurethral insertion of the cystoscope results in extravasation of blood and subsequent clot formation during lithotripsy. If the clot entraps stone fragments that remain adherent to the bladder wall, complete evacuation of stone fragments may not be possible.

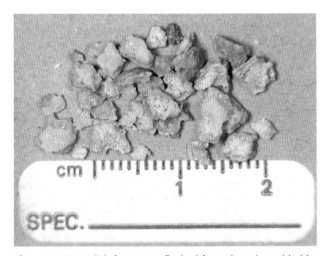

Figure 34.5 Urolith fragments flushed from the urinary bladder of the female Miniature Schnauzer described in Figure 2. The outer layer of the urolith was composed of 100% calcium oxalate monohydrate. The interior of the urolith was composed of 95% magnesium ammonium phosphate and 5% calcium phosphate carbonate.

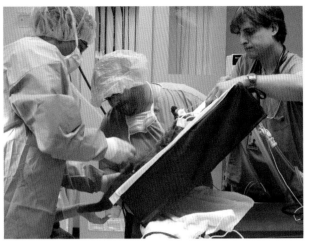

Figure 34.6 Following lithotripsy, the "V" trough is tilted to facilitate positioning of small urolith fragments into the trigone of the urinary bladder. Then, voiding urohydropropulsion is performed to evacuate urolith fragments.

Our experience to date is that most of these fragments are less than 0.2–0.5 mm in diameter. Bleeding and formation of blood clots usually resolve in 24–48 hours. At that time, fragments retained in the bladder can be removed by voiding urohydropropulsion or allowed to pass during the voiding phase of micturition.

Urolith removal via laser lithotripsy may not be possible or ideal in all patients (Table 34.2). For example, cystoscopic evaluation of the urinary tract is not possible in male cats and some small male dogs because the urethra will not permit transurethal passage of a suitable cystoscope. In some cases urolith burden is excessively large, such that surgical cystotomy is likely to be more efficient and cost effective. Although we believe that laser lithotripsy can be quickly learned, the cost of purchasing a Holmium:YAG laser and cystoscopic equipment should be considered in terms of projected patient use. Additional accessories facilitating laser lithotripsy and urolith removal is provided in Table 34.3.

Post-lithotripsy care

Although cystoscopic evaluation of the urinary bladder and urethra with rigid endoscopes is sufficient for assessing complete urolith removal in female patients, the same degree of certainty is not achieved when using flexible fiberoptic endoscopes in males. Visual resolution of the fiberoptic scope is limited due to an image created from multiple individual fibers. In addition, maneuverability within the bladder is limited because the fiberoptic scope only deflects in one visual plane and can only be rotated to a limited degree. For these reasons, we recommend a lateral survey radiograph and a lateral double contrast

Table 34.1 Strategies to improve lithotripsy efficiency

Strategy	Indication	Rationale	Procedure
Sufficiently deep anesthetic plane	Lithotripsy, basket retrieval and voiding urohydropropulsion	Sufficient anesthesia will minimize patient discomfort, and mucosal hemorrhage and inflammation. To avoid urethral spasms which reduce the functional diameter of the urethra.	In addition to providing adequate administration of a moderate level of inhalant anesthetics consider a constant rate of fentanyl (10–25 mcg/hour per kg) Administer Propofol (1–2 mg/kg) as an intravenous bolus just prior to voiding urohydropropulsion.
Clear residual urine from the bladder prior to cystoscopy	Uroliths in male dogs	Reduced optical clarity of urine impedes visual inspection. The working channel of flexible cystoscopes is usually too narrow to rapidly empty and fill the bladder.	Using a large bore transurethral catheter, empty the urinary bladder and rinse 2–3 times with saline. Following the final rinse. Leave the bladder half full.
Use a V trough to position female patients	Uroliths in female dogs and female cats	V trough supports the patient during lithotripsy and voiding urohydropropulsion to remove urolith fragments from the bladder	Position female dogs in dorsal recumbency. Instead of having to lift the dog up in the air, the trough near the head of the patient is tilted upward while keeping the opposite end on the trough stationary allowing gravity to reposition urocystoliths for voiding urohydropropulsion.
Fluoroscopy	Uroliths in male dogs	The optical clarity and limited deflectability of flexible cystoscopes impedes lithotripsy. Fluoroscopy can improve operator orientation and urolith location.	Place dogs in lateral recumbency and center X-ray beam over the urinary bladder. With experience, we find that fluoroscopy is rarely needed.
Fragment bladder stones by first moving them into the urethra	Bladder stones in male dogs Sufficient hematuria to prevent visualization and safe laser fragmentation of bladder stones	Stones lodged in the urethra are held in place more firmly than stones in the urinary bladder. When the laser is activated, they are less likely to be deflected out of the target zone. Because the volume of the urethra is small compared to the urinary bladder, blood can be efficiently cleared from the working area.	Stone baskets and stone grabbers are used to retrieve stones from the urinary bladder and lodge them in the most distal portion of the urethra that could accommodate their size. Voiding urohydropropulsion can also be used to move bladder stones into the urethra.
Occlude urethra proximal to stone	Urethroliths in male dogs	Proximal occlusion of the urethra will prevent stones and stone fragments from returning to the urinary bladder where they are more difficult to retrieve and fragment.	Insert a gloved index finger into the rectum and firmly occlude the lumen of the pelvic urethra by applying digital pressure against the ischium through the ventral wall of the rectum. Gently insert a lubricated catheter with a distensible balloon such that the inflatable balloon is proximal to urethral stones. Distending the balloon will occlude the urethra.

Table 34.2 Relative limitations before considering transurethral laser lithotripsy

Limitation	Rationale
Bleeding disorders	Intravesicular hemorrhage obscures the operator's visibility to accurately aim the laser and retrieve urolith fragments
Small dogs	Although the urethra of most females can accommodate instruments to perform lithotripsy, the urethra of male dogs less than 6 kg may be too narrow for scope insertion or to safely manage uroliths by this technique.
Male cats	The urethra of the male cat is too narrow to accommodate passage of cystoscopes with working channels for laser fibers. However, transurethral laser lithotripsy may be possible in male cats following perineal urethrostomy because the urethral lumen is wider.
Urethral stricture	Urethral strictures may impede the passage of cystoscopes and related equipment used to successfully perform transurethral laser lithotripsy. We commonly encounter urethral strictures in dogs that have undergone urethrostomy surgery or other forms of urethral trauma.
Urinary tract infection	Urinary tract infection increases the propensity for urethral swelling and intravesicular hemorrhage during lithotripsy.
	Infusing the bladder with saline or manually compressing the bladder during voiding urohydropropulsion may cause reflux of bacteria from the urinary bladder into the renal pelvises.
Excessive hematuria	Intravesicular hemorrhage obscures the operator's visibility to accurately aim the laser and retrieve urolith fragments
Large stone burden	Extended procedural time or additional lithotripsy procedures may be required to successfully fragment and remove all uroliths.
Small uroliths	Uroliths likely to pass through the urethral lumen should be managed by voiding urohydropropulsion or basket retrieval.
Equipment Cost	Most veterinary centers purchased either the 20 watt VersaPulse PowerSuite laser sold by Lumenis Inc. or the 30 watt Odyssey 30 manufactured by Convergent Laser Technologies. Costs range from $40,000 to $60,000.

cystogram to assess the lower urinary tract following lithotripsy.

Inspection of the urethra with either type of cystoscope is sufficient to recognize residual urethroliths. Nonetheless, consider a positive contrast urethrogram in cases of considerable urethral trauma or suspected urethral perforation.

We routinely provide antimicrobics (e.g., penicillins, potentiated penicillins, or flouroquinolones) for approximately 4 days to minimize development of iatrogenic urinary tract infection associated with insertion of the cystoscope through the urethra. The need, dose, and duration of prophylactic antimicrobic therapy maybe better determined by the number and magnitude of patient and procedural risk factors that are encountered during lithotripsy. Do not forget that the duration and selection of antimicrobics is best determined by results of follow-up monitoring.

We also administer medication to minimize urinary discomfort (e.g., non-steroidal anti-inflammatory agents or opioids); duration of therapy is variable (e.g., 1–4 days)

and based on the degree of urothelial trauma associated with uroliths and their removal. The need to continue medication to relieve discomfort is based on duration of clinical signs referable to urinary tract pain.

Safety of intracorporeal laser lithotripsy

Bladder and urethral perforation, urethral swelling, hematuria, and leukocyturia have been reported in dogs whose uroliths were managed by laser lithotripsy. (Adams et al. 2008; Grant et al. 2008; Lulich et al. 2008) In one patient, iatrogenic perforation of the urinary tract resolved following transurethral catheterization for 3–7 days. Urethral obstruction due to urethral swelling also resolved following a few days of transurethral catheterization. In a similar manner, hematuria and inflammation abated by the third day following urolith removal. These results indicate that complications are short-lived, and most resolve spontaneously or with medical management. Table 34.4 lists potential complications and strategies to minimize their development.

Table 34.3 Accessories facilitating laser lithotripsy and urolith retrieval

Accessory	Use	Additional information	Source
Biopsy port sealers and adapters	Use to prevent backflow of fluid around laser fibers and other instruments being inserted through the working channel of cystoscopes.	Many types are available. Some are provided with devices such as stone retrieval baskets.	Check-Flow adapter (050885)-Cook Tuohy-Borst Adapter (TBA-6) Cook Urolok II Adapter (730–140) Boston Scientific
Ceramic scissors	Cut off the fractured and frayed end of the laser fiber before each use.	Laser fibers can be reconditioned and used repeatedly.	Ceramic Scissors (C-124) Kyocera Scribe Pen-Lumenis
Inspection scope	Use the inspection scope to evaluate laser fiber integrity prior to fiber sterilization and connection to the laser.	To prevent laser misfiring inspect laser fibers prior to each use.	Inspection Scope-Lumenis
Laser safety goggles	Protective eyewear is needed during laser operation	Laser lithotripsy is relatively safe. However, if the laser is accidentally fired when the tip is not contained within the urinary system, stray laser energy can damage the retina and other tissues in its firing path. Routine corrective lenses will not protect eyes from Holmium: YAG laser energy.	Lumenis Inc. Numerous vendors
Laser ureteral catheter	Insert laser fiber into catheter so the tip of the fiber is not exposed. Insert both into the cystoscope. Before firing the laser, advance the end of the laser fiber out the other end of the protective catheter.	The catheter prevents the sharp end of the laser fiber from damaging the biopsy channel of flexible endoscopes. Catheters also minimize fraying the end of the laser fiber as it is passed through the biopsy channel of cystoscopes.	Laser Ureteral Catheter (022402) Cook
Lithotripsy fibers	Flexible quartz laser fibers transmit laser energy to the surface of the stone.	Laser fibers are available in a variety of diameters (e.g., 200, 365, 550 microns) to accommodate the biopsy channel of any cystoscope. Energy delivered to fragment stones does not vary with fiber diameter; however, smaller fibers can be more expensive.	Laser Fibers (RBLF-200, 365) Laser Peripherals SlimLine 200™, 365™, and 550™. Lumenis ScopeSafe holmium laser fibers, Optical Integrity
Narrow diameter balloon catheters	In male dogs, used to prevent urethroliths and urethrolith fragments from migrating proximally out of the laser field. The balloon at the end of the catheter is positioned in the urethra proximal to the stone prior to its inflation.	Urethroliths are more efficiently fragmented because their movement out of the laser field is limited due to the minimal volume of the urethral lumen.	ClearView Silicon Foley Catheter, SurgiVet Many sizes and vendors
Single action pumping system and tubing.	Attach tubing to flush/biopsy port of flexible endoscope to facilitate administration of flushing solution.	The narrow flush/biopsy channel of flexible endoscopes minimizes adequate flow of flushing solutions. This device overcomes this impediment.	Single Action Pumping System, Boston Scientific

Table 34.3 (*Continued*)

Accessory	Use	Additional information	Source
Stone grasping forceps	In male dogs, some stones can be retrieved and repositioned in the urethra to facilitate lithotripsy.	In general, stone grasping forceps permit easier stone disengagement than stone retrieval baskets.	
Stone retrieval basket	To reposition urocystoliths for fragmentation in the urethra and retrieve stone fragments following lithotripsy	Stone retrieval baskets are available in a variety of sizes and types. Tip-less baskets are preferred because they can retrieve smaller fragments. Many retrieval baskets are marketed for single use, but can be sterilized and reused.	NCircle® Nitinol Tipless Stone Extractors, Cook Urological. Halo Nitinol Tipless Stone Basket, Sacred Heart Medical.
Stripper for laser fiber	Strip approximately 5 mm of plastic coating from the end of laser fibers before each use.	Laser fibers can be reconditioned and used repeatedly. A different gauge stripper is used for each different fiber diameter.	Microstrip precision stripper (Ms1–15 S-18-FS) Slimline
Ureteral access sheath	A human ureteral access sheath is placed in the urethra of male dogs to facilitate clean and rapid access to the urinary bladder. A guide wire is used to facilitate placement of the access sheath.	Lithotripsy is often associated with repeated insertion and repositioning of the endoscope. The access sheath allows clean reinsertions without exteriorizing the penis of male dogs. The sheath protects the urethra from damage during instrumentation and stone retrieval.	Flexor (FUS-095035) Cook
"V" Trough	"V" shaped form padding facilitates positioning female patients in dorsal recumbency.	The trough also facilitates patient repositioning during voiding urohydropropulsion to evacuate stone fragments. Instead of lifting the patient, the trough is tilted such that the head is elevated to position stone fragments in the urethral outflow tract.	

Efficacy of intracorporeal laser lithotripsy

Three studies designed to evaluate the efficacy of the Holmium:YAG laser in dogs with spontaneous uroliths report a complete urolith removal rate of approximately 82% to 84% [6–8]. In all three studies, complete urolith removal was achieved in 100% of dogs with urethroliths. In dogs with urocystoliths, complete urolith removal rate was higher in females (83–96%) than in males (68–81%).

A case-controlled, retrospective study compared 66 dogs whose uroliths were removed with laser lithotripsy to 66 dogs of similar stone burden whose uroliths were removed surgically. (Bevan et al. 2008) Both were equally successful; for every eight procedures, approximately one case required an additional proce-

dure to complete urolith removal. On average, it took 23 minutes longer to manage urinary stones by lithotripsy compared to cystotomy. However, patients undergoing lithotripsy were discharged from the hospital approximately 12 hours sooner. In another report of 23 dogs undergoing laser lithotripsy, 84% were discharged the same day (Grant et al. 2008).

The incorporation of laser lithotripsy epitomizes a paradigm shift in the way uroliths are managed in dogs and cats. With a 100% success rate in the management of urethroliths in dogs, laser lithotripsy abolishes the need to perform disfiguring urethrotomy and urethrostomy surgeries to correct urethral obstruction. Because laser lithotripsy is minimally invasive, patients recover rapidly without the need for restricted activity

Table 34.4 Potential complications when performing transurethral laser lithotripsy

Complication	Occurrence	Avoidance
Bladder rupture	Rare	Bladder perforation is possible during excessive or forced over-distension with fluid, or from direct trauma via careless advancement of cystoscopes and laser fibers. Monitoring bladder fullness and cystoscope position will minimize iatrogenic trauma even in bladders with preexisting weakness.
		Bladder perforation can also occur when incorporating voiding urohydropropulsion to remove urolith fragments. Keeping the size and volume of urolith fragments to a minimum. Insuring adequate anesthesia to promote complete urethral relaxation will minimize excessive intravesical pressure during manual compression. If the integrity of the bladder wall is questionable, remove urolith fragments with a stone retrieval basket.
Cyanide production	Rare	Thermal decomposition of uric acid to cyanide can occur during lithotripsy. However, our attempts to detect cyanide in the effluence during lithotripsy of uroliths composed of purines have been unsuccessful. Nonetheless, continuous irrigation of saline and frequent evacuation of the urinary bladder during lithotripsy is recommended to prevent cyanide from potentially accumulating to harmful concentrations.
Mucosal hemorrhage	Common	Hemorrhage obscures working visibility. In addition to strategies recommended to minimize urethral swelling, use lower laser power settings (0.6 J and 6 watts) to minimize urolith ricocheting during urolith fragmentation
Mucosal perforation	Rare	Mucosal perforation is rare because Holmium: YAG laser energy is delivered in 350 microsecond pulses and is quickly dispersed in fluid surrounding the tip of the laser fiber. Being careful that the laser is activated only when the fiber is in contact with the surface of the stone will avoid urothelial perforation.
Retention of small urolith fragments	Common	Urolith fragments approximately 0.5 mm or less in diameter can become trapped in blood oozing from and attached to denuded urothelium. If not passed, fragments may serve as a nidus for future uroliths. Voiding urohydropropulsion 24 hours or longer following lithotripsy is often sufficient to completely evacuate the bladder. In some cases these minute fragments will spontaneously pass during routine urine voiding
Urethral obstruction	Variable	Complete obstruction is rare because irregular shaped fragments are unlikely to form an occlusive seal within the urethral lumen. However, urethral obstruction may occur when large numbers fragments are voided through the urethra simultaneously. If this occurs, use the laser to break up the fragment conglomeration and reduce fragment size. If anticipated, remove a portion of the fragments with a stone basket prior to voiding urohydropropulsion. Also see urethral swelling below.
Urethral swelling	Common	Urethral swelling impedes evacuation of uroliths and increases the likelihood of urethral obstruction. The degree of swelling is proportional to the frequency with which cystoscopes are passed and urolith fragments removed through the urethral lumen. To minimize this complication, pass well-lubricated scopes gently, select scopes with smaller working diameter than the urethra, fragment stones into smaller fragments before removal, and correct infection prior to lithotripsy. Also consider using a urethral access sheath to protect the urethra. If urethral obstruction is eminent, consider a short period (24 hours) of continuous transurethral catheterization until swelling subsides.

or devices or ointments to prevent premature suture or staple removal. Based on our experience, we recommend that during the initial learning phase, clinicians select female patients because uroliths are easy to target, or dogs with urethroliths because of the short procedure time and extremely high success rate for complete urolith removal. Removal of urethroliths by lithotripsy brings us one step closer to completing our mission of making the surgical removal of uroliths a treatment of historical interest.

References

Adams, L.G., et al. (2008). Use of laser lithotripsy for fragmentation of uroliths in dogs: 73 cases (2005–2006). *J Am Vet Med Assoc* **232**: 1680–1687.

Bevan, J., et al. (2008). Laser lithotripsy and cystotomy are equally effective for management of canine urocystoliths and urethroliths. *J Vet Intern Med* **22**: 732

Chan, K.F., et al. (1999). Holmium: YAG laser lithotripsy: a dominant photothermal ablative mechanism with chemical decomposition of urinary calculia. *Lasers Surg Med* **25**: 22–37.

Dretler, S.P., et al. (1987). Pulsed dye laser fragmentation of ureteral calculi: initial clinical experience. *J Urol* **137**: 386–389.

Grant, D.C., et al. (2008). Holmium: YAG Laser Lithotripsy for urolithiasis in dogs. *J Vet Intern Med* **22**: 534–539.

Lulich, J.P., et al. (2008). Efficacy and safety of laser lithotripsy to manage urocystoliths and urethroliths in dogs: 100 consecutive cases. *J Vet Intern Med* **22**: 732.

Mulvaney, W.P. and C.W. Beck (1968). The laser beam in urology. *J Urol* **99**: 112

Pierre, S. and G.M. Preminger (2007). Holmium laser for stone management. *World J Urol* **25**: 235–239.

Razvi, H.A., et al. (1996). Intracorporeal lithotripsy with the holmium: YAG laser. *J Urol* **156**: 912–914.

35

Canine retrograde urohydropropulsion

Carl A. Osborne, Jody P. Lulich, and David J. Polzin

Overview

Urocystoliths are commonly voided into the urethra of male dogs where they often become lodged adjacent to the caudal aspect of the os penis. On occasion, we have encountered urethroliths in female dogs. If uroliths cause persistent complete obstruction of the urethral lumen, post-renal azotemia will result. If treatment is not provided, death will occur within two to four days. Therefore, safe and cost-effective techniques to restore urine outflow are needed. Refer to the chapter on lithotripsy for details of use of this technique to remove urethroliths.

Once uroliths become lodged in the urethra of male and female dogs, it is very unlikely that they can be removed by the technique of voiding urohydropropulsion. However, in our experience, urethral patency can, with few exceptions, be restored by flushing urethroliths back into the bladder lumen by retrograde urohydropropulsion (Piermattei and Osborne 1971; Osborne and Lees 1995; Osborne et al. 1995; Osborne and Polzin 1999). The efficacy of this technique is related to dilation of a portion of the urethra containing urethroliths with fluid under pressure. However, to be consistently successful, one must be familiar with all aspects of the technique. In our experience, unfamiliarity with the details of this technique is often associated with failure to remove all of the urethroliths. In this chapter, we emphasize aspects of the technique that are frequently overlooked by colleagues who have consulted with us when they were unsuccessful in restoring urethral patency with this procedure. Appropriate care must be taken to minimize trauma and pain to various components of the urinary tract, and iatrogenic urinary tract infection.

Summary of major steps for retrograde urohydropropulsion

1. Verify and localize the urethroliths with the aid of appropriate imaging procedure(s).
2. Decompress the urinary bladder by cystocentesis. Save representative aliquots of pretreatment urine for urinalysis and urine culture.
3. Lubricate the urethral lumen to facilitate retropropulsion of urethroliths.
4. Develop an anesthetic plan based on the overall status of each patient.
5. Perform retrograde urohydropropulsion.
6. Minimize catheter-induced trauma to various components of the urinary tract, and use the appropriate technique to minimize iatrogenic urinary tract infection.
7. Consider an appropriate technique to manage the urocystoliths.

Equipment

Either rigid or flexible urethral catheters may be used. The advantage of using a flexible urethral catheter is that it permits placement of the top of the plunger (aka a piston) on the table so that the barrel of the syringe can be pushed down on the plunger (Figure 35.1). Advancing the syringe barrel over the plunger allows greater pressure to be generated within the isolated segment of the urethral lumen containing the uroliths compared to conventional use of the syringe.

Large capacity syringes, 22-gauge hypodermic needles, and intravenous extension sets will facilitate atraumatic cystocentesis. The length of the 22-gauge needle should be adequate to easily reach a point mid-way between the bladder vertex and the junction of the urethra and the bladder neck. Depending on the size of the patient, and

Nephrology and Urology of Small Animals. Edited by Joe Bartges and David J. Polzin. © 2011 Blackwell Publishing Ltd.

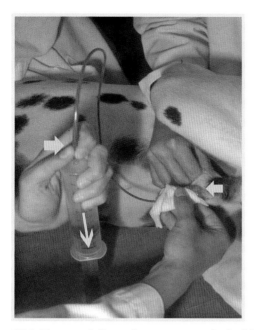

Figure 35.1 Photograph illustrating correct use of a flexible urethral catheter to increase pressure generated with syringe plunger. Arrow heads point to digital pressure applied to junction of catheter with syringe and digital pressure applied to external urethral orifice. Large arrow points to barrel of syringe being advanced over syringe plunger.

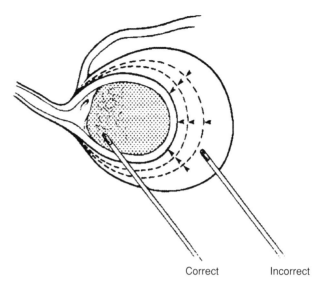

Correct   Incorrect

Figure 35.3 Schematic drawing illustrating correct and incorrect sites of insertion of a needle into the bladder for the purpose of decompressing the overdistended lumen. The needle should be inserted in the ventral or ventrolateral surface of the wall cranial to the junction of the bladder neck with the urethra. This will permit removal of a large volume of urine and decompression of the lumen without need for reinsertion of the needle into the bladder.

the distance of the ventral bladder wall from the ventral abdominal wall, 1.5-inch hypodermic or 3-inch spinal needles may be selected (Figures 35.2 and 35.3).

Two large capacity syringes, a three-way connecting valve, a flexible urethral catheter, sterilized aqueous lubricant, and sterilized isotonic saline (or its equivalent) will be needed to inject a lubricant around the uroliths (Figures 35.4 and 35.5). We recommend that the lubricant

mixture be prepared by connecting the tips of two large-capacity syringes using a three-way valve. One syringe can be partially filled by aseptically removing the syringe plunger and adding an appropriate quantity of sterilized lubricant (such as K-Y Jelly). The other syringe should be partially filled with sterilized saline solution. After closing the outflow port, injection of these solutions back and forth between the syringes will result in a sterilized solution of reduced viscosity that can be readily injected through a urethral catheter.

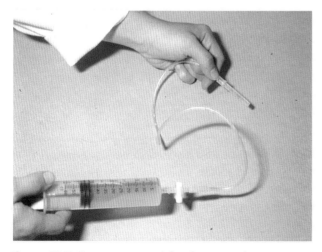

Figure 35.2 Components used for decompressive cystocentesis: Large capacity syringe; Flexible intravenous tubing, 22-gauge needle.

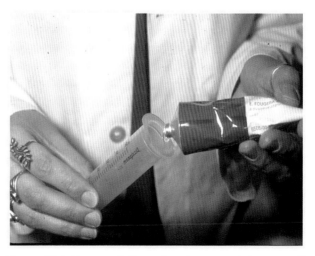

Figure 35.4 Photograph illustrating placement of viscous sterilized aqueous K-Y Jelly into the barrel of a large-capacity syringe.

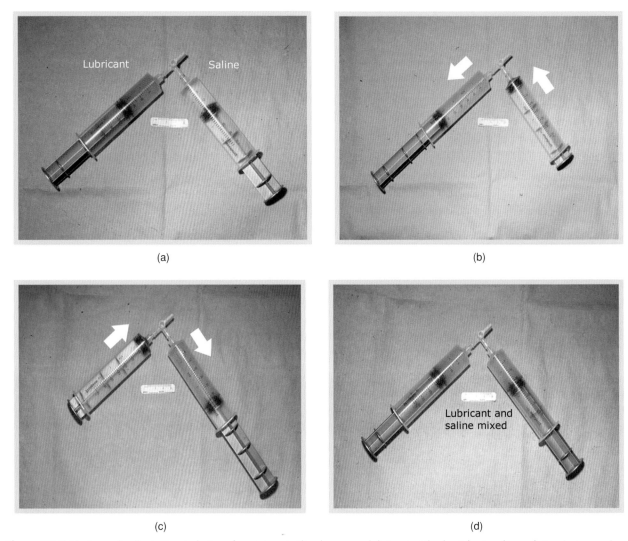

(a)

(b)

(c)

(d)

Figure 35.5 Photographs illustrating technique for mixing sterilized aqueous lubricant with physiologic saline solution in two syringes connected by a three-way valve. (a) Sterile lubricant is contained in syringe on left and sterile physiologic saline solution is contained in syringe on right; (b) the physiologic saline solution is injected into the syringe containing the sterile lubricant; (c) The saline-lubricant mixture is then injected back into the empty syringe; (d) The process is continued until the lubricant and saline are mixed.

Selection of syringe size for urohydropropulsion may substantially affect the volume and pressure of saline in the system. Application of the Law of LaPlace to fluid mechanics indicates that the pressure of a liquid (or gas) within a cylinder is inversely proportional to the radius of the cylinder. Therefore, a 60 milliliter syringe would decrease the pressure that could be created in the system compared to the pressure that could be created with a smaller capacity syringe (i.e., 35 mL or 20 mL capacity syringe). Using this logic, use of a 6- or 12-milliliter syringe could potentially generate more pressure than a 20- or 35-milliliter syringe provided sufficient saline was available to fill the lumen of the catheter and to fill and distend the urethra fluid under pressure. Although adequate pressure may be generated, for most dogs, the volume contained in 6- or 12-milliliter syringes is insufficient to prime the system. Since the 60 mL syringe would likely contain enough saline to fill the lumens of the catheter and urethra, but would be incapable of generating as much pressure as the 20 or 35 milliliter system, while the 12-milliliter syringe would likely generate enough pressure, but contain an insufficient volume of saline to distend the urethra and fill the lumen of the catheter, the 20 or 35 mL syringe system is the compromise likely to be most effective. Compared to the larger and smaller syringes, they have the capacity to generate sufficient pressure and contain an adequate volume of liquid to propel urethroliths back into the bladder lumen (Figure 35.6).

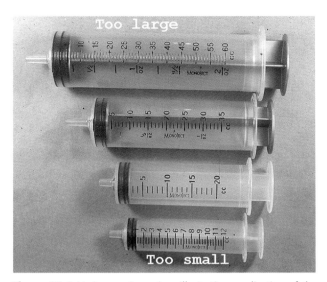

Figure 35.6 Various syringe sizes illustrating application of the Law of LaPlace, which states that pressure is inversely proportional to radius; therefore, syringes with a smaller radius require a higher pressure.

Steps for retrograde urohydropropulsion

Step 1. Verification and localization of urethroliths

Perform appropriate diagnostic procedures to localize the sites of urethrolith(s), and evaluate their number, size, radiodensity, and surface characteristics. Since uroliths rarely form in the urethra, but migrate from the bladder lumen into the urethra be sure to include the urinary bladder in the evaluation. Palpation of the posterior urethra (including palpation of the urethra per rectum) followed by appropriate survey or contrast radiography should be performed to establish the site(s) and cause(s) of outflow obstruction. Ultrasonography may be of value in evaluation of the urinary bladder. If the urethroliths become lodged in an unusual or unexpected location in context of the caudal aspect of the os penis, use contrast urethrography to rule out mural and/or extramural urethral lesions that are contributing to outflow obstruction. If the patient has signs of systemic illness, or if the history suggests prolonged outflow obstruction, pretreatment urine and blood samples should be obtained to assess renal function, and systemic fluid, electrolyte, and acid–base status.

Step 2. Decompressive cystocentesis

Benefits versus risks

If obstruction to urine outflow has already resulted in over-distension of the bladder lumen, it should be decompressed by cystocentesis. To prevent iatrogenic over-distension of the bladder, decompressive cystocentesis should generally be performed prior to urohydropropulsion.

Some *benefits* of performing decompressive cystocentesis prior to performing retrograde urohydropropulsion are: (1) an uncontaminated representative urine sample suitable for analysis and culture is obtained; (2) decompression of an overdistended urinary bladder by removing most (but not all) of the urine provides a mechanism to temporarily ameliorate discomfort and continued adverse effects of obstructive urethropathy (irrespective of cause); and (3) decompression of an overdistended urinary bladder and proximal urethra may decrease resistance to retrograde movement of urethroliths into the bladder lumen. Failure to decompress an overdistended urinary bladder prior to retrograde urohydropropulsion may result in impaired ability to flush urethroliths into the urinary bladder (Table 35.1). If excessive pressure is created in the overdistended bladder lumen, it will rupture.

The potential *risks* of performing decompressive cystocentesis are that: (1) it may result in extravasation of urine into the bladder wall and/or peritoneal cavity, and (2) it may injure the bladder wall or surrounding structures. Although these complications could be severe in patients with a devitalized bladder wall, in our experience this has been a very uncommon exception rather than the rule provided that the majority, but not all, of the urine is removed from the bladder before initiating urohydropropulsion. Intraperitoneal extravasation of a small quantity of urine through the pathway created by 22-gauge hypodermic needle is usually of little consequence. The potential of trauma to the bladder and adjacent structures can be minimized by proper technique.

We are not advocating an "always or never" recommendation regarding decompressive cystocentesis. Clinical judgment is required regarding its use in each patient. However, it is preferable to decompress the urinary bladder by cystocentesis (saving an aliquot for appropriate diagnostic tests) prior to performing retrograde urohydropropulsion in patients: (1) likely to have adequate integrity of the bladder wall, and (2) in which immediate over-distension of the bladder lumen, which predisposes to loss of urine into the bladder wall and peritoneal cavity, is prevented by serially performed decompressive cystocentesis.

Technique of decompressive cystocentesis (Figures 35.2 and 35.3)

We recommend that a 22-gauge needle be attached to a flexible intravenous extension set which in turn is attached to a large-capacity syringe. After the needle is

Table 35.1 Preventable causes of failure of retrograde urohydropropulsion

I. Technique factors:
    A. Failure to lubricate uroliths.
    B. Inadequate pressure/insufficient urethral dilation.
        1. Catheter size too small.
        2. Syringe size too small or too large.
        3. Saline volume too small.
        4. Insufficient pressure applied to syringe plunger.
        5. Lack of complete digital occlusion of urethra.
    C. Resistance to retrograde flushing caused by overdistended bladder.
    D. Lack of coordination between individuals performing technique.
    E. Inadequate pharmacologic control of patient discomfort.
    F. Premature discontinuation of procedure before stones returned to bladder lumen.
II. Patient factors:
    A. Discomfort resulting movement and impaired ability to properly restrain patient.
    B. Rough surface of uroliths (silica; calcium oxalate dihydrate) impairing attempts to move them into the bladder lumen.
    C. Narrowing of urethral lumen (inflammatory swelling; strictures) proximal to site of urethroliths.

inserted into the bladder lumen, one individual should digitally immobilize the urinary bladder containing the tip of the 22-gauge needle, while another aspirates urine from the bladder lumen through the flexible intravenous tubing into a large-capacity syringe. Gentle agitation of the distended bladder in an up-and-down motion *prior* to cystocentesis may disperse particulate matter or crystals throughout the urine, and thus facilitate their aspiration into the collection system.

The bladder should be emptied as completely as is consistent with the atraumatic technique. Attempts to completely evacuate all urine from the bladder lumen is contra-indicated since this mistake predisposes the patient to iatrogenic trauma of the bladder mucosa and underlying tissues with the sharp point of the needle. Depending on the size of the dog, we typically allow about 15–20 mL of urine to remain in the bladder lumen.

In the event patency of the urethra is not established before the bladder fills with urine and fluid is used to back-flush the urethra, decompressive cystocentesis should be repeated before over-distension of the bladder lumen recurs. On occasion, we have used serial decompressive cystocentesis over a span of several days because of problems in restoring urethral patency.

Step 3. Lubrication of urethroliths (Figures 35.4 and 35.5)

Failure to properly lubricate the urethroliths prior to retrograde urohydropulsion may result in inability to flush them into the urinary bladder (Table 35.1).

A liberal quantity of a mixture of one to three parts of sterilized physiologic saline solution (or a comparable parenteral isotonic fluid such as lactated Ringer's solution) to one part of aqueous lubricant should be injected through a catheter into the urethral lumen adjacent to the uroliths (Figures 35.4 and 35.5). This maneuver helps to lubricate the surface of the urolith(s) and the urethral mucosa, which is often inflamed and swollen.

There may be some risk associated with injecting aqueous lubricants into the urinary tract of patients known to have tears in the wall of the urethra or urinary bladder. Aqueous lubricants have been implicated in the formation of periurethral granulomas in human beings (Read et al. 1961) and rabbits (Blaine 1947). However, to date, we have not recognized this problem following use of this technique in hundreds dogs with obstructive urethroliths.

Step 4. Restraint and anesthesia

Some form of sedation or general anesthesia is required for most patients. Pharmacologic agents dependent on renal metabolism or excretion for inactivation and elimination from the body should be avoided. If an uncooperative patient is an anesthetic risk because of a uremic crisis, topical application of lidocaine gel to the urethral mucosa in combination with parenteral administration of a low dose of analgesic may provide adequate patient restraint.

General anesthesia should be used if uroliths cannot be removed from the urethra of non-anesthetized patients by urohydropulsion. Inadequate pharmacologic control of patient discomfort may result in failure to flush the urethroliths into the bladder lumen (Table 35.1). Appropriate precautions should be used for patients in renal failure since they are more sensitive to general anesthesia than normal patients.

A combination of intramuscularly administered oxymorphone (0.1–0.2 mg/kg) followed by slow intravenous administration of propofol (an ultra-short acting anesthetic) with dose titration to effect has been an excellent choice. Propofol is highly protein bound; it is rapidly conjugated in the liver to inactive metabolites. However, neither sedation nor anesthesia produced by propofol is associated with complete relief of pain. Therefore, propofol should be combined with oxymorphone. To avoid apnea, propofol should be slowly administered by the intravenous route. In addition, because propofol administration may be associated with depressant cardiovascular and respiratory effects (especially arterial hypotension), it is imperative that hydration of the patient be adequate prior to anesthesia. If necessary, propofol anesthesia may be prolonged by frequent incremental intravenous injections, or by constant intravenous infusion of low doses. Once urethral patency has been restored, the effects of oxymorphone can be antagonized with nalbuphine HCl (0.03–0.1 mg/kg IV) if continued analgesia is desired, or naloxone (0.002–0.02 mg/kg IV) if respiratory depression is of greater concern.

Inhalant anesthetics may also be considered to anesthetize the patient if the drugs are not dependent on the kidneys for inactivation and excretion from the body.

Step 5. Technique of retrograde urohydropropulsion (Figures 35.7–35.10)

Step 5A procedure for male dogs (Figures 35.7 and 35.8)

To remove uroliths from male dogs by retrograde urohydropropulsion, we recommend the following proce-

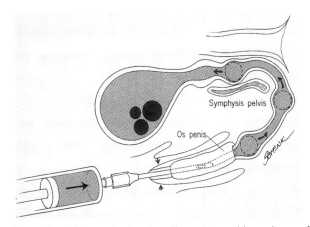

Figure 35.8 Schematic drawing illustrating sudden release of digital pressure at the pelvic urethra and subsequent movement of fluid propelling the urethrolith toward the bladder lumen.

dure: (Osborne and Polzin 1986; Osborne and Lees 1995)

1. Inject a liberal quantity of a mixture of sterilized saline solution and aqueous lubricant through a flexible catheter into the urethral lumen adjacent to the uroliths.

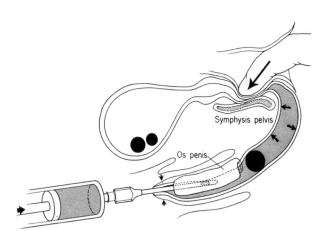

Figure 35.7 Retrograde urohydropropulsion of urethrolith in a male dog. Dilation of the urethral lumen is achieved by injecting fluid with considerable pressure. Digital pressure applied to the external urethral orifice and the pelvic urethra has created a closed system.

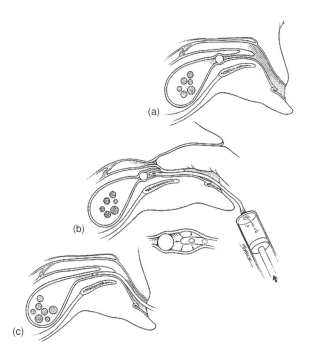

Figure 35.9 Schematic illustration of urohydropropulsion in a female dog with a solitary urethrolith using a conventional urinary catheter. (a) Urolith originating from the bladder has obstructed the urethra. (b) Small portion of the urethral lumen distal to the urethrolith and proximal to a site occluded by digital pressure applied through the vaginal wall has been expanded by injecting saline solution through the catheter. (c) The urolith has been forced back into the bladder lumen, eliminating obstruction to urine outflow.

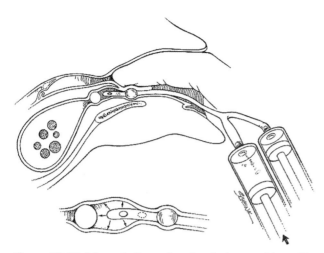

Figure 35.10 Schematic illustration of urohydropropulsion utilizing a Swan-Ganz balloon catheter. Inflation of the balloon with air helps to prevent reflux of saline solution out of the external urethral orifice.

2. Next, an assistant should insert a lubricated gloved index finger into the rectum. Firmly occlude the lumen of the pelvic urethra by applying digital pressure against the ischium through the ventral wall of the rectum (Figure 35.7).

3. A flexible catheter with an attached 20–35 mL syringe filled with sterilized saline should then be inserted into the lumen of the penile urethra via the external urethral orifice and advanced to the site of the urethroliths. The penile urethra should be compressed around the shaft of the catheter by firm digital pressure. As a result of steps 5A-2 and 5A-3, a portion of the urethra from the external urethral orifice to the bony pelvis becomes a closed system. Failure to properly occlude the pelvic and/or the distal-most portion urethral lumen will result in impaired ability to flush the urethroliths into the urinary bladder (Table 35.1; Figure 35.7).

4. Saline should be injected into the urethra until a marked increase in the diameter of the pelvic urethra is perceived by the assistant. Confirmation that the urethra has been markedly distended is important because distention of the urethra to its maximum capacity must be achieved before a sufficient degree of pressure can be created within the urethral lumen to advance the uroliths. Failure to create sufficient pressure in the urethral lumen often results in inability to flush the urethroliths into the urinary bladder (Table 35.1). The likelihood of rupture of the urethral lumen as a result of intraluminal pressure generated by this technique is remote since the path of least resistance for fluid is through the urethra into the bladder lumen and/or out the external

urethral orifice. However, caution must be exercised not to rupture the urinary bladder by over-distending the lumen with the flushing solution. Therefore, the size of the bladder should be monitored at appropriate intervals by abdominal palpation. If and when it becomes full, decompressive cystocentesis should be repeated.

5. At this point, the lumen of all portions of the isolated urethra, except that located in the ventral groove of the os penis, will be markedly dilated (Figure 35.7). Dilation of the lumen of the segment of the urethra located in the ventral groove of the os penis is limited to that caused by stretching of the ventral portion of the urethral wall.

6. Next, digital pressure applied to the pelvic urethra (but not the penile urethra) should be rapidly released (Figure 35.8). Pressure should be maintained in the urethral lumen by continuing to inject saline by pushing the syringe barrel over the syringe plunger after the assistant has released digital pressure applied through the rectal wall. This step requires coordination between the two individuals performing the technique (Table 35.1). When properly coordinated, this step will propel the saline mixture and the urethroliths toward (or into) the bladder lumen (Figure 35.8). Often, especially in cases where the uroliths have recently passed into the urethra, as the digital pressure applied to the intrapelvic urethra wall is released, the urethroliths are easily flushed into the bladder lumen during the first attempt. However, in some situations, the uroliths do not move, or only move a short distance, before the pressure in the urethral lumen has dissipated. If this occurs it may be necessary to repeat the procedure several times before all the uroliths reach the bladder lumen). The position of the urolith(s) may be monitored either by means of palpation of the perineal and pelvic urethra, with the aid of a catheter carefully advanced through, and/or by means of radiography. If it is necessary to repeat the technique, accumulation of large amounts of saline and urine in the lumen of the bladder will necessitate repeating decompressive cystocentesis.

5B Female dogs (Figures 35.9 and 35.10)

Uroliths lodged in the urethra of female dogs may also be returned to the urinary bladder by following a modified procedure of retrograde urohydropropulsion. (Osborne et al. 1983)

1. Inject a liberal quantity of a mixture of sterilized saline solution and aqueous lubricant through a flexible catheter into the urethral lumen adjacent to the uroliths (Figure 35.9). Do not remove the catheter

from the urethra. With a gloved index finger in the rectum or (if the patient is large enough) in the vagina, firmly occlude the lumen of the distal end of the urethra containing the catheter (Figure 35.9). This creates a closed system between the occluding urolith and the site of digital compression of the urethra.

2. After lubrication of the urolith(s), inject saline solution through a catheter to distend the isolated portion of the urethral lumen to its maximum. Dilation of the urethra combined with pressure generated by the intraluminal saline solution usually propels the urolith(s) into the bladder lumen. Gentle digital manipulation of the urolith through the rectal or vaginal wall may aid in moving it toward the bladder.

3. Movement of a large urolith lodged in the neck of the bladder and proximal portion of the urethra may require digital manipulation of the urolith per abdomen by an assistant while saline solution is injected through the catheter.

4. If intraurethral pressure rapidly dissipates because of reflux of saline solution through the external urethral orifice, it may be necessary to repeat the procedure several times before the uroliths reach the urinary bladder. The position of the urolith(s) may be monitored by digital palpation, attempts to advance the catheter, radiography, and/or ultrasonography.

5. If difficulty is encountered in occluding the external urethral orifice around the catheter, a 4–7 Fr balloon catheter (i.e., a flow directed angiographic catheter or a small pediatric Foley catheter) may be used (Figure 35.10). Inflation of the balloon after it has been inserted into the distal urethra combined with firm digital pressure may be effective in minimizing reflux of saline solution through the external urethral orifice.

Step 6. Minimize catheter-induced trauma to the urinary tract, and iatrogenic urinary tract infection

To minimize catheter-associated infection, catheters, lubricants, irrigating solutions, specula, and other instruments should be sterilized. However, because the distal portion of the urethra normally contains a commensal population of bacteria, it is impossible to aseptically catheterize the patient. (Osborne and Lees 1995)

The need for prophylactic antibacterial therapy following retrograde urohydropropulsion must be determined on the basis of the status of the patient and retrospective evaluation of technique. If it is probable that the dog has ongoing UTI, or if restoration of urethral patency is associated with substantial trauma and/ or trauma to

the lower genitourinary tract, appropriate antimicrobial therapy should be considered. Remember to obtain pre-treatment urine samples for urinalysis and bacterial urine culture.

If, following restoration of urethral patency, the decision to use an indwelling transurethral catheter is being considered, the likelihood of inducing an iatrogenic bacterial infection must be considered. Ascending migration of bacteria through the lumen of the catheter may be minimized by use of closed drainage systems that prevent reflux of urine from the collection receptacle back into the urinary tract (Osborne and Lees 1995). However, bacteria may gain access to the bladder lumen by migrating through the space between the outside surface of the indwelling transurethral catheter and the surface of the urethral mucosa. The question is not whether urinary tract infection will occur, but rather when urinary tract infection will occur.

Never forcefully advance the catheter through the lumen of the urethra! Trauma to the urethral wall is the usual consequence of use of excessive force, and may result in acute inflammatory swelling followed by formation of irreversible strictures. Over-insertion of excessive lengths of catheter should also be avoided to minimize trauma to the bladder, and/or to prevent the catheter from becoming knotted or entangled within the bladder and/or urethral lumens.

At one time, a common method used to attempt move urethroliths that occluded the urethra was pushing them back into the bladder with a catheter. However, this technique is not currently recommended because it is associated with: (1) a high risk of urethral trauma (abrasion, contusion, laceration, or puncture); (2) inflammatory constriction of the urethral lumen at the site where the catheter was forced past the urolith; (3) a high risk of secondary urinary tract infection; and; (4) a high rate of failure. If advancement of a catheter beyond a urethrolith cannot be achieved without excessive trauma to the urethra, it should be abandoned in favor of other non-surgical or surgical methods. If the urolith can be moved easily by inserting a catheter into the urethral lumen, our experience has been that it also can be moved readily by retrograde urohydropulsion with far less chance of iatrogenic trauma.

References

Blaine, G. (1947). Experimental observations on absorbable alginale products in surgery. *Ann Surg* **125**: 1022–1114.

Osborne, C.A., et al. (1983). Nonsurgical removal of uroliths from the urethra of female dogs. *J Am Vet Med Assoc* **182**: 47–50.

Osborne, C.A. and D.J. Polzin (1986). Nonsurgical management of canine obstructive urolithopathy. *Vet Clin North Am* **16**: 333–347.

Osborne, C.A. and G.E. Lees (1995). Bacterial infections of the canine and feline urinary tract. In: *Canine and Feline Nephrology and Urology*, edited by C.A. Osborne and D.R. Finco. Baltimore, MD: Williams and Wilkins, pp. 759–797.

Osborne, C.A., et al. (1999). Canine retrograde urohydropropulsion. Lessons from 25 years experience. *Vet Clin North Am* **29**: 267–281.

Piermattei, D.L. and C.A. Osborne (1971). Nonsurgical removal of calculi from the urethra of male dogs. *J Am Vet Med Assoc* **159**: 1755–1757.

Read, R.J., et al. (1961). Granulomas induced by surgical lubricating jelly. *J Clin Pathol* **36**: 41–48.

36

Feline urethral obstruction

Carl A. Osborne, Jody P. Lulich, and David J. Polzin

Overview-diagnostics

Before considering various aspects of treatment designed for urethral obstruction, the fact that obstructive urethropathy can be caused by one or more intra-luminal, mural, or extramural abnormalities, located at one or more sites, should be considered (Table 36.1). Why is this important? Because, techniques designed to eliminate plugs or stones that are obstructing the urethral lumen would likely have little or no effect on correcting obstructive lesions located within the urethral wall or periurethral tissue. Therefore, inability to restore urethral patency by decompressive cystocentesis followed by flushing the urethral lumen should arouse one's suspicion that mural or periurethral lesions are causing outflow obstruction in addition to, or instead of, a firmly lodged urethral plug or urethrolith.

Correcting intraluminal urethral obstructions

Following selection of a method of patient restraint designed to minimize adverse drug reactions and iatrogenic trauma to the lower urinary tract, we recommend a step-by-step priority of procedures to remove matrix-crystalline plugs or uroliths obstructing the urethral lumen (Osborne et al. 1995). In order of priority they are: (1) massage of distal urethra followed by step (2), an attempt to induce voiding by gentle palpation of the urinary bladder (Figure 36.1). If steps 1 and 2 are unsuccessful, proceed to step (3), decompressive cystocentesis (Figures 36.2–36.4), followed by step (4) urethral flushing (Figures 36.5–36.7).

Sometime's we use combinations of steps 1 to 4. If steps 1 to 4 are unsuccessful, the next step is use of appropriate

Nephrology and Urology of Small Animals. Edited by Joe Bartges and David J. Polzin. © 2011 Blackwell Publishing Ltd.

contrast radiology, ultrasonography, and/or endoscopy to determine if the cause of urethral obstruction is intra-luminal, mural, and/or extramural. If irreversible mural or extramural disorders are responsible for persistent or frequently recurrent urethral obstruction, surgical management may be required. Let us consider each of these steps in greater detail.

STEP 1. *Gentle Massage* of the penis between the thumb and fingers may help to dislodge matrix-crystalline plugs located in the distal urethra. If necessary, the penis may be manipulated while it is retracted within the prepuce. Although this step is often ineffective, its simplicity and occasional success make it worth trying prior to consideration of decompressive cystocentesis and urethral catheterization. Massage may disrupt plug material packed into the penile urethra to such a degree that subsequent attempts to induce micturition by gentle palpation of the urinary bladder may result in the plug being voided (Figure 36.1).

STEP 2. Inability of a cat to void urine spontaneously indicates that increasing intraurethral pressure by *digitally compressing +the urinary bladder* is unlikely to be effective. However, if this technique is utilized *following* urethral massage (Bardelli et al. 1999), sufficient intraluminal pressure may be generated to dislodge fragments of urethral precipitates. *Caveat*-Caution must be used to prevent iatrogenic damage to the urinary bladder.

STEP 3. In general, *decompressive cystocentesis* should be performed if steps 1 and 2 are ineffective in re-establishing urethral patency (Table 36.2, Figures 36.2–36.4). The *benefits* of performing decompressive cystocentesis prior to flushing the urethral lumen via a catheter are: (1) a urine sample suitable for analysis and culture may be obtained; (2) decompression of an overdistended urinary bladder by removing most (but not all) of the urine provides a mechanism to temporarily halt the continued adverse effects of obstructive

Table 36.1 Diagnostic rule-outs for urethral obstruction in male cats

Primary causes	Iatrogenic causes	Perpetuating causes
Intraluminal	**Intraluminal**	**Tissue damage**
Urethral plugs (matrix and/or crystals)	Increased production of inflammatory reactants red blood cells, white cells, fibrin, etc.	Reverse flushing solutions
Urethroliths	Sloughed tissue	Catheter-induced trauma
Tissue sloughed from urinary bladder and/or urethra		Catheter-induced foreign body reaction
		Catheter-induced infection
Mural or Extramural	**Mural**	**Postsurgical dysfunction**
Strictures	Inflammatory swelling	Strictures
Urethral neoplasms	Muscular spasm	
Prostate neoplasms	Reflex dyssnergia	
Reflex dyssnergia	Strictures	
Anomalies		
Combinations	**Combinations**	**Combinations**

back-pressure irrespective of cause; (3) the magnitude of pain caused by overdistension of the bladder and urethra may be reduced; (4) decompression of an overdistended urinary bladder and proximal urethra may facilitate repulsion of a urethral plug or urolith into the bladder lumen; and (5) the gross and microscopic character of aspirated urine may provide valuable clues about the nature of the obstructive disorder (intra-luminal precipitates of matrix and crystalline material versus mural or extraluminal compression (Figure 36.4). Urine that contains large quantities of visible precipitates indicates that the patient is at risk of obstruction following subsequent flushing of the urethral lumen (Figure 36.4).

The potential *risks* of performing decompressive cystocentesis are that: (1) it may result in extravasation of urine into the bladder wall and/or peritoneal cavity, (2) it may injure the bladder wall or surrounding structures, and (3) on rare occasions cystocentesis has been associated with sudden collapse in cats. Although a cause and effect relationship has not been established, stimulation of the vagus has been implicated. Acute over-distension of the bladder has been associated with bradycardia in two humans (Koch et al. 2001). In another case report, enhancement of baroreceptor heart-rate

Figure 36.1 Photograph of the external urethral orifice (big arrow) of an obstructed 3-year-old male cat after digital manipulation of the distal portion of the urethra and then manual compression of the urinary bladder. Fragments of a matrix-crystalline plug (small arrows) are visible on the microscope slide.

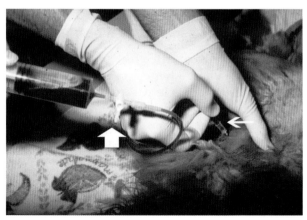

Figure 36.2 A 22-gauge needle has been attached to one end of a flexible intravenous extension set (small arrow), and a three-way valve (large arrow). A large capacity syringe has been attached to the other end of the 3-way valve. The intravenous extension set allows one individual to immobilize the 22-gauge needle inserted into the bladder lumen while the movement associated with aspirating urine into the syringe is unlikely to cause unwanted movement of the sharp tip of the needle in the bladder lumen.

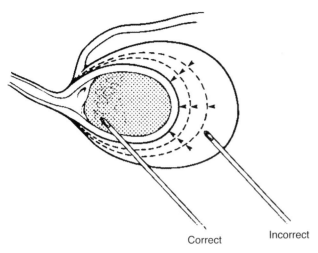

Correct   Incorrect

Figure 36.3 Correct and incorrect sites of insertion of a 22-guage needle into the urinary bladder for the purpose of removing large quantities of urine. The needle should be inserted in the ventral or ventro-lateral surface of the wall cranial to the junction of the bladder neck with the urethra. The correct position permits removal of a large volume of urine and decompression of the lumen without need for reinsertion of the needle into the bladder.

sensitivity occurred following distension of the urinary bladder in patients with essential hypertension. (Bardelli et al. 1999) In our experience, these events have been the rare exception rather than the rule. A key point is the importance of preventing overdistension of the bladder by repeating serial cystocentesis until adequate urine outflow is restored. Loss of a small quantity of urine into the peritoneal cavity has been of little consequence, especially

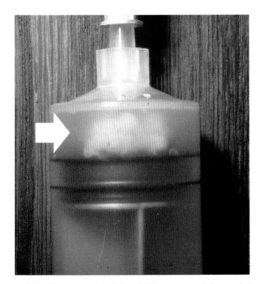

Figure 36.4 Photograph of insoluble material (arrow) in urine aspirated by cystocentesis from the urinary bladder of an obstructed male cat. This type of abnormality is a risk factor for recurrence of obstruction and should be considered in the recommendation for therapy with an indwelling transurethral catheter.

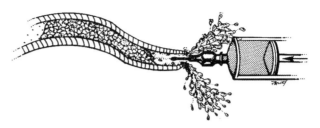

Figure 36.5 Illustration of flushing of a male cat's urethra containing a matrix-crystalline plug. After insertion of a Minnesota olive-tipped catheter, a large quantity of saline is injected the urethral lumen and allowed to reflux out of the distal urethra.

if it does not contain pathogens. The potential of trauma to the bladder and adjacent structures can be minimized by proper technique. In context of minimizing acute collapse, sedating frightened patients to minimize hypertension, and trying to avoid creating excessive pressure caused by overdistending the bladder lumen with fluid used to flush the urethra should be considered.

We do not advocate an "always or never" recommendation regarding decompressive cystocentesis. Clinical judgment is required regarding its use in each patient. However, it is preferable to decompress the urinary bladder by cystocentesis, saving an aliquot of urine for appropriate diagnostic tests, prior to flushing the urethral

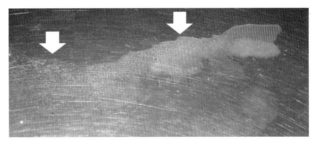

Figure 36.6 Photograph of matrix and crystals on the surface of a stainless steel table-top after flushing the urethral lumen as described in Figure 36.5.

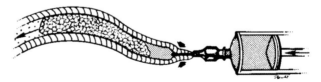

Figure 36.7 Schematic illustration of reverse flushing a male cat's urethral lumen obstructed by a matrix-crystalline plug. After insertion of the Minnesota Olive-Tipped Urethral Catheter (thin long white arrow), digital pressure is used to seal the distal portion of the penile urethra around the olive-tip (fat short white arrows). Then, saline is injected into the urethral lumen with the objective of flushing the plug into the bladder lumen.

Table 36.2 Technique of decompressive cystocentesis

1. Attach a 22-gauge needle to one end of a flexible intravenous extension set, and attach to a three-way valve and large capacity syringe (35–60 mL) to the other end. Use of a large capacity syringe minimizes unnecessary manipulation, and therefore reduces the likelihood of trauma to the bladder wall. The intravenous extension set will allow one individual to immobilize the 22-gauge needle inserted into the bladder lumen while another person aspirates urine into the syringe (Figure 36.1).

2. The 22-gauge needle should be inserted through the ventral or ventrolateral wall of the bladder to minimize trauma to the ureters and adjacent major abdominal vessels (Figure 36.2). The needle should be inserted midway between the vertex of the bladder surface and the junction of the bladder with the urethra. This will permit removal of urine and decompression of the bladder lumen. If the needle is placed in or adjacent to the vertex of the bladder, it may not remain within the lumen as the bladder shrinks in size.

3. Excessive digital pressure should not be applied to the bladder wall while the needle is in its lumen lest urine be forced around the needle into the peritoneal cavity. Caution should also be taken to prevent laceration of the bladder as a result of movement of the needle. The bladder should be emptied as completely as is consistent with atraumatic technique. Attempts to remove all the urine from the bladder lumen is undesirable as the sharp point of the needle may than damage the bladder wall. Allow 15–20 mL of urine to remain in the bladder.

4. In the event patency of the urethra is not established before the bladder refills with urine or solutions used to flush the urethra, decompressive cystocentesis should be repeated. On occasion we have used serial cystocentesis over a span of several days because of problems of restoring urethral patency.

5. The need for prophylactic antibacterial therapy following cystocentesis must be determined on the basis of the status of the patient and retrospective evaluation of technique. If subsequent restoration of urethral patency requires intermittent or indwelling catheterization, preventative antimicrobial therapy should be considered after the catheter is removed. Remember to obtain pre-treatment samples for urinalysis and bacterial culture.

lumen in patients: (1) likely to have adequate integrity of the bladder wall, and (2) in which immediate overdistension of the bladder lumen is not allowed to recur (Osborne et al. 1996).

STEP 4. *Flushing the urethral lumen* with sterilized solutions following urethral catheterization may dislodge urethral plugs and uroliths (Table 36.3). However, it is emphasized that urethral obstruction may be caused by a combination of intra-luminal precipitates (uroliths or matrix-crystalline urethral plugs), swelling of the urethral wall, and/or spasm of urethral musculature (Table 36.1).

Reverse flushing solutions should be selected thoughtfully since accumulation and absorption of large quantities of acid or anesthetic solutions from an inflamed urinary bladder may cause systemic toxicity. In addition, they may damage the coating of glycosaminoglycans (GAGS) that lines the surface of the urothelium. Glycosaminoglycans normally minimize adherence of crystals and microbes to the urethral mucosa (Osborne et al. 1996). Adherence of crystals to the urothelium is most likely to occur if acidic solutions are used in an attempt to dissolve struvite crystals. Pending results of further studies, we prefer physiological saline or lactated Ringer's solution because they are readily available, sterilized, nontoxic, nonirritating, and economical. We do not recommend buffered acetic acid (so-called Walpole's solution).

STEP 5. Inability to establish adequate urethral patency by use of catheters and reverse flushing should arouse a high index of suspicion that the underlying cause is not a urethral plug (Table 36.1). In the interim, appropriate *diagnostic procedures* should be considered. Overdistension of the bladder lumen may be prevented by serial decompressive cystocentesis. We do not recommend *surgical intervention* as a short term solution for correction of obstructive urethropathy in uremic cats unless no reasonable alternative exists.

Immediate considerations following restoration of urethral patency

After urine flow has been established by nonsurgical techniques, most of the urine should be removed from the bladder lumen. However, removing all the urine from the bladder lumen is unnecessary and inadvisable since trauma associated with such efforts may aggravate the severity of bladder lesions. Manual compression may be used provided it does not require substantial pressure to induce voiding. Manual compression of the bladder is not necessarily the procedure of choice if an overdistended bladder has been recently decompressed by cystocentesis, since it may result in extravasation of urine into the bladder wall or peritoneal cavity. Alternative methods include intermittent transurethral catheterization,

Table 36.3 General guidelines for transurethral flushing of obstructed male cats (Figures 36.1–36.7)

1. Protect the patient from iatrogenic complications associated with catheterization of the urethra (especially trauma, and urinary tract infection with bacteria).
2. Strive to use meticulous aseptic "feather-touch" technique.
3. Use only sterile catheters.
4. Cleanse the penis and prepuce with warm water prior to catheterization.
5. Select the shortest Minnesota olive-tipped feline urethral catheter[a] for initial catheterization of the urethra, and attach it to a flexible IV connection set and 35–60 ml syringe.
6. Coat the olive tip with sterile aqueous lubricant.
7. Prior to insertion of the catheter into the external urethral orifice, the extended penis should be displaced dorsally until the long axis of the urethra is approximately parallel to the vertebral column.
8. Carefully advance the catheter to the site of obstruction. If necessary, replace the short olive tipped Minnesota needle with a longer one. Record the site of suspected obstruction, since this information may be of value when considering use of muscle relaxants, and/or when considering urethral surgery to prevent recurrent obstruction. CAUTION: Never use excessive force when advancing the catheter.
9. Next, flush a large quantity of physiological saline or lactated Ringer's solution (as much as several hundred mL) into the urethral lumen, and allow it to reflux out the external urethral orifice. When possible, the catheter may be advanced toward the bladder. As a result of this maneuver, the obstructed urethral plugs may be gradually dislodged and flushed around the catheter and out of the urethral lumen. Application of steady but gentle digital pressure to the bladder wall after the urethra has been flushed with physiological saline or lactated Ringer's solution may result in expulsion of a urethral plug or urolith from the urethral lumen. Excessive pressure should not be used because it may result in: (1) trauma to the bladder, (2) reflux of potentially infected urine into the ureters and renal pelvis, and/or (3) rupture of the bladder wall.
10. If the technique outlined in step 9 is unsuccessful, it may be necessary to attempt repulsion of suspected urethral plugs or uroliths back into the bladder lumen by occluding the distal end of the urethra around the olive tip of the catheter before injecting fluid into the urethra. By preventing reflux of solutions out of the external urethral orifice, this maneuver will tend to dilate the urethral lumen. *Excessive force should not be used.* Failure to decompress an overdistended urinary bladder may result in impaired ability to flush plugs nd uroliths into the urinary bladder. If the obstruction persists, consider further diagnostic evaluation.
11. On occasion, it is advantageous to allow the reverse flushing solution to soften the obstructing urethral plugs (this technique is ineffective for most uroliths) before attempting to propel them back into the bladder. Allowing the lapse of several hours between attempts to remove firmly lodged plugs by reverse flushing has been effective.

[a]Minnesota feline olive-tipped urethral catheters are available from EJAY International, Inc, P. O. Box 1835, Glendora, California 91740.

and/or cystocentesis. Each of these procedures has benefits and risks that must be considered in light of the status of the urinary bladder and urethral of each patient.

If the gross appearance of voided or aspirated urine suggests that obstruction with intra-luminal debris is likely to recur, removal of this material with saline or lactated Ringer's solution flushes of the bladder lumen may be of value. Particulate material that has accumulated in the dependent portion of the bladder may be dispersed throughout the bladder lumen by digitally moving the bladder in an up-and-down fashion, which may in turn facilitate aspiration of crystals, inflammatory reactants, and blood clots into the catheter and syringe.

Local instillation of antimicrobial agents into the bladder lumen in an attempt to prevent or treat urinary tract infection is of unproved value. Unless the bladder wall is hypotonic or atonic, the antimicrobial agent is likely to be voided soon after instillation. In case the circumstances

warrant use of antimicrobial agents, they should be given orally or parenterally to maximize their effectiveness.

The size of the urinary bladder should be periodically evaluated following restoration of adequate urethral patency to ensure that urethral obstruction has not recurred and/or that the detrusor muscle is not hypotonic. Micturition induced by gentle digital compression of the bladder may facilitate evaluation of urethral patency.

Although glucocorticoid therapy has been advocated to minimize inflammatory swelling of the urethra, we do not recommend glucocorticoids in this situation. Why not? Because glucocorticoids may aggravate the severity of uremia by inducing protein catabolism via gluconeogenesis and because they may predispose the patient to nosocomial bacterial UTI.

Following relief of urethral obstruction, a transitory obligatory post-obstructive diuresis may develop. Even though cats with post-obstructive polyuria may

Table 36.4 Guidelines to reduce risk of catheter-induced bacterial UTI

1. Urinary catheterization should only be performed by personnel properly trained and experienced with use of proper aseptic, atraumatic techniques.
2. Select indwelling urethral catheters constructed of materials least likely to cause irritation and inflammation of the adjacent mucosa.
3. Thoroughly cleanse the external genitalia, and insert the catheter using aseptic technique.
4. Avoid overinsertion of catheters to minimize damage to the mucosa of the urinary bladder.
5. Avoid open catheters; maintain a closed system.
6. Avoid prolonged use of indwelling catheters.
7. Prevent retrograde flow of urine from the collection receptacle by positioning it below the level of the patient.
8. Try to avoid inducing unnecessary diuresis during indwelling catheterization, especially if an "open " system is used.
9. Avoid giving prophylactic antimicrobial drugs in attempt to prevent UTI unless the duration of catheterization is less than 2–3 days. Even when indwelling catheters are used for a short period, waiting until the catheter is removed before treating with antimicrobics may be the best strategy.
10. Unless there are specific indications for treatment with corticosteroids where benefits clearly outweigh risks, they should not be given to patients with indwelling catheters. Usually, the risk of UTI outweighs the potential benefit of reducing catheter-induced inflammation with corticosteroids.
11. During longer duration use of indwelling catheters, avoid administration of antibiotics unless evidence of UTI associated with morbidity is detected. Although antibiotics may decrease the frequency and delay the onset of UTI, there is high risk of promoting development of infections with one or more bacteria that are resistant to multiple antimicrobial drugs.
12. Perform urinalyses every 24–48 hours for evidence of infection. Perform culture of urine with susceptibility tests if infection is suspected.
13. If catheter-induced infection develops and remains asymptomatic, treat the infection after removal of the catheter.
14. Remove the catheter as soon as feasible. At the time of catheter removal perform urinalysis, quantitative urine culture, and antimicrobial susceptibility tests.
15. If UTI is confirmed after the catheter is removed, initiate therapy with an appropriate antimicrobial drug and continue giving for at least 10–14 days.
16. If infection with more than one bacterial species occurs, and if the pathogens have different susceptibilities to drugs, first treat the bacteria most likely to be virulent. Then select the drug most likely to eliminate the remaining pathogens.
17. Remove and, if appropriate, replace indwelling catheters that are contaminated.

consume some water, the amount is often insufficient to maintain proper fluid balance. Therefore, supplementing water intake by parenteral administration of rehydrating or maintenance fluids is often advisable.

Risks associated with indwelling transurethral catheters

We do not recommend routine use of indwelling transurethlral catheters in all cats following relief of urethral obstruction because the catheters may induce further damage to the urinary tract. Disruption of the glycosaminoglycan (GAG) coating of the urothelium as a result of indwelling transurethral catheters may promote adherence of microbes to the underlying mucosal epithelial cells and the submucosal tissues resulting in bacterial urinary tract infection. Disruption of the GAG coating may also result in adherence of crystals to the urothelium, facilitating recurrence of obstruction by allowing crystals to grow and/or aggregate.

Catheter-induced nosocomial urinary tract UTIs are common, especially in cats with preexisting disease of the lower tract, Why? Because catheters interfere with host defenses, that normally prevent ascending migration of bacterial pathogens through the urethral lumen. Even when closed catheter systems are used, catheters allow bacteria to ascend the urethral lumen via the interface between the catheter and the mucosal surface. Bacteria may also adhere to the surface of urinary catheters and initiate growth of biofilms composed of bacteria, bacterial glycocalicies, Tamm-Horsfall protein, and struvite crystals. These biofilms may shield bacteria from antimicrobial drugs resulting in treatment failures. (Nikel et al. 1985; Osborne et al. 2000) Ascending bacterial UTI has the potential to cause significant morbidity including pyelonephritis, renal failure, and septicemia. Therefore, unnecessary use of urinary catheters should be avoided. Factors to consider in the prevention and treatment of catheter-induced infections are summarized in Table 36.4.

Using indwelling transurethral catheters

The likelihood of whether or not a cat will voluntarily resume adequate voiding following restoration of urethral patency may be assessed by (1) evaluation (e.g., is the stream of sufficient caliber and force that it could drill a hole in a snow bank?), (2) the abundance of material in urine with the potential to occlude the urethral lumen, and (3) the adequacy of detrusor tone immediately following relief of urethral obstruction. Indwelling transurethral catheters may be indicated following relief of urethral obstruction to: (1) facilitate measurement of the rate of urine formation during intensive care of critically uremic cats, (2) promote recovery of detrusor atony by maintaining an empty bladder, and (3) minimize recurrence of urethral obstruction caused by urine precipitates or mural abnormalities in high risk patients. However, indwelling transurethral catheters are often unnecessary if: (1) the cat has a good urine stream during the voiding phase of micturiton, (2) a functional detrusor muscle, and (3) urine does not contain particulate matter that could reobstruct the urethral lumen.

When use of indwelling transurethral catheters is deemed to be beneficial, several precautions will minimize catheter-induced complications (Table 36.4).

Dysfunctional urinary bladder following relief of urethral obstruction

Severe and/or prolonged distension of the urinary bladder caused by obstruction to urine outflow may cause impaired capacity of the detrusor muscle to contract normally during the voiding phase of micturition. The underlying cause is thought to be related to disruption of specialized portions of bladder smooth muscle cells (so-called tight junctions) that normally transmit neurogenic impulses from smooth muscle pace-maker cells. In this situation, the cat has impaired ability to completely empty the bladder. However, voiding can usually be induced by manual compression applied through the abdominal wall.

Once urethral patency has been reestablished, therapy designed to maintain relatively low pressure within the bladder lumen may be associated with restoration of adequate detrusor function. One therapeutic option consists of trial therapy with bethanachol, a parasympathomimetic (muscarinic) agent. This drug may enhance detrusor contractility. A recommended empirical oral dosage for cats is 1.25–2.5 mg given every 8 hours. If the desired effect does not occur within a few days, the dose may be increased incrementally up to 5–7.5 mg every 8 hours, provided harmful side effects do not occur (e.g., excessive salivation, abdominal cramping, vomiting and/or diarrhea).

Since bethanachol can also increase urethral resistance by its nicotinic effects on urethral smooth muscle located in the proximal urethra, this undesirable action may be given with phenoxybenzamine. Phenoxybenzamine is an alpha adrenergic antagonist which facilitates relaxation of smooth muscle in the proximal urethra (oral dose = 0.25 mg/kg every 12 hours). Alternatively, an indwelling transurethral catheter whose tip is located within the bladder lumen may be utilized. Logic indicates that periodic voiding induced by manual compression of the urinary bladder may also be considered, provided this technique does not enhance detruser muscle atony by increasing intraluminal pressure.

If an indwelling transurethral catheter is utilized to minimize accumulation of urine within the bladder, the previously described precautions designed to prevent catheter-induced injury and infection should be considered. In addition to orally administered antimicrobial agents, irrigation of the bladder lumen with antimicrobial solutions may be considered, provided a sufficient quantity of the bacteriocidal agent remains in the bladder long enough to have a beneficial effect. Only sterilized solutions should be injected in a volume sufficient to allow contact with all portions of the bladder mucosa.

Persistent urethral outflow resistance

Following restoration of urethral patency (as confirmed by transurethral catheterization, induced voiding, or contrast radiography), impaired flow of urine through the urethra may persist. This may be related to one or more primary, predisposing, or perpetuating causes (Table 36.1). One cause is inflammatory swelling induced by trauma during attempts to remove plugs or stones from the urethra. This problem can be expected to resolve within a few days provided there is no persistent periurethral extravasation of urine.

Another possibility is a spasm of smooth or skeletal muscles surrounding the urethra. However, the frequency with which this type of abnormality occurs and its responsiveness to smooth and skeletal relaxants have not been extensively characterized. On the basis of logic, one would predict that striated muscle relaxants would be helpful for cats with obstructions localized to the postprostatic urethra. However, at this time, this hypothesis has not been evaluated. On the basis of current evidence, routine use of smooth and skeletal relaxants in cats following urethral obstruction is not warranted.

Other potential causes of impaired voiding through the urethra include reflex dyssynergia, intra-luminal accumulations of sloughed tissue, inflammatory cells, blood clots, and/or recurrence of matrix-crystalline urethral plugs. Urethral strictures may cause persistent outflow resistance in patients with recurrent urethral obstruction. Urethral strictures usually occur as a sequela to: (1) catheter trauma induced at the time of treatment of urethral plugs or urethroliths, (2) use of indwelling transurethral catheters, especially those constructed of material that stimulates a foreign body response, and (3) self-trauma (Nikel et al. 1985; Osborne et al. 1996). Formation of urethral strictures may be minimized by proper patient restraint during urethral catheterization, avoiding use of indwelling transurethral catheters when possible, and use of restraint devices to minimize self-trauma. If urethral strictures predispose to persistent clinical signs, corrective surgery should be considered, but not before the lower urinary tract has been evaluated by appropriate imaging studies.

Managing post-renal uremia

An in-depth discussion of post-renal uremia caused by urethral obstruction is beyond the scope of this chapter. Briefly, obstructive urethropathy (Chapter 70) that persists longer than about 24 hours usually results in post-renal azotemia. This occurs because back-pressure induced by obstruction of outflow impairs glomerular filtration, renal blood flow, and tubular function. After obstruction of the urethra of otherwise untreated normal cats, death will occur within 3–6 days. Damage to the mucosal surface of the urinary bladder may shorten survival time. Despite the potentially catastrophic outcome of urethral obstruction, the biochemical consequences of this disorder are potentially reversible provided appropriate supportive and symptomatic parenteral therapy is given. In severe cases, supportive therapy to minimize hyperkalemia, metabolic acidosis, hypocalcemia, and extracellular fluid depletion should be given a very high priority.

References

Bardelli, M., et al. (1999). Baroreceptor heart-rate sensitivity enhancement after urinary bladder distension in essential hypertensives. *Urol Res* **27**: 153–156.

Koch, A.J., et al. (2001). Severe bradyarrhythmia in a patient with Alzheimer's disease and a patient with cerebral ischemia, both induced by acute distension of the bladder. *Int J Clin Pract* **55**: 323–325.

Nikel, J.C., et al. (1985). Electron microscopic study of an infected Foley catheter. *Can J Surg* **54**: 50.

Osborne, C.A., et al. (1995). Disorders of the feline lower urinary tract.: *Canine and Feline Nephrology and Urology*, edited by C.A. Osborne and D.R. Finco. Philadelphia, PA: Williams and Wilkens, pp. 625–680.

Osborne, C.A., et al. (1996). Medical management of feline urethral obstruction. *Vet Clin North Am* **26**: 483.

Osborne, C.A., et al. (2000). Feline lower urinary tract diseases. In: *Textbook of Veterinary Internal Medicine*, edited by S.J. Ettinger and E.C. Feldman, Volume **2**, 5th edition. Philaelphia, PA: WB Saunders, pp. 1710–1747.

37

Voiding urohydropropulsion

Jody P. Lulich and Carl A. Osborne

Historically, most uroliths in the urinary bladder were either medically dissolved or surgically removed; however, 15 years ago at the University of Minnesota, we developed an innovative technique to remove urocystoliths, called voiding urohydropropulsion (Table 37.1).

By taking advantage of the effect of gravity on urolith position in the urinary bladder and dilation of the urethral lumen during the voiding phase of micturition, this simple technique allowed uroliths to be rapidly flushed out of the urinary tract. A limitation of this technique is its ineffectiveness to manage uroliths larger than the diameter of the urethral lumen; however, with the introduction of lithotripsy to fragment urocystoliths this hurdle has been overcome. As a result, voiding urohydropropulsion remains an integral component of minimally invasive urolith management of all urocystoliths regardless of size. What follows are answers to clinically relevant questions that we believe are most important to effectively perform voiding urohydropropulsion in dogs and cats.

Uroliths that can be retrieved by voiding urohydropropulsion

The relationship between the size, shape, and surface contour of urocystoliths and the luminal diameter of the urethra is an important factor in the selection of patients for voiding urohydropropulsion. Logically, uroliths larger than the smallest diameter of any portion of the distended urethral lumen cannot pass. Compared to uroliths with an irregular contour, smooth uroliths pass more easily through the urethra. This may be related, at least in part, to the fact that uroliths with sharp or irregular surface projections are more likely to adhere to the urethral mucosa.

In our series of clinical cases, diameters of the largest uroliths expelled from urinary bladders were (1) 7 mm from a 7.4-kg female dog, (2) 5 mm from a 9.0-kg male dog, (3) 5 mm from a 4.6-kg female cat, and (4) 1 mm from a 6.6-kg male cat (Lulich et al. 1993). In male cats, uroliths greater than 1 mm in diameter may be voided through the urethra modified by perineal urethrostomy. As a guideline, smooth urocystoliths less than 5 mm in diameter can usually be removed by voiding urohydropropulsion in dogs weighing more than 16–18 pounds.

Volume of urine of fluid in the urinary bladder to effectively perform voiding urohydropropulsion

Successful voiding urohydropropulsion requires that urinary bladders be maximally distended with urine or sterile isotonic solutions such as lactated Ringer's solution or normal saline solution. Maximal luminal distension facilitates rapid and forceful digital compression of the bladder and thus enhances the intraluminal pressure needed to propel the stones through the urethra. For most dogs, we fill the bladder lumen with saline injected through an 8-Fr flexible rubber transurethral catheter. We determine the degree of bladder distension by abdominal palpation. Sometimes, fluid leaks through the urethra after the catheter is removed. When this occurs, it may be helpful to occlude the distal urethral orifice by digital compression.

Nephrology and Urology of Small Animals. Edited by Joe Bartges and David J. Polzin. © 2011 Blackwell Publishing Ltd.

Table 37.1 Performing voiding urohydropropulsion

1. Anesthetize the patient	The type of anesthesia selected may vary based on the likelihood of success and gender of the patient. Consider reversible short-acting anesthetics (e.g., propofol) for patients with very small uroliths that are easily removed. Patients likely to go to surgery/lithotripsy should be placed under inhalation anesthesia.
2. Attach a three-way stopcock to the end of the urinary catheter	The 3-way stopcock facilitates control of the volume of fluid entering the bladder and containment of fluid once the bladder is filled.
3. Fill the urinary bladder	Sterile physiologic solutions (LRS, normal saline) are injected through a transurethral catheter to distend the bladder. If fluid is expelled prematurely around the catheter prior to adequate bladder filling, the vulva and/or urethra can be gently occluded using your thumb and first finger. Placement of additional fluid may not be needed.
4. Position the patient such that the spine is approximately vertical	Repositioning the patient allows uroliths to accumulate at the neck of the bladder facilitating their expulsion. Anatomically, the urethra does not become vertical until the caudal spine is 20–25° anterior of vertical, but this may not be clinically important.
5. Agitate the bladder	Agitating the urinary bladder left and right is performed to collect uroliths in the trigone and to dislodge uroliths loosely adhered to the bladder mucosa.
6. Express the urinary bladder	Apply steady digital pressure to the urinary bladder to induce micturition. Once voiding begins, the bladder is more vigorously compressed. Compress the urinary bladder dorsally and cranially (toward the back and head of the patient). Movement of the urinary bladder caudally toward the pelvic canal may cause the urethra to kink preventing maximal urethral dilation preventing the passage of stones.
7. Repeat steps 2 through 6	The bladder is flushed repeatedly until no uroliths are expelled.
8. Medical imaging	Radiography provides an accurate method of assessing successful expulsion of uroliths. To enhance detection of remaining small uroliths consider double-contrast cystography (only the lateral view is needed).

Effectiveness of voiding urohydropropulsion with a urethrolith

Voiding urohydropropulsion is not likely to be effective in patients with uroliths lodged in the urethra at the time of diagnosis. Uroliths obstructing the urethral lumen have usually been subjected to considerable pressure during attempts by the patient to void. Therefore, attempts to induce voiding of a fluid-filled urinary bladder via abdominal palpation are unlikely to create additional pressure sufficient to move the obstruction. In addition, if complete urethral obstruction and bladder overdistension are associated with underlying disease that has weakened the bladder wall, digital pressure applied to the bladder could result in bladder rupture. For patients with uroliths lodged in the urethra, we recommend laser lithotripsy to fragment the urolith (see Chapter 34). If lithotripsy is not available, uroliths should be returned to the urinary bladder by retrograde urohydropropulsion (see Chapter 35) (Osborne et al. 1999) and dissolved medically (see Chapter 69), if possible, or removed by cystotomy (see Chapter 83).

Optimal anesthesia for voiding urohydropropulsion

Anesthesia is not necessary to perform voiding urohydropropulsion in all patients. For most patients, however, we recommend anesthesia to facilitate positioning of the patient as well as filling, localization, palpation, and compression of the urinary bladder. When anesthetics are used, we recommend agents that provide analgesia and muscle relaxation. In our experience, voiding urohydropropulsion is easiest and safest to perform in patients receiving inhalation anesthetics (isoflurane or halothane). We generally include a narcotic as one of the preanesthetic drugs to minimize pain. For small urocystoliths unlikely to induce any urethral discomfort, we typically use a combination of intramuscularly administered morphine (1 mg/kg) and acepromazine (0.1 mg/kg) followed by intravenously administered propofol titrated to effect instead of inhalant anesthetics. For cases that are likely to be difficult, we give a small amount of propofol just prior to voiding to insure urethral relaxation. In some dogs, we have used propofol as the sole anesthetic agent.

Propofol-induced anesthesia is easily titrated, and recovery is rapid and smooth (Robinson et al. 1995). Drugs to minimize pain following the procedure are usually not needed, but are provided based on the degree of difficulty and the need for repeated voiding to remove stones.

Voiding urohydropropulsion in male dogs

The success of voiding urohydropropulsion is not dependent on whether patients are male or female but on whether uroliths are of sufficiently small size to pass through the urethral lumen. As the diameter of the urethra in male dogs appears to be smaller than that in female dogs of comparable weight and because the os penis in male dogs restricts expansion of the urethral lumen, larger uroliths can be voided from female dogs compared to male dogs of similar size. For example, we reported that the largest urolith removed from a 9-kg male dog was 5 mm in diameter, whereas the largest urolith removed from a 7.4-kg female dog was 7 mm in diameter.

Performing voiding urohydropropulsion in large dogs

To facilitate vertical positioning of large dogs for voiding urohydropropulsion, we use examination tables designed to tilt. The patient is positioned in lateral recumbency while the urinary bladder is being filled. The patient is then placed on its back. With one person supporting the forelimbs and another person supporting the rear limbs, the table is tilted approximately 55° from horizontal. Once voiding has been completed, the table is returned to a horizontal position, and the patient can rest in lateral recumbency.

Strategy when uroliths become lodged in urethra during voiding urohydropropulsion

If uroliths are too large to easily pass through the urethral lumen, they may become lodged in the urethra during voiding urohydropropulsion. For most patients, when this occurs, uroliths are easily flushed back into the urinary bladder by retrograde hydropropulsion (see Chapter 35). If the urinary bladder is overdistended with the fluid, however, retrograde urohydropropulsion may be difficult. The excessive intravesicular pressure that is created as the bladder is filled with fluid to perform voiding urohydropropulsion forces uroliths to move distally along the urethra. Therefore, successful retrograde urohydropropulsion of uroliths may first require that the bladder be emptied by decompressive cystocentesis.

Once uroliths have been returned to the urinary bladder, determining the need for their surgical removal requires knowledge of the likelihood that uroliths may re-obstruct the urethra, of the degree of patient discomfort, and of urolith composition. Laser lithotripsy or surgery should be considered if repeat re-obstruction follows successful retrograde urohydropropulsion. When surgery is necessary, we recommend that uroliths be removed by cystotomy rather than by urethrotomy, because urethral strictures are likely sequelae to urethrotomies.

Uroliths amenable to medical dissolution that remain in the bladder can be dissolved using medical protocols. Asymptomatic uroliths, not amenable to dissolution that remain in the bladder, usually do not require treatment until they become clinically active.

Complications of voiding urohydropropulsion

If patients are carefully selected and a good technique is used, voiding urohydropropulsion is a safe procedure. Visible hematuria is the most common complication of voiding urohydropropulsion, but it resolves in most dogs within several hours (Lulich et al. 1993). If patients with uroliths have concomitant urinary tract infection, we recommend treatment with antimicrobial drugs for several days prior to performing voiding urohydropropulsion.

Urethral obstruction with uroliths can occur if voiding urohydropropulsion is performed in dogs with uroliths too large to pass through all segments of the urethral lumen. When this occurs, uroliths are easily flushed back into the urinary bladder by retrograde urohydropropulsion. If uroliths cannot be medically dissolved, lithotripsy or cystotomy may be needed to prevent re-obstruction.

Filling the urinary bladder by means of transurethral catheterization is a risk for urinary tract infection; however, we have not observed bacterial urinary tract infection in any of our patients in association with voiding urohydropropulsion. This may result from the fact that we provided prophylactic antimicrobic agents for 3–5 days following urethral catheter placement. Likewise, because uroliths are a risk factor for urinary tract infection, it is logical to assume that urolith removal restores the normal host defenses necessary to prevent bacterial invasion of the urinary tract.

In performing voiding urohydropropulsion for 15 years in over 400 dogs, surgery was needed three times to repair a ruptured urinary bladder. This occurred in a female dog with a recent urethral obstruction. After 24 hours of dysuria, this dog passed the urolith that completely obstructed the urethra. Voiding urohydropropulsion was then attempted to remove the remaining uroliths. During the procedure, another urolith obstructed the urethra; manual compression of an inflamed bladder wall contributed to bladder rupture. Uroliths were surgically removed, the bladder wall was repaired, and the patient made a satisfactory recovery. In the other two cases, the depth of anesthesia was not sufficient to relax the urethra. When the bladder was manually expressed, the bladders ruptured at the apex.

Performing voiding urohydropropulsion for uroliths not removed during surgery

Voiding urohydropropulsion performed within days to weeks of cystotomy is not recommended. Within this period, it is unlikely that the surgical incision site in the bladder wall has regained sufficient integrity to accommodate the intravesicular pressures created during voiding urohydropropulsion. Consider laser or shock wave lithotripsy, or cystotomy to remove residual uroliths. In some cases we have be able to retrieve small uroliths using a stone basket.

Two months after cystotomy, we removed small uroliths by voiding urohydropropulsion in a Dalmatian with recurrent urate uroliths. Double-contrast cystography following voiding urohydropropulsion confirmed that the integrity of the bladder wall was not disrupted. Likewise, excessive hemorrhage did not occur following the procedure.

Role of voiding urohydropropulsion with recurrent urolithiasis

Voiding urohydropropulsion is an effective nonsurgical method for managing recurrent urocystoliths. Voiding urohydropropulsion has been especially useful in managing uroliths for which preventive therapy was not possible and when owner compliance with preventive therapy was less than adequate to prevent recurrence. Likewise, management of highly recurrent uroliths such as those composed of calcium oxalate can be improved by this technique.

Successful management of recurrent urocystoliths by voiding urohydropropulsion requires urolith detection when they are still small enough to pass through the urethral lumen. This is the optimum time to quickly and completely remove urocystoliths by voiding urohydropropulsion. Therefore, we recommend radiographic imaging of the urinary tract every 3–6 month following cystotomy even if patients do not have urinary tract signs. If patients are re-evaluated only when clinical signs associated with uroliths are recognized, the uroliths are often too large to pass through the urethra by that time.

Learning to perform voiding urohydropropulsion

To help minimize the anxiety associated with a new technique, consider performing voiding urohydropropulsion in a dog that you have scheduled for cystotomy. For your first attempt, select a patient that in all probability is likely to have a successful outcome. We recommend a medium-sized female dog with relatively smooth uroliths equal to or less than 5 mm in diameter. Sedate the patient as if a cystotomy is going to be performed; however, first try voiding urohydropropulsion. If difficulty is encountered in catheterizing the urethra or if all the urocystoliths cannot be voided, the patient is already prepared for surgery. Even if the urinary bladder ruptures, which is not likely if the proper technique is used, the patient is prepared for surgery. We also consider lithotripsy or surgical backup for cases in which voiding urohydropropulsion is less likely to be effective. Preparing for such events minimizes veterinarian and owner anxiety about performing this unique minimally invasive procedure.

References

Lulich, J.P., et al. (1993). Nonsurgical removal of uroliths in dogs and cats by voiding urohydropropulsion. *J Am Vet Med Assoc* **203**: 660–663.

Osborne, C.A., et al. (1999). Canine retrograde urohydropropulsion: lessons from 25 years of experience. *Vet Clin North Am Small Anim Pract* **29**(1): 267–281.

Robinson, E.P., et al. (1995). Propofol: a new sedative-hypnotic anesthetic agent. In: *Current Veterinary Therapy XII Small Animal Practice*, edited by J.D. Bonagura and R.W. Kirk. Philadelphia, PA: WB Saunders, pp. 77–80.

38

Urethral bulking for urinary incontinence

Joe Bartges

Urinary incontinence is a common problem, especially in older spayed female dogs with urethral sphincter mechanism incompetency (Chapter 76). Medical therapy using estrogen or phenylpropanolamine alone or in combination can be effective; however, some dogs do not respond to or become unresponsive to medical therapy with time. For these dogs, surgical techniques, such as culposuspension, can be performed; however, success is limited and complication rate can be high. A less invasive technique, urethral bulking, has been used in women and female dogs.

It has been thought that injection of bulking agents into the urethral submucosa creates artificial urethral cushions improving urethral closure (coaptation) and restoring continence. It appears that injection therapy functions as a central filler volume that increases the length of muscle fibers and closure power of the urethral sphincter (Klarskov and Lose 2008). The urethral sphincter consists of muscle fibers, collagen, vessels, and nerves, with a central component compressing the lumen (Schafer 2001). Increasing the central filler volume augments the sarcomere length of muscle fibers, strengthening muscle power up to a sarcomere length of 2.2 μm.

There are many substances that have been evaluated and used for urethral bulking, but collagen has been used predominantly in human and veterinary medicine. Teflon was used for several years, but is no longer available for use due to poor long-term outcome and to migration from injection site with subsequent granuloma formation in human beings (Mittleman and Marraccini 1983; Arnold et al. 1989; Kiilholma et al. 1993).

Carbon-coated zirconium oxide beads (Durasphere, Boston Scientific Corporation, Narick, MA) was approved by the FDA in 1999 for treatment of women

with urinary incontinence. It has a large particle size and chronic loss of material does not occur, it does not provide more durability than collagen (Chrouser et al. 2004) and has been associated with urethral prolapse (Ghoniem and Khater 2006). Ethylene vinyl (Tegress, Bard Urological, Covington, GA) was approved by the FDA in 2004 and has a success rate of 43% at approximately 4 years; (Kuhn et al. 2008), however, there are serious complications associated with its use in some women (Erekson et al. 2007; Hurtado et al. 2007). Polydimethylsiloxane (Macroplastique, Uroplasty, Inc., Minnetonka, MN) has been shown to be more effective than collagen in a prospective randomized controlled clinical trial in women with a success rate of 61% at one year versus 48% success rate at a year with collagen (Ghoniem et al. 2009). It was concluded that polydimethylsiloxane is a safe, efficacious, minimally invasive, injectable silicone material for treating urinary incontinence. Porcine dermal implant (Permacol, Covidien, Dublin, Ireland) appears to have a higher urodynamic success rate than polydimethylsiloxane in women with stress urinary incontinence for up to 6 months; however, longer term studies have not been performed (Bano et al. 2005). Women receiving calcium hydroxyapatite (Coaptite, Boston Scientific Corporation, Narick, MA) injections had better outcomes after a single treatment with a lower volume of injected material when compared with patients treated with collagen (Mayer et al. 2007). Urethral granulomatous reaction and urethral prolapse have been reported with its use (Palma et al. 2006; Ko et al. 2007; Lai et al. 2008). A multi-center study concluded that non-animal stabilized hyaluronic acid/dextranomer copolymer (Zuidex, Q-Med, Uppsala, Sweden) delivered by an Implacer device was an effective treatment for women with stress urinary incontinence (van Kerrebroeck et al. 2004).

Collagen (Contigen, Bard Urological, Covington, GA) has been used the most for urethral bulking in human

Nephrology and Urology of Small Animals. Edited by Joe Bartges and David J. Polzin. © 2011 Blackwell Publishing Ltd.

medicine and is the only reported compound used for urethral bulking in dogs. Collagen is a biocompatible biomaterial with diverse formulations based on its biochemical, biological, and physical properties (DeLustro et al. 1991). There are many genetically distinct types of collagen; however, the availability, versatility, and biocompatibility of dermal collagens have led to their dominance as the primary source. Bovine dermal collagen is immunogenically weak and its natural properties led to the development of highly purified injectable fibrillar suspensions that have been used medically for soft tissue augmentation (DeLustro et al. 1986; DeLustro et al. 1987). Glutaraldehyde cross-linked collagen is composed of >95% type I collagen with the remainder being type III collagen. These biomaterials are highly compatible with and incorporated into the host's connective tissue encouraging fibroblast infiltration, new host collagen deposition, and neovascularization. Glutaraldehyde cross-linking results in fibrillar collagen with resistance to collagenase and enhanced persistence at the site of injection. Furthermore, cross-linking prevents rapid shrinkage of the injected volume (syneresis); therefore, injection of large volumes is not required and the injected cross-linked collagen fibrillar structure is stabilized and maintained. For this reason, glutaraldehyde cross-linked bovine collagen has been used for treatment of urinary incontinence in human beings (Shortliffe et al. 1989; Eckford and Abrams 1991; Herschorn et al. 1992; Kieswetter et al. 1992; Appell 1994; Ben-Chaim et al. 1995; Moore et al. 1995; Nataluk et al. 1995; Bartholomew and Grimaldi 1996; Faerber 1996; Tschopp et al. 1999; Kassouf et al. 2001; Lang et al. 2002; Martins et al. 2007; Sakamoto et al. 2007; Appell 2008; Isom-Batz and Zimmern 2009).

Dogs are placed under general anesthesia and positioned in dorsal recumbency. Peri-vulvar fur is clipped and the area prepared with scrub. A 2.7-mm rigid cystoscope is introduced through the vulva and into the urethra. Diagnostic cystoscopy can be performed (Chapter 19).

For urethral bulking injection, the ureteral orifices, the trigone, and proximal urethra are identified. The cystoscope is withdrawn to the level of the proximal urethra just distal to the trigone, approximately 1–1.5 cm caudal to the urinary bladder neck (Figure 38.1).

During the procedure, sterile fluid is infused at a rate that is equal to the fluid drainage through the cystoscope side port so that the urethral lumen remains dilated facilitating visualization of the urethral lumen. The injection needle with or without the protective sheath, depending on the diameter of the operating port channel, is inserted through the operating port. The coating of the injection needle has a green stripe on the same side as the

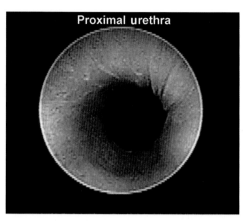

Figure 38.1 Proximal urethra viewed cystoscopically in an 8-year-old, spayed female, border collie with medically unresponsive urinary incontinence. The dog is positioned in dorsal recumbency; therefore, the dorsal urethra is located at the bottom of the photograph.

bevel of the needle tip. Polydimethylsiloxane and non-animal, stabilized hyaluronic acid/dextranomer require a special device for injection. Prior to insertion, the needle is loaded with bulking compound by attaching the syringe containing the compound to the needle and slowly injecting until it is observed in the needle tip.

Urethral bulking agent is injected submucosally in three locations; at approximately the 2, 6, and 10 o'clock positions. I usually inject in two locations; at the 6 and 12 o'clock positions (Figures 38.2 and 38.3).

In women, injections are usually performed at the 3 and 9 o'clock positions. The needle is inserted with visualization at the selected site so that the bevel of the needle is completely inserted submucosally. The bulking agent is injected until a bleb is visualized that approaches midline of the urethral lumen. The amount injected depends

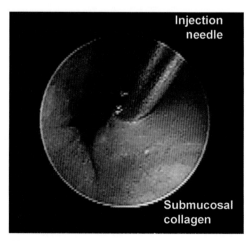

Figure 38.2 Injection needle inserted submucosally with injected collagen, which appears white and glistening. Same dog as in Figure 38.1.

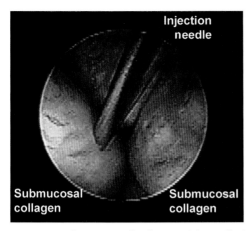

Figure 38.3 Second injection of collagen with needle inserted submucosally. Same dog as in Figures 38.1 and 38.2.

on the size of the dog and the visualization of the size of the bleb. Once the volume has been administered, the injection is stopped, and the needle held in place for 60 seconds to allow the compound to "set up". The needle is removed and one or more additional sites are injected in a similar fashion. The procedure is considered complete when the urethral lumen is closed by deposits when viewing cystoscopically (Figure 38.4). (Arnold et al. 1996; Barth et al. 2005)

It is imperative that the cystoscope not be inserted across the injection sites into the more proximal urethra or bladder as this will result in diffusion of the injected collagen into the submucosal tissue and a decreased bulk-

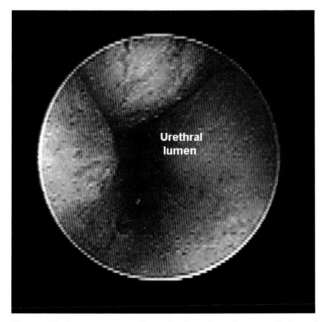

Figure 38.4 Appearance of proximal urethra after completion of collagen injection. Compare the luminal diameter with that seen in Figure 38.1. Same dog as in Figures 38.1–38.3.

ing effect. If cystoscopy cannot be performed, laparotomy and cystotomy can be undertaken for collagen injection. (Barth et al. 2005)

Once the procedure is completed, the dog is recovered. Many dogs can be returned to their owner the same day depending on recovery from anesthesia. Some patients may not be able to urinate following the procedure and may require placement of an indwelling urethral catheter for 1–2 days. When successful, dogs are usually continent within 2–3 days of performing the procedure. Drug therapy can be discontinued at that time. I usually do not treat dogs with peri-procedural antibiotics except for a single dosage of intravenously-administered ampicillin (22 mg/kg) at time of termination of the procedure. A urinalysis and, if necessary, an aerobic bacteriological urine culture is performed approximately 7 days following the procedure.

In the only study published on collagen injection in dogs (Barth et al. 2005), continence was achieved in 27 of 40 dogs for 1–64 months with a mean of 17 months. In 10 dogs, collagen injection improved the urinary incontinence and they received additional medical treatment. Of these, 6 dogs regained continence for a period of 9–47 months (mean, 23 months) and 4 dogs had improvement for 25–78 months (mean, 43 months). In 3 dogs, the collagen injection had no effect. In 16 dogs that were initially continent after treatment, there was deterioration after 1–25 months (mean, 8 months); 12 dogs were then treated medically. Of these, 11 were continent for 2–64 months (mean, 27 months) and 1 dog had improvement of incontinence for 29 months. In 2 dogs, incontinence reoccurred 2 and 12 months after the medical treatment was started. For the remaining 4 dogs, 2 owners refused any further treatment and accepted the urinary incontinence for 42 and 36 months and 2 dogs were treated again with collagen. Collagen injections can be repeated when necessary and there is no limit on how often or when re-treatment may be performed.

Complications occur infrequently and are usually minor in nature including hematuria, dysuria, and pain. Urethral obstruction has occurred in women; however, this has not been observed to occur in dogs injected with collagen. (Barth et al. 2005)

Urethral bulking is a viable treatment for dogs with urinary incontinence that are no longer responsive to medical therapy.

References

Appell, R.A. (1994). Collagen injection therapy for urinary incontinence. *Urol Clin North Am* **21**(1): 177–182.

Appell, R.A. (2008). Transurethral collagen denaturation for women with stress urinary incontinence. *Curr Urol Rep* **9**(5): 373–379.

Arnold, S., et al. (1989). Treatment of urinary incontinence in dogs by endoscopic injection of Teflon. *J Am Vet Med Assoc* **195**(10): 1369–1374.

Arnold, S., et al. (1996). Treatment of urinary incontinence in bitches by endoscopic injection of glutaraldehyde cross-linked collagen. *J Small Anim Pract* **37**(4): 163–168.

Bano, F., et al. (2005). Comparison between porcine dermal implant (Permacol) and silicone injection (Macroplastique) for urodynamic stress incontinence. *Int Urogynecol J Pelvic Floor Dysfunct* **16**(2): 147–150; discussion 150.

Barth, A., et al. (2005). Evaluation of long-term effects of endoscopic injection of collagen into the urethral submucosa for treatment of urethral sphincter incompetence in female dogs: 40 cases (1993–2000). *J Am Vet Med Assoc* **226**(1): 73–76.

Bartholomew, B. and T. Grimaldi (1996). Collagen injection therapy for type III stress urinary incontinence. *Aorn J* **64**(1): 75–83, 85–86.

Ben-Chaim, J., et al. (1995). Submucosal bladder neck injections of glutaraldehyde cross-linked bovine collagen for the treatment of urinary incontinence in patients with the exstrophy/epispadias complex. *J Urol* **154**(2 Pt 2): 862–864.

Chrouser, K.L., et al. (2004). Carbon coated zirconium beads in beta-glucan gel and bovine glutaraldehyde cross-linked collagen injections for intrinsic sphincter deficiency: continence and satisfaction after extended followup. *J Urol* **171**(3): 1152–1155.

DeLustro, F., et al. (1986). A comparative study of the biologic and immunologic response to medical devices derived from dermal collagen. *J Biomed Mater Res* **20**(1): 109–120.

DeLustro, F., et al. (1987). Reaction to injectable collagen: results in animal models and clinical use. *Plast Reconstr Surg* **79**(4): 581–594.

DeLustro, F., et al. (1991). The biochemistry, biology, and immunology of injectable collagens: Contigen TM Bard® collagen implant in treatment of urinary incontinence. *Pediatr Surg Int* **6**: 245–251.

Eckford, S.D. and P. Abrams (1991). Para-urethral collagen implantation for female stress incontinence. *Br J Urol* **68**(6): 586–589.

Erekson, E.A., et al. (2007). Ethylene vinyl alcohol copolymer erosions after use as a urethral bulking agent. *Obstet Gynecol* **109**(2 Pt2): 490–492.

Faerber, G.J. (1996). Endoscopic collagen injection therapy in elderly women with type I stress urinary incontinence. *J Urol* **155**(2): 512–514.

Ghoniem, G., et al. (2009). Cross-linked polydimethylsiloxane injection for female stress urinary incontinence: results of a multicenter, randomized, controlled, single-blind study. *J Urol* **181**(1): 204–210.

Ghoniem, G.M. and U. Khater (2006). Urethral prolapse after dura-sphere injection. *Int Urogynecol J Pelvic Floor Dysfunct* **17**(3): 297–298.

Herschorn, S., et al. (1992). Early experience with intraurethral collagen injections for urinary incontinence. *J Urol* **148**(6): 1797–1800.

Hurtado, E., et al. (2007). The safety and efficacy of ethylene vinyl alcohol copolymer as an intra-urethral bulking agent in women with intrinsic urethral deficiency. *Int Urogynecol J Pelvic Floor Dysfunct* **18**(8): 869–873.

Isom-Batz, G. and P.E. Zimmern (2009). Collagen injection for female urinary incontinence after urethral or periurethral surgery. *J Urol* **181**(2): 701–704.

Kassouf, W., et al. (2001). Collagen injection for treatment of urinary incontinence in children. *J Urol* **165**(5): 1666–1668.

Kieswetter, H., et al. (1992). Endoscopic implantation of collagen (GAX) for the treatment of urinary incontinence. *Br J Urol* **69**(1): 22–25.

Kiilholma, P.J., et al. (1993). Complications of Teflon injection for stress urinary incontinence. *Neurourol Urodyn* **12**(2): 131–137.

Klarskov, N. and G. Lose (2008). Urethral injection therapy: what is the mechanism of action? *Neurourol Urodyn* **27**(8): 789–792.

Ko, E.Y., et al. (2007). Bulking agent induced early urethral prolapse after distal urethrectomy. *Int Urogynecol J Pelvic Floor Dysfunct* **18**(12): 1511–1513.

Kuhn, A., et al. (2008). Long-term results and patients' satisfaction after transurethral ethylene vinyl alcohol (Tegress) injections: a two-centre study. *Int Urogynecol J Pelvic Floor Dysfunct* **19**(4): 503–507.

Lai, H.H., et al. (2008). Large urethral prolapse formation after calcium hydroxylapatite (Coaptite) injection. *Int Urogynecol J Pelvic Floor Dysfunct* **19**(9): 1315–1317.

Lang, J., et al. (2002). Clinical study on collagen and stress urinary incontinence. *Clin Exp Obstet Gynecol* **29**(3): 180–182.

Martins, S.B., et al. (2007). Clinical and urodynamic evaluation in women with stress urinary incontinence treated by periurethral collagen injection. *Int Braz J Urol* **33**(5): 695–702; discussion 702–703.

Mayer, R.D., et al. (2007). Multicenter prospective randomized 52-week trial of calcium hydroxylapatite versus bovine dermal collagen for treatment of stress urinary incontinence. *Urology* **69**(5): 876–880.

Mittleman, R.E. and J.V. Marraccini (1983). Pulmonary Teflon granulomas following periurethral Teflon injection for urinary incontinence [letter]. *Arch Pathol Lab Med* **107**(11): 611–612.

Moore, K.N., et al. (1995). Periurethral implantation of glutaraldehyde cross-linked collagen (Contigen) in women with type I or III stress incontinence: quantitative outcome measures. *Br J Urol* **75**(3): 359–363.

Nataluk, E.A., et al. (1995). Collagen injections for treatment of urinary incontinence secondary to intrinsic sphincter deficiency. *J Endourol* **9**(5): 403–406.

Palma, P.C., et al. (2006). Massive prolapse of the urethral mucosa following periurethral injection of calcium hydroxylapatite for stress urinary incontinence. *Int Urogynecol J Pelvic Floor Dysfunct* **17**(6): 670–671.

Sakamoto, K., et al. (2007). Long-term subjective continence status and use of alternative treatments by women with stress urinary incontinence after collagen injection therapy. *World J Urol* **25**(4): 431–433.

Schafer, W. (2001). Some biomechanical aspects of continence function. *Scand J Urol Nephrol Suppl* (207): 44–60; discussion **35**: 106–125.

Shortliffe, L.M., et al. (1989). Treatment of urinary incontinence by the periurethral implantation of glutaraldehyde cross-linked collagen. *J Urol* **141**(3): 538–541.

Tschopp, P.J., et al. (1999). Collagen injections for urinary stress incontinence in a small urban urology practice: time to failure analysis of 99 cases. *J Urol* **162**(3 Pt 1): 779–782; discussion 782–783.

van Kerrebroeck, P., et al. (2004). Efficacy and safety of a novel system (NASHA/Dx copolymer using the Implacer device) for treatment of stress urinary incontinence. *Urology* **64**(2): 276–281.

39

Laser ablation of ectopic ureter

Joseph W. Bartges

Ectopic ureter is a congenital condition in which one or both ureters insert at a point outside of the trigone of the urinary bladder (Chapter 58). They may be unilateral or bilateral and intramural or extramural. Intramural ureters enter the bladder trigone in the normal position, fail to open into the bladder lumen, tunnel beyond the normal ureteral orifice position, and exit distally at variable locations within the urogenital tract. Extramural ureters bypass the bladder and insert directly into the urethra, vagina, or ductus deferens (Cannizzo et al. 2003; Samii et al. 2004; Sutherland-Smith et al. 2004a).

Traditional treatment for ureteral ectopia includes: neoureterostomy with ligation of the distal ureteric tunnel, neoureterostomy with urethral-trigonal reconstruction, and neoureterocystostomy (McLaughlin and Chew 2000; Sutherland-Smith et al. 2004b; Mayhew et al. 2006). Persistent postsurgical incontinence rate is reported to range from 42% to 78% in dogs (McLaughlin and Chew 2000; Mayhew et al. 2006). Urinary incontinence (Chapter 76) is caused most commonly by concurrent urethral sphincter mechanism incompetency, but can also be caused by re-cannulization of the distal ureteral segment, recurrent urinary tract infections, or a hypoplastic bladder.

Transurethral laser ablation of ectopic ureters can be performed on intramural ectopic ureters to correct the condition. It can only be performed on patients with intramural ectopic ureters because the abdominal cavity would be entered if the procedure were to be used on a patient with an extramural ureter. The procedure utilizes a flexible (Berent et al. 2008) or rigid endoscope (Chapter 19) and a flexible laser fiber (Chapter 34). A laser (an acronym for Light Amplification by Stimulated Emission of Radiation) is a device which transmits light of various frequencies into an extremely intense, small, and nearly non-divergent beam of monochromatic radiation with all waves in phase. Lasers mobilize immense heat and power when focused in close range. The technique was first described by McCarthy in 2006 (McCarthy 2006) using a diode laser; however, a Holmium:YAG laser fiber is used most frequently. A Holmium:YAG laser is a laser whose active medium is a crystal of yttrium, aluminum, and garnet (YAG) doped with holmium (chromium and thulium), and whose beam falls in the near infrared portion of the electromagnetic spectrum (2,100 nm).

The patient is anesthetized and placed in dorsal recumbency if a female and in lateral recumbency if a male. The cystoscope is inserted into the urethra and the normal and ectopic ureters identified. A guide wire or catheter is placed into the ectopic ureter along side of the cystoscope to protect the urethral wall. A laser fiber, typically Holmium:YAG, is inserted through the operating channel of the cystoscope and used to transect the free wall of the ectopic ureters until the opening is as close as possible to the normal anatomic location (Figures 39.1–39.5). Performing the procedure with fluoroscopy availability is preferred as this allows retrograde contrast urethrocystography and ureteropyelography to be performed (Berent et al. 2008).

The benefits of this procedure are elimination of the need for invasive abdominal surgery, shorter recovery time, elimination of the possibility of recannulization of the distal ureter segment, and the procedure is somewhat less expensive than surgical correction. In one report of 11 dogs that had intramural ectopic ureters corrected by this method, 8/11 (72.7%) of dogs were completely continent three months after the procedure without other surgical or medical intervention (Berent and Mayhew 2007). In another report of 4 male dogs with ectopic ureter, all dogs were continent immediately following the procedure and remained continent (Berent et al. 2008).

Nephrology and Urology of Small Animals. Edited by Joe Bartges and David J. Polzin. © 2011 Blackwell Publishing Ltd.

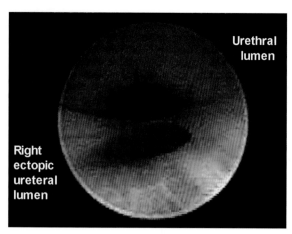

Figure 39.1 Cystoscopic view (2.7 mm, 30-degree rigid cystoscope) of a right intra-mural ectopic ureter in an 8-month old, spayed female, terrier cross.

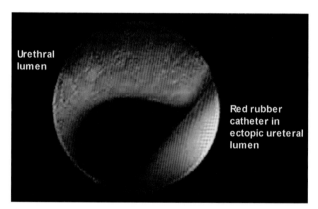

Figure 39.2 Cystoscopic view of dog described in Figure 39.1. A 5-Fr red rubber catheter has been inserted into the lumen of the right intra-mural ectopic ureter.

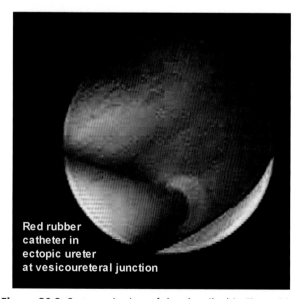

Figure 39.3 Cystoscopic view of dog described in Figure 39.1. The 5-Fr red rubber catheter extends through the lumen of the right intra-mural ectopic ureter and is visualized entering the ureteral orifice at the level of the trigone.

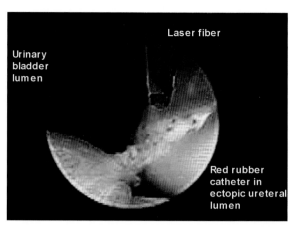

Figure 39.4 Cystoscopic view of laser ablation of the medial wall of the right intra-mural ectopic ureter in dog described in Figure 39.1. The red rubber catheter is present in the lumen of the ectopic ureter in order to protect the urethral wall. The Holmium:YAG laser fiber is visualized exiting the operating channel of the cystoscope.

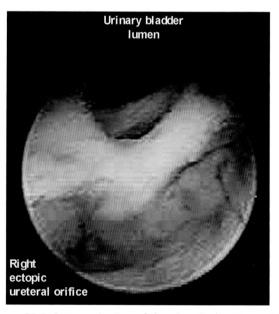

Figure 39.5 Cystoscopic view of dog described in Figure 39.1 following laser ablation of a right intra-mural ectopic ureter. The medial wall of the ectopic ureter has been ablated to the level of the trigone.

References

Berent, A. and P. Mayhew (2007). Cystoscopic-guided laser ablation of intramural ureteral ectopia in 12 Dogs. *J Vet Int Med* **21**: 600.

Berent, A.C., et al. (2008). Use of cystoscopic-guided laser ablation for treatment of intramural ureteral ectopic in male dogs: four cases (2006–2007). *J Am Vet Med Assoc* **232**(7): 1026–1034.

Cannizzo, K.L., et al. (2003). Evaluation of transurethral cystoscopy and excretory urography for diagnosis of ectopic ureters in female dogs: 25 Cases (1992–2000). *J Am Vet Med Assoc* **223**(4): 475–481.

Mayhew, P.D., et al. (2006). Comparison of two surgical techniques for management of intramural ureteral ectopia in dogs: 36 cases (1994–2004). *J Am Vet Med Assoc* **229**(3): 389–393.

McCarthy, T. (2006). Endoscopy brief: transurethral cystoscopy and diode laser incision to correct an ectopic ureter. *Veterinary Medicine* **101**(9): 558–559.

McLaughlin, R. Jr. and C.W. Miller (1991). Urinary incontinence after surgical repair of ureteral ectopia in dogs. *Vet Surg* **20**(2): 100–103.

McLaughlin, M.A. and D.J. Chew (2000). Diagnosis and surgical management of ectopic ureters. *Clin Tech Small Anim Pract* **15**: 17–20.

Samii, V.F., et al. (2004). Digital fluoroscopic excretory urography, digital fluoroscopic urethrography, helical computed tomography, and cystoscopy in 24 dogs with suspected ureteral ectopia. *J Vet Intern Med* **18**(3): 271–281.

Sutherland-Smith, J., et al. (2004a). Ectopic ureters and ureteroceoles in dogs: presentation, cause, and diagnosis. *Compend Contin Educ Vet* **26**(4): 303–310.

Sutherland-Smith, J., et al. (2004b). Ectopic ureters and ureteroceoles in dogs: treatment. *Compend Contin Educ Vet* **26**(4): 311–314.

40

Drug therapy with renal failure

Joe Bartges and Tomas Martin-Jimenez

Many drugs are primarily excreted in urine as unchanged and pharmacologically active drugs and/or as active metabolites. With renal insufficiency, such drugs accumulate in the body; therefore, changes in renal function alters disposition of drugs and dosage regimens require modification. Renal insufficiency may influence drug pharmacokinetics, pharmacodynamics, and toxicity by reduced renal clearance resulting in accumulation of parent drug and/or metabolites, altered rate of biotransformation, decreased protein binding, altered volume of distribution, altered electrolyte status, altered drug disposition and/or activity secondary to acid-base of fluid-balance abnormalities, reduced activity of antimicrobial agents secondary to reduced excretion or dilution with polyuria, and enhanced drug activity or toxicity due to synergistic interaction with uremic complications (Lefebvre et al. 1996; Ritschel and Kearns 1999; Riviere 1999). Renal insufficiency not only affects mean clearance of a drug, but increases individual pharmacodynamics variability.

Pharmacological actions of drugs

Drugs are administered to induce a desired response for a sufficiently long period of time without inducing adverse events. Pharmacologic action is related to the plasma concentration of the drug. Determinants of plasma drug concentration include liberation, absorption, distribution, metabolism, elimination, and response (Figure 40.1). Liberation of the drug is the first step in determining pharmacological effect and is important for all drugs administered by all routes except IV. Following administration and liberation (except for drugs administered

IV), the drug must be absorbed. After absorption (or IV administration), drugs distribute throughout the body and are metabolize (activation or inactivation) and eliminated (via non-renal and renal routes). These processes influence the plasma concentration for a drug and the response observed (Ritschel and Kearns 1999).

The dosing regimen for a drug is based on the dose administered and the interval between administrations (Boothe 2005). The dose of a drug required to achieve a desired plasma concentration is determined by the maximal plasma concentration and the volume of distribution for that drug. The dose of drug must be increased or decreased proportionately with changes in the volume of distribution to achieve the same desired plasma concentration. The volume of distribution of a drug is the sole determinant of the plasma concentration after IV administration for drugs that do not accumulate (i.e., dosing interval is sufficiently long so that each dose is essentially eliminated before administration of the next dose). For drugs that do accumulate, the initial dose must also take into account how much of the drug may accumulate; this is dependent on the elimination half-life (defined as the time required to reduce the plasma concentration by one-half through various elimination processes) of the drug in relation to the dosing interval.

The dosing interval for a drug is determined by the time it takes for maximal plasma concentration to drop to a point below which the desired response no longer occurs. This time depends on how much fluctuation in plasma drug concentration occurs during the dosing interval and its rate of elimination. The longer the elimination of a drug, the longer the time interval can be between doses. Decreasing the dosing interval is of no benefit for drugs with a long half-life. In contrast, increasing a dosing interval may be dangerous for drugs with a short half-life (Hardin et al. 1994). Adding an additional dose (i.e., shortening the dosing interval)

Nephrology and Urology of Small Animals. Edited by Joe Bartges and David J. Polzin. © 2011 Blackwell Publishing Ltd.

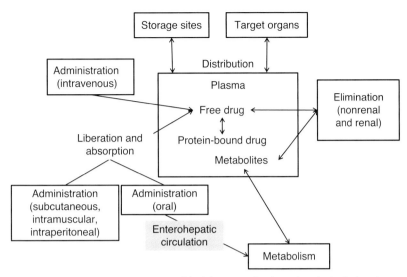

Figure 40.1 Determinants of plasma drug concentration. Modified from Boothe (2005) and Ritschel and Kearns (1999).

is more effective than doubling the dose. Some drugs remain effective despite dosing intervals that are longer than elimination rates due a post-administration killing effect of certain antimicrobial agents, tissue accumulation, active metabolites especially those whose metabolites take longer to eliminate than the parent compound, and drugs that destroy targets that must be re-synthesized before the effect resolves.

For drugs with long elimination half-lives, dosing interval can be correspondingly prolonged. In some situations, the dosing interval is shorter than the elimination half-life, and with each subsequent dose some of the previously administered drug will remain in the body. The amount of drug remaining depends on how much shorter the dosing interval is compared with the half-life. In this situation, the drug begins to accumulate with multiple doses. Eventually, a steady-state is reached for the drug such that the amount of drug administered with each dose equals the amount eliminated during the dosing interval. The amount that a drug accumulates as steady state is reached depends on the difference between drug elimination half-life and dosing interval.

Effects of renal failure on pharmacologic effects

Renal failure may alter pharmacological effects of drugs in many ways. The concentration of a free drug in plasma influences the pharmacological effect of that drug. The degree of protein binding and its alteration with renal insufficiency may affect a drug's disposition and activity. If a drug is normally greater than 90% protein bound and has a small volume of distribution (volume of distribution is defined as the volume in which the amount of drug would need to be uniformly distributed to produce the observed blood concentration), its activity and disposition may be altered with uremia because protein-binding may be decreased.

Protein-losing nephropathy results in hypoalbuminemia and may progress to uremia. Decreased protein binding of drugs in uremia is greater than can be accounted for by hypoalbuminemia in this situation (Rambausek and Ritz 1985). More likely, a conformational change and/or competition for binding sites occur with albumin due to uremic toxins, including free fatty acids, amino acids, and small dialyzable organic acids. The result of increased free drug concentration in blood is an increase in the volume of distribution, which means that with an increase in concentration of drug in blood there is an increase in free drug concentration in blood. Subsequent biotransformation of the drug may be altered, although there are differences in biotransformation among species depending on differences in hepatic metabolism.

With renal failure, there may be a decrease in clearance of the drug if it is primarily cleared by glomerular filtration, although tubular secretory mechanisms may compensate. The elimination of a drug from the body can be thought of in terms of elimination by renal and non-renal routes. Depending on whether a drug is eliminated by renal or non-renal routes or a combination of the two, retention of the drug with a subsequent increase in blood concentrations may occur. If the non-renal elimination of drug is minimal or unchanged in renal insufficiency, then the overall elimination of the drug would be decreased in renal failure due to decreased renal elimination. This may result in drug toxicity.

Patients in renal insufficiency have various alterations in fluid, electrolyte, and acid-base balance that may influence drug choice and dosage regimen. For example, sodium ampicillin contains 3 mEq of sodium per gram and administration could result in sodium imbalances. Administration of antacids or laxatives could result in magnesium imbalances. Compounds that function as non-reabsorbable anions in the distal tubule, such as penicillin, may compete with and cause urinary loss of hydrogen and potassium ions. Metabolic acidosis associated with renal insufficiency may influence dissociation of a drug thereby increasing its free form concentration. Polyuria from renal failure or administration of diuretics may decrease antimicrobial agent concentrations in urine and renal parenchyma to sub-therapeutic levels. Conversely, dehydration is associated with decreased renal perfusion and glomerular filtration rate that can alter drug elimination (Miyazaki et al. 1990).

Drug toxicity may be potentiated if the drug's action is synergistic with uremic complications. Uremia is associated with coagulopathy and administration of drugs that affect platelet function or coagulation may result in hemorrhage. Uremia is also associated with gastrointestinal and neurological complications, and these clinical signs may be exacerbated by drugs with similar adverse reactions. Altered blood–brain barrier may increase blood concentrations in cerebrospinal fluid. Uremic gastroenteritis may alter gastrointestinal motility and absorption of substances; decreased absorption may be markedly impaired with gastrointestinal edema associated with hypoalbuminemia.

Caution should be exercised in patients with renal insufficiency including choice and dosage regimen of drugs. Unfortunately, many drugs have not been evaluated in dogs and cats with renal failure, and while therapeutic monitoring of drugs in patients with renal failure is ideal, it is difficult to implement.

Drug dosage regimens with renal failure

Total body clearance (elimination) of a drug can be divided into non renal and renal routes. During renal failure, predicting drug disposition is based on the assumption that renal clearance is directly correlated to glomerular filtration rate. This assumes the intact nephron hypothesis holds and that a relative glomerulo-tubular balance is present. With these assumptions, renal clearance is linearly related to glomerular filtration rate whether the drug is cleared by glomerular filtration or tubular mechanisms. More practical clinically is to relate elimination half-life to glomerular filtration rate, which when plotted gives a hyperbolic curve (Figure 40.2). If a drug is eliminated primarily by non renal routes, elimination half-life remains relatively constant with renal failure because the drug's elimination is influenced minimally by renal elimination. If the drug is excreted renally, clearance

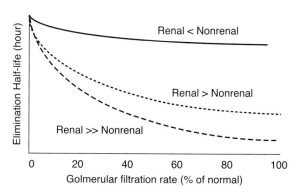

Figure 40.2 Relationship between elimination half-life and renal function (glomerular filtration rate). The three drugs depicted depend on renal elimination to varying degrees and are related to non renal elimination. Modified from Riviere (1999).

is unaffected relatively until glomerular filtration rate is 30–40% of normal. This is the basis for recommendation that dose adjustment in renal failure is only necessary after two-thirds to three-quarters of renal function is lost; in other words, azotemic renal failure. Another approach to relate elimination half-life and glomerular filtration for drugs eliminated primarily by kidneys is through the use of dose fraction where the fraction of dose administered is based on the degree of abnormal renal function divided by normal renal function (abnormal glomerular filtration rate / normal glomerular filtration rate). Because glomerular filtration is not measured directly in most patients although it can, (Miyamoto 2001; Bexfield et al. 2008) glomerular filtration rate is estimated by the inverse of the serum or plasma creatinine concentration; however, this is only a rough guideline.

Calculation of modified dosage regimens with renal failure

Calculated dosage regimens with renal failure will be modified by relating the proportion of decrease in renal function to normal renal function. This method assumes that a standard loading dose is administered; drug absorption, distribution, protein binding, non-renal elimination, and tissue sensitivity are unchanged; creatinine clearance is directly correlated to drug clearance; and renal function is relatively constant over time. When constructing modified dosage regimens for patients with renal failure, both the dose and dosage interval must be modified to achieve a plasma drug concentration-time profile that is similar to a normal situation.

Constant-interval, dose-reduction method

Assuming a safe and effective dosage regimen for a drug has been determined in a patient with normal renal function, the normal dosage regimen may be adjusted according to the dose fraction. One method is to use constant-interval, dose-reduction. With this method, the dose is reduced by a factor of the dose fraction, but the dose interval is not changed. In other words, dose administered with renal failure = dose administered with health multiplied by the dose fraction; the time interval between administered doses is unchanged. This method is used with drugs that have a low therapeutic index.

Constant-dose, interval-extension method

The second method is termed constant-dose, interval-extension. With this method, the dosage interval is extended by the inverse of the dose fraction, but the administered dose is unchanged. In other words, dosage interval time with renal failure = dosage interval time with health divided by the dose fraction; the administered dose is unchanged. This method is used with drugs whose activity persists despite dosing intervals that are longer

than elimination rates (i.e., concentration-dependent bactericidal activity of flouroquinolones) (Lefebvre et al. 1998).

Implementing dose-reduction methods in patients with renal failure

The therapeutic goal of drug administration is to maintain a steady-state plasma concentration of the drug. When repeated doses of a drug are administered, accumulation occurs until steady-state is achieved; this takes approximately four to five half-lives. The prolonged elimination present in patients with azotemic renal failure causes excessive delays in attaining steady state; therefore, an appropriate loading dose should be administered so that therapeutic concentrations of the drug can be attained immediately. If the constant-interval, dose-reduction method is used, give the usual dose initially, followed by the calculated reduced dose. If the

Table 40.1 Suggested dosage regimen adjustments with renal failure (Lefebvre 2002)

Drugs	Comments
Antimicrobial Agents	
Aminoglycosides	Contraindicated because of nephrotoxicity, but can be used cautiously especially with monitoring of plasma concentrations.
Penicillins	Accumulation, but high therapeutic index; therefore, dosages generally are not changed. For dicloxacillin and oxacillin, no change. For others, when GFR<0.5 mL/kg/min, divide the dose by 2 or multiply the dosage interval by 2.
Cephalosporins	Potentially nephrotoxic (especially cephaloridine)
Sulfonamides	Apparently, slightly nephrotoxic in the dog. Dosage regimen adjustment is recommended: for sulfisoxazole, multiply the dosage interval by 2–3 when GFR<1 mL/kg/min.
Tetracyclines	Extensive accumulation, potentially nephrotoxic, exacerbation of azotemia, contraindicated except doxycycline, which is eliminated primarily by non-renal routes.
Fluoroquinolones	No dosage regimen adjusted required for marbofloxacin in dogs.
Lincosamides and macrolides	No dosage regimen adjusted required for erythromycin and clindamycin.
Metronidazole	No dosage regimen adjusted required
Anti-Inflammatory Drugs	
NSAIDs	Nephrotoxic risk. No accumulation observed with tolfenamic acid.
Corticosteroids	Worsens azotemia
Cardiovascular Drugs	
Digitalis glycosides	Accumulation of digoxin, but not digitoxin.
ACE inhibitors	Enalapril and captopril are extensively cleared by the kidney in dogs. Minimal risk of toxicity with benazepril because of non-renal elimination.
Antiarrhythmic drugs	Hepatic elimination, but active metabolites are cleared renally and the therapeutic index is low.
Diuretics	Decreased elimination and diuretic response for furosemide. Furosemide potentiates aminoglycoside nephrotoxicity.
Anesthetics	
Barbiturates	Adverse renal hemodynamic effects and potential increase in sensitivity of the central nervous system.
Ketamine	Reduced risk of adverse effects in renal failure
Gas anesthetics	Isoflurane preferred to halothane and methoxyflurane.

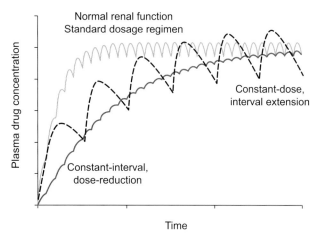

Figure 40.3 Plasma drug concentration-time curves of an orally administered drug to a patient with normal renal function (thin line), a patient with 20% of renal function where the drug dosing regimen was altered using the constant-interval, dose-reduction method (thick line), and a patient with 20% of renal function where the drug dosing regimen was altered using the constant-dose, interval-extension method (thick, dashed line).

constant-dose, interval-extension method is used, give the initial two doses as would be administered to a healthy animal at the normal time interval before extending the interval dosing time (Riviere 1999).

Selecting the appropriate dosage adjustment method (Table 40.1) (Riviere 1999).

- Do not use drugs unless definite therapeutic indications are present.
- If the dosage regimens of a drug in renal failure has been determined by clinical pharmacokinetic studies, this should be followed rather than estimating a modified dosage regimen.
- If an assay procedure for a drug is available, periodic measurement of blood concentrations of the drug can be performed.
- In a situation in which a drug has not been studied but some information on its characteristics are available, it is possible to estimate an appropriate dose in renal failure
  - All estimated modified dosage regimens are approximations because it is impossible to duplicate a normal plasma drug concentration-time profile in a patient in renal failure (Figure 40.3).
  - The constant-dose, interval-extension method produces peak and trough plasma concentrations

similar to those seen in healthy patients; however, there are prolonged periods of potentially sub-therapeutic plasma concentrations. This method is preferred for drugs whose toxicity correlates to high trough rather than peak concentrations (i.e., amino-glycosides) (Riviere et al. 1985).
  - The constant-interval, dose-reduction method produces peak plasma concentrations that are lower and trough concentrations are greater in renal failure patients when compared with healthy patients. There are no periods of sub-therapeutic concentrations.
- Careful clinical monitoring for toxic and pharmacologic effect is important
- Whenever possible, select a drug that is biotransformed by the liver or excreted by non renal routes (e.g., benazepril versus enalapril) (Lefebvre et al. 1999)

References

Bexfield, N.H., et al. (2008). Glomerular filtration rate estimated by 3-sample plasma clearance of iohexol in 118 healthy dogs. *J Vet Intern Med* **22**(1): 66–73.

Boothe, D.M. (2005). Principles of drug therapy. In: *Textbook of Veterinary Internal Medicine*, edited by S.J. Ettinger and E.C. Feldman, 6th edition. St. Louis, MO: Elsevier Saunders, pp. 492–498.

Hardin, T.C., et al. (1994). Comparison of ampicillin-sulbactam and ticarcillin-clavulanic acid in patients with chronic renal failure: effects of differential pharmacokinetics on serum bactericidal activity. *Pharmacotherapy* **14**(2): 147–152.

Lefebvre, H.P. (2002). *Dosage Regimen Adjustment in Renal Failure: Why, When and How*. Grenada: World Small Animal Veterinary Association Congress.

Lefebvre, H.P., et al. (1996). Drug prescription in renal-impaired dogs. *Rev Med Vet* **147**: 757–782.

Lefebvre, H.P., et al. (1999). Effects of renal impairment on the disposition of orally administered enalapril, benazepril, and their active metabolites. *J Vet Intern Med* **13**(1): 21–27.

Lefebvre, H.P., et al. (1998). Effect of experimental renal impairment on disposition of marbofloxacin and its metabolites in the dog. *J Vet Pharmacol Ther* **21**(6): 453–461.

Miyamoto, K. (2001). Clinical application of plasma clearance of iohexol on feline patients. *J Feline Med Surg* **3**(3): 143–147.

Miyazaki, H., et al. (1990). The pharmacokinetics and pharmacodynamics of furosemide in anesthetized dogs with normal and experimentally decreased renal function. *Nippon Juigaku Zasshi* **52**(2): 265–273.

Rambausek, M. and E. Ritz (1985). Digitalis in chronic renal insufficiency. *Blood Purif* **3**(1–3): 4–14.

Ritschel, W.A. and G.L. Kearns (1999). *Handbook of Basic Pharmacokinetics*, 5th edition. Washington, DC: American Pharmaceutical Association.

Riviere, J.E. (1999). *Comparative Pharmacokinetics: Principles, Techniques, and Applications*. Ames, IA: Iowa State Press.

Riviere, J.E., et al. (1985). Decreased fractional renal excretion of gentamicin in subtotal nephrectomized dogs. *J Pharmacol Exp Ther* **234**(1): 90–93.

Section 4

Clinical syndromes

41

Azotemia and uremia

Sheri J. Ross

In 1840, Piorry and L'Heritier introduced the term *uremia*, literally "urine in the blood", based on their hypothesis that clinical signs of kidney failure were the result of reabsorption of urine into the blood stream (Richet 1988). We now know that uremia develops when disturbances in tubular and endocrine functions of the kidney cause retention of toxic metabolites, changes in the volume and composition of the body fluids, and an excess or deficiency of various hormones (Bergstrom and Furst 1978). The many compounds that accumulate in blood and tissues of patients with compromised renal function are referred to as *uremic retention solutes*. If one of these retained solutes affects a biochemical or physiologic function, it is called a *uremic toxin*. In addition to retention of solutes, dysregulation of endocrine and metabolic functions may also lead to uremic toxicity. Although most commonly associated with chronic kidney disease (CKD), uremia may also be the sequela of severe acute kidney injury (AKI) and obstruction or rupture of the urinary tract. Regardless of cause, accumulation of uremic toxins may affect function of every organ system in the body engendering a myriad of clinical signs collectively referred to as the uremic syndrome.

Although the association between clinical deterioration and uremia has been long recognized, our understanding of the specific contributing toxins remains incomplete. Initially, a single yet unidentified retained solute was thought to account for all of the clinical signs associated with uremia. This single molecule concept was later replaced by the hypothesis that each clinical manifestation of uremia has a single, causative, uremic toxin. The current belief is that each metabolic function may be altered in different ways by one or more uremic toxins. This theory better explains the variability in both the diversity and severity of clinical signs that constitute the uremic syndrome.

Before a uremic retention solute may be further classified as a uremic toxin, it must fulfill five criteria proposed by Massry in 1977. These criteria are: (1) the compound should be chemically identified and accurate quantitative analysis in biologic fluids should be possible; (2) total body and plasma concentrations of the compound should be higher in uremic than in non-uremic patients; (3) there should be a relationship between the level of the compound and one or more of the manifestations of uremia; (4) a reduction in the level of the compound must result in amelioration of the clinical manifestation, (5) administration of the compound to otherwise normal patients at a comparable dose should produce the related clinical manifestation (Massry 1977).

A comprehensive review of the literature in 2003 by the European Uremic Toxin Work Group identified 90 known uremic retention solutes (Vanholder et al. 2003a). In the six years since, over 25 additional retention solutes have been identified and the number continues to grow (Vanholder et al. 2008). Despite the rapidly increasing number of identified uremic retention solutes, very few may actually be classified as uremic toxins. This is due largely to difficulty in proving the biological impact of the individual solutes. Additionally, elevated blood concentrations of uremic retention solutes likely occur not only due to impaired renal excretion, but may also result from impaired degradation and/or increased synthesis.

The increased survival of patients associated with the advent of hemodialysis almost 60 years ago, substantiated the theory that much of the uremic syndrome is due to small molecular weight, water-soluble compounds. Although these molecules were efficiently removed with conventional hemodialysis, it was soon recognized that hemodialysis was not true renal replacement therapy, in that an adequate dialysis did not completely eliminate a

Nephrology and Urology of Small Animals. Edited by Joe Bartges and David J. Polzin. © 2011 Blackwell Publishing Ltd.

393

host of clinical signs that did resolve with renal transplantation. This new clinical disorder was termed the "residual syndrome." Although some components of the residual syndrome have been attributed to the deleterious effects of hemodialysis, the majority of the clinical signs have been ascribed to persistent uremic toxins that are not efficiently removed during dialysis due to large size, protein binding or volume of distribution (Depner 2001; Meyer and Hostetter 2008).

Classification of uremic retention solutes

The differential behavior of uremic retention solutes during dialysis is the basis for the most commonly used classification scheme. In general, solutes are categorized into three major groups; (1) small water-soluble compounds, (2) protein-bound compounds, and (3) larger middle molecules (Table 41.1).

The low molecular weight, water-soluble compounds have been most extensively studied. This group generally includes compounds with a molecular weight less than 500 Da that are easily removed by dialysis; this trait has facilitated their identification and characterization. Quantitatively, urea is the most important retained solute in patients with kidney disease. Due to high serum concentrations and ease of measurement, urea is often used as a surrogate low molecular weight uremic toxin, even though the compound itself is not intrinsically toxic. Most of the direct toxic effects of urea have only been proven in vitro at high concentrations. In a classic study by Johnson et al., urea, sufficient to maintain blood urea >200 mg/dl, was added to the dialysate of a cohort of patients. No adverse clinical effects were noted during the 3-month study period (Johnson et al. 1972). Despite the apparent lack of toxicity of the compound itself, blood urea concentrations correlate quite well with clinical signs of uremia. Although greater than 50 low molecular weight, water-soluble, uremic retention solutes have been identified, only a few are known to exert biological effects.

A substantial number of retained uremic retention solutes are protein bound, and are thus not readily removed by dialysis. Most of the solutes in this group are low molecular weight, but some are larger (e.g., leptin). Classic examples of compounds from this group include phenols, indoles, and homocysteine. The protein bound uremic retention solutes have been the focus of a great deal of research since many of these solutes have significant biologic effects. Decreased serum albumin has recently been shown to increase the free fraction, and thus toxicity, of many solutes within this group (DeSmet et al. 2001). This relationship may contribute to the poor clinical outcomes of patients with hypoproteinemia (DeSmet

Table 41.1 Classification of some major uremic retention solutes

Solute	Group
Free water-soluble low-molecular-weight solutes	
ADMA (asymmetrical dimethylarginine)	Guanidines
B-lipoprotein	Peptides
Creatinine	Guanidines
Guanidine	Guanidines
Hypoxanthine	Purines
Malondialdehyde	
Methylguanidine	Guanidines
Osteoprotegerin (OPG)	
Oxalate	
SDMA (symmetric dimethylarginine)	Guanidines
Urea	
Uric acid	Purines
Xanthine	Purines
Middle molecules	
Adrenomedullin	Peptides
Atrial natriuretic peptide	Peptides
B2-microglobulin	Peptides
Complement factor D	
Cystatin C	Peptides
Degranulation inhibiting protein I	Peptides
Endothelin	Peptides
Hyaluronic acid	Peptides
Interleukin 1-β	Cytokines
Interleukin-6	Cytokines
Leptin	Peptides
Parathyroid hormone	Peptides
Retinol binding protein	Peptides
Tumor necrosis factor-α	Cytokines
Protein-bound solutes	
Furan propionic acid	
Hippuric acid	Hippurates
Homocysteine	
Indole-3 acetic acid	Indoles
Indoxyl sulfate (IS)	Indoles
N-carboxymethyllysine	Advanced glycation end products
P-cresol	Phenols
Pentosidine	Advanced glycation end products
Phenol	Phenols
Quinolinic acid	Indoles
Spermidine	Polyamines

et al. 2003). The healthy kidney can clear many of these protein-bound solutes by active tubular secretion; this process cannot be duplicated by currently available renal replacement techniques. Therefore, despite their known toxic effects, the removal of the protein-bound uremic retention solutes remains inadequate.

The term *middle molecules* has been assigned to the group of uremic retention solutes with molecular weights >500 Da. Babb and Scribner first suggested the middle molecule hypothesis in the late 1970s to explain the persistence of certain clinical signs in patients receiving increasing doses of dialysis (Babb 1981). Their hypothesis attributes clinical illness to the retention of molecules, normally cleared by the glomerulus, that are not cleared by the limited permeability of the dialysis membranes. Due to the technical limitations of the day, Babb et al were not able to identify which compounds were causing the clinical illness. Current analytical techniques have facilitated the identification of many middle molecules, some of which have been associated with inflammation, malnutrition, and immune dysfunction. These three clinical problems are common in uremic patients and each contributes significantly to morbidity and mortality.

The prototype middle molecule is β_2-microglobulin; other members of this group include the advanced glycation end products (AGEs), the advanced oxidation protein products (AOPPs), and many complement proteins and cytokines. Since the size of middle molecules precludes their removal by conventional dialysis techniques, increasing the pore size of the dialyzer membrane may facilitate their removal. The removal of middle molecules may also be enhanced by shifting from hemodialysis to hemofiltration or hemodiafiltration. Whilst the chief method of solute removal in hemodialysis is simple diffusion which relies entirely on concentration gradients, hemofiltration and hemodiafiltration utilize convective solute removal. These modalities utilize convection, whereby solutes are carried across the dialyzer membrane in response to a transmembrane pressure gradient (a process known as solvent drag). Recent studies have shown that the mean predialysis serum β_2 microglobulin level over time is predictive of all-cause mortality, independent of the chronicity of dialysis and residual kidney function (Cheung 2006).

Clinical manifestations of uremia

The clinical manifestations of uremia are diverse. The literature describes more than 75 clinical symptoms attributed to uremia, resulting from disturbances in all organ systems of the body. Some of the most common clinical manifestations of uremia observed in veterinary patients are listed in Table 41.2. The number and severity of clinical signs vary from patient to patient, and are partially dependent on the magnitude of the reduction in functioning renal mass, and the rapidity with which renal function is lost. Rapid-onset uremia, resulting from

Table 41.2 Common clinical manifestations associated with uremia

Gastrointestinal system
  Anorexia
  Gastrointestinal ulcers
  Halitosis ("uremic breath")
  Nausea, vomiting
  Oral ulceration/stomatitis/glossitis (Figure 41.1)
  Pancreatitis
Hematological system
  Coagulopathy
  Granulocyte and lymphocyte dysfunction
  Hypoproliferative anemia
  Lymphopenia
  Neutrophilia
  Platelet dysfunction
Cardiopulmonary system
  Cardiomyopathy
  Hypertension
  Pericarditis
  Pleuritis
  Uremic pneumonitis/Pulmonary edema
Skeletal system
  Amyloidosis (β2-microglobulin)
  Defective calcitriol metabolism
  Osteodystrophy
  Osteoporosis
Neuromuscular system
  Depression
  Fatigue
  Muscle twitching
  Muscle weakness
  Peripheral polyneuropathy
  Pruritis
  Uremic encephalopathy
Immunological system
  Inadequate antibody formation
  Stimulation of inflammation (baseline)
  Susceptibility to cancer
  Susceptibility to infection
Endocrinology
  Dyslipidemia, hypertriglyceridemia
  Peripheral insulin resistance and glucose intolerance
  Secondary hyperparathyroidism
Miscellaneous
  Hypothermia
  Increased protein-muscle catabolism
  Thirst
  Weight loss

AKI or post-renal causes, usually results in more severe clinical signs than gradual-onset uremia from progressive CKD. Patients with CKD typically do not exhibit clinically significant symptoms of uremia until they reach

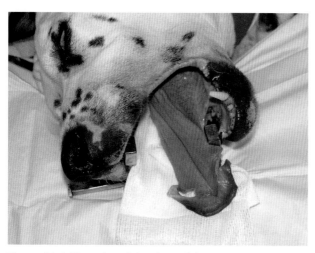

Figure 41.1 Necrosis and sloughing of the anterior portion of the tongue in a severely uremic dog.

stage 3, although some patients may have mild clinical signs with stage 2 CKD (Chapter 48).

Commonly reported clinical manifestations of uremia include gastrointestinal signs, anemia, coagulopathy, acidosis, hyperkalemia, calcium and phosphorous derangements, endocrine abnormalities, malnutrition, and cardiovascular complications. For detailed descriptions of the pathophysiology and management of these uremic manifestations, the reader is directed to the chapters on CKD (Chapter 48) and AKI (Chapter 49) (Table 41.2 and Figure 41.1).

Metabolic effects of uremia

Carbohydrate metabolism

Uremia is typically associated with impaired glucose metabolism and a mild increase in serum glucose levels. Although resistance to insulin at the tissue level is the predominant cause of impaired glucose metabolism, alterations in insulin degradation and insulin secretion may also contribute to this (Adrogué 1992; Mak and DeFronzo 1992; Alvestrand 1997). The healthy kidney plays an important role in the metabolism of insulin (Rabkin 1972; Adrogué 1992; Mak and DeFronzo 1992). Insulin has a molecular weight of 6,000 and is freely filtered at the glomerulus. Once filtered into the tubular lumen, insulin enters proximal tubular cells by carrier-mediated endocytosis, and is then transported into lysosomes where it is metabolized to amino acids (Rabkin 1972). Due to decreased renal clearance, plasma insulin concentrations are often mildly to moderately increased in patients with CKD. Despite this increase in insulin levels, significant peripheral resistance to the action of

insulin results in an overall decrease in tissue glucose utilization.

Impaired glucose metabolism and insulin resistance are associated with an increased risk of cardiovascular complications and death in non-diabetic human CKD patients. Insulin resistance has also been associated with reduced lipoprotein lipase activity resulting in hypertriglyceridemia. Peripheral insulin resistance may contribute to malnutrition in patients with CKD, since insulin deficiency stimulates the breakdown of muscle tissue and activates a common proteolytic pathway via the ubiquitin-proteasome system.

Oxidative stress

Traditionally, the term oxidative stress describes the imbalance between generation of oxidants and antioxidant defense. In the context of uremia, the term implies an imbalance in favor of pro-oxidants, which leads to the oxidation of macromolecules and to tissue damage. Several studies have demonstrated increased in oxidative stress in patients with CKD (Daschner et al. 1996). In human medicine, oxidative stress plays a pivotal role in the pathogenesis of vascular injury, thus contributing to cardiovascular related morbidity and mortality (Beckeer et al. 1997). Cardiovascular disease does not contribute significantly to the clinical course of most veterinary patients with CKD, probably due to the shorter duration of clinical disease.

Oxidants in the plasma are not readily detectable, since they are highly reactive compounds that generally have half-lives of only a few seconds. However, markers of oxidative stress, such as lipid, carbohydrate, and protein oxidation products, have been detected in the plasma and tissues of uremic patients. Many studies have found a positive correlation between increased plasma levels of oxidative stress markers and cardiovascular end-points in human CKD patients (Busch et al. 2004; Deschamps-Latscha et al. 2005).

Since there is mounting evidence that oxidative stress increases long before the onset of end stage kidney disease, antioxidant therapeutic strategies may rationally be employed early as in the course of CKD. Proposed therapeutic antioxidants include enzymes such as superoxide dismutase, as well as vitamins E and C. High-dose vitamin E has been shown to decrease atherosclerosis in rats with CKD, although the same effect has not yet been documented in humans.

Inflammation

Chronic inflammation in patients with CKD is being recognized as a significant predictor of morbidity, mortality, and progression of renal disease. Recent evidence suggests that persistent inflammation (and oxidative stress) starts in the early stages of CKD and increases in severity as the patient becomes uremic (Sela et al. 2005). Low-grade, chronic inflammation, characterized by increased serum levels of C-reactive protein (CRP) and pro-inflammatory cytokines (e.g., tumor necrosis factor (TNF)-a and (IL)-6), contribute significantly to cachexia and cardiovascular disease in human patients with CKD (Stenvinkel et al. 1999). High serum concentrations of CRP and low serum concentrations of albumin are independent risk factors for mortality in human CKD patients (Menon et al. 2005), but IL-6 seems to be the inflammatory marker that best predicts outcome (Honda et al. 2005). Although the underlying cause(s) of this chronic inflammation has not been fully elucidated, the main contributors are believed to be increased serum concentrations of uremic toxins, comorbid diseases, increased serum cytokines, oxidative stress, malnutrition, and increased incidence of infection. One obvious management strategy to minimize systemic inflammation in CKD patients is identification and treatment of any infections. Additionally, various anti-inflammatory nutritional and pharmacological therapies have been recommended.

Uremia and drug metabolism

The physiologic changes associated with uremia may have a profound effect on the absorption, distribution, metabolism, and excretion of drugs and their metabolites (Chapter 40). Indeed, it is quite common for uremia to decrease the gastrointestinal absorption of orally administered drugs. In one of the first studies to demonstrate this phenomenon, the gastrointestinal absorption of d-xylose was shown to be reduced by 30% in dialysis-dependent human patients (Craig et al. 1983). Drug absorption may also be altered by a change in gastric pH. Increased plasma concentrations of urea combine with gastric urease, resulting in the formation of ammonia, which buffers gastric acid. Therefore, the efficacy of many oral phosphate binders may be decreased in patients with CKD, since they rely on the release of phosphorous during the acid hydrolysis of proteins in the stomach (Maton and Burton 1999). In addition to alterations in drug absorption, uremic patients often have reduced serum protein binding of many drugs, due to a decrease in serum albumin concentration and decreased binding affinity of the remaining serum albumin (Boobis 1977; McNamara et al. 1981).

The rate of elimination of drugs excreted by the kidneys is proportional to the glomerular filtration rate (GFR). Ideally, the clinician knows the patient's GFR prior to administering any medication that relies on renal excretion. Several methods utilizing GFR have been developed for human patients to tailor drug dosages to the degree of renal dysfunction. However, GFR measurements are often not performed in veterinary practice since they are time-consuming and can be labor-intensive. We thus often rely on serum creatinine to provide an estimate of renal function on which to base therapeutic decisions. The residual renal function and metabolic condition of the uremic patient must be carefully reviewed prior to the addition of any medication to the treatment regimen. Likewise, interactions between different medications, as well as the metabolic pathways must also be considered, since the excretory capacities of the uremic patient may be easily overwhelmed.

Management of uremia

Extracorporeal removal of uremic toxins

The standard of care for management of the uremic syndrome in humans consists of hemodialysis (Chapters 28 and 29), peritoneal dialysis (Chapter 30), or renal transplantation (Chapter 31). As noted above, removal of uremic toxins by conventional hemodialysis occurs primarily by diffusion across the dialysis membrane, thereby limiting removal to compounds that are less than 500 daltons and less than 90% protein bound (i.e., the small water-soluble compounds) (Vanholder et al. 2003b). The use of large-pored dialysis membranes to perform high-flux dialysis decreases the importance of molecular mass in determining removal during extracorporeal circulation. During high-flux dialysis, the treatment time, flow rates, volume of distribution and percent of protein binding of the uremic toxin are more important determinants of clearance (Schaedeli and Uehlinger 1998). As a consequence, many more of the so-called middle molecules are removed during high-flux dialysis than during conventional hemodialysis (Hakim et al. 1996; Gotch 1998).

Protein-bound uremic toxins are poorly removed by both conventional and high-flux hemodialysis, and many strategies have been used to increase the removal of protein bound solutes. Increasing the pore size of the dialyzer while using albumin-enriched dialysate has shown limited success. Likewise, adsorptive techniques using either charcoal or polymer based sorbets have been used (Dhondt et al. 2000).

As with conventional hemodialysis, solute removal by peritoneal dialysis is most effective for smaller, non-protein bound compounds. However, higher-molecular-weight compounds may be somewhat more effectively removed by peritoneal dialysis because of active secretion into peritoneal lymphatic fluid.

Non-dialytic treatment of uremia

Although dialysis and/or renal transplantation is the standard of care for human patients with advanced uremia, the associated costs and availability limit their use in developing nations. Similar financial and geographical constraints are encountered in the treatment of uremic patients in veterinary medicine. Therefore, therapies designed to prevent or delay the need for dialysis and/or renal transplantation will have significant economic and clinical benefit for both human and veterinary medicine.

Traditionally, non-dialytic management of uremic patients has been symptomatic, with a goal of amelioration of clinical signs. Recently, the emphasis has evolved toward developing therapies that mitigate the clinical manifestations of uremia by interfering with the generation, absorption, or mechanism of action of known uremic toxins. Many uremic toxins are absorbed from the intestinal tract, and may even be produced by intestinal flora. The ingestion of sorbents that bind specific solutes thus preventing their systemic absorption is a commonly used therapeutic modality. For example, enteral aluminum hydroxide is often used to minimize the absorption of ingested phosphorous. A non-selective oral sorbent composed of a high-purity multiporous spherical activated carbon has been shown to decrease the serum concentrations of indoxyl sulfate and p-cresol (Niwa et al. 1992, 1993; Takahashi et al. 2005). Although this approach has theoretical applications for uremia management, most often large quantities of the sorbents must be ingested, rendering clinical use challenging.

The gastrointestinal tract can also be used to mitigate uremia via the ingestion of live bacteria (probiotics) that either naturally, or via genetic engineering, catabolize uremic solutes. Many of the previous logistical problems involved with administration (e.g., protecting the bacteria so that it survives gastric passage) have recently been resolved, greatly improving the therapeutic value of probiotics (Chow 2002). Several studies have demonstrated the safety and efficacy of probiotic therapy in an experimental setting (Hida et al. 1996; Taki et al. 2005; Ranganathan et al. 2006), and a randomized controlled clinical trial assessing probiotic therapy in dogs with naturally occurring stage 3 and 4 CKD is ongoing.

Recent efforts have focused on finding ways to neutralize the toxic effects of uremic retention solutes prior to the appearance of clinical signs. Some uremic toxins have a preferential action on only one or a few systems. However, the majority of the uremic toxins studied to date have effects on multiple systems, most likely resulting from interference with common cellular activities such as changes in receptor activity, alterations of intracellular calcium level, activation/inhibition of transcription factors, and generation of reactive oxygen species. Identification of these common pathways and a more detailed understanding of the pathophysiologic effects of the individual uremic toxins are needed to develop more targeted pharmacologic inhibitors.

The uremic syndrome is characterized by alterations in many biochemical and physiologic processes attributable to declining renal function. Despite recent advances, our knowledge of the nature and biologic behavior of individual uremic retention solutes is incomplete. Extracorporeal renal replacement therapy has been the mainstay of treatment for uremic human patients, but cost and availability have limited its use in veterinary medicine. Many of the non-dialyzable, large and/or protein-bound uremic toxins have been associated with significant toxicity, making them targets for therapeutic intervention. Therapeutic options currently under investigation include oral sorbents and/or probiotics to modify the absorption of many uremic toxins from the intestinal tract, and pharmacologic intervention to inhibit the effects of the uremic toxins. Hopefully, one or more of these new therapies will develop into a readily available and cost-effective management option for uremia, resulting in improved quality and quantity of life for both human and veterinary patients.

References

Adrogué, H.J. (1992). Glucose homeostasis and the kidney. *Kidney Int* **42**: 1266.

Alvestrand, A. (1997). Carbohydrate and insulin metabolism in renal failure. *Kidney Int* **52**(Suppl 62): S48.

Babb, A.L., et al. (1981). The middle molecule hypothesis in perspective. *Am J Kidney Dis* **1**: 46–50.

Beckeer, B.M., et al. (1997). Reassessing the cardiac risk profile in chronic hemodialysis patients: A hypothesis on the role of oxidant stress and other non-traditional cardiac risk factors. *J Am Soc Nephrol* **8**: 475–486.

Bergstrom, J. and P. Furst (1978). Uremic toxins. *Kidney Int* **8**(Suppl): S9–S12.

Boobis, S.W. (1977). Alteration of plasma albumin in relation to decreased drug binding in uremia. *Clin Pharmacol Ther* **22**: 147–153.

Busch, M., et al. (2004). Potential cardiovascular risk factors in chronic kidney disease: AGEs, total homocysteine and metabolites, and the C-reactive protein. *Kidney Int* **66**(1): 338–334.

Cheung, A.K., et al. (2006). Serum beta-2 microglobulin levels predict mortality in dialysis patients: results of the HEMO study. *J Am Soc Nephrol.* **17**(2): 546–55.

Chow, J. (2002). Probiotic and prebiotics: a brief overview. *J Ren Nutr* **12**(2): 76–86.

Craig, R.M., et al. (1983). Kinetic analysis of d-xylose absorption in normal subjects and in patients with chronic renal failure. *J Lab Clin Med* **101**: 496–506.

Daschner, M., et al. (1996). Influence of dialysis on plasma lipid peroxidation products and antioxidant levels. *Kidney Int* **50**: 1268–1272.

De Smet, R., et al. (2001). A decrease of serum albumin increases the free concentration of p-cresol and its toxicity (abstract). *Int J Artif Organs* **24**(8): 544.

De Smet, R., et al. (2003). Toxicity of free *p*-cresol: a prospective and cross-sectional analysis. *Clin Chem* **49**: 470–478.

Depner, T.A. (2001). Uremic toxicity: urea and beyond. *Semin Dial* **14**(4): 246–251.

Deschamps-Latscha, B., et al. (2005). Advanced oxidation protein products as risk factors for atherosclerotic cardiovascular events in nondiabetic predialysis patients. *Am J Kidney Dis* **45**(1): 39–47.

Dhondt, A., et al. (2000). The removal of uremic toxins. *Kidney Int* **58**(suppl 76): S47–S59.

Gotch, F.A. (1998). The current place of urea kinetic modelling with respect to different dialysis modalities. *Nephrol Dial Transplant* **13**(Suppl 6): 10–14.

Hakim, R.M., et al. (1996). Effect of the dialysis membrane on mortality of chronic hemodialysis patients. *Kidney Int* **50**: 566–570.

Hida, M., et al. (1996). Inhibition of the accumulation of uremic toxins in the blood and their precursors in the feces after oral administration of Lebenin, a lactic acid bacteria preparation, to uremic patients undergoing hemodialysis. *Nephron* **74**: 349–355.

Honda, H., et al. (2005). Serum albumin, C-reactive protein, interleukin-6 and feutin-A as predictors of malnutrition, cardiovascular disease, and mortality in patients with end-stage renal disease. *Am J Kidney Dis* **47**: 139–148.

Johnson, W.J., et al. (1972). Effects of urea loading in patients with far advanced renal failure. *Mayo Clin Proc* **47**: 21–29.

Mak, R.H. and R.A. DeFronzo (1992). Glucose and insulin metabolism in uremia. *Nephron* **61**: 377.

Massry, S.G. (1977). Is parathyroid hormone a uremic toxin? *Nephron* **19**: 125–130.

Maton, P.N. and M.E. Burton (1999). Antacids revisited: a review of their clinical pharmacology and recommended therapeutic use. *Drugs* **57**: 855–870.

McNamara, P.J., et al. (1981). Endogenous accumulation products and serum protein binding in uremia. *J Lab Clin Med* **98**: 730–740.

Menon, V., et al. (2005). C-reactive protein and albumin as predictors of all-cause an cardiovascular mortality in chronic kidney disease. *Kidney Int* **68**: 766–772.

Meyer, T.W. and T.H. Hostetter (2008). Uremia. *N Engl J Med* **357**(13): 1316–1325.

Niwa, T., et al. (1992). Suppressed serum and urine levels of indoxyl sulfate by oral sorbent in experimental uremic rats. *Am J Nephrol* **12**: 201–206.

Niwa, T., et al. (1993). Suppressive effect of an oral sorbent on the accumulation of p-cresol in the serum of experimental uremic rats. *Nephron* **65**: 82–87.

Rabkin, R., et al. (1972). Glomerular filtration and proximal tubular absorption of insulin 125 I. *Am J Physiol* **223**: 1093.

Ranganathan, N., et al. (2006). In vitro and in vivo assessment of intraintestinal bacteriotherapy in chronic kidney disease. *ASAIO J* **52**(1): 70–79.

Richet, G. (1988). Early history of uremia. *Kidney Int* **33**: 1013–1015.

Schaedeli, F. and D.E. Uehlinger (1998). Urea kinetics and dialysis treatment time predict vancomycin elimination during high-flux hemodialysis. *Clin Pharmacol Ther* **63**: 26–38.

Sela, S., et al. (2005). Primed peripheral polymorphonuclear leukocyte: a culprit underlying chronic low grade inflammation and systemic oxidative stress in chronic kidney disease. *J Am Soc Nephrol* **16**: 2431–2438.

Stenvinkel, P., et al. (1999). Strong association between malnutrition, inflammation, and atherosclerosis in chronic renal failure. *Kidney Int* **55**: 1899–1911.

Takahashi, N., et al. (2005). Therapeutic effects of long-term administration of an oral adsorbent in patients with chronic renal failure: two-year study. *Int J Urol* **12**(1): 7–11

Taki, K., et al. (2005). Beneficial effects of Bifidobacteria in a gastroresistant seamless capsule on hyperhomocysteinemia in hemodialysis patients. *J Ren Nutr* **15**(1): 77–80.

Vanholder, R., et al. (2003a). Review on uremic toxins: classifications, concentration and interindividual variability. *Kidney Int* **63**: 1934–1943.

Vanholder, R., et al. (2003b). Survival of hemodialysis patients and uremic toxin removal. *Artif Organs* **27**: 218–223.

Vanholder, R., et al. (2008). A bench to bedside view of uremic toxins. *J Am Soc Nephrol* **19**: 863–870.

42

Polyuria and polydipsia

Katherine James

Definition and recognition of a clinical problem

Polyuria refers to formation and voiding of excessive urine volume and polydipsia to excessive voluntary intake of water or other liquids. Polyuria is usually accompanied by increased frequency of voiding, but it is solely the increase in volume that defines polyuria. Thus, when clients report an increased frequency of urination, it is important to refine that observation to whether the medical problem is polyuria or pollakiuria (see Chapter 47) because they require different diagnostic approaches.

Clients may report that their pet has only one or the other, polydipsia or polyuria; however, the two almost invariably present together. Water loss must match water intake to maintain body fluid osmolality within a narrow range that is rapidly and tightly regulated (James and Lunn 2007). Thus, it is clinically appropriate to consider them together as a single medical problem, polyuria/polydipsia (PU/PD). It is possible for polydipsia to exist without polyuria when excessive non-urinary fluid losses exist, such as with diarrhea or respiratory losses in panting dogs; but such situations are recognized easily and rarely persist.

Polyuria is defined as daily urine volume in excess of 50 mL/kg (Feldman and Nelson 2004). Polydipsia is defined as fluid intake exceeding 100 mL/kg per day (Feldman and Nelson 2004). For clinicians, these numerical definitions are rarely useful and it is not necessary for clients to measure their pet's water intake as a means to determine if PU/PD is present. Normal water intake can be variable, particularly in dogs. In part, this is because intake required to compensate for losses changes depending on environmental temperature and their activities. Further, water content and intake from diet varies. The

magnitude of this variability should not be underestimated. In a relatively homogenous group of laboratory dogs, individuals had a tenfold variability in insensible losses due to evaporative respiratory water loss, depending on whether they spent more of their time resting quietly compared to running in circles and barking in their cages (O'Conner and Potts 1969). The myriad of different environments, diets, and activities of pets results in significant variability in required water intake.

There is significant variability in species-typical behavior of dogs and cats. Although healthy cats do not drink much water beyond what is in their diets and the resultant species-typical urine-specific gravity (USG) is considered to be above 1.030–1.040, there are exceptions. Some healthy cats choose to drink more because they enjoy running water from a faucet or fountain. They may even enjoy the social interaction of having the owner turn on the faucet and interact with them while they drink.

For clinicians, water intake is best assessed as appropriate or not appropriate based on that animal's environment, diet, and activities. An alternative approach to use to measure water intake is to place PU/PD on the problem list if the owner reports increased water intake or urine output compared to their normal observations and a substantiating low USG is present. It is the author's observation that USGs of <1.025 are sufficiently low to corroborate an owner report of PU/PD. Clinically, we employ USG as a surrogate test for urine volume. It is quite unusual to have a low USG and low urine volume as this requires ingestion of a low-solute (low protein, low salt) diet (James and Lunn 2007). Thus, for clinical patients, it is sufficient to assume a low USG is associated with a high urine volume. When the solute content of urine is increased by solutes not normally present, for example, glucose, urine volume may be higher than the USG typically reflects. The magnitude of this effect is generally insufficient to

Nephrology and Urology of Small Animals. Edited by Joe Bartges and David J. Polzin. © 2011 Blackwell Publishing Ltd.

lead to a false conclusion that a patient is not PU/PD due to higher USG. Also under such circumstances the USG may be higher than expected; the hypothesis being this reflects glomerulotubular imbalance.

Most patients with PU/PD are persistent throughout the day; however, with primary polydipsia some animals will drink more at certain times of day. Thus USG measurements from different times of day may be required before a client complaint of PU/PD can be entirely dismissed.

Detection of a low USG in a patient when the owner has not observed an increased urine volume or water intake also warrants assessment. In some animals, low USG represents an appropriate renal response to the individual drinking relatively more than the average dog or cat. In other animals, it may be a sign of a medical problem. Determination of USG from samples obtained early in the morning, before the patient drinks, can be helpful in determining if PU/PD is likely to be behavioral or a sign of a medical problem warranting further investigation. Most animals that drink for enjoyment do not do so overnight. Therefore, first morning urine is expected to be the most concentrated of the day. If the USG is sufficiently high, then PU/PD need not be pursued because that demonstrates the kidney can concentrate urine appropriately. Although collecting the urine sample prior to the animal eating or drinking once it has woken is essential, it is neither necessary nor desirable to restrict water access overnight for this assessment. Some patients with PU/PD have a large volume obligate polyuria and will dehydrate rapidly when water is withheld. When the USG is repeatedly low on two or three first morning samples, PU/PD should be pursued even if the client has not noticed it.

Interpretation of USG

The terms *normal* and *abnormal* are not applicable in assessment of USG. For the clinician assessing results of a urinalysis (UA), it is much more helpful to consider whether the USG is *appropriate* or *inappropriate*. If a patient drinks water in excess of what is required to compensate for normal daily losses, it is appropriate for the kidney to excrete extra water as dilute urine. Common examples are a dog that ingests water while playing in a swimming pool or a cat that drinks water from a faucet whenever it is turned on. Production of dilute urine by these animals after water ingestion reflects a normal physiological response. Even extreme hyposthenuria can be appropriate as the normal diluting function of the kidney maintains water balance in the face of an increased water load.

In contrast, if an animal is placed in a hot environment and pants for thermoregulation with resultant insensible respiratory water loss, then the appropriate response is production of concentrated urine if drinking water is not readily available. It is inappropriate to produce dilute urine and a urinary concentrating defect exists.

The range of USG considered typical for dogs is determined by clinical experience and is influenced by the wide variety of canine lifestyles. Dogs appear to be similar to people in that some individuals simply enjoy drinking more than do others. In addition, dogs have a strong thirst response and will not delay water intake if it is available. Thus, it is the opinion of the author that the typical range for canine USG is 1.010–1.040. When a USG above 1.040 is detected persistently, it raises concern for inadequate water intake and may reflect a client withholding water from a pet they perceive as having PU/PD, when in fact it does not.

USGs less than 1.010 in dogs can be appropriate; dogs that engage in water-based games may have USGs as low as 1.000. However such animals are at the limit of renal diluting ability and are at significant risk of clinically important hyponatremia. Generally patients with hyposthenuria require assessment for behaviors that promote high water intake. If none are found, medical evaluation for PU/PD is warranted.

The species-typical anticipated range of USG produced by healthy cats is different. Clinical experience indicates that healthy cats on a dry diet usually have a USG greater than 1.040, and cats on canned diets have USGs of 1.030 or greater. Apart from individual cats that enjoy drinking from a water fountain or a running faucet, most cats do not drink in excess of their needs. Therefore, typical range for feline USG is expected to be 1.040–1.055 for cats on dry food, with a somewhat decreased lower limit for cats fed canned food exclusively. Evaluation for behaviors by an individual cat that promotes higher water intake is warranted when USGs less than 1.030–1.040 are detected depending on diet.

True ranges for isosthenuria, hyposthenuria, and hypersthenuria in an individual animal are defined by the individual's plasma osmolality. As this varies, so will the range of urine osmolalities corresponding to isosthenuria, hyposthenuria, or hypersthenuria. Values of cited USG typically used to describe these ranges correspond to USG values that are observed in normal animals producing urine that is isosthenuric, hyposthenuric, or hypersthenuric with respect to plasma. This distinction becomes important in animals with an abnormally high or low plasma osmolality.

Causes of PU/PD

The ability of the kidney to concentrate urine has three basic requirements (1) presence of ADH, (2) ability of the renal tubules to respond to ADH, and (3) maintenance of high osmolarity of renal medullary interstitial fluid. ADH binds to vasopressin (V2) receptors in the distal renal tubule, which activates intracellular second messenger systems, leading to insertion of water channels (termed aquaporin-2) into the apical membrane of the epithelial cells (Cohen and Post 2002). This allows water to flow along the osmotic gradient between the distal convoluted tubule/collecting duct lumen and the hypertonic renal medulla. Basic understanding of these normal processes allows a classification of causes of PU/PD according to underlying pathophysiology.

Mechanisms leading to PU/PD can be divided into primary polydipsia with compensatory polyuria or primary polyuria with compensatory polydipsia. Disorders leading to primary polyuria can be further subdivided into those associated with reduced or absent ADH synthesis or release, failure of the renal tubule to respond to ADH, or reduction in the osmotic gradient between the filtrate in the distal convoluted tubule and renal medullary interstitium. There are a small number of clinical syndromes capable of causing simultaneous primary polyuria and primary polydipsia.

It is often difficult to distinguish between primary polydipsia and primary polyuria. Water deprivation testing (WDT) cannot be accomplished safely because patients with primary polyuria require polydipsia to prevent hypernatremia. Thus, depriving water to a patient with primary polyuria can have no outcome other than harm to the patient.

Evaluation of serum sodium concentration ($[Na^+]$) in some cases provides an impression which of the two is more likely. A patient with primary polydipsia may have a subnormal or low-normal $[Na^+]$, whereas $[Na^+]$ may be high or high-normal in patients with primary polyuria. Use of serum sodium values cannot make a definitive distinction because low or low-normal $[Na^+]$ may also result from combination of hypovolemia and ongoing water intake (James and Lunn 2007). A classic example is the dog with hypoadrenocorticism that has a primary polyuria, hypovolemia from excess urinary sodium loss, yet a high ADH and intact thirst despite low $[Na^+]$. Finding a low or low-normal $[Na^+]$ in a patient assessed as having a normal ECF volume suggests a primary polydipsia and prioritizes subsequent diagnostic testing. Further, a high or high-normal $[Na^+]$ suggests primary polyuria and serves as a warning that the patient should not be subjected to water restriction. In many PU/PD patients, the $[Na^+]$ will be mid-range normal. This can occur when primary polyuria and polydipsia co-exist. For example, patients with liver failure may have a primary polydipsia associated with hepatic encephalopathy, but may also be polyuric due to low BUN and loss of renal medullary hypertonicity. It also occurs with mild cases of PU/PD

when regulatory processes that maintain the ideal $[Na^+]$ are not challenged.

Table 42.1 provides a list of known and reported causes of PU/PD in dogs and cats (Lunn and James 2007). The mechanism underlying the PU/PD is also listed, if it is known.

Primary polydipsia

Primary polydipsia may be medical or behavioral. It may be a manifestation of hepatic encephalopathy, (Grauer and Nichols 1985) hyperthyroidism, hyperadrenocorticism (Lunn and James 2007), or gastrointestinal disease (Henderson and Elwood 2003). A rare form of primary polydipsia is described in humans resulting from a lesion in the thirst center, but this has not been described in dogs and cats (Feldman and Nelson 2004). Behavioral primary polydipsia represents a range from normal behavior to an overt psychological problem termed "pyschogenic polydipsia." There are few documented cases in the literature, but most clinicians associate this problem with active dogs that have insufficient stimulation or exercise, or with pets in stressful environments (Feldman and Nelson 2004). It is a matter of clinical judgment whether the drinking behavior is within the realm of acceptable variability among dogs or should be labeled as compulsive and warranting behavior modification.

Primary polyuria: Reduced or absent ADH synthesis or release

Reduced or absent ADH synthesis or secretion is termed central diabetes insipidus (CDI). ADH deficiency may be partial or complete, resulting in partial or complete CDI. Causes include head trauma (Rogers et al. 1977; Smith and Elwood 2004; Aroch et al. 2005), neoplasia (Harb et al. 1996), or congenital defects (Ramsey et al. 1999). Many cases are idiopathic (Court and Watson 1983; Harb et al. 1996). Patients with complete CDI are profoundly PU/PD, producing hyposthenuric urine. CDI patients produce so large a urine volume that when they are deprived of water and cannot meet urinary losses for as short a time as two hours, hypernatremia develops. Onset is often acute. Partial CDI results in less severe PU/PD and USG can be isosthenuric.

Primary polyuria: Failure of renal tubules to respond to ADH

Primary (congenital) nephrogenic diabetes insipidus (1°NDI)

This results from a defect in cellular mechanisms that allow renal tubules to respond to ADH. Patients with 1°NDI are unable to concentrate their urine despite

Table 42.1 Causes of polyuria and polydipsia, classification, and underlying mechanism

Cause	Classification	Mechanism(s)
Pyelonephritis	Primary polyuria: 2° NDI	Bacterial endotoxin reduces tubular sensitivity to ADH (Lunn and James 2007) Damaged countercurrent mechanism (Feldman and Nelson 2004)
Pyometra	Primary polyuria: 2° NDI	Bacterial endotoxin reduces tubular sensitivity to ADH (Lunn and James 2007)
Liver failure	Primary polyuria: 2° NDI Primary polydipsia	Loss of medullary hypertonicity (Rogers et al. 1977) Impaired hormone metabolism (Rogers et al. 1977) Psychogenic (Rogers et al. 1977)
Portosystemic shunt	Primary polyuria: 2° NDI Primary polydipsia	Loss of medullary hypertonicity (Deppe et al. 1999) Increased GFR (Deppe et al. 1999) Psychogenic (Grauer and Pitts 1987)
Hyperadrenocorticism	Primary polyuria: CDI Primary polyuria: 2° NDI Primary polydipsia	Impaired release of ADH (Feldman and Nelson 2004) Impaired tubule response to ADH (Cohen and Post 2002) Psychogenic (Nichols 2000)
Hypoadrenocorticism	Primary polyuria: 2° NDI	Loss of medullary hypertonicity
Hyperthyroidism	Primary polyuria: 2° NDI	Loss of medullary hypertonicity (Feldman and Nelson 2004) Psychogenic (Feldman and Nelson 2004)
Acromegaly	Primary polyuria: 2° NDI Primary polyuria: CDI	Osmotic diuresis due to diabetes mellitus (Peterson et al. 1988) Interference with action of ADH? (Schwedes 1999) Partial CDI? (Schwedes 1999)
Pheochromocytoma	Primary polyuria: 2° NDI	Excessive catecholamines (Feldman and Nelson 2004)
Primary hyperaldosteronism	Primary polyuria: CDI Primary polyuria: 2° NDI	Impaired release of ADH (Rijnberk et al. 2001) Impaired tubule response to ADH (Rijnberk et al. 2001)
Hypercalcemia	Primary polyuria: 2° NDI	Interferes with action of ADH on renal tubule (Cohen and Post 2002)
Hypokalemia	Primary polyuria: 2° NDI	Down-regulation of aquaporin-2 (Cohen and Post 2002) Loss of medullary hypertonicity
Hyponatremia	Primary polyuria: 2° NDI	Loss of medullary hypertonicity (Tyler et al. 1987)
Diabetes mellitus	Primary polyuria: 2° NDI	Osmotic diuresis
Primary renal glycosuria	Primary polyuria: 2° NDI	Osmotic diuresis
Fanconi syndrome and other tubulopathies	Primary polyuria: 2° NDI	Osmotic diuresis
Chronic renal failure	Primary polyuria: 2° NDI	Osmotic diuresis
Polyuric acute renal failure	Primary polyuria: 2° NDI	Osmotic diuresis
Postobstructive diuresis	Primary polyuria: 2° NDI	Osmotic diuresis Down-regulation of aquaporin-2 (Cohen and Post 2002)
Chronic partial ureteral obstruction	Primary polyuria: 2° NDI	Down-regulation of aquaporin-2 (Cohen and Post 2002)
Renal medullary solute washout	Primary polyuria: 2° NDI	Decreased renal medullary tonicity with loss of osmotic gradient
Leiomyosarcoma	Primary polyuria: 2° NDI	Impaired tubule response to ADH (Cohen and Post 1999, 2003)
Polycythemia	Primary polyuria: CDI Primary polyuria: 2° NDI	Impaired release of ADH (vanVonderen et al. 1997) Action of atrial natriuretic peptide (vanVonderen et al. 1997)
Leptospirosis	Primary polyuria?	CRF, 2°NDI?
Splenomegaly	Primary polydipsia?	Psychogenic? (Couto 2003)
Primary nephrogenic diabetes insipidus	Primary polyuria: 1° NDI	Congenital inability of nephron to respond to ADH

(Continued)

Table 42.1 (*Continued*)

Cause	Classification	Mechanism(s)
Primary polydipsia	Primary polydipsia	Psychogenic polydipsia (Henderson et al. 2003)
		Hepatic encephalopathy (Rogers et al. 1977)
		Hyperthyroidism (Feldman and Nelson 2004)
		Gastrointestinal disease (Smith and Elwood 2004)
Central diabetes insipidus (CDI)	Primary polyuria: CDI	Antidiuretic hormone deficiency (partial or complete)
Diet, drugs, and toxins	Various	Several mechanisms

Source: From Lunn and James 2007.
Abbreviations: NDI = nephrogenic diabetes insipidus. ADH = antidiuretic hormone. GFR = glomerular filtration rate. CDI = central diabetes insipidus. CRF = chronic renal failure.

adequate blood levels of ADH. Two forms of congenital 1°NDI have been described in humans, but there are very few case reports in dogs or cats (Hoppe and Karlstam 2000; Cohen and Post 2002; Feldman and Nelson 2004).

Secondary (acquired) nephrogenic diabetes insipidus (2°NDI)

It should be apparent from Table 42.1 that this category encompasses the vast majority of causes of PU/PD in dogs and cats. Diseases that lead to loss of renal medullary hypertonicity or osmotic diuresis also cause a 2°NDI, as loss of the normal concentration gradient interferes with effects of ADH. Secondary NDI leads to impaired ability to concentrate urine in the face of water deprivation and impaired response to exogenous ADH.

Renal medullary solute washout

Loss of renal medullary solutes (particularly sodium and urea) leads to reduced medullary hypertonicity, which impairs ability of the nephron to produce concentrated urine. Renal medullary solute washout is rarely a primary cause of PU/PD; the exception being use of very low solute diets. More commonly, it is secondary to prolonged diuresis accompanying marked PU/PD including fluid therapy and diuretic use. For this reason, using abrupt WDT as a means to rule in primary polydipsia is rarely fruitful. Most patients eating appropriate diets replete in salt and protein recover from medullary solute washout rapidly and gradual onset WDTs are better for ruling in primary polydipsia.

Diagnostic approach to PU/PD

Although the list of causes of PU/PD in Table 42.1 is long, many causes can be ruled in or ruled out by obtaining a minimum database and performing additional simple diagnostic tests. This is termed the problem specific database for PU/PD. In addition to complete blood cell counts (CBC), chemistry with electrolytes, and UA, all cats and dogs presenting with PU/PD should have a urine culture. For dogs, leptospirosis titers are also included.

The most common causes of PU/PD in dogs are chronic renal failure (CRF), hyperadrenocorticism, and diabetes mellitus (DM). The most common causes in cats are CRF, hyperthyroidism, and DM. CDI, 1°NDI, and psychogenic polydipsia are uncommon.

PU/PD is in and of itself not particularly detrimental, but some of underling medical syndromes that manifest as PU/PD are. Focus initially on ruling out underlying clinical syndromes or diseases with morbidity and mortality. Most of those diseases, including DM, hypercalcemia, hypokalemia, and renal failure, are detected with a minimum database. Pyelonephritis and leptospirosis are two diseases that may not be revealed by a minimum database as some patients have PU/PD only without organ failure; therefore, they should be tested for. Those PU/PD patients with normal problem-specific database in which the underlying cause of PU/PD is not detected are then evaluated at a slower pace, often necessitated by client constraints.

Signalment and history

The species, age, breed, and sex of the patient may guide initial formulation of a list of differential diagnoses. For example, pyometra is usually a disease of intact females. The patient history may reveal changes that suggest specific causes for PU/PD. For example, a dog with HAC may be polyphagic and lethargic. A careful history of the patient's urinary habits should be obtained in order to confirm the problem is PU/PD and not pollakiuria or inappropriate urination. Polyuric animals may show nocturia or may urinate inappropriately in the house. Previously continent pets with a predisposition to incontinence may develop it associated with increased urine volume. It is essential to obtain a complete medication and diet history in a patient exhibiting PU/PD. Medications associated with PU/PD include glucocorticoids, anticonvulsants, and diuretics. High salt diets may cause PU/PD. Numerous cases of what appears to be a diet-related tubular disease, which may or may not cause PU/PD, have been reported in multiple countries associated with food ingredients from Asia, particularly chicken jerky treats. Urinary tract infection is not a cause for PU/PD unless it is present in the kidneys. Bacterial cystitis does not appear to cause any defect in the renal concentrating ability. It could be hypothesized that discomfort of lower urinary tract inflammation could lead to a primary stress-induced polydipsia but such an occurrence has not been reported in veterinary literature. A positive urine culture in a patient presenting for PU/PD warrants further diagnostic assessment for presence of pyelonephritis.

Working from a complete problem list

When the cause of PU/PD is not immediately evident from the problem specific database, the remainder of the evaluation is often considerably more complicated. Thus, pursue other problems and do not focus solely on the PU/PD problem. Other problems may be additional manifestations of the same underlying disease yet have fewer differential diagnoses and thus lead to a diagnosis more efficiently. It is important to generate a complete problem list for all patients with PU/PD.

A complete physical examination (see Chapter 4) may yield findings suggestive of underlying causes of PU/PD. Examples include coat and skin changes, pot-bellied appearance, and hepatomegaly with HAC. Thyroid nodules or masses may be detected in patients with hyperthyroidism. Enlarged lymph nodes or anal gland mass may suggest presence of neoplasia, which can lead to hypercalcemia. Renal pain suggests obstruction or infection.

Urinalysis

The urinalysis (see Chapter 7) should include physical description, pH, USG, sediment examination, and tests for presence of hemoglobin, protein, glucose, ketones, and bilirubin. The USG can be helpful in the ranking as to likelihood of differential diagnoses for PU/PD. However, for many of the conditions that cause PU/PD, the USG may range between hyposthenuria, isosthenuria, and minimally concentrated, depending on the patient's hydration status, and residual urine concentrating ability. Marked hyposthenuria occurs most likely with DI and psychogenic polydipsia; however, hyposthenuria can occur with HAC, hypercalcemia, and pyometra (examples of secondary nephrogenic DI), and rarely acute renal failure. Detection of hyposthenuria argues against stable

CRF as the *sole* cause of PU/PD. In the latter condition, urine is usually isosthenuric; however, a patient with mild or moderate CRF retains the ability to dilute urine and is able to produce hyposthenuric urine if additional conditions causing PU/PD are present (James and Lunn 2007). For example, a young animal with congenital renal disease may have CRF and 1°NDI and produce hyposthenuric urine (Hoppe and Karlstam 2000).

Do not disregard the role of renal disease in patients with hyposthenuria lacking overt renal failure, as some diseases that inhibit concentrating ability lead to renal failure if not diagnosed and treated. Examples include pyelonephritis, leptospirosis, hypokalemia, or hypercalcemia. While persistent isosthenuria is most suggestive of CRF, intermittent isosthenuria can occur with many causes of PU/PD. A random urine SG of >1.030 means that an obligate polyuria is unlikely to be present because the kidney is capable of producing concentrated urine. Finally, when interpreting USG it is important to consider medical interventions that interfere with the kidney's ability to respond to disorders of fluid balance. Examples include fluid therapy, diuretics, or feeding of markedly protein-restricted diets.

CBC and serum chemistry profile

These tests may reveal evidence of infection or inflammation, liver disease, endocrinopathies, hypercalcemia, and renal failure. Abnormalities on CBC and serum chemistry profile may allow many differential diagnoses for PU/PD to be ruled in or ruled out without further testing. However, subtle changes or values that are technically within normal ranges may provide diagnostic clues suggesting a direction for further investigation. Examples include low blood urea nitrogen (BUN), low-normal albumin and low MCV in liver failure, high-normal BUN and creatinine suggesting early or mild CRF, mild polycythemia and thrombocytosis in HAC, and low-normal $[Na^+]$ with high-normal $[K^+]$ in hypoadrenocorticism. Ensure that serum chemistry profiles are complete with the inclusion of electrolytes as valuable diagnostic clues can be missed if only partial or abbreviated panels are evaluated. When chemistry or CBC values are "borderline" or unexpected, tests should be repeated to verify findings. For example, serum total calcium that is slightly above normal reference range should never be ignored. If it persists, an ionized calcium is obtained.

Urine culture

This is an essential early step in evaluation of PU/PD. Bacterial or fungal pyelonephritis can cause a 2°NDI resulting in PU/PD that may be associated with hyposthenuria (Grauer and Nichols 1985; Newman et al. 2003).

Many causes of PU/PD, such as CRF, HAC, or DM, can predispose to urinary tract infection. If pyelonephritis is suspected but initial urine culture is negative, further tests are indicated, including repeated urine cultures (see Chapter 9), abdominal ultrasonography (see Chapter 16), ultrasound-guided aspiration of the renal pelvis (see Chapter 6), excretory urography (see Chapter 15), and possibly a trial course of antibiotics. With dilute urine the number of inflammatory cells may be low and UTI may be present despite a lack of detectable pyuria. Similarly the absence of microscopically detectable bacteriuria should never be used to rule out UTI.

Leptospirosis serology or polymerase chain reaction (PCR)

Early or mild infection can lead to PU/PD without azotemia (Harkin and Gartrell 1996; Harkin et al. 2003). The mechanism is not known, but as the organisms preferentially localize in the kidney, this could be a form of NDI or a manifestation of early CRF. Leptospirosis may be diagnosed by finding a single high (>1:800) microscopic agglutination test (MAT) titer, by demonstrating a fourfold rise in MAT titer, or by a PCR test on urine (see Chapter 27) (Harkin et al. 2003; Langston and Heuter 2003). As delaying diagnosis of leptospirosis could be harmful and as this is a zoonotic disease, early testing is recommended in dogs with PU/PD in locations where leptospirosis has been reported.

Thyroid hormone assay

This should be performed early in evaluation of any middle-aged or older cat with PU/PD. A total T4 can be obtained initially. If this is normal, yet other clinical problems exist for which hyperthyroidism is a differential, further testing is indicated, with repeated total T4, free T4 or nuclear scintigraphy. Hyperthyroidism in dogs is uncommon and usually associated with a palpable thyroid mass (Peterson et al. 1989), but simply ruled out with a serum total T4. Iatrogenic hyperthyroidism from overtreatment should be ruled out in hypothyroid dogs on supplementation.

Adrenal function testing

The adrenocorticotrophic hormone (ACTH) stimulation test is a useful first-line test of adrenal function in canine PU/PD. Although around 15% of pituitary-dependent and 40% of adrenal-dependent HAC cases will have normal ACTH stimulation test results, (Behrend and Kemppainen 2001) this test is sensitive for diagnosis of hypoadrenocorticism and is the only adrenal function test that will identify iatrogenic HAC (James and Lunn

2007). If there is clinical suspicion of HAC from signalment, history, clinical signs, serum chemistry, UA, and CBC results, a normal ACTH stimulation test should be followed by a low dose dexamethasone suppression test. ACTH stimulation testing is used to rule out hypoadrenocorticism and should be included early in the work-up for any canine patient with even low-normal $[Na^+]$ or high normal $[K^+]$. Electrolyte abnormalities are late-developing manifestations of hypoadrenocorticism and the disease must be suspected while electrolytes are within reference range as long as the trend is in the appropriate direction.

Bile acids

Both acquired liver failure and congenital portosystemic shunts (Rogers et al. 1977; Grauer and Pitts 1987) can be associated with PU/PD. Many patients with these disorders will have other appropriate historical or clinical findings, or provide clues on a serum chemistry panel (low BUN, low albumin, and low cholesterol), but this is not true in all cases. Fasting and post-prandial bile acids are indicated in work-up of PU/PD. Bile acids should be prioritized early in the evaluation for patients with a low BUN:creatinine ratio; although for particularly high urine volume PU/PD, low BUN:creatinine ratios may occur with diuresis.

Imaging studies

Imaging studies are recommended when the history, physical examination, and diagnostic tests discussed above have not identified the cause of PU/PD. Thoracic and abdominal radiographs and abdominal ultrasonography can be used to screen for neoplasia. Contrast studies or ultrasonography may be indicated in pursuit of specific differential diagnoses: examples include excretory urography for pyelonephritis, ultrasonography to rule out "stump" pyometra, and adrenal ultrasound evaluation in suspected HAC or pheochromocytoma. Brain imaging may be indicated if CDI is suspected or diagnosed in an older dog (Court and Watson 1983). Abdominal ultrasonography, portography, or rectal scintigraphy are indicated if portosystemic shunt is suspected.

Assessment of glomerular filtration rate (GFR)

It is possible for a patient to have CRF without demonstrating azotemia because loss of approximately 66% of functional renal mass results in loss of concentrating ability, but more than 75% of functional renal mass must be lost before azotemia develops. This is more likely to occur in dogs because cats maintain enough concentrating ability despite progressive loss of GFR that PU/PD is not noted clinically. Once CRF progresses in a cat to the point of causing detectable PU/PD, azotemia is present, and there is no indication to perform a GFR study. In contrast, it is not unusual to evaluate a dog for PU/PD and detect only isosthenuria without elevated BUN and creatinine. A GFR measurement should be considered in a dog that repeatedly and consistently has isosthenuria or minimally concentrated urine, for which no other explanation is found, particularly when the BUN and creatinine are not at the low end of the reference range. GFR may be assessed by iohexol clearance, exogenous creatinine clearance, or nuclear scintigraphy (see Chapter 14) (Krawiec et al. 1986; Finco et al. 2001; Watson et al. 2002).

Ruling in primary polydipsia

In some patients, primary polydipsia can be diagnosed by obtaining serial USGs and demonstrating production of concentrated urine on at least some occasions (van Vonderen et al. 1999, 2004). This finding rules out primary polyuria as the cause of PU/PD and confirms that the patient is capable of normal urine concentrating ability. As primary polydipsia can be a behavioral problem, increased USG may also be noted when the patient's environment is changed, for example, during hospitalization with free access to water.

When these simple steps fail to rule in primary polydipsia, gradual water deprivation can be used in patients for whom a clinical cause for primary polydipsia has been made. This includes a normal problem-specific database for PU/PD, evaluation to satisfactory explanation of concurrent problems such as hypoalbuminemia or elevated liver enzymes, and a serum $[Na^+]$ that is *not* high or high-normal.

The client should first measure the patient's water consumption over two days to establish free choice daily intake. The water ration at home can then be decreased by 5% per day, while keeping food consumption and activity level constant. The patient should be examined daily, and body weight, USG, BUN, and $[Na^+]$ determined. The test should be discontinued if the patient shows any clinical signs of illness, loses 5% or more of body weight, or develops elevated BUN or $[Na^+]$. If USG increases to 1.030 or greater, diagnosis of primary polydipsia is confirmed. It must be stressed that this approach should only be considered when other common causes of PU/PD have been ruled out, when the client is able to closely monitor the pet, and when the veterinarian is prepared to examine the animal daily.

Classic WDT

With careful patient selection, the WDT can be a useful tool, but in the opinion of this author, its use is rarely justi-fied. Details of the test will not be presented here, but can be obtained from many historical references (Feldman and Nelson 2004). The purpose of the WDT is to determine if an animal can produce a concentrated urine in response to water deprivation. This depends on release of endogenous ADH and ability of the kidneys to respond to ADH. If the patient does not produce concentrated urine, the final part of the WDT involves assessing response to administration of exogenous ADH. The WDT should only be considered when the differential diagnoses for PU/PD have been definitively narrowed down to CDI (partial or complete), primary NDI, and primary polydipsia. All causes of 2°NDI should be fully investigated before a WDT is considered. Although simple in principle, in practice, there are several challenges involved in performing the WDT correctly, and results are often difficult to interpret. This test can also be dangerous if performed incorrectly or if patient selection is inappropriate.

Although it may seem obvious, it is important to remember that "common things are common." The vast majority of cases of PU/PD in dogs and cats are due to HAC, CRF, DM, and hyperthyroidism. CDI, psychogenic polydipsia, and primary NDI are uncommon. A diagnostic plan for any problem should start with tests that are simple, inexpensive, safe, and easy to interpret. A WDT can be expensive, difficult to perform and interpret, and even dangerous. Most cases of PU/PD are due to some form of 2°NDI. This includes HAC, hypoadrenocorticism, hypercalcemia, CRF, liver failure, pyelonephritis, and pyometra. A WDT in these patients would lead to a diagnosis of NDI and the clinician would still then have to test for all the potential acquired causes of NDI. It makes more sense to rule them out first. An animal with pyelonephritis, CRF, hypoadrenocorticism or leptospirosis could potentially decompensate during WDT. Many causes of 2°NDI are harmful if not detected and managed. Examples include pyelonephritis, hypoadrenocorticism, leptospirosis, hypercalcemia, hyperthyroidism, and CRF. Early detection of these diseases may improve survival and prognosis. In contrast, delaying diagnosis of psychogenic polydipsia or CDI is less likely to be harmful provided there is constant access to water.

Some WDT protocols recommend measuring urine and serum osmolality because if a patient is water-deprived but has obligate polyuria a free water deficit occurs leading to elevated serum osmolality. This means that isosthenuria in that patient at that time will be associated with higher urine osmolality. Thus, measuring urine and serum osmolality can be helpful in a WDT when it appears that USG is gradually increasing, but in fact the urine is still isosthenuric for that patient because the patient's serum is hyperosmolar. Classic WDT can be used to rule in partial CDI; however, most work-ups for PU/PD can be safely aborted before this stage as most clients will be comfortable with an assurance that serious causes have been eliminated.

Alternatives to WDT

As an alternative to the WDT, CDI can be diagnosed through use of a DDAVP response trial (Nichols 2000). DDAVP (1-desamino-8-D-arginine vasopressin) is desmopressin, a synthetic analogue of ADH. The DDAVP response trial should only be performed when causes of 2°NDI have been ruled out and when the patient can be closely observed. Prior to starting the trial, the pet owner should measure daily water intake for 2–3 days to establish a baseline. The intranasal preparation of DDAVP is then given into the conjunctival sac (1–4 drops twice daily for 5–7 days) and the patient monitored for reduction in water intake or increase in USG. This is a logical approach because if CDI is ultimately diagnosed it is treated by DDAVP administration (Nichols 2000). If patient signalment, history, or [Na⁺] suggest primary polydipsia, a DDAVP response trial is not recommended due to potential risk of inducing water intoxication.

Interpretation of the DDAVP response trial

1. Patients with CDI would be expected to show a dramatic reduction in water intake, usually of greater than 50%.
2. Patients with HAC can show a variety of responses to DDAVP therapy, which can lead to mistakes in diagnosis. These authors and others (Nichols 2000; James and Lunn 2007) have noted that some dogs with HAC are able to concentrate their urine in response to water deprivation, suggesting that polydipsia may be psychogenic: these patients may not produce concentrated urine during a DDAVP trial. Poor response to DDAVP in a patient with HAC may also be attributed to 2°NDI associated with glucocorticoid excess (Grauer and Nichols 1985). Other patients with HAC may show a partial response to DDAVP suggesting diagnosis of partial CDI (Henderson and Elwood 2003).
3. Failure to concentrate urine in response to a DDAVP trial will occur in both 1°NDI and 2°NDI. The former is a rare condition only likely in very young animals. In a mature dog or cat-acquired causes of NDI are likely and must be investigated.

Creating PU/PD

It is often desirable for clinicians to create PU/PD as an element of a prevention plan for urolithiasis patients. There are several ways that it is accomplished using diet, behavior modification, and diuretics.

Addition of salt or water to the diet can achieve a diuresis and increase urine volume. Addition of salt increases thirst and water intake through associated drinking. The problem with adding salt is that it may decrease palatability and promote nausea particularly in patients that have potassium citrate, also a salt, added to the diet for prevention of certain types of urolithiasis. In some patients, high dietary sodium may worsen hypertension or fluid retention.

Creating a water diuresis increases urine volume. Soup is effective for increasing urine volume in many dogs. Prepare a broth by heating a meat with a high fat content in water such that the fat in the meat creates a highly palatable soup base. Most of the meat can then be discarded if the patient requires a protein-restricted diet. An appropriate kibble is then added. This intervention does not unbalance the diet and preparation time for clients is short such that it can be used as a daily dietary intervention to provide a high water meal.

For some dogs and most cats, liquid-based treats can be used to increase water intake. Recommendations for cats include water in which tuna is packaged, half and half (or commercially available lactose-free milk made for cats), and meat-based broths.

Many cats prefer running water to still water. Thus, addition of regularly cleaned fountains is indicated for cats to increase urine volume. Cats that may have been discouraged from drinking from sink faucets should be encouraged. For some dogs and cats, the taste of the water does seem to make a difference and some will drink more when offered certain brands of bottled water.

For dogs, clicker training to drink on command is also a viable option. It requires an investment in learning the training technique by the client, but once learned, it has many other uses.

Overall success of these interventions depends on quality of monitoring so that clients and clinicians can get regular feedback on what is effective and what is not because the rapidity with which the kidney adjusts urine concentration to match intake. To this end, clients can obtain refractometers for use at home. Inexpensive models are available and allow the client to collect information from all different times in the day. In this way, further changes are precisely made in the management plan. If a urolithiasis patient has dilute urine whenever measured from 10 AM to midnight and yet has concentrated urine at 3 AM, this pinpoints when in the day we need to make further progress to increase urine volume.

References

Aroch, I., et al. (2005). Central diabetes insipidus in 5 cats: clinical presentation, diagnosis and oral desmopressin therapy. *J Feline Med Surg* **7**(6): 333–339.

Behrend, E.N. and R.J. Kemppainen (2001). Diagnosis of canine hyperadrenocorticism. *Vet Clin North Am Small Anim Pract* **31**(5): 985–1001.

Cohen, M. and G.S. Post (1999). Nephrogenic diabetes insipidus in a dog with intestinal leiomyosarcoma. *J Am Vet Med Assoc* **215**(12): 1818–1820.

Cohen, M. and G.S. Post (2002). Water transport in the kidney and nephrogenic diabetes insipidus. *J Vet Intern Med* **16**(5): 510–517.

Cohen, M., et al. (2003). Gastrointestinal leiomyosarcoma in 14 dogs. *J Vet Intern Med* **17**(1): 107–110.

Court, M.H. and A.D. Watson (1983). Idiopathic neurogenic diabetes insipidus in a cat. *Aust Vet J* **60**(8): 245–247.

Couto, C.G. (2003). Lymphadenopathy and splenomegaly. In: *Small Animal Internal Medicine*, edited by R.W. Nelson and C.G. Couto, 3rd edition. pp. 1200–1209.

Deppe, T.A., et al. (1999). Glomerular filtration rate and renal volume in dogs with congenital portosystemic vascular anomalies before and after surgical ligation. *J Vet Intern Med* **13**(5): 465–471.

Feldman, E.C. and R.W. Nelson (2004). *Canine and Feline Endocrinology and Reproduction*. St. Louis, MO: WB Saunders.

Finco, D.R., et al. (2001). Relationship between plasma iohexol clearance and urinary exogenous creatinine clearance in dogs. *J Vet Intern Med* **15**(4): 386–373.

Grauer, G.F. and C.E.R. Nichols (1985). Ascites, renal abnormalities, and electrolyte and acid-base disorders associated with liver disease. *Vet Clin North Am Small Anim Pract* **15**(1): 197–214.

Grauer, G.F. and R.P. Pitts (1987). Primary polydipsia in three dogs with portosystemic shunts. *J Am Anim Hosp Assoc* **23**(2): 197–200.

Harb, F.H., et al. (1996). Central diabetes insipidus in dogs: 20 cases (1986–1995). *J Am Vet Med Assoc* **209**(11): 1884–1888.

Harkin, K.R. and C.L. Gartrell (1996). Canine leptospirosis in New Jersey and Michigan: 17 cases (1990–1995). *J Am Anim Hosp Assoc* **32**: 495–501.

Harkin, K.R., et al. (2003). Clinical application of polymerase chain reaction assay for diagnosis of leptospirosis in dogs. *J Am Vet Med Assoc* **222**(9): 1224–1229.

Henderson, S.M. and C.M. Elwood (2003). A potential causal association between gastrointestinal disease and primary polydipsia in three dogs. *J Small Anim Pract* **44**(6): 280–284.

Hoppe, A. and E. Karlstam (2000). Renal dysplasia in boxers and Finnish harriers. *J Small Anim Pract* **41**(9): 422–426.

James, K.M. and K.F. Lunn (2007). Normal and abnormal water balance: hyponatremia and hypernatremia. *Compend Cont Educ Pract Vet* **29**(10): 589–609.

Krawiec, D.R., et al. (1986). Evaluation of ^{99m}Tc-diethylenetriaminepentaacetic acid nuclear imaging for quantitative determination of the glomerular filtration rate of dogs. *Am J Vet Res* **47**(10): 2175–2179.

Langston, C.E. and K.J. Heuter (2003). Leptospirosis: a re-emerging zoonotic disease. *Vet Clin North Am Small Anim Pract* **33**(4): 791–807.

Lunn, K.F. and K.M. James (2007). Normal and abnormal water balance: polyuria and polydipsia. *Compend Cont Educ Pract Vet* **29**(10): 612–624.

Mulnix, J.A., et al. (1976). Evaluation of a modified water-deprivation test for diagnosis of polyuric disorders in dogs. *J Am Vet Med Assoc* **169**(12): 1327–1330.

Newman, S.J., et al. (2003). Cryptococcal pyelonephritis in a dog. *J Am Vet Med Assoc* **222**(2): 180–183.

Nichols, R. (2000). Clinical use of the vasopressin analogue DDAVP for the diagnosis and treatment of diabetes insipidus. In: *Kirks' Current Veterinary Therapy XIII*, edited by J.D. Bonagura. Philadelphia, PA: WB Saunders, pp. 325–326.

O'Conner, W.J. and D.J. Potts (1969). The external water exchanges of normal laboratory dogs. *Q J Exp Physiol* **54**: 244–265.

Peterson, M.E., et al. (1988). Acromegaly in 14 cats. *J Vet Intern Med* **4**(4): 192–201.

Peterson, M.E., et al. (1989). Radioactive iodine treatment of a functional thyroid carcinoma producing hyperthyroidism in a dog. *J Vet Intern Med* **3**(1): 20–25.

Ramsey, I.K., et al. (1999). Concurrent central diabetes insipidus and panhypopituitarism in a German shepherd dog. *J Small Anim Pract* **40**(6): 271–274.

Rijnberk, A., et al. (2001). Aldosteronoma in a dog with polyuria as the leading symptom. *Domest Anim Endocrinol* **20**: 227–240.

Rogers, W.A., et al. (1977). Partial deficiency of antidiuretic hormone in a cat. *J Am Vet Med Assoc* **170**(5): 545–547.

Schwedes, C.S. (1999). Transient diabetes insipidus in a dog with acromegaly. *J Small Anim Pract* **40**(8): 392–396.

Smith, J.R. and C.M. Elwood (2004). Traumatic partial hypopituitarism in a cat. *J Small Anim Pract* **45**(8): 405–409.

Tyler, R.D., et al. (1987). Renal concentrating ability in dehydrated hyponatremic dogs. *J Am Vet Med Assoc* **191**(9): 1095–1100.

van Vonderen, I.K., et al. (1997). Polyuria and polydipsia and disturbed vasopressin release in 2 dogs with secondary polycythemia. *J Vet Intern Med* **15**(5): 300–303.

van Vonderen, I.K., et al. (1999). Disturbed vasopressin release in 4 dogs with so-called primary polydipsia. *J Vet Intern Med* **13**(5): 419–425.

van Vonderen, I.K., et al. (2004). Vasopressin response to osmotic stimulation in 18 young dogs with polyuria and polydipsia. *J Vet Intern Med* **18**(6): 800–806.

Watson, A.D.J., et al. (2002). Plasma exogenous creatinine clearance test in dogs: comparison with other methods and proposed limited sampling strategy. *J Vet Intern Med* **16**(1): 22–33.

43

Proteinuria and microalbuminuria

Hattie Syme and Jonathon Elliott

When proteinuria is severe, it can result directly in clinical signs. This is discussed in Chapter 44 on nephrotic syndrome and in the chapters dedicated to inherited (see Chapter 56) and acquired (see Chapter 53) glomerular diseases. It is recognised increasingly that proteinuria of lesser magnitude is also of clinical importance due to its prognostic significance. We focus on subnephrotic proteinuria quantified by either measurement of urine protein-creatinine ratio (UPC) or documentation of microalbuminuria.

Origin of proteinuria

Renal proteinuria may result from glomerular or tubular pathology or a combination of the two. The normal glomerulus restricts filtration of most proteins on basis of size, and, to a lesser extent, charge. Thus, in a patient with normal renal function, very few protein molecules of a size equal to or greater than albumin (approximately 69 kDa) appear in urine. Proteins smaller than albumin do traverse the glomerular barrier to a certain extent and some very small proteins will cross the barrier relatively freely. The glomerular basement membrane and slit-diaphragm formed between the interdigitating foot processes of the podocytes provide most of the size and charge selective permeability of the glomerular capillary wall. The endothelial cells, basement membrane, and podocyte foot processes interact with each other to produce a structurally robust and functionally effective glomerular filter. It follows that loss of integrity of any of these structures, either directly or as a result of more generalised glomerular injury, is likely to result in proteinuria and it may be severe. It has also been demonstrated in experimental studies, that increases in glomerular hydrostatic pressure increase the amount of protein that traverses this barrier. Dogs and cats subjected to sub-total nephrectomy, show an increase in glomerular capillary pressure and a corresponding increase in proteinuria (Brown et al. 1990; Brown and Brown 1995). Dogs and cats with systemic hypertension also tend to be more proteinuric than those that are normotensive, (Jacob et al. 2005; Syme et al. 2006) and this is presumed to be caused, at least in part, by transmission of increased systemic arterial pressure to glomerular capillaries. However, an alternative explanation for this association is that patients with hypertension are more likely to have glomerular disease than patients with normotensive chronic kidney disease and thus are more proteinuric. It is proposed that glomerular proteinuria may also occur in animals with systemic illness as a result of generalised endothelial cell dysfunction.

Tubular disease may also result in proteinuria although this is typically of lesser magnitude than in patients with glomerular disease. In the healthy, normally functioning kidney, small amounts of protein, particularly those of low molecular weight but also including small amounts of albumin, traverse the glomerular barrier into the primary glomerular filtrate and are subsequently taken up into tubular epithelial cells for processing. Within the proximal tubule, two multi-ligand receptors, megalin and cubulin, are responsible for endocytotic uptake of a large variety of peptides and proteins including albumin. Proteinuria resulting from specific defects in these tubular transport mechanisms has been reported in humans but is rare. Reduced tubular reabsorption of protein may occur more commonly due to decrease in the number of functioning tubules and increased filtered load per functioning nephron (resulting from adaptive hyperfiltration) in patients with chronic kidney disease.

Nephrology and Urology of Small Animals. Edited by Joe Bartges and David J. Polzin. © 2011 Blackwell Publishing Ltd.

Prognostic significance of proteinuria

Proteinuria has been demonstrated to be of prognostic significance in both dogs (Jacob et al. 2005) and cats (Kuwahara et al. 2006; Syme et al. 2006; King et al. 2007) with chronic kidney disease; with patients that are more proteinuric, in general, having shorter survival times. This holds true even for proteinuria at sub-nephrotic levels with a demonstrable difference in survival with a cut-off point for UPC as low as 0.2 in cats and 1.0 in dogs.

Hypertensive cats and dogs tend to be more proteinuric than their normotensive counterparts even when severity of azotemia is comparable, although, there is a great deal of individual variability (Jacob et al. 2005; Syme et al. 2006). However, diagnosis of hypertension or how well blood pressure is controlled after the instigation of anti-hypertensive therapy, does not appear to predict the survival of cats (Syme et al. 2006; Jepson et al. 2007). This is in contrast to the findings in dogs with chronic kidney disease where hypertension is predictive of reduced survival times (Jacob et al. 2005). The difference between results in these two species may be due to failure to effectively control blood pressure in hypertensive dogs whereas in cats amlodipine is very effective at reducing blood pressure. In hypertensive cats, proteinuria measured either before or after introducing anti-hypertensive therapy is predictive of survival (Jepson et al. 2007) (Table 43.1).

Pathogenesis of renal injury

Proteinuria may have prognostic significance for many different reasons and these are not mutually exclusive. Dogs and cats with proteinuria are more likely to have glomerular disease and that tends to be more rapidly progressive than tubular disease. As discussed above, proteinuria may serve as a marker for glomerular hypertension, generalised endothelial dysfunction, or loss of functioning tubules, any of which may be linked to increased rate of progression of kidney disease through proteinuria-independent mechanisms. Nonetheless, numerous experimental studies provide evidence that proteinuria might also play a direct role in mediating ongoing renal injury.

Table 43.1 Survival of dogs and cats with proteinuria

UPC	Number reaching end-point/Number in group	Relative risk	95% Confidence interval	P	Time to end-point (days)
Feline studies					
Syme et al. (2006)[4], patients included 29 normal, 65 normotensive azotaemic, 15 hypertensive non-azotaemic, and 27 hypertensive azotemic cats					
End point was death due to any cause or euthanasia					
<0.2	17/62	—	—	—	462
0.2–0.4	18/38	2.0	1.0–4.0	0.036	128
≥0.4	26/36	4.7	2.5–8.7	<0.001	98
King et al. (2007), patients all had azotaemic CKD. Known hypertensive patients were excluded					
End point was the need for parenteral fluid administration or euthanasia or death due to renal failure					
<0.2	NR	—	—	—	NR
0.2–0.4	NR	2.2	0.86–5.6	0.10	NR
≥0.4	NR	4.9	2.3–10.6	<0.001	NR
Jepson et al. 2007), all patients were hypertensive, 78 were azotemic, 57 non-azotemic					
End point was death due to any cause or euthanasia					
<0.2	21/36	—	—	—	490
0.2–0.4	24/34	2.2	1.1–4.2	0.018	313
≥0.4	33/48	2.9	1.6–5.4	0.001	162
Canine studies					
Jacob et al. (2005), all patients were azotemic, 7 dogs were also hypertensive at enrollment onto the study					
End point was death due to any cause or euthanasia					
<1.0	12/20	—	—	—	524
≥1.0	20/25	2.9	1.4–6.2	0.004	248

NR-not reported.

Table 43.2 Conditions associated with proteinuria and/or microalbuminuria in dogs and cats

Dogs	Cats
Renal disease	Renal disease
Glucocorticoid therapy (Waters et al. 1997; Schellenberg et al. 2008)	Systemic hypertension (Syme et al. 2006)
Hyperadrenocorticism (Ortega et al. 1996; Hurley and Vaden 1998)	Hyperthyroidism (Syme and Elliott 2001)
Neoplastic disease (Whittemore et al. 2006)	
Lower urinary tract disease (Whittemore et al. 2006)	Lower urinary tract disease (Mardell and Sparkes 2006; Whittemore et al. 2007)
Health status (diseased versus healthy) (Whittemore et al. 2006)	Health status (diseased versus healthy) (Mardell and Sparkes 2006; Whittemore et al. 2007)

Urinary proteins may elicit pro-inflammatory and pro-fibrotic effects that contribute directly to tubulointerstitial damage. Proteinuria may mediate this injury through activation of transcription factors such as NF-κB and up-regulation of various pro-inflammatory and pro-fibrotic genes (reviewed by Abbate et al. 2006). Proteinuria is also associated with transdifferentiation of tubular epithelia cells into myofibroblasts, which is believed to be a crucial step in fibrosis of the kidney. This is mediated, at least in part, by actions of transforming growth factor beta (TGF-β) (Yang and Liu 2001). TGF-β also promotes synthesis of extracellular matrix and is a key promoter of fibrosis (Okuda et al. 1990). Other reported mediators of renal damage in response to proteinuria include, the vasoconstrictive peptide endothelin-1 and molecules that attract monocytes/macrophages such as monocyte chemoattractant protein-1 (MCP-1) and RANTES. The mechanisms by which proteinuria leads to renal injury are multifactorial and involve complex interactions between numerous pathways of cellular damage.

Whether proteins such as albumin are directly responsible for mediating renal injury is controversial, although albumin has been shown to have direct effects in some cell culture models. It has been argued that it may not be directly toxic to tubular epithelial cells but that it is the molecules that bind to it, such as free fatty acids, that perpetrate injury (Thomas et al. 2002). Alternatively, injury could be mediated by other molecules that are of a similar size or smaller than albumin and so are able to traverse the glomerular barrier in settings where proteinuria occurs; circulating cytokines and growth factors may reach tubular cells by this route as may various components of complement (Nangaku et al. 2002).

Proteinuria and albuminuria as predictive markers

The association of proteinuria with progression of renal disease and reduced survival has led to an interest in the use of proteinuria, and often more specifically microalbuminuria, as a screening test for at-risk patients in the general population. This approach has limitations, however, in that in an individual patient it is difficult to predict significance of a positive screening test (Mardell and Sparkes 2006). Proteinuria or microalbuminuria may be detected when any number of renal or extra-renal diseases occur (see Table 43.2). Positive test results are more common with advancing age, presumably due to an increase in the prevalence of systemic diseases (Whittemore et al. 2006, 2007). When dogs or cats are known to be at risk for development of glomerular disease, results of these screening tests may be more meaningfully interpreted, allowing detection of disease at an early stage (Vaden et al. 2001; Grauer et al. 2002; Lees et al. 2002).

Treatment of proteinuria

If proteinuria is directly injurious to the kidney, then interventions to reduce proteinuria should be associated with delayed progression of renal disease. This has resulted in recommendations that reduction in proteinuria be used as a primary therapeutic end-point. It is important to recognize, however, that if proteinuria is simply a marker for some other injurious process (e.g., glomerular hypertension or increased tubular processing) and therapeutic interventions ameliorate that process, a survival benefit may still be evident, even if this is not directly mediated by reduction in proteinuria.

A number of studies have been performed in human patients with chronic kidney disease that indicate treatment with angiotensin converting enzyme (ACE) inhibitors or angiotensin II receptor blockers (ARB) may be superior to treatment with other anti-hypertensive agents, and that this is due to greater reduction in urinary protein excretion that occurs with these drugs (Maschio et al. 1996; Agodoa et al. 2001). The ACE-inhibitor benazepril has been shown to reduce glomerular capillary pressure in cats with experimentally reduced renal mass (Brown et al. 2001). The anti-proteinuric effect of benazepril has been demonstrated in clinical cases of naturally occurring chronic kidney disease (King et al. 2006; Mizutani et al. 2006). As might be expected, reduction in proteinuria is greatest in those patients that are most proteinuric before treatment (King et al. 2006; Mizutani et al. 2006). Unfortunately, despite the demonstrated efficacy of ACE-inhibitors in reducing proteinuria, demonstrable benefit in terms of increased survival times (King et al. 2006), or reduction in the number of cats with an increase in the severity of azotaemia over a follow-up period of 6 months (Mizutani et al. 2006), could not be demonstrated, although favorable trends were evident in both studies. These results are disappointing. It is possible that clear benefit to ACE-inhibitor therapy could be demonstrated by carefully selecting the population that was studied to include only cats that were grossly proteinuric, had mild azotaemia at the study outset and allowing for a prolonged period of follow-up. However, if this were the case, it would not be representative of many cats with chronic kidney disease.

The ACE-inhibitor enalapril has been used in a placebo-controlled study of dogs with biopsy confirmed glomerulonephritis. Dogs treated with enalapril had a reduction in proteinuria compared with those receiving a placebo and progression of renal disease was slowed (Grauer et al. 2000). Although clinical studies have not been performed in dogs with less severe proteinuria, dogs subjected to sub-total nephrectomy and treated with enalapril did show a tendency to a reduction in proteinuria compared to control dogs, and a reduction in glomerular and tubulointerstitial lesions when the study was terminated after 6 months of treatment (Brown et al. 2003).

There are concerns that treatment of hypertension with calcium-channel blockers, such as amlodipine, may exacerbate glomerular hypertension and proteinuria due to afferent arteriolar vasodilation. However, in studies of cats with naturally occurring hypertension, proteinuria was actually reduced when cats were treated with amlodipine (Jepson et al. 2007). This was presumably due to marked reduction in systemic blood pressure that occurred when treatment was implemented. In dogs, where reduction in blood pressure in response to amlodipine treatment is more modest, worsening of proteinuria may be a more realistic concern, but no data exist to substantiate or refute this possibility.

Other potential strategies for reducing urinary protein excretion include, endothelin receptor antagonists, use of calcium channel blockers with selectivity for the efferent arteriole, and dietary therapies. Eicosapentaenoic acid supplementation has been demonstrated to reduce pro-

teinuria and slow renal disease progression in a canine remnant kidney model although the level of supplementation used in these studies was marked (Brown et al. 1998).

References

Abbate, M., et al. (2006). How does proteinuria cause progressive renal damage? *J Am Soc Nephrol* **17**: 2974–2984.

Agodoa, L.Y., et al. (2001). Effect of ramipril vs amlodipine on renal outcomes in hypertensive nephrosclerosis: a randomized controlled trial. *JAMA* **285**: 2719–2728.

Brown, S.A., Brown, C.A. (1995). Single-nephron adaptations to partial renal ablation in cats. *Am J Physiol* **269**: R1002–1008.

Brown, S.A., et al. (1990). Single-nephron adaptations to partial renal ablation in the dog. *Am J Physiol Renal Physiol* **258**: F495–503.

Brown, S.A., et al. (1998). Beneficial effects of chronic administration of dietary [omega]-3 polyunsaturated fatty acids in dogs with renal insufficiency. *J Lab Clin Med* **131**: 447–455.

Brown, S.A., et al. (2001). Effects of the angiotensin converting enzyme inhibitor benazepril in cats with induced renal insufficiency. *Am J Vet Res* **62**: 375–383.

Brown, S.A., et al. (2003). Evaluation of the effects of inhibition of angiotensin converting enzyme with enalapril in dogs with induced chronic renal insufficiency. *Am J Vet Res* **64**: 321–327.

Grauer, G.F., et al. (2000). Effects of enalapril versus placebo as a treatment for canine idiopathic glomerulonephritis. *J Vet Intern Med* **14**: 526–533.

Grauer, G.F., et al. (2002). Development of microalbuminuria in dogs with heartworm disease *J Vet Intern Med* **16**: 352.

Hurley, K.J., Vaden, S.L. (1998). Evaluation of urine protein content in dogs with pituitary-dependent hyperadrenocorticism. *J Am Vet Med Assoc* **212**: 369–373.

Jacob, F., et al. (2005). Evaluation of the association between initial proteinuria and morbidity rate or death in dogs with naturally occurring chronic renal failure. *J Am Vet Med Assoc* **226**: 393–400.

Jepson, R.E., et al. (2007). Effect of control of systolic blood pressure on survival in cats with systemic hypertension. *J Vet Intern Med* **21**: 402–409.

King, J.N., et al. (2006). Tolerability and efficacy of benazepril in cats with chronic kidney disease. *J Vet Intern Med* **20**: 1054–1064.

King, J.N., et al. (2007). Prognostic factors in cats with chronic kidney disease. *J Vet Intern Med* **21**: 906–916.

Kuwahara, Y., et al. (2006). Association of laboratory data and death within one month in cats with chronic renal failure. *J Small Anim Pract* **47**: 446–450.

Lees, G.E., et al. (2002). Persistent albuminuria precedes onset of overt proteinuria in male dogs with X-Linked hereditary nephropathy. *J Vet Intern Med* **16**: 353.

Mardell, E.J., Sparkes, A.H. (2006). Evaluation of a commercial in-house test kit for the semi-quantitative assessment of microalbuminuria in cats. *J Feline Med Surg* **8**: 269–278.

Maschio, G., et al. (1996). Effect of the angiotensin-converting-enzyme inhibitor benazepril on the progression of chronic renal insufficiency. The Angiotensin-Converting-Enzyme Inhibition in Progressive Renal Insufficiency Study Group. *N Engl J Med* **334**: 939–945.

Mizutani, H., et al. (2006). Evaluation of the clinical efficacy of benazepril in the treatment of chronic renal insufficiency in cats. *J Vet Intern Med* **20**: 1074–1079.

Nangaku, M., et al. (2002). C6 mediates chronic progression of tubu-lointerstitial damage in rats with remnant kidneys. *J Am Soc Nephrol* **13**: 928–936.

Okuda, S., et al. (1990). Elevated expression of transforming growth factor-beta and proteoglycan production in experimental glomeru-lonephritis. Possible role in expansion of the mesangial extracellular matrix. *J Clin Invest* **86**: 453–462.

Ortega, T.M., et al. (1996). Systemic arterial blood pressure and urine protein/creatinine ratio in dogs with hyperadrenocorticism. *J Am Vet Med Assoc* **209**: 1724–1729.

Schellenberg, S., et al. (2008). The effects of hydrocortisone on systemic arterial blood pressure and urinary protein excretion in dogs. *J Vet Intern Med* **22**: 273–281.

Syme, H.M., Elliott, J. (2001). Evaluation of proteinuria in hyperthy-roid cats. *J Vet Intern Med* **15**: 299.

Syme, H.M., et al. (2006). Survival of cats with naturally occurring chronic renal failure is related to severity of proteinuria. *J Vet Intern Med* **20**: 528–535.

Thomas, M.E., et al. (2002). Fatty acids exacerbate tubulointerstitial injury in protein-overload proteinuria. *Am J Physiol Renal Physiol* **283**: F640–F647.

Vaden, S.L., et al. (2001). Longitudinal study of microalbuminuria in soft-coated wheaten terriers. *J Vet Intern Med* **15**: 300.

Waters, C.B., et al. (1997). Effects of glucocorticoid therapy on urine protein-to-creatinine ratios and renal morphology in dogs. *J Vet Intern Med* **11**: 172–177.

Whittemore, J.C., et al. (2006). Evaluation of the association between microalbuminuria and the urine albumin-creatinine ratio and sys-temic disease in dogs. *J Am Vet Med Assoc* **229**: 958–963.

Whittemore, J.C., et al. (2007). Association of microalbuminuria and the urine albumin-to-creatinine ratio with systemic disease in cats. *J Am Vet Med Assoc* **230**: 1165–1169.

Yang, J., Liu, Y. (2001). Dissection of key events in tubular epithelial to myofibroblast transition and its implications in renal interstitial fibrosis. *Am J Pathol* **159**: 1465–1475.

44

Nephrotic syndrome

Barrak Pressler

Nephrotic syndrome is an uncommon to rare complication of protein-losing nephropathies in dogs and cats. It refers to the concurrent presence of proteinuria, hypoalbuminemia, extravascular accumulation of fluid, and hyperlipidemia, and when present is pathognomonic for glomerular disease. Evidence in people and laboratory models of glomerular disease have questioned whether these disparate clinicopathologic findings are all direct consequences of massive urinary albumin loss, or whether instead they are distinct manifestations of one or more unidentified disease processes. Patients with hypoalbuminemia, proteinuria, and hyperlipidemia but no third-spacing of fluid are occasionally referred to as having "incomplete" or "incipient" nephrotic syndrome. However, because nephrotic syndrome by definition requires the presence of edema, and many patients with severe hypoalbuminemia will not develop extravascular fluid accumulation, this author does not favor these terms.

Epidemiology

Relative prevalence and causes of nephrotic syndrome in dogs or cats with glomerular disease are unknown. Retrospective studies of dogs with glomerular disease have reported that 5.8–37.5% of these patients are diagnosed with nephrotic syndrome at the time of initial presentation to referral institutions (DiBartola et al. 1980; Jaenke and Allen 1986; Center et al. 1987; Cook and Cowgill 1996). However, true prevalence of this complication is probably less than 10% when considering that patients with nephrotic syndrome are more likely to be referred than those with asymptomatic proteinuria. Nephrotic

syndrome is more likely in cats than in dogs at time of diagnosis of glomerular disease, most likely due to the high prevalence of membranous glomerulopathy with massive proteinuria in cats with glomerular disease (Nash et al. 1979).

Nephrotic syndrome in people is more likely in patients with glomerular diseases associated with large amounts of urine albumin loss (Olson 2006). Adults with primary glomerular diseases and nephrotic syndrome are most likely to have membranous glomerulopathy, followed by minimal change disease and focal segmental glomerulosclerosis. Secondary glomerular diseases, including amyloidosis and diabetic glomerulosclerosis, increase in prevalence in geriatric nephrotic syndrome patients. Pediatric patients with nephrotic syndrome are most commonly diagnosed with minimal change disease. Case series of glomerular disease in dogs and cats have previously suggested nephrotic syndrome may be more common in dogs and cats with membranous glomerulopathy or dogs with amyloidosis; however, in a recent large retrospective study of dogs with nephrotic syndrome, no association was found with the membranoproliferative glomerulonephritis, membranous glomerulopathy, or amyloidosis (Nash et al. 1979; Jaenke and Allen 1986; Center et al. 1987; Cook and Cowgill 1996; Klosterman et al. In press). Therefore, presence of nephrotic syndrome should not increase clinical suspicion of any glomerular disease histologic subtype, including secondary causes of glomerular disease such as drugs, infectious agents, or immune-mediated diseases (Stone et al. 1994; Koutinas et al. 1999; Vasilopulos et al. 2005). This author has treated nephrotic syndrome in dogs with membranous glomerulopathy, membranoproliferative glomerulonephritis, or amyloidosis, and in cats with membranous glomerulopathy or membranoproliferative glomerulonephritis.

Nephrology and Urology of Small Animals. Edited by Joe Bartges and David J. Polzin. © 2011 Blackwell Publishing Ltd.

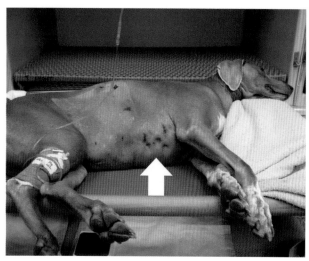

Figure 44.1 Pitting edema in a dog with nephrotic syndrome. This 9-year-old Weimaraner was evaluated for severe hypoalbuminemia, and was diagnosed with nephrotic syndrome. Although no ascites was present, severe pitting edema was noted along the ventral thorax and abdomen. The three depressions on the ventral thorax are pitting areas where digital pressure had been placed while positioning the dog in lateral recumbency.

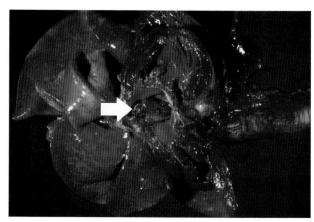

Figure 44.2 Pulmonary arterial thromboembolism (arrow) in a 5-year-old, castrated male Doberman pinscher with nephrotic syndrome that developed dyspnea acutely and was euthanized.

Clinical presentation

Patients with nephrotic syndrome are referred most commonly for abdominal distention secondary to ascites, and in order to be clinically apparent the volume of accumulated abdominal fluid is usually large. However, it is not uncommon for patients who are diagnosed with protein-losing nephropathies in the absence of overt ascites to have some degree of sub-clinical abdominal fluid accumulation evident when diagnostic imaging is performed. Many patients also have pitting subcutaneous edema, particularly in the extremities and ventral abdomen, thorax, and neck (Figure 44.1). Fluid less commonly accumulates in the pleural and pericardial spaces, but dyspnea or tamponade are very rare. Fluid is usually a pure transudate (total nucleated cell count less than 1,000 cells/ul; total protein concentration less than 1.0 g/dL). Finding an increased cell count or protein concentration should likely increase clinical suspicion that an extra-renal disease has resulted in peritoneal effusion and concurrent secondary glomerular disease.

All patients with proteinuria are at increased risk of thromboembolic complications due to urinary loss of anticoagulant proteins, increased synthesis of procoagulant factors, and generalized platelet activation (Olson 2006; Singhal and Brimble 2006). However, human patients with nephrotic syndrome are at increased risk of thromboembolism as compared to those with asymptomatic proteinuria, with renal vein or extra-renal sites

of thrombosis found in 35% and 20% of nephrotic syndrome patients, respectively (Llach 1985; Abrass 1997). This increased incidence may be due to vascular stasis and/or reduced rate of blood flow due to hypovolemia and reduced activity levels in affected patients. Thromboemboli may form in either the arterial or venous systems in people, although emboli of the renal, pulmonary, and deep veins are most common (Llach 1985; Abrass 1997). Limited retrospective studies in dogs with glomerular disease suggest that risk of thromboembolism is not linearly associated with severity of proteinuria, and relationship to nephrotic syndrome in particular has not been examined (Cook and Cowgill 1996). Sites of thrombosis reported by others or encountered by this author include the splenic, hepatic, intestinal and other mesenteric veins, pulmonary vasculature (Figure 44.2), and the renal and adrenal artery and vein (Figure 44.3) (Stone et al. 1994; Cook and Cowgill 1996; Ritt et al. 1997).

Although people with nephrotic syndrome are at increased risk of coronary artery disease, secondary infections, and acute renal failure, these have not been recognized as occurring more frequently in veterinary patients with nephrotic syndrome versus those with asymptomatic proteinuria. Coronary artery disease risk correlates with severity of lipid dysregulation in people (Buemi et al. 2005). Pneumococcal sepsis or peritonitis are the most common secondary infections in people, likely because of the frequent use of immunosuppressive drugs, urinary loss of immunoglobulins, a generalized dysregulation of the immune system, and increased risk of cutaneous infections due to fragility of edematous skin (Soeiro et al. 2004). Risk factors in human nephrotic syndrome patients for development of acute renal failure include chronic hypovolemia, sepsis, thromboembolic

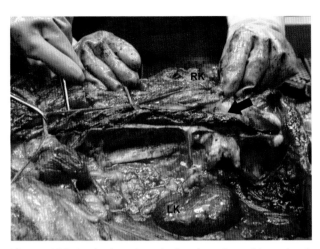

Figure 44.3 Aortic thromboembolism in a dog with nephrotic syndrome. This dog was evaluated for acute renal failure. An aortic thromboembolism (arrow) was diagnosed via abdominal ultrasonography, with suspected bilateral partial occlusion of the renal arteries. Note that the kidneys are normal in size but the surfaces are slightly irregular, a common finding in dogs with glomerular disease. The dog is in left lateral recumbency with the head to the right of the image. LK, left kidney; RK, right kidney.

disease, and increased risk of tubular necrosis due to reduced protein binding of nephrotoxic drugs.

Pathophysiology

Nephrotic syndrome may be solely due to massive urinary loss of albumin and other proteins, with third spacing of fluid and hyperlipidemia being natural pathophysiologic consequences of decreased plasma oncotic pressure. Conversely, growing evidence in people and animal models suggests that these latter components of nephrotic syndrome may only be partially related to hypoalbuminemia, and instead may result from independent pathologic processes that occur concurrently with glomerular damage.

Proteinuria and hypoalbuminemia

Hypoalbuminemia in patients with nephrotic syndrome is a direct consequence of proteinuria. In people, "nephrotic range" proteinuria refers to urine protein loss greater than 3 g/24 hours/1.73 m^2 (in adults), and identifies patients at increased risk for development of nephrotic syndrome (Orth and Ritz 1998). Authors of at least one large retrospective study of nephrotic syndrome in dogs were unable to establish serum albumin concentrations or urine protein:creatinine ratio values that were associated with increased risk of edema formation; dogs with glomerular disease without nephrotic syndrome frequently had serum albumin concentrations as low as those with nephrotic syndrome, and UPC values

were likewise mildly to severely increased in both patient groups (Klosterman et al. In press). Previous studies likewise have reported that dogs with serum albumin concentrations less than 1.5 g/dL or urine protein:creatinine ratios greater than 10.0 are not consistently reported to have third-spacing of fluid (Jaenke and Allen 1986; Center et al. 1987; Cook and Cowgill 1996). Loss of larger serum proteins, particularly globulins, is rarely sufficient to result in hypoglobulinemia in dogs or cats (DiBartola et al. 1980; Jaenke and Allen 1986; Center 1987; Cook and Cowgill 1996; Olson 2006).

Extravascular fluid accumulation

Hypoalbuminemia is necessary for third-spacing of fluid to occur, but the pathogenesis of extravascular fluid accumulation is more complex than simply due to the associated drop in plasma oncotic pressure. Under homeostatic conditions, the sum of Starling's forces favors net movement of fluid out of the proximal capillaries, but edema is prevented by re-uptake of fluid in the distal capillaries and the lymphatic circulation. Hypoalbuminemia results in a decrease in plasma oncotic pressure and thus initially favors greater net outward flow of fluid. However, albumin rapidly equilibrates between the vascular and interstitial spaces, and a given reduction in plasma albumin concentration should result in a near-identical decrease in interstitial albumin concentration (Koomans 2003). Additionally, rodents and dogs with severe, induced hypoalbuminemia fail to develop edema following fluid challenge despite a significant reduction in plasma oncotic pressure (Joles et al. 1988; Doucet et al. 2007).

Several hypotheses exist as to the metabolic derangements which are responsible for edema formation in patients with nephrotic syndrome. The "underfill" hypothesis argues that the initial decrease in plasma oncotic pressure results in up-regulation of the renin-angiotensin-aldosterone system due to the initial increase in fluid extravasation and secondary decrease in circulating blood volume (Rodriguez-Iturbe et al. 2002; Olson 2006). Increased sodium retention therefore maintains near-normal intravascular hydrostatic pressure which is not matched by an increase in interstitial hydrostatic pressure, and edema forms. In people, this hypothesis is not favored in most cases of nephrotic syndrome, as the hypovolemia and hypotension which would be expected in this theory are rare; however, underfill leading to nephrotic syndrome may be more likely in pediatric patients. Alternatively, the "overfill" hypothesis proposes a primary nephron defect that prevents adequate sodium excretion (Rodriguez-Iturbe et al. 2002; Olson 2006). Indeed, human patients diagnosed with protein-losing nephropathies prior to onset of nephrotic syndrome are often sodium avid despite being normoalbuminemic (Doucet et al. 2007). Sodium avidity secondarily results in increased intravascular volume, a rise in hydrostatic pressure, and ultimately fluid extravasation. Hypertension would be expected in these patients, and this indeed occurs in human adults and many veterinary patients with glomerular disease with or without nephrotic syndrome. This unidentified tubular defect may be uniform in all patients with nephrotic syndrome, as albumin directly stimulates the proximal tubular sodium/hydrogen exchanger, many patients with nephrotic syndrome demonstrate up-regulation of the basolateral Na/K-ATPase transporter, and progressive tubulointerstitial disease secondary to proteinuria may non-specifically result in sodium retention (Doucet et al. 2007).

Finally, some evidence suggests that an unidentified "permeability factor," such as an autoantibody or cytokine, may directly alter vascular and glomerular permeability and be the proximate cause of edema in nephrotic syndrome (van den Berg and Weening 2004). Immunosuppressive therapy in people, particularly using drugs which down-regulate T_H2-associated responses, significantly reduces edema formation with a disproportionately milder reduction in proteinuria, as does plasmapheresis (Artero et al. 1994; Dantal et al. 1998; Bussemaker et al. 2001; van den Berg and Weening 2004). Relative percentage of various peripheral circulating T-cell subsets and types and amounts of cytokines produced vary in patients with nephrotic syndrome at the time of diagnosis versus time of remission, arguing that some immune dysregulation accompanies disease (Van den Berg and Weening 2004). Plasma from human patients with some forms of glomerular disease induces proteinuria in rats following intraperitoneal injection, and increases permeability of isolated glomeruli (Sharma et al. 1999 and Sharma et al. 2002). These studies are, of course, complicated by the necessary assumption that all nephrotic syndromes have the same etiopathogenesis; likewise, veterinarians should be cautious in assuming that nephrotic syndrome in veterinary patients has a similar pathogenesis as in people. No studies on immune dysregulation in dogs or cats with nephrotic syndrome have been performed to date.

Hyperlipidemia

Although cholesterol is the only lipid routinely measured in most dogs and cats with nephrotic syndrome, human patients and animal models have both quantitative and qualitative abnormalities in serum lipoprotein profiles. These include an increase in serum total, very low-, low-, and intermediate-density lipoprotein cholesterol, serum triglycerides, and chylomicrons, most of which are inversely proportional to the severity of hypoalbuminemia (Delvin et al. 2003; Kronenberg et al. 2005). A significant correlation between serum cholesterol and albumin has not been found in dogs with glomerular disease in general, but patients with nephrotic syndrome have not been specifically studied (Center et al. 1987; Cook and Cowgill 1996).

Increases in cholesterol and triglycerides are due to both up-regulated activity of enzymes in their synthesis pathways as well as reduced catabolism (Delvin et al. 2003; Kronenberg 2005). 3-hydroxy-3-methyl-glutaryl coenzyme A (HMG-CoA reductase, the rate-limiting enzyme in synthesis of cholesterol) activity is increased in patients with nephrotic syndrome; activity of this enzyme is also increased in animal models with hereditary analbuminemia, arguing that hypercholesterolemia may be a direct consequence of hypoalbuminemia (Vaziri and Liang 1995; Liang and Vaziri 2003; Kronenberg 2005). In addition, culture of hepatic cells in hypoalbuminemic medium results in increased transcription of genes that contribute to nephrotic syndrome-associated dyslipidemia, but not when oncotic pressure is normalized either via addition of albumin or dextrans, a non-albumin high-oncotic pressure molecule (Yamauchi et al. 1992). Reduced catabolism of serum lipids occurs due to decreased hepatic LDL and HDL receptor protein concentrations, preventing reverse cholesterol transport (Delvin et al. 2003; Kronenberg 2005). LDL and VLDL receptors are downregulated in a number of tissues in patients with nephrotic syndrome, also preventing cellular uptake of lipids. Catabolism may be also be decreased due to qualitative differences in lipoprotein concentrations within VLDL molecules; reduced VLDL concentrations of apo E in nephrotic syndrome patients, a ligand for the VLDL receptor, results in impaired VLDL uptake by cells and therefore reduced lipolysis of triglyceride-rich lipoproteins.

Finally, although HDL cholesterol concentrations are usually unremarkable in human patients with nephrotic syndrome, there is nevertheless a disturbed maturation from lipid-poor to lipid-rich HDL particles and a qualitative shift in lipid-rich to lipid-poor HDL molecules (Kronenberg 2005). This is a consequence of urinary loss of lecithin:cholesterol acyltransferase (LCAT), the enzyme responsible for esterification of cholesterol within HDL particles (Vaziri et al. 2001).

Treatment

As with non-nephrotic syndrome-associated glomerular diseases, diagnostic approach and therapy should most importantly focus on identifying and treating any extra-renal causes of disease and maximally reducing proteinuria. Renal-formulated diets are likely important in minimizing fluid accumulation because of their reduced sodium content, and ACE-inhibitors decrease water and sodium retention by inhibition of the renin-angiotensin-aldosterone axis and increase plasma oncotic pressure by reducing proteinuria via decreased intra-glomerular hydrostatic pressure. For a complete review of anti-proteinuric therapy and other adjunctive therapies recommended for treatment of glomerular disease regardless of the presence of nephrotic syndrome, see Chapter XXX.

Removal of fluid is recommended only when patients are in obvious discomfort or presence of fluid may be life-threatening. Indications for abdominocentesis generally include dyspnea due to impaired contraction of the diaphragm during inspiration, reduced appetite, or markedly decreased activity levels. A less common indication for removal of ascites in dogs and cats is severe hypertension, which anecdotally may be aggravated by large volumes of ascites. Removal of large volumes of fluid should be avoided as this may cause further up-regulation of the renin–angiotensin–aldosterone axis due to hypovolemia following increased extravasation of fluid to replace the removed fluid. In addition, although the ascites in patients with nephrotic syndrome is usually a pure transudate, removal of even the small quantities of albumin within this fluid may further aggravate nephrotic syndrome. Repeated removal of fluid and secondary intravascular underfilling and acidosis may result in hyponatremia and hyperkalemia. Pleural or pericardial fluid of sufficient volume to result in noticeable physical examination abnormalities (such as muffled heart or lung sounds or tachypnea) should be removed before they progress to life-threatening volumes.

Diuretic therapy is usually initiated in veterinary patients with nephrotic syndrome and clinical signs severe enough to merit fluid removal. As discussed above, the "overfill" hypothesis argues that a primary sodium hyperavidity defect is partially responsible for development of nephrotic syndrome, and therefore diuretic therapy may be independently indicated regardless of whether or not fluid accumulation is severe. The most commonly used first-line diuretic is furosemide. The dose should be adjusted to minimize fluid accumulation until anti-proteinuric or disease-specific therapy is sufficient to minimize albumin loss; the goal should not be to completely stop fluid extravasation, as the diuretic doses typically required for this outcome lead to hypovolemia and electrolyte abnormalities. In addition, human patients with nephrotic syndrome may be resistant to the loop diuretics, presumptively through a maximally activated renin-angiotensin-aldosterone axis (Doucet et al. 2007). In these cases spironolactone, an aldosterone antagonist, may be more, effective and minimizes the likelihood of electrolyte abnormalities. Patients that require chronic diuretic therapy may respond better to spironolactone monotherapy or a sub-maximal dose of furosemide in conjunction with standard dosing of spironolactone.

Intravenous fluid therapy in patients with nephrotic syndrome is occasionally required when hypovolemia is present or acute renal failure is suspected. Low-sodium isotonic crystalloids or synthetic colloids (which are standardly supplied in 0.9% sodium chloride) are most appropriate. Hypoalbuminemic patients have metabolic alkalosis, and thus 0.9% or 0.45% sodium chloride is more appropriate than alternative buffered solutions. Although in theory a low-sodium fluid should reduce the likelihood of iatrogenic "overfill," patients with nephrotic syndrome are sufficiently sodium avid that decreasing the rate of fluid administration is likely more critical to avoid overhydration and worsening fluid extravasation than the sodium concentration.

Anticoagulant therapy in people and veterinary patients with glomerular disease is usually initiated once serum albumin decreases below 2.0–2.5 g/dL or urine albumin loss is greater than 10 g/24 hours (Singhal and Brimble 2006; Charlesworth et al. 2008). Aspirin is used most commonly in dogs and cats in order to minimize spontaneous platelet aggregation. Although warfarin and heparin are also regularly used in people with documented thromboembolic disease, there is minimal to no experience with these drugs in veterinary patients with nephrotic syndrome. If therapy with either drug is begun, therapeutic monitoring should be intense, as severe hypoproteinemia lowers the recommended starting doses and therapeutic margins for both drugs. Prognosis in people with existing thromboemboli is not improved by fibrinolysis, and there are no good protocols in place for dogs or cats with this complication (Singhal and Brimble 2006; Charlesworth et al. 2008).

Due to the association between hyperlipidemia and coronary artery occlusion by atherosclerotic plaques in people with nephrotic syndrome, treatment with HMG-CoA reductase inhibitors (i.e., "statins") is oftentimes recommended (Buemi et al. 2005; Charlesworth et al. 2008). Other less-effective lipid-lowering treatments may include ACE-inhibitors and diets with increased omega-3:omega-6 polyunsaturated fatty acid ratios (Buemi et al. 2005). Fortunately, there are no documented consequences directly attributed to hyperlipidemia in dogs or cats with nephrotic syndrome. As a result, other than non-specific therapy with a commercial renal-formulated that includes an appropriately modified polyunsaturated fatty acid ratio, no specific lipid-lowering drugs are recommended.

Nephrotic syndrome in people is commonly treated with immunosuppressive drugs, as the most common underlying diseases (membranous glomerulopathy and minimal change disease) are frequently steroid-responsive (Hodson et al. 2005). Unfortunately, prednisone or cyclosporine in dogs with glomerular disease in general have only provided evidence of worsened or at best unaltered prognosis (Center et al. 1987; Vaden et al. 1995; Waters et al. 1997). Anecdotally, some patients with nephrotic syndrome, particularly when secondary to Lyme-associated nephritis or membranous glomerulopathy, have responded to immunosuppressive therapies. Due to the risks associated with these therapies they are only recommended following biopsy-determined glomerular disease subtype, comprehensive extra-renal screening for concurrent diseases, and ideally, consultation with a veterinary nephrologist.

Prognosis

The only retrospective study of dogs with nephrotic syndrome demonstrated shorter median survival time following initial evaluation when compared to dogs with non-nephrotic glomerular disease. Median survival of nephrotic dogs was approximately 13 days after first evaluation at one of eight referral institutions, whereas dogs with glomerular disease but without nephrotic syndrome survived a median of 105 days. When dogs were stratified based on absence or presence of azotemia (defined as a serum creatinine concentration greater than 1.5 mg/dl) this difference in survival was only significant in non-azotemic dogs, implying that the negative effect of azotemia on survival affects prognosis to a far greater degree than the negative effect of nephrotic syndrome alone (Klosterman et al. In press). Similar studies have not been performed in cats, but clinical experience suggests that, as with dogs, the presence of nephrotic syndrome is a negative prognostic indicator.

References

Abrass, C. (1997). Clinical spectrum and complications of the nephrotic syndrome. *J Investig Med* **45**(4): 143–153.

Artero, M., et al. (1994). Plasmapheresis reduces proteinuria and serum capacity to injure glomeruli in patients with recurrent focal glomerulosclerosis. *Am J Kidney Dis* **23**(4): 574–581.

Buemi, M., et al. (2005). Statins in nephrotic syndrome: a new weapon against tissue injury. *Med Res Rev* **25**(6): 587–609.

Bussemaker, E., et al. (2001). Tryptophan immunoadsorption strongly reduces proteinuria in recurrent nephrotic syndrome. *Nephrol Dial Transplant* **16**(6): 1270–1272.

Center, S., et al. (1987). Clinicopathologic, renal immunofluorescent, and light microscopic features of glomerulonephritis in the dog: 41 cases (1975–1985). *J Am Vet Med Assoc* **190**(1): 81–90.

Charlesworth, J., et al. (2008). Adult nephrotic syndrome: non-specific strategies for treatment. *Nephrology (Carlton)* **13**(1): 45–50.

Cook, A. and L. Cowgill (1996). Clinical and pathological features of protein-losing glomerular disease in the dog: a review of 137 cases (1985–1992). *J Am Anim Hosp Assoc* **32**(4): 313–322.

Dantal, J., et al. (1998). Antihuman immunoglobulin affinity immunoadsorption strongly decreases proteinuria in patients with relapsing nephrotic syndrome. *J Am Soc Nephrol* **9**(9): 1709–1715.

Delvin, E., et al. (2003). Dyslipidemia in pediatric nephrotic syndrome: causes revisited. *Clin Biochem* **36**(2): 95–101.

DiBartola, S., et al. (1980). Urinary protein excretion and immunopathologic findings in dogs with glomerular disease. *J Am Vet Med Assoc* **177**(1): 73–77.

Doucet, A., et al. (2007). Molecular mechanism of edema formation in nephrotic syndrome: therapeutic implications. *Pediatr Nephrol* **22**(12): 1983–1990.

Hodson, E., et al. (2005). Evidence-based management of steroid-sensitive nephrotic syndrome. *Pediatr Nephrol* **20**(11): 1523–1530.

Jaenke, R. and T. Allen (1986). Membranous nephropathy in the dog. *Vet Pathol* **23**(6): 718–733.

Joles, J., et al. (1988). Hypoproteinemia and recovery from edema in dogs. *Am J Physiol* **254**(6 Pt 2): F887–F894.

Klosterman, E., et al. Comparison of signalment, clinicopathologic findings, histologic diagnosis, and prognosis in dogs with glomerular disease with or without nephrotic syndrome. *J Vet Intern Med*, in press.

Koomans, H. (2003). Pathophysiology of oedema in idiopathic nephrotic syndrome. *Nephrol Dial Transplant* **18**(Suppl 6): vi30–vi32.

Koutinas, A., et al. (1999). Clinical considerations on canine visceral leishmaniasis in Greece: a retrospective study of 158 cases (1989–1996). *J Am Anim Hosp Assoc* **35**(5): 376–383.

Kronenberg, F. (2005). Dyslipidemia and nephrotic syndrome: recent advances. *J Ren Nutr* **15**(2): 195–203.

Liang, K. and N. Vaziri (2003). HMG-CoA reductase, cholesterol 7alpha-hydroxylase, LCAT, ACAT, LDL receptor, and SRB-1 in hereditary analbuminemia. *Kidney Int* **64**(1): 192–198.

Llach, F. (1985). Hypercoagulability, renal vein thrombosis, and other thrombotic complications of nephrotic syndrome. *Kidney Int* **28**(3): 429–439.

Nash, A., et al. (1979). Membranous nephropathy in the cat: a clinical and pathological study. *Vet Rec* **105**(4): 71–77.

Olson, J. (2006). The nephrotic syndrome and minimal change disease. In: *Heptinstall's Pathology of the Kidney*, edited by J. Charles Jennette et al. Philadelphia PA: Lippincott, Williams and Wilkins, pp. 125–154.

Orth, S. and E. Ritz (1998). The nephrotic syndrome. *N Engl J Med* **338**(17): 1202–1211.

Ritt, M., et al. (1997). Nephrotic syndrome resulting in thromboembolic disease and disseminated intravascular coagulation in a dog. *J Am Anim Hosp Assoc* **33**(5): 385–391.

Rodriguez-Iturbe, B., et al. (2002). Interstitial inflammation, sodium retention, and the pathogenesis of nephrotic edema: a unifying hypothesis. *Kidney Int* **62**(4): 1379–1384.

Sharma, M., et al. (1999). The FSGS factor: enrichment and in vivo effect of activity from focal segmental glomerulosclerosis plasma. *J Am Soc Nephrol* **10**(3): 552–561.

Sharma, M., et al. (2002). Proteinuria after injection of human focal segmental glomerulosclerosis factor. *Transplantation* **73**(3): 366–372.

Singhal, R. and K.S. Brimble (2006). Thromboembolic complications in the nephrotic syndrome: pathophysiology and clinical management. *Thromb Res* **118**(3): 397–407.

Soeiro, E., et al. (2004). Influence of nephrotic state on the infectious profile in childhood idiopathic nephrotic syndrome. *Revista do Hospital das Clinicas Faculdade Medicina Sao Paulo* **59**(5): 273–278.

Stone, M., et al. (1994). Lupus-type anticoagulant in a dog with hemolysis and thrombosis. *J Vet Intern Med* **8**(1): 57–61.

Vaden, S., et al. (1995). The effects of cyclosporine versus standard care in dogs with naturally occurring glomerulonephritis. *J Vet Intern Med* **9**(4): 259–266.

van den Berg, J. and J. Weening (2004). Role of the immune system in the pathogenesis of idiopathic nephrotic syndrome. *Clin Sci (London)* **107**(2): 125–136.

Vasilopulos, R., et al. (2005). Nephrotic syndrome associated with administration of sulfadimethoxine/ormetoprim in a Doberman. *J Small Anim Pract* **46**(5): 232–236.

Vaziri, N., et al. (2001). Acquired lecithin-cholesterol acyltransferase deficiency in nephrotic syndrome. *Am J Physiol Renal Physiol* **280**(5): F823–F828.

Vaziri, N. and K. Liang (1995). Hepatic HMG-CoA reductase gene expression during the course of puromycin-induced nephrosis. *Kidney Int* **48**(6): 1979–1985.

Waters, C., et al. (1997). Effects of glucocorticoid therapy on urine protein-to-creatinine ratios and renal morphology in dogs. *J Vet Intern Med* **11**(3): 172–177.

Yamauchi, A., et al. (1992). Oncotic pressure regulates gene transcriptions of albumin and apolipoprotein B in cultured rat hepatoma cells. *Am J Physiol* **263**(2 Pt 1): C397–C404.

45

Abnormal renal palpation

Claudia Kirk and Joe Bartges

Abdominal palpation is an important part of a complete physical examination, and palpation of the kidneys should be performed when clinical signs of urinary tract disease are present. The kidneys are normally "bean-shaped" organs that lie retroperitoneally ventral to sublumbar musculature. The right kidney lies cranial to the left kidney and is recessed in the renal notch of the liver and medial to the last rib and abdominal wall. The left kidney is positioned more caudally then the right kidney and is caudal to the spleen, caudal to the last rib, and medial to the abdominal wall. In dogs, the left kidney can be palpated normally while the right kidney is palpable uncommonly. Relative to body weight, feline kidneys are larger than canine kidneys and all aspects of both kidneys are readily palpable and moveable.

When normal renal morphology is altered, it is usually associated with a pathological process although it may be secondary to physiological processes. Major palpable abnormalities include change in size, either enlargement (renomegaly) or decrease or a change in shape. Other changes may include change in consistency, less or more than two kidneys, position different than normal, and pain. Changes may be unilateral or bilateral.

Alteration in size

Increased size (renomegaly)

Renomegaly may be due to pathological or physiological processes. Renal compensatory hypertrophy occurs when one kidney is non-functional and small or not present. Examples where compensatory hypertrophy may occur include unilateral nephrectomy, renal agenesis or dysplasia (Figure 45.1), or infarction of one kidney.

Unilateral renomegaly is pathologic when the other kidney is functional. Bilateral renomegaly is common with portovascular anomalies, acromegaly, and bilateral cellular infiltration. Infiltration of renal tissue usually occurs with inflammatory or neoplastic cells (Figures 45.2–45.4).

Decreased size

Reduction in renal size usually reflects chronic disease or developmental problems and can be unilateral or bilateral. Chronic renal disease is the most common cause of reduced renal size (Figure 45.5).

Alteration in shape

Many diseases alter renal shape including renal dysplasia, horseshoe kidney, perinephric pseudocysts, renal neoplasia (Figure 45.3), subcapsular hematomas, or polycystic kidney disease (Figure 45.6).

Alteration in consistency

Palpation of kidneys may reveal a change in consistency including softness due to fluid (such as cystic disease, subcapsular blood or fluid accumulation, or a cystic tumor) or degeneration or firmness due to infiltration by neoplastic or inflammatory cells or fibrosis. Perinephric pseudocysts and polycystic kidney disease have a fluctuant consistency.

Alteration in number

The most common cause of alteration in number of kidneys is congenital disease. Decreased number may occur with renal agenesis or fusion (horseshoe kidney) and increased number may be due to renal duplication. Renal duplication has been reported to occur in Beagles

Nephrology and Urology of Small Animals. Edited by Joe Bartges and David J. Polzin. © 2011 Blackwell Publishing Ltd.

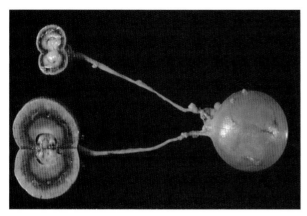

Figure 45.1 Left unilateral renal hypoplasia with compensatory hypertrophy of the right kidney in a cat. Photograph courtesy of Dr. Linden Craig, Department of Pathobiology, College of Veterinary Medicine, The University of Tennessee.

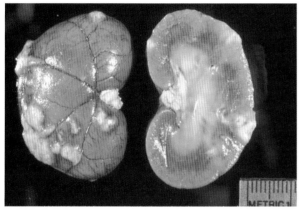

Figure 45.2 Renal involvement with feline infectious peritonitis. Photograph courtesy of Dr. Linden Craig, Department of Pathobiology, College of Veterinary Medicine, The University of Tennessee.

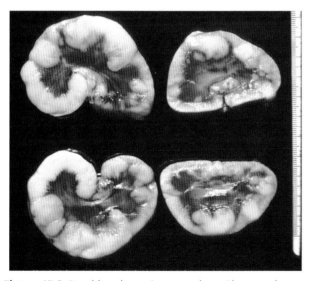

Figure 45.3 Renal lymphoma in an aged cat. Photograph courtesy of Dr. Linden Craig, Department of Pathobiology, College of Veterinary Medicine, The University of Tennessee.

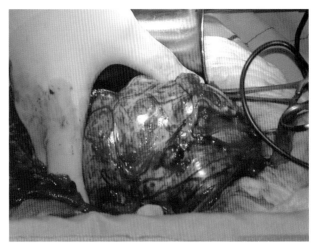

Figure 45.4 Appearance of a nephroblastoma at surgery in a dog.

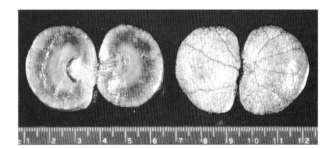

Figure 45.5 Kidneys from a 20-year-old, Siamese cat with chronic renal failure.

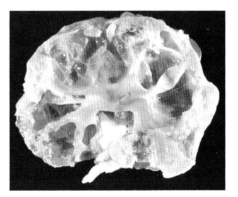

Figure 45.6 Feline polycystic kidney disease.

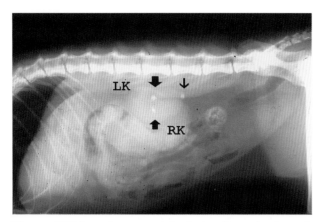

Figure 45.7 Lateral survey abdominal radiograph of an 8-year-old, castrated male domestic shorthaired cat, with bilateral nephroliths (large arrows), small left kidney (LK), right ureterolith (small arrow), and enlarged right kidney (RK) due to hydronephrosis secondary to ureteral obstruction.

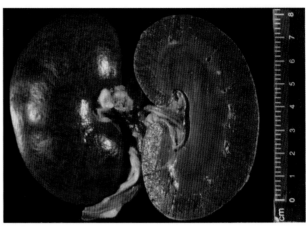

Figure 45.8 Kidneys from dog with leptospirosis. Photograph courtesy of Dr. Linden Craig, Department of Pathobiology, College of Veterinary Medicine, The University of Tennessee.

and English bull terriers. Renal agenesis may be unilateral (often with ipsilateral hypertrophy) or bilateral. Acquired reduction in renal number is usually due to surgical removal (nephrectomy).

Alteration in position

Alteration in renal position may be due to developmental problems (such as renal ectopia) or to acquired conditions (such as displacement by intra-abdominal organomegaly or adipose tissue accumulation or surgical transposition).

Pain

Renal pain occurs with distention of the renal capsule due to cellular infiltration, infection, or fluid accumulation, or to trauma. Examples include ureteral obstruction with hydronephrosis (Figure 45.7), infections such as leptospirosis (Figure 45.8), pyelonephritis, or feline infectious peritonitis (Figure 45.2), acute toxicities such as ethylene glycol, neoplastic infiltration (Figures 45.3 and 45.4)

46

Discolored urine

Joe Bartges

Normal urine

Normal urine is typically transparent and yellow or amber upon visual inspection. Primarily, two pigments impart yellow coloration: urochrome and urobilin. Urochrome is a sulfur-containing oxidation product of colorless urochromogen. Urobilin is a degradation product of hemoglobin. Because the 24-hour urinary excretion of urochrome is relatively constant, highly concentrated urine is amber in color, whereas dilute urine may be transparent or light yellow in color. The intensity of the color is in part related to volume of urine collected and concentration of urine produced; therefore, it should be interpreted in the context of the urine specific gravity. Caution must be exercised not to over-interpret significance of urine color as part of a complete urinalysis. Significant disease may exist when urine is normal in color. Abnormal urine color may be caused by presence of several endogenous or exogenous pigments. Although the abnormal color indicates a problem, it provides relatively nonspecific information. Causes of abnormal coloration should be investigated with appropriate laboratory tests and examination of urine sediment. Detection of abnormal urine color should prompt questions related to diet, administration of medication, environment, and collection technique. Knowledge of urine color may also be important in interpreting colorimetric test results because it may induce interference.

Discolored urine

Urine color that is anything other than yellow or amber is abnormal. There are many potential causes of discolored urine (see Table 46.1). The most common abnormal

urine color in dogs and cats is red, brown, or black, which may be caused by hematuria, hemoglobinuria, myoglobinuria, and bilirubinuria.

Pale yellow urine

Urine that is pale yellow or clear in appearance may be normal or may be indicative of a polyuric state. Urine may be appropriately dilute if it is associated with recent consumption or administration of fluids, consumption of a diet containing low quantities of protein or high quantities of sodium chloride, glucocorticoid excess, or administration of diuretics. Urine is considered to be inappropriately concentrated if it is dilute in presence of dehydration. Diseases associated with persistently dilute urine include diabetes mellitus, diabetes insipidus, hyperadrenocorticism, hypoadrenocorticism, hypercalcemia, hyperthyroidism, and renal failure. If urine is pale yellow or clear, urine specific gravity is often less than 1.015. A simple test to determine whether polyuria is persistent, is to determine the urine specific gravity of a sample collected in the morning. Other tests should include serum biochemical analysis and a complete urinalysis, and possibly measurement of serum thyroxine concentration, adrenal function testing, or monitoring urine specific gravity after several days of vasopressin administration.

Red, brown, or black urine

Presence of red, brown, or black urine suggests blood, hemoglobin, myoglobin, or bilirubin. A positive occult blood reaction is obtained when urine contains any of these substances. Discoloration of urine may also result in false-positive reactions on other urine dipstick test pads. Analysis of urine sediment reveals presence of red blood cells if discoloration is due to hematuria. If no red blood cells are present on microscopic examination of urine sediment, hemoglobin, myoglobin, or bilirubin

Nephrology and Urology of Small Animals. Edited by Joe Bartges and David J. Polzin. © 2011 Blackwell Publishing Ltd.

Table 46.1 Potential causes of discolored urine

Urine color	Causes	Urine color	Causes
Yellow or amber	Urochromes Urobilin	Yellow-brown or green-brown	Bile pigments
Deep yellow	Highly concentrated urine Quinacrine[a] Nitrofurantoin[a] Phenacetin[a] Riboflavin (large quantities)[a] Phenolsulfonphthalein (acidic urine)[a]	Brown to black (brown or red-brown when viewed in bright light in thin layer)	Melanin Methemoglobin Myoglobin Bile pigments Thymol[a] Phenolic compounds[a] Nitrofurantoin[a] Nitrites[a] Naphthalene[a] Chlorinated hydrocarbons[a] Aniline dyes[a] Homogentisic acid[a]
Blue	Methylene blue Indigo carmine and indigo blue dye[a] Indicans[a] Pseudomonas infection[a] Water-soluble chlorophyll[a] Rhubarb[a] Toluidine blue[a] Triamterene[a] Amitriptyline[a] Anthraquinone[a] Blue food dye[a]	Colorless	Very dilute urine (diuretics, diabetes mellitus, diabetes insipidus, glucocorticoid excess, fluid therapy, overhydration)
Green	Methylene blue Dithiazanine Urate crystalluria Indigo blue[a] Evan's blue[a] Bilirubin Biliverdin Riboflavin[a] Thymol[a] Phenol[a] Triamterene[a] Amitriptyline[a] Anthraquinone[a] Green food dye[a]	Milky white	Lipid Pyuria Crystals
Red, pink, red-brown, red-orange, or orange	Hematuria Hemoglobinuria Myoglobinuria Porphyrinuria Congo red Phenolsulfonphthalein (following alkalinization) Neoprontosil Warfarin (orange)[a] Food pigments (rhubarb, beets, blackberries)[a]	Brown	Methemoglobin Melanin Sulfasalazine[a] Nitrofurantoin[a] Phenacetin[a] Naphthalene[a] Sulfonamides[a] Bismuth[a] Mercury[a] Feces (rectal-urinary fistula) Fava beans[a] Rhubarb[a]

Table 46.1 (*Continued*)

Urine color	Causes	Urine color	Causes
	Carbon tetrachloride[a]		Sorbitol[a]
	Phenazopyridine		Metronidazole[a]
	Phenothiazine[a]		Methocarbamol[a]
	Diphenylhydantoin[a]		Anthracin cathartics[a]
	Bromsulphalein (following alkalinization)		Clofazimine[a]
	Chronic heavy metal poisoning (lead, mercury)[a]		Primaquine[a]
	Rifampin[a]		Chloroquine[a]
	Emodin[a]		Furazolidone[a]
	Phenindione[a]		Copper toxicity
	Eosin[a]		
	Rifabutin[a]		
	Acetazolamide[a]		
	Red food dye[a]		
Orange-yellow	Highly concentrated urine		
	Excess urobilin		
	Bilirubin		
	Phenazopyridine		
	Sulfasalazine[a]		
	Fluorescein sodium[a]		
	Flutamide[a]		
	Quinacrine[a]		
	Phenacetin[a]		
	2,4-d[a]		
	Acetazolamide[a]		
	Orange food dye[a]		

[a]Only observed in human beings.

should be suspected. Examination of plasma color may aid in differentiating these. If discolored urine is due to myoglobin, plasma will be clear because myoglobin in plasma is not bound significantly to a carrying protein, which results in filtration and excretion. If plasma is pink, it is suggestive of hemoglobin. If plasma is yellow, it is suggestive of bilirubin; serum bilirubin concentration should also be increased. A positive occult blood test may also occur if red blood cells present in urine lyse. Myoglobinuria is indicative of muscle damage; serum creatine kinase activity is often increased in this setting. Hemoglobinemia is indicative of intravascular hemolysis resulting from immune-mediated, parasite-mediated, or drug-mediated destruction of red blood cells. Hyperbilirubinemia results from liver disease, post-hepatic obstruction, or hemolysis.

Milky white urine

Milky white colored urine may be due to presence of white blood cells (pyuria), lipid, or crystals. The more concentrated the urine sample is, the more opaque it may appear. Presence of pyuria secondary to a bacterial urinary tract infection is the most common cause of milky white urine; however, pyuria may occur due to inflammation without an infection. Lipiduria may be observed in healthy animals, but is frequently observed in cats affected with hepatic lipidosis. Crystalluria if heavy and present in a concentrated urine sample may also result in milky white urine color. Microscopic examination of urine sediment will aid in differentiation of these causes.

47

Clinical signs of lower urinary tract disease

Joe Bartges

Diseases of the lower urinary tract including the prostate or vagina have characteristic clinical signs that are usually, but not always, present (Osborne et al. 1972; Bartges and Osborne 1995; Ling 1995; Watson 2007; van Dongen and L'eplattenier 2009). Oftentimes, multiple clinical signs are present and indicate further evaluation of the patient (Table 47.1).

Alteration in volume or frequency of urination

Polyuria/polydipsia

Polyuria/polydipsia is not typically associated with lower urinary tract disease, but implies either primary renal disease or extra-renal disease influencing urine concentration and/or water intake (see Chapter 42). They may be associated with lower urinary tract signs such as incontinence or periuria, and if associated with bacterial pyelonephritis may be associated with recurrent bacterial cystitis.

Dysuria

Dysuria is difficult urination often associated with pain. Painful urination by dogs and cats is not always easy to discern.

Stranguria

Stranguria refers to slow and painful urination and can be associated with partial urinary outflow obstruction or inflammation of the lower urogenital tract. Causes of stranguria are the same as those for dysuria.

Pollakiuria

Pollakiuria is excessively frequent urination usually associated with passage of small volume. Often, it is associated with inflammatory conditions, but may be associated with decreased urine storage capacity.

Decreased size of urine stream

Decreased size of urine stream is associated with partial urethral obstruction due to scar tissue, masses involving the urethra or impinging on the urethra, urethroliths, prostatic disease, or urethral spasm.

Urinary obstruction (anuresis)

Dogs and cats with urethral obstruction attempt to urinate but are unable to pass urine (see Chapters 35 and 36). It must be differentiated from attempts at defecation (constipation or colitis). Most often, it is due to a mechanical obstruction (e.g., uroliths or neoplasia), but may be due to functional causes (e.g., reflex dyssynergia).

Inappropriate urination (periuria)

Periuria refers to inappropriate urination (literally, urinating around). It occurs with inability to retain urine due to irritation and inflammation or to behavioral conditions.

Incontinence

Urinary incontinence (enuresis) refers to involuntary urination (see Chapter 76). This usually occurs when the animal is relaxed or asleep due to loss of conscious control of urination. While awake, urination occurs normally. There are neurogenic and non-neurogenic causes of urinary incontinence; the most common cause is urethral sphincter mechanism incompetency that occurs in spayed female dogs. Female dogs and cats that leak urine

Nephrology and Urology of Small Animals. Edited by Joe Bartges and David J. Polzin. © 2011 Blackwell Publishing Ltd.

Table 47.1 Problem-oriented rule-outs for diseases of the lower urinary tract and prostate

D	Degenerative	Benign prostatic hypertrophy
		Urethral sphincter mechanism incompetency
A	Anatomic	Congenital malformations of bladder or urethra
		Congenital or acquired urethral stricture
		Ectopic ureter
		Detrusor atony
		Urinary bladder or urethral spasm
		Prostatic cysts
M	Metabolic	Urolithiasis
N	Neoplastic	Urinary bladder, urethra, or prostate – commonly transitional cell carcinoma or adenocarcinoma
B	Behavioral	
I	Inflammatory	Urinary bladder polyps
		Lymphoplasmacytic cystitis or urethritis
		Eosinophilic cystitis
	Infectious	Bacterial or fungal cystitis or prostatitis
		Prostatic abscessation
	Idiopathic	Feline idiopathic cystitis
	Iatrogenic	Complications associated with Cystocentesis, catheterization, endoscopy, or surgery
T	Trauma	Blunt or penetrating trauma
	Toxic	Certain drugs or environmental exposure – e.g., cyclophosphamide-induced sterile cystitis

when sitting but awake may have urethral sphincter dysfunction; however, this implies there is urine pooling in the caudal vagina.

Alteration in urine consistency

Discolored urine

Presence of red blood cells in urine (hematuria) is associated with lower urinary tract disease, but may also occur with upper urinary tract disease (e.g., nephrolithiasis) or disorders of coagulation (e.g., acquired or congenital coagulation factor deficiency). When hematuria occurs due to lower urinary tract disease, usually other clinical signs of lower urinary tract disease are present. Hematuria occuring in the absence of clinical signs of lower urinary tract disease usually localizes the disease to the upper urinary tract or to systemic disorders of coagulation. Dogs with prostatic disease may have hematuria without additional signs of lower urinary tract disease. Urine may differ from normal yellow color with polyuric states (clear to light yellow), lipid or crystals (white), pigmenturia (red, brown, or black), or blue-green (certain bacterial infections) (see Chapters 7 and 46).

Malodorous urine

Urine normally has an ammonia odor that is more intense with concentrated urine. Additionally, cats, especially males, excrete felinine ((R)-2-amino-3-(4-hydroxy-2-methylbutan-2-ylthio)propanoic acid), which is con-

verted by excreted peptidase, cauxin, to the pheromone 3-mercapto-3-methylbutan-1-ol that imparts a pungent odor to urine. A change in urine odor may occur with infection, hematuria, certain drugs (e.g., amoxicillin), and certain foods (e.g., asparagus).

Crystalluria or small uroliths in urine

Microscopic crystalluria may indicate presence of or propensity to form uroliths, but may be normal and does not predict future urolith formation (see Chapter 7). Crystalluria by itself does not cause lower urinary tract disease. Additionally, crystalluria must be interpreted in light of urine sample collection and processing. Cooling urine from core body temperature to ambient or refrigeration temperature promotes in vitro crystal formation and may be merely an artifact. If crystalluria is a concern, then urine should be collected and evaluated within a couple of hours of collection. Passage of sand or small uroliths is abnormal, and should be collected and submitted for quantitative analysis. The animal should be evaluated further for additional uroliths in all parts of the urinary tract by imaging studies.

Other clinical findings that may be associated with lower urinary tract disease

Abdominal fluid

Abdominal effusion should be characterized as transudate, exudate, or modified transudate; however, abdominal effusion may be urine due to leakage from the urinary tract. For example, urinary bladder rupture secondary to urethral obstruction or trauma is associated with uroabdomen (see Chapter 11).

Excessive licking of prepuce or vulva

Excessive licking of the prepuce or vulva may occur with many diseases of the lower urinary tract especially the very distal part, but may also occur habitually. Excessive licking may cause irritation that is irritating, resulting in continued licking and a vicious cycle of cause and effect.

Blood dripping from prepuce or vulva

The appearance of drops of blood or blood fluid from the prepuce or vulva suggests that the source is distal to the bladder. This occurs most commonly with prostatic disease (male dogs) or with estrous (females), but may occur with diseases of the distal urethra, penis, prepuce, or vagina.

Prostatomegaly

In intact male dogs, prostatomegaly most often occurs due to benign prostatic hypertrophy and/or bacterial prostatitis (see Chapter 78). In this situation, the prostate is typically symmetrically enlarged and not painful unless acute bacterial prostatitis is present. With asymmetric prostatomegaly, prostatic cysts, or neoplasia may be present. Prostatomegaly in male dogs castrated at least six months prior to examination nearly always have prostatic neoplasia with or without associated bacterial infection.

Pus dripping from prepuce or vulva

Pus dripping from the prepuce usually occurs from balanoposthitis, but may be observed with prostatitis. Pus exuding from the vulva occurs most commonly in prepuberal female dogs due to puppy vaginitis. In adult female dogs or cats, purulent vaginal discharge may indicate infectious vaginitis or pyometra.

Painful rectal examination

Pain during digital examination of the rectum is usually caused by disease of the rectum, anus, peri-anal area, bony pelvis, caudal lumbar vertebrae, lumbosacral area, or coxofemoral joints. Occasionally, it may be related to prostatic or intra-pelvic urethral disease.

Painful defecation

Pain during defecation is usually caused by disease of the rectum, anus, peri-anal area, bony pelvis, caudal lumbar vertebrae, lumbosacral area, or coxofemoral joints. It may occur with prostatic disease especially with inflammation secondary to inflammation. Passage of ribbon-like stools is observed with narrowing of the descending colon and may occur with prostatomegaly especially if prostatic neoplasia is present and has metastasized to iliac lymph nodes resulting in dorsal and ventral compression of the colon.

Painful or abnormal gait of rear limbs

Painful or abnormal gait in rear limbs is associated usually with musculoskeletal or neurological disease, especially lumbosacral disease or coxofemoral or stifle arthritis. It may occur with lower urinary tract disease such as prostatic or urinary bladder neoplasia that has metastasized to iliac lymph nodes or caudal lumbar vertebrae or with iliac lymphadenopathy due to extension of infection or inflammation from the urinary bladder or prostate.

Fever

Diseases of the lower urinary tract are uncommonly associated with fever; however, it may be present with infection (prostatitis or pyelonephritis with cystitis).

References

Bartges, J.W. and C.A. Osborne (1995). Clinical algorithms and data bases for urinary tract disorders. In: *Canine and Feline Urology and Nephrology*, edited by C.A. Osborne and D.R. Finco. Philadelphia, PA: Lea & Febiger, pp. 68–99.

Ling, G.V. (1995). *Lower Urinary Tract Diseases of Dogs and Cats.* St. Louis, MO: Mosby.

Osborne, C.A., et al. (1972). *Canine and Feline Urology.* Philadelphia, PA: WB: Saunders.

van Dongen, A.M. and H.F. L'eplattenier (2009). Kidneys and urinary tract. In: *Medical History and Physical Examination in Companion Animals*, edited by A. Rijnberk and F.J. Van Sluijs. Edinburgh: Saunders Elsevier, pp. 101–107.

Watson, A.D.J. (2007). Dysuria and haematuria. In: *BSAVA Manual of Canine and Feline Nephrology and Urology*, edited by J. Elliott and G.F. Grauer. Gloucester: BSAVA, pp. 1–7.

Section 5

Upper urinary tract disorders

48

Chronic kidney disease

David J. Polzin

Characteristics of chronic kidney disease

Chronic kidney disease (CKD) is the most commonly recognized form of kidney disease in dogs and cats. It is defined as any structural and/or functional abnormality of one or both kidneys that has been continuously present for three months or longer. Kidneys of dogs and cats with CKD are typically characterized by a permanent reduction in the number of functioning nephrons. Although renal structure and function do not consistently parallel one another, primary kidney diseases usually display evidence of both structural and functional derangements. The rare exceptions to this generality would include patients that have relatively limited structural lesions (e.g., renal cysts or a nephrolith) with essentially normal overall renal function or patients with specific renal tubular disorders (e.g., renal glucosuria) with essentially normal renal structure. In general, the clinical impact of CKD on the patient reflects the extent of reduction in renal function rather than the impact of structural lesions.

In most instances, CKD is an irreversible and typically progressive disease. Once a patient is diagnosed with CKD, the condition can usually be expected to be a lifelong condition, even with treatment. However, in some patients CKD may be complicated by concurrent prerenal and postrenal components or active kidney diseases that may be reversible (e.g., pyelonephritis or acute-on-CKD). After correcting reversible primary diseases and/or prerenal or postrenal components of renal dysfunction, further improvement in kidney function should not be expected because compensatory and adaptive changes designed to sustain kidney function have largely already occurred.

In most patients, a slow but inexorable progressive decline in kidney function typically follows diagnosis.

It is not necessary for the disease process responsible for initiating CKD to persist, for this progressive loss of renal function to occur. In some patients, this pattern follows an almost linear decline in renal function, while in others the pattern is characterized by a period of relatively stable renal function followed by a precipitous decline in renal function. Some patients may have multiple periods of stable renal function and precipitous declines before succumbing to CKD. However, there are exceptions to this progressive pattern, particularly among cats. Some cats have stable renal function for years and may die of other diseases before their CKD becomes terminal.

Since the progression of CKD is often relatively slow, patients with CKD often survive for many months to years with a good quality of life. Although as yet no treatment can correct existing irreversible kidney lesions of CKD, the clinical and biochemical consequences of reduced kidney function can often be ameliorated by supportive and symptomatic therapy. In addition, the spontaneously progressive course of CKD may be slowed by therapeutic intervention.

Although frequently considered a disease of older animals, CKD occurs with varying frequency in dogs and cats of all ages. One estimate of the incidence of CKD in the general population of dogs and cats is 0.5–1.5% of dogs and 1–3% of cats (Brown et al. 2007a). Although a somewhat higher prevalence of CKD occurs in young dogs due to the occurrence of congenital renal disease, the greatest prevalence is in geriatric dogs. At the University of Minnesota Veterinary Medical Center, in excess of 10% of dogs and 30% of cats over 15 years of age have a diagnosis of CKD. One retrospective study reported that 53% of cats with CKD were over seven years old, but animals ranged in age from 9 months to 22 years (DiBartola et al. 1987). In a study on age distribution of kidney disease in cats based on data submitted from 1980 to 1990 to the Veterinary Medical Data Base at Purdue

Nephrology and Urology of Small Animals. Edited by Joe Bartges and David J. Polzin. © 2011 Blackwell Publishing Ltd.

University, 37% of cats with the diagnosis of "renal failure" were less than ten years old, 31% of cats were between the ages of 10 and 15, and 32% of cats were older than 15 years of age (Lulich et al. 1992). Similarly, in a study of cats with CKD reported in 1998, the mean age was 12.6 years with a range of 1–26 years (Elliot and Barber 1998). Mean age among 45 control cats in this study was 10.0 years. During the year 1990, the prevalence of kidney disease was reportedly 16 cases for every 1,000 cats of all ages, 77 cases per 1,000 cats over age 10 years, and 153 per 1,000 among cats older than 15 years (DiBartola et al. 1987). Maine Coon, Abyssinian, Siamese, Russian Blue, and Burmese cats were disproportionately reported as affected.

Pathophysiology of CKD

The loss of kidney function that occurs in CKD typically is characterized by a progressive decline in the number of surviving nephrons. This decline in the number of functioning nephrons, at least initially, is presumed to be the result of the patient's primary kidney disease. However, once the number of surviving nephrons declines below some critical mass, surviving nephrons continue to be damaged and lost even if the primary kidney disease is no longer active. This ongoing loss of nephrons that occurs subsequent to the decline in the number of surviving nephrons is called "spontaneous progression of CKD." Spontaneous progression of CKD occurs as a consequence, at least in part, of the adaptive processes that mitigate the decline in renal function that accompanies loss of nephrons. Thus, the renal adaptive responses to the loss of nephrons, while advantageous in the short-term because it helps to sustain overall renal function, is deleterious in the long-term because it leads to additional nephron loss and a progressive decline in renal function.

The kidneys adapt to loss of nephrons by recruitment of the surviving nephrons to recoup much of the function lost. Overall renal function is the sum of the function of the individual nephrons. In terms of glomerular filtration rate (GFR), the kidneys' total GFR is the sum of the GFR of each individual nephron, called the single nephron GFR or SNGFR. In this way, the kidneys are able to adapt to CKD by minimizing the functional losses associated with structural loss. However, there are consequences or "trade-offs" to be paid for these adaptations. One trade-off from the perspective of the nephrologist is that in many cases functional deterioration in CKD lags well behind structural injury, thus confounding early diagnosis of CKD. More ominous, however, is that the surviving nephrons function at a much higher level which ultimately contributes to their demise, thus leading to spontaneous progression of CKD.

Pathophysiology of CKD

Consequences of nephron loss

Kidney function typically declines progressively over months to years in dogs and cats with naturally occurring CKD (Elliot and Barber 1998; Jacob et al. 2002). Typically, the decline in kidney function occurs in association with a progressive decline in the number of functioning nephrons. At least initially, reduction in kidney function is presumed to be a consequence of the patient's primary kidney disease. However, studies in several species suggest that loss of a critical mass of functional renal tissue invariably leads to failure of the remaining nephrons, suggesting that CKD may progress through mechanisms independent of the initiating cause (Brenner et al. 1982; Hostetter et al. 2001a; Rennke and Denker 2007). Regardless of where renal injury begins, if it persists, the kidneys will gradually self-destruct through a final common pathway involving interstitial nephritis and fibrosis (Harris and Neilson 2006). This process is called "spontaneous progression of CKD."

Spontaneous progression of CKD in rodent models is characterized by progressive azotemia, proteinuria, arterial hypertension, and, eventually, death due to uremia. Renal lesions observed in this process include focal segmental glomerulosclerosis and tubulointerstitial lesions, including tubular dilation and interstitial inflammation and fibrosis (Hostetter et al. 2001a). Results of several studies suggest that the findings obtained in rodents are likely to be applicable to dogs and cats (Polzin et al. 1988; Adams et al. 1994, 1992). Surgical reduction of renal mass in dogs and cats results in proteinuria, glomerulopathy, and tubulointerstitial renal lesions. While these findings are consistent with observations in rats, reducing renal mass by 7/8 or less does not consistently result in a progressive decline in renal function in dogs or cats. However, progressive decline in renal function has been reported to occur in dogs when renal mass is reduced by 15/16 (Finco et al. 1992). The renal lesions observed in these experimental studies are similar to lesions described in humans, dogs, and cats with spontaneous progressive nephropathies of diverse origins. Lesions observed in spontaneous diseases typically include focal and segmental glomerulosclerosis and tubulointerstitial lesions characterized by fibrosis and a sterile inflammatory infiltrate. The preponderance of clinical and experimental evidence suggests that in dogs and cats with stages 2 and 3 CKD, progression of renal disease may result, at least in part, from factors unrelated to the activity of the inciting disease.

It appears that progression of CKD occurs, at least in part, as a consequence of the adaptive processes that mitigate the decline in renal function accompanying loss of nephrons. Thus, the renal adaptive responses to the loss of nephrons, while advantageous in the short-term because they help sustain total renal function, is deleterious in the long-term because it leads to additional loss of nephron and a progressive decline in renal function.

The kidneys adapt to loss of nephrons by recruitment of the surviving nephrons to recoup much of the function lost. Overall renal function is the sum of the function of the individual nephrons. In terms of GFR, the kidneys' total GFR is the sum of the GFR of each individual nephron, called the single nephron GFR or SNGFR. In this way, the kidneys are able to adapt to CKD by minimizing the functional losses associated with structural loss. However, there are consequences or "trade-offs" to be paid for these adaptations. One trade-off from the perspective of the nephrologist is that in many cases functional deterioration in CKD lags well behind structural injury, thus confounding early diagnosis of CKD. More ominous, however, is that the surviving nephrons function at a much higher level which ultimately contributes to their demise, thus leading to spontaneous progression of CKD.

One proposed model of the final common pathway leading to progression of CKD involves six sequential steps (Harris and Neilson 2006). In the first step, persistent glomerular injury leads to local hypertension in the glomerular tufts, increased SNGFR, and proteinuria. In the second step, proteinuria accompanied by increased local production of angiotensin II facilitates a downstream cytokine bath that induces accumulation of interstitial mononuclear cells. Step three begins with the appearance of interstitial neutrophils, but is rapidly replaced by a nephritogenic immune response characterized by macrophages and T lymphocytes producing interstitial nephritis. In step four, inflammation affects the tubular epithelia inducing disaggregation of cells from basement membranes and adjacent sister cells. In addition, epithelial-mesenchymal transition occurs where tubular epithelial cells transform into fibroblasts. In step five, fibroblasts lay down a collagenous matrix, disrupting vasa recti and surviving tubules. In the sixth and final stage, an acellular scar results from cells being trapped away from local survival factors that provided a supportive microenvironment.

Glomerular hypertension

The increase in SNGFR that occurs as nephrons are lost, results largely from a marked reduction in glomerular arteriolar resistance with greater vasodilation of the afferent arteriole. As renal mass is reduced, the ability of the surviving nephrons to autoregulate is lost, thereby transmitting systemic arterial pressure to the glomerulus (Brown et al. 1995). Preferential vasodilation of the afferent arteriole results in (1) elevation in intraglomerular capillary pressure as a consequence of increased transmission of systemic arterial pressure to the glomerulus (intraglomerular hypertension), (2) marked increase in effective renal plasma flow (glomerular hyperperfusion), and (3) increased production of glomerular filtrate (glomerular hyperfiltration). These increases in pressure, flow, and filtration may be exacerbated by elevations in systemic arterial pressure.

Intraglomerular hypertension, with consequent glomerular hyperfiltration, occurs as a compensatory event designed to maintain the total GFR as nephrons are lost to disease. In primary glomerulopathies, intraglomerular hypertension may also occur as a compensatory adaptation to reduction in permeability of the glomerular capillary wall to small solutes and water. In this setting, the fall in GFR is minimized by elevating intraglomerular pressure (Rennke and Denker 2007). Persistent elevations in intraglomerular pressure appear to be deleterious over time.

Glomerular hypertrophy and intraglomerular hypertension promote cell injury and the glomerular structural and functional derangements associated with progression of CKD. There is evidence that (1) epithelial cell injury is a major factor in hyaline accumulation within the glomerular capillary wall, (2) mesangial dysfunction results in matrix accumulation and microaneurysm formation, and (3) endothelial cell injury leads to thrombosis (Rennke and Denker 2007).

Glomerular hypertension and hyperperfusion are associated with an increase in the volume and surface area of the glomerular tuft. Expansion in surface area of the glomerulus accompanying the enhanced glomerular volume occurs without a corresponding increase in the number of terminal visceral glomerular epithelial cells (podocytes) covering the glomeruli. As the glomerulus enlarges and the filtration surface expands, hypertrophy, but not hyperplasia of the podocytes occurs. The resulting reduction in glomerular podocyte cell density likely contributes to the glomerular injury and proteinuria that accompanies loss of renal mass. Podocytes contribute importantly to the integrity of the glomerular filtration barrier through a complex series of interdigitating cell foot processes between adjacent podocytes connected by structures called "slit diaphragms." The slit diaphragms are part of the small pore system of filtration that is a major component of the resistance to filtration of water and limits trafficking of macromolecules including albumin across the capillary wall. As expansion of the filtration surface exceeds the ability of hypertrophied podocytes to maintain the integrity of all interdigitating foot processes and filtration slit diaphragms, focal and segmental areas of epithelial simplification (effacement or "fusion" of foot processes) and focal loss and denudation of epithelial cells occur leading to local increases in flow of ultrafiltrate and increased convection of albumin. Proteinuria occurs only in nephrons with damaged podocytes and represents the earliest sign of renal hemodynamic injury. The consequence of loss of podocyte structural integrity is loss of glomerular hydraulic conductivity, proteinuria and, ultimately, focal and segmental glomerulosclerosis.

Portions of glomeruli denuded by loss of podocytes allow increased flux of water, small solutes and some macromolecules across the capillary wall (hyperfiltration). Increased glomerular capillary pressure combined with decreased hydraulic conductivity facilitates accumulation of large macromolecules in the subendothelial space since they are too large to pass the glomerular basement membrane. Accumulation of this amorphous hyaline material narrows glomerular capillary lumens exacerbated by expansion of mesangial matrix and infiltrating cells due to influx of macromolecules into the mesangial areas.

Segmental and sometimes nodular sclerosis may develop subsequent to microaneurysm formation in glomerular capillaries. Microaneurysms may develop as a consequence of increases in glomerular capillary diameter and intraglomerular pressure leading to increased tension exerted on the glomerular capillary walls. These microaneurysms usually thrombose as a consequence of exposure of platelets to mesangial components; a local inflammatory response develops following thrombosis. Segmental and nodular sclerosis follows as these lesions organize and capillaries collapse trapping cellular debris. Local generation of cytokines and growth factors and influx of macrophages stimulate mesangial matrix overproduction leading to expansion of the mesangium, further promoting glomerulosclerosis.

Endothelial dysfunction appears to promote development of thrombi in glomerular capillaries, although the mechanism is not completely understood. Increased shear stress from intraglomerular hypertension may cause endothelial cells to lose their thromboresistance leading to platelet adhesion.

The relative contribution of each of these factors to development of glomerulosclerosis is unknown. However, these processes are associated with progressive injury to and further loss of nephrons. This loss of nephrons and the associated progression of CKD occurs independent of the underlying disease processes responsible for the initial renal injury.

Role of angiotensin II and aldosterone

Angiotensin II is an important mediator of intraglomerular capillary pressure because it selectively increases efferent arteriolar vasoconstriction. Although angiotensin type 1 receptors are present on both afferent and efferent arterioles, afferent vasoconstriction is mitigated selectively by vasodilatory agonists such as nitric oxide and prostaglandins (Harris and Neilson 2006). Preferential vasoconstriction of the efferent arteriole under the influence of angiotensin II increases glomerular capillary hypertension, thus promoting renal injury.

In addition to its hemodynamic effects on the glomerulus, angiotensin II impairs glomerular size-selectivity and has been shown to induce proteinuria in absence of any structural glomerular damage (Harris and Neilson 2006). In addition, angiotensin II induces cytoskeletal changes and alters podocyte function by increasing intracellular calcium levels in podocytes.

Glomerular expression of cytokines and chemokines can be directly stimulated by angiotensin II (Harris and Neilson 2006). Further, activation of the local renin-angiotensin system, as well release of proinflammatory and profibrotic factors may result from shear stress to endothelial cells and mechanical stress to mesangial cells and podocytes.

Aldosterone increases renal vascular resistance and glomerular capillary pressure and may complement the detrimental activity of angiotensin II (Harris and Neilson 2006). In addition, there are many potential mechanisms by which aldosterone may mediate fibrosis, collage formation, and an inflammatory response including increased expression of proinflammatory molecules, stimulation of TGF-β_1 synthesis, generation of reactive oxygen species, up-regulation of angiotensin II receptors, and others (Epstein 2004).

Proteinuria and tubulointerstitial disease

Proteinuria is a strong, independent risk factor for progression to end-stage CKD in humans (Iseki et al. 2003). It has also been shown to be related to progression of renal disease in dogs and cats (Finco et al. 1999; Jacob et al. 2005; Syme et al. 2006). It is unclear whether proteinuria itself contributes to progressive renal injury or is just a marker of the process leading to progression.

Proteinuria may promote progressive renal injury in several ways. Some proposed mechanisms include mesangial toxicity, tubular overload and hyperplasia, toxicity from specific proteins such as transferrin/iron, and induction of pro-inflammatory molecules such as monocyte chemoattractant protein-1. Excessive proteinuria may injure renal tubules via toxic or receptor-mediated pathways or via an overload of lysosomal degradative mechanisms. Abnormally filtered proteins accumulate in the renal proximal tubular lumens where, after endocytosis into proximal tubular cells, they contribute to renal tubulointerstitial injury through a complex cascade of intracellular events. These events include up-regulation of vasoactive and inflammatory genes such as the endothelin-1 (ET-1) gene, the monocyte chemoattractant protein 1 (MCP-1) gene which encodes for an inflammatory peptide involved in macrophage and T-lymphocyte recruitment, and the RANTES (regulated on activation, normal T-cell expressed and secreted) that encodes for a chemotactic molecule for monocytes and memory T-cells (Pisoni and Remuzzi 2001). Formed in excessive amounts, these molecules are secreted toward the basolateral side of tubular cells and incite an inflammatory reaction within the interstitium. In addition, complement components escaping through glomerular capillary walls may initiate interstitial injury. Small lipids bound to filtered proteins may also be liberated during resorption. Inflammatory or chemotactic properties of these lipids may promote tubulointerstitial disease. Finally, inspissation of filtered proteins due to tubular reabsorption of water in the distal nephron may lead to formation of casts that obstruct nephrons.

In humans, conditions that are associated with relatively selective albuminuria rarely induce significant tubulointerstitial injury, even when the quantity of proteinuria is great. In contrast, glomerular injury associated with nonselective proteinuria (a combination of larger and small albumin-sized molecules) incites substantial tubulointerstitial injury (Harris and Neilson 2006). This finding suggests that filtered moieties other than or in addition to albumin may induce tubular injury and dysfunction.

Renal secondary hyperparathyroidism

Incidence and pathophysiology

Renal secondary hyperparathyroidism develops early in the course of CKD, so it may be present in many dogs and cats at the time of initial diagnosis of CKD. The overall prevalence of renal secondary hyperparathyroidism in cats was reported to be 84% in one study (Barber and Elliot 1998). Hyperparathyroidism was present in all cats with "end-stage" CKD and 47% of asymptomatic cats with only biochemical evidence of CKD. It may be present in patients with normal serum calcium and phosphorus concentrations (Nagode et al. 1996). In general, plasma PTH levels increase as serum creatinine concentration increases (Nagode et al. 1996).

Hyperparathyroidism in CKD is multifactorial in origin. Recent studies have suggested that fibroblast growth factor-23 (FGF-23) may be involved in its origin (Gutierrez et al. 2005). Phosphorous retention occurs as GFR declines in early renal failure and is intimately related to development of renal secondary hyperparathyroidism. Fibroblast growth factor-23 is a phosphaturic hormone that mitigates phosphorus retention early in the course of CKD, but it also appears to inhibit renal 1α-hydroxylase activity, thus potentially contributing to decreased calcitriol levels (Gutierrez et al. 2005). The decline in calcitriol levels is one of the earliest identifiable changes that occurs in the development of renal secondary hyperparathyroidism.

A relative deficiency of calcitriol has been described in dogs with CKD, although absolute values were within the normal range (Gerber et al. 2003). Relative or absolute deficiency of calcitriol is believed to play a pivotal role in development of renal secondary hyperparathyroidism. Calcitriol, the most active form of vitamin D, is formed by 1α-hydroxylation of 25–hydroxycholecalciferol in renal tubular cells. Parathyroid hormone (PTH) promotes renal 1α-hydroxylase activity and formation of calcitriol. In turn, calcitriol limits PTH synthesis by feedback inhibition. Phosphorus retention and FGF-23 inhibit renal 1α-hydroxylase activity. Early in the course of CKD, these inhibitory effects on renal tubular 1α-hydroxylase activity limit calcitriol production. As calcitriol normally inhibits PTH synthesis, reduced calcitriol synthesis promotes renal secondary hyperparathyroidism. Initially, the resultant hyperparathyroidism increases 1α-hydroxylase activity despite continued phosphorous retention, thereby restoring calcitriol production toward normal. However, normalization of calcitriol production occurs at the expense of persistently elevated plasma PTH activities – a classic example of the "trade-off hypothesis." As CKD progresses, loss of viable renal tubular cells ultimately limits renal calcitriol synthetic capacity and calcitriol levels subsequently remain low. Deficiency of calcitriol leads to skeletal resistance to the action of PTH and elevates the set-point for calcium-induced suppression of PTH secretion. Skeletal resistance to PTH limits skeletal release of calcium, while elevating the set-point for PTH secretion allowing hyperparathyroidism to persist even when plasma ionized calcium concentrations are normal or elevated (Nagode et al. 1996).

Recent evidence suggests that phosphorous retention may also play a primary role in directly promoting hyperparathyroidism. Phosphorous has been shown to stimulate PTH secretion in parathyroid cultures (Almaden et al. 1996). Further, phosphorous restriction in dogs and humans with CKD has been shown to decrease

PTH secretion without changing serum calcitriol levels (Lopez-Hilker et al. 1990; Combe and Aparicio 1994). In untreated human patients with mild to moderate CKD (serum creatinine concentration ≤ 3.0 mg/dL), serum phosphorus concentrations correlated directly with PTH, independent of serum calcium and 1,25-dihydroxyvitamin D levels (Kates et al. 1997). Interestingly, this correlation was present despite the fact that most patients had serum phosphorous concentrations within the normal range. Importantly, overt hyperphosphatemia may not be a prerequisite for phosphorous to have an effect on PTH secretion (Kates et al. 1997; Barber and Elliot 1998). It has been suggested that high phosphorous intake may accentuate uremia-induced abnormal phosphorous metabolism causing increased parathyroid cell phosphorous concentration. In vitro studies have suggested that parathyroid glands exposed to elevated phosphorous levels respond by increasing PTH secretion (Almaden et al. 1996). Reduced calcitriol levels may have a permissive effect and/or an additional direct effect on PTH secretion in this setting (Kates et al. 1997).

In more advanced CKD, the presence of uremic toxins appears to prevent the inhibition of parathyroid cell proliferation induced by calcitriol (Canalejo et al. 2003). At this point, only serum calcium concentration correlates with serum PTH activity (Kates et al. 1997). Impaired intestinal absorption of calcium due to low serum calcitriol levels likely plays an important role in hyperparathyroidism in these advanced CKD patients. Blood ionized calcium concentrations are often reduced in cats with CKD; in one study, over 50% of cats with advanced end-stage CKD were hypocalcemic (Barber and Elliot 1998). Ionized calcium concentration has been reported to range from low to high in dogs with CKD (Schenck and Chew, 2003).

Clinical consequences

Although renal secondary hyperparathyroidism and renal osteodystrophy, are well-documented effects of CKD, clinical signs associated with renal osteodystrophy are uncommon in dogs and cats. In dogs, it most often occurs in immature patients, presumably because metabolically active growing bone is more susceptible to the adverse effects of hyperparathyroidism. For unexplained reasons, bones of the skull and mandible may be the most severely affected and may become so demineralized that the teeth become moveable and fibrous changes are obvious, particularly in the maxilla. Marked proliferation of connective tissue associated with the maxilla may cause distortion of the face. Jaw fractures can occur but are uncommon. Other possible but uncommon clinical

manifestations of severe renal osteodystrophy include, cystic bone lesions, bone pain, and growth retardation.

Although excessive levels of PTH affect bones and kidneys, it may also affect the function of other organs and tissues, including brain, heart, smooth muscles, lungs, erythrocytes, lymphocytes, pancreas, adrenal glands, and testes as well (Bro and Olgaard 1997). Toxicity of PTH appears to be mediated through enhanced entry of calcium into cells with PTH or PTH2 membrane receptors. Sustained PTH-mediated calcium entry leads to inhibition of mitochondrial oxidation and production of ATP. Extrusion of calcium from cells is reduced because of the impairment in ATP production and disruption of the sodium-calcium exchanger. Persistently increased basal cytosolic calcium levels promote cellular dysfunction and death (Nagode et al. 1996).

Potential non-skeletal clinical consequences of hyperparathyroidism include mental dullness and lethargy, weakness, anorexia, and an increased incidence of infections due to immunodeficiency (Nagode et al. 1996). Hyperparathyroid-induced cellular dysfunction may lead to carbohydrate intolerance, platelet dysfunction, impaired cardiac and skeletal muscle function (due to impaired mitochondrial energy metabolism and myofiber mineralization), inhibition of erythropoiesis, altered red cell osmotic resistance, altered B cell proliferation, synaptosome and T-cell dysfunction, and defects in fatty acid metabolism (Nagode et al. 1996; Vanholder, 1998). Excess PTH levels may also promote nephrocalcinosis and consequent progressive loss of renal function.

Renal secondary hyperparathyroidism may be associated with substantial enlargement of the parathyroid glands. This finding may be of clinical importance in cats because of frequent coincident hyperthyroidism that may be suggested by the presence of a thyroid nodule palpable in the cervical region. In a recent report, hyperplastic parathyroid glands were palpable as paratracheal masses in 11 of 80 cats with spontaneous CKD (Elliot and Barber 1998). Care should be taken to confirm hyperthyroidism prior to treatment as both hyperparathyroidism and hyperthyroidism can lead to paratracheal masses.

Causes of CKD

Conceptual model for development of CKD

A conceptual model for the course of CKD has been proposed which includes initiation and progression of CKD (Stevens and Levey 2005). It begins with antecedent conditions (i.e., risk factors for renal disease), followed by stages of kidney damage and decreased GFR, ultimately leading to kidney failure and renal death. Antecedent conditions or susceptibility factors are conditions that put patients at increased risk to develop kidney damage. These factors are not well understood in dogs and cats. Presumably, factors such as older age, preexisting renal impairment (e.g., reduced numbers of nephrons at birth), and as yet undefined genetic factors may predispose to renal injury. Recognizing such factors would potentially be of great value in preventing development of kidney damage and the later stages of CKD.

Initiating factors which directly lead to kidney damage may include a diversity of factors such as immune-mediated diseases, systemic infections, urinary tract infections, nephrolithiasis, urinary tract obstruction, drug or other nephrotoxicity, systemic and glomerular hypertension, chronic hypoperfusion, developmental disorders, amyloidosis, and others. The relative contribution of these factors to the overall incidence of CKD in dogs and cats has not been well established, partly because the underlying causes of CKD are often not recognized. However, individuals with recognized susceptibility factors or initiation factors for CKD should be tested for kidney injury on an ongoing basis (i.e., screening efforts). Ideally, diagnosis and treatment of CKD would commence during this phase of CKD. Treatments should be directed toward the primary disease process, managing comorbid conditions and slowing progression of CKD.

In patients with kidney damage, progression factors cause worsening of kidney damage and thereby promote or accelerate a progressive decline in GFR. In dogs and cats these factors may include higher levels of proteinuria, elevated phosphorous concentrations and possibly higher blood pressure. Kidney disease may progress because of the initial damage or as a result of pathways independent of the initial damage (i.e., spontaneous progression). Efforts should be made to assess the rate of progression of CKD and attempt intervention to slow progression.

The patient enters end stage kidney disease or kidney failure at the point where symptomatic and supportive care becomes the focus of management. In humans with end-stage kidney failure, this is the stage where replacement by dialysis and transplantation are initiated (see Chapters 27–30). Options for successful management of canine and feline patients with end-stage kidney failure are seriously limited and uremic death or euthanasia may become inevitable. As such, delaying or preventing progression to this stage is a priority in the management of all dogs and cats with CKD.

Pursuit of the causes for CKD

It appears plausible that early recognition of kidney disease will provide an opportunity to treat the primary diseases underlying CKD. Because early detection and treatment directed toward an etiologic cause is thought likely to result in the most desirable clinical outcome, recognition of the many potential causes of CKD is important. Early detection and confirmation of many of these disorders is challenging and requires careful screening of patients with a judicious application of appropriate diagnostic tools as indicated, including kidney function tests, urinalysis, imaging of the urinary system, serologic screening for predisposing diseases, urine cultures, and renal biopsy.

CKD may be initiated by a variety of different acquired, familial, or congenital, diseases. In a study of biopsy findings in 37 dogs with primary renal azotemia, chronic tubulointerstitial nephritis was observed in 58%, glomerulonephropathy occurred in 28%, and amyloidosis was observed in 6% (Minkus et al. 1994). In cats, tubulointerstitial nephritis was observed in 70%, glomerulonephropathy occurred in 15%, and lymphoma was observed in 11%, and amyloidosis occurred in 2%. Unfortunately, the initiating cause(s) of CKD often cannot be identified at the time of diagnosis. The initiating causes of diseases thought to originate in the tubulointerstitium have been especially elusive. Glomerulonephropathies have been linked to a variety of neoplastic, metabolic, and infectious and noninfectious inflammatory processes (see Chapters 26, 52, and 53) (Cook and Cowgill 1996).

Several systemic causes for CKD have been proposed. Among the more intriguing proposals is that vaccines may play a role in development of the tubulointerstitial renal disease so often recognized in cats with CKD. Subcutaneous administration of feline herpesvirus 1, calicivirus, and panleukopenia virus vaccines grown on Crandell Rees feline kidney (CRFK) cells to kittens have been shown to induce production of anti-feline renal tissue antibodies in serum (Lappin et al. 2005). Further, immunologic sensitization of cats against CRFK lysates has been shown to induce an acute lymphocytic-plasmacytic interstitial nephritis (Lappin et al. 2006). While these observations prompt serious questions as to whether repeated administration of feline vaccines grown in CRFK cell cultures may play a role in development of the tubulointerstitial CKD in cats, it remains to be demonstrated that the antibodies and acute lesions reported so far will in fact progress to CKD. Nonetheless, the potential for vaccines playing a role in initiating kidney damage can not yet be excluded, and the incidence of CKD in older cats is substantial. As a consequence, a recommendation to consider monitoring kidney function in geriatric cats for evidence of kidney damage may be warranted.

It has also been suggested that periodontal disease may be linked to microscopic renal lesions in dogs, but a cause and effect relationship has yet to be confirmed (DeBowes et al. 1996). In a fashion similar to the association reported in humans with HIV, feline immunodeficiency virus (FIV) has been linked to renal disease in cats (Thomas et al. 1993; Poli et al. 1995). However, few cats with CKD are FIV positive, thus raising doubt as to the overall contribution of FeLV-associated nephritis to CKD.

While early recognition of CKD is a critical step in recognizing the primary diseases responsible for CKD, early diagnosis is the exception rather than the rule. Most patients with CKD are diagnosed relatively late in the course of their disease and the primary cause of CKD is typically not identified. Difficulty in detecting the inciting cause of CKD is associated with three phenomena related to the evolution of progressive renal diseases. First, various components of nephrons (glomeruli, peritubular capillaries, tubules, and interstitial tissue) are functionally interdependent. Second, the functional and morphologic responses of tissues comprising the kidneys to different etiologic agents are limited in number. Third, after maturation of nephrons, which occurs at approximately one month of age, new nephrons cannot be formed to replace others irreversibly destroyed by disease. Progressive irreversible lesions initially localized to one portion of the nephron are eventually responsible for development of lesions in the remaining but initially unaffected portions of nephrons. For example, progressive lesions (such as amyloid or immune complex disease) confined initially to glomeruli will subsequently decrease peritubular capillary perfusion. Reduced peritubular capillary perfusion will in turn result in tubular epithelial cell atrophy, degeneration, and necrosis. There is also evidence that tubular epithelial cells may also be damaged as a consequence of proteinuria. As described previously, proteinuria damages tubules by release of cytokines and chemokines that promote inflammation and fibrosis. Ultimately nephron destruction initiated by glomerular proteinuria will simulate repair by substitution of functioning nephrons with nonfunctional connective tissue.

Similarly, generalized progressive interstitial disease initially caused by bacteria eventually destroys tubules and glomeruli and stimulates inflammation and fibrosis. Thus, irrespective of the initiating cause, replacement of the majority of the damaged nephrons with collagenous connective tissue results in overall reduction in kidney size and impaired renal function.

Because of the structural and functional interdependence of various components of nephrons, differentiation of different progressive renal diseases that have reached an advance stage is often difficult. Functional and structural changes prominent during earlier phases of progressive generalized renal diseases may permit iden-

tification of a specific cause and/or localization of the initial lesion to glomeruli, tubules, interstitium, or vessels. With time, however, destructive changes of varying severity (atrophy, inflammation, fibrosis, and mineralization of diseased nephrons), superimposed on compensatory and adaptive morphologic and functional adaptations of remaining partially and totally viable nephrons, provide a functional and morphologic similarity to the findings associated with these diseases.

Despite the irreversibility of generalized renal lesions associated with CKD, it is important to formulate diagnostic plans to try to identify the underlying cause and to determine if it is still active. Although specific therapy directed at eliminating or controlling the primary cause will usually not substantially alter existing renal lesions, it is important in context of minimizing further nephron damage. Renal diseases potentially amenable to specific therapy include bacterial pyelonephritis, obstructive uropathy, nephrolithiasis, renal lymphoma (particularly in cats), hypercalcemic nephropathy, perinephric psuedocysts, and some glomerulopathies.

Acute onset of non-urinary disorders, especially those that promote substantial fluid losses or interfere with compensatory polydipsia, may precipitate a uremic crisis in patients with compensated CKD (so-called "acute-on-chronic"). However, if acute decompensation of CKD has been caused by reversible factors, correction of them will often result in recompensation of the CKD.

Clinical signs of CKD

Early clinical signs of CKD

Among the first clinical signs to be noticed by owners of pets with CKD are polyuria, polydipsia, progressive weight loss, muscle wasting, and a decline in appetite that sometimes manifests as selectivity in appetite. Of these signs, those most likely to prompt consideration of CKD are polyuria and polydipsia. Polydipsia may be recognized by owners who find that the water bowls must be filled more often or that pets may seek more water from new or unusual sources. Some dogs will begin to exhibit urinary incontinence with the onset of polyuria due to increased filling of the bladder. Another common observation by owners is that the urine appears to be clear or less yellow. In cats, polyuria is often recognized when the litter box appears to be wetter, heavy, or have more litter "clumps" present.

While these signs are often among the first signs that owners recognize, they actually occur only after a substantial loss of renal function has already occurred. Loss of urine concentrating ability, and the subsequent polyuria and polydipsia, usually occurs only after a 75% or greater decline in renal function. Thus, while these signs date the onset of the clinical phase of CKD, they may not reflect the actual onset of the disease.

In some diseases, clinical signs specific to the primary disease may present before the onset of clinical signs that result from the loss of renal function. For example, polycystic kidney disease or renal neoplasia may be recognized by owners or veterinarians as a mass or masses within the abdomen. Nephroliths associated with ureteroliths may be recognized as abdominal pain, vomiting or licking at the flank. Pyelonephritis may be recognized as pollakiuria, foul-smelling and/or cloudy urine, polyuria, polydipsia, nausea, anorexia, or pyrexia. Glomerular diseases may be recognized by edema. Congenital or familial renal failure may be recognized as impaired growth, polyuria and difficult house training.

Clinical signs of advanced CKD

As renal function continues to decline, the clinical signs of the polysystemic clinical syndrome known as uremia (see Chapter 39) dominate the clinical presentation of the patient. Uremia is the clinical syndrome that results from loss of kidney functions. Impaired renal glomerular, tubular and endocrine functions lead to retention of toxic metabolites, changes in the volume and composition of body fluids, and excess or deficiency of various hormones. Presumably, the clinical signs of uremia reflect the sum effect of these derangements on organ systems throughout the body. The most prominent clinical signs of uremia are related to the gastrointestinal tract (described below). Other clinical findings may include weight loss, muscle wasting, hypothermia, lethargy, weakness, muscle tremors, uremic pericarditis and pneumonitis, hypertension, altered behavior or neuropathies (uremic or hypertensive encephalopathy), renal osteodystrophy, anemia, and a hemorrhagic diathesis.

Gastrointestinal signs in CKD

Gastrointestinal manifestations remain among the most prominent and vexing clinical signs of uremia. Decreased appetite and weight loss are non-specific findings that often precede other gastrointestinal signs of uremia. The appetite may be selective for certain foods and wax and wane throughout the day. The decline in appetite appears to be multifactorial in origin. Studies using a rodent model has suggested that an "anorectic factor" in the plasma of uremic patients that can suppress appetite (Anderstam et al. 1996). This factor appears to be middle molecule in size and may be a peptide. Elevated serum leptin concentrations have also been implicated as a factor contributing to anorexia (Wolf et al. 2002). Nausea and altered taste sensation due to increased levels of urea,

ammonia and other retained toxins in saliva may also contribute to anorexia.

In one study of cats with spontaneous CKD, dysphagia and oral discomfort was observed in 7.7% of uremic cats and 38.5% of cats with end-stage CKD (Elliot and Barber 1998). Periodontal disease was observed in 30.8% of uremic and 34.6% of end-stage CKD cats in the same study. Halitosis was reported in 7.7% of cats in both groups. Moderate to severe CKD may result in uremic stomatitis characterized by oral ulcerations (particularly located on the buccal mucosa and tongue), brownish discoloration of the dorsal surface of the tongue, necrosis and sloughing of the anterior portion of the tongue (associated with fibrinoid necrosis and arteritis; Figure 48.1), and uriniferous breath. The mucous membranes may also become dry (xerostomia). Degradation of urea to ammonia by bacterial urease may contribute to many of these signs. Poor oral hygiene and dental disease may exacerbate the onset and severity of uremic stomatitis.

Vomiting is a frequent, but inconsistent finding in uremia resulting from the effects of as yet unidentified uremic toxins on the medullary emetic chemoreceptor trigger zone and from uremic gastroenteritis. The severity of vomiting correlates variably with the magnitude of azotemia. Because uremic gastritis may be ulcerative, hematemesis may occur. Although vomiting has generally been thought to be a more frequent complaint among uremic dogs, vomiting reportedly occurs in about one-quarter to one-third of uremic cats (Elliot and Barber 1998). Vomiting may impair compensatory polydipsia enhancing the risk of dehydration and exacerbating prerenal azotemia and clinical signs of uremia.

In dogs, uremic gastropathy is characterized microscopically by mineralization of the mucosa and of submucosal blood vessels, edema, vasculopathy, and glandular atrophy (Peters et al. 2005). Gastric mineralization appears to be related to the calcium-phosphate product. In addition, elevated gastrin levels have been implicated in development of uremic gastropathy. Gastrin, a hormone that induces gastric acid secretion directly by stimulating receptors located on gastric parietal cells as well as by increasing histamine release from mast cells in the gastric mucosa, is normally excreted by the kidneys and elevated blood levels may develop as kidney function declines. Indeed, elevated blood gastrin levels have been documented in cats with spontaneous CKD (Goldstein et al. 1998). Elevated gastrin levels may promote gastric hyperacidity and possible gastric irritation and ulceration. Enhanced histamine release may also promote gastrointestinal ulceration and ischemic necrosis of the mucosa through a vascular mechanism characterized by small venule and capillary dilatation, increased endothelial permeability, and intravascular thrombosis (Lemarié et al. 1995). However, gastric hyperacidity has not been documented in uremic dogs or cats, and mucosal necrosis and ulceration appear to be uncommon findings in uremic gastropathy in dogs (Peters et al. 2005). Lesions of uremic gastropathy have not been described in cats. Uremic gastropathy and its associated clinical signs appear to be more common in dogs than cats.

Uremic enterocolitis, manifest as diarrhea, may occur in dogs and cats with severe uremia, but it is typically less dramatic and less common than uremic gastritis. In one study, diarrhea was not reported by owners of 80 cats with spontaneous CKD (Elliot and Barber 1998). However, when present, uremic enterocolitis is often hemorrhagic. Considerable gastrointestinal hemorrhage may initially escape clinical detection. Intussusception may occasionally complicate uremic enterocolitis. In contrast, constipation is a relatively common complication of CKD, particularly in cats. However, it appears to be primarily a manifestation of dehydration rather than gastrointestinal dysfunction. It may also occur as a complication of intestinal phosphate binding agents.

Laboratory abnormalities in CKD

Multiple hematological and biochemical abnormalities may be found in patients with CKD (Table 48.1). These abnormalities vary greatly in their clinical significance to the patient. A complete picture of the patient's clinical condition is best achieved by a complete evaluation of the hematological and biochemical condition of the patient.

Azotemia

Azotemia is defined as an excess of urea, creatinine, and other non-protein nitrogenous compounds in the blood (see Chapter 39). Since urea nitrogen, creatinine, and many other non-protein nitrogenous compounds are excreted largely by glomerular filtration, a decline in glomerular filtration leads to accumulation of a wide variety of non-protein nitrogen-containing

Table 48.1 Principal laboratory abnormalities in chronic kidney disease

Azotemia
Hyperphosphatemia
Hypokalemia and hyperkalemia
Metabolic acidosis
Hypercalcemia and hypocalcemia
Hypermagnesemia
Anemia (normocytic, normochromic)
Hypoalbuminemia

compounds, including urea and creatinine. Retention of some of these metabolic wastes may be further aggravated by catabolism of body tissues and extrarenal factors that promote renal hypoperfusion. Since these compounds are derived almost entirely from protein degradation, their production may increase when dietary protein increases.

While BUN is present in higher concentrations than other non-nitrogenous waste products, it is generally thought to be relatively nontoxic. Regardless of whether urea per se is toxic, BUN concentrations nonetheless tend to correlate reasonably well with clinical signs of uremia. Therefore, BUN is often viewed as a surrogate marker of retained "uremic toxins." Urea is synthesized using nitrogen derived from amino acid catabolism. It may then be excreted by the kidneys, retained in body water, or metabolized to ammonia and amino acids plus carbon dioxide by bacteria in the gastrointestinal tract. Ammonia produced in the gastrointestinal tract is recycled to urea in the liver yielding no net loss of nitrogen or urea. The concept of "trapping" nitrogenous wastes in the gut by enhancing anabolic microbial uptake of intestinal ammonia and urea with subsequent excretion from the body via the feces is currently being examined as a possible means of using the gastrointestinal tract to eliminate nitrogenous waste products.

In addition to increasing protein intake and declining renal function, BUN concentrations may also be increased by gastrointestinal hemorrhage, enhanced protein catabolism, decreasing urine volumes (due to pre-renal factors such as dehydration), and certain drugs (e.g., glucocorticoids). Urea nitrogen concentrations may decline with portosystemic shunts, hepatic failure, and low protein diets. It is important to interpret changes in BUN in the clinical context of the patient. While a reduced BUN may be accompanied by improved clinical signs in some clinical settings (e.g., feeding a reduced protein diet), reduced BUN concentration may in other settings be an undesirable finding. For example, it may also indicate protein calorie malnutrition due to inadequate protein intake as a consequence of improperly formulated diets or failure of the patient to consume adequate amounts of food. Because many extrarenal factors influence BUN concentration, creatinine is preferred to evaluate kidney function because it is a more reliable measure of GFR.

Hyperphosphatemia

Hyperphosphatemia is common in patients with azotemic CKD, but unexpected in patients with non-azotemic renal disease. In general, serum phosphorus concentrations parallel BUN concentrations in patients with CKD. Nonetheless, derangements in body phosphorus metabolism begin very early in the course of CKD.

The kidneys play a central role in phosphorus metabolism because phosphorus excretion occurs primarily via the kidneys. Phosphorus is freely filtered by the glomerulus and reabsorbed in the renal tubules. Thus, phosphorus excretion is the net of glomerular filtration less tubular reabsorption of phosphorus. If dietary phosphorus intake remains constant, a decline in glomerular filtration rate will lead to phosphorus retention and ultimately hyperphosphatemia. However, during the early stages of CKD, serum phosphorus concentrations remain well regulated because of a compensatory decrease in renal tubular phosphorous reabsorption. Renal tubular adaptation occurs as a consequence of the phosphaturic effects of FGF-23 and PTH. Renal excretion of phosphorous is enhanced by reducing the tubular transport maximum for phosphorous reabsorption in the proximal tubule via the adenyl cyclase system. However, when glomerular filtration rates decline below about 20% of normal, this adaptive effect reaches its limit and hyperphosphatemia ensues.

The primary consequences of phosphorus retention and hyperphosphatemia are progression of CKD, renal secondary hyperparathyroidism, and the associated renal osteodystrophy. Hyperphosphatemia per se does not appear to cause any clinical signs. As described previously, elevated serum phosphorus concentrations have been shown to be directly linked to increased mortality in humans, cats, and dogs with CKD (Finco et al. 1992; Block et al. 1998; King et al. 2007; Boyd et al. 2008). Renal secondary hyperparathyroidism and renal osteodystrophy occur in dogs and cats, but the clinical implications of these complications appear to be relatively limited. Young dogs seem to be at increased risk for developing clinical signs of renal osteodystrophy, primarily of the bones of the skull. The result is deformation of the skull and mandible, sometimes associated with substantial pain. The term "rubber jaw" has been applied to some dogs that develop fibrous skeletal changes in the mandible. However, most adult dogs either do not survive sufficiently long or do not have sufficient elevations in PTH to develop clinical signs associated with renal osteodystrophy, even though skeletal lesions can be demonstrated histologically in many dogs and cats with CKD.

Hyperphosphatemia combined with even a normal plasma calcium concentration can produce an elevated calcium-phosphate product (Ca X PO$_4$ in units of mg/dL). When the calcium-phosphate product exceeds approximately 70, calcium phosphate tends to precipitate in blood vessels, joints, and soft tissues. This process, called metastatic calcification, is especially prominent in

proton-secreting organs, such as the stomach and kidneys, in which basolateral bicarbonate secretion results in an increase in pH that promotes calcium hydrogen phosphate (brushite) precipitation (Brushinsky 2005). However, myocardium, lung, and liver are also commonly mineralized in patients with CKD.

Increasing calcium X phosphorous product was found to have a mortality risk trend similar to that seen for phosphate (Block et al. 1998). The risk of mortality associated with hyperphosphatemia appeared to be independent of elevated PTH levels, which alone appeared to have only a weak association with mortality. However, the statistical association between PTH and mortality may have been impaired by use of multiple methods for PTH assay in the patients studied. Analysis of calcium revealed no correlation with relative risk of death.

Metabolic acidosis

The kidneys eliminate acid by recapturing filtered bicarbonate and secreting hydrogen ions in urine buffered as titratable acids (primarily phosphate) or ammonium. Since essentially all filtered bicarbonate is successfully reclaimed and the quantity of phosphate available for urinary buffering is limited to the quantity that is excreted, the only option for increasing renal acid excretion is increasing renal ammoniagenesis. The kidneys generate ammonia via metabolism of glutamine to glutamate and alpha-ketoglutarate in the renal tubules. However, the number of functioning renal tubules becomes limited as CKD progresses. As a consequence, metabolic acidosis develops in CKD primarily because the ability to increase renal ammonia production, and thus excrete hydrogen ions, is limited by loss of functional renal mass. Decreased medullary recycling of ammonia due to structural renal damage may also contribute to impaired ammonium excretion.

Retention of phosphorous and organic acid (uric acid, hippuric acid, and lactic acid) in CKD promotes an increase in the anion gap. However, hyperchloremic acidosis (normal anion gap), high anion gap or mixed hyperchloremic-high anion gap acidoses may all occur in patients with CKD. Hyperchloremic acidosis is more likely in less severely azotemic patients. Hyperchloremic acidosis also occurs in patients with renal tubular acidosis (RTA). Fanconi syndrome in Basenji dogs is an example of a CKD characterized by impaired ability to reabsorb bicarbonate by the proximal tubules (proximal or type 2 RTA—see Chapter 54).

Metabolic acidosis is a common manifestation of advanced CKD, but is relatively uncommon among cats with less severe CKD (IRIS CKD stages II and III) (Elliot et al. 2003a). A cross-sectional study of 59 cats with CKD revealed that a blood pH below 7.27 was found in 10 of 19 cats with severe azotemia, 3 of 20 cats with moderate azotemia, and none of 20 cats with mild azotemia. A subsequent longitudinal study indicated that metabolic acidosis usually developed late in the course of CKD and is more likely a consequence of advanced CKD than the cause of progression to the advanced stages of CKD (Elliot et al. 2003b). Metabolic acidosis was not found to be a prognostic factor in cats with CKD (King et al. 2007; Boyd et al. 2008).

Chronic metabolic acidosis may promote a variety of adverse clinical effects including anorexia, nausea, vomiting, lethargy, weakness, muscle wasting, weight loss, and malnutrition. Alkalization therapy is often of value in reversing these signs. In addition, chronic metabolic acidosis may increase urinary calcium excretion and promote progressive bone demineralization. Studies on the effects of dietary acidification in cats have revealed that chronic metabolic acidosis can cause negative calcium balance and bone demineralization or negative potassium balance which may in turn promote hypokalemia, renal dysfunction, and taurine depletion (Fettman et al. 1992).

Chronic metabolic acidosis may impair adaptation to protein restriction and promote protein malnutrition in patients with CKD. Protein catabolism is increased in patients with acidosis to provide a source of nitrogen for hepatic glutamine synthesis, glutamine being the substrate for renal ammoniagenesis (Mitch 1997). The combined effects of reduced protein synthesis due to uremia and accelerated proteolysis due to acidosis promote elevations in blood urea nitrogen, increased nitrogen excretion, and negative nitrogen balance typical of uremic acidosis. Altered branched chain amino acid metabolism appears to be involved. Chronic metabolic acidosis increases the activity of muscle branched chain keto acid dehydrogenase, the rate-limiting enzyme in branched chain amino acid catabolism. This is important in that branched chain amino acids are rate limiting in protein synthesis and play a role in regulation of protein turnover. Alkalization therapy effectively reverses acidosis-associated protein breakdown. There is speculation that changes in intracellular pH accompanying acidosis lead to alterations in gene transcription which increase the activity of the cytosolic, ATP- and ubiquitin-dependent protein degradation pathway. Severe chronic metabolic acidosis has the potential to induce a cycle of progressive protein malnutrition and metabolic acidosis. Excessive protein catabolism may lead to protein malnutrition despite adequate dietary intake. This process may then accelerate breakdown of endogenous cationic and sulfur-containing amino acids, thus promoting further acidosis.

Acidosis poses a particularly vexing problem for CKD patients consuming protein-restricted diets. Dietary protein requirements appear to be similar for normal humans and humans with CKD unless uremic acidosis is present. When acid-base status is normal, adaptive reductions in skeletal muscle protein degradation protect patients consuming low-protein diets from losses in lean body mass. Metabolic acidosis blocks the metabolic responses to dietary protein restriction in two ways (1) it stimulates irreversible degradation of the essential, branched chain amino acids and (2) it stimulates degradation of protein in muscle (Mitch 1997). Thus, acidosis may limit the ability of patients to adapt to dietary protein restriction. Metabolic acidosis also suppresses albumin synthesis in humans and may reduce the concentration of serum albumin. These findings have yet to be been confirmed in dogs and cats.

Calcium disorders

Classically, serum calcium levels have been described as declining in patients with CKD. However, serum total calcium concentration is the sum of serum protein-bound calcium, ionized calcium and complexed calcium, and the concentrations of total, ionized, complexed, and protein-bound calcium vary widely in dogs and cats with CKD (Schenck and Chew, 2003). Ionized hypercalcemia was reportedly found in 6% and ionized hypocalcemia in 26% of 80 cats with spontaneous CKD (Barber et al. 1998). Further, mean blood ionized calcium concentration was significantly lower in CKD cats in this study than in normal control cats, and over half of the cats with advanced (stage IV) CKD were hypocalcemic when evaluated using ionized calcium measurements. However, when these same 80 cats were evaluated using total serum calcium concentrations, hypercalcemia was found in 21% of the cats, while hypocalcemia was detected in only 8%. Clearly, serum total calcium concentrations do not reliably reflect ionized calcium concentrations in cats with CKD.

Similar discrepancies have been observed in dogs with CKD (Kruger et al. 1996; Schenck and Chew, 2003). While metabolic acidosis is known to influence the relative ratio of ionized to bound calcium, metabolic acidosis does not appear to explain the discrepancies between ionized and total calcium concentrations in dogs with CKD (Kogika et al. 2006). Elevated serum total calcium concentrations in patients with CKD occurs predominantly as a consequence of increased complexing of calcium to retained organic and inorganic anions such as citrate, phosphate, or sulfate (Schenck and Chew, 2003).

Hypercalcemia of CKD should be carefully discriminated from hypercalcemic nephropathy or renal damage induced by ionized hypercalcemia. Hypercalcemia due to malignancy or hypervitaminosis D is most often linked to hypercalcemic nephropathy. Both of these conditions may elevate the calcium X phosphorus product leading to renal mineralization, inflammation, and fibrosis. Primary hyperparathyroidism is typically characterized by hypercalcemia and hypophosphatemia. Because phosphorus concentrations are typically lower with this condition, it appears less likely to induce hypercalcemic nephropathy. One way of discriminating the cause–effect relationship between hypercalcemia and kidney disease is to determine the patient's blood ionized calcium concentration. Only ionized hypercalcemia promotes kidney injury. However, true ionized hypercalcemia and hypercalcemic renal damage may occur in patients with CKD as a consequence of excessive dosages of calcitriol or calcium-containing intestinal phosphate-binding agents, or, rarely, in patients with severe renal hyperparathyroidism with marked hyperplasia of the parathyroid glands. We have also observed small increases in ionized calcium concentrations in dogs and cats with early to moderate CKD that are not receiving calcitriol or calcium therapy and do not have advanced hyperparathyroidism. The mechanism of ionized hypercalcemia in these animals is unclear.

Hypermagnesemia

The kidneys are responsible for magnesium excretion. Therefore, hypermagnesemia is common in azotemic CKD (Barber et al. 1998). Protein binding of magnesium is usually normal, while complexed magnesium is usually increased and ionized magnesium may be increased, normal or decreased in patients with CKD. Although the homeostatic mechanisms involved in the control of magnesium are not well documented, they appear to rely on the bone, gut, and kidney.

Hypoproliferative anemia

As renal function declines in patients with CKD, a normochromic, normocytic hypoproliferative anemia typically develops. Typically, the severity of anemia is roughly proportional to the loss of kidney function. Examination of the bone marrow of patients with CKD usually reveals hypoplasia of the erythroid precursors with little or no interference with normal leukopoiesis and megakaryocytopoiesis. Spiculed and deformed red cells (burr cells or echinocytes) may be observed in the peripheral blood. The factors responsible for formation of these burr cells is not known, but their prevalence does not appear to correlate with the severity of CKD.

The clinical signs of anemia contribute importantly to the clinical effects of CKD and include pallor of the mucous membranes, fatigue, listlessness, lethargy, weak-ness, and anorexia. These signs can be ameliorated by correcting anemia by hormone replacement. While the hematocrit may become quite low in patients with CKD, compensatory mechanisms such as increased levels of 2,3 DPG, lowered peripheral vascular resistance, and an elevated cardiac output (in the absence of previous cardiac disease) help maintain tissue oxygenation.

The primary mechanism underlying anemia of CKD is inadequate renal production of the hormone erythropoietin (EPO). EPO is a circulating glycoprotein produced in renal peritubular fibroblast-like type-1 interstitial cells (Weidemann and Johnson 2009). EPO stimulates red blood cell production in the bone marrow by enhancing survival of certain erythrocyte progenitor cells. Deficiency of EPO in CKD results from a reduction in the overall number of peritubular interstitial cells available to produce the hormone. Organs other than the kidneys appear to have the capability to produce EPO. Although the kidneys produce approximately 90% of systemic EPO in adults, around 10% of circulating EPO is of nonrenal origin. In addition to the kidneys, EPO mRNA expression has been found in the liver, brain, spleen, lung, and testis, although the levels of expression are low in lung and spleen. The reason why alternate sources of EPO such as liver and brain cannot compensate for the impairment in renal EPO production has not been resolved. Current research is directed at identifying novel means of enhancing endogenous nonrenal production of EPO as a treatment for anemia of CKD.

Although EPO deficiency is the principal cause for anemia in CKD, the anemia is multifactorial in origin and may be exacerbated by concurrent illness and poor nutrition. Experimental and clinical evidence exists for a supporting role for shortened red cell life span, nutritional abnormalities, and erythropoietic inhibitor substances in uremic plasma, blood loss, and myelofibrosis. Anemic CKD patients have a relative rather than absolute EPO deficiency in that plasma levels typically exceed the normal range, but are low relative to the severity of anemia (King et al. 1992). Anemic CKD cats have been reported to have plasma EPO concentrations similar to normal cats (Cook and Lathrop 1994).

Other clinically important causes for anemia in dogs and cats with CKD are iron deficiency and chronic gastrointestinal blood loss. In most patients, iron deficiency can only be detected by measuring serum iron, staining bone marrow biopsy samples for iron content, or through response to iron supplementation. Chronic gastrointestinal hemorrhage may occur even in the absence of characteristic color changes in the feces. It can be suspected on the basis of a hematocrit level that is unexpectedly low relative to the magnitude of renal dysfunction, and an elevation in the serum urea nitrogen to serum creatinine

Table 48.2 Comorbid conditions in CKD

Hyperthyroidism (cats)
Urinary tract infections
Nephroliths and ureteroliths
Hypertension
Cardiac disease
Degenerative joint disease
Dental and oral diseases

ratio. Diagnosis is usually confirmed by improvement in anemia following therapy with famotidine and sucralfate.

Diagnosis of CKD

In order to facilitate optimum patient management and provide an accurate prognosis, the diagnostic evaluation should achieve six goals. These goals are to (1) confirm the presence of kidney disease, (2) differentiate acute from chronic disease, (3) stage CKD, (4) identify clinical, biochemical, and hematological complications of CKD, (5) determine the primary renal diagnosis (i.e., type and/or cause of kidney disease), and (6) identify the presence of any comorbid conditions that may be present in the patient (Table 48.2).

Kidney disease may be suspected on the basis of "markers" of kidney disease or a reduction in kidney function. Markers of kidney disease may be recognized from hematologic or serum biochemical evaluations, urinalysis or imaging or pathology studies (Table 48.3).

Findings suggesting kidney disease may also be found by physical examination or from the medical history. For example, abnormal renal size or shape on physical examination suggests kidney disease, while the medical history may reveal early signs consistent with kidney disease. Markers of kidney disease should be viewed as hints that kidney disease may be present and should be pursued diagnostically; they do not necessarily confirm the presence of kidney disease.

In most patients, diagnosing kidney disease requires consideration of multiple pieces of evidence to develop a confirmed diagnosis. Table 48.4 provides a summary of diagnostics required in initial evaluation of a patient with suspected kidney disease.

Interpretation of serum creatinine concentration

Serum creatinine is a relatively insensitive estimate of glomerular filtration rate until a substantial reduction in overall kidney function has already occurred. It requires about a 75% reduction in GFR before serum creatinine values consistently exceed the upper limit of normal for many laboratories. The insensitivity of serum creatinine results from at least two important factors. The first is the innate relationship between GFR and serum creatinine and the second is that factors other than intrinsic renal disease can cause serum creatinine concentration to increase.

The relationship between serum creatinine and GFR is such that every time the GFR declines by half, the serum creatinine concentration doubles. For example, if

Table 48.3 Markers of kidney damage

Blood markers[a]	Urine markers
Azotemia	Impaired urine concentration
Hyperphosphatemia	Impaired urine dilution
Hypoalbuminemia	Proteinuria
Hyperkalemia	Cylinduria
Hypokalemia	Hematuria
Metabolic acidosis	Pyuria
Hypocalcemia	Inappropriate urine pH
Hypercalcemia	Inappropriate urine glucose
Hypoproliferative anemia	Cystinuria
Imaging markers—abnormalities in kidney:	
Increased or decreased kidney size	
Renal mineralization, nephroliths, or ureteroliths	
Abnormal renal shape	
Absence of a kidney	
Abnormal renal echo texture by ultrasonography	

[a]Markers must be confirmed to be of renal origin to be evidence of kidney damage.

Table 48.4 Initial diagnostic database for patients with CKD

Medical history
Physical examination
Arterial blood pressure
Renal function tests
    Serum creatinine concentration
    Serum urea nitrogen concentration
    Estimation of GFR by plasma disappearance of exogenous substances (optional)
Urinalysis (including urine sediment)
Measurement of proteinuria
    Urine protein: creatinine ratio
    Species-specific test for albuminuria (optional)
Aerobic urine culture (prefer by cystocentesis)
Serum electrolytes: Serum sodium, potassium, chloride, calcium, magnesium, and phosphorus concentrations
Measurement of acid-base status
    Serum bicarbonate or total CO_2 concentration
    Blood gas analysis (optional)
Serum albumin and globulin concentrations
Survey abdominal radiographs
Abdominal ultrasound
Renal biopsy if proteinuric (optional)

a dog has a baseline creatinine of 0.5 mg/dL and its GFR declines by 50%, the serum creatinine only increases to 1.0 mg/dL, still well within the normal range. If a further reduction of 50% in GFR occurs (to 25% of the original GFR), the creatinine will rise to 2.0 mg/dL where it might begin to be recognized as elevated. A further decline of 50% in GFR (to 12.5% of normal) and the creatinine increases to 4.0 mg/dL. As can be seen by this example, the slope of the rise in serum creatinine concentration becomes much more acute after a substantial loss of GFR has already occurred, but the slope is flat over most of the range of GFR. It follows that the wider the normal range is for serum creatinine concentration, the less sensitive it is for intrinsic kidney disease. However, if the range becomes too narrow, serum creatinine will lose specificity because other factors may influence the creatinine value including body muscle mass, breed of dog, and other factors. This conundrum is intrinsic to the nature of serum creatinine and limits its utility in diagnosis of early CKD.

In addition to intrinsic kidney disease, prerenal and postrenal factors may cause serum creatinine concentration to increase. As a consequence, whenever serum creatinine is elevated, it is necessary to sift out prerenal, intrinsic renal and postrenal azotemia with the recognition that they may occur together in the same patient. In most instances, postrenal contributions are clinically obvious

from the physical examination (distension of the urinary bladder, inability to detect an intact bladder, inability to void normally) and medical history (anuria, stranguria, and dysuria). However, when urinary obstruction occurs above the urinary bladder, imaging studies may be necessary to detect the problem.

In most patients, the difficulty is in differentiating prerenal and intrinsic renal azotemia. In most instances, this decision will be based on examination of the urine concentration. As a consequence, serum creatinine concentration must *always* be interpreted in light of knowledge of the concurrent urine concentration. Most commonly, prerenal causes for azotemia reflect reduced perfusion of the kidneys. When systemic conditions lead to hypoperfusion of the kidneys, the normal physiologic response is for the kidneys to produce concentrated urine in order to preserve salt and water. As a consequence, prerenal azotemia should be associated with relatively concentrated urine. In dogs, the urine specific gravity should exceed 1.030, while in cats the urine specific gravity should exceed 1.035–1.040. If the urine specific gravity is below these cut-off points, intrinsic renal azotemia is likely. Of course, if there is another disease process causing impaired urine concentration, this rule-of-thumb may be inaccurate. Therefore, it is important to consider whether the clinical picture suggests the possibility of an alternate explanation for dilute urine. It should also be remembered that very dilute urine (less than about 1.006–1.007) suggests urine-diluting capacity is intact and should be interpreted as evidence of adequate intrinsic renal function. In instances where urine concentration is not available for comparison (e.g., the patient has received fluid therapy), prerenal azotemia may be established on the basis of response to treatment.

While a single measure of serum creatinine concentration may correlate poorly with GFR, serial evaluation of serum creatinine concentrations within the same individual can be quite sensitive in detecting progressive changes in GFR. As a consequence, serially evaluating serum creatinine concentrations at regular intervals in patients suspected as being at risk for CKD may increase the sensitivity of this test.

Differentiating acute from CKD

It is important to differentiate acute and CKD from one another because management and the short- and long-term consequences of acute and CKD are potentially very different. The term "chronic" in the clinical context of CKD means that kidney disease has been present long enough that the resulting condition is usually an irreversible and often progressive loss of kidney function. In contrast, acute kidney disease (or acute kidney injury) implies that the loss of kidney function is of recent onset and has the potential for reversibility of the renal injury.

Recovery of kidney function following injury to the kidneys may reflect reversibility of the primary renal injury and/or compensatory adaptations that allow surviving nephrons to increase their function (described above in the section on response to loss of nephrons). In patients with CKD, adaptive compensatory enhancements in kidney function have already become fully engaged, so further improvement in intrinsic kidney function should not be expected (although correction of prerenal and postrenal conditions may lead to improvement in renal function). Since it typically takes approximately 3 months or longer for these compensatory adaptations to completely evolve, it is reasonable to consider kidney disease that has been present for approximately 3 months or longer to define CKD.

In most patients, the duration of CKD may be estimated from the medical history or inferred from physical examination findings or renal structural changes identified through imaging studies or renal pathology. Presence of clinical signs such as weight loss, polyuria, polydipsia, decreased appetite and others for approximately three months or longer provides substantial evidence of chronicity. Physical examination findings of poor nutritional status and hair coat quality are more typical of chronic as opposed to acute kidney disease. Small kidneys provide strong support of CKD because irreversible loss of nephrons is usually associated with replacement by fibrosis. Physical examination may provide a clue as to kidney size, but reduced kidney size confirmed by imaging studies confirms the diagnosis of CKD. Although uncommon, radiographic evidence of renal osteodystrophy confirms the presence of CKD because of the time required for such lesions to develop.

Laboratory findings are typically less reliable in confirming chronicity of kidney disease. However, when available, documented persistence of abnormalities in kidney function such as persistently elevated serum creatinine concentrations or proteinuria over three or more months is conclusive support for diagnosis of CKD. While the magnitude of increase in serum creatinine or urea nitrogen concentrations is not useful for differentiating acute from CKD, the relationship between clinical signs and magnitude of renal dysfunction may be helpful. At any given level of azotemia, patients with acute kidney failure are likely to show more severe clinical signs because of the rapidity of increase in azotemia as well as the lack of time to adapt to the azotemic environment. Dogs or cats that have marked azotemia but have only mild clinical signs are likely to have CKD. Other laboratory findings that may provide evidence support-

Table 48.5 Stages of chronic kidney disease in dogs and cats

Stage	Serum creatinine values (mg/dL/μmol/L)	
	Dogs	Cats
Stage 1	<1.4/<125	<1.6/<140
Stage 2	1.4–2.0/125–179	1.6–2.8/140–249
Stage 3	2.1–5.0/180–439	2.9–5.0/250–439
Stage 4	>5.0/>440	>5.0/>440

ing chronicity are hypoproliferative anemia and greater magnitude of hyperphosphatemia.

Staging CKD

The International Renal Interest Society (IRIS) has proposed a 4-tier system for staging CKD in dogs and cats based on their renal function, proteinuria, and blood pressure (Tables 48.5–48.7). Staging CKD in this fashion facilitates application of appropriate clinical practice guidelines for diagnosis, prognosis, and treatment. This system has been accepted by the American and European Societies of Veterinary Nephrology and Urology. Although the specific values used to categorize patients with CKD into these stages are based largely on observational data, staging is nonetheless useful for establishing prognosis and managing patients with CKD.

The stage of CKD is based on the level of kidney function as measured by the patient's serum creatinine concentration. As described above, serum creatinine remains the most commonly used estimate of GFR in dogs, cats, and humans. However, the limited specificity and sensitivity of serum creatinine concentration as an estimate of GFR can lead to misclassification. Therefore, staging should be based on a minimum of two serum creatinine values obtained when the patient is fasted and well hydrated. Creatinine values should ideally be determined over several weeks to assess stability of CKD.

Table 48.6 Classification of proteinuria by urine protein:creatinine ratio[a]

Classiciation	Urine protein:Creatinine ratio	
	Dogs	Cats
Proteinuric (P)	>0.5	>0.4
Borderline proteinuric (BP)	0.2–0.5	0.2–0.4
Non-proteinuric (NP)	<0.2	<0.2

[a]Based on ACVIM consensus statement on proteinuria (Lees et al. 2005).

Table 48.7 IRIS[a] blood pressure stages for dogs and cats

	Arterial pressure (AP)	
	Systolic blood pressure (mmHg)	Diastolic blood pressure (mmHg)
Stage 0	<150	<95
Stage I	150–159	95–99
Stage II	160–179	100–119
Stage III	≥180	≥120

[a]IRIS: International Renal Interest Society (www.iris-kidney.com).

The patient's overall clinical status should be considered when interpreting serum creatinine concentrations and other laboratory tests and when planning patient management. Inter-laboratory variations, patient-specific characteristics (e.g., breed, age, gender, body condition, and lean body mass), and transient prerenal and postrenal events may influence serum creatinine values. Reduced muscle mass is a common manifestation of advanced CKD and may result in a substantial reduction in serum creatinine concentration relative to true GFR, particularly in cats. In addition, published reference ranges for serum creatinine are often broad. Therefore, using the staging system described here, some patients classified as having mild renal azotemia (stage 2) may have serum creatinine values within published reference ranges. To avoid misdiagnosis, it is important that evidence of CKD beyond the serum creatinine value be sought. In addition, recent evidence suggests that some breeds of dogs may normally have higher normal values for serum creatinine. In general, larger body size may be associated with a higher upper limit of serum creatinine in dogs (see Chapter 13).

According to the IRIS classification system, the stage of CKD is further qualified by the magnitude of proteinuria, as measured by the urine protein-to-creatinine ratio (UPC), and arterial blood pressure. Before performing a UPC, a urinalysis and urine culture should be performed to rule-out hemorrhage, inflation or infection as the cause for an increased UPC value. The urine sediment should be determined to be inactive before performing the UPC (Lees et al. 2005). Unless the UPC is markedly elevated or less than 0.2, it is recommended that proteinuria be confirmed to be persistent by reexamining the UPC 2–3 times over at least 2 weeks. The average of these determinations should be used to classify the patient as non-proteinuric; borderline proteinuric or proteinuric (Table 48.6). Patients with borderline proteinuria should be re-evaluated after two months to reassess their classification. In some patients, classification of proteinuria

may change due to the natural course of their disease or in response to therapy.

As with proteinuria, arterial pressure should be determined several times, over several weeks, to establish the blood pressure classification. Consult Chapter 12 for additional information on determining blood pressure.

Management of CKD

A clinical action plan should be developed for each patient based on their diagnosis, stage of CKD, existing complications and comorbid conditions, and risk factors for progression of their kidney. In general, treatment of CKD includes (1) specific therapy, (2) prevention and treatment of complications of decreased kidney function ("conservative medical management"), (3) management of comorbid conditions, and (4) therapy designed to slow loss of kidney function.

It is only possible to provide specific therapy for kidney disease when a specific diagnosis of the responsible underlying disease(s) has been identified. This is one of the reasons why a thorough diagnostic evaluation must be performed prior to initiating therapy. Specific therapy is directed at the etiopathogenic processes responsible for the patient's primary renal disease. Because the renal lesions of CKD are irreversible, they usually cannot be completely reversed or eliminated by specific therapy. Nonetheless, progression of renal lesions may be slowed or stopped by therapy designed to eliminate active renal diseases. Specific therapies are described in the chapters of this text on the various types of primary kidney disease.

Unfortunately, a primary renal diagnosis amenable to specific therapy is not identified for many patients. In such instances, the primary thrust of therapy is directed at the clinical and biochemical complications of decreased kidney function. Conservative medical management of CKD consists of supportive and symptomatic therapy designed to correct deficits and excesses in fluid, electrolyte, acid-base, endocrine, and nutritional balance thereby minimizing the clinical and pathophysiologic consequences of reduced renal function. Conservative medical management also includes therapy designed to limit the progressive loss of renal function.

The goals of conservative medical management of patients with CKD are to ameliorate clinical signs of uremia, minimize disturbances associated with excesses or losses of electrolytes, vitamins, and minerals, support adequate nutrition by supplying daily protein, calorie, and mineral requirements, and modify progression of CKD. In order to optimally meet these goals, treatment recommendations must be individualized to patients' needs based on their unique clinical and laboratory finding. Because CKD is progressive and dynamic, serial clinical and laboratory assessment of the patient, and modification of the therapy in response to changes in the patient's condition, is an integral part of conservative medical management. It is also essential that the response to treatment be monitored to make sure that the treatments successfully achieve their goals.

Nutritional therapy

Diet therapy was among the earliest treatments used in managing CKD in dogs and cats. The approach to diet therapy has changed greatly over the decades, but nonetheless, diet therapy remains a mainstay in the management of canine and feline CKD. At one time, reducing dietary protein content was central to the dietary approach to treating CKD; however, it is now recognized that other diet modifications are probably as or more important and effective. As a consequence, substituting maintenance or senior diets that are lower in protein content than the pet's usual diet is not a satisfactory substitute for feeding diets specifically formulated for dogs and cats with CKD. Diets specifically designed for dogs and cats with CKD are modified from typical maintenance diets in several ways including reduced protein, phosphorus, and sodium content, increased B-vitamin content, caloric density and soluble fiber, a neutral effect on acid-base balance, supplementation of omega-3-polyunsaturated fatty acids and the addition of antioxidants. In addition, feline renal diets are typically supplemented with additional potassium. Of these diet modifications, only phosphate, omega-3 PUFA, antioxidants, and protein have been examined individually for effectiveness.

Renal diets

The effectiveness of diet therapy in minimizing uremic episodes and mortality in dogs and cats with naturally occurring stages 2 and 3 CKD has been established in double-masked, randomized, controlled clinical trials (Jacob et al. 2002; Ross et al. 2006). These studies compared a renal diet to a prototypical maintenance diet. The renal diets were characterized by reduced quantities of protein, phosphorus, and sodium compared to the maintenance diet, and were supplemented with omega-3 PUFA.

In dogs, the risk of developing a uremic crisis was reduced by approximately 75% for dogs consuming the renal diet, as compared to dogs consuming an adult maintenance diet. The median symptom-free interval in dogs fed the renal diet was 615 days compared to 252 days in dogs consuming the maintenance diet. Further, the risk of death irrespective of the cause was reduced by 66% and the risk of death due to renal causes was reduced by 69% for dogs consuming the renal diet. Median sur-

vival time for dogs consuming the renal diet was 594 days compared to 188 days for dogs consuming the maintenance diet. Owners of dogs fed the renal diet reported significantly higher quality of life scores for their dogs than owners of dogs consuming the maintenance diet. The renoprotective effects of the renal diet appeared be associated, at least in part, with reduction in the rate progression of CKD.

In a masked, controlled clinical trial, 22 cats were randomized to a manufactured renal diet and 23 cats were randomized to a prototypical maintenance diet (Ross et al. 2006). Cats in this study were mid-IRIS CKD stage II through stage III CKD with serum creatinine concentrations ranging from 2.0 mg/dL to 4.5 mg/dL, or. The risks of uremic crises and renal deaths were significantly reduced when the renal diet was fed. Among the 22 cats fed the renal diet, there were no uremic crises or renal deaths and only 3 deaths due to non-renal causes over the two years of study. By contrast, among the 23 cats consuming the maintenance diet, 6 developed uremic crises, 5 died of renal causes and 5 died of non-renal causes.

Two additional trials, a non-randomized study and a retrospective study, further support the effectiveness of renal diets in cats with CKD (Elliot and Barber 1998; Plantinga et al. 2005). In the non-randomized clinical trial, a manufactured renal diet was compared to no diet change (Elliot and Barber 1998). Cats that would not accept the renal diet, either due to pet or owner issues, continued to eat their regular diet. Therefore, this study was neither randomized nor blinded, but nonetheless yielded results strongly indicating that the renal diet was associated with a significant improvement in survival. Cats fed the renal diet (mean survival time = 633 days) survived substantially longer than cats that ate their regular diet (mean survival time = 264 days). Serum urea nitrogen, and phosphorus concentrations and PTH activities were lower in cats consuming the renal diet. The second study was a retrospective study performed in 31 first-opinion veterinary practices in The Netherlands. Survival times for cats fed one or more of 7 feline renal diets were compared to cats not fed a renal diet (Plantinga et al. 2005). The median survival time for cats fed a renal diet was 16 months compared to 7 months for cats consuming a standard diet.

All clinical studies performed to date clearly support recommending renal diets for dogs with IRIS CKD stages III and IV and cats with IRIS CKD stages II through IV. Renal diets are not currently recommended in IRIS CKD stage II dogs because they have not been critically evaluated in this population. However, any patient with IRIS CKD stage II that persistently has serum phosphorus values exceeding 4.5 mg/dL may benefit from dietary therapy to reduce the serum phosphorus concentration (see the section below on serum phosphorus guidelines). Further, renal diets appear to reduce the magnitude of proteinuria in proteinuric dogs and are advocated for all dogs with proteinuric kidney disease (Burkholder, 2004; Lees et al. 2005). All of these studies were not designed to selectively determine the benefits of modifying individual dietary components, but rather report the results of a "diet effect." While studies on individual dietary components have been reported in dogs and cats with induced CKD, the potential interactions between components have not been examined, nor have the results of these studies on individual dietary components been confirmed in patients with spontaneous CKD.

It is important to evaluate the nutritional response to diet therapy. Body weight, body condition score, food intake (calorie intake), serum albumin concentration, packed cell volume and quality of life should be monitored. The primary goal is to assure adequate food intake, stable body weight, and a body condition score at or near 5/9. If the patient is not meeting nutritional goals, the patient should be evaluated for uremic complications, dehydration, and progression of CKD, metabolic acidosis, anemia, electrolyte abnormalities, UTI, and non-urinary tract diseases. In addition, feeding practices should be examined to rule out management errors in feeding.

Specific dietary components

As described above, renal diets differ from manufactured maintenance diets in several fundamental ways. While the therapeutic value of specific dietary components has not been well studied in clinical trials, there have been multiple studies performed in dogs and cats with induced kidney disease. Dietary components that have received the greatest attention include protein, phosphorus, lipids and antioxidants. The principal focus of these studies has been on the renoprotective effects of the dietary modifications.

The initial interest in protein restriction in CKD was based on the now well-accepted association between dietary protein intake, retention of non-nitrogenous waste products of protein catabolism, and development of clinical signs of uremia. It is generally believed that waste products of protein catabolism contribute to at least some of the clinical signs of uremia (see Chapter 41). The ideal quantity of protein to feed dogs and cats with CKD remains unresolved; however, there is a general consensus of opinion, that limiting dietary protein intake for the purpose of ameliorating clinical signs of uremia is indicated for dogs and cats with IRIS CKD stages 3 and 4. While not generally regarded as an important uremic toxin, BUN is a surrogate marker for these retained non-protein nitrogenous waste products and typically correlates better with clinical signs than serum creatinine concentration. Blood urea nitrogen can also be used as a crude measure of dietary compliance; while it declines as dietary protein intake is reduced, inadequate food consumption may also be associated with reduced BUN concentrations.

Later, based on studies in rats, dietary protein was proposed as a major cause for development and progression of CKD in humans (Brenner, 1982). This association formed the basis of the "hyperfiltration theory" of progressive renal disease which sought to link excessive protein restriction to glomerular hyperperfusion, hyperfiltration, proteinuria and a progressive structural and function decline in the kidneys. Based on this theory, several studies have attempted to examine the role of protein intake on progression of CKD in dogs and cats.

The concept of reducing dietary protein intake in CKD patients in the absence of clinical signs of uremia has been questioned. Instead, it has been argued that limiting protein intake in these patients is justified on the basis of slowing progression of CKD. This suggestion derives from studies in rats indicating that dietary protein restriction limits glomerular hyperfiltration and hypertension and slows the spontaneous decline in kidney function that follows reduction in kidney mass (Hostetter et al. 2001a). Studies in humans have supported the concept that protein restriction may slow progression of CKD, albeit this effect may be small (Levey et al. 1999). A recent study of very low-protein diet therapy of CKD in humans indicated that it was ineffective in slowing progression of kidney disease and increased the risk of death (Menon et al. 2009). Multiple studies have failed to confirm a beneficial role for protein restriction in limiting progression of CKD in dogs or cats. When not excessive, limiting protein intake does not appear to have any adverse effects. It may be easier to initiate treatment with renal diets before the onset of clinical signs of uremia. In addition, as renal disease progresses, protein restriction may delay onset of clinical signs of uremia. While a role for protein restriction in slowing progression of canine and feline CKD has not been entirely excluded, available evidence fails to support a recommendation for or against protein restriction in patients with stage 2 CKD. However, studies examining high dietary protein intake by dogs with normal kidneys do not appear to lead to CKD (Polzin, unpublished data; Churchill, unpublished data).

Diet phosphorus

Phosphorus restriction is one of the core characteristics of renal diets. As protein is a major source of phosphorus, phosphorus restricted diets are usually protein restricted as well. Phosphorus content is restricted in order to limit phosphorus retention, hyperphosphatemia, renal secondary hyperparathyroidism, and progression of renal disease. While phosphorus retention and hyperphosphatemia are unlikely to directly cause clinical signs, they may promote increased levels of FGF-23, renal secondary hyperparathyroidism, reduced levels of calcitriol, and renal mineralization, some or all of which may contribute to progression of CKD. It is still unclear whether the salutary effects of phosphate restriction is mediated via changes in renal hemodynamics, via reduced renal mineralization, or changes of cellular calcium/phosphate concentrations, respectively, or via other factors (Ritz et al. 2005). Several lines of evidence have linked phosphorus restriction and control of serum phosphorus concentrations to slowing the progression of CKD. In studies performed in dogs with induced CKD, dietary phosphorus restriction improved survival and slowed the decline in renal function characteristic of CKD (Finco et al. 1992). In studies performed in cats with induced CKD, dietary phosphorus restriction limited renal mineralization. Two recent clinical studies in cats with spontaneous CKD have linked increased serum phosphorus concentrations to decreased survival (King et al. 2007; Boyd et al. 2008). Taken together, these observations suggest phosphorus restriction is an important dietary component supporting the renoprotective effects of diet therapy of CKD.

Omega-3 PUFA and antioxidants

In dogs with induced CKD, dietary omega-3 PUFA supplementation has been shown to be renoprotective. Dietary supplements rich in omega-3 PUFA reduce the concentrations of 2-series prostaglandins (PG) and increase the synthesis of 3-series PG (e.g., PGE3), which are believed to be less inflammatory (Bagga, 2003). Compared to dogs fed diets high in saturated fats or omega-6 PUFA, dogs consuming a diet supplemented with omega-3 PUFA had lower mortality, better renal function, fewer renal lesions, less proteinuria, and lower cholesterol levels (Brown et al. 1998). In dogs fed the omega-3 PUFA diet, renal function actually increased and remained above baseline over 20 months of study. Glomerulosclerosis, tubulointerstitial fibrosis, and interstitial inflammatory cell infiltrates were diminished among dogs fed the omega-3 PUFA diet. The renoprotective effects observed with dietary omega-3 PUFA enhancement included their tendency to reduce hypercholesterolemia, suppress inflammation and coagulation (by interfering with the production of proinflammatory, procoagulant prostanoids, thromboxanes, and/or leukotrienes), lower blood pressure, favorably influence renal hemodynamics,

provide antioxidant effects, or limit intrarenal calcification (Brown 2008).

Preliminary findings suggest that effects of dietary supplementation with antioxidants in the form of vitamin E, carotenoids, and lutein may be similar to omega-3 PUFA in slowing progression of induced CKD in dogs. Further, the combination of omega-3 PUFA (omega-6:omega-3 ratio of 5:1) with antioxidants appeared to be more effective than either omega-3 PUFA or antioxidants alone (Brown 2008).

Taken together, these findings justify a recommendation for dietary supplementation with omega-3 PUFA and antioxidants as appropriate for at least dogs with CKD for the purpose of slowing progression of CKD. While the ideal quantity of omega-3 PUFA to supplement and the optimum ratio of omega-3 to omega-6 PUFA for renal diets has yet to be conclusively established, one gram of omega-3 PUFA per 10 kg or an omega-6:omega-3 ratio of 5:1 may be reasonable. The dietary content of omega-3 PUFA should be considered when establishing an appropriate supplemental dosage for omega-3 PUFA.

Studies on the effects of omega-3 PUFA and antioxidants have not been reported for cats; however, a retrospective study on the effects of several renal diets did find that survival was greatest among cats fed the diet containing the highest omega-3 PUFA content (Plantinga et al. 2005). Unfortunately, this study was retrospective and it is not possible to accurately assess the effects of dietary omega-3 PUFA levels from this data.

Meeting nutritional needs

It is common for pet owners to consider food consumption to be a premier indicator of their pet's quality of life. When pets are ill, owners may be happy when their pet shows any interest in food. However, it is inappropriate to accept the pet's consumption of "some" food as a goal of therapy. Malnutrition resulting from inadequate attention to nutrition is a major cause for morbidity and mortality in dogs and cats with IRIS CKD stages 3 and 4. Specific nutritional goals for maintaining body weight and body condition score should be set at the outset of nutritional therapy. Many dogs and cats with CKD have body condition scores below 4/9. Optimally, patients should consume sufficient calories *from an appropriate diet* to maintain a body condition score of 4 to 5/9. It is particularly important to assure sufficient calorie intake for patients with body condition scores of 3/9 or lower or when patients fail to consume adequate calories to maintain a stable, appropriate body weight. Factors promoting weight loss and malnutrition include anorexia, nausea, vomiting and the subsequent reduction in nutrient intake, hormonal and metabolic derangements, and catabolic factors related to uremia, particularly acidosis. Failure to adequately address uremic gastroenteritis, uremic stomatitis and dental health can promote anorexia. Metabolic acidosis can impair adaptation to limited protein diets, thereby promoting protein catabolism and malnutrition.

It is appropriate to consider placing a feeding tube when patients fail to spontaneously consume adequate food. Feeding via a gastrostomy or an esophagostomy tube is a simple and effective way to provide an adequate intake of calories and water. In addition, feeding tubes simplify drug administration. Based on this line of reasoning, use of feeding tubes has been recommended for CKD patients. Although there is only weak evidence supporting the effectiveness of feeding tubes in achieving nutritional goals of dogs and cats with CKD, there is no proven effective alternative to this intervention. It is important to emphasize to pet owners that the goal of placing feeding tubes is to improve nutrition and thus improve the quality of life for the patient, not just to keep the patient alive.

Managing gastrointestinal signs of uremia

Gastrointestinal complications of CKD, including reduced appetite with reduced food intake, nausea, vomiting, uremic stomatitis and halitosis, gastrointestinal hemorrhage, diarrhea, and hemorrhagic colitis, are not uncommon in dogs and cats with IRIS CKD stages 3 and 4. Treatment for these gastrointestinal signs is largely symptomatic. As described above, reducing dietary protein intake may be beneficial in ameliorating many of the gastrointestinal signs of uremia. Although a link between the products of protein metabolism/catabolism and clinical signs of uremia is clear, the precise "toxins" causing the clinical signs remain unknown. Nonetheless, improvement in clinical signs often correlates with a reduction in BUN as protein intake is reduced. Thus, the presence of gastrointestinal complications of CKD signs is sufficient justification to warrant limiting protein intake.

Oral rinses with dilute (0.1%) chlorhexidine have been recommended for uremic stomatitis, but the effectiveness of such therapy has yet to be established. Good dental hygiene including dental scaling (when possible) may be helpful in minimizing oral lesions. Patient undergoing anesthesia for dental cleaning should be pre-loaded with fluids and the depth of anesthesia with particular emphasis on maintaining acceptable blood pressure and tissue perfusion is essential in these patients.

Management of anorexia, nausea, and vomiting typically includes (1) limiting gastric acidity using H_2 blockers, (2) suppressing nausea and vomiting using antiemetics, and (3) providing mucosal protection using sucralfate. Of these treatments, H_2 blockers are most commonly employed and few adverse effects have been attributed to their use. The most commonly used H_2 blockers include famotidine and ranitidine. However, their efficacy remains unproven. The lack of evidence of gastric hyperacidity in dogs and cats with CKD raises concern regarding their effectiveness.

Antiemetics are typically added when anorexia, nausea or vomiting persist despite the use of an H_2 blocker. The antiemetics most commonly used in patients with CKD include metoclopramide, 5-HT_3 receptor antagonists such as ondansetron HCl or dolasetron mesylate, and the neurokinin (NK_1) receptor antagonist maropitant citrate. Questions have been raised concerning the appropriateness of using metoclopramide in patients with CKD because metoclopramide, a dopamine antagonist, has been shown to reduce renal blood flow in humans (Israel et al. 1986). Studies in uremic humans have shown the 5-HT_3 receptor antagonist ondansetron to be twice as effective as metoclopramide in reducing the clinical signs of uremic nausea and vomiting (Perkovic et al. 2002). Maropitant may also be more effective than metoclopramide because it may suppress both the vomiting center and the chemoreceptor trigger zone. Sucralfate is added when gastrointestinal ulcerations and hemorrhage are suspected.

Treatment of phosphorus retention and hyperphosphatemia

Clinical importance on managing serum phosphorus concentrations

The kidneys play a pivotal role in regulating phosphorus balance because they are the primary route of phosphorus excretion. Renal phosphorus excretion is the net of glomerular filtration less tubular reabsorption of phosphorus. If dietary phosphorus intake remains constant, a decline in glomerular filtration rate will lead to phosphorus retention and ultimately hyperphosphatemia. However, during the early stages of CKD, serum phosphorus concentrations typically remain within the normal range because of a compensatory decrease in phosphorous reabsorption in the surviving nephrons. This renal tubular adaptation is a consequence of the phosphaturic effects of FGF-23 and PTH. Renal excretion of phosphorous is enhanced by reducing the tubular transport maximum for phosphorous reabsorption in the proximal tubule via the adenyl cyclase system. When glomerular filtration rates decline below about 20% of normal, this adaptive effect reaches its limit and hyperphosphatemia ensues. However, before hyperphosphatemia develops, the trade-off for maintaining serum phosphorus within normal limits is persistent elevations in FGF-23 and PTH.

Further, substantial phosphorus retention occurs in tissues before serum phosphorus levels exceed the upper limit of normal. These trade-offs may have serious consequences including progressive loss of renal function and impaired production of calcitriol.

The most important clinical consequence of phosphorus retention and hyperphosphatemia is progression of CKD. Elevated serum phosphorus concentrations have been shown to be predictive of increased mortality in humans, cats, and dogs with CKD (Finco et al. 1992; Block et al. 1998; King et al. 2007; Boyd et al. 2008). In dogs with induced CKD, consuming a diet high in phosphorus has been shown to be associated with increased mortality (Brown, 1991; Finco et al. 1992). In cats, hyperphosphatemia has been found to predict shorter survival (King et al. 2007; Boyd et al. 2008). In humans with CKD, the adjusted relative risk of mortality has been shown to progressively increase as serum phosphorous concentrations increase (Block et al. 1998). However, in this study, the mortality risk associated with hyperphosphatemia appeared to be independent of elevated PTH levels, which alone appeared to have only a weak association with mortality. Further, in humans with mild to moderate CKD plasma fibroblast growth factor 23 concentrations, an early measure of phosphorus retention has been shown to predict progression of CKD (Fliser et al. 2007).

Hyperphosphatemia may be associated with an elevated calcium-phosphate product (Ca X PO_4 in units of mg/dL) even when serum calcium concentration remains within normal limits, thus increasing the risk of mineralization of blood vessels, joints, and soft tissues. This process, called metastatic calcification, is especially prominent in proton-secreting organs, such as the stomach and kidneys, in which basolateral bicarbonate secretion results in an increase in pH that promotes calcium hydrogen phosphate (brushite) precipitation (Brushinsky, 2005). However, myocardium, lung, and liver may also be mineralized in patients with CKD.

Without treatment, phosphorus retention, and subsequently hyperphosphatemia and renal secondary hyperparathyroidism, occur early in the course of renal failure (in most dogs and cats with IRIS CKD stages 2–4) (Nagode et al. 1996; Ritz et al. 2005; Brown et al. 2007b). Although hyperphosphatemia has been linked to pruritus, conjunctivitis, renal osteodystrophy, and soft-tissue calcification in humans, hyperphosphatemia per se has not been conclusively linked to any clinical signs in dogs and cats with CKD. Rather, minimizing phosphorus retention and hyperphosphatemia is an important therapeutic goal in patients with CKD primarily because it appears to slow progression of CKD and prolong survival (Finco et al. 1992; Barber et al. 1999).

Methods of limiting hyperphosphatemia and phosphorus retention

Impaired renal perfusion (prerenal azotemia) promotes increased serum phosphorus concentrations, so the first step in correcting hyperphosphatemia is to assure that the patient is well hydrated. Minimizing long-term phosphorus retention and hyperphosphatemia may be accomplished by limiting dietary phosphorus intake, oral administration of agents that bind phosphorus within the lumen of the intestines, or a combination of these methods. The usual approach is to start with diet therapy, and add phosphorous binding agents if diet therapy alone fails to bring the serum phosphorous concentration into the target range.

Intervention to manage serum phosphorus concentration is indicated for dogs and cats with IRIS CKD stages 2–4 when serum phosphorus concentration rises above the therapeutic target concentration. The goal of therapy is to reduce serum phosphorus concentrations into the recommended therapeutic range. Ideally, serum phosphorus concentration should be maintained within the target range of 3.5–4.5 mg/dL in IRIS CKD stage II, 3.5–5.0 mg/dL in IRIS CKD stage III, and 3.5–6.0 mg/dL in CKD stage IV. These targets were established based on expert opinion and have not been evaluated in clinical trials (Elliot et al. 2006). They are often below the upper limits of many established laboratory normal ranges because the stated goal is to limit phosphorus retention even before the onset of overt hyperphosphatemia.

Simply reducing serum phosphorus concentration into the normal range may fail to normalize serum PTH levels (Nagode et al. 1996; Barber et al. 1999). However, current available evidence suggests that limiting phosphorus retention and minimizing hyperphosphatemia is the most important therapeutic goal. Other than preventing development of the skeletal lesions of renal osteodystrophy, it has yet to be established whether normalization of PTH levels is an important therapeutic goal in dogs and cats with CKD.

Dietary phosphorus restriction

Serum phosphorus concentrations result from the net balance between dietary intake and renal excretion of phosphorus. Therefore, maintaining serum phosphorus concentrations within the normal range as renal function declines requires modification of phosphorus intake. In theory, optimum control of hyperphosphatemia would be achieved by reducing dietary phosphorus intake "in proportion" to the decrease in glomerular filtration rate. However, there is a limit to the extent to which dietary phosphorus can be reduced. Nonetheless, the first step in managing phosphorus balance in dogs and cats with CKD is to initiate diet therapy with a phosphorus-restricted diet when serum phosphorus concentrations exceed the target concentration for the patient's IRIS CKD stage.

Manufactured renal diets are substantially reduced in phosphorus content and are often successful in achieving serum phosphorus targets into CKD stage 3. Typical commercial dog foods contain approximately 1–2% phosphorus on a dry matter basis and provide about 2.7 mg/kcal or more phosphorus. Modified protein diets designed for dogs with CKD may contain as little as 0.13–0.28% phosphorus on a dry matter basis and provide about 0.3–0.5 mg/kcal of phosphorus. Typical commercial cat foods contain from 1 to 4% phosphorus on a dry matter basis and provide about 2.9 mg/kcal or more. Modified protein diets designed for cats with CKD may contain as little as 0.5% phosphorous on a dry matter basis and provide about 0.9 mg/kcal of phosphorus.

Approximately 4–6 weeks after imitating dietary phosphorus restriction, the serum phosphorus concentration should be reassessed to determine whether the treatment target has been met. Serum phosphorus levels typically decline gradually as phosphorus leaches out of multiple tissues in the body. Thus, the overall efficacy of dietary phosphorus restriction in reducing serum phosphorus concentrations may not occur until the patient has been consuming the phosphorus-restricted diet for several weeks. In a study in cats with CKD, the effect of restricting dietary phosphorus intake was apparent after 28–49 days (Barber et al. 1999). Samples obtained for determinations of serum phosphorus concentration should be collected after a 12-hour fast to avoid postprandial hyperphosphatemia. Sample hemolysis should be avoided because red blood cells contain substantial quantities of phosphorus. If after 4–8 weeks, diet therapy alone fails to maintain the serum phosphorus concentrations below the target value, addition of an intestinal phosphate binding agent should be considered to reduce serum phosphorus concentration below the target concentration.

Intestinal phosphorus binding agents

Intestinal phosphate binding agents induce formation of nonabsorbable salts of phosphorus within the lumen of the gastrointestinal tract. The goal of such therapy is to bind phosphorus contained in the diet, thus effectively lowering the absorbable phosphorus content of the ingested food. Because the target of such therapy is diet phosphorus, it is essential that phosphate binding agents be given at or about meal time. If the patient is fed more than one daily, the total daily dose of the phosphate binder should be divided and a portion adminis-

tered with every meal. Administering the binders away from meal time markedly reduces their effectiveness. In addition, calcium-based phosphate-binding agents that are given between meals function primarily as calcium supplements rather than as a phosphate binder.

Phosphate binders typically release constituents in the process of binding phosphorus. For example, aluminum-based phosphorus binders release aluminum, calcium-based phosphorus binders release calcium, lanthanum-based phosphorus binders release lanthanum and sevelamer (Renagel) may release hydrochloric acid and nitrogen compounds. Because some of these substances may lead to toxicity, caution is advised when administering these agents at dosages above the recommended dose range.

The most commonly used intestinal phosphate binding agents in dogs and cats contain aluminum as hydroxide, oxide or carbonate salts. Because of concern about aluminum toxicity in humans, aluminum-containing binding agents are becoming more difficult to obtain. Although aluminum-containing binding agents usually appear to be well tolerated and safe in dogs and cats, aluminum toxicity has been reported in dogs with advanced CKD treated with high doses of aluminum-containing phosphate binding agents (Segev et al. 2008). The presenting signs in these dogs were severe neuromuscular in nature and were localized as a cerebral and peripheral neuropathy and junctionopathy. Clinical signs included decreased menace response, weakness, and ataxia, absence of patellar reflexes, decreased pelvic limb withdrawal, obtundation, tetraparesis, and lateral recumbency. Microcytosis was also noted in these dogs and may be potentially useful in early detection of aluminum toxicity in dogs. Chelation therapy was necessary to correct aluminum toxicity in these dogs.

In order to minimize the risk of inducing aluminum toxicity, alternate drugs that do not contain aluminum may be used or added to the aluminum-based phosphorus binding agents. These products include calcium carbonate, calcium acetate, sevalamer hydrochloride, or lanthanum carbonate. Sucralfate, a complex polyaluminum hydroxide salt of sulfate used primarily for treatment of gastrointestinal ulcerations may also be effective in binding phosphorus within the intestine. Experience with these drugs in dogs and cats are limited, but hypercalcemia may be a problem with the calcium-based products, particularly when administered with calcitriol or between meals. The newest product, lanthanum carbonate and other salts of lanthanum appear to be quite effective and are associated with minimal side-effects. Lanthanum is reportedly minimally absorbed from the intestinal tract, thus may be of reduced toxicity risk compared to aluminum salts. Lanthanum salts and sevalemer hydrochloride are substantially more expensive than calcium or aluminum salts at the time of this writing.

Dosing of phosphorus binders is "to effect", which means that the dose is adjusted to assure that the serum phosphorus target is achieved (see above). Therapy is usually begun at a dose at the lower end of the recommended dose range and adjusted upward as needed every 4–6 weeks until the therapeutic target is reached. Different types of phosphate binding agents (i.e., aluminum-based, calcium-based, lanthanum-based, or sevalemer) may be combined in order to minimize the risk of overdosage or toxicity. If dosage substantially exceeds the dosage range recommended for the binding agent, it is best to add a different phosphorus binding agent rather than risk inducing toxicity.

Aluminum-containing intestinal phosphorus binding agents include aluminum hydroxide, aluminum carbonate, and aluminum oxide. The recommended dose range for these compounds is 30–100 mg/kg/day. They are available over-the-counter in liquid, tablet, or capsule forms from most pharmacies as antacid preparations. In humans, capsules and tablets are less effective than liquids, but liquid preparations may be quite unpalatable to some dogs and cats. Chemical formulations of aluminum hydroxide (USP) have also been used in powder form. This approach has the advantage of being relatively free from taste or texture that might adversely affect the patient's appetite.

Calcium-based phosphorus-binding agents include calcium acetate, calcium carbonate, or calcium citrate. Because calcium-based products may promote clinically significant hypercalcemia, it is recommended that serum calcium concentrations be monitored intermittently when using these drugs. They should generally not be used in hypercalcemic patients. When indicated, they may be used between meals as a source of additional dietary calcium. As mentioned above, reduced dosages of calcium carbonate and calcium acetate may be used concurrent with aluminum-based binding agents to limit risks of both hypercalcemia and aluminum toxicity. However, calcium citrate may promote absorption of aluminum and should therefore not be used in concert with aluminum-based binding agents. Calcium acetate is the most effective calcium-based phosphorus-binding agent as well as the agent least likely to induce hypercalcemia because it releases the least amount of calcium compared to the amount of phosphorus it binds (Yudd and Llach 2000). Doses from 60 to 90 mg/kg/day have been recommended for calcium acetate and 90 to 150 mg/kg/day for calcium carbonate. Some calcium carbonate preparations may not be effective because they fail to dissolve well in the gastrointestinal tract; this may be investigated by examining the stool or obtaining radiographs of the abdomen for evidence of radiodense tablets that have failed to dissolve.

While the dosage of lanthanum carbonate has not been reported for dogs and cats, a reasonable starting dose would be about 30 mg/kg/day divided with meals. Since it is thought that lanthanum largely remains within the lumen of the gut and is not absorbed, increasing dosage to achieve the therapeutic target seems to be a reasonable goal. Until more information on use of these products in dogs and cats with CKD become available, substantial increases in dosage should probably be avoided. In Europe, lanthanum carbonate is available in a flavored liquid form intended for cats with CKD.

Like lanthanum-based binders, the therapeutic advantage of sevelamer hydrochloride (Renagel® Tablets and Capsules, Genzyme Corp.) is that it does not promote hypercalcemia or absorption of aluminum. However, it is more expensive than older phosphorus binding agents. In addition, concerns have been raised over its potential for inducing vitamin-K deficiency and hemorrhage. In preclinical studies in rats and dogs, sevelamer hydrochloride reduced vitamin D, E, K, and folic acid levels when given at doses of 6–100 times the recommended human dose. In clinical trials in humans, there has been no evidence of reduction in serum levels of vitamins in patients receiving vitamin supplements. There is scant information on the safety, effectiveness or dosage of sevelamer in dogs and cats. On the basis of extrapolating the recommended dosage from humans, an initial dose of 30–135 mg/kg/day divided and given with meals may be considered. Because the contents of Renagel expand in water, the manufacturer recommends that tablets and capsules should be swallowed intact and should not be crushed, chewed, broken into pieces, or taken apart prior to administration. Sevelamer reportedly lowers total and low-density lipoprotein cholesterol concentrations and elevated high-density lipoprotein cholesterol levels in humans (Akizawa et al. 2003).

Calcitriol therapy

Rationale for calcitriol therapy

Patients with CKD typically have reduced levels of calcitriol. Calcitriol (1,25-dihydroxyvitamin D), the most active metabolite of vitamin D, results from hydroxylation of 25 hydroxycholecalciferol in the kidneys. As kidney function declines in patients with CKD, phosphate retention, increased levels of fibroblast growth factor-23, and hyperphosphatemia impair renal 1α-hydroxylase activity, thus reducing production of calcitriol (Kazama et al. 2005). To some degree, this functional decline in calcitriol production may be ameliorated by limiting phosphorus intake. However, as CKD progresses reduced renal mass further limits the number of cells available to undertake the hydroxylation of 25-hydroxyvitamin D resulting in calcitriol deficiency (Gutierrez et al. 2005).

Calcitriol enhances intestinal calcium and phosphorus uptake, inhibits PTH synthesis and release, and activates receptors on many cells in the body. Calcitriol is very effective in reducing PTH levels in dogs and cats with CKD (Nagode et al. 1996). Although PTH has been proposed as a potential uremic toxin responsible for many constitutional signs or uremia, the clinical benefits of reducing PTH levels remains unclear. It has been suggested that patients receiving calcitriol therapy may (1) be brighter and more alert and interactive with owners, (2) show an improvement in appetite, (3) be more physically active than before treatment, and (4) have longer life-spans (Nagode et al. 1996). Further, these authors provide pathophysiological support for the purported benefits of calcitriol therapy through referenced studies from multiple species. In contrast, Finco and colleagues, using parathyroidectomy combined with an experimental model of CKD, concluded that increased PTH levels do not contribute importantly to clinical signs of uremia in dogs (Finco et al. 1997). However; this study was not designed to directly address the effectiveness of calcitriol therapy in managing clinical signs of dogs and cats with CKD.

A masked, randomized, controlled clinical trial performed at the University of Minnesota Veterinary Medical Center confirmed the value of calcitriol in reducing mortality in dogs with IRIS CKD stages III and IV (Polzin, unpublished data). The survival benefit appeared to result from reduced progression of CKD. These findings are consistent with results of recent studies in human patients with CKD which confirmed a similar survival benefit of calcitriol therapy (Cheng and Coyne 2007; Shoben et al. 2008). Further, studies in humans have shown that calcitriol deficiency may predict shorter survival in humans with CKD (Ravani, 2009). However, a randomized clinical trial performed in cats revealed equivocal benefits for calcitriol in altering the course of CKD (Polzin, unpublished data). Neither the dog nor cat study could confirm nor refute the proposed clinical benefits of calcitriol therapy beyond enhanced survival in dogs. Possible mechanisms by which calcitriol may influence progression of CKD include systemic activation of vitamin D receptors, downregulation of the renin angiotensin system, and reducing podocyte loss associated with glomerular hypertrophy (Andress 2006; Freundlich et al. 2008; Pörsti 2008).

Guidelines for using calcitriol

Calcitriol therapy is indicated for dogs with IRIS CKD stages III and IV and possibly IRIS CKD stage II to slow progressive deterioration in renal function. A recommen-

dation for or against use of calcitriol in cats with CKD cannot be made at this time.

Prior to initiating calcitriol therapy, serum phosphorus should be managed to achieve treatment targets described previously. In addition, ionized calcium levels should be confirmed to be within or below the normal range. Since calcitriol may increase intestinal absorption of both phosphorus and calcium, it is recommended to monitor serum phosphorus and ionized calcium concentrations during calcitriol therapy to avoid hyperphosphatemia and ionized hypercalcemia. If serum albumin concentrations are within normal limits, total serum calcium may cautiously be used to monitor for hypercalcemia, but any increase in serum calcium concentration should be evaluated by measuring ionized calcium. Total serum calcium values may not accurately portray ionized calcium levels in dogs with CKD (Schenck and Chew, 2003). It is unclear whether renoliths containing calcium constitute a relative contraindication to calcitriol therapy.

Calcitriol should initially be provided at a dose of 2–3 ng/kg every 24 hours. Life-long treatment will be necessary to achieve the desired effect of reduced renal mortality. Because it enhances intestinal absorption of calcium and phosphorus, calcitriol should not be given with meals; administration of calcitriol in the evening on an empty stomach reduces the risk of inducing hypercalcemia. Available dose forms are designed for humans and contain relatively very large doses of calcitriol. A compounding pharmacy is necessary to prepare formulations in appropriate dosages for use in dogs and cats. Overdosage of calcitriol is potentially dangerous and should be avoided due to the induction of hypercalcemia with possible renal injury (hypercalcemic nephropathy).

Early detection of hypercalcemia, should it occur, is important to limit the extent of renal injury. However, the onset of hypercalcemia after initiation of vitamin D therapy is unpredictable (i.e., it may occur after days to months of treatment). Therefore, continued monitoring of serum calcium, phosphorus, and creatinine concentrations are necessary to detect hypercalcemia, hyperphosphatemia, or deteriorating renal function before irreversible renal damage ensues. Serum creatinine, phosphorus and ionized calcium concentrations should be measured 2, 5, and 8 weeks after initiating therapy to assure appropriate dosing, stable renal function and the absence of hyperphosphatemia and hypercalcemia. Use of calcium-containing phosphorus binding agents, particularly calcium carbonate, and other oral calcium supplements predispose to hypercalcemia in patients receiving calcitriol. If serum phosphorus and ionized calcium concentrations are well controlled after 8 weeks of calcitriol therapy, serum creatinine, phosphorus, and ionized calcium concentrations should ideally be monitored every 1–2 months throughout calcitriol therapy. The product of serum calcium and phosphorus concentrations (in mg/dL) should not exceed 60; the goal is to attain values between 42 and 52 (Kates et al. 1997).

Calcitriol's rapid onset (about 1 day) and short duration of action (half-life less than 1 day) permits rapid control of unwanted hypercalcemia. If hypercalcemia develops, it is advisable to stop treatment completely rather than reduce the dose. Therapy may be re-instituted with a reduced dosage or altered dosing strategy when serum calcium concentration returns to normal and serum phosphorus concentration returns to target concentration. When calcitriol therapy is associated with hypercalcemia, the daily dose may be doubled and given every other day (Hostutler et al. 2006). This approach is thought to be less likely to induce hypercalcemia because the effect of calcitriol on intestinal calcium absorption is related to the duration of exposure of intestinal cells to calcitriol.

Pulse therapy has been advocated to control renal secondary hyperparathyroidism when plasma PTH concentration is markedly elevated or when standard therapy with calcitriol fails to normalize plasma PTH levels (Nagode et al. 1996). In this approach, patients are given 20 ng/kg of calcitriol twice per week in the evening on an empty stomach. Pulse therapy is usually used no longer than 1–2 months to suppress resistant hyperparathyroidism. If successful, calcitriol may then be given at the standard daily dose.

Although suppression of hyperparathyroidism has been suggested as one of the possible justifications for calcitriol therapy, the value of monitoring serum PTH activity during calcitriol therapy is unclear because the clinical benefits of suppressing hyperparathyroidism remain unproven. In the Minnesota canine study that confirmed a survival benefit arising from therapy with calcitriol, dosage of calcitriol was increased up to 5 ng/kg/day to lower PTH values into the normal range, unless hypercalcemia ensued. If hypercalcemia developed, the dosage of calcitriol was reduced. On the basis of this schema for establishing a dosage for calcitriol, the mean calcitriol dosage used in this clinical trial was 1.9 ng/kg/day.

Treating metabolic acidosis

Minimizing metabolic acidosis by the administration of alkali and/or feeding diets that do not produce an acid effect may play an important role in management of patients with CKD. Minimizing renal acidosis may benefit patients with CKD in several ways, including (1) ameliorating signs of uremic acidosis, including anorexia, lethargy, nausea, vomiting, muscle weakness, and weight loss, (2) minimizing the catabolic effects of metabolic acidosis on protein metabolism, (3) enhancing the patient's capacity to adapt to additional acid stress resulting from such factors as diarrhea, dehydration, or respiratory acidosis, (4) limiting skeletal damage (demineralization and inhibited skeletal growth) resulting from bone buffering, and (5) rectifying adverse effects of severe acidosis on the cardiovascular system (impaired myocardial contractility and enhanced venoconstriction) (Mitch 1997; Adrogue and Madias 1998). In addition, evidence in rodents suggest that limiting metabolic acidosis may slow down the progression of CKD (Nath 1998; Wesson and Simoni 2009).

Studies in rodents with reduced renal mass have shown that consuming an acid-inducing diet may promote progressive renal injury (Nath 1998; Wesson and Simoni 2009). This progressive renal injury is accompanied by increased renal cortical H^+ content, and may occur in this model even when the increased acid load does not alter systemic acid-base measurements. Administration of alkali has been shown to correct the progressive decline in renal function. A possible mechanism underlying progressive renal injury in this model is that increased renal ammoniagenesis occurring consequent to the increased acid load may activate the alternative complement pathway, leading to tubulointerstitial injury (Nath 1998). However, the applicability of this model to canine and feline renal diseases is unclear. When cats with induced renal disease were fed an acidifying diet, evidence of progressive renal disease was not apparent (James, unpublished data).

In a study in cats with naturally occurring CKD, metabolic acidosis reportedly occurred in less than 10% of cats with stages 2 and 3 CKD, but approached 50% of cats with overt signs of uremia (Elliot and Barber 1998). Based on these findings, it appears that only a minority of cats with clinically stable IRIS CKD stages 2 and 3 are likely to require routine alkalinization therapy. However, the decision to intervene with alkalinization therapy should be based on a laboratory assessment of the patient's acid-base status. Unfortunately, no evidence-based intervention threshold for treating metabolic acidosis is available for dogs and cats. In studies performed at the University of Minnesota we have been unable to demonstrate adverse clinical effects of mild to moderate chronic metabolic acidosis in cats with induced CKD (James, unpublished data). In absence of clear clinical evidence, we recommend considering alkalinization therapy when blood gas analysis confirms plasma bicarbonate values remain below 15 mmol/L in well hydrated dogs and cats with CKD. However, for patients with metabolic acidosis associated with a blood pH below 7.10, more immediate parenteral intervention with sodium bicarbonate should be considered to increase the blood pH above 7.20 (Sabatini and Kurtzman 2009). Low serum or plasma total CO_2 values obtained by autoanalyzer techniques should be confirmed by blood gas analysis because falsely low total CO_2 readings may occur when blood collection tubes are not fully filled or are exposed to air while awaiting analysis (James et al. 1997).

Treatment options for alkalinization therapy include feeding a pH-neutral renal diet and/or oral administration of sodium bicarbonate or potassium citrate. Most renal diets are neutral to slightly alkalinizing in effect and are an appropriate first step in mitigating metabolic acidosis. When several weeks of diet therapy alone fails to ameliorate the metabolic acidosis, alkalinization therapy should be considered. In general, alkali should be administered as several smaller doses over the day rather than a single large daily dose in order to minimize fluctuations in blood pH.

Sodium bicarbonate is the most commonly used alkalinizing agent for patients with metabolic acidosis. Because the effects of gastric acid on oral sodium bicarbonate are unpredictable, the dosage should be individualized for each patient. Unfortunately, many dogs and cats find sodium bicarbonate powder distasteful when administered in food or water. A more acceptable solution is to administer alkali in tablet form. Sodium bicarbonate is available as 5 and 10 grain tablets.

Potassium citrate may offer the advantage, especially in cats, of allowing for the simultaneous treatment of both hypokalemia and acidosis with a single drug. Metabolic acidosis when accompanied by potassium depletion or magnesium depletion may respond poorly to alkali therapy alone. However, in that potassium doses required for adequate correction of hypokalemia may exceed the citrate dose required to correct acidosis, the response to therapy should be monitored to avoid excessive alkalinization. Starting doses of 40–60 mg/kg every 8–12 hours are recommended.

The response to alkalinization therapy should be determined by performing blood gas analysis 10–14 days after initiating therapy. Ideally, blood should be collected just prior to administration of the drug. Plasma bicarbonate or blood gas analysis should be used to assess response to treatment 2–4 weeks after initiating therapy. Therapy should be adjusted to maintain serum bicarbonate levels ideally between 18 and 25 in dogs and 15 and 22 in cats. A suggested initial dose of sodium bicarbonate is 8–12 mg/kg body weight given every 8–12 hours. Urine pH is an unreliable means of assessing the need for or response to treatment and is not recommended for this purpose.

Treating potassium disorders

Although rare in dogs, potassium depletion and hypokalemia are relatively common in cats with IRIS CKD stages 2 and 3. Hypokalemia becomes less of an issue in cats with IRIS CKD stage 4 because the marked reduction in GFR is more likely to promote potassium retention and hyperkalemia. Estimates of the prevalence of hypokalemia in IRIS CKD stages 2 and 3 cats are in the range of 20–30% (DiBartola et al. 1987; Lulich et al. 1992; Elliot and Barber 1998). Since potassium leaves the cells as hypokalemia develops, total body potassium depletion is likely to be at least as common as hypokalemia (Theisen et al. 1997). The mechanisms underlying development of hypokalemia in cats with CKD remain unclear, but inadequate potassium intake, increased urinary loss, and enhanced activation of the renin-angiotensin-aldosterone system due to dietary salt restriction may play a role (Buranakarl et al. 2004). While increasing the potassium content of renal diets has reduced the incidence of overt clinical signs of hypokalemia, hypokalemia remains a common laboratory finding in cats with CKD. In addition, the antihypertensive agent amlodipine may promote hypokalemia in cats with CKD (Henik et al. 1997).

Hypokalemia and potassium depletion may affect the kidneys or muscles of cats with CKD. Diets low in potassium and high in acid content have been implicated in impairing renal function and promoting development of lymphoplasmacytic tubulointerstitial lesions in cats (Dow et al. 1987; Dow et al. 1990; DiBartola et al. 1993; Adams et al. 1994; Theisen et al. 1997). Potassium depletion may result in reduced renal blood flow and GFR as a consequence of angiotensin II and thromboxane-mediated renal vasoconstriction. In addition, hypokalemia may promote polyuria by impairing renal responsiveness to antidiuretic hormone, and by stimulating the brain thirst centers through increased levels of angiotensin II. Hypokalemic polymyopathy, characterized by generalized muscle weakness and cervical ventroflexion, is a well-recognized, although increasingly less common complication of CKD in cats.

While there is a consensus of opinion that cats with hypokalemia should receive potassium supplementation, the value of "prophylactic" potassium supplementation in normokalemic cats yet to be established. Higher potassium diets combined with oral potassium supplementation has been advocated for cats with CKD in order to prevent or treat hypokalemia and the renal and muscular consequences of potassium depletion. While potassium supplementation is unlikely to be medically harmful to polyuric, normokalemic cats, administration of an oral medication may impose an unnecessary burden on both the cat and the cat owner. Potassium supplementation may be inappropriate for cats with IRIS CKD stage 4, particularly in cats receiving angiotensin-converting enzyme inhibitors or other drugs that may promote hyperkalemia.

In general, oral replacement is the safest and preferred route for administering potassium. Parenteral therapy is generally reserved for patients requiring emergency reversal of hypokalemia or for patients that cannot or will not accept oral therapy. Up to 30 mEq/L of potassium chloride may be added to fluids to be administered subcutaneously.

Gluconate or citrate salts of potassium may be used for oral supplementation. However, potassium chloride is not recommended because of its lack of palatability and acidifying nature. Potassium gluconate may be administered orally as tablets, flavored gel, or in a palatable powder form (Tumil-K, Daniels Pharmaceuticals, Inc.). Depending on the size of the cat and severity of hypokalemia, potassium gluconate is usually provided at a dose of 2–6 mEq per cat per day. Acidosis is a major risk factor for development of hypokalemia and therefore acid-base status should be determined and normalized early in the management of hypokalemia. Potassium citrate solution (Polycitra®-K Syrup, Baker Norton) is an excellent alternative that has the advantage of providing simultaneous alkalinization therapy. Potassium citrate is initially given at a dose of 40–60 mg/kg/day divided into 2 or 3 doses. If muscle weakness is present, it usually resolves within 1–5 days after initiating parenteral or oral potassium supplements. Thereafter, potassium dosage should be adjusted based on the clinical response of the patient and serum potassium determinations. Serum potassium concentration should initially be monitored every 7–14 days and the dosage adjusted accordingly to establish the final maintenance dosage. In patients with hypokalemic polymyopathy, it may be necessary to monitor serum potassium concentrations every 24–48 hours during the initial phase of therapy. It is unclear whether all cats require long-term potassium supplementation; however, preliminary evidence suggests that such therapy may be required by at least some older cats with CKD.

Prophylactic supplementation of low oral daily doses of potassium (2 mEq/day) has been recommended for cats with CKD (Dow and Fettman 1992). This recommendation appears to be based on the as yet unproved hypothesis that in some cats with CKD, hypokalemia and potassium depletion might promote a self-perpetuating cycle of declining renal function, metabolic acidosis, and continuing potassium losses. It is proposed that supplementation may stabilize renal function before potassium depletion exacerbates the disease. However, results of a recent clinical trial suggested that in cats that initially had normal serum potassium concentrations but depleted muscle potassium pools, daily supplementation for 6 months with 4 mEq of potassium gluconate was not demonstrably superior to providing sodium gluconate in restoring muscle potassium stores (Theisen et al. 1997).

However, this study was limited by the small number of cats enrolled. In addition, median muscle potassium content did increase in the potassium supplemented cats from 328 to 402 mEq/kg, a value close to the value of 424 mEq/L established for normal cat muscle. While the value of providing supplemental potassium to cats with normal serum potassium concentrations has not been established, it is clear that muscle potassium and probably total body potassium stores are likely to be reduced in cats with CKD. On the basis of current data, neither a recommendation for nor against routine supplementation of potassium can be supported.

Hypokalemia may be more likely to develop when diets that are acidifying and restricted in magnesium content are fed. Therefore, they should generally be avoided in cats with CKD. In addition, intensive fluid therapy during uremic crises, particularly with potassium deficient fluids, may promote hypokalemia in cats or dogs that were not previously hypokalemic. Therefore, serum potassium concentrations should be monitored during fluid therapy and maintenance fluids should be supplemented with potassium chloride to prevent iatrogenic hypokalemia (concentrations of 13–20 mEq/L are appropriate for maintenance fluids). Care should be taken to assure that potassium is not administered intravenously at a rate exceeding 0.5 mEq/kg/hour.

Maintaining hydration

Fluid balance in patients with polyuria is maintained by compensatory polydipsia. If water consumption is insufficient to compensate for polyuria, dehydration will result. Dehydration is a relatively common complication of CKD and in patients with clinical evidence of dehydration, intervention to correct and prevent dehydration is indicated. Cats with CKD appear to be particularly susceptible to chronic dehydration, perhaps because the magnitude of compensatory polydipsia is inadequate. However, lack of adequate access to good quality drinking water, certain environmental conditions and intercurrent illnesses that limit fluid intake or promote fluid losses (e.g., pyrexia, vomiting, or diarrhea) may also promote dehydration.

Chronic dehydration may promote decreased appetite, lethargy, weakness, constipation, and prerenal azotemia, and predispose to acute kidney injury. Additional loss of kidney function due to acute kidney injury is a potentially important cause for progression of CKD. Owners of pets with CKD should be warned that fluid losses due to vomiting or diarrhea that might not present a threat to an animal with normal kidneys, could lead to a deterioration in kidney function or precipitate uremic crisis in a patient with CKD.

The goal of therapy is to correct and prevent dehydration and its clinical effects. Acute correction of fluid needs may be administered intravenously or subcutaneously, depending of the severity of dehydration and specific needs of the individual patient. Long-term administration of subcutaneous fluid therapy may be considered for patients with signs consistent with chronic or recurrent dehydration. The principal benefits of subcutaneous fluid therapy include improved appetite and activity and reduced constipation. The decision to recommend administration of subcutaneous fluids should be made on a case-by-case basis. Not every patient with CKD requires or will benefit from fluid therapy. While a substantial number of cats with CKD appear to benefit from subcutaneous fluid therapy, proportionately fewer dogs require fluid therapy. The owner's comfort with home administration of subcutaneous fluids should also be considered. While inexpensive, administration of fluids subcutaneously at home does require time and may cause stress on the owner-pet relationship. Inappropriate fluid administration also has the potential to promote hypernatremia, hypokalemia, hypertension and fluid overload.

For long-term administration, a balanced electrolyte solution (e.g., lactated Ringer's solution) is administered subcutaneously every one to three days as needed. The volume to be administered depends upon patient size with a typical cat receiving about 75–100 mL per dose. If the clinical response of the patient is suboptimal, the dose may cautiously be increased. However, it is possible to induce fluid overload patients with excessive administration of fluids. In addition, sodium-containing fluids used for subcutaneous therapy do not provide electrolyte-free water. A more physiologically appropriate approach is to provide water via a feeding tube. This approach may also be easier for clients. Because the bulk of evidence suggests excessive sodium intake may be harmful to the kidneys, recommendations for long-term sodium administration in any form should be carefully considered (Weir and Fink 2005). Further, excessive salt intake may reduce the effectiveness of antihypertensive therapy.

Response to long-term subcutaneous fluid therapy should be monitored by serially assessing hydration status, clinical signs, and renal function. If a detectable improvement in clinical signs and or renal function does not accompany fluid therapy, the need for long-term therapy should be re-assessed.

Angiotensin converting enzyme inhibitors (ACEI) and managing proteinuria in patients with CKD

Proteinuria is recognized as an important factor promoting progression of CKD in dogs and cats. Clinical studies in both species have identified the presence of proteinuria as an indicator of increased mortality (Jacob et al. 2005; Syme et al. 2006). Studies in humans have consistently found that reduction in proteinuria is associated with a slowing of the progression of CKD (Abbate et al. 2006). However, evidence that reducing proteinuria slows progression of CKD in dogs and cats is scant (Grodecki et al. 1997; Grauer et al. 2000; King et al. 2006). Nonetheless, current standards of care suggest that dogs and cats in IRIS CKD stages 2, 3, and 4 with urine protein:creatinine ratios greater than 0.5 and 0.4, respectively, and dogs and cats with IRIS CKD stage 1 and protein:creatinine ratios greater than 2.0 should be treated for proteinuria (Lees et al. 2005).

Standard management for proteinuria in dogs and cats with CKD has been to initiate therapy with a renal diet and administer an ACEI with the therapeutic goal of reducing the urine protein:creatinine ratio at least in half or, ideally, into the normal range. Dosage for the ACE inhibitors enalapril and benazepril in dogs and cats with CKD is 0.25–0.5 mg/kg given orally every 12–24 hours (Plumb 2008). Benazepril has been advocated preferentially over enalapril because benazepril's biliary excretion may compensate somewhat for reduced renal clearance in patients with CKD.

In proteinuric humans, therapy of proteinuria may be enhanced by addition of angiotensin II receptor blockers and/or anti-aldosterone drugs such as eplerenone or spironolactone to ACEI therapy (Campbell et al. 2003; Remuzzi et al. 2005; Sato et al. 2005). Angiotensin receptor blockers and ACEI differ in the mechanism by which they inhibit angiotensin II. The ACEI block conversion of angiotensin I to angiotensin II. However, angiotensin II formation is not completely inhibited because it can also be generated by a non-ACE-dependent pathway such as by the enzyme chymase. Also, because bradykinin is normally degraded by ACE, ACEI therapy is associated with elevated bradykinin levels. Bradykinin is a vasodilator that may have renoprotective effects by stimulating nitric oxide production. Angiotensin receptor antagonists block the type 1 receptor, but leave type 2 receptor effects unopposed, which appears to be important in vasodilation. In rats with nephropathy, angiotensin II antagonism has been reported to normalize proteinuria, eliminate inflammatory cell infiltration, and ameliorate glomerular and tubular structural changes (Remuzzi et al. 2002). A combination of an angiotensin receptor antagonist and ACEI has been suggested as a way to maximize blockade of the renin-angiotensin system by affecting both the bioavailability of angiotensin II and also by affecting its activity at the receptor level (Hilgers and Mann 2002). Each type of drug has been shown to be effective in reducing proteinuria and slowing progression of renal disease. However, in experimental models and clinical models in humans, combination therapy has proven more effective than either drug alone (Campbell et al. 2003). In humans, there does not appear to be an increase in toxicity or adverse events with combination therapy (Rosenberg 2003). Whether combination therapy is safe, effective, and provides a therapeutic advantage needs to be determined for dogs and cats with CKD. However, the angiotensin II receptor blocker losartan is not metabolized to the active metabolite and therefore has little activity in dogs (Papich 2007). It is not known whether the same is true of irbesartan, but recommended dosages for irbesartan are much higher than those recommended for humans, suggesting a potential problem with conversion of this drug as well.

Blockade of the renin-angiotensin system limits both angiotensin II and aldosterone while retarding progression of renal disease. Recent studies have implicated aldosterone as an important pathogenic factor in this process (Epstein 2001; Hostetter et al. 2001b). Selective blockade of aldosterone, independent of renin-angiotensin blockade, reduces proteinuria and glomerular lesions in rats with experimental kidney disease. Where blockade of the renin-angiotensin system ameliorates proteinuria and glomerular injury, selective reinfusion of aldosterone restores proteinuria and glomerular lesions despite continued blockade of the renin-angiotensin system. This observation suggests an independent pathogenic role for aldosterone as a mediator of progressive renal disease. Aldosterone appears to promote progressive renal injury through both hemodynamic effects and direct cellular actions (Epstein 2001). It appears to have fibrogenic properties in the kidneys, perhaps in part by promoting production of the profibrotic cytokine TGF-β (Hostetter et al. 2001b). Experimental studies have shown that the aldosterone-receptor antagonist eplerenone may attenuate proteinuria and renal damage, independent of its effect on blood pressure. While ACEI initially causes an acute reduction in aldosterone concentration, this effect is not sustained. It has been proposed that use of aldosterone-receptor antagonists in addition to ACEI will have additional benefits toward protecting the kidneys (Epstein 2001). However, the role of this form of therapy has yet to be established in dogs and cats.

Consult Chapter 42 entitled "Proteinuria" for additional information on management of proteinuria in dogs and cats with CKD.

Managing hypertension in patients with CKD

Rationale for treatment

Arterial hypertension is a relatively common complication of CKD in dogs and cats and has been linked to renal, ocular, neurological and cardiac complications. The importance of hypertension in patients with kidney disease is that preexisting CKD increases the vulnerability of the kidneys to hypertensive injury (Bidani and Griffin 2004). Elevated blood pressure has been reported to be an independent risk factor for progression of CKD in dogs; although proteinuria was not included in the statistical model used to confirm this association (Jacob et al. 2003). In general, proteinuria appears to increase the risk of adverse outcomes associated with arterial hypertension (Syme et al. 2006; Jepson et al. 2007).

While reduction in blood pressure reduces the risk of hypertensive organ injury in hypertensive humans, firm evidence that lowering blood pressure will prevent or ameliorate the renal and extrarenal complications of arterial hypertension in dogs is lacking. However, the clinical benefit of limiting arterial blood pressure has been demonstrated in cats. Subcutaneous administration of the antihypertensive drug hydralazine reduced the prevalence of seizures developing as a consequence of hypertension following renal transplantation in cats (Kyles et al. 1999). Further, in an induced model of hypertensive renal kidney disease, only 2 of 10 cats receiving the antihypertensive agent amlodipine developed evidence of hypertensive retinal lesions compared to 7 of 10 cats that received placeboes (Mathur et al. 2002). Higher blood pressure is associated with increased proteinuria in dogs, cats and humans with CKD, and, since proteinuria appears to promote progressive renal injury, this association may provide a valid justification for lowering blood pressure.

Indications for treatment

Unless there is evidence for hypertension-related organ injury (e.g., retinal lesions or neurological signs) or the systolic blood pressure is greater than 200 mmHg, the decision to initiate anti-hypertensive therapy should generally not be considered an emergency. Before initiating therapy for arterial hypertension, the elevation in blood pressure should be confirmed on the basis of at least three distinct determinations of blood pressure, ideally collected over several days to several weeks. Every effort should be made to minimize the risk that measured elevations in blood pressure represent a transient "white coat" effect, rather than a sustained elevation in blood pressure (Belew et al. 1999). Consult Chapter 13 for information on how to obtain accurate blood pressure measurements.

Patients with IRIS CKD stage 2–4 having arterial blood pressures persistently exceeding 160/100 (arterial pressure stage II) should be considered for treatment because available evidence suggests that their concurrent azotemic CKD may place them at increased risk for sustaining additional renal injury or developing complications associated with elevated blood pressure (Stiles et al. 1994; Kyles et al. 1999; Mathur et al. 2002; Jacob et al. 2003; Lees et al. 2005; Brown et al. 2007b). In patients with IRIS CKD stage I and blood pressure values persistently exceeding 180/120 mmHg (arterial pressure stage III), antihypertensive therapy should be considered (Brown et al. 2007b).

General goals and guidelines for treatment of elevated blood pressure in patients with CKD

The optimum endpoint for antihypertensive therapy has not been established for dogs and cats with CKD. In the absence of such information, treatment for arterial hypertension should be initiated cautiously with the goal of reducing blood pressure to at least below 150/95 mmHg. Except in patients with acute, severe ocular or neurological lesions, rapid reduction in blood pressure may not be not necessary. Satisfactory blood pressure control is often achieved quickly in cats; however, it may take weeks to months to achieve satisfactory blood pressure control in dogs.

ACEI such as enalapril and benazepril, and the calcium channel blocker amlodipine are the mainstays of antihypertensive therapy in dogs and cats. These drugs may have unique renoprotective benefits and are therefore appropriate initial options for managing hypertensive renal patients.

Activation of the renin-angiotensin system and impaired renal autoregulation are characteristic of most generalized renal diseases. In this setting, activation of the renin-angiotensin system is associated with preferential vasoconstriction of the postglomerular arterioles. While this enhances GFR, it also promotes intraglomerular hypertension and hyperperfusion as well as proteinuria. Further, exposure of glomerular capillaries to increases in systemic arterial blood pressure can exacerbate these adverse effects of activation of the renin-angiotensin system. While ACEI generally produce a relatively limited reduction in blood pressure in dogs and cats (Brown et al. 2001, 2003), they are renoprotective by virtue of reducing intraglomerular pressure and proteinuria and by limiting the profibrotic actions of angiotensin II on the kidneys. The ACEI enalapril has been reported to reduce severity of renal lesions that develop in dogs with surgically reduced renal mass (Brown et al. 2003). Further, in dogs with a form of hereditary nephritis, a glomerulopathy, enalapril significantly reduced proteinuria and increased survival (Grodecki et al. 1997). In a group of dogs with diverse glomerulopathies, enalapril significantly reduced proteinuria (Grauer et al. 2000).

ACEI should probably always be included in the treatment of hypertension in dogs with CKD and dogs and cats with proteinuria. In proteinuric patients, their dosing should largely be managed according to their effectiveness in reducing proteinuria. It is unclear whether they should routinely be included in management of hypertension in non-proteinuric cats. Dosage for the ACE inhibitors enalapril and benazepril in dogs and cats with CKD is 0.25–0.5 mg/kg given orally every 12–24 hours (Plumb 2008). Benazepril has been advocated preferentially over enalapril because benazepril's biliary excretion may compensate somewhat for reduced renal clearance in patients with CKD. Additionally, use of vasodilators in management of hypertension may result in reflex activation of the renin angiotensin system. Minimizing the effects of an activated renin angiotensin system using agents such as ACE inhibitors or anti-aldosterone drugs such as spironolactone may be useful in promoting effectiveness of vasodilator therapy.

Amlodipine, a dihydropyridine calcium channel blocker, preferentially vasodilates preglomerular renal arterioles which theoretically could increase glomerular hypertension. However, CCB have additional renoprotective properties. They may prevent renal injury by limiting renal growth, by reducing mesangial entrapment of macromolecules, and by attenuating the mitogenic effects of diverse cytokines and growth factors (e.g., platelet-derived growth factor and platelet-activating factor). Further, in vitro amlodipine has been shown to inhibit proliferation of mesangial cells. However, clinical trials in humans have provided conflicting results as to the renoprotective effect of CCB beyond their antihypertensive effects. In addition, studies on amlodipine administered to normal dogs suggests that it may activate the renin-angiotensin system (Atkins et al. 2007). Controlled studies on the renoprotective effects of amlodipine in dogs and cats have not been published. However, clinical experience indicates that they are effective antihypertensive agents in dogs and cats with CKD. However, in contrast to observations in other species, amlodipine appears to reduce proteinuria in hypertensive cats with CKD, presumably due to the profound reduction in blood pressure that typically accompanies their use in cats (Jepson et al. 2007).

Amlodipine is the antihypertensive of choice for most cats with CKD because it is usually highly effective, has few side-effects, and has a relative rapid onset. Dosage for cats less than 5 kg is 0.625 mg/day and 1.25 mg/day for cats greater than 5 kg. These dosages may be doubled (or given twice daily) if further reduction in blood pressure is required. Amlodipine typically reduces systolic blood pressure by about 30–50 mmHg within the first 1–2 months of therapy in cats with CKD (Elliot et al. 2001; Mathur et al. 2002).

Managing hypertension in dogs is more challenging than in cats. Dogs typically require two or more drugs for adequate control of hypertension. In most instances, combination therapy is initiated with an ACEI (dosage above) and amlodipine. The starting dosage for amlodipine is 0.1–0.2 mg/kg given once daily. Dosage may be increased as needed up to 0.6 mg/kg daily (once per day or divided q 12 hours). If this combination fails to maintain the systolic blood pressure below 150 mmHg, adding a third drug to this combination may be considered. While there is no uniform consensus as to which drug or drugs to use next, a variety of options exist (consult the chapter of this text entitled "Hypertension"). Hydralazine has been effective in some dogs in this setting.

Upon initiating antihypertensive therapy, blood pressure should generally be measured every 1–2 weeks to assess response to therapy and to determine if dosage adjustments may be needed. Upon reaching the therapeutic endpoint, blood pressure should be monitored at least every three months to assess continued response and compliance with treatment recommendations. Monitoring also minimizes the risk that hypotension will occur; however, hypotension is an uncommon complication of therapy for arterial hypertension. Clinical signs of hypotension in dogs and cats may include somnolence, lethargy, weakness, and decreased responsiveness to commands or stimulation. Impaired renal blood flow and prerenal azotemia may also develop. Development of these signs in a patient receiving antihypertensive therapy should prompt evaluation of arterial blood pressure.

Consult Chapter 68, "Hypertension" for additional information on management of arterial hypertension.

Managing Anemia in CKD

General guidelines for minimizing anemia of CKD

Multiple factors may contribute to development of anemia in CKD, including iatrogenic and spontaneous blood loss, poor nutrition, reduced red blood cell lifespan, and inadequate renal production of EPO. Optimum therapeutic response results from addressing all of the factors that contribute to the patient's anemia.

Chronic low-grade gastrointestinal blood loss can promote moderate to severe anemia in patients with CKD that otherwise may have sufficient endogenous EPO production to maintain their hematocrit values at a higher value. These patients may have overt gastrointestinal signs or melena, but they are not consistently present. The decline in hematocrit is typically much more rapid than with other causes for anemia of CKD. Iron deficiency and an elevation in BUN/creatinine ratio above what is expected in context of the patient's diet may provide indirect evidence of occult gastrointestinal blood loss. Confirming gastrointestinal hemorrhage is often best achieved by assessing the response to a therapeutic course with histamine H2-receptor antagonists and sucralfate. Improvement in hematocrit and reduction in BUN concentration are consistent with reduced gastrointestinal blood loss as a contributor to the patient's anemia.

Iron deficiency is relatively common in dogs and cats with CKD. In a recent study, the serum iron concentrations of 3 of 6 CKD dogs and 3 of 7 CKD cats were below the reference range; transferrin saturations were less than 20% (Cowgill et al. 1998). Whether this is related primarily to inadequate intake and absorption of iron or increased losses of iron due to gastrointestinal blood loss is unclear. Unfortunately, iron status can be difficult to assess in dogs and cats. Serum iron levels can be used to screen for both iron deficiency and anemia of chronic inflammatory disease as contributing factors in the diagnostic evaluation of anemia.

Administration of iron may be appropriate for iron deficiency and when administering EPO to enhance red blood cell production. Ferrous sulfate may be administered orally or iron dextran may be administered by intramuscular injection. While parenteral administration of iron may be associated with a small risk of anaphylaxis, shunting of iron to reticuloendothelial storage, and iron overload, it is likely the most effective way to rapidly restore iron levels when beginning EPO therapy. Although serum iron levels and transferrin saturation should be monitored to adjust therapy, starting doses of iron sulfate of 50–100 mg/day for cats and 100–300 mg/day for dogs have been recommended. Oral iron supplements may be associated with gastrointestinal upset and diarrhea, so small divided doses may be preferable.

In addition to iron deficiency, other nutritional abnormalities may promote anemia. Protein malnutrition, and its attendant changes in plasma amino acid and hormone concentrations, is known to cause suboptimal erythropoiesis and anemia. Similar changes occur in human patients and may reflect mild protein/calorie malnutrition commonly present in advanced CKD. Although they have not been examined in dogs and cats, deficiencies in riboflavin (vitamin B2), cobalamin (vitamin B12), folate, niacin or pyridoxine (vitamin B6) might theoretically induce nutritional anemia. Vitamin status cannot be easily determined in dogs and cats; however, deficiencies should be suspected in patients with persistent anorexia, protein/calorie malnutrition or gastrointestinal malabsorption. In addition, some drugs may predispose the patient to nutritional anemia even when dietary intake is normal. For example, therapy with trimethoprim or methotrexate may interfere with cellular folate metabolism. Hypersegmentation of the polymorphonuclear leukocytes may provide a clinical indication of vitamin B12 or folate deficiency.

Nutritional deficiencies can be minimized through timely initiation of proper diet modifications and, if necessary, use of dietary supplements. In addition to minimizing renal anemia, preventing protein/calorie malnutrition may reduce morbidity. B vitamins, folate, and niacin can be provided as an oral supplement often with iron. Evidence of a therapeutic benefit in dogs and cats with CKD has not been demonstrated.

Patients with CKD may have shortened red blood cell life span. Proposed mechanisms for this mild hemolytic tendency include a malfunctioning of the membrane Na+−K+−ATPase pump and impaired regeneration of reduced glutathione needed to prevent hemoglobin oxidation. Cat hemoglobin appears to be especially prone to oxidative stress as evidenced by the frequent observation of Heinz bodies in their red blood cells. Cats with large numbers of Heinz bodies tend to be more anemic. Drugs and foods (e.g., onions, propylene glycol, methylene blue, sulfonamides) that promote formation of Heinz bodies should be avoided in uremic pets whenever possible.

The hyperphosphatemia commonly observed in patients with CKD may have a favorable effect in oxygen transport because the associated increase in intracellular red cell phosphorus increases red cell 2,3 DPG levels. Increased 2,3 DPG levels promote a rightward shift in the oxyhemoglobin dissociation curve, thereby improving tissue oxygenation and decreasing the stimulus for EPO synthesis.

Anabolic steroids

Anabolic steroids were at one time the mainstay of therapy for anemia associated with CKD. Controlled safety and efficacy studies in dogs and cats are lacking, and clinical experience with anabolic steroids has generally been seen as disappointing as a treatment for anemia of CKD. Empirically, anabolic steroids appear to produce a small increase in hematocrit in some patients. However, in one study in humans on dialysis, results approaching those achieved with EPO replacement therapy were reported with the anabolic steroid nandrolone decanoate in older male patients with CKD (Teruel et al. 1996).

Blood transfusion

For patients with CKD, blood transfusions are primarily indicated when there is a need for rapid correction of anemia or when no other treatment option is available. In selected patients, repeated transfusions have been used for long-term maintenance of hematocrit; however, transfusion-related complications are common among these patients. In general, limited availability and expense of blood products, increased risk of transfusion reactions with multiple transfusions, immunosuppression, trans-

fer of infectious agents, and decreased life span of transfused.

Hormone replacement therapy

The most effective means of correcting anemia of CKD is hormone replacement therapy. However, a major obstacle to EPO replacement therapy in dogs and cats has been the development of anti-EPO antibodies. These antibodies develop because recombinant human erythropoietin (rHuEPO) differs structurally from canine and feline EPOs. Development of anti-EPO antibodies renders administered rHuEPO ineffective and, with continued administration of the hormone, may render the patient's remaining endogenously produced EPO largely ineffective leaving the patient markedly anemic and often transfusion-dependent. Because of this significant drawback, the recommendation to use rHuEPO is usually reserved for patients with advanced CKD that require correction of anemia to maintain a satisfactory quality of life. Premature initiation of EPO therapy with subsequent development of anti-EPO antibodies may deprive the patient of the clinical benefits of this therapy when clinical signs of anemia eventually do develop and EPO can be of greatest clinical benefit. Thus, EPO therapy is usually not recommended until hematocrit values decline below about 20% to 22% and clinical signs attributable to anemia are present.

With the intent of preventing and correcting anemia associated with development of anti-EPO antibody formation, recombinant canine and feline EPO have been evaluated. Therapy with recombinant canine EPO was effective in correcting anemia of CKD in dogs without the apparent risk of antibody formation; however, it was ineffective in correcting the red cell aplasia that resulted from anti-EPO antibodies directed against rHuEPO (Randolph et al. 2004a). Unfortunately, therapy with the feline recombinant EPO product evaluated was also associated with development of anti-EPO antibodies (Randolph et al. 2004). Neither canine nor feline recombinant EPO is currently available commercially.

Recombinant EPO products usually correct the anemia of CKD and ameliorate the clinical signs associated with the anemia. A dose-dependent increase in hematocrit usually follows administration of rHuEPO (Cowgill et al. 1998). Correction of hematocrit to low normal typically takes approximately 2–8 weeks depending on the starting hematocrit and dose given. As anemia resolves, most dogs and cats have increases in appetite, body weight, energy level and sociability (Cowgill et al. 1998). In human CKD patients, partial correction yields substantial improvement in quality of life and correction of most anemia-related symptoms (Paoletti and Cannella

2006). While the optimum therapeutic target hematocrit has not been established for dogs and cats with CKD, a reasonable cost-effective target would be to target the lower end of the normal range.

EPO products currently used in dogs and cats include rHuEPO and darbepoetin (DPO). DPO has the advantage of having a duration of action approximately 3 times longer than EPO so it may be administered weekly rather than 3 times weekly. While it has also been suggested that the structural modifications responsible for the longer duration may reduce the likelihood of anti-EPO antibody formation, no evidence is available to confirm or deny this.

Induction therapy with EPO is begun with a dosage of 50–150 units/kg subcutaneously three times weekly, with most dogs and cats receiving 100 units/kg administered three times weekly. Higher doses may accelerate the response to therapy, while lower doses may slow the response. Thus, when anemia is severe (hematocrit <14%) but not requiring transfusion, daily therapy with 150 units/kg may be preferred for the first week to expedite response. In contrast, when hypertension is present, a dosage of 50 units/kg three times per week may be considered, as too rapid an increase in hematocrit is thought to promote hypertension.

During induction therapy, hematocrit should be monitored weekly or biweekly until the target hematocrit of approximately 30–35% for cats and 37–42% for dogs is achieved (Cowgill et al. 1998). When a hematocrit at the low end of the target range is reached, the dosing interval may be decreased to twice weekly. Many animals require 50–100 units/kg two to three times weekly to maintain their hematocrit in the target range; however, the dose and dosing interval required to maintain individual patients in the normal range is highly variable. Ongoing monitoring of hematocrit will be necessary to allow adjustments in dose and dosing interval. Animals requiring more than 150 units/kg three times weekly should be evaluated for EPO resistance. Due to the lag time between dosage adjustment and effect on hematocrit, patience must be exercised so as not to adjust the dose too frequently. Frequent dose adjustments will result in rapid, unpredictable changes in hematocrit and an inability to find a stable dosing regimen. In general, dosage should not be changed any more often than once monthly. Avoiding iatrogenic polycythemia is especially important.

DPO is supplied in μg rather than units; 1 μg DPO = 200 units of EPO. It is administered at a dosage equivalent to EPO (consult the product package insert for details), but the dosing interval is extended three-fold. For example, a 10 kg dog that would receive 1,000 IU EPO (100 U/kg EPO) three times weekly for a total weekly dose of 3,000 IU EPO, would receive 3,000 IU EPO × 1 μg DPO/200 IU EPO = 15 μg DPO per week during induction. Thus, the induction dosage for DPO in most dogs and cats is approximately 1.5 μg/kg weekly. Once the target hematocrit is achieved (treatment targets for EPO and DPO are the same), the frequency of administration of DPO may be decreased to every other week. The dosage thereafter should be adjusted to maintain the target hematocrit either by adjusting frequency of administration, dosage or both in a fashion similar to that described for EPO. Empirical evidence suggests that dogs and cats with CKD respond to DPO in a fashion similar to EPO.

Individuals may differ in their response to EPO therapy. The basis for individual differences in response to EPO therapy is not fully understood. Several causes of blunted response or failure to resolve renal anemia with EPO therapy have been identified including functional or absolute iron deficiency, anti-EPO antibody formation, ongoing gastrointestinal blood loss or hemolysis, concurrent inflammatory or malignant disease, and aluminum overload. Owner errors related to drug storage, handling, or administration may account for some instances of poor response to EPO therapy. The demand for iron associated with stimulated erythropoiesis is high, and human patients without preexisting iron overload will exhaust iron storage during EPO therapy. The same appears true of dogs and cats. Iron supplementation is therefore recommended for all patients receiving EPO therapy. At a minimum, an intramuscular injection of iron dextran (50–300 mg) should be provided at the time EPO or DPO are initiated.

A variety of mostly minor adverse effects related to EPO therapy in dogs and cats may include systemic hypertension, seizures, local reactions at the injection site, and development of antibodies directed at EPO (Cowgill et al. 1998). Seizures have been observed in human, canine, and feline patients being treated with EPO that have no prior history of seizure a disorder (Cowgill et al. 1998). In dogs and cats, they have been reported in the setting of moderate to severe azotemia. Although hypertension, anemia, and uremic encephalopathy may be contributory, in humans, seizures are thought to be related to compensatory adaptations to increases in red blood cell mass. Seizures are not thought to be directly related to EPO. Allergic reactions including cutaneous or mucocutaneous reactions or cellulitis sometimes with fever and arthralgia were uncommonly observed in both dogs and cats early in the course of EPO therapy (Cowgill et al. 1998). Lesions generally resolved within a few days and some did not recur when therapy was reinstated.

As described previously, the most important complication associated with use of hormone replacement therapy is refractory anemia and hypoplasia of the erythroid bone marrow associated with formation of neutralizing anti-EPO antibodies (Cowgill et al. 1998). The severity of anemia may be worse than before initiation of EPO treatment, suggesting that the anti-EPO antibodies may interfere with both administered and endogenous EPO. The EPO protein appears unpredictably immunogenic in many, affecting some but not all dogs and cats, with antibody titers developing at variable times from several weeks to months after onset of therapy. Typically, antibody titers will decline with cessation of therapy, but persistent administration of EPO despite formation of antibodies may result in persistence of antibodies. A test for anti-EPO antibodies is not currently available. However, failure of an increase in EPO or DPO dosage to increase hematocrit in absence of an identifiable cause for treatment failure, (described above) strongly suggests development of anti-EPO antibody formation. Demonstrating an increase in the bone marrow myeloid/erythroid ratio provides further support that EPO resistance results from antibody formation. If anti-EPO antibody formation is suspected, EPO or DPO therapy should be terminated immediately. After therapy is stopped and antibody titers decline, suppressed erythropoiesis may be reversible and pre-treatment levels of erythropoiesis may be attained.

While regulation of RBC production is the principal function of EPO in the hematopoietic system, a growing body of evidence indicates that the therapeutic benefits of rHuEPO could extend far beyond correction of anemia (Bahlmann and Fliser 2009). Studies have also identified a tissue-protective effect of rHuEPO that prevents ischemia-induced tissue damage in several organ systems including the kidneys. This tissue-protective action of rHuEPO is not the result of improved tissue oxygenation associated with of anemia correction. The ultimate clinical therapeutic applications, if any, of these findings have yet to be determined.

Medication review and dose modification

Current medications should be reviewed at each clinic visit (Board 2002). It should be confirmed that current and new medications have specific appropriate indications, dosages are correct for the level of renal function, and do not pose a risk of drug interaction. Also consider whether the owner is being asked to administer an excessive number of medications, because this can affect compliance and the owner's perception of quality of life.

As the kidneys are responsible for elimination of many drugs from the body, renal drug clearance may be reduced as renal function declines causing the half-life of the drug to be prolonged. In addition, distribution, pro-

tein binding, and hepatic biotransformation of drugs may be altered. The sum effect of these changes is that for many drugs normally excreted by the kidneys, there is a tendency for drugs to accumulate in patients with reduced kidney function. Excessive drug accumulation promotes an increased rate of adverse drug reactions and nephrotoxicity. If drugs requiring renal excretion must be administered to patients with impaired kidney function, dosage regimens should be adjusted to compensate for decreased organ function. However, dosage adjustments may not be appropriate for drugs that are administered to a physiologic endpoint or effect such as antihypertensive agents.

Patients with preexisting CKD may also be predisposed to nephrotoxicity. For this reason, nephrotoxic drugs and drugs requiring renal excretion should generally be avoided in patients with kidney disease. Where possible, less nephrotoxic drugs should be chosen. If nephrotoxic drugs are unavoidable, therapeutic drug monitoring or serial evaluation of renal function is essential.

So-called "complementary medications" (sometimes called herbal medicines, naturopathic remedies, and phytomedicines) should be used with caution in patients with CKD. Their potential for interactions with prescribed medications or simple adverse consequences in patients with reduced kidney function should be considered. Herbal products to be avoided in patients with renal dysfunction include aristolochic acid, barberry, buchu, Chinese herbal drugs, juniper, licorice, and noni juice (Kappel and Piera 2002).

Patient follow-up and monitoring

In order to successfully individualize treatment to meet the specific, and often changing, needs of the patient, regular monitoring of patients is an essential component of the treatment plan. Treatment goals should be clearly recorded and compared to regular measurement of the patient's progress. Evaluations every 2–4 weeks are suggested until the initial response to therapy can be established. In general, patients in IRIS CKD stages III and IV should thereafter be evaluated about every 2–4 months. Patients in IRIS CKD stages I and II generally require less frequent monitoring, typically about every 4–6 months once they have been established to have stable renal function. Patients with progressive CKD, proteinuria or arterial hypertension generally require more frequent monitoring. In addition, the frequency of evaluation may vary depending on severity of renal dysfunction, complications present in the patient, treatments being used and response to treatment. Patients receiving therapy with EPO or calcitriol require frequent monitoring lifelong. A typical monitoring visit would include at least a medical history with medication review, physical examination, body weight and nutritional assessment, hematocrit, chemistry profile, urinalysis, and blood pressure. Depending on the patient and results of the urinalysis, the urine protein:creatinine ratio and a urine culture may also be included. Additional specific recommendations for monitoring are described in the various treatment sections.

References

Abbate, M., et al. (2006). How does proteinuria cause progressive renal damage? *J Am Soc Nephrol* **17**: 2974–2984.

Adams, L., et al. (1994). Influence of dietary protein/calorie intake on renal morphology and function in cats with 5/6 nephrectomy. *Lab Invest* **70**: 347–357.

Adams, L., et al. (1992). Correlation of urine protein/creatinine ratio and twenty-four-hour urinary protein excretion in normal cats and cats with surgically induced chronic renal failure. *J Vet Intern Med* **6**: 36–40.

Adrogué, H. and N. Madias (1998). Management of life-threatening acid-base disorders. *N Engl J Med* **338**: 26–34.

Akizawa, T., et al. (2003). New strategies for treatment of secondary hyperparathyroidism. *Am J Kidney Dis* **41**: S100–S103.

Almaden, Y., et al. (1996). Direct effect of phosphorus on PTH secretion from whole rat parathyroid glands in vitro. *J Bone Miner Res* **11**: 970–976.

Anderstam, B., et al. (1996). Middle-sized molecule fractions isolated from uremic ultrafiltrate and normal urine inhibit ingestive behavior in the rat. *J Am Soc Nephrol* **7**: 2453–2460.

Andress, D.L. (2006). Vitamin D in chronic kidney disease: a systemic role for selective vitamin receptor activation. *Kidney Int* **69**: 33–43.

Atkins, C.E., et al. (2007). The effect of amlodipine and the combination of amlodipine and enalapril on the renin-angiotensin-aldosterone system in the dog. *J Vet Pharmacol Ther* **30**: 394–400.

Bagga, D., et al. (2003). Differential effects of prostaglandin derived from omega-6 and omega-3 polyunsaturated fatty acids on COX-2 expression and IL-6 secretion. *Proc Natl Acad Sci U S A* **100**: 1751–1756.

Bahlmann, F.H. and D. Fliser (2009). Erythropoietin and renoprotection. *Curr Opin Nephrol Hypertens* **18**: 15–20.

Barber, P., et al. (1999). Effect of dietary phosphate restriction on renal secondary hyperparathyroidism in the cat. *J Small Anim Pract* **40**: 62–70.

Barber, P. and J. Elliot (1998). Feline chronic renal failure: calcium homeostasis in 80 cases diagnosed between 1992 and 1995. *J Small Anim Pract* **39**: 108–116.

Belew, A., et al. (1999). Evaluation of the white-coat effect in cats. *J Vet Intern Med* **13**: 134–142.

Bidani, A.K. and K.A. Griffin (2004). Pathophysiology of hypertensive renal damage. Implications for therapy. *Hypertension* **44**: 595–601.

Block, G., et al. (1998). Association of serum phosphorus and calcium X phosphate product with mortality risk in chronic hemodialysis patients: a national study. *Am J Kidney Dis* **31**: 607–617.

Board, NKFKDOQIA. (2002). Clinical practice guidelines for chronic kidney disease: evaluation, classification, and stratification. Part 4. Definition and classification of stages of chronic renal failure. *Am J Kidney Dis* **39**: S46–S75.

Boyd, L.M., et al. (2008). Survival in cats with naturally occurring chronic kidney disease (2000–2002). *J Vet Intern Med* **22**: 1111–1117.

Brenner B.M., et al. (1982). Dietary protein intake and the progressive nature of kidney disease: the role of hemodynamically mediated glomerular injury in the pathogenesis of progressive glomerular sclerosis in ageing, renal ablation, and intrinsic renal disease. *N Engl J Med* **307**: 652–659.

Bro, S. and K. Olgaard (1997). Effects of excess PTH on nonclassical target organs. *Am J Kidney Dis* **30**: 606–620.

Brown, S.A., et al. (1991). Beneficial effects of dietary mineral restriction in dogs with marked reduction of functional renal mass. *J Am Soc Nephrol* **1**: 1169–1179.

Brown, S.A. (2008). Oxidative stress and chronic kidney disease. *Vet Clin North Am Small Anim Pract* **38**: 157–166.

Brown, S.A. (2007a). In: *BSAVA Manual of Canine and Feline Nephrology and Urology*, edited by J. Elliott and G.F. Grauer, 2nd edition. Gloucester, England: British Small Animal Veterinary Association, pp. 223–230.

Brown, S.A., et al. (2007b). Guidelines for the identification, evaluation, and management of systemic hypertension in dogs and cats. *J Vet Intern Med* **21**: 542–558.

Brown, S.A., et al. (2003). Evaluation of the effects of inhibition of angiotensin converting enzyme with enalapril in dogs with induced chronic renal insufficiency. *Am J Vet Res* **64**: 321–327.

Brown, S.A., et al. (1998). Beneficial effects of chronic administration of dietary omega-3 polyunsaturated fatty acids in dogs with renal insufficiency. *J Lab Clin Med* **131**: 447–455.

Brown, S.A., et al. (2001). Effects of the angiotensin converting enzyme inhibitor benazepril in cats with induced renal insufficiency. *Am J Vet Res* **62**: 375–383.

Brown, S.A., et al. (1995). Impaired renal autoregulatory ability in dogs with reduced renal mass. *J Am Soc Nephrol* **5**: 1768–1774.

Brushinsky, D. (2005). Disorders of calcium and phosphorus homeostasis. In: *Primer on Kidney Diseases*, edited by A. Greenberg, 4th edition. San Diego, CA: Academic Press, pp. 120–130.

Buranakarl, C., et al. (2004). Effects of dietary sodium chloride intake on renal function and blood pressure in cats with normal and reduced renal function. *Am J Vet Res* **65**: 620–627.

Burkholder, W.J., et al. (2004). Diet modulates proteinuria in heterozygous female dogs with X-linked hereditary nephropathy. *J Vet Intern Med* **18**: 165–175.

Campbell, R., et al. (2003). Effects of combined ACE inhibitor and angiotensin II antagonist treatment in human chronic nephropathies. *Kidney Int* **63**: 1094–1103.

Canalejo, A., et al. (2003). Effects of uremic ultrafiltrate on the regulation of the parathyroid cell cycle by calcitriol. *Kidney Int* **63**: 732–737.

Cheng, S. and D. Coyne (2007). Vitamin D and outcomes in chronic kidney disease. *Curr Opin Nephrol Hypertens* **16**: 77–82.

Combe, C. and M. Aparicio (1994). Phosphorus and protein restriction and parathyroid function in chronic renal failure. *Kidney Int* **46**: 1381–1386.

Cook, A. and L. Cowgill (1996). Clinical and pathological features of protein-losing glomerular disease in the dog: a review of 137 cases (1985–1992). *J Am Anim Hosp Assoc* **32**: 313–322.

Cook, S. and C. Lathrop (1994). Serum erythropoietin concentrations measured by radioimmunoassay in normal, polycythemic, and anemic dogs and cats. *J Vet Intern Med* **8**: 18–25.

Cowgill, L., et al. (1998). Use of recombinant humans erythropoietin for management of anemia in dogs and cats with renal failure. *J Am Vet Med Assoc* **212**: 521–528.

DeBowes, L., et al. (1996). Association of periodontal disease and histologic lesions in multiple organs from 45 dog. *J Vet Dent* **13**: 57–60.

DiBartola, S., et al. (1993). Development of chronic renal disease in cats fed a commercial diet. *J Am Vet Med Assoc* **202**: 744–751.

DiBartola, S., et al. (1987). Clinicopathologic findings associated with chronic renal disease in cats: 74 cases (1973–1984). *J Am Vet Med Assoc* **190**: 1196–1202.

Dow, S. and M. Fettman (1992). Renal disease in cats: the potassium connection. In: *Current Veterinary Therapy XI*, edited by R. Kirk. Philadelphia, PA: WB Saunders, pp. 820–822.

Dow, S., et al. (1990). Effects of dietary acidification and potassium depletion on acid-base balance, mineral metabolism and renal function in adult cats. *J Nutr* **120**: 569–578.

Dow, S., et al. (1987). Potassium depletion in cats: renal and dietary influences. *J Am Vet Med Assoc* **191**: 1569–1575.

Elliot, J. et al. (2006). *Symposium on Phosphatemia Management in the Treatment of Chronic Kidney Disease*. Louisville, KY: Vetoquinol.

Elliott, J., et al. (2003a). Assessment of acid-base status of cats with naturally occurring chronic renal failure. *J Small Anim Pract* **44**: 65–70.

Elliott, J., et al. (2003b). Acid-base balance of cats with chronic renal failure: effect of deterioration in renal function. *J Small Ani Pract* **44**: 261–268.

Elliot, J., et al. (2001). Feline hypertension: clinical findings and response to antihypertensive treatment in 30 cases. *J Small Anim Pract* **42**: 122–129.

Elliot, J. and P. Barber (1998). Feline chronic renal failure: clinical findings in 80 cases diagnosed between 1992 and 1995. *J Small Anim Pract* **39**: 78–85.

Epstein, M. (2004). Aldosterone as a determinant of progressive renal dysfunction: a paradigm shift. *Nephrol Self Assess Program* **3**: 285–295.

Epstein, M. (2001). Aldosterone as a mediator of progressive renal disease: pathogenic and clinical implications. *Am J Kid Dis* **37**: 677–688.

Fliser, D., et al. (2007). Fibroblast growth factor 23 (FGF23) predicts progression of chronic kidney disease: the mild to moderate kidney disease (MMKD) study. *J Am Soc Nephrol* **18**: 2601–2608.

Finco, D., et al. (1999). Progression of chronic renal disease in the dog. *J Vet Intern Med* **13**: 516–528.

Finco, D., et al. (1997). Effects of parathyroidectomy on induced renal failure in dogs. *Am J Vet Res* **58**: 188–195.

Finco, D., et al. (1992). Effects of dietary phosphorus and protein in dogs with chronic renal failure. *Am J Vet Res* **53**: 2264–2271.

Fettman, M., et al. (1992). Effect of dietary phosphoric acid supplementation on acid-base balance and mineral and bone metabolism in adult cats. *Am J Vet Res* **53**: 2125–2135.

Freundlich, M., et al. (2008). Suppression of renin-angiotensin gene expression in the kidney by paracalcitol. *Kidney Int* **74**: 1394–1402.

Gerber, B., et al. (2003). Serum concentrations of 1,25-dihydroxycholecalciferol and 25-hydroxycholecalciferol in clinically normal dogs and dogs with acute and chronic renal failure. *Am J Vet Res* **64**: 1161–1166.

Goldstein, R., et al. (1998). Gastrin concentrations in plasma of cats with chronic renal failure. *J Am Vet Med Assoc* **213**: 826–828.

Grauer, G., et al. (2000). Effects of enalapril versus placebo as a treatment for canine idiopathic glomerulonephritis. *J Vet Intern Med* **14**: 526–533.

Grodecki, K.M., et al. (1997). Treatment of X-linked hereditary nephritis in Samoyed dogs with angiotensin converting enzyme (ACE) inhibitor. *J Comp Pathol* **117**: 209–225.

Gutierrez, O., et al. (2005). Fibroblast growth factor-23 mitigates hyperphosphatemia but accelerates calcitriol deficiency in chronic kidney disease. *J Am Soc Nephrol* **16**: 2205–2215.

Harris, R.C. and E.G. Neilson (2006). Toward a unified theory of renal progression. *Annu Rev Med* **57**: 365–380.

Henik, R., et al. (1997). Treatment of systemic hypertension in cats with amlodipine besylate. *J Am Anim Hosp Assoc* **33**: 226–234.

Hilgers, K. and J. Mann (2002). ACE inhibitors versus AT1 receptor antagonists in patients with chronic renal disease. *J Am Soc Nephrol* **13**: 1100–1108.

Hostetter, T., et al. (2001a). Hyperfiltration in remnant nephrons: a potentially adverse response to renal ablation. *J Am Soc Nephrol* **12**: 1315–1325.

Hostetter, T., et al. (2001b). Aldosterone in renal disease. *Curr Opin Nephrol Hypertens* **10**: 105–110.

Hostutler, R.A., et al. (2006). Comparison of the effects of daily and intermittent-dose calcitriol on serum parathyroid hormone and ionized calcium concentrations in normal cats and cats with chronic renal failure. *J Vet Intern Med* **20**: 1307–1313.

Iseki, K., et al. (2003). Proteinuria and the risk of developing end-stage renal disease. *Kidney Int* **63**: 1468–1474.

Israel, R., et al. (1986). Metoclopramide decreases renal plasma flow. *Clin Pharmacol Ther* **39**: 261–264.

Jacob, F., et al. (2005). Evaluation of the association between initial proteinuria and morbidity rate or death in dogs with naturally occurring chronic renal failure. *J Am Vet Med Assoc* **226**: 393–400.

Jacob, F., et al. (2003). Association between initial systolic blood pressure and risk of developing a uremic crisis or of dying in dogs with chronic renal failure. *J Am Vet Med Assoc* **222**: 322–329.

Jacob, F., et al. (2002). Clinical evaluation of dietary modification for treatment of spontaneous chronic renal failure in dogs. *J Am Vet Med Assoc* **220**(8): 1163–1170.

James, K., et al. (1997). Serum total carbon dioxide concentrations in canine and feline blood: the effect of underfilling blood tubes and comparisons with blood gas analysis as an estimate of plasma bicarbonate. *Am J Vet Res* **58**: 343–347.

Jepson, R.E., et al. (2007). Effect of control of systolic blood pressure on survival in cats with systemic hypertension. *J Vet Intern Med* **21**: 402–409.

Kappel, J. and C. Piera (2002). Safe drug prescribing for patients with renal insufficiency. *Can J Med* **166**: 473–477.

Kates, D., et al. (1997). Evidence that serum phosphate is independently associated with serum PTH in patients with chronic renal failure. *Am J Kidney Dis* **30**: 809–813.

Kazama, J.J., et al. (2005). Role of circulating fibroblast growth factor 23 in the development of secondary hyperparathyroidism. *Ther Apher Dial* **9**: 328–330.

King, J.N., et al. (2006). Tolerability and efficacy of benazepril in cats with chronic kidney disease. *J Vet Intern Med* **20**: 1054–1064.

King, J.N., et al. (2007). Prognostic factors in cats with chronic kidney disease. *J Vet Intern Med* **21**: 906–916.

King, L., et al. (1992). Anemia of chronic renal failure in dogs. *J Vet Intern Med* **6**: 264–270.

Kogika, M.M., et al. (2006). Serum ionized calcium in dogs with chronic renal failure and metabolic acidosis. *Vet Clin Pathol* **35**: 441–445.

Kruger, J., et al. (1996). Hypercalcemia and renal failure. *Vet Clin North Am* **26**: 1417–1445.

Kyles, A., et al. (1999). Management of hypertension controls postoperative neurological disorders after renal transplantation in cats. *Vet Surg* **28**: 436–441.

Lappin, M.R., et al. (2005). Investigation of the induction of antibodies against Crandell-Rees feline kidney cell lysates and feline renal cell lysates after parenteral administration of vaccines against feline viral rhinotracheitis, calicivirus, and panleukopenia in cats. *Am J Vet Res* **66**: 506–511.

Lappin, M.R., et al. (2006). Interstitial nephritis in cats inoculated with crandell rees feline kidney cell lysates. *J Feline Med Surg* **8**: 353–356.

Lees, G.E., et al. (2005). Assessment and management of proteinuria in dogs and cats: 2004 ACVIM forum consensus statement (small animal). *J Vet Intern Med* **19**: 377–385.

Lemarié, R., et al. (1995). Mast cell tumors: clinical management. *Compend Cont Educ Pract Vet* **17**: 1085–1101.

Levey, A., et al. (1999). Dietary protein restriction and the progression of chronic renal disease: what have all the resuts of the MDRD study shown? *J Am Soc Nephrol* **10**: 2426–2439.

Lopez-Hilker, S., et al. (1990). Phosphorus restriction reverses hyperparathyroidism in uremia independent of changes in calcium and calcitriol. *Am J Physiol* **259**: F432–F437.

Lulich, J., et al. (1992). Feline renal failure: questions, answers, questions. *Compend Cont Educ Pract Vet* **14**: 127–153.

Menon, V., et al. (2009). Effect of a very-low protein diet on outcomes: long-term follow-up of the modification of diet in renal disease (MDRD) study. *Am J Kidney Dis* **53**: 208–217.

Mathur, S., et al. (2002). Effects of the calcium channel antagonist amlodipine in cats with surgically induced hypertensive renal insufficiency. *Am J Vet Res* **63**: 833–839.

Minkus, G., et al. (1994). Evaluation of renal biopsies in cats and dogs – histopathology in comparison with clinical data. *J Small Anim Pract* **35**: 465–472.

Mitch, W. (1997). Mechanisms causing loss of lean body mass in kidney disease. *Am J Clin Nutr* **67**: 359–366.

Nagode, L., et al. (1996). Benefits of calcitriol therapy and serum phosphorus control in dogs and cats with chronic renal failure: both are essential to prevent or suppress toxic hyperparathyroidism. *Vet Clin North Am* **26**: 1293–1330.

Nath, K. (1998). The tubulointerstitium in progressive renal disease. *Kidney Int* **54**: 992–994.

Paoletti, E. and G. Cannella (2006). Update on erythropoietin treatment: should hemoglobin be normalized in patients with chronic kidney disease? *J Am Soc Nephrol* **17**: S74–S77.

Papich, M.G. (2007). Saunders *Handbook of Veterinary Drugs*, 2nd edition. St. Louis, MO: WB Saunders, pp. 379–380.

Perkovic, L.D., et al. (2002). Comparison of ondansetron with metoclopramide in the symptomatic relief of uremia-induced nausea and vomiting. *Kidney Blood Press Res* **25**: 61–64.

Peters, R.M., et al. (2005). Histopathologic features of canine uremic gastropathy: a retrospective study. *J Vet Intern Med* **19**: 315–320.

Pisoni, R. and G. Remuzzi (2001). Pathophysiology and management of progressive chronic renal failure. In: *Primer on Kidney Diseases*, edited by A. Greenberg, 3rd edition. San Diego, CA: National Kidney Foundation, pp. 385–396.

Plantinga, E.A., et al. (2005). Retrospective study of the survival of cats with acquired chronic renal insufficiency offered different commercial diets. *Vet Rec* **157**: 185–187.

Plumb, D.C. (2008). *Plumb's Veterinary Drug Handbook*, 6th edition. Ames, IA: Blackwell Publishing, pp. 130–131

Poli, A., et al. (1995). Renal involvement in feline immunodeficiency virus infection: p24 antigen detection, virus isolation, and PCR analysis. *Vet Immunol Immunopathol* **46**: 13–20.

Polzin, D., et al. (1988). Development of renal lesions in dogs after 11/12 reduction of renal mass: influence of dietary protein intake. *Lab Invest* **58**: 172–183.

Pörsti, I.H. (2008). Expanding targets of vitamin D receptor activation: downregulation of several RAS components in the kidney. *Kidney Int* **74**: 1371–1373.

Randolph, J.E., et al. (2004). Expression, bioactivity, and clinical assessment of recombinant feline erythropoietin. *Am J Vet Res* **65**: 1355–1366.

Randolph, J.E., et al. (2004a). Clinical efficacy and safety of recombinant canine erythropoietin in dogs with anemia of chronic renal failure and dogs with recombinant human erythropoietin-induced red cell aplasia. *J vet Intern Med* **18**: 81–91.

Ravani, P., et al. (2009). Vitamin D level and patient outcome in chronic kidney disease. *Kidney Int* **75**: 88–95.

Remuzzi, G., et al. (2005). The role of renin-angiotensin-aldosterone system in the progression of chronic kidney disease. *Kidney Int* **68**(Suppl 99): S57–S65.

Remuzzi, A., et al. (2002). Effect of angiotensin II antagonism on the regression of kidney disease in the rat. *Kidney Int* **62**: 885–894.

Rennke, H.G. and B.M. (2007). *Renal Pathophysiology: The Essentials*, 2nd edition. Philadelphia, PA: Lippincott, Williams & Wilkins.

Ritz, E., et al. (2005). Role of calcium-phosphorus disorders in the progression of renal failure. *Kidney Int* **68** (Suppl 99): S66–S70.

Rosenberg, M. (2003). Chronic kidney disease: progression. *Nephrol Self Assess Program* **2**: 89–103.

Ross, S.J., et al. (2006). Clinical evaluation of dietary modification for treatment of spontaneous chronic kidney disease in cats. *J Am Vet Med Assoc* **229**: 949–957.

Sabatini, S. and N.A. Kurtzman (2009). Bicarbonate therapy in severe metabolic acidosis. *J Am Soc Nephrol* **20**: 692–695.

Sato, A., et al. (2005). Antiproteinuric effects of mineralcorticoid receptor blockade in patients with chronic renal disease. *Am J Hypertens* **18**: 44–49.

Segev, G., et al. (2008). Aluminum toxicity following administration of aluminum-based phosphate binders in 2 dogs with renal failure. *J Vet Intern Med* **22**: 1432–1435.

Schenck, P.A. and D.J. Chew (2003). Determination of calcium fractionation in dogs with chronic renal failure. *Am J Vet Res* **64**: 1181–1184.

Shoben, A.B., et al. (2008). Association of oral calcitriol with improved survival in nondialyzed CKD. *J Am Soc Nephrol* **19**: 1613–1619.

Stevens, L.A. and A.S. Levey (2005). Chronic kidney disease: staging and principles of management. In: *Primer on Kidney Diseases*, edited by A. Greenberg, 4th edition. San Diego, CA: Academic Press, pp. 455–463.

Stiles, J., et al. (1994). The prevalence of retinopathy in cats with systemic hypertension and chronic renal failure or hyperthyroidism. *J Am Anim Hosp Assoc* **30**: 564–572.

Syme, H.M., et al. (2006). Survival of cats with naturally occurring chronic renal failure is related to severity of proteinuria. *J Vet Intern Med* **20**: 528–535.

Teruel, J., et al. (1996). Androgen versus erythropoietin for the treatment of anemia in hemodialyzed patients: a prospective study. *J Am Soc Nephrol* **7**: 140–144.

Theisen, S., et al. (1997). Muscle potassium content and potassium gluconate supplementation in normokalemic cats with naturally occurring chronic renal failure. *J Vet Intern Med* **11**: 212–217.

Thomas, J., et al. (1993). Association of renal disease indicators with feline immunodeficiency virus infection. *J Am Anim Hosp Assoc* **29**: 320–326.

Vanholder, R. (1998). The uremic syndrome. In: *Primer on Kidney Diseases*, edited by A. Greenberg, 2nd edition. San Diego, CA: Academic Press, pp. 403–407.

Weidemann, A. and R.S. Johnson (2009). Nonrenal regulation of EPO synthesis. *Kidney Int* **75**: 682–688.

Weir, M. and J.C. Fink (2005). Salt intake and progression of chronic kidney disease: an overlooked modifiable exposure? A commentary. *Am J Kidney Dis* **45**: 176–188.

Wesson, D.E. and J. Simoni (2009). Increased tissue acid mediates a progressive decline in glomerular filtration rate of animals with reduced nephron mass. *Kidney Int* **75**: 929–935.

Wolf, G., et al. (2002). Leptin and renal disease. *Am J Kidney Dis* **39**: 1–11.

Yudd, M. and F. Llach (2000). Current medical management of secondary hyperparathyroidism. *Am J Med Sci* **320**: 100–106.

49

Acute kidney insufficiency

Larry D. Cowgill and Cathy Langston

Introduction

Acute kidney disease represents a spectrum of disease associated with a sudden onset of renal parenchymal injury most typically characterized by generalized failure of the kidneys to meet the excretory, metabolic, and endocrine demands of the body, that is, acute renal failure. Acute renal failure (ARF) is associated with rapid hemodynamic, filtration, tubulointerstitial, or outflow injury to the kidneys and subsequent accumulation of metabolic toxins (uremia toxins) and dysregulation of fluid, electrolyte, and acid-base balance. ARF reflects only a subset of patients with the highest morbidity and mortality. The term "acute kidney injury" (AKI) has been adopted in human medicine to better reflect the broad spectrum of acute diseases of the kidney and to reinforce the concept that AKI encompasses a continuum of functional and parenchymal damage (Kellum et al. 2007b; Himmelfarb et al. 2008). These conditions may be imperceptible clinically at early stages and culminate with patients requiring renal replacement therapy (RRT) (Bellomo et al. 2004; Kellum et al. 2007b; Mehta et al. 2007; Kellum 2008).

The clinical presentation of AKI includes prerenal and postrenal conditions which may be independent or combined with intrinsic renal injury depending on the functional origin, extent, and duration of the conditions inciting the disease. Animal patients most often are recognized with an acute uremia which must be differentiated subsequently into its prerenal, intrinsic renal parenchymal, and/or postrenal components for proper diagnostic evaluation, management, and staging. AKI conceptually is a disease affecting intrinsically normal kidneys, but events predisposing to AKI frequently are superimposed on preexisting chronic kidney disease (CKD) to produce

a seemingly acute uremia with similar clinical features. Currently there are no discrete markers to define or stage the conditions that represent AKI, although some urine biomarkers are showing promise (Bonventre 2007; Bagshaw and Gibney 2008; Coca et al. 2008; Ferguson et al. 2008; Vaidya et al. 2008). There also is no formal categorization of the spectrum of the functional deficiencies to standardize its classification, severity, stage, clinical course, response to therapy, or prognosis for recovery (Kellum et al. 2002; Mehta and Chertow 2003; Bagshaw and Gibney 2008).

Precise definitions for AKI have not been established in veterinary medicine. A myriad of definitions have been proposed in both human medicine and veterinary medicine based on sequential changes in glomerular filtration rate (GFR), azotemia, or urine production to provide objective criteria for the diagnosis (Mehta and Chertow 2003; Cowgill and Francey 2005; Langston 2010). To emphasize the concept that AKI represents a continuum of renal injury, staging schemes recently have been proposed for human patients to stratify the extent and duration of renal injury and the potential for recovery. One staging system is categorized progressively into **R**isk, **I**njury, **F**ailure, **L**oss, and **E**SKD (RIFLE) (Bellomo et al. 2004; Hoste et al. 2006; Hoste and Kellum 2007; Kellum 2008). A second slightly more restricted staging system emerged as an expert consensus from the Acute Kidney Injury Network (AKIN) in an attempt to reproducibly identify early AKI and classify its course with regard to prognosis and appropriate diagnostic and therapeutic interventions (Mehta et al. 2007; Molitoris et al. 2007). There is considerable overlap between both systems, and criteria for each staging category are based ostensibly on insensitive markers of renal injury including abrupt changes in GFR, serum creatinine, urine output, and duration of signs. Preliminary validation of these staging concepts to predict morbidity

Nephrology and Urology of Small Animals. Edited by Joe Bartges and David J. Polzin. © 2011 Blackwell Publishing Ltd.

and outcome have been encouraging; however, the criteria which define these staging schemes are rarely applicable in animal patients in which the abruptness of the disease and the magnitude of changes in GFR, azotemia, or urine production are rarely known or quantitated (Hoste and Kellum 2007; Kellum 2008). To date, no formal staging system has been established for AKI in animals to stratify or characterize the severity of the renal impairment as has been established recently for CKD in dogs and cats and AKI in humans (Polzin et al. 2005; Hoste et al. 2006; Hoste and Kellum 2006; IRIS 2006; Uchino et al. 2006; Lopes et al. 2008; Cruz et al. 2009; Elliott and Watson 2009). The International Renal Interest Society (IRIS) staging system for CKD was developed as a consensus scheme to promote the more uniform characterization and recognition of CKD in animals with the goal to better understand its pathophysiology and to facilitate its evaluation and rational management. It seems tenable to adapt this same schematic approach to classify and stratify the severity of AKI in dogs and cat. Unlike the IRIS staging for CKD, the staging of AKI would not imply the kidney disease is stable or at steady-state. On the contrary, the "stage" represents a moment in the course of the disease and is predicted to change as the condition worsens or improves or transitions to CKD. Table 49.1 outlines an arbitrary staging scheme for AKI in dogs and cats based on serum creatinine, urine formation, and requirement for RRT which is intended to facilitate classification, functional stratification, and therapeutic decision making. This scheme should be considered as preliminary and remains subject to consensus revision and modification as appropriate biomarkers are validated to provide greater specificity and sensitivity to the staging of AKI.

AKI Stage I defines animals with historical, clinical, laboratory (biomarker, glucosuria, cylinduria, inflammatory sediment, microalbuminuria, etc.), or imaging evidence of AKI that are non-azotemic and/or whose clinical presentation is readily fluid volume-responsive. Stage I also includes animals with progressive (hourly or daily) increases in serum creatinine within the non azotemic range (or laboratory reference range). Presumptive guidelines could include a 0.3 mg/dL increase in serum creatinine within a 48 hour interval. AKI Stage II defines animals with documented AKI characterized by mild azotemia in addition to other historical, biochemical, or anatomic characteristics of AKI. This would include animals that have an increase from their baseline serum creatinine associated with preexisting CKD. AKI Stages III, IV, and V define animals with documented AKI and progressively greater degrees of parenchymal damage and functional failure (uremia). Each stage of AKI is further substaged on the basis of current urine production as oligoanuric (O) or non-oliguric (NO) and on the requirement for RRT. The inclusion of substaging by urine production is based on the importance of the interrelationship of urine production to the pathological or functional contributions to the renal injury and its influence on the clinical presentation, therapeutic options, and outcome of AKI. Substaging on the requirement for RRT is established on the need to correct life-threatening iatrogenic or clinical consequences of AKI including severe azotemia, hyperkalemia, acid-base disorders, overhydration, oliguria, or anuria, or the need to eliminate nephrotoxins. The requirement for RRT could occur at any of the proposed stages. Substaging on the requirement for RRT has similar clinical, therapeutic, and prognostic implications as for urine production to

Table 49.1 Proposed staging system for acute kidney injury in dogs and cats

AKI stage[a]	Serum creatinine (mg/dL)	Clinical description
Stage I	<1.6	[b]Non azotemic AKI or volume-responsive AKI [c]Historical, clinical, laboratory, or imaging evidence of renal injury [d]Progressive non azotemic increase in serum creatinine; ≥0.3 mg/dL within 48 hours
Stage II	1.6–2.5	Mild AKI: Historical, clinical, laboratory, or imaging evidence of AKI and mild static or progressive azotemia
Stage III	2.6–5.0	Moderate to severe AKI: Documented AKI and increasing severities of azotemia and functional renal failure
Stage IV	–10.0	
Stage V	>10.0	

[a]Each stage of AKI is further substaged on the basis of current urine production as oligoanuric (O) or non oliguric (NO) and on the requirement for renal replacement therapy (RRT); (see text)

categorize the severity of the renal injury as well as its influence on outcome.

AKI is associated with a rapid (hours to days) and progressive increase in serum urea nitrogen (BUN), creatinine and phosphate, and variable hyperkalemia, metabolic acidosis, and urine formation (Cowgill and Francey 2005; Grauer 2009; Langston 2010). The progression of azotemia may not be recognized in animals presented late in the course of the disease or in those without serial blood chemistry determinations. Oliguria and anuria are characteristic features of severe forms of AKI, but this classic presentation is unpredictable. Nonoliguric forms of AKI are common and must be differentiated from the azotemia and polyuria associated with CKD. In contrast to CKD, AKI is potentially reversible in its earliest stages before the development of renal failure. It may also be reversible at advanced stages if the animal survives the life-threatening consequences of AKI, the predisposing conditions resolve, and the imposed renal injury repairs. There are intervention points and degrees of severity where specific and supportive therapy may alter the natural behavior of the disease. If, however, these intervention opportunities are missed or the injury is too severe, the pathological damage is likely to progress, and the injury becomes less capable of morphologic and functional repair. With delays to initiate therapy or failure to provide appropriate supportive therapy at these critical points, the outcome may be irreversible renal damage or death of the animal.

Etiology of AKI

The etiology of AKI is multifactorial according to the origin, extent, and duration of the conditions that incite the injury or alter renal function. Singular or a combination of hemodynamic (prerenal) disturbances, intrinsic parenchymal injury, and postrenal disorders contribute to the structural and/or functional derangements of AKI. The traditional categorical contributors (prerenal, intrinsic renal, postrenal) to AKI are neither discrete nor clinically definable. It is also important to recognize that the etiologies of AKI vary geographically and between species, and their relative prevalence changes over time.

Hemodynamic failure (prerenal azotemia) is a functional decline in glomerular filtration resulting from deficiencies in renal blood flow, perfusion pressure, or excessive vasoconstriction of the renal vasculature. Hemodynamic failure is a common cause of early stages of AKI (See above), but it can coexist with other causes of excretory failure and more severe stages of AKI. It is not associated with structural damage to the kidney and is reversible with timely correction of the underlying hemodynamic or volume deficiencies. This cat-

egory of AKI is currently termed volume-responsive AKI (Kellum 2007). Hemodynamic failure is a coordinated neural and humoral response of the kidneys to imposed hemodynamic deficiencies, hypotension, and hypovolemia to preferentially preserve perfusion to vital organs like the heart and brain. At the onset of these hemodynamic deficiencies, GFR decreases, and renal salt and water conservation and urine concentration increase through activation of the sympathetic nervous system, the renin-angiotensin-aldosterone system (RAAS), and the release of antidiuretic hormone. Consequently, nitrogenous excretory products are retained producing azotemia, and urine formation is reduced promoting oliguria (Himmelfarb et al. 2008; Kellum 2008). Although these hemodynamic-induced manifestations represent appropriate physiologic responses to renal hypoperfusion, they are, by themselves, rarely of just physiologic significance in patients who are being evaluated or hospitalized for AKI.

Severe hypotension (mean arterial blood pressure <80 mmHg) falls below the autoregulatory capacity for glomerular filtration, and GFR decreases in proportion to the hypotension (Badr and Ichikawa 1988). Azotemia and increased urine specific gravity are hallmarks of hemodynamic failure but may be masked by underlying conditions (e.g., CKD, adrenal insufficiency, hepatic insufficiency, hypercalcemia, and diuretic administration) that impair renal solute reabsorption and concentrating ability. Hemodynamically-mediated azotemia may develop with mild degrees of hypotension in animals with preexisting heart failure or CKD when renal function is maintained by activated autoregulatory mechanisms through the RAAS to preserve basal filtration pressure. Similarly, nonsteroidal anti-inflammatory drugs (NSAIDs) and angiotensin converting enzyme (ACE) inhibitors may induce hemodynamic failure by decompensating glomerular function in animals whose filtration is dependent on prostaglandin or angiotensin II-mediated regulation of glomerular vasculature (Hirsch 2007). Azotemia may develop also in conditions of volume overload in which renal perfusion is compromised by poor cardiac output (congestive heart failure), decreased effective intravascular volume (nephritic syndrome) or excessive vascular resistance and reduced renal perfusion pressure (sepsis, hepatic failure) (Himmelfarb et al. 2008).

Clinical conditions causing direct structural injury to the vasculature, glomeruli, tubular epithelium, or interstitium of the kidney can cause the entire spectrum of AKI. Intrinsic structural injury to the kidney generally promotes more severe AKI and will not be reversed completely by restoration of fluid volume or hemodynamic deficiencies. Renal injury can develop as a continuation of functional hemodynamic deficiencies, overt ischemic events, or exposure to exogenous drugs or toxins that directly target the kidney. Intrinsic renal diseases or systemic diseases with secondary renal manifestations also promote AKI (Table 49.2). The hemodynamic insults that promote intrinsic renal injury are identical to those promoting hemodynamic failure; but the hypovolemia,

Table 49.2 Causes of acute kidney injury in dogs and cats

Hemodynamic causes
  Hypovolemia
  Hypotension
  Shock (hypovolemic, hemorrhagic, hypotensive, septic)
  Decreased cardiac output (congestive heart failure,
    arrhythmias, cardiac arrest, cardiac tamponade)
  Deep anesthesia/extensive surgery
  Trauma (renal avulsion)
  Hyperthermia/hypothermia
  Extensive cutaneous burns
  Transfusion reaction
  Hyperviscosity/polycythemia
  Adrenal insufficiency
  NSAIDs
  Diuretic abuse

Primary renal diseases
  Large vessels:
    Renal vessel thrombosis or stenosis, DIC
  Glomeruli and small vessels:
    Hemolytic uremic syndrome, Alabama rot
    Immune-mediated (acute glomerulonephritis, systemic
      lupus erythematosus, vasculitis)
  Tubules:
    Heme pigmenturia—crush syndrome, oxalate nephrosis
    Ischemia
    Toxins: Endogenous toxins, exogenous toxins, drugs
  Interstitium:
    Infectious (pyelonephritis, leptospirosis, borreliosis,
      infectious canine hepatitis)
    Neoplasia (lymphoma) renal transplant rejection

Outflow obstruction
  Ureteral obstruction
  Urethral obstruction
  Uroabdomen

Systemic diseases with renal manifestations
  Infectious: feline infectious peritonitis, babesiosis,
    leishmaniasis, bacterial endocarditis
  Systemic inflammatory response syndrome, sepsis, multiple
    organ failure
  Pancreatitis
  Hepatorenal syndrome
  Malignant hypertension
  SLE
  Peritonitis
  Vasculitis
  Hypercalcemia

hypotension, or hypoperfusion have been sustained or increased in severity to induce ischemic damage to the kidney that cannot be reversed readily with volume restoration. Renal ischemia also develops with thrombosis of renal arteries and veins, disseminated intravascular coagulation, incompatible blood transfusions, or septic thrombi. Vasculitis, pancreatitis, hypoproteinemia, heat stroke, and gastric torsion pose a high risk for development of hemodynamically-mediated ischemic injury (Lane et al. 1994; Behrend et al. 1996; Vaden et al. 1997; Cowgill and Francey 2005; Langston 2010). Age, sepsis, gender, breed, preexisting renal disease, dehydration, electrolyte abnormalities, and poor tissue perfusion may impose additional risks of AKI (Vaden et al. 1997; Grauer 1998; Leblanc et al. 2005; Grauer 2009).

Hemodynamically-mediated causes account for approximately 40% of AKI in human patients (Palevsky 2004). Hemodynamically-mediated AKI is reported variably but appears to be less common in animals. In a large series of reported cases with severe uremia (all receiving RRT), hemodynamic etiologies represented less than 10% of identified causes in dogs (Segev et al. 2008b). In dogs with a broader spectrum of AKI, the incidence was greater than 30% (Vaden et al. 1997). In cats, hemodynamic causes were recognized in only 13% of cases (Worwag and Langston 2008). This difference in incidence between animals and people may reflect inadequate capture of volume responsive AKI that weren't categorized as AKI in animal studies.

AKI is frequently caused by exposure to exogenous or endogenous toxins. Nephrotoxins include environmental chemicals, pharmaceutical agents, and biotoxins that produce direct sublethal injury, apoptosis, or necrosis of the tubular epithelium. Some nephrotoxins incite interstitial inflammation or tubular obstruction by intraluminal precipitation (Taber and Mueller 2006; Clarkson et al. 2008; Pannu and Nadim 2008; Rumbeiha and Murphy 2009). Alternatively, nephrotoxins may decrease renal perfusion leading to ischemic cell injury and death. Similarly, many pharmaceuticals used routinely in clinical practice have potential nephrotoxicity if dosed excessively or administered to animals with overt risks for AKI (e.g., hypotension, advanced age, hypovolemia, sepsis, concomitant drug therapy, renal insufficiency). Nephrotoxins may react directly with apical, basolateral or subcellular membranes of tubular cells to alter their permeability, disrupt their protein makeup, or activate phospholipases. They may promote free radical generation, interfere with lysosome function, activate cellular endonucleases and proteinases, interference with oxidative phosphorylation, and shut down energy dependent cellular processes (Taber and Mueller 2006; Pannu and Nadim 2008). Nephrotoxins are diverse chemically, but are most commonly associated with organic compounds and solvents, antimicrobials, vasoactive drugs, plant toxins, miscellaneous therapeutics, or dietary adulterants (Table 49.3) (Vaden et al. 1997; Dobson and Kell 2008; Segev et al. 2008b; Worwag and Langston 2008).

Ethylene glycol intoxication is one of the most common causes of AKI and the second most common intoxication recognized in companion animals (Grauer and Lane 1995; Grauer and Lane 1995; Vaden et al. 1997; Thrall et al. 1998; Segev et al. 2008b; Worwag and Langston 2008; Grauer 2009; Rumbeiha and Murphy 2009). Automobile antifreeze is the usual source of exposure, but a history of exposure to antifreeze is often denied and alternative sources of ethylene glycol exposure should be considered. Glycoaldehyde, glyoxylic acid, glycolate, and oxalic acid, the major metabolites of ethylene glycol, promote the specific nephrotoxicity, so timely recognition and decontamination of ethylene glycol from the patient is important to prevent or minimize the renal injury (Thrall et al. 1998; Cowgill and Francey 2005; Rumbeiha and Murphy 2009).

Aminoglycoside antimicrobials (neomycin, gentamicin, tobramycin, amikacin, netilmicin, and streptomycin) are polycations with low protein-binding capacity and are freely filtered at the glomerulus. They demonstrate hierarchical nephrotoxicity (as above) according to the number of cationic groups and ability to be transported across the cell (Kaloyanides 1984; Kaloyanides 1997; Pannu and Nadim 2008). Aminoglycosides interact with the negatively charged phospholipids on the brush border membrane of the proximal tubule and concentrate in proximal epithelium by pinocytosis (Molitoris et al. 1993; Pannu and Nadim 2008). Once internalized, aminoglycosides accumulate in subcellular organelles and disrupt cytosolic, mitochondrial, and lysosomal function to promote cell death (Molitoris et al. 1993; Ward et al. 2005; Pannu and Nadim 2008). Aminoglycosides also induce free radical injury and alter the ultrafiltration coefficient of glomerular capillaries to further decrease GFR. The nephrotoxicity of aminoglycosides is enhanced by reabsorption and concentration in the proximal tubule, high peak serum concentrations, prolonged cumulative dosing, preexisting kidney disease, advanced age, volume depletion, renal ischemia, or concurrent exposure to other nephrotoxins (Taber and Mueller 2006; Clarkson et al. 2008; Pannu and Nadim 2008). Extracellular fluid (ECF) volume expansion prior to aminoglycoside administration and once-daily dosing reduces drug accumulation in the renal cortex and decreases nephrotoxicity (Pannu and Nadim 2008).

Amphotericin B is a polyene antibiotic that disrupts the integrity of cell membranes and increases their permeability. It also reduces renal blood flow and GFR due to arterial vasoconstriction. The altered membrane permeability increases cellular metabolism and promotes oxygen deprivation leading to cellular necrosis. The toxicity of amphotericin B is potentiated by the dose and duration of therapy, preexisting renal disease, sodium depletion, hypovolemia, and concomitant use of nephrotoxic drugs (Taber and Mueller 2006). Its toxicity is lessened by sodium loading, ECF volume expansion prior to drug administration, and administration of liposome encapsulated formulations (Greene 2006; Taber and Mueller 2006).

NSAIDs have become a mainstay therapy for animals with chronic pain or inflammation due to the availability of efficacious veterinary products, convenient administration, and marketing claims of safety. Consequently, NSAIDs-induced AKI has increased in incidence in dogs and cats that have multiple predispositions for AKI as well as in animals with unsupervised consumption of toxic amounts of palatable preparations. NSAIDs either nonselectively or selectively inhibit renal cyclooxygenases which mediate production of prostaglandins to maintain afferent arteriolar blood flow and GFR during states of hypoperfusion (Palevsky 2004; Cheng and Harris 2005; Harris 2006; Taber and Mueller 2006). Prostaglandins are of little physiologic or regulatory significance during euvolemic states, but prostaglandin synthesis (via cyclooxygenase up-regulation) is increased when renal blood flow is compromised (dehydration, hypovolemia, congestive heart failure, dietary salt restriction, surgery, or diuretic use) and when renal water and solute reabsorption is regulated by heightened renin, angiotensin II, vasopressin, and catecholamine-mediated events (Cheng and Harris 2005; Harris 2006; Taber and Mueller 2006). The regionally generated vasodilatory prostaglandins, PGE_2 and PGI_2, antagonize the increased vascular resistance induced by angiotensin II, norepinephrine, vasopressin, and endothelin and preserve renal blood flow and glomerular filtration during these hemodynamic stresses (Taber and Mueller 2006). By disrupting these effects, NSAIDs administration shifts the circulatory balance, predisposing the renal vasculature to unopposed vasoconstriction which constitutes an adverse effect. Prostaglandins also participate in counterregulatory control of salt and water reabsorption and renin synthesis (Palevsky 2004; Cheng and Harris 2005; Harris 2006; Taber and Mueller 2006). NSAID inhibition of these prostaglandin effects increase vascular tone and promote antinatriuretic, antireninemic, and antidiuretic effects.

The principal renal toxicity associated with NSAID use and overdosage in animals is renal ischemia and rarely papillary necrosis secondary to their hemodynamic effects. An allergic tubulointerstitial nephritis and a syndrome of proteinuria with hypertension

Table 49.3 Nephrotoxins and mechanism of nephrotoxicity

Class of agent	Examples
Antimicrobials	Aminoglycosides (ATN, AIN), aztreonam (AIN), bacitracin (ATN), carbapenems (AIN), cephalosporins (AIN), colistin (ATN), penicillins (AIN), polymixin (ATN), quinolones (AIN), rifampin(AIN), sulfonamides (AIN, Cry), tetracyclines (AIN, Fanconi), vancomycin (AIN, ATN),
Antiprotozoals	Dapsone (AIN), pentamidine (ATN), sulfadiazine (AIN, Cry), thiacetarsamide, trimethoprim-sulfamethoxazole (AIN, Cry)
Antifungals	Amphotericin B (ATN, HD)
Antivirals	Acyclovir (Cry, ATN), foscarnet (Cry, ATN), indivir (Cry), cidofovir (ATN)
Chemotherapeutics	Azathioprine (AIN), cis- or carboplatin (ATN), cytosine arabinoside (AIN), doxorubicin, gemcitabine (Vasc), ifosfamide (ATN), methotrexate (Cry), mitomycin (Vasc), oxaliplatin (ATN), pentostatin (ATN), anti-vascular endothelial growth factor (bevacizumab and others)
Immunosuppressives	Cyclosporine (HD, ATN, CIN, Vasc), interleukin (IL) 2, rapamycin (Vasc), tacrolimus (HD, ATN, CIN, Vasc)
Nonsteroidal anti-inflammatory drugs	All (HD, AIN, GN)
Angiotensin-converting enzyme inhibitors, angiotensin receptor antagonists	All (HD, GN), captopril (also AIN)
Diuretics	All (HD), furosemide (AIN), thiazides (AIN), triamterene (Cry), acetazolamide (AIN)
Diagnostic agents	Radiocontract agents (ATN, HD, Osm), gadolinium (high dose), oral sodium phosphate solution
Miscellaneous therapeutics	Acetaminophen (AIN), allopurinol (nephrolithiasis, AIN), carbamazepine (AIN, ATN), cimetidine (AIN), clopidogrel (vasc), deferoxamine, dextran (Osm), dopamine (HD), ε-aminocaproic acid, epinephrine (HD), hydralazine (GN), hydroxyethyl starch (Osm), IVIg (Osm), lipid lowering agents (AIN), lithium, mannitol (Osm, HD), methoxyflurane, methyldopa (AIN), pamidronated (GN), penicillamine (GN), phenobarbitol (AIN), phenytoin (AIN), phosphorus-containing urinary acidifiers, propanolol (HD), propylthiouracil (GN), proton-pump inhibitors (AIN), ranitidine(AIN), streptokinase (AIN), ticlopidine (Vasc), topiramate (nephrolithiasis), quinine/quinidine (Vasc), vitamin D3 analogs (psoriasis medications), warfarin (AIN), zoledronate
Heavy metals	Antimony, arsenic (ATN), bismuth salts, cadmium, chromium, copper, gold (GN), lead, mercury (HD), nickel, silver, thallium, uranium
Organic compounds	Carbon tetrachloride and other chlorinated hydrocarbons, chloroform, ethylene glycol (ATN), herbicides, pesticides, solvents
Miscellaneous toxins	Bee venom (ATN), disphosphonates, gallium nitrate, lilies, germanium, grapes and raisins, melamine cyanurate (Cry), mushrooms, silicon, snake venom (HD), sodium fluoride, superphosphate fertilizer, vitamin D3-containing rodenticides (HD)
Endogenous toxins	Hemoglobin, myoglobin
Illicit drugs	Amphetamines[a], cocaine[a] (HD), heroin[a], barbiturates[a], phencyclidine[a] [a]AKI from rhabdomyolysis
Alternative products	Herbal: *Akebia* sp, Aristolchic acid (fibrosis), *Ephedra* sp (ma huang), Cape aloes, *Taxus celebica*, *Uno degatta*, *Glycyrrhiza* sp, *Datura* sp Adulterants: mefenamic acid, dichromate, cadmium, phenylbutazone

Source: Compiled from (Cowgill and Francey 2005; Taber and Mueller 2006; Langston and Boyd 2007; Evenepoel 2009; Perazella 2009; Rumbeiha and Murphy 2009; Langston 2010).

Abbreviations: ATN, acute tubular necrosis; AIN, acute interstitial nephritis; HD, hemodynamic; GN, glomerular; Cry, obstructive nephropathy (crystal formation); ON, osmotic nephrosis; Vas, Vascular; CIN, chronic interstitial nephritis.

and hyporeninemic-hypoaldosteroneism have been described in humans (Harris 2006; Taber and Mueller 2006; Pannu and Nadim 2008). The nephrotoxicity of NSAIDs is exacerbated in animals with congestive heart failure, nephrotic syndrome, AKI or CKD, hypertension, cirrhosis, and anesthesia in which blood volume is compromised and renal vascular tone is increased. Despite early claims of lessened nephrotoxicity for the COX-2 selective NSAIDs, these agents have similar renal toxicity in susceptible patients and should be used with similar precautions to the non-selective or COX-1 selective inhibitors.

Angiotensin-converting enzyme (ACE) inhibitors and angiotensin receptor blockers (ARBs) blunt angiotensin II-mediated vasoconstriction of the efferent arteriole resulting in decreased efferent arteriolar resistance, glomerular capillary pressure, and GFR (Lefebvre et al. 2007; Pannu and Nadim 2008). Azotemia and acute decompensation of underlying kidney disease are seen in dogs and cats following ACE inhibitor administration. The severity of the change in kidney function is variable and typically occurs in animals with existing CKD or hemodynamic predispositions (e.g., sodium depletion, congestive heart failure, and diuretic use) when the maintenance of basal GFR is dependent on angiotensin II-mediated vasoconstriction (Atkins et al. 2002; Lefebvre et al. 2006; Lefebvre et al. 2007).

Toxicity associated with ingestion of plant material has become an important cause of nephrotoxicity in dogs and cats over the past 10 years. Both lily poisoning in cats and grape/raisin toxicity in dogs appear to be immerging etiologies for AKI (Brady and Janovitz 2000; Gwaltney-Brant et al. 2001; Langston 2002; Mazzaferro et al. 2004; Rumbeiha et al. 2004; Eubig et al. 2005; Morrow et al. 2005; Berg et al. 2007). AKI associated with lily ingestion has been documented for decades but was not specifically identified as a common etiology for AKI in cats in published reviews prior to 2000 (Grauer and Lane 1995; Langston et al. 1997; Brady and Janovitz 2000; Cowgill and Elliott 2000). More recently, lily poisoning has become a prominent etiology for cats presenting with acute azotemia (Brady and Janovitz 2000; Langston 2002; Rumbeiha et al. 2004; Berg et al. 2007). Essentially all species of the genus *Lillium* including Easter lilies, Tiger lilies, Asiatic hybrid lilies, Japanese lilies, and Stargazer lilies and the genus *Hemerocallis* including Day lily, Orange day lily, Red lily, and Western lily are nephrotoxic to cats (Hadley et al. 2003; Means 2007; Hovda 2010). Lily poisoning causes a very acute onset of anorexia, depression, vomiting, polydipsia, marked azotemia, and severe uremic signs associated with extensive toxic necrosis of the proximal tubular epithelium and pancreas (Brady and Janovitz 2000; Langston 2002; Rumbeiha et al. 2004). Any environmental exposure to lily plants should raise suspicion of intoxication as consumption of even small segments of the leaves or especially the flowers can prove fatal. The toxicity is reproducible with a water-soluble extract from the leaves and flowers, but the precise identity of the toxin remains uncharacterized (Rumbeiha et al. 2004).

Ingestion of grapes and raisins were first noted to be associated with AKI in 1999 (Gwaltney-Brant et al. 2001). Vomiting is a common feature that occurs within hours of ingestion (Gwaltney-Brant et al. 2001; Campbell and Bates 2003; Penny et al. 2003; Mazzaferro et al. 2004; Eubig et al. 2005; Stanley and Langston 2008). Undigested grapes or raisins may be seen in the vomitus or in diarrheal contents. Azotemia develops in some dogs within 24 hours. Hypercalcemia was present in 63% of dogs in one series (Eubig et al. 2005). Proximal tubular degeneration and necrosis were noted on renal histopathology, with intracellular pigment noted in 6 of 10 cases. The chemical composition of the pigment is undetermined (Morrow et al. 2005). Approximately 50% of dogs that developed azotemia survived, of which 65% had complete resolution of azotemia (Eubig et al. 2005). Not all grape or raisin ingestion leads to clinical signs, and the amount of ingestion leading to intoxication is reported variably. The toxic principle causing the tubular degeneration also is unknown.

Over the past decade the most significant new cause of AKI in both dogs and cats was caused by nephrotoxic and obstructive injury resulting from ingestion of pet foods manufactured with sourced ingredients from China that were adulterated with melamine and cyanuric acid (Cianciolo et al. 2008; Dobson et al. 2008; Yhee et al. 2009). Two widespread incidences involving thousands of animals have been documented in Asia in 2003 and 2004 and North America in 2007 (Brown et al. 2007; Thompson et al. 2008; Osborne et al. 2009; Yhee et al. 2009). The underlying cause of these disasters was ultimately unraveled through a remarkable epidemiologic process following massive recalls of suspected pet foods following both outbreaks (Brown et al. 2007; Puschner et al. 2007; Cianciolo et al. 2008; Dobson et al. 2008; Yhee et al. 2009). In 2008, widespread outbreaks of urolithiasis and renal death were also reported affecting greater than 50,000 children exposed to powdered formula or milk powder from China adulterated with melamine (Bhalla et al. 2009; Hau et al. 2009). Melamine is an organic base derived from urea which is used commercially in the manufacture of plastic products and as a fertilizer (Dobson et al. 2008; Hau et al. 2009; Yhee et al. 2009). Melamine and a variety of similar triazine compounds, including cyanuric acid, are nonprotein nitrogen chemicals with no known nutritional value. They have been nefariously added as adulterants to sourced ingredients of manufactured pet foods and human foods to falsely bolster the measured or apparent nitrogen content (Burns 2007; Hau et al. 2009).

Individually, melamine and cyanuric acid have minimal acute *in vivo* renal toxicity in cats and dogs when ingested up to 1% of the diet or in vitro cytotoxicity at even very high concentrations (Puschner et al. 2007; Dobson et al. 2008). In combination, these chemicals interact to form a melamine–cyanurate complex which is highly ordered and ostensibly insoluble in acidic urine, predisposing to crystal deposition and urolith formation throughout the kidney (Puschner et al. 2007; Dobson et al. 2008; Thompson et al. 2008; Hau et al. 2009; Osborne et al. 2009). When coingested in the diet, clinical signs of depression, anorexia, vomiting, polydipsia, polyuria, and azotemia are seen acutely in experimental cats consuming diets containing 0.2% melamine and cyanuric acid or with ingestion of as little as 32 mg/kg body weight of each substance (Puschner et al. 2007; Cianciolo et al. 2008). Similar signs and clinical courses are seen in dogs and cats exposed naturally to food contaminated to a similar extent (Puschner et al. 2007; Hau et al. 2009). Natural exposure causes variable and progressive azotemia and most dogs and cats die of acute uremia (Burns 2007; Yhee et al. 2009). The majority of exposed animals develop characteristic fan-shaped, refractile, birefringent crystals distributed throughout the cortex, medulla, and pelvis of the kidney and in urine. Green-yellowish uroliths are an additional distinguishing feature that can cause outflow obstruction at the renal pelvis, ureter or urethra (Cocchi et al. 2009; Hau et al. 2009; Osborne et al. 2009; Yhee et al. 2009). The melamine-cyanurate complex also causes dose dependent necrosis of the distal tubular epithelium by undefined effects (Brown et al. 2007; Puschner et al. 2007; Yhee et al. 2009).

Melamine-cyanuric acid intoxication promotes AKI (and CKD) in both dogs and cats; however, the prevalence of disease and demonstrated mortality has been disproportionate between the reported outbreaks in Asia and North America for undetermined reasons (Yhee et al. 2009) (Cowgill, personal observations, 2008). The nearly instantaneous and continuous reporting of the initial and subsequently observed cases throughout North America by informal listserves and internet communication is likely responsible in part for the rapid recognition of the 2007 outbreak as well as its relative containment in scope compared to the 2003–2004 outbreaks in Asia.

Another recently recognized food-related nephrotoxicity in dogs is thought to be associated with consumption of chicken jerky treats imported from China or a vegetarian dental chew treat distributed in Australia

(Anonymous 2007; FDA 2008; Lau 2009). Ingestion of these treats led to an acquired form of Fanconi syndrome, including glucosuria with normoglycemia, aminoaciduria, cylindiuria, hypokalemia, metabolic acidosis, and frequently azotemia. Gastrointestinal signs (vomiting and anorexia) and elevated liver enzymes were commonly reported. Small breed dogs are more commonly affected. Most dogs recover, although permanent renal damage or death is possible. After recognition of the problem and voluntary recall of the suspected products, the number of cases seems to have declined (Lau 2009). Acquired Fanconi syndrome also has been associated with copper storage hepatopathy. (Appleman et al. 2008; Hill et al. 2008b)

Acquired infectious, immune-mediated, neoplastic, or degenerative diseases expressed primarily in the kidney may cause intrinsic renal failure (Table 49.2). If fulminating and extensive, they produce AKI that must be differentiated from ischemic or nephrotoxic etiologies.

Leptospirosis is a worldwide zoonotic disease that affects many organ systems in infected dogs. It has been reported to occur rarely in domestic cats (Carlos et al. 1971; Bryson and Ellis 1976; Dickeson and Love 1993; Agunloye and Nash 1996; Mylonakis et al. 2005). Renal, hepatic, pulmonary, vascular, and hematologic manifestations are common; and involvement of any of these organ systems in isolation or combination should prompt suspicion of leptospirosis (Rentko et al. 1992; Harkin and Gartrell 1996; Birnbaum et al. 1998; Adin and Cowgill 2000; Ward 2002; Ward 2002; Ward et al. 2002; Boutilier et al. 2003; Greenlee et al. 2005; Geisen et al. 2007).

The disease is caused by pathogenic strains of a gram-negative motile spirochete from the genomospecies, *Leptospira* (Greene et al. 2006; Levett 2001; Guerra 2009). Identification of causative organisms in the clinical setting has become confused as there is transition of the taxonomy from the clinically familiar phenotypic classification of species, serogroups, and serovars based primarily on pathogenicity, culture, and serology to a genotypic classification of genomospecies based on DNA identification (Greene et al. 2006; Levett 2001). Unfortunately, the molecular methods for genotypic classification of leptospires are not routine, necessitating continued clinical application of serological classification. Both the presence of leptospirosis as well as the prevalence of pathogenic serovars in dogs maintains tremendous geographic variability. The most commonly reported serovars in dogs over the past 10 years in the United States included autumnalis, grippotyphosa, bratislava, and pomona (Adin and Cowgill 2000; Boutilier et al. 2003; Goldstein et al. 2006; Moore et al. 2006; Stokes et al. 2007). The prevalence of leptospirosis has recognized seasonality. It is most typically diagnosed from July through

December in the Northern Hemisphere and from January through June in the Southern Hemisphere, corresponding to warm and wet weather conditions that are favorable for persistence of the organism in the environment (Greene et al. 2006; Rentko et al. 1992; Harkin and Gartrell 1996; Birnbaum et al. 1998; Adin and Cowgill 2000; Levett 2001; Ward 2002; Ward 2002; Ward et al. 2002; Goldstein et al. 2006; Miller et al. 2007).

Leptospiral organisms colonize renal tubules of maintenance hosts and are excreted in the urine to establish a reservoir in the environment. Incidental hosts, like the dog, are exposed to the organism by direct contact with urine, by indirect exposure to urine-contaminated water or soil, or by contact with infected blood or tissues (Levett 2001; Guerra 2009). The organism gains access to the blood stream through mucous membranes or abraded skin. Once they have penetrated, leptospires attach to endothelial cells promoting vascular damage, vasculitis, vascular leakage and hemorrhage, inflammation, and dysregulation of the coagulation system (Guerra 2009). Leptospires circulating in renal capillaries migrate into the interstitium and subsequently invade the tubular epithelial cells. The organism can be detected within tubular epithelium or the tubular lumen by silver staining or immunohistochemical techniques (Wild et al. 2002). Subcellular injury from putative leptospiral toxins causes hepatic dysfunction without major histologic lesions (Greene et al. 2006). The incubation period is approximately 7 days to the onset of early signs which include fever, stiffness, myalgia, vomiting, dehydration, pulmonary fluid exudation or hemorrhage (Figure 49.1),

or shock (Greene et al. 2006). In subacute to chronic stages of the disease, additional signs can include conjunctivitis, uveitis, rhinitis, meningitis, as well as hepatic and renal dysfunction (Adin and Cowgill 2000; Langston and Heuter 2003; Greenlee et al. 2004; Greenlee et al. 2005; Goldstein et al. 2006; Geisen et al. 2007; Mastrorilli et al. 2007; Guerra 2009). The onset of clinical signs can vary depending on host susceptibility and the infecting serovar.

In most studies, the infecting serovar did not determine the spectrum of clinical signs or outcome for survival. In a single study, dogs naturally infected with serovar pomona were more likely to demonstrate vomiting, thrombocytopenia, worse azotemia, and greater mortality than dogs infected with other serovars (Goldstein et al. 2006; Geisen et al. 2007).

Bacterial infection of the kidney (nephritis, pyelonephritis) is caused either by ascending infection from the lower urogenital tract or by hematogenous distribution to the kidneys. Acute pyelonephritis is a bacterial or fungal infection causing patchy or diffuse interstitial inflammation and tubular epithelial necrosis. The most common infecting organism is *E.coli*, but other major isolates include *Staph.* spp., *Proteus*, *Strep.* spp., *Enterococcus* spp., *Klebsiella* spp., and Pseudomonas (Barsanti et al. 1994; Norris et al. 2000; Barsanti 2006; Labato 2009). Host factors that increase the risk for pyelonephritis include structural and anatomic abnormalities of the urinary tract, instrumentation (e.g., catheterization) of the urinary tract, disorders of micturition, impaired immune defenses (e.g.,

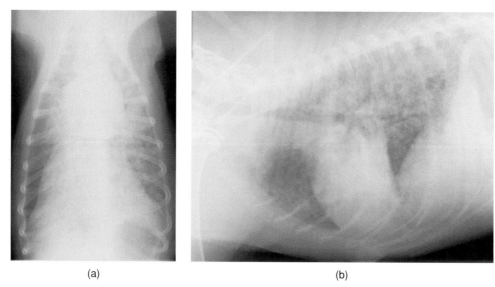

(a)   (b)

Figure 49.1 Uremic lung ventral dorsal (left) and lateral (right) thoracic radiographs of a dog with progressing AKI (Stage IV, O, RRT) secondary to leptospirosis (16-fold increase in MAT titer @ >1:3200 to L. pomona). The radiographic features include diffuse, patchy, heavy, and nodular pulmonary infiltrates with a predominate peribronchial distribution and air brochograms.

diabetes mellitus, hyperadrenocorticism, and immuno-suppressive drug therapy) (Langston and Boyd 2007; Tolkoff-Rubin et al. 2009). Fungal pyelonephritis is less common and may be identified by the presence of yeast or hyphae in the urine, fungal culture, or fungal serology (Day and Holt 1994; Starkey and McLoughlin 1996; Newman et al. 2003; Pressler et al. 2003; Coldrick et al. 2007).

AKI associated with significant proteinuria can occur from a variety of causes. Proteinuria may be renal in origin (i.e., acute tubular injury, or glomerular disease) or from concurrent lower urinary tract infection or inflammation. Chronic glomerular disease is commonly diagnosed only when signs of acute uremia become apparent in later stages, but acute glomerular disease with renal failure can occur with several infectious or inflammatory diseases. *Borrelia burgdorferi* has been associated with a syndrome of glomerular proteinuria and ARF that is often fatal within 1–2 weeks (Dambach et al. 1997; Littman 2003; Hutton et al. 2008). Although Borrelia organisms have not been definitively identified in the kidney, an antibody-antigen immune reaction may be involved in the pathogenesis (Hutton et al. 2008). The cause of cutaneous and glomerular vasculopathy in Greyhounds ("Alabama Rot") is unknown; the renal lesions are similar to hemolytic-uremic syndrome in humans which is caused by shiga-toxin producing strains of *E. coli* (Cowan et al. 1997). Acute infection with *Ehrlichia canis* can cause proteinuria and minimal change glomerulopathy (Codner et al. 1992; Cohn 2003). A severe acute glomerulonephritis can be seen in dogs with Leishmaniasis, a protozoan infection transmitted by bites of the sand fly. The organism invades macrophages, and the disease involves multiple organs such as spleen, liver, lymph nodes, bone marrow, kidneys, and skin (Lopez-Pena et al. 2009). Moderate to severe proteinuria and glomerular lesions are encountered commonly, although tubular and interstitial lesions may also be seen (Zaragoza et al. 2003; Zatelli et al. 2003). Death from renal failure is a common outcome (Zatelli et al. 2003).

Obstruction or diversion of urine flow can lead to acute azotemia. Urinary obstruction decreases GFR by a combination of neurohumoral events and increased back-pressure in the kidney. An increase in intratubular pressure from the obstruction disrupts the balance of hydrostatic and oncotic pressures that determine glomerular ultrafiltration leading to the decrease in GFR. The azotemia usually resolves promptly after reestablishing urine flow, but temporary or permanent renal damage may develop if repair is delayed. Common causes of urethral obstruction include urolithiasis, mucus plugs, blood clots, neoplasia, or stricture and may be treated on an emergency basis by placement of a urethral catheter

or cystostomy tube. Rupture of the urinary system also causes azotemia that rapidly reverses if managed by correction or urinary diversion (i.e., urethral catheter to bypass the rupture, peritoneal drain, or surgical repair). Ureteral obstruction may cause acute severe azotemia, and currently it is the most common etiology of AKI in cats treated with hemodialysis. The incidence of ureteral calculi in cats has increased over the past decade, and the majority (98%) of these calculi are composed of calcium oxalate (Kyles et al. 2005; Kyles and Westropp 2009). Other causes of ureteral obstruction include dried solidified blood clots, pyelonephritis debris, and stricture formation (Westropp et al. 2006; Kyles and Westropp 2009). For acute azotemia to develop, there must be bilateral obstruction, obstruction of a solitary kidney, or unilateral ureteral obstruction and a contralateral nonfunctional kidney (either from preexisting chronic disease or acute concurrent disease such as pyelonephritis).

Pathophysiology of AKI

Phases of AKI

AKI can be categorized into four pathophysiologic phases: the initiation phase, the extension phase, the maintenance phase, and recovery. The **initiation phase** begins with the renal insult (e.g., ischemic, nephrotoxic, obstructive) and continues until there is a definable change in renal function such as decreased urine output or azotemia. The length of time necessary to develop a recognizable clinical change is variable and depends on the nature and severity of the insult (Finn 2001). During this phase, early intervention has the greatest potential to alter the progression and severity of the renal injury, but clinical signs are often not apparent and conventional biomarkers are too insensitive to reveal the injury or to prompt intervention.

Next is the **extension phase**, during which the injury is perpetuated by inducible events associated with continued hypoxia or inflammatory responses that propagate damage to the kidney in concert with or independently of the initiating insult (Figure 49.2 and 49.3) (Sutton et al. 2002). Cortical (proximal tubules) and outer medullary (pars recta, medullary thick ascending limb of Henle's loop) structures are predisposed to toxic and ischemic damage because they receive 90% of renal blood flow, are highly metabolic, and have high energy requirements. Intrarenal vasoconstriction and capillary obstruction, hypoperfusion, and hypoxia in the extension phase decrease ATP concentration in sensitive epithelia, impair Na^+K^+ ATPase activity, and trigger cellular swelling and apoptotic and necrotic cell death (Padanilam 2003). Less severely affected epithelial cells undergo loss of the

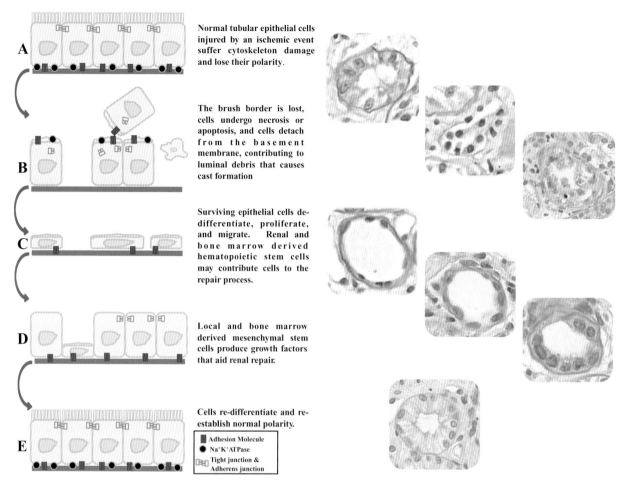

Figure 49.2 (Left) Schematic representation of the progressive pathophysiologic events affecting renal tubular epithelial cells during ischemic acute kidney injury. (Right) Renal histopathological in a dog with acute kidney injury of undetermined cause in various stages of injury and repair demonstrating each category of events portrayed in the schematic illustration (PAS, magnification 40×).

brush border at the apical cell surface, loss of cellular polarization, and cellular detachment from the basement membrane (Racusen 2001; Padanilam 2003). These sublethal cellular injuries may trigger intrinsic pathways to initiate necrotic or apoptotic cell death or intrinsic cellular protections may block these programmed events and spare the cell. Intervention during this phase may or may not be successful depending on the extent of epithelial damage, cellular targets for the intervention, and the timing of the pathologic events.

The third phase is the *maintenance phase,* which generally lasts from 1 to 3 weeks but varies greatly in duration (Finn 2001; Clarkson et al. 2008). Urine output during this phase can be increased or decreased, and the urine resembles the glomerular ultrafiltrate with little modification by tubular processes. In this phase, a critical amount of parenchymal damage has occurred which may not be reversible.

The fourth phase, the *recovery phase*, is the interval in which the renal parenchymal damage is being repaired (Figure 49.2). In oliguric or anuric animals, this phase is heralded by an increase in urine output that is accompanied variably by a decrease in urine sodium concentration. In these animals, sodium losses may be extreme causing profound volume depletion which can delay or interrupt renal recovery or even cause additional renal injury (Finn 2001; Cowgill and Francey 2005; Liu and Brakeman 2008; Langston 2010). In nonoliguric animals, a change in urine output may not be a useful indicator of recovery. Instead, decreases in BUN, creatinine, or urea appearance as predictors of improved renal clearance, or increases in urine concentration and decreases in sodium excretion, as evidence of improved tubular function, mark the recovery phase. Regeneration and repair of the renal damage may take weeks to months.

Cellular mechanisms of ischemic AKI

Cellular damage involves three forms of injury: sublethal damage, apoptosis, and necrosis (Padanilam 2003; Liu and Brakeman 2008). Although AKI is commonly called acute tubular necrosis, necrosis is not the prominent

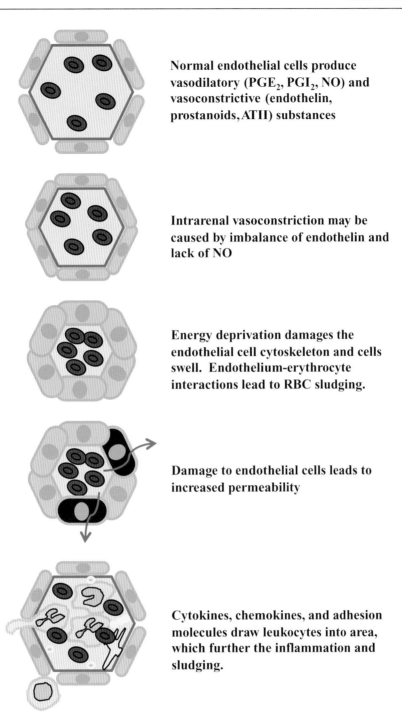

Normal endothelial cells produce vasodilatory (PGE_2, PGI_2, NO) and vasoconstrictive (endothelin, prostanoids, ATII) substances

Intrarenal vasoconstriction may be caused by imbalance of endothelin and lack of NO

Energy deprivation damages the endothelial cell cytoskeleton and cells swell. Endothelium-erythrocyte interactions lead to RBC sludging.

Damage to endothelial cells leads to increased permeability

Cytokines, chemokines, and adhesion molecules draw leukocytes into area, which further the inflammation and sludging.

Figure 49.3 Schematic representation of the responses of renal vascular endothelial cells to ischemic acute kidney injury; see text for detailed discussion.

histologic feature (Racusen 2001; Padanilam 2003). A patchy distribution of tubular foci with degenerative and apoptotic, and less commonly necrotic, damage occurs throughout the kidney with minimal interstitial inflammatory infiltrates (Racusen 2001). Proximal tubular cells at the corticomedullary junction and outer medulla and are most severely affected by ischemia and hypoxia. These cells are at greatest risk because of their high oxygen and energy requirements and the marginal perfusion of the microvasculature in this region during the initiation and extension phases of AKI (Padanilam 2003; Clarkson et al. 2008). The vulnerability of different nephron segments to energy deprivation varies along the nephron causing some segments to undergo necrotic cell death, others to undergo apoptosis, and still others to be only sublethally injured. A variety of disorders of cellular metabolism contribute to the mechanisms promoting irreversible cell death or sublethal epithelial and endothelial damage.

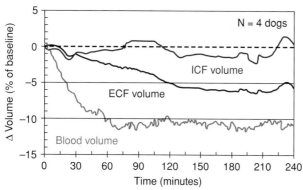

Figure 49.4 Effects of furosemide on changes in fluid volume in normal dogs. Mean changes (% of baseline) in blood volume (red), extracellular fluid volume (ECF volume, blue), and intracellular fluid volume (ICF volume, magenta) in response to intravenous administration of furosemide at 4 mg/kg (time, 0) to 4 clinically normal dogs. Change in blood volume was measured b optically every 20 seconds by an in-line hematocrit monitor, and ECF and ICF volumes were determined every 5–10 seconds with multifrequency bioimpedance spectroscopy. Blood volume is affected disproportionately and most severely by the diuretic response during the 4 hours of observation.

Under conditions of oxygen deprivation, ATP is depleted leading to an energy deficit in the cell and disruption of ATP mediated processes. Prolonged ischemia and depletion of ATP will cause relocation of membrane-associated proteins and transporters, alterations in cellular polarity, perturbations in cytosolic composition, and mitochondrial damage further impairing the ability to regenerate ATP (Bonventre 2003; Devarajan 2006; Bonventre 2007; Kosieradzki and Rowinski 2008). Decreased activity of Na^+K^+ ATPase dissipates the Na^+ and K^+ concentration gradients across the cell. The accumulation of cytosolic Na^+ and water causes cellular swelling which can initiate necrotic cell death (Padanilam 2003). Swelling of the tubular epithelium and vascular endothelium causes tubular obstruction and vascular congestion, respectively (Figure 49.3 and 49.4). These events compromise tubular fluid flow and reperfusion of the oxygen-sensitive parenchyma (Bonventre and Weinberg 2003; Goligorsky et al. 2004; Versteilen et al. 2004; Tumlin 2009).

The role of increased cytosolic free calcium in the cellular events of AKI is multifactorial. Cytosolic calcium concentration increases substantially in energy depleted states because of impaired activity of intracellular calcium transporters (Finn 2001). This promotes mitochondria uptake of calcium, leading to mitochondrial swelling and uncoupling of oxidative phosphorylation. Calcium channel blockers, especially diltiazem and verapamil, ameliorate AKI if given to kidney transplant donor and recipient (Finn 2001). The effects of calcium channel blockers

are not due entirely to preservation of cytosolic calcium. They improved renal hemodynamics and stabilized cell membranes. Other factors that contribute to ischemic damage on a cellular basis are reperfusion injury, oxidant injury, intracellular acidosis, phospholipase activation, and protease activation (Racusen 2001; Padanilam 2003; Devarajan 2006; Clarkson et al. 2008; Garwood 2009).

Ischemia leads to an inflammatory response in the kidney by three mechanisms: ATP depletion, increased hypoxia inducible factor (HIF), and increased reactive oxygen molecule species (Bonventre and Weinberg 2003; Bonventre and Zuk 2004; Furuichi et al. 2009). Depletion of ATP during renal ischemia causes mitochondrial damage and a resultant increase in production of inflammatory cytokines and reactive oxygen species (Figure 49.2) (Segerer et al. 2000; Bonventre and Zuk 2004; Clarkson et al. 2008; Andreoli 2009). These cytokines induce chemokines which attract macrophages, polymorphonuclear leukocytes, and T lymphocyte cells. In a positive feedback loop, the recruited inflammatory cells then generate more cytokines and reactive oxygen species, exacerbating the inflammatory response and causing further tissue injury to both tubular epithelial cells and the vascular endothelium (Heinzelmann et al. 1999; Nath and Norby 2000; Bonventre and Zuk 2004; Grigoryev et al. 2008; Garwood 2009).

Ischemic vascular endothelial cells express a variety of adhesion molecules including intercellular adhesion molecule-1 (ICAM-1), P-selectin, and E-selectin. These events lead to adhesion of leukocytes and platelets to the endothelium, which further diminishes flow in the peritubular capillaries and promotes further ischemia and hypoxia in the oxygen deprived and metabolically sensitive regions of the outer medulla. Disruption of endothelial integrity may also account for fibrin deposits in the renal microvasculature (Devarajan 2006; Devarajan 2009). Endothelium-erythrocyte interactions lead to sludging of red blood cells in peritubular capillaries, further limiting the delivery of oxygen to the tubules (Mason et al. 1987; Hellberg et al. 1991; Yamamoto et al. 2002; Clarkson et al. 2008).

Normal cells have poised apoptotic machinery which is disengaged by regulatory survival factors. If no survival factors are present due to cellular injury, apoptosis is triggered to promote cell death (Liu and Brakeman 2008). In response to ischemia, hypoxic renal tubular cells upregulate HIF genes in addition to other cell survival gene targets to oppose apoptotic damage. Failure of the upregulation of HIF is associated with lethal cellular damage (apoptotic cell death). Erythropoietin (EPO) is one of the transcriptional gene targets of stabilized HIF which is responsible in part for its anti-apoptotic effects. It is therefore possible that therapeutic intervention with HIF or EPO can ameliorate apoptotic damage to the tubular epithelium and protect the kidney against ischemic injury (Gong et al. 2004; Patel et al. 2004; Sharples et al. 2004; Clarkson et al. 2008; Hill et al. 2008a; Rosen and Stillman 2008; Weidemann et al. 2008; Lee et al. 2009).

Tubular epithelial dysfunction and endothelial dysfunction both contribute to the reduction in GFR and renal blood flow associated with ischemic renal injury. Under normal circumstances, tubular production of prostaglandins (such as prostacyclin) mediates vasodilatation of the afferent arteriole, which decreases renal vascular resistance and helps maintain renal blood flow (Andreoli 2009). In addition tubular generation of angiotensin II increases efferent arteriolar resistance to maintain intraglomerular pressure and ultrafiltration. (Andreoli 2009) Renal vascular endothelial cells release a variety of counter-regulatory vasoactive products including vasodilatory factors (nitric oxide, prostaglandin E2, and prostacyclin) and vasoconstrictive factors (endothelin, prostanoids, and components of the renin-angiotensin system) capable of overriding the normal regulation of vascular tone. The increased vascular resistance, characteristic of AKI, may be due to an imbalance in these opposing factors to favor vasoconstriction (Garwood 2009). Endothelial nitric oxide synthase (eNOS) function is decreased with hypoxic/ischemic renal damage reducing nitric oxide-mediated vasodilation and facilitating vasoconstriction. In contrast, inducible nitric oxide synthase (iNOS) is increased. iNOS generates reactive oxygen and nitrogen molecules that may participate in toxic damage to the tubules (Goligorsky et al. 2002; Goligorsky et al. 2004; Andreoli 2009). Some agents, such as endothelin, angiotensin-II, and adenosine, have diverse effects promoting cortical vasoconstriction and vasodilation in the medullary microcirculation, depending on the type and density of their vascular receptors (Ruschitzka et al. 1999; Wilhelm et al. 1999; Conger 2001; Sutton et al. 2002).

Changes in vasomotor tone of the vasculature impact oxygen delivery to regional tubular segments. The proximal tubule has a constant workload and constant energy and oxygen requirement is normally supplied with a high pO_2 content (Brezis and Rosen 1995). Damage to the proximal tubule is related to decreased oxygen delivery rather than increased metabolic demand. The outer medulla normally exists in a state of chronic oxygen deprivation, despite the high metabolic demands and energy expenditure of this region due to the activity of the basolateral Na^+K^+ ATPase pumps in the pars recta (S3 segment) of the proximal tubule and medullary ascending thick loop of Henle (mTAL) (Brezis and Rosen 1995; Lameire et al. 2005; Clarkson et al. 2008). The distal tubule also operates in a quasi-oxygen deprived setting and has a variable workload dependent on GFR, proximal tubule solute reabsorption, and distal delivery of solute. The disproportionate ischemic damage to tubular segments in the outer medulla including the pars recta and the mTAL and distal tubule reflects this regional imbalance of oxygen delivery and oxygen demand during ischemia.

The actin cytoskeleton plays an important role in renal cell function and cytoskeletal injury during energy depletion and is an important and consistent feature of ischemic AKI (Racusen 2001; Devarajan 2006). The normal reabsorption and unidirectional transport of sodium depends on cell polarity. With ATP depletion, disruption of actin cytoskeleton impairs the fence function of junctional complexes which normally prevent migration of certain membrane-imbedded structures including solute transporters and pumps and integrins (molecules that mediate cell-cell and cell-basement membrane adhesion). This membrane disorientation results in loss of polarity of epithelial cells in the proximal tubule which may be reversible with reestablishment of the cytoskeleton. Sodium/potassium ATPase pumps remain functional but are redistributed from basolateral to apical membrane disrupting transepithelial solute and sodium reabsorption from the tubular lumen.

The structural integrity of the microvilli of the proximal tubular brush border is disrupted by damage to the actin core bundle. This causes sloughing of the microvilli and intrabubular obstruction by fragments of brush border in more distal segments. The actin cytoskeleton also plays an important role to limit paracellular reabsorption at the junction complexes between epithelial cells. Ischemic injury to the cytoskeleton increases permeability of tight junctions permitting back-leakage of glomerular filtrate which contributes to the oliguria. Disrupted cell-substrate attachment from damage to the cytoskeleton and integrins leads to denudement of cells from basement membrane (Figure 49.2). This allows more back-leakage of glomerular filtrate, loss of tight junction complex function, sloughing of cells into the tubular lumen, and necrotic cell death. Adhesion of detached renal epithelial cells to sublethally injured cells still attached to basement membrane causes aggregation of detached cells within the lumen, causing cast formation and tubular obstruction (Devarajan 2006).

In addition to the fall in GFR, the ability of the kidney to concentrate urine diminishes during ischemic AKI due to loss of aquaporin water channels and dissipation of the medullary solute gradient. Treatment with EPO or alpha-melanocyte stimulating hormone has been shown to help normalize aquaporin expression (Kwon et al. 1999; Gong et al. 2004).

Pathophysiology of nephrotoxic AKI

The kidney is predisposed to nephrotoxic damage because its rich blood supply enhances delivery of toxins for filtration and exposure to the tubular epithelium. In addition, the kidney metabolizes many drugs and xenobiotics (i.e., ethylene glycol) and in the process may transform a relatively harmless parent compound into a toxic metabolite (Clarkson et al. 2008). Nephrotoxic acute injury can be mediated via altered renal hemodynamics, allergic interstitial inflammation, direct tubular epithelial toxicity, vascular injury, intratubular obstruction, or osmotic nephrosis. The toxicity of many substances is increased in the presence of borderline or overt renal ischemia (Clarkson et al. 2008; Evenepoel 2009). NSAIDs inhibit prostaglandin mediated dilation of the afferent arteriole and cause a functional increase in renal vascular resistance and decrease in renal blood flow and GFR. In contrast, ACE inhibitors and angiotensin receptor antagonists alter renal hemodynamics primarily by promoting efferent arteriolar vasodilation, decreased glomerular capillary hydrostatic pressure and GFR. Calcineurin inhibitors (e.g., cyclosporine) cause afferent arteriolar constriction through a vasoconstrictive imbalance of prostaglandin E2 (vasodilation) and thromboxane A2 (vasoconstriction) mediated vascular resistances (Olyaei et al. 2001). Radiocontrast agents are postulated to cause AKI by a combination of vasoconstriction and direct tubular toxicity due to generation of reactive oxygen species (Solomon 1998; Heyman and Rosen 2003; Heyman et al. 2008). Hypercalcemia and amphotericin causes vasoconstriction (Deray 2002; Schenck et al. 2006). Acute allergic interstitial nephritis is an idiosyncratic, hapten-mediated allergic reaction to a wide variety of drugs that is typically not dose related. Mechanisms include production of antibodies that cross-reacts with intrinsic ligands in the kidney or deposition of antibody-antigen complexes in the renal interstitium (Michel and Kelly 1998). Acute interstitial nephritis is rarely recognized in veterinary patients (Hadrick et al. 1996).

Direct toxic effect to tubular cell function by the nephrotoxin or the formation of reactive oxygen species is the major mechanism of nephrotoxic injuries (Nath and Norby 2000; Rumbeiha and Murphy 2009). Intracellular concentrations of the toxic substance determine toxicity. Small, poorly protein bound toxins such as aminoglycosides or ethylene glycol are freely filtered at the glomerulus and are typically eliminated in the urine. The proximal tubular reabsorption of toxins or drugs by the brush border leads to their intracellular accumulation. The proximal tubule also actively secretes many protein-bound substances via various transcellular organic anion or cation transport mechanisms which leads to their cellular accumulation.

Some drugs including antineoplastics, immunotherapeutics, and antiplatelet agents induce a thrombotic microangiopathy causing embolic ischemia in the kidney (Medina et al. 2001; Dlott et al. 2004; Zakarija and Bennett 2005). Intratubular obstruction from solute precipitation or crystal formation may occur with acyclovir, sulfonamides, methotrexate, indinavir, triamterene, and melamine/cyanuric acid (Perazella 1999; Cianciolo et al. 2008). Single nephron glomerular filtration is impaired in the obstructed tubules causing cumulative filtration failure of the entire kidney. The intraluminal compound may secondarily induce localized toxicity to the tubular epithelium (i.e., calcium oxalate and melamine-cyanuric acid). Osmotic nephrosis occurs when a hyperoncotic substance is transported into the proximal tubule cells by pinocytosis and induces severe cellular swelling. It has been recognized in humans exposed to sucrose, mannitol, intravenous immunoglobulin, radiocontrast agents, dextran, and hydroxyethyl starch (Markowitz and Perazella 2005; Evenepoel 2009).

Renal recovery

Renal recovery depends on the normalization of sublethally injured cells with realignment of polarity, migration of viable cells to gaps on the basement membrane, removal of necrotic cells and intratubular casts, and regeneration of renal cells and repopulation of the tubular epithelium (Racusen 2001; Clarkson et al. 2008). Why some cells escape lethal damage from apoptosis and necrosis is unclear, but may be mediated by heat shock proteins in addition to up-regulation of other cellular protections (Kelly 2005; Riordan et al. 2005; Devarajan 2009). Dedifferentiation of surviving renal tubular epithelial cells that subsequently proliferate and migrate to the denuded areas of the basement membrane is the main method of renal repair (Bonventre 2003; Duffield et al. 2005; Clarkson et al. 2008; Devarajan 2009). These "recovery cells" express vimentin, which is normally found in undifferentiated mesenchymal cells but not differentiated kidney cells, and proliferating cell nuclear antigen, a marker of mitogenic activity (Liu and Brakeman 2008; Devarajan 2009).

These intrinsic surviving cells are crucial to tubular regeneration, but undifferentiated stem cells may also participate in tubular regeneration. Renal progenitor stem cells potentially reside in the renal papillae and can migrate, proliferate, differentiate, and contribute to renal repair (Oliver et al. 2004; Clarkson et al. 2008). Bone marrow-derived hematopoietic stem cells have been shown to migrate from the bone marrow and differentiate into renal tubular cells, but their exact role in renal recovery is uncertain (Kale et al. 2003; Lin et al. 2003; Clarkson et al. 2008). Infusion of mesenchymal stem cells can provide renoprotection (Lange et al. 2005). However, the effects may be related to beneficial paracrine effects (i.e., production of survival or growth factors) rather than direct contribution to the repopulation of new epithelial cells (Krause and Cantley 2005; Togel et al. 2005; Lin 2006; Liu and Brakeman 2008). Epidermal growth factor, insulin-like growth factor-1, α-melanocyte stimulating hormone, EPO, hepatocyte growth factor, bone morphogenetic protein-7, and transforming growth factor-β play undefined roles in renal recovery and are under active investigation as interventions to treat AKI.

Instead of regeneration of the tubular epithelium and renal recovery, the pathologic events can progress to interstitial fibrosis, the prominent feature of the transition to CKD. Transforming growth factor (TGF)-β and platelet derived growth factor (PDGF) are known to induce fibrosis in a variety of organs including the kidney. Tubular epithelial cells, fibroblasts, and infiltrating inflammatory cells provide rich sources of TGF-β and PDGF (Furuichi et al. 2009).

Diagnosis of AKI

The clinical presentation of AKI is influenced by the underlying etiology and severity of the renal injury, the duration of the disorder, previous therapy, and comorbid diseases predisposing or complicating the renal injury. The spectrum of clinical signs ranges from inapparent to profound. The diagnosis is generally founded on the finding of progressive azotemia, alterations of urine composition, and altered renal imaging. As currently conceived, AKI spans a spectrum of conventional syndromes including (1) hemodynamic failure (prerenal azotemia), (2) hemodynamic failure complicating CKD, (3) acute (parenchymal or intrinsic) renal failure, (4) hemodynamic failure complicating ARF, (5) acute exacerbation of CKD, and (6) postrenal azotemia. Each of these disparate azotemic conditions may appear quite similar and must be further differentiated on the basis of a comprehensive clinical assessment which includes: past and present history of the illness, physical examination, laboratory testing, diagnostic imaging, histopathology, and special diagnostic testing.

History

AKI is characterized by a sudden onset of azotemia or illness of less than a week's duration; however, animals with acute uremia secondary to underlying urinary or systemic diseases may have a longer duration of documented ill-

ness. It is rare to capture the onset of AKI in animals prior to development of overt azotemia unless a progressive increase in serum creatinine or decrease in urine output develops in a hospital setting. Signs consistent with AKI include: listlessness, depression, anorexia, vomiting, diarrhea, and weakness. Less commonly, seizures, syncope, bradycardia, ataxia, and dyspnea may be reported. Thorough questioning of owners may reveal relevant exposure to nephrotoxic chemicals or plants, new environments, ill animals, traumatic events, recent surgery, diagnostic testing, newly prescribed medications, supplements and diets, or blood loss (Table 49.2). Owners should be questioned about the use of holistic and herbal therapies that may contain nephrotoxic substances. Oliguria or anuria are seminal features of some stages of AKI, but a history of normal or increased urine production does not exclude its diagnosis. Historical weight loss, polyuria, polydipsia, nocturia or isosthenuria, or laboratory evidence of preexisting azotemia suggests underlying CKD. It is common for animals with asymptomatic stages of CKD to decompensate suddenly, following subtle insults including fever, concomitant disease, vomiting, diarrhea, congestive heart failure, hypovolemia, hypotension, and drug administration, resulting in an uremic crisis that appears acute in onset and course.

Physical examination

Physical examination provides an important window to the localization, extent, and cause of AKI. Due to the sudden onset of the disease, most animals have good body composition and coat condition. Poor body composition should raise suspicion for decompensation of preexisting kidney disease (acute-on-chronic kidney disease). In the absence of hemorrhage or hemolysis, mucous membrane color is pink in contrast to animals with CKD or acute-on-chronic disease who may have pale mucous membranes. Dehydration is common at first presentation and may manifest as prolonged capillary refill time, dry mucous membranes, decreased skin turgor, sunken eyes, tachycardia, poor pulse quality, and hypotension. Animals who have received parenteral fluid therapy are often overhydrated with characteristic wet mucous membranes, serous nasal discharge, increased skin turgor and weight, peripheral edema, tachypnea, dyspnea, muffled heart sounds, hypertension, chemosis, and ascites. Measurement of arterial blood pressure is essential in every animal with AKI to determine if hypotension that demands immediate attention is a cause or contributor to the onset of kidney injury.

Depression, hypothermia, oral ulceration, "uremic breath", bile-stained fur, scleral injection, cutaneous bruising, discoloration or necrosis of the tongue, tachycardia or bradycardia, tachypnea, muscle fascicu-lations, and seizures are consistent findings in animals with advanced stages of AKI. These signs become more profound as the severity of azotemia and stage of AKI increases. Hypothermia that is inversely proportional to the degree of azotemia is an expected finding in animals with BUN concentrations greater than 100 mg/dL (Ash 1991). A normal or slightly elevated body temperature is inappropriate for azotemic animals and should be con-sidered a fever, prompting evaluation for an underlying infectious or inflammatory condition.

Asymmetric kidneys (either enlarged or small) are consistent features of ureteral obstruction in cats. Bilater-ally enlarged, firm, slightly resilient, and/or painful kid-neys may be indicative of acute nephritis or nephrosis or bilateral ureteral obstruction. Enlarged kidneys must be differentiated from neoplasia, amyloidosis, perinephric pseudocysts, or polycystic kidney disease.

The size of the urinary bladder varies depending on urine production and the integrity of the outflow tract. An undetectable urinary bladder may indicate oliguria or anuria from severe AKI, bilateral ureteral obstruc-tion, or rupture of the bladder. An enlarged, firm, and painful bladder is indicative of lower urinary outflow obstruction.

AKI often occurs in animals with comorbid condi-tions that contribute to the presenting clinical signs and may over shadow the characteristic signs of AKI. Lame-ness, icterus, fever, discolored urine, back or flank pain, petechiae, dyspnea, edema, and dysuria are associated with some etiologies of AKI.

Laboratory assessment

The initial laboratory assessment should include a com-plete blood count, comprehensive biochemical profile (serum creatinine, urea, phosphate, calcium, bicarbon-ate, sodium, potassium, chloride, glucose, albumin, glob-ulin, hepatic transaminases, and bilirubin), complete urinalysis, urine protein/creatinine ratio, and urine cul-ture. The laboratory features of AKI change rapidly and selected chemistries should be evaluated daily to iden-tify new clinical problems, reassess the stage of AKI, and direct therapy.

Complete blood count

The complete blood count may reflect abnormalities caused by primary or comorbid conditions which have diagnostic relevance, but the findings are rarely specific to AKI. Typically, the complete blood count reveals nor-mal red cell parameters (RBC count, hematocrit or PCV, hemoglobin concentration) unless influenced by con-current hydration or acute blood loss (e.g., gastrointesti-nal hemorrhage). Dehydration and hemoconcentration will overestimate actual RBC mass, and overhydration and excessive fluid administration cause hemodilution which underestimates RBC mass (Chew 2000). An ane-mia that is non-regenerative suggests underlying CKD, but patients with AKI that are anemic may not have evi-dence of regeneration due to the lag time (3–5 days) for reticulocytes to appear in the circulation after acute blood loss. Erythropoietic response may be blunted from the AKI or coexisting inflammatory conditions (Eckardt 2002; Liangos et al. 2003; Hoste and De Waele 2005).

Serum chemistry profile

Progressive (and often subtle) azotemia is the hallmark of AKI, but the progressive component is observed incon-sistently in animals because of variations in the stage and chronicity of disease at presentation. Serum crea-tinine increases proportionally with the severity of the renal injury or completeness of urinary outflow obstruc-tion. Reductions in lean body mass, creatinine gener-ation, and overhydration can lower the serum creati-nine concentration and over estimate true renal func-tion (Braun et al. 2003; Laroute et al. 2005; Le Garreres et al. 2007). There is a curvilinear inverse relationship between serum creatinine and GFR (Finco 1995; Braun et al. 2003). Incremental changes in serum creatinine are small in AKI Stage I and II despite significant changes in GFR (Lees 2004). Notwithstanding the insensitivity and limitations of serum creatinine as a biomarker of kidney injury, it currently stands as the best, most time-tested, and most familiar clinical marker of AKI. BUN concen-tration increases with decreases in renal function, but unlike creatinine, urea is influenced by numerous extra renal factors which make its concentration less specific as a marker of kidney damage.

Urea appearance, the net rate of urea accumulation in the body from its generation, distribution and removal, is influenced by exogenous and endogenous protein metabolism, hepatic function, hydration status, urine production, and diuretic therapy in addition to its resid-ual renal clearance (Depner 2005; Israni and Kasiske 2008). These global influences on serum urea concen-tration make it a useful predictor of the overall clinical severity of the uremic state (renal function, catabolism, nutritional adequacy). Urea also functions as a surrogate marker for the production and removal of a variety of low molecular weight nitrogenous uremia toxins which contribute to uremia (Depner 2001).

AKI produces characteristic perturbations in serum phosphate, calcium, electrolytes, and bicarbonate as the stage of the disease increases; however, for compara-ble degrees of azotemia the changes are usually more profound than seen with CKD. Over 75% of dogs and cats with AKI are hyperphosphatemic at presentation (Vaden et al. 1997; Worwag and Langston 2008). Total serum calcium concentrations are below the reference range in 25% of dogs with AKI, but the proportion with hypocalcemia increases to 50% in animals with acute ethylene glycol intoxication (Thrall et al. 1984; Vaden et al. 1997). Signs of hypocalcemia (i.e., muscle fasciculation, and tetany) rarely develop or require treatment with calcium. Total calcium is a poor predictor of ionized calcium in dogs with CKD, and approximately 1/3 of dogs with CKD have ionized hypocalcemia (Schenck and Chew 2005; Kogika et al. 2006). Reports of ionized calcium concentrations are not available for dogs and cats with AKI.

Serum potassium concentration varies with the stage and etiology of the disease, the extent of vomiting, and fluid and diuretic administration. Serum potassium is typically increased (between 5.5 and 9.0 mEq/L) in proportion to the stage of AKI, and tends to be higher in animals with anuric AKI or urinary outflow obstruction compared to those with nonoliguric AKI. Serum bicarbonate concentration generally decreases, and the bicarbonate deficit increases with increasing stages of AKI. Profuse vomiting, dehydration, or previous bicarbonate administration may cause metabolic alkalosis that is atypical for the severity of disease.

Urine evaluation

A complete urinalysis should be performed on every patient at initial presentation. Both renal concentrating and diluting capabilities become impaired in the early phases of intrinsic AKI, and urine specific gravity becomes "fixed" in the range between 1.008 and 1.018. A urine specific gravity >1.030 for dogs or >1.035 for cats in the presence of azotemia indicates hemodynamic (prerenal) failure (Osborne et al. 1995). A urine specific gravity between 1.012–1.029 (dogs) or 1.012–1.034 (cats) associated with azotemia is consistent with a hemodynamic component superimposed on intrinsic renal insufficiency or an underlying urine concentrating defect. Glucosuria in the absence of hyperglycemia is an important sign of proximal tubular dysfunction. It predicts tubular necrosis and is a useful discriminator between intrinsic AKI and other types of acute or chronic uremia (Vaden et al. 1997). Qualitative (dipstick) proteinuria is detected in most uremic animals but has little discriminatory importance (Vaden et al. 1997). Overt proteinuria associated with a urine protein:creatinine ratio greater than six alerts to the possibility of a primary glomerular injury.

The urine sediment examination may demonstrate red blood cells, white blood cell, casts, crystals, yeast, fungi, or bacteria that identify the etiology of the uremia and should be performed routinely on freshly obtained urine. Urinary casts are formed within the tubular lumen and are indicative of tubular injury. Urinary casts are classified according to their material content and state of maturation (or decomposition) as: hyaline, epithelial, granular, fatty, waxy, or red or white blood cell. Granular and hyaline casts document active renal pathology with epithelial cell shedding or necrosis and protein (glomerular) leakage, respectively. Casts are detected in approximately 30% of dogs with AKI, but their absence does not exclude the diagnosis of acute parenchymal injury (Vaden et al. 1997). A variety of crystals are found in the urine sediment of dogs and cats, and most urinary crystals can be identified in clinically normal animals. Heavy calcium oxalate crystalluria is highly suggestive of ethylene glycol intoxication, calcium oxalate urolithiasis, or oxalate nephrosis in cats. (Grauer et al. 1984; Thrall et al. 1984; Gregory et al. 1993; Osborne et al. 1995; Thrall et al. 1998; Cianciolo et al. 2008; Langston et al. 2008) Green-brown globular crystals have been recognized in animals' exposure to melamine and cyanuric acid (Cianciolo et al. 2008).

The tubular epithelial enzymes, gamma-glutamyl transpeptidase (GGT) and N-acetyl-beta-D-glucosaminidase (NAG), have been measured in canine urine to predict cellular leakage and early tubular injury or necrosis (Grauer et al. 1995; Rivers et al. 1996; Palacio et al. 1997; Clemo 1998; Heiene et al. 2001; Brunker et al. 2009). Of these, NAG appears to be more sensitive and specific for epithelial injury and early recognition of renal damage, but neither has been adopted widely in veterinary or human diagnostics. Newer and more specific biomarkers, including urine kidney injury molecule (KIM)-1, interleukin-18, and neutrophil gelatinase associated lipocalin (NGAL) are under evaluation and may prove to be of more diagnostic utility (Bonventre 2008; Coca et al. 2008; Waikar and Bonventre 2008; Haase et al. 2009; Vaidya et al. 2009).

Renal imaging

Radiography and ultrasonography are highly complementary imaging modalities, and both are indicated in the evaluation of AKI. Ultrasonography provides greater delineation of renal structure, intrarenal architecture, parenchymal consistency, and outflow integrity than survey radiography. Ultrasonic imaging facilitates percutaneous needle aspiration and biopsy procedures for collection of specimens for cytology, culture, biochemical analysis, and histopathology (Borjesson 2003). Duplex

Doppler ultrasonography can be used to verify regional blood flow in the kidney and to predict changes in vascular impedance which may correspond to stages in the pathogenesis or repair of renal injury or outflow obstruction (Rivers et al. 1997; Rivers et al. 1997; Choi et al. 2003; Novellas et al. 2007). Ultrasographic imaging can provide immediate confirmation of ureteral obstruction or pre-existing renal disease.

For the diagnosis of ureteral obstruction in cats, good quality survey radiographs may be more sensitive and predictive than ultrasonography by revealing discrete radiodensities in the retroperitoneal space and should be performed in all cats with unexplained AKI. In 20–30% of cats with ureteral obstruction, no calcific material is identified with either ultrasound or survey radiographs (Kyles et al. 2005). For these circumstances and for cases with multiple sites of obstruction or stenosis, antegrade pyelography or computed tomography with contrast can be used to define the indication and location for surgical intervention. Antegrade pyelography combines ultrasound or fluoroscopic-guided pyelocentesis and antegrade injection of positive radiographic contrast media into the renal pelvis and ureter to delineate the size and patency of the ureter. Antegrade pyelograpy reliably confirms the presence, degree and location of ureteral obstructions (Rivers et al. 1997; Adin et al. 2003). Computed tomography with contrast is less invasive than antegrade pyelography and is potentially superior at confirming mineralized uroliths and the differential patency of the ureters. This is especially useful for cats with bilateral ureteroliths or multiple sites of obstruction along a ureter which antegrade pyelography would fail to document. Other imaging modalities including excretory urography, renal scintigraphy, and magnetic resonance imaging may have indications in selected patients but are not used routinely for AKI.

Renal pathology

Percutaneous or laparoscopic needle biopsy techniques can be performed in both dogs and cats with sedation or light anesthesia (Osborne et al. 1996; Rawlings et al. 2003; Vaden et al. 2005). However, routine kidney biopsy of patients presenting with AKI is likely unjustified to establish a diagnosis. Renal biopsy should be considered if the definitive cause, extent, and chronicity of the renal injury cannot be established with noninvasive diagnostic methods (described above) or if therapeutic or life-ending decisions are predicated on this information. The short-term reversibility and long-term outcome of AKI may not, however, be predictable on the basis of morphologic findings at the outset of the disease. Many animals with extensive pathologic changes recover if supported with renal replacement therapies for sufficient time to allow regeneration and repair of the kidneys to proceed fully.

Other diagnostic tests

Differentiating hemodynamic causes or contributions from intrinsic renal causes of azotemia is important. Clinical signs of dehydration or hypotension, increased urine specific gravity, or partial or complete resolution of azotemia following restoration of fluid balance and blood pressure indicates hemodynamic causes or component of the azotemia. A BUN/creatinine ratio >20 also suggests a hemodynamic component, but this is neither a sensitive nor specific sign and can result from gastrointestinal hemorrhage or hypercatabolism. Avid sodium reabsorption and a urinary fractional excretion of sodium less than 1% can distinguish animals with hemodynamic azotemia and functional oliguria from those with intrinsic azotemia in which fractional sodium excretion (FE_{Na}) usually is greater than 1%. This distinction is discussed consistently in the human literature, but it has limited discriminatory power and rarely has been advocated or utilized in veterinary diagnostics. Urinary fractional excretion of urea is better at discriminating hemodynamic from intrinsic AKI than FE_{Na} when diuretics have been used, but it has not been evaluated in dogs or cats (Anderson and Barry 2004; Bagshaw et al. 2007c; Pepin et al. 2007; Clarkson et al. 2008; Diskin et al. 2008; Fahimi et al. 2009; Macedo and Mehta 2009).

Serologic testing for leptospirosis should be performed on all dogs evaluated for AKI without a confirmed etiology. A suspicion of leptospirosis is heightened by the presence of leukocytosis, thrombocytopenia, increased liver transaminases, and hyperbilirubinemia. Serologic evaluation should be broad-based and include titers to serovars canicola, icterohemorrhagiae, pomona, bratislava, grippotyphosa, autumnalis, and hardjo. Additional testing should be performed for serovars in any regionally specific serogroups as the distribution of infecting serovars changes with time and differs regionally throughout the world (Birnbaum et al. 1998; Adin and Cowgill 2000; Ward 2002; Ward 2002; Ward et al. 2002; Boutilier et al. 2003; Harkin et al. 2003; Goldstein et al. 2006; Moore et al. 2006; Stokes et al. 2007; Zwijnenberg et al. 2008). Strict serologic criteria to distinguish an active leptospiral infection from previous or vaccinal exposure have not been established. Moreover, the recent introduction of multivalent vaccines makes interpretation of serologic results more difficult. A microscopic agglutination titer (MAT) >1:100 indicates positive serology, and a two-fold to four-fold or greater change (increase or decrease) in titer between paired sera separated by 7–14 days predicts active infection (Greene et al. 2006; Heath and Johnson 1994; Levett 2001; Goldstein et al. 2006). Ambiguity in the diagnosis arises when only a single titer is available for evaluation. Previous retrospective studies arbitrarily established single titers of >1:800–>1:3200 to nonvaccinal serogroups as criteria for a positive diagnosis of active leptospirosis in dogs (Rentko et al. 1992; Harkin and Gartrell 1996; Birnbaum et al. 1998; Goldstein et al. 2006; Moore et al. 2006; Geisen et al. 2007). However, laboratory variation, differences in humoral responses, immunologic response to individual serovars, vaccination, background (asymptomatic) exposure, and time of sampling post exposure make strict serologic criteria difficult to assign.

Vaccination with serovars icterohemorrhagiae and canicola can produce titers to those serogroups greater than 1:1250 (Kerr and Marshall 1974). Vaccination with serovars pomona and grippotyphosa can produce titers up to 1:3200 to serogroup pomona and 1:400 to serogroup grippotyphosa. Interestingly, current vaccines can cause very high titers (1:12,800) to the serogroup autumnalis, although that serogroup is not included in the vaccine (Barr et al. 2005). High vaccinal titers dissipate rapidly and should be below suggested cutoff criteria within several months of vaccination (Barr et al. 2005). Surveys of non selected and asymptomatic dogs revealed a surprisingly high percentage that had not been vaccinated who had positive serology to leptospirosis serogroups indicating background population exposure (Harkin et al. 2003; Stokes et al. 2007; Zwijnenberg et al. 2008). Shedding of leptospiral DNA has been recognized using sensitive polymerase chain reaction assays in seronegative dogs who were either symptomatic or asymptomatic (Harkin et al. 2003; Harkin et al. 2003). These observations suggested some dogs have delayed seroconversion or fail to seroconvert despite being actively infected, and some serovars appear to induce a strong and persistent serologic response despite the absence of active infection (Greenlee et al. 2004). The infecting leptospiral organism is generally regarded to be the same as the serogroup producing the highest MAT titer. This distinction is problematic as there is considerable immunologic cross reactivity among infecting serogroups (Levett 2001). The highest initial titers may not correspond to the infecting serovars or the highest titer which persists in the subacute or convalescent phase of the disease due to cross reactivity among serogroups. In some cases, paradoxical reactions produce the highest titer to organisms to which the animal had never been exposed (Levett 2001; Barr et al. 2005).

Given the limitations of current diagnostic methods, consensus guidelines for a diagnosis of an active leptospirosis could include (1) a single elevated MAT titer >1:800 to vaccinal serogroups accompanied by clinical signs consistent with leptopsirosis; (2) a single MAT titer ≥1:400 for non-vaccinal serogroups; (3) evidence of seroconversion in paired acute and convalescent sera; (4) a four-fold or greater change in MAT titer (increase or decrease) in paired serologic sampling; (5) positive culture for *Leptospira* organisms, (6) positive direct fluorescent antibody reaction on infected tissue or urine; and (7) presence of typical clinical signs of leptospirosis followed by a response to appropriate antimicrobial therapy (Adin and Cowgill 2000; Goldstein et al. 2006; Geisen et al. 2007). The utility, availability, sensitivity, and specificity of PCR-based diagnostic testing may provide an additional approach in the future.

Ethylene glycol intoxication can be diagnosed presumptively by a history of possible or definitive exposure and presence of typical clinical signs. Presumptive diagnostic findings include an increased serum osmolality and osmolal gap, profound metabolic acidosis, increased anion gap, hypocalcemia, the presence of calcium oxalate crystalluria, and characteristic sonographic appearance of the kidneys (Grauer et al. 1984; Thrall et al. 1984; Thrall et al. 1998). Cageside tests are available to test for ethylene glycol in blood but they lack adequate sensitivity and specificity and should be combined with appropriate history and clinical parameters (Acierno et al. 2008). Confirmation of the diagnosis, the degree of intoxication, and response to decontamination therapy is best performed by chemical analysis of gastric fluid, serum, or urine for the presence of ethylene glycol or its toxic metabolites by commercial laboratories. Toxic concentrations of ethylene glycol and glycolic acid may persist for days in oliguria or anuria animals despite therapy with alcohol or 4-methylpyrazole (Cowgill and Langston 1996; Cowgill and Francey 2005). Samples should be obtained prior to administration of products containing propylene glycol to avoid false-positive results.

Testing for other nephrotoxins is generally based on knowledge of potential exposure or specific clinical signs. The most appropriate samples to collect depend on the suspected toxin. In general, whole blood in EDTA (lead, arsenic), serum (trace elements, drugs, ethylene glycol), urine (drugs, some metals), or gastric contents (pesticides, plants, metals, feed-associated toxicants) can be collected antemortem. Kidney and liver tissue (wrapped in plastic; if suspected organic toxin – wrap in aluminum foil) can be collected postmortem for pesticides (liver) or metals (liver, kidney). All samples except blood should be submitted frozen (Galey 1992).

Clinical consequences of AKI

AKI produces a variable admixture of clinical signs that change in spectrum and intensity with the stage, duration, etiology, and course of the disease. In the earliest stages of AKI, clinical signs are likely to be few and non specific, whereas at advanced stages they are multisystemic and life-threatening. Azotemia; fluid, electrolyte, and acid-base imbalances; metabolic and endocrine disturbances; and nutritional deficiencies contribute to the expression of advanced AKI. In animals with predisposing or comorbid medical conditions or multiple organ dysfunctions, it may be difficult to distinguish if the clinical problems relate specifically to the renal dysfunction or to the coexisting conditions. Nearly all clinical consequences of AKI (e.g., vomiting, hyperkalemia, metabolic acidosis, bleeding) become more profound as the stage of disease worsens. If the observed clinical or laboratory signs are inappropriate for the stage of AKI, other predisposing or comorbid conditions are likely contributing to the clinical appearance. Although common clinical threads exist for all stages, AKI represents multiple clinically distinct syndromes predicated on the etiology, severity, and functional integrity of the kidneys and urinary outflow system.

Alterations in body fluid volume–dehydration and hypervolemia

Alterations of fluid balance are common and significant therapeutic targets for all stages of AKI. Both the state of hydration (the overall loss or gain of fluid) and volemia (the relative volume of the vasculature) must be estimated at presentation and reassessed at regular intervals to direct the therapeutic plan. Under most circumstances, fluid balance is judged on the basis of clinical assessments (Mathews 2006). Most causes of AKI cause reductions of fluid intake and/or excessive fluid losses through vomiting, diarrhea, or polyuria leading to dehydration, hypovolemia and hypotension at initial presentation (Grauer 1998). Dehydration and hypovolemia exacerbate the azotemia by superimposing hemodynamic contributions to the underlying uremia and predisposing the kidneys to additional ischemic injury and decreased urine output (Sutton et al. 2002; Bonventre and Weinberg 2003). In contrast, overhydration and hypervolemia are common complications of hospitalization and aggressive fluid management (Cowgill and Francey 2005). Hypervolemia imposes a risk of pulmonary and peripheral edema, pleural effusion, systemic hypertension, and congestive heart failure (Figure 49.4).

Many clinical parameters are at the clinician's disposal to assess the initial and ongoing fluid status of uremic animals including: body weight, heart rate, pulse character, capillary refill time, mucous membrane wetness, chest auscultation, skin turgor, tear production, serous nasal discharge, blood pressure, central venous pressure, plasma proteins and hematocrit. Technologies including multifrequency bioimpedance spectroscopy provide additional options to quantitate noninvasively and sequentially static or real-time changes in ECF volume, intracellular fluid volume, and total body water (Figure 49.5) (Elliott et al. 2002; Elliott et al. 2002; Cowgill 2004; Cowgill and Francey 2006).

Inadequate urine production

Oliguria and anuria are life-threatening features of AKI. Oliguria often is defined as urine production of less than 0.27 mL/kg/hour (<6.5 mL/kg/day), whereas anuria constitutes essentially no urine formation

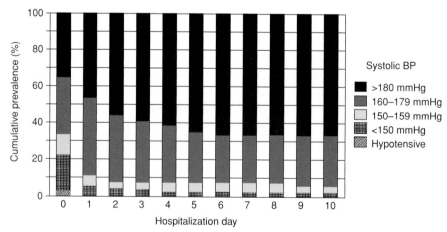

Figure 49.5 Distribution of systolic blood pressures in dogs with acute kidney injury during the first 10 days of hospitalization and management. There is a dramatic redistribution of blood pressure during hospitalization and a marked rise in the prevalence of dogs with severely increased pressure (>180 mmHg) from 35% at admission to 76% on day 10. (Courtesy, Dr. Thierry Francey.)

(<0.08 mL/kg/hour) (Cowgill and Francey 2005). An assessment of bladder size and urethral patency should be performed to determine if the oliguria or anuria is secondary to post renal causes. Oliguria induced from hemodynamic failure should be volume-responsive and resolve with restoration of systemic blood pressure and ECF volume. Approximately 30–60% of animals with parenchymal AKI have oliguria or anuria at initial presentation (Vaden et al. 1997; Francey and Cowgill 2004; Cowgill and Francey 2005). Solute retention, overhydration, hyperkalemia, and metabolic acidosis quickly become life-threatening if the oliguria or anuria is not corrected. Administration of all enteral and parenteral fluids, blood products, and maintenance fluids become problematic or contraindicated in oliguric or anuric animals despite an ongoing need for these therapies. Fluid overload, hypertension, congestive heart failure, and pulmonary edema become risks for aggressive fluid therapy in oliguric animals. The conversion from an oliguric to a nonoliguric state becomes a therapeutic goal to facilitate use of these essential therapies but may not correspond with improvement in GFR or the prognosis for recovery (Shilliday et al. 1997; Nolan and Anderson 1998; Vijayan and Miller 1998; Finn 2001; Mehta et al. 2002; De Vriese 2003).

Cardiovascular complications

Cardiovascular disorders develop from the underlying cause of the AKI, the uremia per se, or as a result of certain therapies. Abnormalities in myocardial contractility and excitability may be triggered or worsened by hypervolemia, acidosis, hyperkalemia, and uremic toxins. Bradycardia, supraventricular or ventricular premature contractions, and paroxysmal ventricular tachycardia are common electrocardiographic abnormalities. Cardiac arrest is a complication of severe hyperkalemia or the collective metabolic, acid-base, and electrolyte disturbances of acute uremia. Some normokalemic animals develop bradycardia (heart rates <80/minutes) which is presumed to be secondary to increased vagal tone associated with uremic gastroenteritis. An acute episode of vomiting will promote further vagal stimulation, worsening bradycardia, and cardiac arrest. The condition is prevented with anticholingeric drugs, which should be given prophylactically to uremic animals that are vomiting and demonstrate bradycardia (Cowgill and Elliott 2000). Congestive heart failure is an attendant risk of uremia or its fluid management. Volume overload may mimic congestive heart failure, by development of biventricular dilation, pulmonary edema, pleural effusion, or pericardial effusion and tamponade. Animals with severe AKI rarely develop pericardial effusion secondary to ure-

mic pericarditis, but it is seldom recognized or of clinical significance (Madewell and Norrdin 1975; Berg and Wingfield 1984; Rush et al. 1990; Davidson et al. 2008; Nelson and Ware 2009).

Hypertension was present in approximately 80% of dogs presented to the Veterinary Medical Teaching Hospital of University of California for hemodialysis for AKI. Overhydration was present in 65% of these dogs at the time of initial blood pressure measurement (Francey and Cowgill 2004). Target organs most at risk for hypertensive damage are the kidneys, heart, eyes, and brain. Manifestations include progressive renal injury, acute blindness, hyphema, retinal hemorrhage, retinal detachment, left ventricular hypertrophy, myocardial ischemia, hypertensive encephalopathy (intermittent confusion, depression and collapse), dementia, and cerebrovascular hemorrhage causing seizures, coma and death (Brown et al. 2005; Stepien and Henik 2009). Systemic hypertension is exacerbated iatrogenically during the management of AKI and must be closely monitored and prevented (Figure 49.4).

Pulmonary complications

Respiratory complications include pleural effusion, pulmonary edema, aspiration pneumonia, uremic pneumonitis, pulmonary artery thromboembolism and pulmonary hemorrhage (Rivers and Johnston 1996; Baumann and Fluckiger 2001; Greenlee et al. 2005). In a retrospective review, respiratory disease was present in 1/3 of dogs with AKI Stage IV, RRT and AKI Stage V, RRT at hospital presentation, and the prevalence of respiratory complications increased during hospitalization to affect half of the dogs (Thierry Francey, personal observations, 2004). In humans with AKI, 55–86% had respiratory failure, and respiratory involvement was a significant risk factor for death (Mehta et al. 2002; Bouchard and Mehta 2009). There are four predispositions to pulmonary edema in AKI: volume overload (cardiogenic edema), left ventricular dysfunction (cardiogenic edema), increased pulmonary capillary permeability (noncardiogenic edema), and acute lung injury (noncardiogenic edema with inflammation) (Faubel 2008). Fluid overload is the most common contributor to overt pulmonary edema (and pleural effusion) in animals with AKI, but interstitial edema develops even in the absence of an acute gain in body water (Kramer et al. 1999; Klein et al. 2008; Scheel et al. 2008; Bouchard and Mehta 2009). Dysregulation of lung salt and water transporters and increased levels of interleukin-6 contribute to increased lung permeability (Rabb et al. 2003; Klein et al. 2008; Scheel et al. 2008). Interstitial pulmonary edema can be identified on thoracic radiographs as a manifestation of uremia. A condition known as "uremic lung" is a well established complication of acute uremia of varied etiologies. It is often mistaken for pulmonary edema from fluid overload, but, distinct from volume overload, it develops from increased vascular permeability in the lung, leakage of albumin (and possibly RBCs) into the interstitium, erythrocyte sludging in pulmonary capillaries, and interstitial edema and inflammation as distant-organ casualty of acute uremia (Figure 49.1) (Scheel et al. 2008). The pathological events in the lung are evident within hours of the initiation of AKI. They appear to be associated with transcriptional events activating severity-dependent proinflammatory and proapoptotic processes in the kidney which invoke sequential and analogous transcriptional and inflammatory events in the lung (Hassoun et al. 2007; Grigoryev et al. 2008; Scheel et al. 2008). The pulmonary changes are mediated by interleukin-6 and facilitated by up-regulation of local chemokines induced by the transcriptional activity (Hoke et al. 2007; Grigoryev et al. 2008; Klein et al. 2008; Scheel et al. 2008). The pathogenesis of uremic lung serves as an example of the emerging concept of "distant organ damage". Presumptively, the coordinated (genomic, humoral, and cellular) and exuberant inflammatory response propagated in the kidney by AKI is transferred to distant organs (lung, brain, gut) that are recruited incidentally to contribute to the multisystemic inflammatory manifestations of AKI (Hassoun et al. 2007; Grigoryev et al. 2008; Scheel et al. 2008). Clinically, uremic lung is recognized in animals with severe AKI analogous to the severity-dependent changes seen in experimental settings, and it is frequently associated with leptospirosis and lily intoxication (Figure 49.1) Pulmonary hemorrhage contributes to the pulmonary pattern seen in dogs with leptospirosis which may represent a more severe variation of uremic lung (Baumann and Fluckiger 2001; Niwattayakul et al. 2002; Dolhnikoff et al. 2007; Andrade et al. 2008; Dall'Antonia et al. 2008; Gouveia et al. 2008).

Neurologic disorders

The brain is one of several distant organs that become dysfunctional or damaged by AKI. The encephalopathy noted in animals with acute uremia may be due to uremia per se, hypertension, fluid or electrolyte disturbance, dialysis, transplant rejection, drug toxicity, or induced inflammatory responses. Clinical signs of uremic encephalopathy include: dullness, lethargy, impaired mentation, altered behavior, confusion, stupor, coma, fatigue, sleep disturbances, anorexia, nausea, myoclonus, tremors, cramps, and seizures (Wolf 1980; Vanholder et al. 2003a; Vanholder et al. 2003b; Brouns and De Deyn 2004; Arieff 2008; Clarkson et al. 2008; Meyer and

Hostetter 2008; Raff et al. 2008; Vanholder et al. 2008; Lacerda et al. 2010). Electroencephalogram findings generally are abnormal by the time AKI is diagnosed and worsen as the severity of uremia progresses. (Brouns and De Deyn 2004; Arieff 2008) Neurologic signs are more severe and progress more rapidly in AKI compared to CKD (Brouns and De Deyn 2004; Arieff 2008). The cause of uremic encephalopathy is undetermined but is likely multifactorial. The response to dialysis suggests that uremic encephalopathy is caused or influenced by retained uremic solutes, but no singular solute or pathogenesis has been shown to account for the disorder (Brouns and De Deyn 2004). Recent experimental studies in mice with ischemic AKI revealed wide spread cellular inflammation, increased soluble proinflammatory mediators, disruption of the blood-brain barrier, and decreased locomotor activity. These findings suggested that the functional abnormalities of uremic encephalopathy have, in part, an inflammatory foundation as seen in other distant organ damage (Liu et al. 2008). Parathyroid hormone has been implicated and is supported by findings of neurologic disorders in human patients with primary hyperparathyroidism and by improvement of neurologic signs in human patients with CKD after parathyroidectomy (Arieff 2008). Parathyroid hormone facilitates entry of calcium into cells, and the increase in brain calcium content may contribute to the neurologic signs (Brouns and De Deyn 2004; Arieff 2008). Other central nervous system disorders associated with uremia include cerebrovascular disease (e.g., ischemia, and hemorrhage), central pontine myelinolysis (from rapid correction of hyponatremia), and movement disorders (characterized by multifocal action-induced jerks) (Brouns and De Deyn 2004).

A progressive peripheral polyneuropathy, indistinguishable from other metabolic polyneuropathies (i.e., diabetes mellitus), can occur with CKD, but it rarely develops acutely or subacutely with acute uremic presentations. (Brouns and De Deyn 2004; Arieff 2008) Aluminum toxicity from aluminum containing phosphate binders or dialysis water contamination can cause diffuse encephalopathic signs or neuromuscular disorders including profound weakness (Alfrey 1993; Segev et al. 2008a). Drugs including H2-receptor blockers (i.e., famotidine) and metoclopramide can induce CNS dysfunction in uremic animals when given at conventional doses. These findings reinforce the need to modify the dosage or frequency of administered medications that undergo renal excretion.

Electrolyte and acid base disturbances

Electrolyte imbalances occur frequently and are often the earliest life-threatening complications for animals with AKI. Hyperkalemia is the most problematic electrolyte abnormality and develops from the reduced renal clearance of potassium or imposed therapies. Over 90% of ingested potassium is excreted by the kidneys, with the remaining 10% excreted in feces. Potassium excretion is impaired if there is diminished sodium and water delivery to the distal nephron, which can occur in the presence of diminished renal blood flow or glomerular filtration or inadequate tubular fluid flow. Potassium excretion is also impaired if aldosterone concentration is decreased (e.g., NSAIDs, ACEi, ARB) or in the presence of aldosterone resistance (e.g., spironolactone). Diuretics that block sodium channels (i.e., triamterene, amiloride) can also decrease renal excretion of potassium (Schaefer and Wolford 2005; DiBartola and de Morais 2006). Hyperkalemia develops from transcellular shifts of potassium from the intracellular compartment, where the concentration is normally high, to the extracellular compartment, where potassium concentration is normally low. These changes occur with insulin deficiency, transcellular fluid shifts, acidemia, crush injuries or other causes of cellular lysis, acidosis, hypertonicity, and certain drugs (e.g., beta-blockers, digitalis, succinylcholine). Metabolic acidosis from mineral acids (i.e., $NH_4^+Cl^-$ or H^+Cl^-) causes hyperkalemia, but organic metabolic acidosis is not associated with hyperkalemia (Schaefer and Wolford 2005; DiBartola and de Morais 2006; Mount and Zandi-Nejad 2008). Hyperkalemia may occur from increased potassium intake in conjunction with potassium supplementation, potassium penicillin, or enteral or parenteral nutritional support (Schaefer and Wolford 2005; DiBartola and de Morais 2006; Mount and Zandi-Nejad 2008; Segev et al. 2010).

The major adverse effects of hyperkalemia stem from reduction of the transmembrane potassium gradient and changes in cell membrane excitability, increased resting membrane potential, and persistent depolarization of resting membrane potential (Schaefer and Wolford 2005; Parham et al. 2006; Mount and Zandi-Nejad 2008). Peripheral conducting and contractile cells are the most significantly impacted by these changes producing generalized muscular weakness, reduced cardiac contractility, disturbed cardiac conduction, cardiac arrhythmias, and neurologic abnormalities (Schaefer and Wolford 2005; DiBartola and de Morais 2006; Parham et al. 2006; Mount and Zandi-Nejad 2008).

The electrocardiographic abnormalities of the hyperkalemia commence at serum potassium concentrations greater than 6.5 mEq/L but are influenced further by the rate of rise of serum potassium and co-existent hyponatremia, hypocalcemia, and acidemia. Sequential abnormalities with moderate hyperkalemia (serum potassium concentration 6.5–8.0 mEq/L) include bradycardia, heightening and peaking of the T-wave, diminution in the P-wave and R-wave amplitudes, prolongation of the PR interval, absence of the P-wave, widening of the QRS complex, and ST segment depression. As the serum potassium concentrations exceed 8.0 mEq/L, potentially fatal arrhythmias associated with idioventricular complexes, ventricular escape beats, paroxysmal ventricular tachycardia, sine wave QRS complexes, heart block and ventricular fibrillation or asystole prevail (Schaefer and Wolford 2005; Parham et al. 2006; Mount and Zandi-Nejad 2008). Although these ECG changes are well described, many animals with hyperkalemia will have normal ECG findings or other electrocardiographic abnormalities (Parham et al. 2006; Tag and Day 2008).

Neuromuscular abnormalities associated with hyperkalemia include paresthesia, hyporeflexia, weakness, ascending flaccid paralysis and respiratory failure (Schaefer and Wolford 2005; DiBartola and de Morais 2006; Mount and Zandi-Nejad 2008).

Dysnatremias are less common and generally represent disturbances in water metabolism. Administration of maintenance or sodium free fluids for volume restoration or maintenance requirements may cause iatrogenic hyponatremia. Hyponatremia is associated with excessive losses of sodium in vomitus, stool, or urine associated with pancreatitis-induced vomiting, adrenal insufficiency, renal salt wasting, or diuretic administration. Transient hyponatremia may be seen following the administration of mannitol or synthetic colloid solutions as a result of free water shifts from the cellular to the extracellular space. Excessive free water loads can also be supplied with enteral administration of nutritional supplements to animals with limited excretory capacity. Hypernatremia usually indicates excessive free water loss from heat prostration or diabetes insipidus. In hospitalized animals, it is a common complication of replacement crystalloid fluid administration without provision for insensible free water losses. Also commonly, hypernatremia is an iatrogenic complication of excessive administration of sodium bicarbonate or hypertonic saline.

The kidneys are the major site for the regulation of acid-base homeostasis and development of metabolic acidosis proportional to the stage of AKI is predictable. Metabolic acidosis develops from the ongoing or excessive production of non volatile metabolic acids, the impaired filtration of the acid load, and decreased reabsorption of bicarbonate and generation of ammonia to facilitate net acid excretion (Rose 2001; DiBartola 2006; de Morais et al. 2008; Dubose 2008). The severity of the acidosis is influenced by concurrent acid loads accompanying diabetic ketoacidosis, lactic acidosis (decreased tissue perfusion), or ethylene glycol or salicylate intoxication (DiBartola 2006). Severe metabolic acidosis produces tachypnea, decreased cardiac contractility, decreased arterial blood pressure, decreased hepatic and renal blood flow, decreased myocardial contractility, cardiac arrhythmias, peripheral arterial vasodilation and venous vasoconstriction (DiBartola 2006). It contributes to the depression, lethargy, stupor or coma seen in AKI (DiBartola 2006). Metabolic acidosis induces insulin resistance and increases amino acid oxidation and protein catabolism which contribute to the azotemia and protein-energy wasting (see below).

Metabolic alkalosis occurs in animals with ECF volume contraction, intractable vomiting, or those receiving sodium bicarbonate and may predominate other metabolic disturbances. A respiratory component (acidosis or alkalosis) may be mixed with the metabolic acid-base disturbance in animals with concurrent pulmonary edema or hemorrhage, pleural effusion, pneumonia, aspiration pneumonia, hyperventilation, or pulmonary thromboemboli. The respiratory component of these disturbances will only be evident on blood gas analysis (DiBartola 2006).

Uremic Intoxications

A myriad of ill-defined "uremic toxins" of diverse molecular size and chemical classification accumulate in uremic animals due to excretory failure of the kidneys or altered metabolism (Vanholder et al. 2003a; Vanholder et al. 2003b; Yavuz et al. 2005). Collectively, "uremic toxins" contribute towards many of the classical complications of acute uremia in direct proportion to the severity of the azotemia and stage of AKI. Many uremic intoxications and their attributable signs can be ameliorated by renal replacement therapies including hemodialysis predicting they are of reasonably small molecular size (i.e., <1500 D).

Gastrointestinal disorders include: anorexia, nausea, vomiting, fetid breath, stomatitis, oral ulcerations, necrosis of the tip and lateral margins of the tongue, gastritis, gastrointestinal ulcers, hematemesis, gastrointestinal bleeding, enterocolitis, diarrhea, intussusception, and ileus (Krawiec 1996; Antoniades et al. 2006). Gastritis and gastric ulceration exacerbates the anorexia, nausea and vomiting associated with acute uremia. Gastric lesions are often associated with hypergastrinemia from increased gastrin secretion or its reduced renal clearance (Goldstein et al. 1998). Hypersecretion of gastric acid and direct damage by uremia toxins to the gastric mucosa, submucosal, and vasculature contribute further to the gastritis (Goldstein et al. 1998). Esophagitis develops secondary to gastric reflux from severe and persistent vomiting and as a complication of esophageal feeding tubes. Acute pancreatitis is recognized more commonly as an etiology as well as a complication of AKI, and the associated severe and protracted vomiting is an important cause of esophagitis and aspiration pneumonia (Vaden et al. 1997; Langston 2002; Cowgill and Francey 2005).

Uremic bleeding manifests as purpura, petechia, ecchymosis, bruising, bleeding from gum margins and venipuncture sites, epistaxis, and gastrointestinal blood loss. The gastrointestinal blood loss can be occult or overt and contribute to anemia. Impaired platelet-platelet and platelet-vessel wall interaction induced by uremia toxins are the major cause of uremic bleeding (Hedges et al. 2007; Galbusera et al. 2009). Other hematologic manifestations include anemia from decreased EPO production, blood loss, shortened RBC life span, and impaired immunity (Vanholder et al. 2003a; Vanholder et al. 2003b; Clarkson et al. 2008; Meyer and Hostetter 2008; Raff et al. 2008; Vanholder et al. 2008).

In addition to these major morbidities, "uremia toxins" cause or contribute to endocrine, metabolic, and other manifestations of the uremia (Cowgill and Francey 2005; Meyer and Hostetter 2008). Reduced resting energy expenditure leads to hypothermia, which is most pronounced in animals with severe uremia where body temperature may approach 96°F or lower (Ash 1991; Meyer and Hostetter 2008). Hypothermia resolves with correction of the azotemia by dialysis predicting the cause to be a low molecular weight solute. A normal temperature in animals with moderate azotemia (BUN >100 mg/dL) suggests the presence of fever and an underlying infectious or inflammatory process. Other manifestations of uremia described in people include pruritis, hiccups, serositis, diminution in taste and smell, oxidant stress, inflammation, and insulin resistance (Vanholder et al. 2003a; Clarkson et al. 2008; Meyer and Hostetter 2008; Raff et al. 2008; Vanholder et al. 2008).

Nutritional complications

Protein-energy wasting constitutes the loss of lean body mass and fat reserves and is common in both humans and animals with AKI. It contributes to many of the comorbidities of AKI including: impaired immune function, increased susceptibility to infection, delayed wound healing, decreased strength, poor quality of life, and mortality (Fouque et al. 2008; Fiaccadori and Cremaschi 2009). The imposed catabolism associated with multiple organ dysfunction exacerbates the hyperkalemia, hyperphosphatemia, acidosis and azotemia, increases morbidity and mortality, and negatively influences the outcome of AKI (Mitch 1993; Druml 1998; Chan 2004; Fouque et al. 2008; Fiaccadori and Cremaschi 2009). Anorexia, nausea and vomiting, comorbid catabolic illnesses, uremic toxins, oxidative stress, inflammation, and endocrine abnormalities including insulin resistance and hyper-parathyroidism contribute cumulatively to the nutritional inadequacies (Fouque et al. 2008; Fiaccadori and Cremaschi 2009). Metabolic acidosis is a major stimulus for breakdown of muscle protein in acute uremia and increases the ongoing catabolism (Mitch 1981; Mitch et al. 1989).

An accurate assessment of the nutritional status of uremic animals is necessary to guide nutritional therapy (Delaney et al. 2006). Currently, there are no clinically applicable tools with appropriate sensitivity and specificity to precisely define nutritional status and ongoing protein-energy wasting (Delaney et al. 2006; Fiaccadori and Cremaschi 2009). A recent consensus has established four categorical abnormalities for human patients to define protein-energy wasting associated with AKI that appear applicable in animals. The categorical diagnosis of protein-energy wasting includes (1) biochemical criteria including hypoalbuminemia or hypocholesterolemia, (2) reduced body weight or fat mass, (3) decreased muscle mass, and (4) low protein or energy intake (Fouque et al. 2008).

Serum albumin has been shown to be a strong outcome predictor for a variety of kidney syndromes in humans and animals (Iseki et al. 1993; Mastrorilli et al. 2007; Fouque et al. 2008; Segev et al. 2008b; Worwag and Langston 2008; Kovesdy et al. 2009). Low or decreasing serum albumin is highly correlated with mortality independent of nutritional state and is appropriately predictive for protein-energy wasting which includes both nutritional inadequacy as well as inflammatory induced wasting (Fouque et al. 2008). Change in body weight, seemingly the simplest means to document nutritional status and wasting, can be flawed by increases in hydration which mask significant losses of fat stores or lean body mass (categories 2 and 3, above). Body condition scoring has proven to be a useful index to assess nutritional status, and sequential changes in the body condition score can serve as an integrated surrogate for changes in body fat mass or lean mass (Laflamme 1997; Son et al. 1998). A body condition score below "ideal" is a predictor of protein-energy wasting in dogs or cats with AKI. Bioelectrical impedance analysis is a safe, noninvasive, and reproducible method to quantitate changes in total body water, ECF volume, body cell mass and fat free mass which may have future application for serial assessment of body composition in uremic animals (Elliott et al. 2002; Elliott et al. 2002; Chanchairujira and Mehta 2005). (Cowgill, personal observation, 2005) Dietary protein and energy intake can be readily evaluated by a comprehensive dietary history and feeding practices. Partial or complete anorexia can be associated with protein-energy wasting. The consensus recommendation suggests that if three or more of the categories are fulfilled, a diagnosis of protein-energy wasting can be ascribed to the AKI and nutritional support is essential (Fouque et al. 2008).

Medical management of AKI

Management strategies for AKI in animals are designed to correct documented or predicted clinical consequences of the presenting or evolving stages of AKI. Therapeutic recommendations are based on historical convention in animal patients, recommendations extrapolated from human therapeutics, and results of experimental animal models of AKI (Chew 2000; Cowgill and Francey 2005; Jo et al. 2007; Clarkson et al. 2008; Langston 2010). Medical approaches have changed very little over the past 20 years; nor have outcomes changed for specific etiologies and stages of AKI (Vaden et al. 1997; Cowgill 2004; Cowgill and Francey 2005; Segev et al. 2008b). Renal replacement therapies have provided the most significant advancement for resolution of clinical signs, but improvement in outcomes may only follow wider availability of these therapies in veterinary practice. Medical recommendations are prioritized to prevent development of AKI in animals that are highly predisposed and at high risk for renal injury. For animals with established AKI, therapy is directed to eliminate initiating or ongoing renal insults and to ameliorate identified circulatory, biochemical, metabolic, and clinical abnormalities associated with the renal injury.

The pathophysiologic mechanisms that mediate AKI have been characterized in great detail in recent years (see Pathogenesis of AKI, above). Cellular energetics, vascular congestion, cytosolic calcium, oxidant stress, necrosis, apoptosis, nitric oxide, epithelial cytoskeleton, growth promoters, and inflammatory cytokines are but a few participants recognized to participate in its pathogenesis (Kellum 2008). Novel therapies have emerged from scientifically crafted experimental models of AKI for each of these specific pathophysiologic events. Yet, despite the promise of these targeted therapies, none have become established in clinical therapeutics. This is to be expected for a disease process with diverse and multifactorial predispositions, etiologies, and stages. Consequently, specific approaches to the management of AKI remain supportive for the predicted and documented clinical consequences.

Prevention of acute renal injury

The highest therapeutic priority for AKI is to intervene preventatively in patients with recognized predispositions to renal injury. Preexisting kidney disease, advanced age, dehydration, hypovolemia, hypotension, sepsis, fever, prolonged anesthesia/surgery, trauma, systemic disease, use of vasoactive or nephrotoxic drugs, high environmental temperatures, and nephrolithiasis are predisposing risks (Grauer 1996; Lameire et al. 2008; Lameire et al. 2008; Murrary and Palevsky 2009; Langston 2010). Risk factors are cumulative and impose additive potential for kidney injury. When any of these conditions coexist with ongoing or projected therapy that has the potential to injure the kidney, exposure to ischemic or nephrotoxic events must be prevented or eliminated, ECF volume and renal hemodynamics must be preserved, and adequate urine flow and solute excretion should be maintained. Specifically, dehydration, hypovolemia, hypotension, hypertension, systemic infections, thrombosis, and environmental nephrotoxins (e.g., antifreeze, contaminated food, and nephrotoxic plants) should be avoided. Nephrotoxic or vasoactive drugs should be discontinued or their dosage should be modified to nontoxic levels. Dehydration, ECF volume depletion, hypovolemia, and decreased renal perfusion represent some of the most formidable predispositions for AKI (Bellomo et al. 2005; Lameire et al. 2005; Lameire et al. 2008; Lameire et al. 2008; Venkataraman 2008). Hemodynamic adequacy must be established, and recognized fluid, electrolyte, and acid-base imbalances must be corrected in the course of emergent or ongoing medical care. Induced vomiting, gastric lavage, administration of activated charcoal and cathartics, and provision of specific antidotes should be instituted following exposure to nephrotoxins. Extracorporeal therapies including hemodialysis, hemoperfusion, and therapeutic plasma exchange may be indicated to promote elimination of specific nephrotoxins once renal exposure is established (Cowgill and Francey 2005; Shalkham et al. 2006; Smith and Chang 2008).

To date, the best overall protection from events that promote AKI is the establishment and maintenance of normal hydration, intravascular volume, systemic hemodynamics, and adequate urine formation. In usual clinical settings, there are few opportunities to intervene with preventative strategies. However, when animals with predisposing risk factors are scheduled for high risk diagnostic or therapeutic procedures (e.g., radiocontrast imaging, anesthesia, or surgery) or prescribed potentially renal compromising drugs (e.g., aminoglycosides, ACE inhibitors, NSAIDs, Amphotericin B, diuretics, or antithyroid drugs), proactive attention to hydration status and systemic hemodynamics is warranted. Correction of existing fluid deficits and administration of saline or balanced replacement fluids throughout and following renal compromising procedures is the best insurance to prevent or moderate the severity of AKI (Bellomo et al. 2005; Licari et al. 2007; Himmelfarb et al. 2008; Kellum

et al. 2008c; Lameire et al. 2008; Lameire et al. 2008; Townsend and Bagshaw 2008; Venkataraman 2008). Mild to moderate ECF volume expansion with saline or balanced electrolyte fluids is beneficial before the administration of known nephrotoxic drugs (aminoglycosides, cis-platinum, amphotericin B), anesthesia, or surgical intervention. Mannitol administered (see details, below) prior to exposure to hemodynamic or nephrotoxic insults will promote urine formation and a natriuresis. It has shown efficacy to prevent the induction of AKI in only limited clinical settings in human patients (crush injury, renal transplantation, and surgery) and has little generic indication (Duke 1999; Venkataram and Kellum 2001; Kellum et al. 2008b). Recently, the use of colloidal starch solutions for hemodynamic stabilization have been criticized and shown in certain settings to contribute to AKI (Lameire et al. 2008; Townsend and Bagshaw 2008). The preventative use of other therapies has consistently failed to provide any advantage over judicious management with crystalloid fluids (Lameire et al. 1995; Kellum 1997; Duke 1999; Lameire and Vanholder 2001; Gambaro et al. 2002; Lameire et al. 2002; Bellomo et al. 2005; Himmelfarb et al. 2008; Kellum et al. 2008a).

Conventional management of established AKI

As for prevention of AKI, conventional strategies for the management of existing AKI involve elimination of identified causes of the renal injury and goal–directed supportive therapy specific to the life-threatening and morbid consequences of acute uremia. In many cases the inciting event has passed or cannot be identified at initial presentation. In circumstances where the etiology persists, every effort should be made to eliminate continued exposure. The administration of nephrotoxic drugs should be discontinued or modified to safe dosages. Systemic infections (e.g., Leptospirosis) should be aggressively treated with appropriate antimicrobial therapy, and hemodynamic deficiencies must be resolved rapidly to promote euvolemia, normotension, and adequate renal perfusion. The goals of conventional therapy are to correct existing and ongoing hemodynamic deficiencies and alleviate abnormalities in body fluid volume and composition. Concurrent goals are to promote urine formation and correct biochemical abnormalities and manifestations of uremia until compensatory adaptations to the renal damage have occurred (Bellomo et al. 2005; Lameire et al. 2005; Kellum et al. 2008a; Mehta et al. 2008; Pinsky et al. 2008). Animals with AKI Stages I and II may regain adequate renal function within 2–5 days, forestalling life-threatening azotemia and electrolyte disorders and need only short-term support. Those with higher stages of AKI may require weeks of supportive care before the onset of renal repair. Animals with severe kidney failure, AKI Stage IV or V, may die within 5–10 days despite appropriate conventional management unless supported with RRT for an indefinite time. This disparity between the window of survival with conventional supportive therapy and the extended time required to repair severe acute renal injury underlies, in part, the poor prognosis and outcomes associated with severe stages of AKI.

Alterations in systemic hemodynamics and body fluid volume

Deficiencies in body fluid volumes are classic causes and consequences of AKI, and fluid therapy remains the foundation of medical management (Bellomo et al. 2005; Cowgill and Francey 2005; Licari et al. 2007; Himmelfarb et al. 2008; Lameire et al. 2008; Townsend and Bagshaw 2008; Langston 2010). The fluid prescription must be goal-directed to correct the specific alterations in fluid volume and composition, to restore systemic and renal hemodynamic adequacy, and to promote urine formation. Replacement fluids should mimic the composition of fluid losses and be formulated to restore depleted fluid compartments. Priority is given to restoration of intravascular and interstitial volume in the extracellular compartment, normalization of arterial blood pressure and renal perfusion, and balancing ongoing fluid losses. Dehydration, depletion of the ECF volume, and hypovolemia are present in most animals at initial presentation due to nausea, vomiting, and diarrhea. Occasionally, hemorrhage is the prevailing disorder. In the absence of hypovolemic shock or cardiovascular compromise, these fluid deficits should be corrected with normal saline or balanced crystalloids administered intravenously within the first 2–4 hours of presentation (Licari et al. 2007; Kellum et al. 2008a). The initial replacement volume is calculated from clinical estimates of dehydration according to the formula:

Volume replacement (mL) = [body weight (kg)]

    ×[estimated deficit (%)] × 1000

The estimated deficit is a value between 5 and 15% determined from history, physical examination, blood pressure and laboratory information or computed from known deviations from historical or ideal dry (non volume expanded) weight. A 5% deficit may not be clinically apparent and can be replaced routinely to assure adequate hydration and to provide a mild fluid challenge to animals with oliguria and volume-responsive azotemia (Himmelfarb 2009). Bolus replacement of an estimated 8% deficit with crystalloid fluids increases blood volume transiently (10–30 minutes) by approximately 75%. With subsequent distribution out of the vasculature or slower administration over an hour, the same replacement volume expands the intravascular and ECF compartments by approximately 20% (Silverstein et al. 2005). Aggressive fluid replacement must be tempered in animals with oliguria, sepsis, or cardiovascular disease to prevent fluid overload, circulatory congestion, and incipient heart failure. There is clear evidence in human patients with AKI that over aggressive or excessive fluid resuscitation is associated with worse morbidity, mortality, and poorer outcomes (Bagshaw et al. 2008; Kellum et al. 2008a; Townsend and Bagshaw 2008; Bouchard and Mehta 2009; Bouchard and Mehta 2009; Bouchard et al. 2009). Serial monitoring of central venous pressure (CVP) can facilitate safe and efficient fluid administration to these animals. An increase in CVP of 5–7 cm H_2O above baseline or an absolute CVP greater than 10 cm H_2O may indicate an excessive rate or volume of fluid administration and warrants slowing or discontinuing further fluid delivery. However, there are suggestions that CVP and other ventricular preload indicators may not be predictive of compromised cardiovascular and hemodynamic function and thus potentiate fluid accumulation (Townsend and Bagshaw 2008). It is important to assess and monitor fluid balance of the patient frequently and judiciously resist overhydration. Five percent dextrose in water or maintenance formulations (including 0.45% saline/2.5% dextrose solutions) are not appropriate or effective formulations to replace ECF volume deficits and should be reserved for insensible or maintenance fluid requirement later in the course of treatment (Cowgill and Francey 2005; Kellum et al. 2008a). The volume status of the animal should be re-evaluated once the estimated deficit has been replaced to insure the therapeutic goals for restoration of hydration and blood pressure were achieved. Additional fluid may be administered cautiously if the initially estimated deficit was insufficient to restore hydration or promote normotension and urine formation.

Fluid deficits associated with profound hypovolemia and hypotension or severe blood loss must be replaced rapidly with crystalloid solutions up to or greater than 90 mL/kg in dogs and up to 60 mL/kg in cats (Day and Bateman 2006; Langston 2008). Perhaps more appropriately, synthetic colloid solutions targeted for blood volume expansion or a combination of balanced crystalloid and colloid solutions should be administered when oxygen carrying capacity is less critical than volume restoration. Hydroxyethyl starch (hetastarch) is recommended at 10–20 mL/kg in dogs and 10–15 mL/kg in cats as a rapid or incremented intravenous bolus infusion. Dextran-70 or Hetastarch administered at 20 mL/kg to normal dogs will expand blood volume immediately following bolus administration by 17–24% and by approximately 35% by

60 minutes post administration (Silverstein et al. 2005). Recent evidence suggests high molecular weight starch solutions may promote renal injury and low molecular weight solutions are more appropriate for septic AKI (Licari et al. 2007; Murray and Palevsky 2009). Fluid replacement for hypotensive shock should be administered aggressively (but not excessively) until blood pressure and vascular volume have stabilized. Synthetic colloid solutions provide no restoration of extravascular volume necessitating concurrent administration of saline or balanced crystalloid solutions to replace interstitial volume. Hemorrhagic hypotension may require administration of compatible whole blood, packed red blood cells, or synthetic hemoglobin products (Oxyglobin, BioPure, Cambridge, MA) (Belgrave et al. 2002; Driessen et al. 2003; Driessen et al. 2006; Weingart and Kohn 2008). Synthetic hemoglobin preparations may be suitable to restore systemic hemodynamic parameters and tissue oxygen debt when blood products are not available (Belgrave et al. 2002; Driessen et al. 2003).

The onset or an increase in urine production of greater than 0.5 mL/kg/hour with fluid volume replacement predicts a significant volume-responsive (prerenal) contribution to the oliguria and azotemia (Himmelfarb 2009). Failure to induce a significant diuresis after volume replacement indicates either the initial fluid deficit was underestimated or the parenchymal damage is severe and volume-unresponsive. An additional 3–5% volume expansion (30–50 mL/kg) may be attempted in an effort to induce a diuresis, taking care to promote only mild volume expansion without overhydration.

After the fluid deficits have been corrected, subsequently administered fluid must reflect the maintenance requirements and ongoing losses. Maintenance fluid requirements are composed of insensible (free water) losses comprising primarily obligatory respiratory losses and sensible losses including urinary losses and ongoing electrolyte-containing losses from vomiting, diarrhea, wound drainage, and bleeding. Maintenance fluids must reflect both the volume of all ongoing outputs as well as their composition. Failure to replace the obligatory free water losses is a common therapeutic error. Maintenance fluid should be composed of 5% dextrose in water to replace insensible free water losses (15–20 mL/kg/day) and balanced electrolyte solutions to replace measured or estimated urine, gastrointestinal, and other sensible losses. Commercial maintenance formulations can be supplied if the sensible losses are proportionate to those of normal animals at 25–40 mL/kg/day. However, the sensible losses of animals with AKI rarely approximate those of normal animals, and usually it is better to prescribe the sensible and insensible requirements independently. Animals provided only replacement solutions

(saline, balanced electrolyte solutions) for maintenance fluid requirements will become depleted of free water and develop hypernatremia within 2–3 days. The severity of the hypernatremia is amplified in animals with appreciable urinary free water losses during the diuretic phase of AKI, during post obstructive diuresis, or subsequent to administration of osmotic diuretics like mannitol. Modifications to the daily free water requirement of maintenance fluids should be determined according to changes in serum sodium concentration during the course of management. The free water deficit or excess can be estimated according to the formula:

Free Water deficit (+volume, mL) or excess (−volume, mL) = [body wt (kg)] × [(measured serum Na−145)/145] × 1000, where 145 represents a normal serum sodium concentration of 145 mmol/L (DiBartola 2006). A positive volume reflects a free water deficit which should be provided to replete the deficiency and correct the hypernatremia. A negative volume predicts a free water excess which should be subtracted from the standard insensible requirement until the excess is eliminated and the hyponatremia is resolved.

The urinary component of the sensible maintenance fluid requirement will be negligible in oliguric and anuric animals and should not be prescribed at a standard rate used for animals with normal urine production. Urinary losses should be measured or accurately estimated in nonoliguric animals to prevent under evaluation of the urine replacement volume. Nonoliguric animals in the diuretic phase of AKI or following relief of a postrenal obstruction may produce 5–30 mL/kg/hour of urine which will not be matched using standard estimates of normal urine production.

Supplementation of potassium in replacement or maintenance fluids must be prescribed on an individual case basis. Fluids containing supplemental potassium are generally contraindicated in oliguric animals or during initial fluid replacement. If the supplemental load of potassium has no effective elimination route, it will quickly promote hyperkalemia. Excessive loads of potassium can be provided inadvertently with use of pre-formulated maintenance solutions containing supplemental concentrations of potassium greater than 5–10 mEq/L. In contrast, animals in the diuretic phase of AKI may excrete exaggerated amounts of potassium and require supplementation to prevent potassium wasting. Potassium supplementation should always be provided cautiously to uremic animals and only with daily monitoring of serum potassium concentrations.

All fluids must be administered cautiously to oliguric and anuric animals. Hypervolemia is a common complication of aggressive fluid administration or inattentive monitoring of fluid balance. Animals with AKI

Stage III–V become increasingly hypervolemic during hospitalization at primary or specialty referral hospitals (Figure 49.4). If initial administration of the estimated fluid deficit and additional mild volume expansion fail to induce an effective diuresis within the first 6–12 hours of therapy, it must be presumed the animal has volume-unresponsive AKI. Further fluid loading will not be beneficial and predisposes life-threatening overhydration (Cowgill and Francey 2005).

Progressive increases in body weight, tachypnea, increased breath sounds, increased skin turgor, chemosis, serous nasal discharge, peripheral or pulmonary edema, circulatory congestion, ascites, and systemic hypertension are predictive of overhydration in animals receiving fluids. Oral mucous membrane wetness does not reflect hydration status in uremic animals due to decreased salivary secretion (xerostomia). Reliance on this sign often causes an erroneous underestimation of the true hydration status and inappropriate administration of additional fluid to overhydrated animals.

Fluid overload may be impossible to correct in animals with oliguric stages of AKI. Consequently, and contrary to a nearly universal clinical temptation, all fluid delivery should be curtailed or discontinued at the first evidence of overhydration. If the fluid burden cannot be corrected with diuretic administration, there are no conventional therapeutic options to resolve it. The consequences of the circulatory overload (systemic hypertension, peripheral and pulmonary edema, plural effusion, congestive heart failure, and ascites) must be managed supportively. Fluid ultrafiltration with hemodialysis or peritoneal dialysis is the only alternative for life-threatening overhydration. Ultrafiltration can reestablish the animal's ideal dry weight or facilitate delivery of fluid-intense treatments like parenteral nutrition that would exceed the animal's excretory capacity (Cowgill and Francey 2005). The rate and volume of fluid removal with hemodialysis is contingent upon the hemodynamic stability of the animal. Slow rates of ultrafiltration at 5–10 mL/kg/hour are readily tolerated. Increased rates of fluid removal up to 20 mL/kg/hour can be prescribed with caution for animals that are markedly overhydrated.

Inadequate urine production

The conversion of anuric or oliguric stages of AKI to a non-oliguric state is been an important early goal for the medical management of AKI (Venkataram and Kellum 2001; Cowgill and Francey 2005; Townsend and Bagshaw 2008; Karajala et al. 2009). The priority to establish a diuresis is less critical for patients managed with RRT where the consequences of inadequate urine production can be corrected during the dialysis sessions. Induction of an effective diuresis has potential to improve fluid and electrolyte imbalances, promote clearance of endogenous and exogenous toxins, and facilitate delivery of adjunctive therapies (Karajala et al. 2009). Theoretically, the diuresis augments intratubular fluid flow and removal of luminal debris, necrotic epithelial remnants, and obstructions promoting and extending the tubular injury.

Oliguric stages of AKI generally are associated with less favorable outcomes than non-oliguric conditions. The desire to promote a diuresis has solidified the empirical use of diuretics (mannitol and furosemide) and renal vasodilators (dopamine and fenoldopam) when fluid therapy alone was ineffective (Kellum 1997; Kellum 1997; Kellum and Decker 2001; Labato 2001; Lameire and Vanholder 2001; Gambaro et al. 2002; Cowgill and Francey 2005). More recently, the validity of these empirical practices has been disputed, and the routine use of these medications in moderate to severe forms of acquired AKI in human beings and animals is losing credibility. The basis for this reversal of position is the accumulating evidence exposing the lack of efficacy or imposed risks associated with diuretic and vasoactive drug use in clinical practice (Kellum 1997; Kellum 1997; Kellum 1998; Dishart and Kellum 2000; Kellum and Decker 2001; Lameire and Vanholder 2001; Venkataram and Kellum 2001; Gambaro et al. 2002; Lameire et al. 2002; Bagshaw et al. 2007; Bagshaw et al. 2007; Jo et al. 2007; Bagshaw et al. 2008; Townsend and Bagshaw 2008; Karajala et al. 2009; Lameire et al. 2009). If delayed beyond a few hours from the initiation phase of the renal insult, the efficacy of pharmacologic agents to alter the course, morphology, or outcome of AKI becomes negligible (Kellum 1997; Shilliday et al. 1997; Kellum and J 2001; Lameire and Vanholder 2001; Gambaro et al. 2002; Jo et al. 2007).

Nevertheless, pharmacologic treatments to promote a diuresis continue to dominate the practice pattern for acute oliguric renal failure in both human and animal patients. Their risks and contraindications are considered to be small, and they often are justified for management of other complications attending the AKI (Bagshaw et al. 2007). Their use should never supplant judicious fluid and hemodynamic support, nor should they be provided as a rescue for excessive fluid administration. In established AKI, potential benefits to an individual animal include (1) conversion from an oliguric or anuric to a nonoliguric state, (2) disclosure of less severe renal injury, (3) better regulation of fluid and electrolyte balance, and (4) opportunity to provide parenteral nutrition.

Mannitol

Hypertonic mannitol (an osmotic diuretic) is used commonly for the prevention and management of oliguric forms of AKI. Putative therapeutic effects include expansion of ECF volume; decreased vascular resistance; increased RBF and GFR; reduced hypoxic cellular swelling; prevention of vascular congestion and erythrocyte aggregation; increased solute excretion, osmotic tubular fluid flow and dispersion of tubular debris; and scavenging of toxic free-radicals (Behnia et al. 1996; Better et al. 1997; Finn 2001; Lameire and Vanholder 2001; Venkataram and Kellum 2001; Gambaro et al. 2002; McClellan et al. 2006; Karajala et al. 2009). The use of mannitol in human patients with oliguric AKI is considerably less than the use of other diuretics (Bagshaw et al. 2007c). In most clinical settings, mannitol is unlikely to have therapeutic efficacy in the prevention or outcome of AKI (Venkataram and Kellum 2001; Kellum et al. 2008b). It also imposes potential adverse effects including fluid overload, hyperosmolality, increased renal oxygen consumption, volume depletion and hypernatremia (Lameire et al. 2009; Redfors et al. 2009).

Despite the absence of evidence-based justification for the use of mannitol in oliguric AKI, it has gained empirical recommendation when fluid therapy alone has failed to promote urine formation (Cowgill and Elliott 2000; Elliott and Cowgill 2000; Labato 2001; Grauer 2009). Conventional practice patterns are to administer mannitol (20–25% solution) at 0.25–1.0 g/kg to fluid replete animals as a slow intravenous bolus. If an effective diuresis results within 30–60 minutes, a maintenance infusion at 1.0–2.0 mg/kg/minute or intermittent boluses of 0.25–0.5 g/kg IV every 4–6 hours can be continued to promote the diuresis as required. If an adequate diuresis is not established by 60 minutes, an additional 0.25–0.5 gm/kg intravenous bolus can be repeated cautiously, but further administration is contraindicated due to the risks of ECF volume expansion, hemodilution, hypervolemia, and mannitol toxicity (Grauer 1995; Grauer and Lane 1995; Visweswaran et al. 1997; Cowgill and Elliott 2000; Elliott and Cowgill 2000; Langston 2010). Mannitol should not be given to animals with severe fluid overload, pulmonary edema, or congestive heart failure. The more established the onset of the uremia, the lower the expectation mannitol therapy will promote a diuresis or favorably influence the course of the disease.

Loop diuretics

Loop diuretics are used nearly universally as a practice pattern in human patients with oliguric or anuric AKI, also without established evidence of their efficacy or benefit to improve outcome with few clinical exceptions (Mehta et al. 2002; Uchino et al. 2004; Bagshaw et al. 2007; Kellum et al. 2007a; Uchino et al. 2007; Townsend and Bagshaw 2008; Karajala et al. 2009). A

similar practice pattern is evident in veterinary medicine. The use of loop diuretics, like furosemide, have evolved from early experimental studies in animals and nonrandomized and uncontrolled clinical trials in humans documenting improvements in urine formation (Lindner et al. 1979; Townsend and Bagshaw 2008). When coupled with the perception and limited evidence that nonoliguric patients have a better prognosis than those who are oliguric, loop diuretics have become a staple in the management of AKI.

Furosemide is a potent natriuretic agent which inhibits active sodium and chloride reabsorption at the $Na^+K^+2Cl^-$ cotransporter in the luminal membrane of the thick ascending limb of the loop of Henle. In addition to promoting increased urine formation, furosemide is a modest vasodilator and can increase renal blood flow by PGE2-mediated events. It has the potential to decrease tubular oxygen consumption and energy requirements in oxygen sensitive tubular segments (Finn 2001; Lameire and Vanholder 2001; Venkataram and Kellum 2001; Gambaro et al. 2002; Abbott and Kovacic 2008; Townsend and Bagshaw 2008). Despite these effects and despite their potential to increase urine formation, the administration of loop diuretics to human patients in the clinical phases of AKI has yet to demonstrate any significant benefit in patient outcomes including mortality, duration of hospitalization, or requirement for RRT (Mehta et al. 2002; Uchino et al. 2004; Bagshaw et al. 2007; Townsend and Bagshaw 2008; Lameire et al. 2009).

In veterinary medicine, there are no observational, prospective, or randomized trials addressing the benefits and/or efficacy of loop diuretics in established AKI. Moreover, here is a dearth of antidotal experience or opinion to justify the current practice pattern for oliguric animals. Recent studies in normal cats, demonstrated furosemide combined with dopamine induced a pronounced increase in urine production and fractional sodium excretion but no significant effect on renal blood flow and GFR compared to fluid therapy alone. Moreover, there was a trend for furosemide-dopamine administration to decrease GFR compared to fluid therapy or fluid therapy and mannitol (McClellan et al. 2006). It is not possible to extrapolate these observations to animals with AKI, but they confirm observations in human patients with AKI in which furosemide alone or combined with dopamine promotes only inconsistent improvement in urine formation.

Furosemide has potential for adverse effects when given to oliguric animals. If effective at establishing a diuresis, furosemide can decrease effective blood volume (Figure 49.5) and cardiac output and activate the renin-angiotensin system which can adversely alter corticomedullary blood flow. It disrupts tubuloglomerular feedback mechanisms and can compromise the tenuous perfusion and oxygen balance in the medulla and promote additional injury (Karajala et al. 2009). Furosemide induced urine production may mislead the clinician about the functional status of the kidney and divert attention from fundamental therapeutic needs or delay initiation of supportive RRT. Current experience and evidence would challenge the rational use of furosemide or other loop diuretic to prevent or benefit the course of AKI or to improve outcomes for animals with oliguric forms of the disease.

Furosemide effectively increases urine output in some animals with AKI, which may be appropriate and beneficial to manage overhydration and to facilitate delivery of large-volume therapies like parenteral nutrition. The conversion from an oliguric to a nonoliguric state may facilitate some aspects of patient management; however, furosemide therapy should not be regarded as a "backup" or "bailout" for overaggressive or inattentive fluid management resulting in volume overload. When prescribed to manage fluid overload, furosemide is given initially at 2–4 mg/kg IV with appropriate monitoring of fluid balance and blood pressure. If an adequate diuresis of greater than 1 mL/kg/hour is not achieved within 30 minutes, the initial dose can be repeated. If a diuresis is achieved, the dosage can be repeated every 6–8 hours or given as a constant rate infusion at 0.25–1.0 mg/kg/hour to extend the diuresis as required. Fluid balance must be monitored carefully to prevent volume contraction which may further impair renal function. (Figure 49.5) There is no indication for the use of furosemide or loop diuretics in animals with nonoliguric AKI except to manage overhydration, hyperkalemia, or toxin elimination.

Dopamine agonists

Dopamine is a catecholamine with multiple physiologic, receptor specific, and dose dependent actions in the kidney with the potential to induce a diuresis in dogs with AKI (Venkataram and Kellum 2001; Sigrist 2007). The major physiologic actions of dopamine affect the renal vasculature to alter renal vascular resistance, renal blood flow and distribution, and GFR and modulate sodium and water reabsorption along the nephron (Fink et al. 1985; Schaer et al. 1985; Furukawa et al. 2002; Tobata et al. 2004; Sigrist 2007). The pharmacologic effects of dopamine are dose dependent and differentially mediated through dopaminergic (DA1-like and DA2-like) and adrenergic receptors. In dogs, DA1-like mediated vascular responses promote pre-glomerular vasodilation, decreased renal vascular resistance, and increased renal blood flow (Fink et al. 1985; Schaer et al. 1985; Furukawa et al. 2002; Tobata et al. 2004; Sigrist 2007). DA1-like

tubular effects inhibit sodium reabsorption along the nephron. DA1-like "renal responses" occur at doses of dopamine between 0.5 and 3 µg/kg/minute.

DA2-like receptors on postganglionic sympathetic nerves inhibit norepinephrine-mediated effects of sympathetic stimulation leading to vasodilatation and reduced sympathetic tone and increased PGE$_2$ production. Activation of DA2-like receptors facilitates the intrarenal DA1-mediated vascular effects and may have direct inhibitory effects on sodium reabsorption on renal tubular cells. DA2-like receptors are activated at doses between 2 and 3 µg/kg/minute, overlapping the effects of the DA1-like receptors.

Activation of β-1 adrenergic receptors occurs at slightly higher dosages between 3 and 10 µg/kg/minute. At this dosage, dopamine has positive inotropic effects on the heart which promotes increased cardiac output and perfusion to the kidney and increased urine formation (Furukawa et al. 2002; Tobata et al. 2004; Sigrist 2007). At doses higher than 10 µg/kg/minute, dopamine activates α-adrenergic receptors. The intrarenal effects at this dosage range include vasoconstriction, increased vascular resistance, decreased GFR, increased sodium reabsorption, and decreased urine formation, which are contrary to therapeutic goals in AKI (Furukawa et al. 2002; Tobata et al. 2004; Sigrist 2007).

Studies in anesthetized and conscious cats document a different spectrum and sensitivity of dopaminergic effects (Wassermann et al. 1980; Clark et al. 1991b; Flournoy et al. 2003; Simmons et al. 2006). Low-dose dopamine infusion (up to 3 µg/kg/minute) caused no significant changes in mean arterial blood pressure, heart rate, urine output, or sodium excretion (Wassermann et al. 1980; Clark et al. 1991b). Only at doses greater than 10 µg /kg/minute did dopamine infusion result in dose-dependent increases in urine output and sodium excretion; however, the diuretic response was associated with variable decreases in GFR, renal vasoconstriction, and inconsistent changes in mean arterial blood pressure and renal blood flow which would be contraindicated in AKI. These findings are most consistent with effects induced by stimulation of α-adrenergic receptors by the higher dopamine doses (Clark et al. 1991b). These differences in the actions of dopamine in cats make the therapeutic administration of dopamine to stimulate a diuresis and natriuresis in oliguric cats conceptually inappropriate and potentially detrimental to renal recovery.

Recently, DA1-like receptors with a high affinity to fenoldopam, a pure DA1 agonist, were identified in the kidney cortex of cats (Flournoy et al. 2003). Fenoldopam administration to conscious cats also has been shown to promote a delayed DA1-mediated diuresis and naturiuresis with variable and inconsistent effects on GFR (Clark et al. 1991a; Clark et al. 1991b; Simmons et al. 2006). Low dosage administration of fenoldopam (<2 µg/kg/minute) or selective DA-1 receptor agonist (YM435) to anesthetized dogs shows similar effects to promote increases in renal blood flow, diuresis and natriuresis with variable and dose dependent influences on systemic hemodynamics and GFR (Yatsu et al. 1997a; Yatsu et al. 1997b; Yatsu et al. 1997c; Halpenny et al. 2001; Murray et al. 2003). Administration of fenoldopam or selective DA-1 receptor agonists to experimental dogs subjected to endotoxic shock, renal ischemia, angiotensin II, Amphotericin B, and other vasoconstricting stimuli have shown significant acute increases in renal blood flow, urine formation, sodium excretion, and improved glomerular filtration (Fink et al. 1985; Nichols et al. 1992; Yatsu et al. 1997c; Yatsu et al. 1998).

Administration of dopaminergic drugs is not without risk. At a range of doses, dopamine can cause renal vasoconstriction, ventricular tachyarrhythmias, medullary hypoxia, and potential for myocardial, intestinal and renal ischemia. Fenoldopam can promote decreased systemic vascular resistance and hypotension. The narrow therapeutic margin and overlap in dosage effects, variable and uncertain elimination kinetics in AKI, and the variable sensitivity and binding affinities for catecholamines in uremic animals make their use risky (Venkataram and Kellum 2001; Sigrist 2007).

Effect of diuretic use on outcome

Despite the early observational and experimental benefits ascribed to diuretic agents and dopaminergic drugs in oliguric forms of AKI that have fostered the generalized use of these agents using urine output as a surrogate for outcome, there has been little documented benefit for their use to attenuate the renal injury, improve mortality, or requirement for RRT (Venkataram and Kellum 2001). Their specific benefits are to increase urine formation and for pressor control. Consensus opinion in human medicine states the use of diuretics or vasoactive drugs in the treatment of AKI should be based exclusively on the need for fluid management and they have no rational indication for the treatment of AKI per se (Venkataram and Kellum 2001; Mehta et al. 2002; Uchino et al. 2004; Bagshaw et al. 2007; Jo et al. 2007; Townsend and Bagshaw 2008; Karajala et al. 2009). Outcomes analysis has not been performed in veterinary patients with naturally acquired AKI to confirm or refute a benefit for the use of diuretics and vasoactive drugs. It is likely that the timing of the renal insult and injury will never be optimal for interventional strategies in the majority of animals. Until conclusive evidence is available, fluid therapy remains the most efficacious therapeutic approach

and the use of diuretics and vasoactive drugs should be reserved to facilitate management of excessive fluid burdens and hyperkalemia. If oliguria or anuria persists following fluid resuscitation, therapeutic efforts should be directed to starting renal replacement therapies.

Management of electrolyte and acid base disorders

Hyperkalemia

Hyperkalemia is a common and life-threatening electrolyte complication of AKI. The severity of the hyperkalemia and the impending or persisting cardiac and neuromuscular disturbances predicate the therapeutic approach. Hyperkalemia is more prevalent and generally more severe in oliguric and anuric animals and is usually proportional to the stage of AKI. Therapy is prioritized according to the severity to (1) antagonize the increased resting potential in the heart, (2) redistribute potassium from the extracellular to the intracellular fluid compartment, and (3) remove the potassium load from the body.

Severe hyperkalemia (>8 mEq/L) is associated with life threatening cardiac arrhythmias and conduction disturbances that are accentuated by how quickly the hyperkalemia developed and the degree of hyponatremia, hypocalcemia and acidosis. For immediate resolution of these signs, calcium gluconate (10% solution) is administered at 0.5–1.0 mL/kg as a slow intravenous bolus to effect to increase the threshold potential for cardiac excitation and correct the bradycardia and ECG abnormalities (Ahmed and Weisberg 2001; Cowgill and Francey 2005; DiBartola and de Morais 2006; Putcha and Allon 2007; Schaer 2008; Willard 2008). Calcium chloride is not recommended due to its potency, acidifying tendency, and irritation if injected extravascularly. Rapid injection of calcium solutions may cause hypotension and cardiac arrhythmias; therefore, arterial blood pressure and an electrocardiogram should be monitored during treatment. The infusion should be halted temporarily if S-T segment elevation, Q-T interval shortening, progressive bradycardia, or hypotension is observed. The effects of calcium infusion are rapid in onset but of short duration (approximately 30–60 minutes). Calcium administration does not lower the serum potassium concentration or resolve the excessive potassium burden. It provides a finite, life-saving reprieve until longer-lasting therapies to control the hyperkalemia can be initiated.

Serum potassium concentrations can be lowered in animals with non life-threatening hyperkalemia or following treatment with calcium salts by increasing the renal or extrarenal clearance of potassium or by the intracellular translocation of potassium. Mild and moderate hyperkalemia (<7.0 mEq/L) may resolve spontaneously with the induction of a diuresis. All potassium containing fluid used to support the diuresis should be replaced with solutions devoid of potassium. The renal elimination of potassium can be increased with furosemide administration at 1–2 mg/kg IV each 6–12 hours in non oliguric and fluid replete animals with mild hyperkalemia. Serum potassium and fluid balance should be monitored closely to prevent dehydration and to insure the hyperkalemia is controlled.

If a diuresis cannot be established or serum potassium cannot be controlled with fluid and furosemide administration, other measures should be instituted to lower serum potassium. Regular insulin at 0.25–1.0 units/kg IV in combination with intravenous dextrose at 1–2 gm/unit of administered insulin is used for the rapid correction of hyperkalemia (Ahmed and Weisberg 2001; Cowgill and Francey 2005; DiBartola and de Morais 2006; Putcha and Allon 2007; Schaer 2008; Willard 2008; Langston 2010). Insulin activates Na^+K^+-ATPase activity promoting the direct cellular uptake of potassium which is uninfluenced by other drugs and clinical conditions. Hypoglycemia is the most common side effect and the blood glucose concentration should be monitored closely to adjust the concurrent dextrose administration. Hypertonic (20%) dextrose can be administered singularly at 0.5–1.5 gm/kg intravenously if the hyperkalemia is not severe. Glucose stimulates insulin release which secondarily increases the uptake of potassium into the cells.

The administration of sodium bicarbonate to lower serum potassium had been accepted widely in the past, but recently its benefit has undergone reconsideration. The influence of alterations of acid-base on changes in serum potassium may be affected considerably by the duration of the hyperkalemia and the clinical conditions predisposing the disturbance (Ahmed and Weisberg 2001; Putcha and Allon 2007). Sodium bicarbonate has shown anecdotal benefits to alleviate the cardiac conduction disturbances and lower serum potassium in animals with AKI in the authors' experience, but there is little immediate efficacy to bicarbonate administration on serum potassium in human patients with end-stage renal disease (Gutierrez et al. 1991; Blumberg et al. 1992; Allon and Shanklin 1996; Kaplan et al. 1997; Ahmed and Weisberg 2001; Putcha and Allon 2007). Under conditions in which the metabolic acidosis associated with AKI warrants correction, sodium bicarbonate can be given to correct an existing bicarbonate deficit. Bicarbonate administration increases extracellular pH which translocates potassium into cells in exchange for hydrogen ions (Cowgill and Francey 2005; DiBartola and de Morais 2006; Schaer 2008). Sodium bicarbonate administration is contraindicated in animals with metabolic alkalosis or hypercapnia and may exacerbate overhydration and hypertonicity. Sodium bicarbonate administration can lower serum calcium concentrations and must be used cautiously in animals with preexisting hypocalcemia. Compelling studies in experimental dogs with induced hyperkalemia demonstrated hypertonic sodium chloride administration to be equally effective as sodium bicarbonate administration to reduce serum potassium concentration and alleviate the cardiac conduction disturbances (Kaplan et al. 1997; Kaplan et al. 2000). The effects of bicarbonate and glucose/insulin are more sustained than calcium gluconate but must be repeated as clinical circumstances dictate until the potassium load is alleviated.

Beta-2 adrenergic stimulation facilitates potassium influx into cells and has been exploited to treat hyperkalemia (Ahmed and Weisberg 2001; Putcha and Allon 2007; Mount and Zandi-Nejad 2008). Albuterol and terbutaline have been used for the management of hyperkalemia in human patients but experience in animals with AKI is lacking.

Mild hyperkalemia (<6.0 mEq/L) is rarely problematic but should be monitored at 8–12 hours intervals. Mild hyperkalemia generally resolves with initial (potassium free) replacement fluids alone or with furosemide and/or bicarbonate administration. For long-term control in refractory cases, sodium polystyrene sulfonate resin (Kayexalate) may be given orally at 2 g/kg in 3–4 divided doses suspended in water or 20% sorbitol to prevent constipation. This resin exchanges sodium for potassium across intestinal mucosa promoting intestinal potassium clearance. Exchange resins are variably effective for sustained control of low grade hyperkalemia, but have little indication for the management of life-threatening hyperkalemia. The administration of Kayexalate is facilitated by use of an esophageal feeding tube, but its acceptability is influenced by side-effects including nausea, constipation, gastrointestinal ulceration and necrosis.

If conventional therapy fails to provide an immediate or lasting resolution for the hyperkalemia, peritoneal or hemodialysis are indicated as the only alternative therapies. For all degrees of hyperkalemia associated with AKI, the most effective and persisting treatment is hemodialysis which achieves whole body clearance of the excessive potassium load. Serum potassium concentration is generally normalized by the end of the dialysis session but undergoes a variable rebound after dialysis influenced by its compartmentalization and transference form the intracellular compartment. Life-threatening cardiac conduction disturbances and ECG abnormalities improve dramatically within minutes of starting hemodialysis without perceptible changes in peripheral blood potassium concentrations (Cowgill and Francey 2005; DiBartola and de Morais 2006). It is plausible the markedly reduced potassium concentration, blood pH, or sodium concentration returning from the dialyzer via the dialysis catheter to the patient's right atrium provides sufficient alteration to coronary circulation to stabilize the myocardium and correct the ECG abnormalities.

Potassium laden fluids and parenteral nutrition solutions with high potassium concentrations can promote hyperkalemia and must be avoided. Similarly, commercial diets high in potassium can cause hyperkalemia. An appropriate diet for hyperkalemic patients may require formulation by a veterinary nutritionist (Segev et al. 2010). Drugs including potassium-sparing diuretics, ACE inhibitors, angiotensin-receptor blockers, and β-2 blocking drugs may promote hyperkalemia and should be used cautiously.

Hypokalemia

Hypokalemia can develop at all stages of AKI if renal potassium losses exceed exogenous inputs. The use of diuretics, inadequate dietary potassium intake, vomiting and diarrhea, and post obstructive diuresis may contribute to the development of hypokalemia. Hypokalemia is usually a laboratory abnormality but clinical signs may be noted if the serum potassium concentration is less than 2.5 mEq/L. Muscle weakness, fatigue, vomiting, anorexia, gastrointestinal ileus, and cardiac dysrhythmias may be seen in affected animals (Schaer 2008; Willard 2008). Ventroflexion of the neck is commonly observed in cats.

Oral potassium supplementation at 1–3 mEq/kg/day is given to animals that are able to eat or being fed through a feeding tube. Even in animals that require parenteral supplementation, serum potassium is rarely less than 2.0 mEq/L, and increasing the potassium concentration of maintenance solutions to 20–30 mEq/L is usually sufficient to restore normokalemia. Potassium supplementation of maintenance solutions should be prescribed cautiously in uremic animals with normal serum potassium concentrations, and serum potassium should be evaluated frequently to avoid hyperkalemia.

Acid-base imbalances

Acid-base disorders are common in animals with AKI. They are often mixed and must be treated on the basis of measured serum bicarbonate concentrations and blood gas analysis. Metabolic acidosis is the most consistent acid-base disturbance. Mild to moderate metabolic acidosis (serum bicarbonate >15 mEq/L) will often resolve following fluid replacement with re-establishment of tissue perfusion and the onset of a diuresis. More severe (serum bicarbonate <15 mEq/L) or persisting metabolic acidosis warrants treatment with intravenous sodium bicarbonate. The initial goal of bicarbonate replacement is to ameliorate, not necessarily resolve, the metabolic acidosis. Serum pH should be corrected to approximately 7.2 and serum bicarbonate to 14–16 mEq/L to stabilize cardiac conduction and contractility and serum potassium. The initial bicarbonate replacement dose (mEq) = [body weight (kg) × 0.3 × bicarbonate deficit], where 0.3 represents the early volume of distribution for bicarbonate, and the bicarbonate deficit is the desired bicarbonate—measured bicarbonate. One-half the calculated replacement is administered intravenously over 30 minutes, and the remainder is provided with intravenous fluids during the following 2–4 hours, if arterial pH has not increased to a value greater than 7.2 following initial distribution (30–60 minutes) of the first dosage (Cowgill and Francey 2005; DiBartola 2006; de Morais et al. 2008; Langston 2008; Langston 2010). Full equilibration of the initial bicarbonate dose requires 2–4 hours, but most uremic animals have an ongoing requirement for sodium bicarbonate of approximately 80–90 mg/kg/day to offset production of metabolic acids. Serum bicarbonate (blood gases and electrolytes) should be reassessed following the estimated initial replacement and at least daily to determine if the deficit is replete or additional therapy is required. Excessive sodium bicarbonate administration can promote metabolic alkalosis, ECF fluid volume overload, pulmonary edema and hypertension. Serum potassium and ionized calcium concentrations may fall with over-correction of the acidemia causing secondary hypoventilation, hypercapnia, shift in oxy-hemoglobin dissociation, reduced tissue oxygen delivery, and paradoxical cerebral acidosis (DiBartola 2006).

The therapeutic goal for bicarbonate replacement is the maintenance of serum bicarbonate between 18 and 20 mEq/L. Ongoing bicarbonate requirements can be supplied with sodium bicarbonate administered per os or via a feeding tube at 30–40 mg/kg every 12 hours to achieve this goal once the animal tolerates oral medication. Alternately, potassium citrate (75 mg/kg per os each 12 hours) can be used if potassium supplementation is needed concurrently. Each citrate molecule is converted into three bicarbonate molecules in the liver. The dosage of the alkalinizing drug is adjusted as necessary according to subsequent bicarbonate measurements to maintain the therapeutic goal.

Mild to moderate metabolic alkalosis (serum bicarbonate between 25 and 35 mEq/L) usually resolves with administration of normal saline or balanced electrolyte solutions to correct ECF volume and chloride deficits and with the onset of diuresis. Persistent vomiting must be controlled with antiemetics (see below) to prevent ongoing metabolic alkalosis. RRT with intermittent or continuous modalities can correct either metabolic acidosis or metabolic alkalosis within the first day of therapy (Cowgill and Francey 2006; Ronco and Ricci 2008). Long-term control of metabolic acid-base disorders by RRT is required until the kidneys are able to regulate acid-base metabolism. The rate and degree of correction is predicated on the frequency and duration of dialysis, the dialysis modality, and the dialysate bicarbonate prescription.

Respiratory acid-base disorders may predominate or contribute to the acid-base profile of animals with concurrent pulmonary complications (see Clinical Consequences, above). Management of the respiratory components of the acid-base disorders requires correction of the underlying pulmonary and/or plural disease and appropriate regulation of ventilation and oxygenation. Sodium bicarbonate is not an appropriate therapy for the acidemia of respiratory origin.

Uremia intoxications

Retained solutes normally removed by the kidneys contribute to the clinical expression of AKI and must be cleared from the body by restoration of excretory function, intensive fluid diuresis, or renal replacement therapies to resolve the signs attributable to these "uremic intoxication". Immediate recovery of excretory function is possible only with volume-responsive and obstructive forms of AKI. In advanced stages of AKI, the symptomatology of the uremia increases with advancing stage, and supportive therapies must be provided to control these manifestations until the injury is repaired.

Oral and gastrointestinal

Oral hygiene, uremic stomatitis, and oral ulceration can be improved dramatically by rinsing the oral cavity with solutions or gels containing 0.1–0.2% chlorhexidine every 8–12 hours. This therapy reduces the bacterial contamination of the oral cavity, helps prevent and heal oral ulcers, and relieves the discomfort associated with the stomatitis and lingual necrosis.

Antiemetic therapy is required to manage the fluid, electrolyte, and acid-base imbalances, nutritional requirements, and the discomfort associated with protracted nausea and vomiting. All oral fluids, medications, and food should be withheld initially until vomiting has been ameliorated at least partially with antiemetic therapy. H2-receptor antagonists such as ranitidine and famotidine are used commonly for the management of gastritis, vomiting, gastric erosion, gastric ulceration, and esophagitis which often accompany uremia. These drugs are not likely to be effective or indicated for vom-

iting of purely central origins in the absence of gastritis (Table 49.4). They reduce gastric acid production by blocking the histamine receptor on gastric parietal cells. They also reduce pepsin production which may promote gastric ulcers formation. H2-receptor antagonists undergo 50–70% renal elimination, and their dose should be reduced in proportion to the degree excretory failure to prevent CNS mediated side-effects. Omeprazole is a potent inhibitor of gastric acid secretion, and acts by irreversible inactivation of H^+/K^+-ATPase activity preventing secretion of hydrogen ions into the stomach (Washabau and Elie 1995; Abelo et al. 2002; Bersenas et al. 2005). Omeprazole reduces acid secretion in the dog for up to 24 hours. Pantaprazole is an injectable proton-pump blocker that can be used in animals unable to tolerate oral omeprazole.

Sucralfate and prostaglandin analogues may be used to manage gastric erosion, ulceration and hemorrhage. Sucralfate is a basic aluminum salt of sucrose octasulfate which binds tightly to exposed protein in gastric ulcers to form a protective barrier to the ulcerogenic and inflammatory effects of gastric acid, pepsin, bile, or pancreatic secretions. Sucralfate also stimulates mucus and bicarbonate secretion and mucosal prostaglandin production with the potential to improve microvascular integrity and mucosal blood flow. Sucralfate is also useful for the management of esophagitis associated with gastric reflux and irritation from esophageal feeding tubes. The efficacy of sucralfate may be limited until active vomiting is controlled with concurrent antiemetic therapy. Misoprostol is a synthetic PGE1 analogue that stimulates the mucus and bicarbonate content of the mucosal barrier. It increases epithelial cell renewal, maintains mucosal blood flow, and stabilizes tissue lysozymes. Misoprostol also reduces gastric acid secretion by binding to an E-receptor on the basolateral aspect of parietal cells. Medical therapy for vomiting and the gastrointestinal complications of AKI are usually continued for 2–3 weeks but may need extension in animals with severe gastritis following some etiologies, that is, antifreeze ingestion or with severe uremia.

Centrally acting antiemetics should be used if vomiting cannot be controlled by local treatments for the gastritis (Table 49.4). Metoclopramide is a D2-dopaminergic antagonist that directly suppresses the chemoreceptor trigger zone (Washabau and Elie 1995; Brown and Otto 2008; Willard 2009). It also has prokinetic effects on the stomach to promote gastric emptying which is often delayed in uremic animals. Metoclopramide can be provided by either oral or parenteral routes and is most effective when administered as a constant intravenous infusion (Table 6). Metoclopramide is excreted by the kidneys and the dosage needs modification in animals

Table 49.4 Drugs used for treating gastrointestinal manifestations of uremia

Indication	Mechanism	Drug	Dose–dog	Dose–cat	Comments
Stomatitis or oral ulceration	Bacteriocidal agent	Chlorhexidine			
Esophagitis, gastritis, gastric ulceration/hemorrhage	H_2-receptor antagonist	Famotidine (Pepcid® *Merck Sharp Dohme*)	0.5–1.0 mg/kg PO, IM, IV q 12–24 hours	0.25–0.5 mg/kg PO, SQ q 24 hours	
		Ranidtidine Zantac® *Glaxo*)	0.5–2.0 mg/kg PO, IV q 8–12 hours	0.5–2.5 mg/kg PO, SQ, IM, IV q 12 hours	
		Cimetidine (Tagamet® *Smith Kline*)	5–10 mg/kg PO, IM, IV q 4–6 hours	5–10 mg/kg PO, IM, IV (slow) q 6–8 hours	
	Proton pump blocker	Omeprazole (Prilosec® *Merck Sharp Dohme*)	0.5–1.0 mg/kg PO q 24 hours	0.7 mg/kg PO q 24 hours	Do not open capsules
		Panteprazole (Protoxix® *Wyeth*)	0.5–1.0 mg/kg IV (over 15 minutes) q 24 hours	0.5–1.0 mg/kg IV (over 15 minutes) q 24 hours	
	Cytoprotective agent	Sucralfate (Carafate® *Marion*)	0.5–1.0 g PO q 6–8 hours	0.25–0.5 g PO q 8–12 hours	Give 30 minutes prior to antacid
Prevention of NSAID GI toxicity	PGE_1 analogue	Misoprostol (Cytotec® *Searle*)	1–3 mcg/kg PO q 6–12 hours		
Antiemetic—CRTZ, emetic center	α_2-adrenergic, D_2-dopaminergic, H_1-histaminergic, M_1-cholinergic antagonists	Chlorpromazine (Thorazine® *Smith Kline*)	0.2–0.5 mg/kg IM, SQ q 6–8 hours	0.2–0.5 mg/kg IM, SQ q 8 hours	
		Prochlorperazine (Compazine® *Smith Kline*)	0.1–0.5 mg/kg IM, SQ q 8–12 hours		
		Acepromazine (PromAce® *Fort Dodge*)	0.01–0.05 mg/kg IM, SQ q 8–12 hours		
Antiemetic—CRTZ, peripheral vagal nerve 0.1–0.3 mg/kg IV q 8–12 hours	$5\text{-}HT_3$ receptor antagonist 0.1 mg/kg PO q 6–8 hours, 0.1–0.3 mg/kg IV q 6–8 hours	Ondansetron (Zofran® *Glaxo Wellcome*)	0.1 mg/kg PO q 12–24 hours		
		Dolasetron (Anzemet® *Hoechst Marion Russel*)	0.5 mg/kg PO, SQ, IV q 24 hours	0.5 mg/kg PO, SQ, IV q 24 hours	
Antiemetic—emetic center, peripheral vagal nerve	Neurokinin receptor antagonist	Maropitant (Cerenia® *Pfizer*)	2 mg/kg PO for 2 days or 1 mg/kg SQ q 24 hours for 5 days	0.5 mg/kg SQ q 24 hours for 5 days	
Antiemetic, prokinetic agent 0.01–0.02 mg/kg/hour CRI	D_2-dopaminergic antagonist, $5\text{-}HT_3$-serotonergic antagonist 0.2–0.4 mg/kg SQ q 6–8 hours or 0.01–0.02 mg/kg/hour CRI	Metoclopramide (Reglan® *Robins*)	0.1–0.5 mg/kg PO, IM, SQ q 6–8 hours		
Prokinetic agent	$5\text{-}HT_4$ receptor agonist, $5\text{-}HT_1/5\text{-}HT_2$ receptor antagonist	Cisapride® (Propulsid *Jansen Pharmceutica Inc*)	0.1–0.5 mg/kg PO q 8–12 hours	2.5–5 mg/cat PO q 8–12 hours	

with severe uremia. Phenothiazine derivative antiemetics (chlorpromazine, prochloroperazine, acepromazine) antagonise α_2-adrenergic receptors at the CRTZ and the emetic center. They are effective antiemetics in uremic animals but are prone to sedative and hypotensive side-effects. They should be considered for animals with intractable vomiting in whom the adverse effects can be accepted. The 5-hydroxytryptamine serotonergic antiemic, ondansetron, has central antiemetic effects at both the CRTZ and emetic center. It is highly effective for chemotherapy-induced vomiting and has shown efficacy for vomiting in animals with AKI. Maropitant is a newly developed class of antiemetic that is gaining favor in uremic animals. Maropitant is a highly specific neurokinin receptor antagonist that blocks the actions of substance P in the emetic center preventing neurotransmission of central or peripheral efferent emetic signals (de la Puente-Redondo et al. 2007; Sedlacek et al. 2008). Maropitant has shown excellent efficacy to prevent acute vomiting induced by a broad spectrum of etiologies including uremia (de la Puente-Redondo et al. 2007; Sedlacek et al. 2008). Although only recently approved for use in dogs, Maropitant has generally replaced the use of other antiemetics for severe and protracted vomiting in both dogs and cats with AKI.

Hematologic and immune disorders

Uremic bleeding intensifies with the stage of AKI and can be life-threatening if associated with CNS or pulmonary hemorrhage (Sohal et al. 2006; Brophy et al. 2007). More commonly uremia is associated with gastrointestinal hemorrhage and anemia or bleeding subsequent to invasive procedures, that is, percutaneous renal biopsies (Sohal et al. 2006). Uremic bleeding improves with resolution of the azotemia following intensive diuresis or dialysis (Boccardo et al. 2004; Galbusera et al. 2009). Transfusion of packed red blood cells is indicated for animals with active bleeding which may reduce the bleeding time through effects on some platelet functions (Livio et al. 1982; Galbusera et al. 2009). Transfusion of platelet rich plasma does not improve platelet function or reduce bleeding time because the function of the transfused cells is altered upon exposure to uremic plasma. Desmopressin administration may be warranted in uremic animals with prolonged bleeding times and active bleeding or prior to performing invasive procedures (Galbusera et al. 2009). The effects are seen within an hour of administration and may persist for 4–8 hours (Galbusera et al. 2009).

EPO replacement therapy is indicated for animals with anemia due to acute-on-chronic AKI or hemorrhage or those expected to develop anemia due to a protracted recovery period, ongoing hemorrhage or excessive blood sampling, blood product incompatibilities, or in animals started on RRT. Darbepoetin (Aranesp™, Amgen, Thousand Oaks, Ca) should be used preferentially to EPOGEN due to its reduced likelihood to induce anit-r-HuEPO antibodies. EPO replacement therapy is divided into an initiation phase to activate erythropoiesis and a maintenance phase to perpetuate the response. The treatment target is a hematocrit of 37–45% for dogs and 30–40% for cats. The initial recommended dose for darbopoetin is 0.45 mcg/kg body weight administered SC once weekly. As the hematocrit reaches the bottom of the respective target range, the dosing interval is decreased to once every 2 weeks. As the hematocrit approaches the upper target value, the dosage interval is reduced further to once every 3 weeks to prevent polycythemia. The dosage schedule is modified as required every 1–3 weeks to maintain the hematocrit within the target range.

The maintenance dosage to sustain the hematocrit within the target range must be established according to the responses of individual animals by frequent monitoring of the hematocrit and adjustment of the dosage interval. Generally, 0.25–0.5 mcg/kg of darbepoetin subcutaneously every 2–3 weeks is sufficient. EPO replacement therapy is discontinued when renal function is recovered sufficiently to maintain erythropoiesis. Animals with partial recovery of renal function that develop CKD may require EPO replacement indefinitely. Progressive decreases in hematocrit, red blood cell count, and hemoglobin concentration secondary to development of anti-r-HuEPO antibodies are the most problematic complications of darbepoetin administration in animals. Aplastic anemia has been recognized in a limited number of dogs and cats treated with darbepoetin, but the incidence is considerably less than recognized with EPOGEN.

Impaired immunity

Uremic animals have increased susceptibility to infection due to accumulation of uremia toxins which impair immunity and cellular host defenses (Haag-Weber and Horl 1993; Horl 2001; Raff et al. 2008; Vanholder et al. 2008). The deficiencies in host defenses are compounded by widespread breaches of mucosal integrity associated with gastrointestinal ulceration, intravenous and bladder catheterization, parenteral medications and nutrition, and intervention with hemodialysis, peritoneal dialysis, and immunosuppressive drugs (Haag-Weber and Horl 1993; Clarkson et al. 2008). Primary sites of infection include the urinary tract, catheter-sites, and the respiratory tract. Infection may be difficult to identify as uremia dampens the febrile response. Strict asepsis during catheter placement and meticulous catheter-site care are mandatory, and the length of time for catheterizations should be minimized. If infection is suspected, blood, urine, and catheter tip cultures should be obtained and broad spectrum antibiotic therapy instituted while awaiting qbacterial identification. Prophylactic use of antibiotics may foster development of bacterial resistance and superinfections and should be prescribed with caution.

Respiratory disorders

Patients with respiratory compromise may require therapies to improve oxygenation. Treatment of the proximate cause of respiratory dysfunction is the first line of defense, but this is not always possible. Pleural effusion (especially in cats) is a common consequence of volume overload and is most directly controlled by thoracocentesis. Correction of volume overload, by fluid restriction, diuretic administration, or ultrafiltration via dialysis (hemo or peritoneal), is necessary if hydrostatic pulmonary edema is present. Cardiac medications may be indicated if cardiogenic pulmonary edema is present from left ventricular dysfunction. Treatment of noncardiogenic edema (i.e., adult respiratory distress syndrome, and uremic lung) is based on controlling the underlying uremic state, which may require aggressive dialytic therapy. Pulmonary hemorrhage, commonly associated with leptospirosis infection (Figure 49.1), may not respond to any therapy, but restriction of anticoagulation in the setting of extracorporeal RRT (i.e., hemodialysis or continuous renal replacement therapy (CRRT)) seems prudent to avoid exacerbating the bleeding. Bacterial and aspiration pneumonia should be treated with appropriate broad-spectrum antibiotic therapy, and aspiration pneumonia should be treated additionally with aggressive antiemetic therapy.

In conjunction with specific therapy, supportive respiratory care may be needed, including oxygen supplementation through an oxygen enriched environment, nasal oxygen, or mechanical ventilation.

Nutritional management

The goals of nutritional therapy are to meet the energy and nutrient requirements of the animal, correct protein-energy wasting, alleviate the azotemia, minimize disturbances in fluid, electrolyte, vitamin, mineral, and acid base balance, and aid renal regeneration and repair. It is clearly established that enteral or parenteral nutritional support should be instituted at the earliest opportunity to prevent ongoing protein-energy wasting and support renal regeneration and repair (Druml 2001; Druml 2001; Fiaccadori and Cremaschi 2009). Enteral therapy or combined enteral and parenteral delivery of nutrition is currently recommended over entirely parenteral delivery to support enterocyte viability and the mucosal barrier functions of the gut (Marks 1998). As a departure from historical practice, enteral nutrition is also recommended in animals in which vomiting has not been resolved completely.

The optimal nutritional regime for dogs and cats with AKI has not been defined, but a high energy and moderated protein, potassium and phosphate formulation as prescribed for CKD is logical and historically advocated. Sufficient energy must be supplied to prevent catabolism of endogenous protein to spare lean body mass and to minimize the azotemia. Animals that have been anorexic for as little as three days are already malnourished and should be provided nutritional support. The resting energy requirement provides an approximation of the energy requirement for animals with AKI and can be estimated from the following formulae:
$[RER (kcal/day) = 70(wt\,kg)0.75$ or $RER (kcal/day) = 70 + (30 \times wt\,kg)]$, where, RER is the resting energy requirement; Wtkg is the body weight in kilograms (Marks 1998; Delaney et al. 2006). The RER is only an approximation of the animal's actual energy needs and requires adjustment as clinical and catabolic conditions change or if body mass falls progressively. Carbohydrates and fats provide the non protein sources of energy required in the diet. Commercial therapeutic renal diets, liquid enteral formulations, parenteral solutions designed for the management of renal failure, or diets formulated by a veterinary nutritionist can be provided per os or through a feeding tube. Most dietary formulations contain a relatively high fat content to maximize the energy density and should be fed cautiously to minimize development of pancreatitis to which animals with AKI are predisposed.

Controlled reduction of non essential protein in the nutritional formulation is required to minimize urea appearance while avoiding protein malnutrition. The optimal protein requirement for animals with AKI is not known and is likely influenced by coexisting clinical conditions, the stage of AKI, and the requirement for RRT (Chan 2004; Fiaccadori and Cremaschi 2009; Valencia et al. 2009). Consequently, the minimum protein requirements for normal dogs [1.25–1.75 g/kg/day; 8–10% protein on a metabolizable energy basis] and cats [3.8–4.4 g/kg/day; 20–25% protein on a metabolizable energy basis] are generally applied to animals with AKI Stage III or greater. This degree of restriction may not be necessary or desired in animals with AKI Stage II or III, and more liberal protein prescriptions may be appropriate. Protein delivery can also be increased if the animal is treated with dialysis to prevent development of excessive azotemia. Phosphorus, sodium, potassium, and magnesium intake should be minimized to prevent accumulation of these minerals and electrolytes; however, intakes must be modified according to the clinical and biochemical dictates of the animal. Commercial therapeutic renal diets may promote hyperkalemia and hyponatremia when fed to dogs with AKI Stage III or greater which should be monitored (Segev et al. 2010).

Delivery of adequate nutrition is constrained by inappetence of the animal, the gastrointestinal manifestations of the uremia, and obtundation. Oral or enteral feeding may not be possible or recommended in the initial management of AKI due to gastritis, pancreatitis, uncontrolled vomiting, or mental status. Peripheral or central parenteral nutrition is indicated for these animals to provide interim nutritional support (Druml 2001, Delaney et al. 2006; Campbell et al. 2006). Peripheral parenteral nutrition is formulated with isotonic solutions administered through a peripheral vein. However, complete nutritional requirements cannot be met by this technique, and it should be used only as an adjunct to oral or enteral feeding or to supply partial nutritional support not in excess of five days. Central parenteral nutrition is formulated to provide all essential nutrients for indefinite periods but requires central venous administration due to the hypertonicity of the nutrient solutions (Campbell et al. 2006; Delaney et al. 2006).

Enteral tube feeding is the preferred route of nutritional support and is recommended in animals whose gastrointestinal health will tolerate feeding but fail to meet nutritional goals voluntarily (Marks 1998; Delaney et al. 2006). Esophageal feeding tubes are the most effective and safe enteral feeding device and are generally preferred over nasoesophageal or percutaneous gastrostomy tubes. Esophageal feeding tubes can be placed quickly under short general anesthesia and facilitate either short-term or indefinite feeding for dogs or cats with AKI (Fischer et al. 2004). Caloric and protein goals can be achieved by the administration of blended therapeutic diets, liquid enteral preparations, or individually formulated diets for the management of uremia. The clinical benefits of enteral or parenteral nutritional support cannot be over emphasized, but it may not be possible to supply the volume load required for the nutritional goals in oliguric animals without dialysis to alleviate overhydration.

Other therapies

Some new therapies including naturetic peptides (ANP and BNP), EPO, and stem cell therapy are under investigation, but their benefit remains to be proven (Bahlmann and Fliser 2009; Bussolati et al. 2009; Nigwekar et al. 2009; Schrier 2009).

Renal replacement therapy

RRT comprises modern extracorporeal techniques including intermittent hemodialysis and CRRT and peritoneal dialysis. The principles and techniques for these therapies have been reviewed extensively (Fischer et al. 2004; Cowgill and Francey 2006; Ross and Labato 2006; Acierno and Maeckelbergh 2008). and elsewhere in this book) Over the past 20 years, extracorporeal RRT has progressed from clinically obscure to mainstream and has now become the advanced standard for the management of uremia in animals. Despite the expanding interest and development of extracorporeal therapies, their availability remains regional and limited. AKI is the most common indication for RRT in dogs and cats (Cowgill and Langston 1996; Langston et al. 1997; Cowgill and Elliott 2000; Langston 2002; Fischer et al. 2004; Cowgill and Francey 2006; Ross and Labato 2006; Acierno and Maeckelbergh 2008; Langston 2008). Without some form of replacement therapy, animals who fail to respond to medical therapies are destined to die from complications of the uremia, precluding regeneration or repair of the renal injury.

The incontrovertible indications for RRT include severe volume overload, hyperkalemia, severe electrolyte and acid-base disturbances, anuria, toxin removal, and overt uremia. What remains equivocal is the timing to initiate RRT and the appropriate modality to institute (Fischer et al. 2004; Cowgill and Francey 2006; Palevsky 2008; Rauf et al. 2008; Ricci and Ronco 2008; Uchino 2008; Fieghen et al. 2009). The regional accessibility and cost of RRT forecast that animals generally will access these therapies at a late stage of disease when more practical medical therapies have been exhausted and failed. Belaboring ineffective conventional therapies often delays referral to a dialysis center and the timely initiation of RRT. As a guideline, RRT should be initiated in animals prior to development of overt uremia associated with AKI Stage IV and Stage V. Delay in therapy leads to greater uremic symptomology, morbidity, and recruitment of additional organ dysfunction. RRT should be considered an immediate therapeutic requirement when the clinical consequences of the azotemia, inadequate urine production, and the fluid, the electrolytes, and acid-base disturbances cannot be managed with medical therapy alone. Oliguric or anuric animals at any stage of AKI in which an effective diuresis cannot be maintained with initial replacement fluids and diuretics should be transferred immediately to an experienced referral center where RRT can be performed. Delays imposed by prolonged and ineffective medical therapy result in deterioration of the animal's condition and further predisposition to life-threatening azotemia, hypervolemia, hyperkalemia, and metabolic acidosis.

These guidelines are made on empirical foundations and clinical experience as no comparisons of early vs late timing to RRT have been reported for animals. They are consistent with observational comparisons of early vs late initiation of RRT in human patients with AKI, but currently there are no evidence-based recommendations on timing supported by outcomes assessments (Palevsky 2008; Fieghen et al. 2009). There are no specific contraindications to starting RRT in animals at milder but progressing stages of AKI as a prophylactic strategy to circumvent the overt morbidity of uremia and aggressive medical therapy.

Intermittent hemodialysis has increased efficiency and reduced labor intensity compared to both peritoneal dialysis and CRRT. It is also a more established extracorporeal modality than CRRT in animals (Cowgill and Langston 1996; Langston et al. 1997; Langston 2002; Fischer et al. 2004; Cowgill and Francey 2006; Ross and Labato 2006; Acierno and Maeckelbergh 2008). In appropriately trained and experienced hands, each is capable of resolving the life-threatening and morbid consequences of acute uremia (Ricci and Ronco 2008; Ronco and Ricci 2008; Uchino 2008; Fieghen et al. 2009). Intermittent hemodialysis techniques have been adapted to embrace some of the physiologic and therapeutic attraction of slow solute and fluid removal and greater hemodynamic stability attached to CRRT. Conversely, CRRT techniques have evolved to balance the labor intensiveness and expense associated with continuous management (Fischer et al. 2004; Cowgill and Francey 2006; Cruz et al. 2008; Ricci and Ronco 2008; Ronco and Ricci 2008). Continuous modalities are often provided over the initial 48–72 hours of RRT. Beyond this time, the vast majority of animals with AKI will require additional dialytic support until renal function returns. The equipment designed for continuous therapy may not be able to provide the kinetic efficiency required for alternate day or outpatient management. The regional center providing CRRT may not be equipped to provide the transition to intermittent therapy, necessitating referral to another regional center providing hemodialysis.

Failure to recover renal function following 2–4 weeks of conventional medical management has been used as a benchmark to predict irreversible from reversible renal failure in animals with AKI Stage III or greater and recommendations for euthanasia. However, these criteria required redefinition with the availability of hemodialysis. Many animals with seemingly irreversible disease at the outset of medical management can recover renal function if supported with hemodialysis beyond the 4-week benchmark. Animals with toxic insults usually have more protracted recovery times than animals with infectious, hemodynamic, or obstructive causes of AKI (Fischer et al. 2004; Cowgill and Francey 2006). In some instances complete or adequate partial recovery of renal function may require 2–6 months of RRT. This revised understanding of the reversibility of AKI has made it impossible to accurately predict outcome at initial presentation or during the early course of management. Pet owners must gamble and balance against the time and expense of RRT that the outcome will be favorable. There are no validated biomarkers of recovery to forecast individual outcomes, but it is often possible to document improvement in renal function from simple kinetic assessments of urea or creatinine during the course of dialysis to help gauge the prospects for recovery (Figure 49.6). Recently, a sensitive and specific scoring system was devised to quantitate the severity and to help predict outcome for recovery of dogs with AKI at presentation for hemodialysis (Segev et al. 2008b). These predictive tools require further prospective validation but may also facilitate outcome prediction in animals with AKI who do not require hemodialysis.

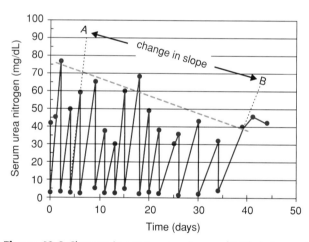

Figure 49.6 Changes in serum urea nitrogen (BUN) during and between hemodialysis sessions in a dog with AKI (Stage III, O, RRT) secondary to ethylene glycol intoxication. BUN drops dramatically during the hemodialysis session then increases during the interdialysis interval before the next treatment. The decrease in SUN during the hemodialysis session reflects the increased "intermittent" clearance of urea by the hemodialyzer. Recovery of residual renal function is identified by the progressive decrease in the predialysis SUN on subsequent days (dashed line), and the change in slope of the increase in SUN in the interdialysis interval (A and B, dotted lines). The change in slope represents a decrease in urea appearance associated with increasing "continuous" urea clearance by the injured kidneys.

Prognosis and outcome of AKI

The prognosis for recovery from acute uremia depends on the underlying cause, extent of the renal injury, the presence of comorbid diseases, degree of multiple organ involvement, and the availability of diagnostic and therapeutic services. The survival rate of AKI in people is about 50% (Ympa et al. 2005). Survival rates for AKI in dogs and cats are highly variable, but range from 20–60% in most large studies that include multiple etiologies (Behrend et al. 1996; Langston et al. 1997; Vaden et al. 1997; Forrester et al. 2002; Francey and Cowgill 2002; Pantaleo et al. 2004; Worwag and Langston 2008). When evaluated by etiology, some general differences in outcomes become apparent (Table 49.5). Survival rates of patients with AKI from a nephrotoxic cause are generally lower, whereas survival rates for infectious diseases and obstructive etiologies are generally more favorable. Dogs with leptospirosis infected with serogroup pomona suffered a worse prognosis for survival than infections with other serogroups. In a study of 20 dogs infected with various serogroups, mortality was correlated to increased cardiac troponin, and the ratio of C-reactive protein to haptoglobin (but not C-reactive protein or haptoglobin individually), which may prove to be useful for predicting outcome for recovery (Mastrorilli et al. 2007). Mortality was increased in dogs with icterus in one study (Miller et al. 2007).

No single parameter has been shown to be consistently prognostic. The degree of azotemia was not predictive of survival in most studies, but was predictive in one study of dogs with AKI from various etiologies and in two studies of dogs with leptospirosis. It is notable, however, that azotemia influenced the prognosis only in dogs treated with conventional therapy, but not in dogs treated with hemodialysis in which the azotemia can be controlled (Behrend et al. 1996; Langston et al. 1997; Vaden et al. 1997; Adin and Cowgill 2000; Forrester et al. 2002; Pantaleo et al. 2004; Mastrorilli et al. 2007; Miller et al. 2007; Worwag and Langston 2008). Azotemia in part may be a marker of the severity of renal damage, but all studies evaluated BUN and serum creatinine at presentation, and thus part of the azotemia may include the rapidly reversible hemodynamic component. Further, the severity of azotemia does not provide an indication of the reversibility of the underlying renal disease, so it is not surprising that etiology appears to play more of a role in predicting outcome than degree of azotemia. Urine volume was predictive in two studies, but not in a third (Behrend et al. 1996; Forrester et al. 2002; Worwag and Langston 2008). An elevated anion gap, hypoalbuminemia, proteinuria, and metabolic acidosis were predictive in two studies but not universally. (Behrend et al. 1996; Vaden et al. 1997; Forrester et al. 2002; Mastrorilli et al. 2007; Miller et al. 2007; Worwag and Langston 2008) Other parameters that were predictive of survival in isolated studies but not confirmed in others include hypocalcemia, hyperphosphatemia, and hyperkalemia (Behrend et al. 1996; Vaden et al. 1997; Worwag and Langston 2008).

Renal recovery may take up to 6 months, and long-term dialytic support during the recovery phase can improve survival rates. A clinical scoring system for outcome prediction of dogs with AKI receiving hemodialysis

Table 49.5 Survival rates for dogs and cats with AKI treated with conventional therapy or dialysis (Rentko et al. 1992; Behrend et al. 1996; Harkin and Gartrell 1996; Langston et al. 1997; Vaden et al. 1997; Adin and Cowgill 2000; Forrester et al. 2002; Francey and Cowgill 2002; Langston 2002; Fischer et al. 2004; Pantaleo et al. 2004; Rollings et al. 2004; Beckel et al. 2005; Eubig et al. 2005; Kyles et al. 2005; Francey 2006; Goldstein et al. 2006; Berg et al. 2007; Geisen et al. 2007; Mastorelli et al. 2007; Miller et al. 2007; Worwag and Langston 2008; Dorval and Boysen 2009)

Category	Dogs		Cats	
	Conventional (%)	Dialysis (%)	Conventional (%)	Dialysis (%)
Combined causes[a]	20–44	33–41	54	25–100
Infectious		70	—	58–100
Leptospirosis	52–82	76–86	—	—
Toxic	43	18	69	0–35
Ethylene glycol	0–8	12–20		44
Lily	—	—	75	33
Obstructive	—	—	75	70
Other[b]	25–37	56	55	29–72

[a]Data from series of AKI from various causes.
[b]Includes hemodynamic, ischemic, metabolic, and undetermined causes.

has been developed and will hopefully help in determining appropriate candidates for dialysis (Segev et al. 2008b). As the variables used for predicting outcome in dogs managed with hemodialysis are common to those with less severe AKI, similar predictive scoring systems may facilitate outcome prediction in other populations of animals with AKI (Segev et al. 2008b). Studies assessing survival in animals treated with conventional therapy cannot be compared to those managed with renal replacement therapies. There are often large disparities in the severity of the renal injury for animals managed with these respective approaches, and the window for survival is finite for animals treated conventionally and indefinite for animals treated with RRT. Severity scoring and staging of AKI will likely provide more precise understanding of outcomes of AKI.

Surviving patients tend to have a longer duration of hospitalization compared to non-survivors (Behrend et al. 1996; Vaden et al. 1997; Worwag and Langston 2008).

Incomplete resolution of azotemia and progression to CKD occurs in approximately 50% of animals that survive the initial AKI (Vaden et al. 1997; Kyles et al. 2005; Worwag and Langston 2008). However, some studies have found much better renal outcomes (Adin and Cowgill 2000; Dorval and Boysen 2009). These divergent observations regarding the residual renal function may reflect the underlying causes of the AKI or the therapeutic approaches employed to support survival. Patients discharged with normal renal parameters tend to maintain normal BUN and serum creatinine concentrations when monitored long-term.

References

Abbott, L.M. and J. Kovacic (2008). The pharmacologic spectrum of furosemide. *J Vet Emerg Crit Care* **18**(1): 26–39.

Abelo, A., et al. (2002). Gastric acid secretion in the dog: a mechanism-based pharmacodynamic model for histamine stimulation and irreversible inhibition by omeprazole. *J Pharmacokinet Pharmacodyn* **29**(4): 365–382.

Acierno, M.J. and V. Maeckelbergh (2008). Continuous renal replacement therapy. *Compend Contin Educ Pract Vet* **30**(5): 264–280.

Acierno, M.J., et al. (2008). Preliminary validation of a point-of-care ethylene glycol test for cats. *J Vet Emerg Crit Care* **18**(5): 477–479.

Adin, C.A. and L.D. Cowgill (2000). Treatment and outcome of dogs with leptospirosis: 36 cases (1990–1998). *J Am Vet Med Assoc* **216**(3): 371–375.

Adin, C.A., et al. (2003). Antegrade pyelography for suspected ureteral obstruction in cats: 11 cases (1995–2001). *J Am Vet Med Assoc* **222**(11): 1576–1581.

Agunloye, C.A. and A.S. Nash (1996). Investigation of possible leptospiral infection in cats in Scotland. *J Small Anim Pract* **37**(3): 126–129.

Ahmed, J. and L.S. Weisberg (2001). Hyperkalemia in dialysis patients. *Semin Dial* **14**(5): 348–356.

Alfrey, A.C. (1993). Aluminum Neurotoxicity. In: *Dialysis Therapy*, edited by A.R. Nissenson and R.N. Fine. Philadelphia, PA: Hanley & Belfus, pp. 275–277.

Allon, M. and N. Shanklin (1996). Effect of bicarbonate administration on plasma potassium in dialysis patients: interactions with insulin and albuterol. *Am J Kidney Dis* **28**(4): 508–514.

Anderson, R.J. and D.W. Barry (2004). Clinical and laboratory diagnosis of acute renal failure. *Best Pract Res Clin Anaesthesiol* **18**(1): 1–20.

Andrade, L., et al. (2008). Leptospiral nephropathy. *Semin Nephrol* **28**(4): 383–394.

Andreoli, S.P. (2009). Acute kidney injury in children. *Pediatr Nephrol* **24**: 253–263.

Anonomous (2007). Jerky treats from China could be causing illness in pets. *J Am Vet Med Assoc* **231**(8): 1183.

Antoniades, D.Z., et al. (2006). Ulcerative uremic stomatitis associated with untreated chronic renal failure: report of a case and review of the literature. *Oral Surg Oral Med Oral Pathol Oral Radiol Endod* **101**(5): 608–613.

Appleman, E.H., et al. (2008). Transient acquired Fanconi syndrome associated with copper storage hepatopathy in 3 dogs. *J Vet Intern Med* **22**(4): 1038–1042.

Arieff, A.I. (2008). Neurologic aspects of kidney disease. In: *Brenner & Rector's The Kidney*, edited by B.M. Brenner, Volume **2**. Philadelphia, PA: Saunders Elsevier, pp. 1757–1783.

Ash, S.R. (1991). An explanation for uremic hypothermia. *Int J Artif Organs* **14**(2): 67–69.

Atkins, C.E., et al. (2002). Effects of long-term administration of enalapril on clinical indicators of renal function in dogs with compensated mitral regurgitation. *J Am Vet Med Assoc* **221**(5): 654–658.

Badr, K.F. and I. Ichikawa (1988). Prerenal failure: a deleterious shift from renal compensation to decompensation. *N Engl J Med* **319**: 623–629.

Bagshaw, S.M., et al. (2008). Oliguria, volume overload, and loop diuretics. *Crit Care Med* **36**(4(Suppl)): S172–S178.

Bagshaw, S.M., et al. (2007a). Loop diuretics in the management of acute renal failure: a systematic review and meta-analysis. *Crit Care Resusc* **9**(1): 60–68.

Bagshaw, S.M., et al. (2007b). Diuretics in the management of acute kidney injury: a multinational survey. *Contrib Nephrol* **156**: 236–249.

Bagshaw, S.M. and R.T.N. Gibney (2008). Conventional markers of kidney function. *Crit Care Med* **36**(Suppl): S152–S158.

Bagshaw, S.M., et al. (2007c). A systematic review of urinary findings in experimental septic acute renal failure. *Crit Care Med* **35**(6): 1592–1598.

Bahlmann, F.H. and D. Fliser (2009). Erythropoietin and renoprotection. *Curr Opin Nephrol Hypertens* **18**(1): 15–20.

Barr, S.C., et al. (2005). Serologic responses of dogs given a commercial vaccine against *Leptospira interrogans* serovar pomona and *Leptospira kirschneri* serovar grippotyphosa. *Am J Vet Res* **66**(10): 1780–1784.

Barsanti, J.A. (2006). Genitourinary infections. In: *Infectious Diseases of the Dog and Cat*, edited by C.E. Greene. St. Louis, MO: Saunders Elsevier, pp. 935–961.

Barsanti, J.A., et al. (1994). Disease of the lower urinary tract. In: *The Cat: Diseases and Clinical Management*, edited by R.G. Sherding, Volume **2**. New York, NY: Churchill Livingstone, pp. 1769–1823.

Baumann, D. and M. Fluckiger (2001). Radiographic findings in the thorax of dogs with leptospiral infection. *Vet Radiol Ultrasound* **42**(4): 305–307.

Beckel, N.F., et al. (2005). Peritoneal dialysis in the management of acute renal failure in 5 dogs with leptospirosis. *J Vet Emerg Crit Care* **15**(3): 201–205.

Behnia, R., et al. (1996). Effects of hyperosmotic mannitol infusion on hemodynamics of dog kidney. *Anesth Analg* **82**(5): 902–908.

Behrend, E., et al. (1996). Hospital-acquired acute renal failure in dogs: 29 cases (1983–1992). *J Am Vet Med Assoc* **208**(4): 537–541.

Belgrave, R.L., et al. (2002). Effects of a polymerized ultrapurified bovine hemoglobin blood substitute administered to ponies with normovolemic anemia. *J Vet Intern Med* **16**(4): 396–403.

Bellomo, R., et al. (2005). Management of early acute renal failure: focus on post-injury prevention. *Curr Opin Crit Care* **11**: 542–547.

Bellomo, R., et al. (2004). Acute renal failure – definition, outcome measures, animal models, fluid therapy and information technology needs: the Second International Consensus Conference of the Acute Dialysis Quality Initiative (ADQI) Group. *Crit Care* **8**: R204–R212.

Berg, R.I., et al. (2007). Resolution of acute kidney injury in a cat after lily (*Lilium lancifolium*) intoxication. *J Vet Intern Med* **21**(4): 857–859.

Berg, R.J. and W. Wingfield (1984). Pericardial effusion in the dog: a review of 42 cases. *J Am Anim Hosp Assoc* **20**: 721–730.

Bersenas, A.M.E., et al. (2005). Effects of ranitidine, famotidine, pantoprazole, and omeprazole on intragastric pH in dogs. *Am J Vet Res* **66**(3): 425–431.

Better, O.S., et al. (1997). Mannitol therapy revisited (1940–1997). *Kidney Int* **51**: 866–894.

Bhalla, V., et al. (2009). Melamine nephrotoxicity: an emerging epidemic in an era of globalization. *Kidney Int* **75**(8): 774–779.

Birnbaum, N., et al. (1998). Naturally acquired leptospirosis in 36 dogs: serological and clinicopathological features. *J Small Anim Pract* **39**: 231–236.

Blumberg, A., et al. (1992). Effect of prolonged bicarbonate administration on plasma potassium in terminal renal failure. *Kidney Int* **41**(2): 369–374.

Boccardo, P., et al. (2004). Platelet dysfunction in renal failure. *Semin Thromb Hemost* **30**(5): 579–589.

Bonventre, J.V. (2003). Dedifferentiation and proliferation of surviving epithelial cells in acute renal failure. *J Am Soc Nephrol* **14**: S55–S61.

Bonventre, J.V. (2007). Diagnosis of acute kidney injury: from classic parameters to new biomarkers. *Contrib Nephrol* **156**: 213–219.

Bonventre, J.V. (2008). Kidney injury molecule-1 (KIM-1): a specific and sensitive biomarker of kidney injury. *Scand J Clin Lab Invest Suppl* **241**: 78–83.

Bonventre, J.V. and J.M. Weinberg (2003). Recent advances in the pathophysiology of ischemic acute renal failure. *J Am Soc Nephrol* **14**: 2199–2210.

Bonventre, J.V. and A. Zuk (2004). Ischemic acute renal failure: an inflammatory disease? *Kidney Int* **66**(2): 480–485.

Borjesson, D.L. (2003). Renal cytology. *Vet Clin North Am Small Anim Pract* **33**(1): 119–134.

Bouchard, J. and R.L. Mehta (2009a). Fluid accumulation and acute kidney injury: consequence or cause. *Curr Opin Crit Care* **15**(6): 509–513.

Bouchard, J. and R.L. Mehta (2009b). Volume management in continuous renal replacement therapy. *Semin Dial* **22**(2): 146–150.

Bouchard, J., et al. (2009). Fluid accumulation, survival and recovery of kidney function in critically ill patients with acute kidney injury. *Kidney Int* **76**(4): 422–427.

Boutilier, P., et al. (2003). Leptospirosis in dogs: a serologic survey and case series 1996 to 2001. *Vet Ther* **4**(4): 387–396.

Brady, M.A. and E.B. Janovitz (2000). Nephrotoxicosis in a cat following ingestion of Asiatic hybrid lily (*Lilium* sp.). *J Vet Diagn Invest* **12**: 566–568.

Braun, J.P., et al. (2003). Creatinine in the dog: a review. *Vet Clin Pathol* **32**(4): 162–179.

Brezis, M.L. and S. Rosen (1995). Hypoxia of the renal medulla – its implications for disease. *N Engl J Med* **332**(10): 647–655.

Brophy, D.F., et al. (2007). The effect of uremia on platelet contractile force, clot elastic modulus and bleeding time in hemodialysis patients. *Thromb Res* **119**(6): 723–729.

Brouns, R. and P.P. De Deyn (2004). Neurological complications in renal failure: a review. *Clin Neurol Neurosurg* **107**: 1–16.

Brown, A.J. and C.M. Otto (2008). Fluid therapy in vomiting and diarrhea. *Vet Clin North Am Small Anim Pract* **38**(3): 653–675.

Brown, C.A., et al. (2007). Outbreaks of renal failure associated with melamine and cyanuric acid in dogs and cats in 2004 and 2007. *J Vet Diagn Invest* **19**(5): 525–531.

Brown, C.A., et al. (2005). Hypertensive encephalopathy in cats with reduced renal function. *Vet Pathol* **42**: 642–649.

Brunker, J.D., et al. (2009). Indices of urine N-acetyl-beta-D-glucosaminidase and gamma-glutamyl transpeptidase activities in clinically normal adult dogs. *Am J Vet Res* **70**(2): 297–301.

Bryson, D.G. and W.A. Ellis (1976). Leptospirosis in a British domestic cat. *J Small Anim Pract* **17**(7): 459–465.

Burns, K. (2007). Events leading to the major recall of pet foods. *J Am Vet Med Assoc* **230**(11): 1600–1620.

Bussolati, B., et al. (2009). Contribution of stem cells to kidney repair. *Curr Stem Cell Res Ther* **4**(1): 2–8.

Campbell, A. and N. Bates (2003). Raisin poisoning in dogs. *Vet Rec* **152**: 376.

Campbell, S.J., et al. (2006). Central and peripheral parenteral nutrition. *Waltham Focus* **16**(3): 1–10.

Carlos, E.R., et al. (1971). Leptospirosis in the Philippines: feline studies. *Am J Vet Res* **32**(9): 1455–1456.

Chan, L.N. (2004). Nutritional support in acute renal failure. *Curr Opin Clin Nutr Metab Care* **7**(2): 207–212.

Chanchairujira, T. and R.L. Mehta (2005). Bioimpedance and its application. *Saudi J Kidney Dis Transpl* **16**(1): 6–16.

Cheng, H.F. and R.C. Harris (2005). Renal effects of non-steroidal anti-inflammatory drugs and selective cyclooxygenase-2 inhibitors. *Curr Pharm Des* **11**: 1795–1804.

Chew, D.J. (2000). Fluid therapy during intrinsic renal failure. In: *Fluid Therapy in Small Animal Practice*, edited by S.P. DiBartola. Philadelphia, PA: WB Saunders, pp. 410–427.

Choi, H., et al. (2003). Effect of intravenous mannitol upon the resistive index in complete unilateral renal obstruction in dogs. *J Vet Intern Med* **17**(2): 158–162.

Cianciolo, R.E., et al. (2008). Clinicopathologic, histologic, and toxicologic findings in 70 cats inadvertently exposed to pet food contaminated with melamine and cyanuric acid. *J Am Vet Med Assoc* **233**(5): 729–737.

Clark, K.L., et al. (1991a). Effects of dopamine DA1-receptor blockade and angiotensin converting enzyme inhibition on the renal actions of fenoldopam in the anaesthetized dog. *J Hypertens* **9**(12): 1143–1150.

Clark, K.L., et al. (1991b). Do renal tubular dopamine receptors mediate dopamine-induced diuresis in the anesthetized cat? *J Cardiovasc Pharmacol* **17**(2): 267–276.

Clarkson, M.R., et al. (2008). Acute kidney injury. In: *Brenner & Rector's The Kidney*, edited by B.M. Brenner, Volume **1**. Philadelphia, PA: Saunders Elsevier, pp. 943–986.

Clemo, F.A. (1998). Urinary enzyme evaluation of nephrotoxicity in the dog. *Toxicol Pathol* **26**(1): 29–32.

Coca, S.G., et al. (2008). Biomarkers for the diagnosis and risk stratification of acute kidney injury: a systematic review. *Kidney Int* **73**(9): 1008–1016.

Cocchi, M., et al. (2009). Renal failure in dogs in Italy associated with melamine-contaminated pet food. *Vet Rec* **164**(13): 407–408.

Codner, E.C., et al. (1992). Investigation of glomerular lesions in dogs with acute experimentally induced Ehrlichia canis infection. *Am J Vet Res* **53**(12): 2286–2291.

Cohn, L.A. (2003). Ehrlichiosis and related infections. *Vet Clin North Am Small Anim Pract* **33**: 863–884.

Coldrick, O., et al. (2007). Fungal pyelonephritis due to Cladophialophora bantiana in a cat. *Vet Rec* **161**(21): 724–727.

Conger, J.D. (2001). Vascular alterations in acute renal failure: roles in initiation and maintenance. In: *Acute Renal Failure: A Companion to Brenner & Rector's The Kidney*, edited by B.A. Molitoris and W.F. Finn. Philadelphia, PA: WB Saunders, pp. 13–29.

Cowan, L.A., et al. (1997). Clinical and clinicopathologic abnormalities in greyhounds with cutaneous and renal glomerular vasculopathy: 18 cases (1992–1994). *J Am Vet Med Assoc* **210**(6): 789–793.

Cowgill, L. and D. Elliott (2000). Acute renal failure. In: *Textbook of Veterinary Internal Medicine*, edited by S.J. Ettinger and E.C. Feldman, Volume **2**. Philadelphia, PA: WB Saunders, pp. 1615–1633.

Cowgill, L.D. (2004). *Dialysis Tools and Toys*. Advanced Renal Therapies Symposium, New York, NY: Animal Medical Center.

Cowgill, L.D. and T. Francey (2005). Acute uremia. In: *Textbook of Veterinary Internal Medicine*, edited by S.J. Ettinger and E.C. Feldman, Volume **2**. Philadelphia, PA: Elsevier Saunders, pp. 1731–1751.

Cowgill, L.D. and T. Francey (2006). Hemodialysis. In: *Fluid, Electrolyte, and Acid-Base Disorders in Small Animal Practice*, edited by S.P. DiBartola. Philadelphia, PA: Saunders Elsevier, pp. 650–677.

Cowgill, L.D. and C.E. Langston (1996). Role of hemodialysis in the management of dogs and cats with renal failure. *Vet Clin North Am Small Anim Pract* **26**(6): 1347–1378.

Cruz, D., et al. (2008). The future of extracorporeal support. *Crit Care Med* **36**(Suppl): S243–S252.

Cruz, D., et al. (2009). Clinical review: RIFLE and AKIN – time for reappraisal. *Crit Care* **13**: 211–219.

Dall'Antonia, M., et al. (2008). Leptospirosis pulmonary haemorrhage: a diagnostic challenge. *Emerg Med J* **25**(1): 51–52.

Dambach, D.M., et al. (1997). Morphologic, immunohistochemical, and ultrastructural characterization of a distinctive renal lesion in dogs putatively associated with Borrelia burgdorferi infection: 49 cases (1987–1992). *Vet Pathol* **34**(2): 85–96.

Davidson, B.J., et al. (2008). Disease association and clinical assessment of feline pericardial effusion. *J Am Anim Hosp Assoc* **44**(1): 5–9.

Day, M.J. and P.E. Holt (1994). Unilateral fungal pyelonephritis in a dog. *Vet Pathol* **31**(2): 250–252.

Day, T.K. and S. Bateman (2006). Shock syndromes. In: *Fluid, Electrolyte, and Acid-Base Disorders in Small Animal Practice*, edited by S.P. DiBartola. Philadelphia, PA: Saunders Elsevier, pp. 540–564.

de la Puente-Redondo, V.A., et al. (2007). The anti-emetic efficacy of maropitant (Cerenia) in the treatment of ongoing emesis caused by a wide range of underlying clinical aetiologies in canine patients in Europe. *J Small Anim Pract* **48**(2): 93–98.

de Morais, H.A., et al. (2008). Metabolic acid-base disorders in the critical care unit. *Vet Clin North Am Small Anim Pract* **38**(3): 559–574.

De Vriese, A.S. (2003). Prevention and treatment of acute renal failure in sepsis. *J Am Soc Nephrol* **14**: 792–805.

Delaney, S.J., et al. (2006). Critical care nutrition of dogs. In: *Encyclopedia of Canine Clinical Nutrition*, edited by P. Pibot, V. Biourge, and D. Elliott. Aimargues, France: Aniwa SAS, pp. 426–450.

Depner, T.A. (2001). Uremic toxicity: urea and beyond. *Semin Dial* **14**(4): 246–251.

Depner, T.A. (2005). Hemodialysis adequacy: basic essentials and practical points for the nephrologist in training. *Hemodial Int* **9**(3): 241–254.

Deray, G. (2002). Amphotericin B nephrotoxicity. *J Antimicrob Chemother* **49**(Suppl S1): 37–41.

Devarajan, P. (2006). Update on mechanisms of ischemic acute kidney injury. *J Am Soc Nephrol* **17**: 1503–1520.

Devarajan, P. (2009). Pathophysiology of pediatric acute kidney injury. In: *Critical Care Nephrology*, edited by C. Ronco, R. Bellomo, and J.A. Kellum. Philadelphia, PA: Saunders Elsevier, pp. 1581–1588.

DiBartola, S.P. (2006a). Disorders of sodium and water: hypernatremia and hyponatremia. In: *Fluid, Electrolyte, and Acid-Base Disorders in Small Animal Practice*, edited by S.P. DiBartola. St. Louis, MO: Saunders Elsevier, pp. 47–79.

DiBartola, S.P. (2006b). Metabolic acid-base disorders. In: *Fluid, Electrolyte. and Acid-Base Disorders in Small Animal Practice*, edited by S.P. DiBartola. St. Louis, MO: Saunders Elsevier, pp. 251–282.

DiBartola, S.P. and H.A. de Morais (2006). Disorders of potassium: hypokalemia and hyperkalemia. In: *Fluid, Electrolyte, and Acid-Base Disorders in Small Animal Practice*, edited by S.P. DiBartola. St. Louis, MO: Saunders Elsevier, pp. 91–121.

Dickeson, D. and D.N. Love (1993). A serological survey of dogs, cats and horses in south-eastern Australia for leptospiral antibodies. *Aust Vet J* **70**(10): 389–390.

Dishart, M.K. and J.A. Kellum (2000). An evaluation of pharmacological strategies for the prevention and treatment of acute renal failure. *Drugs* **59**(1): 79–91.

Diskin, C.J., et al. (2008). The evolution of the fractional excretion of urea as a diagnostic tool in oliguric states. *Am J Kidney Dis* **51**(5): 869–870; author reply 871.

Dlott, J.S., et al. (2004). Drug-induced thrombotic thrombocytopenic purpura/hemolytic uremic syndrome: a concise review. *Ther Apher Dial* **8**(2): 102–111.

Dobson, P.D. and D.B. Kell (2008). Carrier-mediated cellular uptake of pharmaceutical drugs: an exception or the rule? *Nat Rev Drug Discov* **7**: 205–220.

Dobson, R.L., et al. (2008). Identification and characterization of toxicity of contaminants in pet food leading to an outbreak of renal toxicity in cats and dogs. *Toxicol Sci* **106**(1): 251–262.

Dolhnikoff, M., et al. (2007). Pathology and pathophysiology of pulmonary manifestations in leptospirosis. *Braz J Infect Dis* **11**(1): 142–148.

Dorval, P. and S.R. Boysen (2009). Management of acute renal failure in cats using peritoneal dialysis: a retrospective study of six cases (2003–2007). *J Feline Med Surg* **11**(2): 107–115.

Driessen, B., et al. (2003). Arterial oxygenation and oxygen delivery after hemoglobin-based oxygen carrier infusion in canine hypovolemic shock: a dose-response study. *Crit Care Med* **31**(6): 1771–1779.

Driessen, B., et al. (2006). Effects of isovolemic resuscitation with hemoglobin-based oxygen carrier hemoglobin glutamer-200 (bovine) on systemic and mesenteric perfusion and oxygenation in a canine model of hemorrhagic shock: a comparison with 6% hetastarch solution and shed blood. *Vet Anaesth Analg* **33**(6): 368–380.

Druml, W. (1998). Protein metabolism in acute renal failure. *Miner Electrolyte Metab* **24**(1): 47–54.

Druml, W. (2001a). Nutritional management of acute renal failure. *Am J Kidney Dis* **37**(1, Suppl 2): S89–S94.

Druml, W. (2001b). Nutritional support in patients with acute renal failure. In: *Acute Renal Failure: A Companion to Brenner and Rector's*

The Kidney, edited by B.A. Molitoris and W.F. Finn. Philadelphia, PA: WB Saunders, pp. 465–489.

Dubose, T.D. Jr. (2008). Disorders of acid-base balance. In: *Brenner and Rector's The Kidney*, edited by B.M. Brenner, Volume **1**. Philadelphia, PA: Saunders Elsevier, pp. 505–546.

Duffield, J.S., et al. (2005). Restoration of tubular epithelial cells during repair of the postischemic kidney occurs independently of bone marrow-derived stem cells. *J Clin Invest* **115**(7): 1743–1755.

Duke, G.J. (1999). Renal protective agents: a review. *Crit Care Resusc* **1**(3): 265–275.

Eckardt, K. (2002). Anaemia of critical illness – implication for understanding and treating rHuEPO resistance. *Nephrol Dial Transplant* **17**(Suppl 5): 48–55.

Elliott, D.A., et al. (2002a). Evaluation of multifrequency bioelectrical impedance analysis for the assessment of extracellular and total body water in healthy cats. *J Nutr* **132**(6 Suppl 2): 1757S–1759S.

Elliott, D.A., et al. (2002b). Extracellular water and total body water estimated by multifrequency bioelectrical impedance analysis in healthy cats: a cross-validation study. *J Nutr* **132**(6 Suppl 2): 1760S–1762S.

Elliott, D.A. and L.D. Cowgill (2000). Acute renal failure. In: *Current Veterinary Therapy XIII Small Animal Practice*, edited by J.D. Bonagura. Philadelphia, PA: WB Saunders, pp. 173–178.

Elliott, J. and A.D.J. Watson (2009). Chronic kidney disease: staging and management. In: *Kirk's Current Veterinary Therapy XIV*, edited by J.D. Bonagura and D.C. Twedt. St. Louis, MO: Saunders Elsevier, pp. 883–892.

Eubig, P.A., et al. (2005). Acute renal failure in dogs after the ingestion of grapes or raisins: a retrospective evaluation of 43 dogs (1992–2002). *J Vet Intern Med* **19**: 663–674.

Evenepoel, P. (2009). Toxic acute renal failure. In: *Critical Care Nephrology*, edited by C. Ronco, R. Bellomo, and J.A. Kellum. Philadelphia, PA: Saunders Elsevier, pp. 168–171.

Fahimi, D., et al. (2009). Comparison between fractional excretions of urea and sodium in children with acute kidney injury. *Pediatr Nephrol* **24**(12): 2409–2412.

Faubel, S. (2008). Pulmonary complications after acute kidney injury. *Adv Chronic Kidney Dis* **15**(3): 284–296.

FDA. (2008). Caution in feeding chicken jerky to dogs. Available at: http://www.fda.gov/ForConsumers/ConsumerUpdates/ucm048178.htm (accessed December 17, 2009).

Ferguson, M.A., et al. (2008). Biomarkers of nephrotoxic acute kidney injury. *Toxicology* **245**: 182–193.

Fiaccadori, E. and E. Cremaschi (2009). Nutritional assessment and support in acute kidney injury. *Curr Opin Crit Care* **15**(6): 474–480.

Fieghen, H., et al. (2009). Renal replacement therapy for acute kidney injury. *Nephron Clin Pract* **112**(4): c222–c229.

Finco, D.R. (1995). Evaluation of renal functions. In: *Canine and Feline Nephrology and Urology*, edited by C.A. Osborne and D.R. Finco. Baltimore, MD: Williams & Wilkins, pp. 216–229.

Fink, M.P., et al. (1985). Low-dose dopamine preserves renal blood flow in endotoxin shocked dogs treated with ibuprofen. *J Surg Res* **38**(6): 582–591.

Finn, W.F. (2001). Recovery from acute renal failure. In: *Acute Renal Failure: A Companion to Brenner & Rector's The Kidney*, edited by B.A. Molitoris and W.F. Finn. Philadelphia, PA: WB Saunders, pp. 425–450.

Fischer, J.R., et al. (2004a). Clinical and clinicopathological features of cats with acute ureteral obstruction managed with hemodialysis between 1993 and 2004: a review of 50 cases (abstract).

Fischer, J.R., et al. (2004b). Veterinary hemodialysis: advances in management and technology. *Vet Clin North Am Small Animal Pract* **34**(4): 935–967.

Flournoy, W.S., et al. (2003). Pharmacologic identification of putative D1 dopamine receptors in feline kidneys. *J Vet Pharmacol Therap* **26**: 283–290.

Forrester, S.D., et al. (2002). Retrospective evaluation of acute renal failure in dogs. *J Vet Intern Med* **16**(3): 354.

Fouque, D., et al. (2008). A proposed nomenclature and diagnostic criteria for protein-energy wasting in acute and chronic kidney disease. *Kidney Int* **73**(4): 391–398.

Francey, T. (2006). *Outcome of Dogs and Cats Treated with Hemodialysis*. Advanced Renal Therapies Symposium, New York, NY: Animal Medical Center.

Francey, T. and L.D. Cowgill (2002). Use of hemodialysis for the management of ARF in the dog: 124 cases (1990–2001) (abstract). *J Vet Intern Med* **16**(3): 352.

Francey, T. and L.D. Cowgill (2004). Hypertension in dogs with severe acute renal failure (abstract). *J Vet Intern Med* **18**(3): 418.

Furuichi, K., et al. (2009). Chemokine/chemokine receptor-mediated inflammation regulates pathologic changes from acute kidney injury to chronic kidney disease. *Clin Exp Nephrol* **13**: 9–14.

Furukawa, S., et al. (2002). Effects of dopamine infusion on cardiac and renal blood flows in dogs. *J Vet Med Sci* **64**(1): 41–44.

Galbusera, M., et al. (2009). Treatment of bleeding in dialysis patients. *Semin Dial* **22**(3): 279–286.

Galey, F.D. (1992). Effective use of an analytical laboratory for toxicology problems. In: *Kirk's Current Veterinary Therapy XI: Small Animal Practice*, edited by R.W. Kirk and J.D. Bonagura. Philadelphia, PA: WB Saunders, pp. 168–172.

Gambaro, G., et al. (2002). Diuretics and dopamine for the prevention and treatment of acute renal failure: a critical reappraisal. *J Nephrol* **15**(3): 213–219.

Garwood, S. (2009). Ischemic acute renal failure. In: *Critical Care Nephrology*, edited by C. Ronco, R. Bellomo, and J.A. Kellum. Philadelphia, PA: Saunders Elsevier, pp. 157–162.

Geisen, V., et al. (2007). Canine leptospirosis infections – clinical signs and outcome with different suspected *Leptospira* serogroups (42 cases). *J Small Anim Pract* **48**: 324–328.

Goldstein, R.E., et al. (2006). Influence of infecting serogroup of clinical features of leptospirosis in dogs. *J Vet Intern Med* **20**: 489–494.

Goldstein, R.E., et al. (1998). Gastrin concentrations in plasma of cats with chronic renal failure. *J Am Vet Med Assoc* **213**(6): 826–828.

Goligorsky, M.S., et al. (2002). Nitric oxide in acute renal failure: NOS versus NOS. *Kidney Int* **61**: 855–861.

Goligorsky, M.S., et al. (2004). NO bioavailability, endothelial dysfunction, and acute renal failure: new insights into pathophysiology. *Semin Nephrol* **24**(4): 316–323.

Gong, H., et al. (2004). EPO and a-MSH prevent ischemia/reperfusion-induced down-regulation of AQPs and sodium transporters in rat kidney. *Kidney Int* **66**: 683–695.

Gouveia, E.L., et al. (2008). Leptospirosis-associated severe pulmonary hemorrhagic syndrome, Salvador, Brazil. *Emerg Infect Dis* **14**(3): 505–508.

Grauer, G. (1998). Fluid therapy in acute and chronic renal failure. *Vet Clin North Am Small Animal Pract* **28**(3): 609–622.

Grauer, G.F. (1995). Prevention of hospital-acquired acute renal failure. In: *Current Veterinary Therapy XII*, edited by J.D. Bonagura. Philadelphia, PA: WB Saunders, pp. 943–945.

Grauer, G.F. (1996). Prevention of acute renal failure. *Vet Clin North Am Small Anim Pract* **26**: 1447–1459.

Grauer, G.F. (2009). Acute renal failure and chronic kidney disease. In: *Small Animal Internal Medicine*, edited by R.W. Nelson and C.G. Couto. St. Louis, MO: Mosby Elsevier, pp. 645–659.

Grauer, G.F., et al. (1995). Estimation of quantitative enzymuria in dogs with gentamicin-induced nephrotoxicosis using urine enzyme/creatinine ratios from spot urine samples. *J Vet Intern Med* **9**(5): 324–327.

Grauer, G.F. and I.F. Lane (1995a). Acute renal failure. In: *Textbook of Veterinary Internal Medicine*, edited by S.J. Ettinger and E.C. Feldman. Philadelphia, PA: WB Saunders, pp. 1720–1733.

Grauer, G.F. and I.F. Lane (1995b). Acute renal failure: ischemic and chemical nephrosis. In: *Canine and Feline Nephrology and Urology*, editded by C.A. Osborne and D.R. Finco. Philadelphia, PA: Williams & Wilkins, pp. 441–459.

Grauer, G.F., et al. (1984). Early clinicopathologic findings in dogs ingesting ethylene glycol. *Am J Vet Res* **45**(11): 2299–2303.

Greene, C.E. (2006). Antifungal chemotherapy. In: *Infectious Diseases of the Dog and Cat*, edited by C.E. Greene. St. Louis, MO: Saunders Elsevier, pp. 542–550.

Greene, C.E., et al. (2006). Leptospirosis. In: *Infectious Diseases of the Dog and Cat*, edited by C.E. Greene. St. Louis, MO: Saunders Elsevier, pp. 402–417.

Greenlee, J.J., et al. (2005). Experimental canine leptospirosis caused by Leptospira interrogans serovars pomona and bratislava. *Am J Vet Res* **66**(10): 1816–1822.

Greenlee, J.J., et al. (2004). Clinical and pathologic comparison of acute leptospirosis in dogs caused by two strains of *Leptospira kirschneri* serovar grippotyphosa. *Am J Vet Res* **65**(8): 1100–1107.

Gregory, C.R., et al. (1993). Oxalate nephrosis and renal sclerosis after renal transplantation in a cat. *Vet Surg* **22**(3): 221–224.

Grigoryev, D.N., et al. (2008). The local and systemic inflammatory transcriptome after acute kidney injury. *J Am Soc Nephrol* **19**(3): 547–558.

Guerra, M.A. (2009). Leptospirosis. *J Am Vet Med Assoc* **234**(4): 472–478.

Gutierrez, R., et al. (1991). Effect of hypertonic versus isotonic sodium bicarbonate on plasma potassium concentration in patients with end-stage renal disease. *Miner Electrolyte Metab* **17**(5): 297–302.

Gwaltney-Brant, S.M., et al. (2001). Renal failure associated with ingestion of grapes or raisins in dogs. *J Am Vet Med Assoc* **218**(10): 1555–1556.

Haag-Weber, M. and W.H. Horl (1993). Uremia and infection: mechanisms of impaired cellular host defense. *Nephron* **63**(2): 125–131.

Haase, M., et al. (2009). Accuracy of neutrophil gelatinase-associated lipocalin (NGAL) in diagnosis and prognosis in acute kidney injury: a systematic review and meta-analysis. *Am J Kidney Dis* **54**(6): 1012–1024.

Hadley, R., et al. (2003). A retrospective study of day lily toxicosis in cats. *Vet Hum Toxicol* **45**(1): 38–39.

Hadrick, M.K., et al. (1996). Acute tubulointerstitial nephritis with eosinophiluria in a dog. *J Vet Intern Med* **10**(1): 45–47.

Halpenny, M., et al. (2001). Effects of prophylactic fenoldopam infusion on renal blood flow and renal tubular function during acute hypovolemia in anesthetized dogs. *Crit Care Med* **29**(4): 855–860.

Harkin, K.R. and C.L. Gartrell (1996). Canine leptospirosis in New Jersey and Michigan: 17 cases (1990–1995). *J Am Anim Hosp Assoc* **32**: 495–501.

Harkin, K.R., et al. (2003a). Clinical application of a polymerase chain reaction assay for diagnosis of leptospirosis in dogs. *J Am Vet Med Assoc* **222**(9): 1224–1229.

Harkin, K.R., et al. (2003b). Comparison of polymerase chain reaction assay, bacteriologic culture, and serologic testing in assessment of prevalence of urinary shedding of leptospires in dogs. *J Am Vet Med Assoc* **222**(9): 1230–1233.

Harris, R.C. (2006). COX-2 and the kidney. *J Cardiovasc Pharmacol* **47**(Suppl 1): S37–S42.

Hassoun, H.T., et al. (2007). Ischemic acute kidney injury induces a distant organ functional and genomic response distinguishable from bilateral nephrectomy. *Am J Physiol Renal Physiol* **293**(1): F30–F40.

Hau, A.K., et al. (2009). Melamine toxicity and the kidney. *J Am Soc Nephrol* **20**(2): 245–250.

Heath, S.E. and R. Johnson (1994). Leptospirosis. *J Am Vet Med Assoc* **205**(11): 1518–1523.

Hedges, S.J., et al. (2007). Evidence-based treatment recommendations for uremic bleeding. *Nat Clin Pract Nephrol* **3**(3): 138–153.

Heiene, R., et al. (2001). Calculation of urinary enzyme excretion, with renal structure and function in dogs with pyometra. *Res Vet Sci* **70**(2): 129–137.

Heinzelmann, M., et al. (1999). Neutrophils and renal failure. *Am J Kid Dis* **34**(2): 384–399.

Hellberg, P.O.A., et al. (1991). Red cell trapping and postischemic renal blood flow. Differences between the cortex, outer and inner medulla. *Kidney Int* **40**: 625–631.

Heyman, S.N. and S. Rosen (2003). Dye-induced nephropathy. *Semin Nephrol* **23**(5): 477–485.

Heyman, S.N., et al. (2008). Renal parenchymal hypoxia, hypoxia adaptation, and the pathogenesis of radiocontrast nephropathy. *Clin J Am Soc Nephrol* **3**: 288–296.

Hill, P., et al. (2008a). Inhibition of hypoxia inducible factor hydroxylases protects against renal ischemia-reperfusion injury. *J Am Soc Nephrol* **19**: 39–46.

Hill, T.L., et al. (2008b). Concurrent hepatic copper toxicosis and Fanconi's syndrome in a dog. *J Vet Intern Med* **22**(1): 219–222.

Himmelfarb, J. (2009). Acute kidney injury in the elderly: problems and prospects. *Semin Nephrol* **29**(6): 658–664.

Himmelfarb, J., et al. (2008). Evaluation and initial management of acute kidney injury. *Clin J Am Soc Nephrol* **3**: 962–967.

Hirsch, S. (2007). Prerenal success in chronic kidney disease. *Am J Med* **120**: 754–759.

Hoke, T.S., et al. (2007). Acute renal failure after bilateral nephrectomy is associated with cytokine-mediated pulmonary injury. *J Am Soc Nephrol* **18**(1): 155–164.

Horl, W.H. (2001). Neutrophil function in renal failure. *Adv Nephrol Necker Hosp* **31**: 173–192.

Hoste, E.A. and J.A. Kellum (2007). Incidence, classification, and outcomes of acute kidney injury. *Contrib Nephrol* **156**: 32–38.

Hoste, E.A.J., et al. (2006). RIFLE criteria for acute kidney injury are associated with hospital mortality in critically ill patients: a cohort analysis. *Crit Care* **10**: R73.

Hoste, E.A.J. and J.J. De Waele (2005). Physiologic consequences of acute renal failure on the critically ill. *Crit Care Clin* **21**(2): 251–260.

Hoste, E.A.J. and J.A. Kellum (2006). RIFLE criteria provide robust assessment of kidney dysfunction and correlate with hospital mortality. *Crit Care Med* **34**(7): 2016–2017.

Hovda, L.R. (2010). Plant toxicities. In: *Textbook of Veterinary Internal Medicine*, edited by S.J. Ettinger and E.C. Feldman, Volume 1. St. Louis, MO: Saunders Elsevier, pp. 561–565.

Hutton, T.A., et al. (2008). Search for Borrelia burgdorferi in kidneys of dogs with suspected "Lyme nephritis". *J Vet Intern Med* **22**(4): 860–865.

IRIS. (2006). *International Renal Interest Society*. Available at: http://www.iris-kidney.com/index.shtml (accessed January 7, 2010).

Iseki, K., et al. (1993). Serum albumin is a strong predictor of death in chronic dialysis patients. *Kidney Int* **44**(1): 115–119.

Israni, A.K. and B.L. Kasiske (2008). Laboratory assessment of kidney disease: clearance, urinalysis, and kidney biopsy. In: *Brenner & Rector's The Kidney*, edited by B.M. Brenner, Volume **1**. Philadelphia, PA: Saunders Elsevier, pp. 724–756.

Jo, S.K., et al. (2007). Pharmacologic treatment of acute kidney injury: why drugs haven't worked and what is on the horizon. *Clin J Am Soc Nephrol* **2**(2): 356–365.

Kale, S., et al. (2003). Bone marrow stem cells contribute to repair of the ischemically injured renal tubule. *J Clin Invest* **112**: 42–49.

Kaloyanides, G. (1984). Renal pharmacology of aminoglycoside antibiotics. *Contrib Nephrol* **42**: 148–167.

Kaloyanides, G. (1997). Antibiotic and immunosuppression-related renal failure. In: *Diseases of the Kidney*, edited by R.W. Schrier and C. Gottschalk. Boston, MA: Little, Brown and Company, pp. 1115–1151.

Kaplan, J.L., et al. (1997). Alkalinization is ineffective for severe hyperkalemia in nonnephrectomized dogs. Hyperkalemia Research Group. *Acad Emerg Med* **4**(2): 93–99.

Kaplan, J.L., et al. (2000). Hypertonic saline treatment of severe hyperkalemia in nonnephrectomized dogs. *Acad Emerg Med* **7**(9): 965–973.

Karajala, V., et al. (2009). Diuretics in acute kidney injury. *Minerva Anestesiol* **75**(5): 251–257.

Kellum, J., et al. (2007a). Acute renal failure. *Am Fam Physician* **76**(3): 418–422.

Kellum, J.A. (1997a). Diuretics in acute renal failure: protective or deleterious. *Blood Purif* **15**(4–6): 319–322.

Kellum, J.A. (1997b). The use of diuretics and dopamine in acute renal failure: a systematic review of the evidence. *Crit Care* **1**(2): 53–59.

Kellum, J.A. (1998). Use of diuretics in the acute care setting. *Kidney Int Suppl* **66**: S67–S70.

Kellum, J.A. (2007). Prerenal azotemia: still a useful concept? *Crit Care Med* **35**(6): 1630–1631.

Kellum, J.A. (2008). Acute kidney injury. *Crit Care Med* **36**(Suppl): S141–S145.

Kellum, J.A., et al. (2007b). The concept of acute kidney injury and the RIFLE criteria. *Contrib Nephrol* **156**: 10–16.

Kellum, J.A., et al. (2008a). Fluids for the prevention and management of acute kidney injury. *Int J Artif Organs* **31**(2).

Kellum, J.A. and J.M. Decker (2001). Use of dopamine in acute renal failure: a meta-analysis. *Crit Care Med* **29**(8): 1526–1531.

Kellum, J.A., et al. (2008b). Acute renal failure. *Clin Evid (Online)*.

Kellum, J.A., et al. (2002). Developing a consensus classification system for acute renal failure. *Curr Opin Crit Care* **8**: 509–514.

Kellum, J.A., et al. (2008c). Fluid management in acute kidney injury. *Int J Artif Organs* **31**(2): 94–95.]

Kelly, K.J. (2005). Heat shock (stress response) proteins and renal ischemia/reperfusion injury. *Contrib Nephrol* **148**: 86–106.

Kerr, D.D. and V. Marshall (1974). Protection against the renal carrier state by a canine leptospirosis vaccine. *Vet Med Small Anim Clin* **69**(9): 1157–1160.

Klein, C.L., et al. (2008). Interleukin-6 mediates lung injury following ischemic acute kidney injury or bilateral nephrectomy. *Kidney Int* **74**(7): 901–909.

Kogika, M.M., et al. (2006). Serum ionized calcium in dogs with chronic renal failure and metabolic acidosis. *Vet Clin Pathol* **35**: 441–445.

Kosieradzki, M. and W. Rowinski (2008). Ischemia/reperfusion injury in kidney transplantation: mechanisms and prevention. *Transplant Proc* **40**(10): 3279–3288.

Kovesdy, C.P., et al. (2009). Outcome predictability of biomarkers of protein-energy wasting and inflammation in moderate and advanced chronic kidney disease. *Am J Clin Nutr* **90**(2): 407–414.

Kramer, A.A., et al. (1999). Renal ischemia/reperfusion leads to macrophage-mediated increase in pulmonary vascular permeability. *Kidney Int* **55**(6): 2362–2367.

Krause, D.S. and L.G. Cantley (2005). Bone marrow plasticity revisited: protection or differentiation in the kidney tubule? *J Clin Invest* **115**(7): 1705–1708.

Krawiec, D.R. (1996). Managing Gastrointestinal complications of uremia. *Vet Clin North Am Small Anim Pract* **26**(6): 1287–1292.

Kwon, T.-H., et al. (1999). Reduced abundance of aquaporins in rats with bilateral ischemia-induced acute renal failure: prevention by a-MSH. *Am J Physiol Renal Physiol* **277**: 413–427.

Kyles, A.E., et al. (2005). Clinical, clinicopathologic, radiographic, and ultrasonographic abnormalities in cats with ureteral calculi: 163 cases (1984–2002). *J Am Vet Med Assoc* **226**(6): 932–936.

Kyles, A.E. and J.L. Westropp (2009). Management of feline ureteroliths. In: *Kirk's Current Veterinary Therapy XIV*, edited by J.D. Bonagura and D.C. Twedt. St. Louis, MO: Saunders Elsevier, pp. 931–936.

Labato, M.A. (2001). Strategies for management of acute renal failure. *Vet Clin North Am Small Animal Pract* **31**(6): 1265–1287.

Labato, M.A. (2009). Uncomplicated urinary tract infection. In: *Kirk's Current Veterinary Therapy XIV*, edited by J.D. Bonagura and D.C. Twedt. St. Louis, MO: Saunders Elsevier, pp. 918–921.

Lacerda, G., et al. (2010). Neurologic presentations of renal diseases. *Neurol Clin* **28**(1): 45–59.

Laflamme, D.P. (1997). Development and validation of a body condition score system for dogs. *Canine Pract* **22**: 10–15.

Lameire, N., et al. (2008a). The prevention of acute kidney injury: an in-depth narrative review Part 1: volume resuscitation and avoidance of drug-and nephrotoxin-induced AKI. *NDT Plus* **1**: 392–402.

Lameire, N., et al. (2009). The prevention of acute kidney injury: an in-depth narrative review: Part 2: drugs in the prevention of acute kidney injury. *NDT Plus* **2**: 1–10.

Lameire, N., et al. (2005). Acute renal failure. *Lancet* **365**: 417–430.

Lameire, N., et al. (2008b). Acute kidney injury. *Lancet* **372**(9653): 1863–1865.

Lameire, N. and R. Vanholder (2001). Pathophysiologic features and prevention of human and experimental acute tubular necrosis. *J Am Soc Nephrol* **12**: S20–S32.

Lameire, N., et al. (2002). Loop diuretics for patients with acute renal failure: helpful or harmful? *J Am Med Assoc* **288**(20): 2599–2601.

Lameire, N., et al. (1995). Prevention of clinical acute tubular necrosis with drug therapy. *Nephrol Dial Transplant* **10**(11): 1992–2000.

Lane, I.F., et al. (1994). Acute renal failure. Part I. risk factors, prevention, and strategies for protection. *Compend Contin Educ Pract Vet* **16**(1): 15–18, 20–23, 26–29.

Lange, C., et al. (2005). Administered mesenchymal stem cells enhance recovery from ischemia/reperfusion-induced acute renal failure in rats. *Kidney Int* **68**: 1613–1617.

Langston, C.E. (2002a). Acute renal failure caused by lily ingestion in six cats. *J Am Vet Med Assoc* **220**(1): 49–52.

Langston, C.E. (2002b). Hemodialysis in dogs and cats. *Compend Contin Educ Pract Vet* **24**(7): 540–549.

Langston, C.E. (2008). Managing fluid and electrolyte disorders in renal failure. *Vet Clin North Am Small Animal Pract* **38**(3): 677–697.

Langston, C.E. (2010). Acute uremia. In: *Textbook of Veterinary Internal Medicine*, edited by S.J. Ettinger and E.C. Feldman, Volume **2**. Philadephia, PA: Saunders Elsevier, pp. 1969–1984.

Langston, C.E. and L.M. Boyd (2007). Diseases of the kidney. In: *Handbook of Small Animal Practice*, edited by R.V. Morgan. Philadephia, PA: Elsevier, pp. 500–527.

Langston, C.E., et al. (1997). Applications and outcome of hemodialysis in cats: a review of 29 cases. *J Vet Intern Med* **11**(6): 348–355.

Langston, C.E., et al. (2008). Diagnosis of Urolithiasis. *Compend Contin Educ Pract Vet* **30**(8): 447–455.

Langston, C.E. and K.J. Heuter (2003). Leptospirosis: a re-emerging zoonotic disease. *Vet Clin North Am Small Anim Pract* **33**: 791–807.

Laroute, V., et al. (2005). Quantitative evaluation of renal function in healthy Beagle puppies and mature dogs. *Res Vet Sci* **79**(2): 161–167.

Lau, E. (2009). *Virbac Recalls Veggiedent Chews in Australia.* Available at: http://news.vin.com/VINNews.aspx?articleId = 13071 (accessed December 17, 2009).

Le Garreres, A., et al. (2007). Disposition of plasma creatinine in non-azotaemic and moderately azotaemic cats. *J Feline Med Surg* **9**(2): 89–96.

Leblanc, M., et al. (2005). Risk factors for acute renal failure: inherent and modifiable risks. *Curr Opin Crit Care* **11**: 533–536.

Lee, D.W., et al. (2009). Post-treatment effects of erythropoietin and nordihydroguaiaretic acid on recovery from cisplatin-induced acute renal failure in the rat. *J Korean Med Sci* **24**(Suppl 1): S170–S175.

Lees, G.E. (2004). Early diagnosis of renal disease and renal failure. *Vet Clin North Am Small Anim Pract* **34**(4): 867–886.

Lefebvre, H.P., et al. (2007). Angiotensin-converting enzyme inhibitors in veterinary medicine. *Curr Pharm Des* **13**: 1347–1361.

Lefebvre, H.P., et al. (2006). Pharmacokinetic and pharmacodynamic parameters of ramipril and ramiprilat in healthy dogs and dogs with reduced glomerular filtration rate. *J Vet Intern Med* **20**: 499–507.

Levett, P.N. (2001). Leptospirosis. *Clin Microbiol Rev* **14**(2): 296–326.

Liangos, O., et al. (2003). Anemia in acute renal failure: role for erythropoiesis-stimulating proteins? *Artif Organs* **27**(9): 786–791.

Licari, E., et al. (2007). Fluid resuscitation and the septic kidney: the evidence. *Contrib Nephrol* **156**: 167–177.

Lin, F. (2006). Stem cells in kidney regeneration following acute renal injury. *Pediatr Res* **59**(4 Pt 2): 74R–78R.

Lin, F., et al. (2003). Hematopoietic stem cells contribute to the regeneration of renal tubules after renal ischemia-reperfusion injury in mice. *J Am Soc Nephrol* **14**: 1188–1199.

Lindner, A., et al. (1979). Synergism of dopamine plus furosemide in preventing acute renal failure in the dog. *Kidney Int* **16**(2): 158–166.

Littman, M.P. (2003). Canine borreliosis. *Vet Clin North Am Small Anim Pract* **33**: 827–862.

Liu, K.D. and P.R. Brakeman (2008). Renal repair and recovery. *Crit Care Med* **36**(Suppl): S187–S192.

Liu, M., et al. (2008). Acute kidney injury leads to inflammation and functional changes in the brain. *J Am Soc Nephrol* **19**(7): 1360–1370.

Livio, M., et al. (1982). Uraemic bleeding: role of anaemia and beneficial effect of red cell transfusions. *Lancet* **2**(8306): 1013–1015.

Lopes, J.A., et al. (2008). Acute kidney injury in intensive care unit patients: a comparison between the RIFLE and the acute kidney injury network classifications. *Crit Care* **12**: R110–R117.

Lopez-Pena, M., et al. (2009). Visceral leishmaniasis with cardiac involvement in a dog: a case report. *Acta Vet Scand* **51**: 20.

Macedo, E. and R.L. Mehta (2009). Prerenal failure: from old concepts to new paradigms. *Curr Opin Crit Care* **15**(6): 467–473.

Madewell, B.R. and R.W. Norrdin (1975). Renal failure associated with pericardial effusion in a dog. *J Am Vet Med Assoc* **167**(12): 1091–1093.

Markowitz, G.S. and M.A. Perazella (2005). Drug-induced renal failure: a focus on tubulointerstitial disease. *Clin Chim Acta* **351**: 31–47.

Marks, S.L. (1998). The principles and practical application of enteral nutrition. *Vet Clin North Am Small Anim Pract* **28**(3): 677–708.

Mason, J., et al. (1987). The contribution of vascular obstruction to the functional defect that follows renal ischemia. *Kidney Int* **31**: 65–71.

Mastrorilli, C., et al. (2007). Clinicopathologic features and outcome predictors of leptospira interrogans Australis serogroup infection in dogs: a retrospective study of 20 cases (2001–2004). *J Vet Intern Med* **21**(1): 3–10.

Mathews, K.A. (2006). Monitoring fluid therapy and complications of fluid therapy. In: *Fluid, Electrolyte, and Acid-Base Disorders in Small Animal Practice*, edited by S.P. DiBartola. St. Louis, MO: Saunders Elsevier, pp. 377–391.

Mazzaferro, E.M., et al. (2004). Acute renal failure associated with raisin or grape ingestion in 4 dogs. *J Vet Emerg Crit Care* **14**(3): 203–212.

McClellan, J.M., et al. (2006). Effects of administration of fluids and diuretics on glomerular filtration rate, renal blood flow, and urine output in healthy awake cats. *Am J Vet Res* **67**: 715–722.

Means, C. (2007). Lily toxicosis. In: *Clinical Veterinary Advisor Dogs and Cats*, edited by E. Cote. St. Louis, MO: Mosby Elsevier, pp. 638–639.

Medina, P.J., et al. (2001). Drug-associated thrombotic thrombocytopenic purpura-hemolytic uremic syndrome. *Curr Opin Hematol* **8**: 286–293.

Mehta, R.L., et al. (2008). Pharmacologic approaches for volume excess in acute kidney injury (AKI). *Int J Artif Organs* **31**(2): 127–144.

Mehta, R.L. and G. Chertow (2003). Acute renal failure definitions and classification: time for change? *J Am Soc Nephrol* **14**: 2178–2187.

Mehta, R.L., et al. (2007). Acute kidney injury network: report of an initiative to improve outcomes in acute kidney injury. *Crit Care* **11**(2): R31.

Mehta, R.L., et al. (2002a). Refining predictive models in critically ill patients with acute renal failure. *J Am Soc Nephrol* **13**(5): 1350–1357.

Mehta, R.L., et al. (2002b). Diuretics, mortality, and nonrecovery of renal function in acute renal failure. *J Am Med Assoc* **288**(20): 2547–2553.

Meyer, T.W. and T.H. Hostetter (2008). Pathophysiology of uremia. In: *Brenner & Rector's The Kidney*, edited by B.M. Brenner, Volume **2**. Philadelphia, PA: Saunders Elsevier, pp. 1681–1696.

Michel, D.M. and C.J. Kelly (1998). Acute interstitial nephritis. *J Am Soc Nephrol* **9**(3): 506–515.

Miller, R.I., et al. (2007). Clinical and epidemiological features of canine leptospirosis in North Queensland. *Aust Vet J* **85**(1): 13–19.

Mitch, W.E. (1981). Amino acid release from the hindquarter and urea appearance in acute uremia. *Am J Physiol* **241**(6): E415–E419.

Mitch, W.E. (1993). Nutritional influences on changes in kidney growth and function and the responses to kidney diseases. *Semin Nephrol* **13**(5): 503–507.

Mitch, W.E., et al. (1989). Protein and amino acid metabolism in uremia: influence of metabolic acidosis. *Kidney Int Suppl* **27**: S205–S207.

Molitoris, B.A., et al. (2007). Improving outcomes of acute kidney injury report of an initiative. *Nat Clin Pract Nephrol* **3**(8): 439–442.

Molitoris, B.A., et al. (1993). Mechanism of ischemia-enhanced aminoglycoside binding and uptake by proximal tubule cells. *Am J Physiol* **264**(5 Pt2): F907–F916.

Moore, G., et al. (2006). Canine leptospirosis, United States, 2002–2004. *Emerg Infect Dis* **12**(3): 501–503.

Morrow, C.M.K., et al. (2005). Canine renal pathology associated with grape or raisin ingestion: 10 cases. *J Vet Diagn Invest* **17**: 223–231.

Mount, D.B. and K. Zandi-Nejad (2008). Disorders of potassium balance. In: *Brenner & Rector's The Kidney*, edited by B.M. Brenner, Volume **1**. Philadelphia, PA: Saunders Elsevier, pp. 547–587.

Murrary, P.T. and P.M. Palevsky (2009). Acute kidney injury and critical care nephrology. *Nephrol Self Assess Program* **8**(3): 173–226.

Murray, C., et al. (2003). Effects of fenoldopam on renal blood flow and its function in a canine model of rhabdomyolysis. *Eur J Anaesthesiol* **20**: 711–718.

Murray, P.T. and P.M. Palevsky (2009). Acute kidney injury and critical care nephrology. *Nephrol Self Assess Program* **8**(3): 173–226.

Mylonakis, M.E., et al. (2005). Leptospiral seroepidemiology in a feline hospital population in Greece. *Vet Rec* **156**(19): 615–616.

Nath, K.A. and S.M. Norby (2000). Reactive oxygen species and acute renal failure. *Am J Med* **109**: 655–678.

Nelson, O.L. and W.A. Ware (2009). Pericardial effusion. In: *Kirk's Current Veterinary Therapy XIV*, edited by J.D. Bonagura and D.C. Twedt. St. Louis, MO: Saunders Elsevier, pp. 825–831.

Newman, S.J., et al. (2003). Cryptococcal pyelonephritis in a dog. *J Am Vet Med Assoc* **222**(2): 180–183, 174.

Nichols, A.J., et al. (1992). Effect of fenoldopam on the acute and subacute nephrotoxicity produced by amphotericin B in the dog. *J Pharmacol Exp Ther* **260**(1): 269–274.

Nigwekar, S.U., et al. (2009). Atrial natriuretic peptide for management of acute kidney injury: a systematic review and meta-analysis. *Clin J Am Soc Nephrol* **4**(2): 261–272.

Niwattayakul, K., et al. (2002). Hypotension, renal failure, and pulmonary complications in leptospirosis. *Ren Fail* **24**(3): 297–305.

Nolan, C.R. and R.J. Anderson (1998). Hospital-acquired acute renal failure. *J Am Soc Nephrol* **9**(4): 710–718.

Norris, C.R., et al. (2000). Recurrent and persistent urinary tract infections in dogs: 383 cases (1969–1995). *J Am Anim Hosp Assoc* **36**: 484–492.

Novellas, R., et al. (2007). Doppler ultrasonographic estimation of renal and ocular resistive and pulsatility indices in normal dogs and cats. *Vet Radiol Ultrasound* **48**(1): 69–73.

Oliver, J.A., et al. (2004). The renal papilla is a niche for adult kidney stem cells. *J Clin Invest* **114**(6): 796–804.

Olyaei, A.J., et al. (2001). Nephrotoxicity of immunosuppressive drugs: new insight and preventive strategies. *Curr Opin Crit Care* **7**: 384–389.

Osborne, C.A., et al. (1996). Percutaneous needle biopsy of the kidney. Indications, applications, technique, and complications. *Vet Clin North Am Small Anim Pract* **26**(6): 1461–1504.

Osborne, C.A., et al. (2009). Melamine and cyanuric acid-induced crystalluria, uroliths, and nephrotoxicity in dogs and cats. *Vet Clin North Am Small Anim Pract* **39**(1): 1–14.

Osborne, C.A., et al. (1995). A clinician's analysis of urinalysis. In: *Canine and Feline Nephrology and Urology*, edited by C.A. Osborne and D.R. Finco. Baltimore, MD: Williams & Wilkins, pp. 136–205.

Padanilam, B.J. (2003). Cell death induced by acute renal injury: a perspective on the contributions of apoptosis and necrosis. *Am J Physiol Renal Physiol* **284**(4): F608–F627.

Palacio, J., et al. (1997). Enzymuria as an index of renal damage in canine leishmaniasis. *Vet Rec* **140**(18): 477–480.

Palevsky, P.M. (2004). Acute renal failure. *Nephrol Self Assess Program* **3**(5): 239–277.

Palevsky, P.M. (2008). Indications and timing of renal replacement therapy in acute kidney injury. *Crit Care Med* **36**(Suppl): S224–S228.

Pannu, N. and M.K. Nadim (2008). An overview of drug-induced acute kidney injury. *Crit Care Med* **36**(Suppl): S216–S223.

Pantaleo, V., et al. (2004). Application of hemodialysis for the management of acute uremia in cats: 119 cases (1993–2003) (abstract). *J Vet Intern Med* **18**(3): 418.

Parham, W.A., et al. (2006). Hyperkalemia revisited. *Tex Heart Inst J* **33**: 40–47.

Patel, N.S.A., et al. (2004). Pretreatment with EPO reduces the injury and dysfunction caused by ischemia/reperfusion in the mouse kidney in vivo. *Kidney Int* **66**: 983–989.

Penny, D., et al. (2003). Raisin poisoning in a dog. *Vet Rec* **152**: 308.

Pepin, M.-N., et al. (2007). Diagnostic performance of fractional excretion of urea and fractional excretion of sodium in the evaluation of patients with acute kidney injury with or without diuretic treatment. *Am J Kidney Dis* **50**(4): 566–573.

Perazella, M.A. (1999). Crystal-induced acute renal failure. *Am J Med* **106**: 459–465.

Pinsky, M., et al. (2008). Fluid and volume monitoring. *Int J Artif Organs* **31**(2): 111–126.

Polzin, D.J., et al. (2005). Chronic kidney disease. In: *Textbook of Veterinary Internal Medicine*, edited by S.J. Ettinger and E.C. Feldman, Volume **II**. St. Louis, MO: Elsevier Saunders, pp. 1756–1785.

Pressler, B.M., et al. (2003). Candida spp. urinary tract infections in 13 dogs and seven cats: predisposing factors, treatment, and outcome. *J Am Anim Hosp Assoc* **39**(3): 263–270.

Puschner, B., et al. (2007). Assessment of melamine and cyanuric acid toxicity in cats. *J Vet Diagn Invest* **19**(6): 616–624.

Putcha, N. and M. Allon (2007). Management of hyperkalemia in dialysis patients. *Semin Dial* **20**(5): 431–439.

Rabb, H., et al. (2003). Acute renal failure leads to dysregulation of lung salt and water channels. *Kidney Int* **63**(2): 600–606.

Racusen, L.C. (2001). The morphologic basis of acute renal failure. In: *Acute Renal Failure: A Companion to Brenner & Rector's The Kidney*, edited by B.A. Molitoris and W.F. Finn. Philadelphia, PA: WB Saunders, pp. 1–12.

Raff, A.C., et al. (2008). New insights into uremic toxicity. *Curr Opin Nephrol Hypertens* **17**(6): 560–565.

Rauf, A.A., et al. (2008). Intermittent hemodialysis versus continuous renal replacement therapy for acute renal failure in the intensive care unit: an observational outcomes analysis. *J Intensive Care Med* **23**(3): 195–203.

Rawlings, C.A., et al. (2003). Use of laparoscopic-assisted cystoscopy for removal of urinary calculi in dogs. *J Am Vet Med Assoc* **222**(6): 759–761.

Redfors, B., et al. (2009). Effects of mannitol alone and mannitol plus furosemide on renal oxygen consumption, blood flow and glomerular filtration after cardiac surgery. *Intensive Care Med* **35**(1): 115–122.

Rentko, V.T., et al. (1992). Canine leptospirosis: a retrospective study of 17 cases. *J Vet Intern Med* **6**: 235–244.

Ricci, Z. and C. Ronco (2008). Dose and efficiency of renal replacement therapy: continuous renal replacement therapy versus intermittent hemodialysis versus slow extended daily dialysis. *Crit Care Med* **36**(Suppl): S229–S237.

Riordan, M., et al. (2005). HSP70 binding modulates detachment of Na-K-ATPase following energy deprivation in renal epithelial cells. *AM J Physiol Renal Physiol* **288**: F1236–F1242.

Rivers, B.J. and G.R. Johnston (1996). Diagnostic imaging strategies in small animal nephrology. *Vet Clin North Am Small Anim Pract* **26**(6): 1505–1517.

Rivers, B.J., et al. (1996). Evaluation of urine gamma-glutamyl transpeptidase-to-creatinine ratio as a diagnostic tool in an experimental model of aminoglycoside-induced acute renal failure in the dog. *J Am Anim Hosp Assoc* **32**(4): 323–336.

Rivers, B.J., et al. (1997a). Duplex Doppler estimation of resistive index in arcuate arteries of sedated, normal female dogs: implications for use in the diagnosis of renal failure. *J Am Anim Hosp Assoc* **33**(1): 69–76.

Rivers, B.J., et al. (1997b). Ultrasonographic-guided, percutaneous antegrade pyelography: technique and clinical application in the dog and cat. *J Am Anim Hosp Assoc* **33**(1): 61–68.

Rivers, B.J., et al. (1997c). Duplex Doppler estimation of intrarenal pourcelot resistive index in dogs and cats with renal disease. *J Vet Intern Med* **11**(4): 250–260.

Rollings, C.E., et al. (2004). Use of hemodialysis in uremic and non-uremic dogs with ethylene glycol toxicity (abstract). *J Vet Intern Med* **18**(3): 416.

Ronco, C. and Z. Ricci (2008). Renal replacement therapies: physiological review. *Intensive Care Med* **34**: 2139–2146.

Rose, B.D. (2001). Metabolic acidosis. In: *Clinical Physiology of Acid-Base and Electrolyte Disorders*, edited by B.D. Rose and T.W. Post. New York, NY: McGraw-Hill, pp. 578–646.

Rosen, S. and I.E. Stillman (2008). Acute tubular necrosis is a syndrome of physiologic and pathologic dissociation. *J Am Soc Nephrol* **19**: 871–875.

Ross, L.R. and M.A. Labato (2006). Peritoneal dialysis. In: *Fluid, Electrolyte, and Acid-Base Disorders in Small Animal Practice*, edited by S.P. DiBartola. St. Louis, MO: Saunders Elsevier, pp. 635–649.

Rumbeiha, W.K., et al. (2004). A comprehensive study of Easter lily poisoning in cats. *J Vet Diagn Invest* **16**: 527–541.

Rumbeiha, W.K. and M.J. Murphy (2009). Nephrotoxicants. In: *Kirk's Current Veterinary Therapy XIV*, edited by J.D. Bonagura and D.C. Twedt. St. Louis, MO: Saunders Elsevier, pp. 159–164.

Ruschitzka, F., et al. (1999). Endothelial dysfunction in acute renal failure: role of circulating and tissue endothelin-1. *J Am Soc Nephrol* **10**: 953–962.

Rush, J.E., et al. (1990). Pericardial disease in the cat: a retrospective evaluation of 66 cases. *J Am Anim Hosp Assoc* **26**: 39–46.

Schaefer, T.J. and R.W. Wolford (2005). Disorders of potassium. *Emerg Med Clin North Am* **23**: 723–747.

Schaer, G.L., et al. (1985). Norepinephrine alone versus norepinephrine plus low-dose dopamine: enhanced renal blood flow with combination pressor therapy. *Crit Care Med* **13**(6): 492–496.

Schaer, M. (2008). Therapeutic approach to electrolyte emergencies. *Vet Clin North Am Small Anim Pract* **38**(3): 513–533.

Scheel, P.J., et al. (2008). Uremic lung: new insights into a forgotten condition. *Kidney Int* **74**(7): 849–851.

Schenck, P.A. and D.J. Chew (2005). Prediction of serum ionized calcium concentration by use of serum total calcium concentration in dogs. *Am J Vet Res* **66**: 1330–1336.

Schenck, P.A., et al. (2006). Disorders of calcium: hypercalcemia and hypocalcemia. IN: *Fluid, Electrolyte, and Acid-Base Disorders in Small Animal Practice*, edited by S.P. DiBartola. St. Louis, MO: Saunders Elsevier, pp. 122–194.

Schrier, R.W. (2009). AKI: fluid overload and mortality. *Nat Rev Nephrol* **5**(9): 485.

Sedlacek, H.S., et al. (2008). Comparative efficacy of maropitant and selected drugs in preventing emesis induced by centrally or peripherally acting emetogens in dogs. *J Vet Pharmacol Ther* **31**(6): 533–537.

Segerer, S., et al. (2000). Chemokines, chemokine receptors, and renal disease: from basic science to pathophysiologic and therapeutic studies. *J Am Soc Nephrol* **11**: 152–176.

Segev, G., et al. (2008a). Aluminum toxicity following administration of aluminum-based phosphate binders in two dogs with renal failure. *J Vet Intern Med* **22**(6): 1432–1435.

Segev, G., et al. (2010). Correction of hyperkalemia in dogs with chronic kidney disease consuming commercial renal therapeutic diets by a potassium-reduced home prepared diet. *J Vet Intern Med.* (in press.)

Segev, G., et al. (2008b). A novel clinical scoring system for outcome prediction in dogs with acute kidney injury managed by hemodialysis. *J Vet Intern Med* **22**(2): 301–308.

Shalkham, A.S., et al. (2006). The availability and use of charcoal hemoperfusion in the treatment of poisoned patients. *Am J Kidney Dis* **48**(2): 239–241.

Sharples, E.J., et al. (2004). Erythropoietin protects the kidney against the injury and dysfunction caused by ischemia-reperfusion. *J Am Soc Nephrol* **15**: 2115–2124.

Shilliday, I.R., et al. (1997). Loop diuretics in the management of acute renal failure: a prospective, double-blind, placebo-controlled, randomized study. *Nephrol Dial Transplant* **12**: 2592–2596.

Sigrist, N.E. (2007). Use of dopamine in acute renal failure. *J Vet Emerg Crit Care* **17**(2): 117–126.

Silverstein, D.C., et al. (2005). Assessment of changes in blood volume in response to resuscitative fluid administration in dogs. *J Vet Emerg Crit Care* **15**(3): 185–192.

Simmons, J.P., et al. (2006). Diuretic effects of fenoldopam in healthy cats. *J Vet Emerg Crit Care* **16**(2): 96–103.

Smith, J.P. and I.J. Chang (2008). Extracorporeal treatment of poisoning. In: *Brenner & Rector's The Kidney*, edited by B.M. Brenner, Volume **2**. Philadelphia, PA: Saunders Elsevier, pp. 2081–2100.

Sohal, A.S., et al. (2006). Uremic bleeding: pathophysiology and clinical risk factors. *Thromb Res* **118**(3): 417–422.

Solomon, R. (1998). Contrast-medium-induced acute renal failure. *Kidney Int* **53**: 230–242.

Son, H.R., et al. (1998). Comparison of dual-energy x-ray absorptiometry and measurement of total body water content by deuterium oxide dilution for estimating body composition in dogs. *Am J Vet Res* **59**(5): 529–532.

Stanley, S.W. and C.E. Langston (2008). Hemodialysis in a dog with acute renal failure from currant toxicity. *Can Vet J* **49**: 63–66.

Starkey, R.J. and M.A. McLoughlin (1996). Treatment of renal aspergillosis in a dog using nephrostomy tubes. *J Vet Intern Med* **10**(5): 336–338.

Stepien, R.L. and R.A. Henik (2009). Systemic hypertension. In: *Kirk's Current Veterinary Therapy XIV*, edited by J.D. Bonagura and D.C. Twedt. St. Louis, MO: Saunders Elsevier, pp. 713–717.

Stokes, J.E., et al. (2007). Prevalence of serum antibodies against six *Leptospira* serovars in healthy dogs. *J Am Vet Med Assoc* **230**(11): 1657–1664.

Sutton, T.A., et al. (2002). Microvascular endothelial injury and dysfunction during ischemic acute renal failure. *Kidney Int* **62**: 1539–1549.

Taber, S.S. and B.A. Mueller (2006). Drug-associated renal dysfunction. *Crit Care Clin* **22**: 357–374.

Tag, T.L. and T.K. Day (2008). Electrocardiographic assessment of hyperkalemia in dogs and cats. *J Vet Emerg Crit Care* **18**(1): 61–67.

Thompson, M.E., et al. (2008). Characterization of melamine-containing and calcium oxalate crystals in three dogs with suspected pet food-induced nephrotoxicosis. *Vet Pathol* **45**(3): 417–426.

Thrall, M.A., et al. (1998). Advances in therapy for antifreeze poisoning. *Calif Vet* **52**(6): 18–22.

Thrall, M.A., et al. (1984). Clinicopathologic findings in dogs and cats with ethylene glycol intoxication. *J Am Vet Med Assoc* **184**(1): 37–41.

Tobata, D., et al. (2004). Effects of dopamine, dobutamine, amrinone and milrinone on regional blood flow in isoflurane anesthetized dogs. *J Vet Med Sci* **66**(9): 1097–1105.

Togel, F., et al. (2005). Administered mesenchymal stem cells protect against ischemic acute renal failure through differentiation-independent mechanisms. *AM J Physiol Renal Physiol* **289**: F31–F42.

Tolkoff-Rubin, N.E., et al. (2009). Urinary tract infection, pyelonephritis, and reflux nephropathy. In: *Brenner & Rector's The Kidney*, edited by B.M. Brenner, Volume **1**. Philadelphia, PA: Saunders Elsevier, pp. 1203–1238.

Townsend, D.R. and S.M. Bagshaw (2008). New insights on intravenous fluids, diuretics, and acute kidney injury. *Nephron Clin Pract* **109**: 206–216.

Tumlin, J.A. (2009). Impaired blood flow in acute kidney injury: pathophysiology and potential efficacy of intrarenal vasodilator therapy. *Curr Opin Crit Care* **15**(6): 514–519.

Uchino, S. (2008). Choice of therapy and renal recovery. *Crit Care Med* **36**(Suppl): S238–S242.

Uchino, S., et al. (2006). An assessment of the RIFLE criteria for acute renal failure in hospitalized patients. *Crit Care Med* **34**(7): 1913–1917.

Uchino, S., et al. (2007). Patient and kidney survival by dialysis modality in critically ill patients with acute kidney injury. *Int J Artif Organs* **30**(4): 281–292.

Uchino, S., et al. (2004). Diuretics and mortality in acute renal failure. *Crit Care Med* **32**(8): 1669–1677.

Vaden, S.L., et al. (1997). A retrospective case-control of acute renal failure in 99 dogs. *J Vet Intern Med* **11**(2): 58–64.

Vaden, S.L., et al. (2005). Renal biopsy: a retrospective study of methods and complications in 283 dogs and 65 cats. *J Vet Intern Med* **19**: 794–801.

Vaidya, V.S., et al. (2008). Biomarkers of acute kidney injury. *Annu Rev Pharmacol Toxicol* **48**: 463–493.

Vaidya, V.S., et al. (2009). A rapid urine test for early detection of kidney injury. *Kidney Int* **76**(1): 108–114.

Valencia, E., et al. (2009). Nutrition therapy for acute renal failure: a new approach based on 'risk, injury, failure, loss, and end-stage kidney' classification (RIFLE). *Curr Opin Clin Nutr Metab Care* **12**(3): 241–244.

Vanholder, R., et al. (2003a). Review on uremic toxins: classification, concentration, and interindividual variability. *Kidney Int* **63**: 1934–1943.

Vanholder, R., et al. (2003b). New insights in uremic toxins. *Kidney Int* **63**(Suppl 84): S6–S10.

Vanholder, R., et al. (2008). What is new in uremic toxicity? *Pediatr Nephrol* **23**(8): 1211–1221.

Venkataram, R. and J.A. Kellum (2001). The role of diuretic agents in the management of acute renal failure. *Contrib Nephrol* (132): 158–170.

Venkataraman, R. (2008). Can we prevent acute kidney injury? *Crit Care Med* **36**(Suppl): S166–S171.

Versteilen, A.M.G., et al. (2004). Molecular mechanims of acute renal failure following ischemia/reperfusion. *Int J Artif Organs* **27**(12): 1019–1029.

Vijayan, A. and S.B. Miller (1998). Acute renal failure: prevention and nondialytic therapy. *Semin Nephrol* **18**(5): 523–532.

Visweswaran, P., et al. (1997). Mannitol-induced acute renal failure. *J Am Soc Nephrol* **8**(6): 1028–1033.

Waikar, S.S. and J.V. Bonventre (2008). Biomarkers for the diagnosis of acute kidney injury. *Nephron Clin Pract* **109**(4): c192–c197.

Ward, D.T., et al. (2005). Aminoglycosides induce acute cell signaling and chronic cell death in renal cells that express the calcium-sensing receptor. *J Am Soc Nephrol* **16**: 1236–1244.

Ward, M.P. (2002a). Clustering of reported cases of leptospirosis among dogs in the United States and Canada. *Prev Vet Med* **56**(3): 215–226.

Ward, M.P. (2002b). Seasonality of canine leptospirosis in the United States and Canada and its association with rainfall. *Prev Vet Med* **56**: 203–213.

Ward, M.P., et al. (2002). Prevalence of and risk factors for leptospirosis among dogs in the United States and Canada: 677 cases (1970–1998). *J Am Vet Med Assoc* **220**(1): 53–58.

Washabau, R.J. and M.S. Elie (1995). Antiemetic therapy. In: *Kirk's Current Veterinary Therapy XII*, edited by J.D. Bonagura. Philadelphia, PA: WB Saunders, pp. 679–685.

Wassermann, K., et al. (1980). Dopamine-induced diuresis in the cat without changes in renal hemodynamics. *Naunyn Schmiedebergs Arch Pharmacol* **312**(1): 77–83.

Weidemann, A., et al. (2008). HIF activation protects from acute kidney injury. *J Am Soc Nephrol* **19**: 486–494.

Weingart, C. and B. Kohn (2008). Clinical use of a haemoglobin-based oxygen carrying solution (Oxyglobin) in 48 cats (2002–2006). *J Feline Med Surg* **10**(5): 431–438.

Westropp, J.L., et al. (2006). Dried solidified blood calculi in the urinary tract of cats. *J Vet Intern Med* **20**: 828–834.

Wild, C.J., et al. (2002). An improved immunohistochemical diagnostic technique for canine leptospirosis using antileptospiral antibodies on renal tissue. *J Vet Diagn Invest* **14**: 20–24.

Wilhelm, S.M., et al. (1999). Endothelin up-regulation and localization following renal ischemia and reperfusion. *Kidney Int* **55**: 1011–1018.

Willard, M. (2008). Therapeutic approach to chronic electrolyte disorders. *Vet Clin North Am Small Anim Pract* **38**(3): 535–541, x.

Willard, M.D. (2009). Digestive system disorders: general therapeutic principles. In: *Small Animal Internal Medicine*, edited by R.W. Nelson and C.G. Couto. St. Louis, MO: Mosby Elsevier, pp. 395–413.

Wolf, A.M. (1980). Canine uremic encephalopathy. *J Am Anim Hosp Assoc* **16**: 735–738.

Worwag, S. and C.E. Langston (2008). Feline acute intrinsic renal failure: 32 cats (1997–2004). *J Am Vet Med Assoc* **232**(5): 728–732.

Yamamoto, T., et al. (2002). Intravital videomicroscopy of peritubular capillaries in renal ischemia. *Am J Physiol Renal Physiol* **282**: F1150–F1115.

Yatsu, T., et al. (1997a). Renal effect of YM435, a new dopamine D1 receptor agonist, in anesthetized dogs. *Eur J Pharmacol* **322**(1): 45–53.

Yatsu, T., et al. (1998). Effect of YM435, a dopamine DA1 receptor agonist, in a canine model of ischemic acute renal failure. *Gen Pharmacol* **31**(5): 803–807.

Yatsu, T., et al. (1997b). Pharmacological and pharmacokinetic characteristics of YM435, a novel dopamine DA1-receptor agonist, in anaesthetized dogs. *J Pharm Pharmacol* **49**(9): 892–896.

Yatsu, T., et al. (1997c). Dopamine DA1 receptor agonist activity of YM435 in the canine renal vasculature. *Gen Pharmacol* **29**(2): 229–232.

Yavuz, A., et al. (2005). Uremic toxins: a new focus on an old subject. *Semin Dial* **18**(3): 203–211.

Yhee, J.Y., et al. (2009). Retrospective study of melamine/cyanuric acid-induced renal failure in dogs in Korea between 2003 and 2004. *Vet Pathol* **46**(2): 348–354.

Ympa, Y.P., et al. (2005). Has mortality from acute renal failure decreased? A systematic review of the literature. *Am J Med* **118**(8): 827–832.

Zakarija, A. and C.L. Bennett (2005). Drug-induced thrombotic microangiopathy. *Semin Thromb Hemost* **31**(6): 681–690.

Zaragoza, C., et al. (2003). SDS-PAGE and Western blot of urinary proteins in dogs with leishmaniasis. *Vet Res* **34**(2): 137–151.

Zatelli, A., et al. (2003). Glomerular lesions in dogs infected with Leishmania organisms. *Am J Vet Res* **64**(5): 558–561.

Zwijnenberg, R.J.G., et al. (2008). Cross-sectional study of canine leptospirosis in animal shelter populations in mainland Australia. *Aust Vet J* **86**(8): 317–323.

50

Prognosis of acute renal failure

Gilad Segev

Accumulation of uremic toxins, due to acute kidney injury (AKI), may lead to a variety of clinical signs and clinicopathological abnormalities, some of which are life-threatening. Multiple factors determine the outcome and long term prognosis of canine and feline AKI. These include the reversibility of the injury (which mostly depends on its severity and the underlying cause), comorbid disorders, concurrent complications, and the medical management available. Occasionally, the kidney has the potential to recover; however, severe uremia may lead to death before recovery can occur. Medical management provides only a narrow window of opportunity for the kidney to recover, although in some cases recovery may take even months. Dialysis can expand this window to an unlimited period, in the absence of fatal complications or financial constraints. Thus, the availability of therapeutic options should be considered in the assessment of the prognosis.

The overall mortality in dogs with AKI was 44% and 41% of dogs managed medically or with hemodialysis, respectively, (Vaden et al. 1997; Francey and Cowgill 2002) and 44% and 52–60% of cats managed medically or with hemodialysis, respectively (Langston et al. 1997; Pantaleo et al. 2004; Worwag and Langston 2004). The long-term outcome of patients with AKI mostly depends on the degree of reversibility. In one study, 55% of AKI survivors sustained chronic kidney disease (CKD) (Vaden et al. 1997). Euthanasia is a factor that influences the reported mortality rate in veterinary medicine. Euthanized animals with no significant attempt for intervention may be reported as non survivals; therefore, the reported mortality rates may be an overestimation for aggressively managed patients.

As the ability of the kidney to recover is highly dependent on the inciting cause, different etiologies convey different prognoses. While some are associated with reversible injury and favorable outcome, others have been linked to irreversible damage and poor outcome. Limited number of studies has investigated the association of specific AKI etiologies with their outcome (Table 50.1). Selected and common etiologies are discussed below.

Leptospirosis is associated with reversible injury and high survival rates, even when the injury is severe enough to necessitate dialytic intervention (Adin and Cowgill 2000; Segev et al. 2008). In a recent study, only 3/56 dogs diagnosed with leptospirosis and managed with hemodialysis died or were euthanized due to lack of renal improvement (Segev et al. 2008). Pyelonephritis is another etiology that is associated with a favorable outcome as the damage is usually reversible and the underlying cause can be eliminated (Langston et al. 1997). The prognosis of nephrotoxicity, a common etiology of AKI in companion animals, is highly dependent on the toxin. Ischemic injury (e.g., NSAID, ACE inhibitors) is usually reversible, while direct renal damage (e.g., ethylene glycol) is often irreversible. Ethylene glycol intoxication, for example, has a poor outcome even when dialysis is employed (Adin and Cowgill 2000; Francey and Cowgill 2002; Pantaleo et al. 2004; Worwag and Langston 2004). Grapes and raisin intoxication, a recently recognized cause of canine AKI, may result in proximal renal tubule degeneration and necrosis (Eubig et al. 2005; Morrow et al. 2005). Recovery occurs in approximately half of the patients and is typically complete (Eubig et al. 2005). Lily toxicity is a severe often irreversible intoxication in cats resulting in a high mortality rate and CKD in survivors; yet, complete clinical recovery has been described (Berg et al. 2007).

AKI is also a potential complication of hospitalized patients. In a study of hospital acquired canine renal

Nephrology and Urology of Small Animals. Edited by Joe Bartges and David J. Polzin. © 2011 Blackwell Publishing Ltd.

Table 50.1 Association of different etiologies and survival in dogs and cats with acute kidney injury

Etiology	Survival (%)	Comments
Infectious		
Leptospirosis	56–85 (Brown et al. 1996; Harkin and Gartrell 1996; Adin and Cowgill 2000; Goldstein et al. 2006; Mastrorilli et al. 2007)	In most studies, survival rate is approximately 80%. The infecting serovar may influence the survival
Pyelonephritis	Cats, 57–100 (Langston et al. 1997; Pantaleo et al. 2004)	For cats managed with hemodialysis
Toxicosis		
Ethylene glycol	Dogs, 5–20 (Connally et al. 1996; Vaden et al. 1997; Francey and Cowgill 2002; Rollings et al. 2004)	After AKI has been established. 20% survival rate in dogs and 31% in cats were reported for patients managed with hemodialysis
	Cats, 4–31 (Thrall et al. 1984; Pantaleo et al. 2004)	
Lily toxicity	0–50 (Langston 2002; Hadley et al. 2003; Pantaleo et al. 2004)	Typically, survivors sustain CKD, but clinical recovery has been documented (Berg et al. 2007)
Grapes and raisins	50–75 (Gwaltney-Brant et al. 2001; Campbell and Bates 2003; Eubig et al. 2005)	The basement membrane remains intact (Morrow et al. 2005)
Gentamicin	20 (Brown et al. 1985)	In human patients, gentamicin toxicity is often reversible but recovery may be prolonged. In the referenced study 7/8 non-survivors were euthanized
Other		
Hospital acquired renal failure	Dogs, 38 (Behrend et al. 1996)	Older patients were more prone to develop AKI and less likely to survive
Metabolic and hemodynamic	Dogs, 56 (Francey and Cowgill 2002)	For dogs and cats managed with hemodialysis
	Cats, 72 (Pantaleo et al. 2004)	
Ureteral obstruction	Cats, 70–75 (Fischer et al. 2004; Kyles et al. 2005)	The majority of the survivors sustain CKD

Table 50.2 Risk factors for mortality in dogs with AKI

Risk factor
↑Age (Behrend et al. 1996)
↓Body weight (Fischer et al. 2004)
Anemia (Vaden et al. 1997; Segev et al. 2008)
Lymphopenia (Segev et al. 2008)
↑Serum creatinine (Vaden et al. 1997; Segev et al. 2008)
Hyperphosphatemia (Behrend et al. 1996; Segev et al. 2008)
Hypocalcemia (Vaden et al. 1997; Segev et al. 2008)
Increased anion gap (Behrend et al. 1996; Segev et al. 2008)
Hypoalbuminemia (Segev et al. 2008)
↓Urine production (Behrend et al. 1996; Segev et al. 2008)
Respiratory involvement (Segev et al. 2008)
Neurological involvement (Segev et al. 2008)
Presence of DIC[a] (Vaden et al. 1997; Segev et al. 2008)

[a]Disseminated intravascular coagulation.
Risk factors above were identified in a univariate analysis based on retrospective studies of AKI of various etiologies.

Table 50.3 Outcome prediction models using a scoring system in dogs with AKI managed with hemodialysis

Variables	Range		
	Weighting factor		
Body weight (kg)	>36	27.2–36.0	≤27.1
	1.00	1.61	2.73
Red blood cells (10^6cells/μL)	>4.93	3.54–4.93	≤3.53
	1.00	1.51	3.61
Lymphocyte count (cells/μL)	>1000	509–999	≤509
	1.00	1.69	3.44
Creatinine (mg/dL)	≤13.2	>13.2	
	1.00	2.26	
Phosphorous (mg/dL)	≤18.2	18.2	
	1.00	3.13	
Ionized calcium (mmol/L)	>1.1	0.87–1.1	≤0.86
	1.00	1.99	4.16
Anion gap (mmol/L)	≤18.2	>18.2	
	1.00	2.74	
Albumin (g/dL)	>1.9	≤1.9	
	1.00	2.52	
Alanine aminotransferase (U/L)	<210	>210	
	1.00	−2.43	
Urine production (mL/kg/hour)	>1.31	0.1–1.31	0
	1.00	1.44	5.55
Respiratory system involvement	No	Yes	
	1.00	2.48	
Neurological involvement	No	Yes	
	1.00	3.76	
DIC[a]	No	Yes	
	1.00	2.3	

When leptospirosis and EG status are known, the final predictive score is adjusted as follows: leptospirosis, −8.46; EG, +2.47; neither, +1.00.

Cutoff points for models

Diagnosis is unknown			Diagnosis is known		
Cutoff	Sensitivity	Specificity	Cutoff	Sensitivity	Specificity
18.44	52	98	13.39	56	97
19.68	73	88	17.01	67	92
20.51	**81**	**85**	**19.92**	**83**	**90**
21.96	88	73	22.49	90	75
26.29	96	34	24.31	96	70

The clinical value of each individual patient should be compared to the ranges of each variable to assign a weighting factor for the variable. All weighting factors should be summed to a final predictive score. When leptospirosis and EG status are known, an adjustment to the final score is made. The final score is compared to the different cutoff points to predict survival. Dogs with a predictive score below the cutoff point are expected to survive with the corresponding sensitivities and specificities.

[a]Disseminated intravascular coagulation. Optimal cutoff points are bolded.

failure, survival rate was only 38% (Behrend et al. 1996). Old dogs were more likely to develop AKI and less likely to survive (Behrend et al. 1996). In cats, ureteral obstruction has become a common cause for acute uremia. Survival rates with aggressive medical and surgical intervention are high (~75%), but most survivors sustain CKD (Fischer et al. 2004; Kyles et al. 2005).

Although etiology is a major determinant of the prognosis, it is often unknown at presentation and remains unknown throughout the disease course, thus frequently cannot facilitate prognostic projections. Kidney biopsy (see Chapter 23) and histopathology may disclose the underlying etiology, assess the kidney injury severity, and the basement membrane integrity. The latter has a crucial role in the recovery potential of the kidney (Oliver 1953; Vracko 1974).

Based on a limited number of large-scale retrospective studies of dogs and cats with AKI of various etiologies, several risk factors for mortality have been identified, mainly in dogs; however, those were not consistent throughout the studies (Table 50.2).

Persistent anuria/oliguria is the most consistent risk factor among studies of AKI in dogs and cats and is considered a major negative prognostic indicator. The presence or absence of risk factors may aid in the overall assessment, but cannot be translated into an accurate prognosis. Since the 1980s, scoring systems have evolved in the human literature to assess disease severity and to forecast outcomes, mostly in emergency and critically ill patients. Recently, scoring systems were developed to aid in outcome prediction for canine AKI managed with hemodialysis (Segev et al. 2008). These can also be used as an objective tool to assess the severity of the renal injury. Few models were developed with a high sensitivity, specificity and correct classification (Table 50.3). Yet, these models need to be prospectively validated in an independent cohort before their true accuracy and usefulness can be determined. In addition, caution should be exerted when applying such models to individual patients. Scoring systems should not replace proper clinical assessment nor should they serve as a sole prognostic tool.

References

Adin, C.A. and L.D. Cowgill (2000). Treatment and outcome of dogs with leptospirosis: 36 cases (1990–1998). *J Am Vet Med Assoc* **216**: 371–375.

Behrend, E.N., et al. (1996). Hospital-acquired acute renal failure in dogs: 29 cases (1983–1992). *J Am Vet Med Assoc* **208**: 537–541.

Berg, R.I., et al. (2007). Resolution of acute kidney injury in a cat after lily (*Lilium lancifolium*) intoxication. *J Vet Intern Med* **21**: 857–859.

Brown, C.A., et al. (1996). Leptospira interrogans serovar grippotyphosa infection in dogs. *J Am Vet Med Assoc* **209**: 1265–1267.

Brown, S.A., et al. (1985). Gentamicin-associated acute renal failure in the dog. *J Am Vet Med Assoc* **186**: 686–690.

Campbell, A. and N. Bates (2003). Raisin poisoning in dogs. *Vet Rec* **152**: 376.

Connally, H.E., et al. (1996). Safety and efficacy of 4-methylpyrazole for treatment of suspected or confirmed ethylene glycol intoxication in dogs: 107 cases (1983–1995). *J Am Vet Med Assoc* **209**: 1880–1883.

Eubig, P.A., et al. (2005). Acute renal failure in dogs after the ingestion of grapes or raisins: a retrospective evaluation of 43 dogs (1992–2002). *J Vet Intern Med* **19**: 663–674.

Fischer, J.R., et al. (2004). Clinical and clinicopathological features of cats with acute ureteral obstruction managed with hemodialysis between 1993 and 2004: a review of 50 cases. *J Vet Intern Med* **18**: 777.

Francey, T. and L.D. Cowgill (2002). Use of hemodialysis for the treatment of acute renal failure (ARF) in the dog: 124 cases (1990–2001). *J Vet Intern Med* **16**: 352.

Goldstein, R.E., et al. (2006). Influence of infecting serogroup on clinical features of leptospirosis in dogs. *J Vet Intern Med* **20**: 489–494.

Gwaltney-Brant, S., et al. (2001). Renal failure associated with ingestion of grapes or raisins in dogs. *J Am Vet Med Assoc* **218**: 1555–1556.

Hadley, R.M., et al. (2003). A retrospective study of daylily toxicosis in cats. *Vet Hum Toxicol* **45**: 38–39.

Harkin, K.R. and C.L. Gartrell (1996). Canine leptospirosis in New Jersey and Michigan: 17 cases (1990–1995). *J Am Anim Hosp Assoc* **32**: 495–501.

Kyles, A.E., et al. (2005). Management and outcome of cats with ureteral calculi: 153 cases (1984–2002). *J Am Vet Med Assoc* **226**: 937–944.

Langston, C.E., et al. (1997). Applications and outcome of hemodialysis in cats: a review of 29 cases. *J Vet Intern Med* **11**: 348–355.

Langston, C.E. (2002). Acute renal failure caused by lily ingestion in six cats. *J Am Vet Med Assoc* **220**: 49–52, 36.

Mastrorilli, C., et al. (2007). Clinicopathologic features and outcome predictors of Leptospira interrogans Australis serogroup infection in dogs: a retrospective study of 20 cases (2001–2004). *J Vet Intern Med* **21**: 3–10.

Morrow, C.M., et al. (2005). Canine renal pathology associated with grape or raisin ingestion: 10 cases. *J Vet Diagn Invest* **17**: 223–231.

Oliver, J. (1953). Correlations of structure and function and mechanisms of recovery in acute tubular necrosis. *Am J Med* **15**: 535–557.

Pantaleo, V., et al. (2004). Application of hemodialysis for the management of acute uremia in cats: 119 cases (1993–2003). *J Vet Intern Med* **18**: 418.

Rollings, C.E., et al. (2004). Use of hemodialysis in uremic and non-uremic dogs with ethylene glycol toxicity. *J Vet Intern Med* **18**: 416.

Segev, G., et al. (2008). A novel clinical scoring system for outcome prediction in dogs with acute kidney injury managed by hemodialysis. *J Vet Intern Med* **22**: 301–308.

Thrall, M.A., et al. (1984). Clinicopathologic findings in dogs and cats with ethylene glycol intoxication. *J Am Vet Med Assoc* **184**: 37–41.

Vaden, S.L., et al. (1997). A retrospective case-control of acute renal failure in 99 dogs. *J Vet Intern Med* **11**: 58–64.

Vracko, R. (1974). Basal lamina scaffold-anatomy and significance for maintenance of orderly tissue structure. *Am J Pathol* **77**: 314–346.

Worwag, S. and C.E. Langston (2004). Retrospective, acute renal failure in cats: 25 cases (1997–2002). *J Vet Intern Med* **18**: 416.

51

Prognosis of renal failure–chronic

David J. Polzin

Chronic kidney disease (CKD) is typically a progressive and fatal disease. As described elsewhere, in most patients, progression of CKD is thought to occur largely as an adverse consequence or "trade-off" of renal adaptations to the loss of renal function rather than progression of the disease process that initiated the kidney disease. Although progress has been made in understanding and managing many of the processes that lead to progression of CKD, most dogs and cats with IRIS CKD stage II and higher will progress to end-stage renal failure regardless of the inciting cause. Dogs with CKD usually have progressive loss of kidney function and die of complications of kidney disease within months to a year or two of diagnosis. In contrast, cats with CKD have a more unpredictable disease course and may survive substantially longer than dogs. It has been observed that some cats have extended periods of stable renal function lasting months to years. It is not uncommon for these cats to appear to suddenly decompensate after extended periods of seemingly stable renal function (Elliott and Barber 1998; Elliott et al. 2003; Ross et al. 2006). The reason for these species-related differences is not completely understood; however, the renal lesions typically observed in cats appear to differ considerably from those observed in dogs. Proteinuric kidney disease associated with glomerular lesions is more common in dogs, while the lesions observed in cats' with CKD are most often primarily tubulointerstitial lesions with limited proteinuria (Syme et al. 2006). As a generality, glomerular diseases in humans tend to be more progressive compared to tubulointerstitial disease. Thus one factor that may explain the more aggressive course of CKD in dogs is the greater incidence of proteinuric glomerulopathies.

When applied to CKD, prognosis does not generally imply the likelihood of return of adequate kidney function[1] since CKD is irreversible. Short-term prognosis refers to the probability that the patient will achieve a satisfactory quality of life with therapy over the subsequent weeks to months. Long-term prognosis refers to the probability that a satisfactory quality of life can be achieved over many months to years, thus implying an extended period of survival.

A host of factors influence prognosis of CKD, both favorably and unfavorably (Table 51.1). Included among these factors are the quality of medical care provided to the patient and the level of owner's commitment. Because the estimate of prognosis often influences the owner's decisions about treatment options in complying with recommendations for management of the patient, the prognosis provided can influence patient outcome. A comprehensive evaluation of the patient is the best way to establish a reasonably accurate prognosis.

Factors to be considered in establishing meaningful prognoses for patients with CKD include (1) severity of intrinsic renal functional impairment, (2) probability of improving renal function (reversibility, primarily of prerenal, postrenal, and recently acquired primary renal conditions), (3) rate of progression of renal dysfunction with or without therapy, (4) severity and duration of clinical signs and complications of uremia, (5) the nature of the primary renal disease, and (6) age of the patient. In addition, the magnitude of proteinuria and possibly blood pressure appear to be important risk factors that may influence prognosis (Jacob et al. 2003, 2005; Syme et al. 2006).

Severity of uremic signs is often a relatively good predictor of short-term prognosis. Patients with stable CKD with minimal or no clinical signs of uremia usually have a good short-term prognosis. However, it is difficult to provide an accurate prognosis for untreated patients with

Nephrology and Urology of Small Animals. Edited by Joe Bartges and David J. Polzin. © 2011 Blackwell Publishing Ltd.

Table 51.1 Factors influencing prognosis in CKD

Clinical signs
Response to therapy
Rate of progression of CKD
Cause of kidney disease
IRIS stage
Magnitude of Proteinuria
Serum phosphorus concentration
Blood pressure (dogs)

severe clinical signs of uremia because it has yet to be established whether renal function and clinical signs can be improved by treatment. Uremic crisis often occurs in patients with CKD as a consequence of superimposed acute renal failure or prerenal or postrenal conditions (so-called acute-on-chronic uremic crisis). Although CKD is an irreversible condition, improvement of renal function may be possible when uremia results from the sum effects of CKD and a potentially reversible cause of azotemia. If treatment results in improved renal function and ameliorates clinical signs of uremia, the short-term prognosis may substantially improve.

Severity of renal dysfunction as determined by serum creatinine concentration or measurement of glomerular filtration rate (GFR) provides a less accurate means of assessing short-term prognosis than does the clinical condition of the patient. The relationship between magnitude of renal dysfunction and clinical signs of uremia may be highly variable and unpredictable. In addition, these renal function tests reflect the sum effect of renal, prerenal, and postrenal events and cannot establish reversibility of renal impairment. Therefore, short-term prognosis should not be established on the basis of a single measurement of renal function. Changes in renal function that occur in response to treatment provide greater insight into reversibility of renal functional impairment and thus prognosis.

Assessment of the severity of renal dysfunction is typically more useful in establishing long-term prognoses. In general, severe, irreversible renal dysfunction is associated with shorter long-term survival and, often, a lower quality of life. Higher serum creatinine values were reported to be associated with a greater risk of death within one month of diagnosis in cats with CKD; however, no specific value of serum creatinine concentration reliably predicts survival (Kuwahara et al. 2006). In a recent retrospective study of 733 feline patients with CKD and serum creatinine values greater than 2.3 mg/dL, IRIS stage of CKD at the time of initial diagnosis was found to be strongly predictive of survival duration (Boyd et al. 2008). Median survival times for cats in IRIS stages

II, III, and IV at the time of diagnosis were 1,151 days (range 2–3,107), 778 days (range 22–2,100), and 103 days (range 1–1,920), respectively. These survival times differed significantly (p<0.001) by IRIS stage. However, as shown by the wide range of survival times in each group, survival time cannot be accurately determined for an individual cat based solely on IRIS stage, but nonetheless the IRIS stage is predictive of the general trend for survival. Serum phosphorus concentration was the only other factor found to be related to prognosis in this study (Boyd et al. 2008). Phosphorus retention and hyperphosphatemia have both been linked to progression of CKD, but also are related to the magnitude of renal dysfunction (see Chapter 48).

In a recent clinical trial in dogs with spontaneous CKD, mean serum creatinine concentration did not appear to influence survival when dogs were fed a renal diet (Jacob et al. 2002). However, the majority of dogs in this study were CKD stage III. It is possible that the patient's IRIS stage may be more predictive of outcome than variations in serum creatinine values within a stage of CKD. Median survival for 21 dogs with a mean serum creatinine concentration of 3.3 mg/dL was 615 days. Median survival for a subpopulation of dogs in this group with serum creatinine values between 2.0 and 3.1 mg/dL was also 615 days. However, among 17 dogs fed a maintenance diet in this study, median survival for dogs with a mean serum creatinine of 3.7 mg/dL was 252 days, while survival for the subpopulation with serum creatinine values between 2.0 and 3.1 mg/dL was 461 days. Thus, other factors, such as therapeutic intervention, may substantially influence survival. The impact of therapeutic intervention should be considered when providing prognosis estimates.

Studies in dogs, cats, and humans have confirmed that proteinuria is a negative prognostic indicator in patients with CKD (Jacob et al. 2005; Abbate et al. 2006; Syme et al. 2006; King et al. 2007). The adverse effect of proteinuria increases as the magnitude of proteinuria increases. The greater the amount of protein excreted in urine, the more negative the prognosis. In a recent clinical trial, proteinuria was shown to be a risk factor for uremia and death in dogs with CKD (Jacob et al. 2005). In this study, the risk of death associated with CKD increased by 60% for each unit of urine protein-to-creatinine ratio above 1.0. Even small increases in proteinuria above the normal urine protein-to-creatinine ratio of 0.2 appear to be associated with increased risk of mortality in cats with CKD. In another study, elevated protein-to-creatinine ratios were found to be significantly associated with increased risk of mortality within the first month following initial evaluation (King et al. 2007). While the current dominant view is that proteinuria infers a more negative prognosis because it promotes renal injury and thus progression of CKD, an alternate view held by some is that proteinuria may only be a marker linked to progression of CKD (Abbate et al. 2006). Based on studies in humans and rodents, therapeutic amelioration of proteinuria using angiotensin converting enzyme inhibitors may slow progression of CKD, thus improving prognosis (Abbate et al. 2006).

Systemic hypertension has been linked to progression of CKD in humans for decades (El-Nahas and Tamimi 1999). Higher systolic blood pressure at the time of diagnosis is reportedly associated with increased risk of uremic crises and death in dogs with CKD (Jacob et al. 2003). In cats, elevated blood pressure does not appear to be an independent risk factor for progression of CKD; any adverse effect of elevated blood pressure is likely attributable to proteinuria (Jepson et al. 2007).

Endnote

1. Adequate kidney function in this context means sufficient kidney function to prevent retention of waste products in blood (i.e., azotemia) and maintain normal fluid and electrolyte homeostasis.

References

Abbate, M., et al. (2006). How does proteinuria cause progressive renal damage? *J Am Soc Nephrol* **17**: 2974–2984.

Boyd, L.M., et al. (2008). Survival in cats with naturally occurring chronic kidney disease (200–2002). *J Vet Intern Med* **22**: 1111–1117.

Elliot, J. and P. Barber (1998). Feline chronic renal failure: clinical findings in 80 cases diagnosed between 1992 and 1995. *J Small Anim Pract* **39**: 78–85.

Elliott, J., et al. (2003). Acid-base balance of cats with chronic renal failure: effect of deterioration in renal function. *J Small Anim Pract* **44**: 261–268.

El-Nahas, A. and N. Tamimi (1999). The progression of chronic renal failure: a harmful quartet. *Q J Med* **92**: 421–424.

Jacob, F., et al. (2002). Clinical evaluation of dietary modification for treatment of spontaneous chronic renal failure in dogs. *J Am Vet Med Assoc* **220**: 1163–1170.

Jacob, F., et al. (2003). Association between initial systolic blood pressure and risk of developing a uremic crisis or of dying in dogs with chronic renal failure. *J Am Vet Med Assoc* **222**: 322–329.

Jacob, F., et al. (2005). Evaluation of the association between initial proteinuria and morbidity rate or death in dogs with naturally occurring chronic renal failure. *J Am Vet Med Assoc* **226**: 393–400.

Jepson, R.E., et al. (2007). Effect of control of systolic blood pressure on survival in cats with systemic hypertension. *J Vet Intern Med* **21**: 402–409.

King, J.N., et al. (2007). Prognostic factors in cats with chronic kidney disease. *J Vet Intern Med* **21**: 906–916.

Kuwahara, Y., et al. (2006). Association of laboratory data and death within one month in cats with chronic renal failure. *J Small Anim Pract* **47**: 446–450.

Ross, S.J., et al. (2006). Clinical evaluation of dietary modification for treatment of spontaneous chronic kidney disease in cats. *J Am Vet Med Assoc* **229**: 949–957.

Syme, H.M., et al. (2006). Survival of cats with naturally occurring chronic renal failure is related to severity of proteinuria. *J Vet Intern Med* **20**: 528–535.

52

Renal manifestations of systemic disease

Linda Ross

Primary renal disease and renal failure are common causes of morbidity and mortality in dogs and cats. However, renal dysfunction or pathology may also be the result of systemic disease. The signs and laboratory abnormalities associated with renal disease may be the initial reason for presentation, or renal disease may be recognized during a diagnostic workup for seemingly unrelated clinical signs or laboratory abnormalities. It is important for the clinician to recognize these systemic diseases in order to institute appropriate therapy and give an accurate prognosis.

Infectious diseases

Renal pathology has been reported as the result of a variety of infectious diseases in animals. Associated clinical or laboratory abnormalities may be uncommon, such as granulomatous renal lesions with blastomycosis, cryptococcosis, and aspergillosis. In other infections, renal disease or failure is a common or predominant feature of clinical disease; these are discussed below (Table 52.1).

Leptospirosis

Leptospirosis is caused by infection with bacterial spirochetes of the species *Leptospira interrogans* (see Chapters 27 and 49). There are a number of different serovars of leptospirosis that may infect dogs. In the United States, the most common infecting serovars are *L. grippotyphosa* and *pomona* (Ross et al. 2000). Laboratory abnormalities in dogs with leptospirosis can include mild to moderate thrombocytopenia, azotemia, isosthenuria, proteinuria, and glucosuria. The urine sediment frequently contains erythrocytes, leukocytes, and granular casts. Histopathologic changes in acute leptospirosis have been described

as diffuse interstitial inflammation with infiltration primarily of lymphocytes, plasma cells, and less frequently neutrophils; mild scattered renal tubular necrosis; and interstitial edema (Figure 52.1). In chronic cases, the predominant change is interstitial fibrosis with mild, scattered inflammation (Greene et al. 2006; Prescott 2007).

Borreliosis

Borrelia burgdorferri is a spirochete bacterium that infects animals via the bite of an infected tick. In contrast to many other infections, clinical disease occurs not directly as the result of infection, but rather from the host's immune response to the organism (Greene and Straubinger 2006), and this pathogenesis likely applies to the associated renal disease as well. Acute, rapidly progressive renal failure in 49 dogs has been described in a retrospective study and attributed to infection with *Borrelia* (Dambach et al. 1997). Forty-three of these dogs had membranoproliferative glomerulonephritis, five had membranous glomerulonephritis, and one had amyloidosis. Most dogs also had renal tubular necrosis, and all had interstitial lymphoplasmocytic inflammation. Labrador and Golden retriever dogs were at increased risk.

Rocky mountain spotted fever

Rocky Mountain Spotted Fever (RMSF) is caused by infection with the rickesttsial bacteria *Rickettsia rickettsii*. Fever and generalized necrotizing vasculitis are responsible for most of the clinical signs. While acute renal failure is common in people with RMSF, it is less common in dogs, although vascular lesions are seen in the kidneys (Greene and Breitschwerdt 2006).

Feline immunodeficiency virus infection

Cats infected with feline infectious immunodeficiency virus have an increased risk of chronic renal disease,

Nephrology and Urology of Small Animals. Edited by Joe Bartges and David J. Polzin. © 2011 Blackwell Publishing Ltd.

Table 52.1 Infectious diseases associated with renal disease

Leptospirosis
Borreliosis
Rocky mountain spotted fever
Feline immunodeficiency virus infection
Feline infectious peritonitis
Feline leukemia virus infection
Leishmaniasis
Babesiosis
Hepatozoonosis
Sepsis

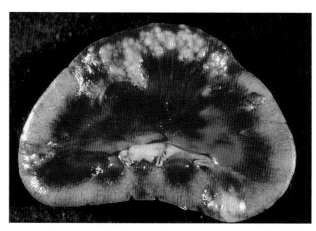

Figure 52.2 Multifocal pyogranulomas in the kidney of a cat with feline infectious peritonitis.

azotemia, and proteinuria (Levy et al. 2000). Renal lesions include thickened Bowman's membrane, segmental to diffuse glomerulosclerosis, amyloidosis, microscopic tubular dilatation and cytoplasmic vacuolization, mononuclear tubulointerstitial inflammation, and interstitial fibrosis (Poli et al. 1993; Poli et al. 1995; Levy et al. 2000).

Feline infectious peritonitis

Feline infectious peritonitis (FIP) is caused by a coronavirus. The non-effusive form of FIP is associated with pyogranulomatous lesions in many organs, including the kidneys (Figure 52.2). The kidneys may be grossly enlarged and irregular. Histologically, multiple pyogranulomas characterized by infiltration of macrophages, lymphocytes, plasma cells, and neutrophils are seen

(Addie and Jarrett 2006). Cats with FIP usually present for signs of systemic illness, including fever, weight loss, and lethargy. However, if renal lesions are extensive, the cat may present for signs of renal disease such as polydipsia, polyuria, and vomiting.

Feline leukemia virus infection

Cats infected with the feline leukemia virus are at increased risk for developing a variety of immune-mediated disorders, including glomerulonephritis. (Anderson and Jarrett 1971). Those with glomerulonephritis have been reported to have higher circulating viral (antigen) loads than those without renal lesions (Poli et al. 1995).

Leishmaniasis

The protozoan genus *Leishmania* includes numerous species that infect dogs and rarely cats. Infection in dogs results in a chronic systemic disease characterized by both cutaneous (exfoliative and ulcerative dermatitis) and visceral lesions. Renal involvment is common. Clinical and laboratory abnormalities include renal pain, polydipsia/polyuria, and azotemia (Nieto et al. 1992; Ciaramella et al. 1997). Proteinuria and hematuria occur in most infected dogs (Nieto et al. 1992; Zatelli et al. 2003). Mesangial, membranous, membranoproliferative, and focal segmental glomerulonephritis have been described in infected dogs (Zatelli et al. 2003).

Babesiosis

Several species of *Babesia* are known to infect dogs. The clinical presentation of infected dogs varies from subclinical to peracute, and is somewhat dependent upon the infecting species (Taboada et al. 2006). Approximately

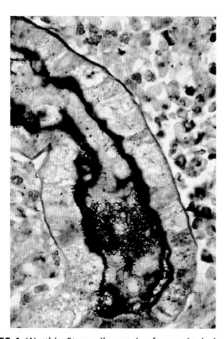

Figure 52.1 Warthin-Starry silver stain of a renal tubule showing numerous leptospires in the lumen.

1/3 of dogs in Spain infected with a *Babesia microti*-like organism (tentatively identified as identical to *Theileria annae*) were azotemic at the time of diagnosis, and azotemia was the main cause of death in infected dogs (Camacho et al. 2004). Acute renal failure appears to be less common in dogs infected with other species of *Babesia*. While many dogs with babesiosis have an elevated blood urea nitrogen concentration, it has been shown not to be due to renal dysfunction, but more likely catabolism of lysed red blood cells (de Scally et al. 2006). However, dogs infected with *Babesia canis* that had renal involvement had a fivefold greater risk of dying than those with other organ damage. It has been suggested that the renal failure seen in dogs with severe babesiosis represents a manifestation of the systemic inflammatory response syndrome (SIRS) and multiple organ dysfunction syndrome (MODS) (Welzl et al. 2001). Membranoproliferative glomerulonephritis has been described in dogs infected with *Babesia gibsoni* (Wozniak et al. 1997).

Hepatozoonosis

Hepatozoonosis in dogs is caused by infection with the protozoan *Hepatozoon canis* in South America, Africa, the Mediterranean countries, and some Asian countries, and by *Hepatozoon americanum* in the United States. *H. canis* is most often associated with clinical disease in dogs with high levels of parasitemia. While clinical signs of renal disease are not a common part of the clinical presentation, glomerulonephritis, interstitial nephritis, and multifocal necrosis have been described (Baneth and Weigler 1997). In contrast, infection with *H. americanum* usually causes severe illness characterized primarily by fever, muscle pain and atrophy, and hyperesthesia. Renal involvement is common, and reported lesions include multifocal pyogranulomatous inflammation with glomerulonephritis, lymphoplasmacytic interstitial nephritis, and mesangioproliferative glomerulonephritis. Renal amyloidosis may also occur in conjunction with systemic amyloidosis. The renal lesions are associated with clinically significant proteinuria, and may contribute to hypoalbuminemia (Macintire et al. 2006).

Sepsis

The term "sepsis" is now considered to represent not just generalized bacterial infection, but the systemic inflammatory response to that infection and subsequent multiple organ dysfunction (Barton 2005). In humans, acute renal failure occurs in up to 51% of patients with sepsis, and is associated with increased mortality (Schrier et al. 2004). Most of the data on the pathogenesis of sepsis-associated acute renal failure is derived from experimen-

tal studies, and the degree to which the same changes occur in clinical disease in humans or animals is not known. The most commonly accepted mechanism is ischemic acute tubular necrosis (Schrier et al. 2004; Klenzak and Himmelfarb 2005). Sepsis does not always result in hypotension. Hyperdynamic septic shock has been associated with increased renal blood flow, but may also result in acute renal failure. Apoptosis of renal tubular cells, rather than necrosis, may be the mechanism for renal injury in these situations. Various cytokines, endotoxin, as well as short periods of ischemia have all been shown to lead to apoptosis of renal tubular cells (Wan 2003; Guo 2004; Wang 2005).

Endocrine disorders

Polyuria and polydipsia are common manifestations of several endocrine disorders (see Chapter 42 on polyuria/polydipsia). However, renal pathology and alterations in renal function also occur as the result of some endocrinopathies (Table 52.2).

Hyperadrenocorticism

Glomerulonephritis and proteinuria occur in many dogs with hyperadrenocorticism. In a clinical study of 41 dogs with glomerulonephritis, an association was found between glomerular lesions and a history of excess endogenous or exogenous glucocorticoids (Center et al. 1987). An experimental study demonstrated that clinically normal dogs developed glomerular lesions and proteinuria after being given immunosuppressive doses of prednisone for 42 days (Waters et al. 1997). In one study, the urine protein:creatinine ratio (UPC) was elevated above normal (1.0) in 46% of dogs with untreated pituitary-dependent hyperadrenocorticism (mean 1.47 ± 1.69) and in 63% of dogs with untreated adrenal tumors (mean 2.7 ± 2.8). The amount of proteinuria was associated with the degree of elevation in arterial blood pressure. Renal histopathology was performed on seven dogs in this study, of which five had glomerulosclerosis and two had glomerulonephritis. UPC ratios decreased significantly in seven dogs after adequate control of hyperodrenocorticism, but not in eight dogs

Table 52.2 Endocrine disorders associated with renal disease or dysfunction

Hyperadrenocorticism
Hypoadrenocorticism
Diabetes mellitus
Hyperthyroidism

in which treatment was not successful in controlling cortisol levels (Ortega 1996). In another study, UPC ratios were found to be elevated (>1.0, range 1.06–4.16) in 1 of 16 (44%) of dogs with untreated pituitary-dependent hyperadrenocorticism. UPC ratios were not significantly different in dogs before or 2 weeks after adequate adrenal suppression with mitotane (Hurley and Vaden, 1998).

The mechanism of proteinuria (see Chapters 8 and 43) and the pathogenesis of glomerular lesions associated with hyperadrenocorticism are not completely understood. Glucocorticoid-induced systemic and glomerular hypertension likely plays a role, and may lead to glomerulosclerosis (Ortega 1996).

Hypoadrenocorticism

Azotemia is commonly found in dogs and cats with untreated hypoadrenocorticism. Decreased renal perfusion secondary to the lack of glucocorticoids and hypovolemia from mineralocorticoid-induced natriuresis causes this pre-renal azotemia. Correction of fluid abnormalities and appropriate mineralo- and glucocorticoid administration results in rapid resolution of azotemia.

Diabetes mellitus

Diabetic nephropathy, characterized by thickening of the glomerular and tubular basement membranes, glomerular mesangial expansion (diffuse glomerulosclerosis), interstitial expansion by extracellular matrix material, and proteinuria, is a common and serious late complication of diabetes mellitus in people (Parving et al. 2008). Similar glomerular lesions have been reported in dogs with diabetes mellitus, (Steffes et al. 1982; Jeraj et al. 1984) as has proteinuria (Kirsch and Reusch 1993). However, clinical renal disease associated with these pathophysiologic abnormalities appears to be rare. This may be because the length of time necessary for clinically significant renal disease to develop (12–20 years in people) exceeds the lifespan of dogs (Muñana 1995).

Hyperthyroidism

Elevated circulating levels of thyroid hormone can increase renal blood flow and glomerular filtration rate (Adams et al. 1997a). This effect can artifactually "mask" renal dysfunction, an effect seen most commonly in geriatric cats with hyperthyroidism. Treatment that restores euthyroidism may result in decreased renal blood flow and glomerular filtration rate, "unmasking" or worsening preexisting azotemia (Adams et al. 1997b).

Table 52.3 Miscellaneous disorders associated with renal disease

Dirofilariasis
Immune-mediated disorders
Systemic lupus erythematosus
Polyarteritis nodosa
Pancreatitis
Pyometra
Disseminated intravascular coagulation
Neoplasia

Miscellaneous disorders associated with renal disease (Table 52.3)

Dirofilariasis

Glomerular pathology has been described in dogs infected with *Dirofilaria immitis* (Klei et al. 1974; Casey and Splitter 1975; Abramowsky et al. 1981; Aikawa et al. 1981; Grauer et al. 1987; Grauer et al. 1989; Nakagaki et al. 1990; Paes-de-Almeida 2003), although clinically significant decreases in renal function are uncommon (Dalton et al. 1971; Osborne et al. 1981). Membranoproliferative glomerulonephritis is the most common lesion (Aikawa et al. 1981; Grauer et al. 1987; Nakagaki et al. 1990) but membranous glomerulonephritis (Casey and Splitter 1975) has also been reported. The pathogenesis of the glomerulopathy has been reported to be in situ formation in the glomerular basement membrane of immune complexes to antigens from adult *Dirofilaria immitis* worms (Aikawa et al. 1981; Grauer et al. 1987; Grauer et al. 1989).

Pancreatitis

Acute pancreatitis, especially in dogs, is frequently associated with azotemia. In mild or early stages of pancreatitis, the azotemia is primarily pre-renal as the result of hypovolemia. However, more severe pancreatitis can result in SIRS and MODS, of which acute renal failure is one manifestation (Ruaux 2000; Whittemore et al. 2005).

Pyometra

Renal dysfunction is common in dogs, (De Schepper et al. 1987; Stone et al. 1988), and to a lesser extent in cats (Kenney et al. 1987), with pyometra. Polydipsia and polyuria occur as the result of decreased urine concentrating ability, which is believed to be a form of nephrogenic diabetes insipidus secondary to endotoxin (Asheim 1965). Azotemia has been reported in 15–37% of dogs (Stone et al. 1988) and 12% of cats (Kenney et al. 1987) with pyometra; enzymuria and urine casts may be seen (De Schepper et al. 1987; Heine 2001). Although some studies have described membranoproliferative glomerulonephritis in dogs with pyometra (Obel 1964; Asheim 1965; Slauson 1979; Johnston 2001), other studies have found mild interstitial nephritis and tubular atrophy without significant glomerular lesions (Stone et al. 1988; Heiene et al. 2001; Heiene et al. 2004; Heiene 2007). In most cases, renal dysfunction is transient, and resolves following ovariohysterectomy or medical treatment of the pyometra (Heiene 2007).

Immune-mediated disorders

Systemic lupus erythematosus

Systemic lupus erythematosus (SLE) is an immune-mediated disease in which deposition of antigen-antibody complexes containing antibodies against a variety of cellular antigens results in inflammation and tissue damage. Renal involvement is common, and has been reported in approximately 55% of dogs and 40% of cats with SLE (Stone 2005). Glomerular lesions, characterized as membranous or membranoproliferative glomerulonephritis in dogs (Lewis 1972; Slauson and Lewis 1979) and membranous glomerulonephritis in cats (Werner et al. 1984; Thompson 1994) have been described (see Chapter 53). Protein-losing nephropathy and azotemia may be a minor or predominant component of the overall clinical manifestation of SLE.

Polyarteritis nodosa

Polyarteritis nodosa (periarteritis nodosa, panarteritis nodosa) is a rare disorder characterized by generalized necrotizing vasculitis affecting primarily small and medium-sized muscular arteries (Thompson 1994; Fox et al. 2005). The pathogenesis of this disorder is unknown, although it is believed to be immune-mediated. The vascular damage results in thrombosis, vascular occlusion, and ischemic damage to various tissues, including the kidneys. Reported renal lesions include fibrinoid necrosis of the tunica media of renal arterioles with infiltration by neutrophils and mononuclear cells, resulting in partial or complete occlusion of the vessel, thrombosis, and associated infarction. Azotemia may occur as the result of these lesions (Lucke 1968; Campbell et al. 1972; Thompson 1994). Fibrinoid necrosis has also been reported in glomeruli (Curtis 1979).

Disseminated intravascular coagulation

Disseminated intravascular coagulation (DIC) is a disorder in which microvascular thrombi are associated with consumption of platelets and clotting factors, resulting in simultaneous hemorrhage and thrombosis, ischemia,

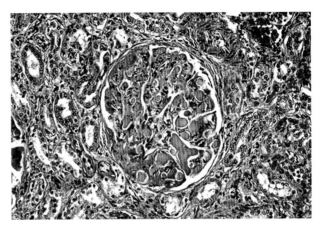

Figure 52.3 Fibrin thrombi occluding dilated glomerular capillaries in a dog with disseminated intravascular coagulation.

and multiple organ failure (Figure 52.3) (Fox et al. 2005). Acute renal failure is one of the most devastating complications of DIC.

Neoplasia

Neoplasia has been associated with glomerulonephritis in dogs and cats (Murray and Wright 1974; Glick et al. 1978; Jeraj et al. 1985; Center et al. 1987). The actual incidence is unknown; one study reported 40% of dogs with glomerulonephritis had neoplasia (Murray and Wright 1974), while another found that 69% of dogs with mastocytosis had glomerulitis (Hottendorf and Nielsen 1968).

References

Abramowsky, C.R., et al. (1981). *Dirofilaria immitus*: 5. Immunopathology of filarial nephropathy in dogs. *Am J Pathol* **104**: 1–12.

Adams, W.H., et al. (1997a). Investigation of the effects of hyperthyroidism on renal function in the cat. *Can J Vet Res* **61**: 53–56.

Adams, W.H., et al. (1997b). Changes in renal function in cats following treatment of hyperthyroidism using [131]I. *Vet Radiol Ultrasound* **38**(3): 231–238.

Addie, D.D. and O. Jarrett (2006). Feline coronavirus infections. In: *Infectious Diseases of the Dog and Cat*, edited by C.E. Greene, 3rd edition. St. Louis, MO: Saunders Elsevier, pp. 88–102.

Aikawa, M., et al. (1981). Dirofilariasis. IV. Glomerulonephropathy induced by *Dirofilaria immitis* infection. *Am J Trop Med Hyg* **30**(1): 84–91.

Anderson, L.J. and W.F.H. Jarrett (1971). Membranous glomerulonephritis associated with leukemia in cats. *Res Vet Sci* **12**: 179–180.

Asheim, A. (1965). Pathogenesis of renal damage and polydipsia in dogs with pyometra. *J Am Vet Med Assoc* **147**(7): 736–745.

Baneth, G. and B. Weigler (1997). Retrospective case-control study of hepatozoonosis in dogs in Israel. *J Vet Intern Med* **11**: 365–370.

Barton, L. (2005). Sepsis and the systemic inflammatory response syndrome. In: *Textbook of Veterinary Internal Medicine*, edited by S.J. Ettinger and E.C. Feldman, 6th edition. St. Louis, MO: Saunders Elsevier, pp. 452–454.

Camacho, A.T., et al. (2004). Azotemia and mortality among Babesia microti-like infected dogs. *J Vet Intern Med* **18**(2): 141–146.

Campbell, L.H., et al. (1972). Ocular and other manifestations of periarteritis nodosa in a cat. *J Am Vet Med Assoc* **161**(10): 1122–1126.

Casey, H.W. and G.A. Splitter (1975). Membranous glomerulonephritis in dogs infected with *Dirofilaria immitus*. *Vet Pathol* **12**(2): 111–117.

Center, S.H., et al. (1987). Clinicopathologic, renal immunofluorescent, and light microscopic features of glomerulonephritis in the dog: 41 cases (1975–1985). *J Am Vet Med Assoc* **190**: 81–90.

Ciaramella, P., et al. (1997). A retrospective clinical study of canine leishmaniasis in 150 dogs naturally infected with L. infantum. *Vet Rec* **141**: 539–543.

Curtis, R. (1979). Polyarteritis in a cat. *Vet Rec* **105**: 354.

Dalton, G.O., et al. (1971). Effect of Dirofilaria immitus on renal function in the dog. *Am J Vet Res* **32**(12): 2087–2089.

Dambach, D.M., et al. (1997). Morphologic, immunohistochemical, and ultrastructural characterization of a distinctive renal lesion in dogs putatively associated with *Borrelia burgdorferi* infection: 49 cases (1987–1992). *Vet Pathol* **34**: 85–96.

de Scally, M.P., et al. (2006). The elevated serum urea:creatinine ratio in canine babesiosis in South Africa is not of renal origin. *J S Afr Vet Assoc* **77**(4): 175–178.

De Schepper, J., et al. (1987). Renal injury in dogs with pyometra. *Tijdschr Diergeneeskd* **112**(Suppl 1): 124S–126S.

Fox, P.R., et al. (2005). Peripheral vascular disease. In: *Textbook of Veterinary Internal Medicine*, edited by S.J. Ettinger and E.C. Feldman, 6th edition. St. Louis, MO: Saunders Elsevier, pp. 1145–1165.

Glick, A.D., et al. (1978). Characterization of feline glomerulonephritis associated with viral-induced hematopoietic neoplasms. *Am J Pathol* **92**: 321–327.

Grauer, G.F., et al. (1987). Clinicopathologic and histologic evaluation of *Dirofilaria immitus*-induced nephropathy in dog. *Am J Trop Med Hyg* **37**(3): 588–596.

Grauer, G.F., et al. (1989). Experimental Dirofilaria immitis-associated glomerulonephritis induced in part by in situ formation of immune complexes in the glomerular capillary wall. *J Parasitol* **75**(4): 585–593.

Greene, C.E. and E.B. Breitschwerdt (2006). Rocky Mountain spotted fever, murine typhuslike disease, rickettsialpox, typhus, and Q fever. In: *Infectious Diseases of the Dog and Cat*, edited by C.E. Greene, 3rd edition. St. Louis, MO: Saunders Elsevier, pp. 232–245.

Greene, C.E. and R.K. Straubinger (2006). Borreliosis. In: *Infectious Diseases of the Dog and Cat*, edited by C.E. Greene, 3rd edition. St. Louis, MO: Saunders Elsevier, pp. 417–435.

Greene, C.E., et al. (2006). Leptospirosis. In: *Infectious Diseases of the Dog and Cat*, edited by C.E. Greene, 3rd edition. St. Louis, MO: Saunders Elsevier, pp. 402–417.

Guo, R., et al. (2004). Acute renal failure in endotoxemia is dependent on caspase activation. *J Am Soc Nephrol* **15**(12): 3093–3102.

Heiene, R., et al. (2001). Calculation of urinary enzyme excretion, with renal structure and function in dogs with pyometra. *Res Vet Sci* **70**(2): 129–137.

Heiene, R., et al. (2004). Vasopressin secretion in response to osmotic stimulation and effects of desmopressin on urinary concentrating capacity in dogs with pyometra. *Am J Vet Res* **65**(4): 404–408.

Heiene, R., et al. (2007). Renal histomorphology in dogs with pyometra and control dogs, and long term outcome with respect to signs of kidney disease. *Acta Vet Scand* **49**(1): 13.

Hottendorf, G.H. and S.W. Nielsen (1968). Pathologic report of 29 necropsies on dogs with mastocytoma. *Vet Pathol* **5**: 102–121.

Hurley, K.J. and S. L. Vaden (1998). Evaluation of urine protein content in dogs with pituitary-dependent hyperadrenocorticism. *J Am Vet Med Assoc* **212**(3): 369–373.

Jeraj, K., et al. (1984). Immunofluorescence studies on renal basement membranes in dogs with spontaneous diabetes. *Am J Vet Res* **45**: 1162–1165.

Jeraj, K.P., et al. (1985). Immune complex glomerulonephritis in a cat with renal lymphosarcoma. *Vet Pathol* **22**(3): 287–290.

Johnston, S.D., et al. (2001). Disorders of the canine uterus and uterine tubes (Oviducts). In: *Canine and Feline Theriogenology*. Philadelphia, PA: WB Saunders, pp 206–224.

Kenney, K.J., et al. (1987). Pyometra in cats: 183 cases (1979–1984). *J Am Vet Med Assoc* **191**(9): 1130–1132.

Kirsch, M. and C. Reusch (1993). Urine characteristics in dogs with diabetes mellitus. Is there a diabetic nephropathy in the dog? *Tierzrztl Prax* **21**(4): 345–348.

Klei, T.R., et al. (1974). Ultrastructural glomerular changes associated with filariasis. *Am J Trop Med Hyg* **23**(4): 608–618.

Klenzak, J. and J. Himmelfarb (2005). Sepsis and the kidney. *Crit Care Clin* **21**: 211–222.

Levy, J.K. (2000). Feline immunodeficiency virus. In: *Current Veterinary Therapy XIII*, edited by J.D. Bonagura. Philadelphia, PA: WB Saunders, pp 284–288.

Lewis, R.M. (1972). Canine systemic lupus erythematosus. *Am J Pathol* **69**: 537–540.

Lucke, V.M. (1968). Renal polyarteritis nodosa in the cat. *Vet Rec* **82**: 622–624.

Macintire, D.K., et al. (2006). *Hepatozoon Americanum* infection. In: *Infectious Diseases of the Dog and Cat*, edited by C.E. Greene, 3rd edition. St. Louis, MO: Saunders Elsevier, pp. 705–711.

Muñana, K.R. (1995). Long-term complications of diabetes mellitus, Part I: Retinopathy, nephropathy, neuropathy. *Vet Clin North Am Small Anim Pract* **25**(3): 715–730.

Murray, M. and N.G. Wright (1974). A morphologic study of canine glomerulonephritis. *Lab Invest* **30**(2): 213–221.

Nakagaki, K., et al. (1990). Histopathological and immunopathological evaluation of filarial glomerulonephritis in *Dirofilaria immitis* infected dogs. *Jpn J Exp Med* **60**(4): 179–186.

Nieto, C.G., et al. (1992). Pathological changes in kidneys of dogs with natural Leishmania infection. *Vet Parasitol* **45**: 33–47.

Obel, A.L., et al. (1964). Light and electron microscopical studies of the renal lesions in dogs with pyometra. *Acta Vet Scand* **5**: 146–178.

Ortega, T.M., et al. (1996). Systemic arterial blood pressure and urine protein/creatinine ratio in dogs with hyperadrenocorticism. *J Am Vet Med Assoc* **209**(10): 1724–1729.

Osborne, C.A., et al. (1981). Renal manifestations of canine dirofilariasis. In: *Proceedings of the Heartworm Symposium '80*, edited by G.F. Otto. Edwardsville, KS: Veterinary Medicine Publishing Company, pp. 67–92.

Paes-de-Almeida, E.C., et al. (2003). Kidney ultrastructural lesions in dogs experimentally infected with *Dirofilaria immitis* (Leidy, 1856). *Vet Parasitol* **113**(2): 157–168.

Parving, H.H., et al. (2008). Diabetic nephropathy. In: *The Kidney*, edited by B.M. Brenner, 8th edition. Philadelphia, PA: Saunders Elsevier, pp. 1265–1298.

Poli, A., et al. (1993). Renal involvement in feline immunodeficiency virus infection: a clinicopathologic study. *Nephron* **64**: 282–288.

Poli, A., et al. (1995). Renal involvement in feline immunodeficiency virus infection: p24 antigen detection, virus isolation and PCR analysis. *Vet Immunol Immunopathol* **46**: 13–20.

Prescott, J.F. (2007). Leptospirosis. In: *Pathology of Domestic Animals*, edited by M.G. Maxie, 5th edition. Philadelphia, PA: Saunders Elsevier, pp. 481–490.

Ross, L.A. and V. Rentko (2000). Canine leptospirosis: Update. In: *Current Veterinary Therapy XIII*, edited by J. Bonagura. Philadelphia, PA: WB Saunders, pp. 308–310.

Ruaux, C.G. (2000). Pathophysiology of organ failure in severe acute pancreatitis in dogs. *Compend Cont Educ Pract Vet* **22**(16): 531–542.

Schrier, R.W. and W. Wang (2004). Acute renal failure and sepsis. *N Engl J Med* **351**(2): 159–169.

Slauson, D.O. and R.M. Lewis (1979). Comparative pathology of glomerulonephritis in animals. *Vet Pathol* **16**: 135–164.

Steffes, M.W., et al. (1982). Diabetic nephropathy in the uninephrectomized dog: microscopic lesions after one year. *Kidney Int* **21**(5): 721–724.

Stone, E.A., et al. (1988). Renal dysfunction in dogs with pyometra. *J Am Vet Med Assoc* **193**(4): 457–464.

Stone, M. (2005). Systemic lupus erythematosus. In: *Textbook of Veterinary Internal Medicine*, edited by S.J. Ettinger and E.C. Feldman, 6th edition. St. Louis, MO: Saunders Elsevier, pp. 1952–1957.

Taboada, J. and R. Lobetti (2006). Babesiosis. In: *Infectious Diseases of the Dog and Cat*, edited by C.E. Greene, 3rd edition. St. Louis, MO: Saunders Elsevier, pp. 722–736.

Thompson, J.P. (1994). Disorders of the immune system. In: *The Cat: Diseases and Clinical Management*, edited by R.G. Sherding, 2nd edition. New York: Churchill Livingstone, pp. 647–670.

Wan, L., et al. (2003). The pathogenesis of septic acute renal failure. *Curr Opin Crit Care* **9**: 496–502.

Wang, W., et al. (2005). Endotoxemic acute renal failure is attenuated in caspase-1-deficient mice. *Am J Physiol Renal Physiol* **288**(5): F997–1004.

Waters, C.B., et al. (1997). Effects of glucocorticoid therapy on urine protein-to-creatinine ratios and renal morphology in dogs. *J Vet Intern Med* **11**(3): 172–177.

Welzl, C., et al. (2001). Systemic inflammatory response syndrome and mutiple-organ damage/dysfunction in complicated canine babesiosis. *J S Afr Vet Assoc* **72**(3): 158–162.

Werner, L.L. and N.T. Gorman (1984). Immune-mediated disorders of cats. *Vet Clin North Am Small Anim Pract* **14**: 1039–1064.

Whittemore, J.C. and V.L. Campbell (2005). Canine and feline pancreatitis. *Compend Cont Educ Pract Vet* **27**(10): 766–776.

Wozniak, E.J., et al. (1997). Clinical, anatomic, and immunopathologic characterization of *Babesia gibsoni* infection in the domestic dog (*Canis familiaris*). *J Parasitol* **83**(4): 692–699.

Zatelli, A., et al. (2003). Glomerular lesions in dogs infected with *Leishmania* organisms. *Am J Vet Res* **64**(5): 558–561.

53

Glomerular disease

Shelly L. Vaden and Gregory F. Grauer

Etiology and prevalence

Glomerular diseases are a leading cause of renal disease and kidney failure in dogs but appear to be less common in cats (MacDougall et al. 1986). The true prevalence of glomerular disease in dogs or cats remains unknown. However, the incidence of glomerular lesions in randomly selected dogs with and without evidence of renal disease is as high as 43–90% (Muller-Peddinghaus and Trautwein 1977; Rouse and Lewis 1975). Glomerular diseases can develop in dogs of any age but appear to be most common in middle-aged to older dogs. The average age of 375 dogs with a variety of glomerular diseases reported in 5 studies was 8.3 years (Murray and Wright 1974; MacDougall et al. 1986; Center et al. 1987; Cook and Cowgill 1996; Vilafranca et al. 1994). Males and females were equally represented.

While dogs and cats with glomerular-range proteinuria can be classified as having a glomerular disease, a renal biopsy (see Chapter 23) is needed to determine the specific disease (Chapter 240) that is present (Table 53.1). The three most common forms of glomerular disease in dogs are membranoproliferative glomerulonephritis (MPGN), membranous nephropathy (MN), and amyloidosis whereas MN is the most common glomerular disease in cats. The recent movement to improve the evaluation of renal biopsy specimens will eventually help clarify the specific glomerular diseases in dogs and cats as well as differences in clinical findings that may be present among the different diseases.

Familial glomerulopathies have been reported in several breeds of dog (Table 53.2). Acquired glomerular injury is the result of damage sustained following immune complex formation or deposition (e.g., MN,

Nephrology and Urology of Small Animals. Edited by Joe Bartges and David J. Polzin. © 2011 Blackwell Publishing Ltd.

MPGN, proliferative glomerulonephritis) or due to damage by systemic factors affecting the glomerulus (e.g., amyloidosis, focal segmental glomerulosclerosis, minimal change disease). Many of the glomerular diseases that occur in dogs and cats are believed to develop secondary to a systemic neoplastic, infectious, or noninfectious-inflammatory (NIN) disease process (Tables 53.3 and 53.4). Infectious diseases may be the most common underlying diseases for dogs and cats with glomerular diseases. A NIN disease may not be obvious at first presentation because it is either resolved or it is occult. In a recent retrospective study of 106 dogs with GN, 43% had no identifiable concurrent disease or disorder and 19% had neoplasia (Cook and Cowgill 1996). Because occult diseases may become overt months after initial presentation, continued observation and scrutiny are necessary.

Membranoproliferative glomerulonephritis

Accounting for 20–60% of cases in various studies, MPGN is probably the most common form of glomerulonephritis (GN) in dogs but is rare in cats (MacDougall et al. 1986; Koeman et al. 1987). The mean age of dogs with MPGN was 10.5 years with males and females equally affected (Vilafranca et al. 1994). MPGN has been identified as a familial disease in Bernese mountain dogs. A unique rapidly progressive form of MPGN, which is accompanied by tubular necrosis and interstitial inflammation and is often fatal, has been reported in association with *Borrelia burgdorferi* in dogs. Although an underlying disease may not be identified during patient evaluation, most cases of MPGN probably develop secondary to a NIN process.

Membranous nephropathy

Although the mean age of dogs with MN, from 4 studies, was 8 years, there was a considerable range (1–14 years)

Table 53.1 Glomerular diseases in dogs

Amyloidosis
Focal segmental glomerulosclerosis
Glomerulonephritis
   Crescentic (rare)
   Membranoproliferative
      Type I (mesangiocapillary) – most common
      Type II (dense deposit disease) – rare, if at all
   Proliferative (mesangial and endocapillary)
      IgA nephropathy
Glomerulosclerosis
   Focal segmental glomerulosclerosis
Hereditary nephritis
Lupus nephritis
Membranous Nephropathy[a]
Minimal change glomerulopathy

[a]Membranous nephropathy is the most common glomerular disease in cats; other forms of glomerular disease appear to be uncommon in cats.

(Lewis 1976; Muller-Peddinghaus and Trautwein 1977; Wright et al.; Jaenke and Allen, 1986; Vilafranca et al. 1994). The mean age of affected cats was only 3.6 years (range 1–7 years). MN appears to be more common in males than in female (males: females: dogs, 1.75:1, cats 6:1).

Proliferative glomerulonephritis

Proliferative GN, due to endocapillary or mesangial proliferation, accounted for only 2–16% of the glomerular lesions in dogs of two studies (Koeman et al. 1987; Vilafranca et al. 1994). The mean age of affected dogs

Table 53.2 Breeds of dogs with familial glomerulopathies

Beagles, amyloidosis, membranoproliferative glomerulonephritis
Bernese mountain dog, mesangiocapillary glomerulonephritis
Bull terrier, hereditary nephritis
Cocker spaniel (especially English), hereditary nephritis
Dalmatian, hereditary nephritis
Doberman pinscher, glomerulosclerosis, cystic glomerular atrophy
English foxhound, amyloidosis
Greyhound, glomerular vasculopathy and necrosis
Newfoundland, glomerulosclerosis
Pembroke Welsh corgi, cystic glomerular atrophy
Rottweiler, atrophic glomerulopathy
Samoyed, hereditary nephritis (rare)
Shar Pei, amyloidosis
Soft-coated wheaten terrier, proliferative and sclerosing glomerulonephritis

Table 53.3 Diseases reported in association with glomerular diseases in dogs

Systemic disease (glomerular disease)
  Neoplastic
    Leukemia (G)
    Lymphosarcoma (A, G)
    Mastocytosis (G)
    Primary erythrocytosis (MCD?)
    Systemic histiocytosis (G)
    Other neoplasms (A, G, MN)
  Infectious
    Bacterial: Borreliosis (MPGN)
    Bartonellosis (G)
    Brucellosis (G)
    Endocarditis (G)
    Pyelonephritis (A)
    Pyometra (A, G)
    Pyoderma (A, G)
    Other chronic bacterial infections (A, G)
    Protozoal: Babesiosis (MPGN)
    Hepatozoonosis (G)
    Leishmaniasis (A, MPGN, MN, P-E, and M)
    Trypanosomiasis (G)
    Rickettsial: Ehrlichiosis (G)
    Viral: Canine adenovirus type 1 (P-M)
    Parasitic: Dirofilariasis (A, MPGN, MN)
    Fungal: Blastomycosis (A)
    Coccidiomycosis (A, G)
  Non-Infectious Inflammatory
    Chronic dermatitis (A, G)
    Inflammatory bowel disease (G)
    Pancreatitis (A, G)
    Periodontal disease (A, G)
    Polyarthritis (A, G)
    Systemic lupus erythematosis (A, MPGN, MN, P-E, and M)
    Other immune-mediated diseases (G)
  Miscellaneous
    Corticosteroid excess (G)
    Trimethoprim-sulfa (G)
    Hyperlipidemia (?)
    Chronic insulin infusion (A)
    Congenital C3 deficiency (MPGN)
    Cyclic hematopoiesis in grey collies (A)
    Idiopathic (A, G, MPGN, MN, MCD, P-E, or M)

A, amyloidosis; G, glomerulonephritis, uncharacterized; MPGN, membranoproliferative (mesangiocapillary) glomerulonephritis; MN, membranous nephropathy; MCD, minimal change disease; P, proliferative (E, endocapillary or M, mesangial).

was between 7 and 9 years. IgA nephropathy is a form of mesangioproliferative GN that probably occurs rarely in dogs. In one study, dogs with enteric or hepatic diseases had the highest incidence of IgA deposition (Miyauchi et al. 1992).

Table 53.4 Diseases reported in association with glomerular diseases in cats

---

Systemic disease (Glomerular disease)
  Neoplastic
    Leukemia (MN)
    Lymphosarcoma (MN)
    Mastocytosis (G)
    Other neoplasms (G)
  Infectious
    Bacterial
    Chronic bacterial infections (G)
    Mycoplasmal polyarthritis (G)
    Viral
    Feline immunodeficiency virus (G)
    Feline infectious peritonitis (MN)
    Feline leukemia virus (G, MN)
  Noninfectious inflammatory
    Pancreatitis (G)
    Cholangiohepatitis (G)
    Chronic progressive polyarthritis (G)
    Systemic lupus erythematosus (MN)
    Other immune-mediated diseases (G)
  Miscellaneous
    Acromegaly (?)
    Mercury toxicity (MN)
    Idiopathic (MN)

G, glomerulonephritis, uncharacterized; MN, membranous nephropathy.

Amyloidosis

Amyloidosis accounts for approximately one-fourth of dogs with glomerular disease; glomerular amyloidosis is uncommon in cats. With the exception of the Chinese Shar Pei, amyloid is deposited primarily in the glomeruli of affected dogs. Reactive amyloidosis is the most common form of amyloidosis in dogs and cats, and older animals are more commonly affected. Females appear to be affected more often than males. Beagles, English Foxhounds, collies and Walker hounds may be at increased risk for amyloidosis, which may be familial in Beagles and English Foxhounds (see Chapter 54).

Hereditary nephritis

Hereditary nephritis (HN) refers to a diverse group of inherited glomerular diseases that are the result of a genetic mutation or deletion in basement membrane collagen (type IV). The presence of defective collagen leads to premature deterioration of the glomerular basement membrane and progressive glomerular disease and renal failure. HN has been reported in several breeds of dogs. An autosomal recessive form occurs in English cocker spaniels, whereas bull terriers and Dalmatians develop an autosomal dominant form. An X-linked dominant form of HN has been described in Samoyeds and mixed breed dogs; carrier females may have mild disease. The report in the Samoyeds is of a single kindred; the disease is not common in this breed.

Glomerulosclerosis

Glomerulosclerosis often develops as an end-stage lesion in response to glomerular injury or decreased functioning nephron mass. The incidence of glomerulosclerosis increases with age, although the percent of glomeruli expected to be sclerotic in dogs grouped by advancing age has not been characterized. Glomerulosclerosis is a common finding in diabetic nephropathy of people. Although glomerulosclerosis and proteinuria can develop in dogs with diabetes mellitus, the clinical relevance of this is unknown. Glomerulosclerosis can also develop following hypertensive renal damage. Focal segmental glomerulosclerosis (FSGS) is a specific glomerular disease that has been identified, but poorly characterized, in dogs. In people, this disease is considered to be a very difficult category of glomerular disease to diagnose pathologically. This disease is most likely under-diagnosed in dogs and may be mischaracterized as MPGN. FSGS was the diagnosis rendered in 10% of dogs with glomerular disease in one study (Vilafranca et al. 1994). Males and females were equally represented and the average age was 8.5 years.

Clinical signs

The clinical signs associated with glomerular disease vary considerably, depending on the severity of proteinuria and the presence or absence of renal failure. Many animals with glomerular disease are asymptomatic, with proteinuria detected during routine health screening. Alternatively, animals may manifest specific signs related to an underlying NIN process. Signs of glomerular disease may be non-specific (e.g., weight loss, lethargy) or consistent with chronic kidney disease or uremia (polyuria, polydipsia, anorexia, vomiting, and malodorous breath). Acute kidney injury is a less common presentation for dogs and cats with glomerular disease.

Physical examination is often unremarkable in dogs and cats with glomerular disease. Non-specific evidence of systemic disease (e.g., poor body condition or poor hair coat) may be present. Dogs with advanced renal failure may have oral ulcerations, pale mucous membranes, or dehydration. Evidence of a predisposing NIN disease may be detected during physical examination. The kidneys of affected animals are variable in size. Animals with chronic kidney disease often have small, firm, and irregularly shaped kidneys while those with milder disease often have normal-sized kidneys and occasionally have enlarged kidneys. Cats with MN may have enlarged kidneys early in the disease process.

As in people, it is likely that the specific glomerular diseases in dogs will differ with respect to the expected clinical signs and associated NIN processes but this has not been fully studied. Persistent proteinuria may lead to the development of nephrotic syndrome (i.e., proteinuria, hypoalbuminuria, hypercholesterolemia, and fluid retention) in some dogs and cats (see Chapter 44). Because amyloidosis and membranous nephropathy are common glomerular diseases that may result in heavy magnitude of proteinuria, these should be considered the top differentials for a dog that presents with the nephrotic syndrome.

When urinary protein losses are severe, decreases of plasma oncotic pressure allow for transudation of fluid into the interstitial space. The resultant decrease in effective plasma volume leads to increased renin-angiotensin-aldosterone activity and retention of water and sodium and worsening of edema. Primary sodium retention may also be involved in the retention of fluid in some patients. Once the serum albumin concentrations are below 1.5 g/dL, fluid retention may occur which is usually manifested as abdominal enlargement consistent with ascites or peripheral edema.

Thromboembolic disease has been reported in 5–14% of dogs with glomerular disease (Center et al. 1987; DiBartola et al. 1989; Cook and Cowgill 1996). Severe protein losses increase the risk of thromboembolic disease. The pathogenesis of the hypercoagulable state is multifactorial; hyperfibrinogenemia, excess urinary losses of antithrombin III, and thrombocytosis accompanied by increased platelet adhesion and aggregation are contributory factors (Green and Kabel 1982; Green et al. 1985). Pulmonary thromboembolism is most common, resulting in dyspnea and hypoxia. Emboli can lodge in other arteries (e.g., mesenteric, renal, iliac, brachial, coronary, splenic) or the portal vein resulting in a variety of accompanying signs.

Systemic hypertension may occur in up to 80% of dogs with glomerular disease (Cowgill 1991). Hypertensive damage to the kidneys, central nervous system, eyes, or heart may induce a variety of other clinical signs but also exacerbation of proteinuria and progressive renal injury (see Chapter 68). A combination of activation of the renin-angiotensin-aldosterone system and decreased renal production of vasodilators, coupled with increased responsiveness to normal vasopressor mechanisms is probably involved in the pathogenesis of hypertension in animals with glomerular disease.

Hypercholesterolemia was reported in 79% of dogs with GN and 86% of dogs with amyloidosis (Center et al. 1987; DiBartola et al. 1989). Increases in total plasma cholesterol, very-low-density lipoprotein (VLDL), and low-density lipoprotein (LDL) cholesterol occur in people but have not been as thoroughly studied in dogs (Wheeler et al. 1989).

Although somewhat controversial in dogs, there is mounting evidence to support that proteinuria induces tubular damage leading to progressive nephron loss in people and rodents. The reports that proteinuria was associated with a greater risk of uremic crisis or death in dogs with chronic kidney disease and a shortened survival in cats with chronic kidney disease may offer indirect evidence that this occurs in dogs and cats (Jacob et al. 2005; Syme et al. 2006). Potential mechanisms of tubulointerstitial damage associated with proteinuria include excessive lysosomal processing leading to activation of nuclear factor $\kappa\beta$ resulting in secretion of cytokines and growth factors (e.g., transforming GF ß1, platelet derived GF, monocyte chemoattractant protein-1, endothelin-1), tubular obstruction with hyaline casts, absorption of transferrin, complement, and lipoproteins leading to immune-mediated and peroxidative damage, and trans-differentiation of tubular cells to myoepithelial cells that can produce collagen and promote fibrosis (Harris et al. 1996; Johnson 1997; Remuzzi 1995; Tang et al. 1999).

Diagnosis

Persistent proteinuria is the hallmark of glomerular disease (see Chapters 8 and 43). The magnitude of proteinuria can range from very low-grade (e.g., microalbuminuria) to heavy, as occurs in nephrotic syndrome. Glomerular disease should be suspected as the cause of persistent proteinuria when other causes of proteinuria have been excluded (i.e., prerenal, postrenal, and functional-, tubular-, or interstitial-renal) and the urine protein:creatinine ratio (UPC) is >2.0 (Lees et al. 2005).

The first step in the diagnostic evaluation of dogs and cats with persistent proteinuria should be a thorough evaluation for underlying NIN diseases. This should include a thorough physical examination; diseases of the oral cavity and skin should not be overlooked as potential underlying diseases. Aspiration cytology should be evaluated on all cutaneous and subcutaneous masses that are present. Serologic testing for regional infectious diseases as well as antinuclear antibodies should be performed (see Chapter 27). During radiographic or ultrasonographic evaluation of the abdomen, attention should also be given to other organs in search of another disease process. Thoracic radiographs should also be evaluated in middle- to advanced-aged dogs.

Renal biopsy (see Chapter 23) provides a definitive diagnosis of glomerular disease but may not be needed if treatment of a potential underlying disease leads to resolution of the proteinuria or if end-stage renal disease is already present. When evaluated appropriately, renal biopsy specimens can provide important clinical information about the type and severity of lesions in dogs and cats with glomerular disease (see Chapter 24). In fact, obtaining an accurate histologic diagnosis may be one of the more important factors in successful management of the dog or cat with glomerular disease. Clinical decisions regarding diagnosis, therapy, and prognosis can be made from the information obtained through renal biopsy. Appropriate evaluation of a renal biopsy specimen from a dog or cat with glomerular disease includes light microscopy with special stains and, in most cases, electron and immunofluorescent microscopy.

Membranoproliferative glomerulonephritis

MPGN is characterized by the light-microscopic findings of thickening of the glomerular capillary walls and increased glomerular cellularity. The most common form, type I MPGN, is caused by the presence of immune complexes on the subendothelial aspect of the glomerular basement membrane. Type II MPGN, also called dense deposit disease, is characterized by intramembranous dense deposits. This is not associated with infectious disease and is probably uncommon in dogs.

Membranous nephropathy

MN results from immune deposits on the subepithelial aspect of the glomerular basement membrane. The capillary loops are thickened and spikes may be evident with periodic acid-Schiff hematoxylin stain as the basement membrane begins to extend between and engulf the deposits. Membranous nephropathy has four ultrastructural stages that correlate with temporal evolution of the disease and clinical presentation in dogs, cats and people. Deposition of immune complexes, progressive engulfment of the complexes by the glomerular basement membrane, and eventual resolution of the complexes characterize these stages. More advanced stages in cats and dogs have been shown to correlate with more severe azotemia, whereas animals with milder disease were more likely to have nephrotic syndrome. In cats, stages III and IV MN may be associated with a poorer prognosis (Nash et al. 1979).

Proliferative glomerulonephritis

Mesangial proliferative GN is characterized by mesangial cell hyperplasia, defined as 4 or more cells per mesangial area. This is often accompanied by an increase in mesangial matrix. Endocapillary proliferative GN occurs when there is a proliferation of glomerular endothelial cells and may be accompanied by an increase in mesangial cellularity. Proliferative GN is an immune-complex mediated disease and deposits can be identified in the mesangium, or subepithelial in the capillary walls.

Amyloidosis

Amyloid is first deposited in mesangial areas, with eventual subendothelial deposition. In hematoxylin and eosin-stained slides, glomerular amyloid appears as eosinophilic nodular deposits that expand the mesangium and glomerular capillary walls. Interstitial amyloid may be present as perivascular and peritubular deposits throughout the medulla. When stained with Congo red and evaluated by conventional light microscopy, amyloid deposits take on various shades of red, depending upon the amount of amyloid and the thickness of the section. Deposits stained with Congo red and evaluated by polarizing microscopy are birefringent and have an apple green color (see Chapter 54).

Hereditary nephritis

Electron microscopy is required to make the diagnosis of HN. Prior to electron micrographic studies of English cocker spaniels, the renal lesions were described as renal cortical hypoplasia, or membranoproliferative or sclerosing GN. The ultrastructural lesions consist of multilaminar splitting and fragmentation of the glomerular basement membrane, often with intramembranous electron-dense deposits.

Glomerulosclerosis

FSGS is diagnosed in the proteinuric patient that has segmental glomerulosclerosis in a glomerulus that is otherwise normal, without other glomerular lesions present to explain the sclerosis. In a biopsy specimen from a patient with FSGS, it would be expected that some of the glomeruli would be normal and some show segmental sclerotic lesions. The sclerotic lesions show solidification of tuft segments and are composed of collapsed capillary basement membranes, increased collagenous matrix, and few viable cells. Some of the affected segments may have large hyaline deposits. IFM should be negative in unaffected areas; however, nonspecific trapping of immunoglobulins and C3 can occur in sclerotic areas.

Treatment

Even though glomerular disease is a major cause of chronic kidney disease in the dog, its treatment has received substantially less attention in veterinary medicine than has the treatment of chronic kidney disease. Inasmuch as systemic disease usually initiates the glomerular injury, primary treatment objectives

Table 53.5 Treatment guidelines for GN

1. Identify and correct any underlying disease processes[a]
2. Immunosuppressive treatment
3. Hemodynamic/antiproteinuric treatment (angiotensin-converting enzyme inhibitors)[a]
4. Antiplatelet-hypercoagulability treatment: Aspirin 0.5 mg/kg every 12–24 hours[a]
5. Supportive care
    a. Dietary: sodium reduced, high quality-low quantity protein, with n-3 fatty acid supplementation[a]
    b. Hypertension:
        Dietary sodium reduction
        Angiotensin-converting enzyme inhibition (e.g., enalapril 0.5 mg/kg every 12–24 hours)[a]
    c. Edema/ascites:
        Dietary sodium reduction
        Cage rest
        Furosemide 1–2 mg/kg as needed if necessary-caution: volume contraction and reduced GFR may result
        Paracentesis for patients with tense ascites and/or respiratory distress
        Plasma transfusions

[a]Denotes those treatments thought to be most important.

include (1) identification and elimination of causative or associated antigens and (2) reduction of the glomerular response to injury (Table 53.5).

Elimination of the source of antigenic stimulation is the treatment of choice for glomerular disease. For example, proteinuria associated with dirofilariasis in dogs often improves or resolves after successful treatment of parasitic infection (Grauer et al. 1989). Unfortunately, elimination of the antigen source often is not possible because the antigen source or underlying disease may not be identified or may be impossible to eliminate (e.g., certain neoplasias).

Based on results in human beings, immunosuppressive drugs have been recommended in dogs with GN. Despite widespread use of immunosuppressive agents, there has only been one controlled clinical trial in veterinary medicine assessing the effects of immunosuppressive treatment. In this study, cyclosporine treatment was found to be of no benefit in reducing proteinuria associated with idiopathic GN in dogs (Vaden et al. 1995). The association between hyperadrenocorticism or long-term exogenous corticosteroid administration and GN and thromboembolism in the dog as well as the lack of consistent therapeutic response to corticosteroids raise questions about use of corticosteroids in dogs with GN. In a retrospective of study of dogs with naturally occurring GN, treatment with corticosteroids may have been detrimental, leading to azotemia and worsening of proteinuria (Center et al. 1987). Similarly, prednisone increased the UPC from 1.5 to 5.6 in carrier female dogs with X-linked hereditary nephropathy (Lees et al. 2002). Consequently, routine use of corticosteroids to treat GN in dogs is not recommended. Treatment with corticosteroids would be indicated, however, if the underlying disease process were known to be steroid-responsive (e.g., systemic lupus

erythematosus). As in human, beings it is also possible that there are specific subtypes of canine glomerular disease (e.g., minimal change glomerulopathy) that will be shown to be steroid responsive as they are appropriately identified and treated.

If an underlying or concurrent disease process cannot be identified and treated, or if immunosuppressive treatment is deemed inappropriate, treatment may be aimed at decreasing glomerular injury. Increased urinary excretion of thromboxane has been detected in dogs with experimentally induced GN (Longhofer et al. 1991; Grauer et al. 1992a). Thromboxane is thought to arise primarily from platelets that are attracted to the glomerulus in immune complex disease. Furthermore, platelet survival is decreased in several types of GN in human patients, and platelet depletion attenuates GN (Clark et al. 1976). These findings suggest that platelets and thromboxane have an important role in the pathogenesis of GN, particularly MPGN. Thromboxane synthetase inhibitors decreased proteinuria, glomerular cell proliferation, neutrophil infiltration, and fibrin deposition in dogs with experimental GN (Longhofer et al. 1991; Grauer et al. 1992a). In the absence of specific thromboxane synthetase inhibitors, aspirin may be a valuable substitute (Grauer et al. 1992b). Appropriate dosage is probably important if nonspecific cyclooxygenase inhibitors such as aspirin are used to decrease glomerular inflammation and platelet aggregation. An extremely low dosage of aspirin (0.5 mg/kg orally once a day) may selectively inhibit platelet cyclooxygenase without preventing the beneficial effects of prostacyclin formation (e.g., vasodilatation, inhibition of platelet aggregation). Low-dose aspirin is easily administered on an outpatient basis and does not require extensive monitoring, as does coumadin treatment. Because fibrin accumulation within the glomerulus is a frequent and irreversible consequence of GN, antiplatelet or anticoagulant treatment may serve a dual purpose.

Evidence is accumulating in dogs with glomerular disease indicating that angiotensin-converting enzyme inhibitors (ACEIs) not only reduce proteinuria but also slow disease progression. In dogs with unilateral nephrectomy and experimentally induced diabetes mellitus, ACEI administration reduced glomerular transcapillary hydraulic pressure and glomerular cell hypertrophy as well as proteinuria (Brown et al. 1993). In another study, ACEI treatment of Samoyed dogs with X-linked hereditary nephritis decreased proteinuria, improved renal excretory function, decreased glomerular basement membrane splitting, and prolonged survival compared with control dogs (Grodecki et al. 1997). A double-blinded, multicenter, prospective clinical trial assessed the effects of enalapril (EN) versus standard care in dogs with naturally occurring, idiopathic glomerular disease (Grauer et al. 2000). Twenty-nine adult dogs with MN (16) or MPGN (13) were identified for study. Dogs were randomly assigned to receive either EN (0.5 mg/kg PO 12–24 hours) ($n = 16$) or placebo ($n = 14$) for six months (one dog was treated first with the placebo and then with EN). All dogs were treated with low-dose aspirin (0.5–5 mg/kg PO 12–24 hours) and fed Hills k/d diet. After six months of treatment, the change in UPC from baseline was different between groups with the EN treatment group having significantly reduced UPCs. When data was adjusted for changes in GFR (UPC × serum creatinine) a similar significant reduction was noted. The change in systolic blood pressure after six months of treatment was also significantly different between groups. Response to treatment was categorized as (a) improvement (>50% reduction in UPC with stable serum creatinine), (b) no progression (<50% reduction in UPC with stable serum creatinine), and (c) progression (>50% increase in UPC and/or serum creatinine or euthanasia due to renal failure). Response to treatment was significantly better in the EN treated dogs compared with the placebo treated dogs (Grauer et al. 2000).

Treatment with ACEI probably decreases proteinuria and preserves renal function associated with glomerular disease by several mechanisms. In dogs, administration of lisinopril decreases efferent glomerular arteriolar resistance, which results in, decreased glomerular transcapillary hydraulic pressure and decreased proteinuria (Brown et al. 1993). In rats, administration of EN prevents the loss of glomerular heparan sulfate that can occur with glomerular disease (Reddi et al. 1991). Administration of ACEI also is thought to attenuate proteinuria by decreasing the size of glomerular capillary endothelial cell pores in people (Wiegmann et al. 1992). In addition, the antiproteinuric and renal protective effects of ACEI in people may be, in part, associated with improved lipoprotein metabolism (Keilani et al. 1993). Decreased production of angiotensin and aldosterone may also result in decreased renal fibrosis (Epstein 2001). Finally, administration of ACEI in dogs slows glomerular mesangial cell growth and proliferation that can alter the permeability of the glomerular capillary wall and lead to glomerulosclerosis (Brown et al. 1993).

Supportive therapy is important in the management of dogs with glomerular disease and should be aimed at alleviating systemic hypertension, decreasing edema or ascites, and reducing the tendency for thromboembolism to occur. Angiotensin converting enzyme inhibitors are recommended as the first line of defense for proteinuric, hypertensive dogs. In those cases where systemic hypertension is refractory to ACEI treatment, a calcium channel blocker should be added to the antihypertensive regimen.

Dietary sodium reduction should be the primary treatment consideration for animal patients with edema or ascites. Paracentesis and diuretics should be reserved for those dogs with respiratory distress or abdominal discomfort. Overzealous use of diuretics may cause dehydration and acute renal decompensation. Plasma transfusions will provide only temporary benefit. In the past, dietary protein supplementation has been recommended to offset the effects of proteinuria and reduce edema and ascites; however, recent studies in proteinuric heterozygous female dogs with X-linked nephropathy suggest that, reduced dietary protein is associated with reduced proteinuria (Burkholder et al. 2004). N-3 fatty acid supplementation may also be beneficial: in dogs with surgically reduced remnant kidneys, dietary supplementation with fish oil reduced proteinuria, intraglomerular pressures, and glomerular lesion and maintained glomerular filtration rate (Brown et al. 1998).

Prevention

It is unlikely that all glomerular diseases can be prevented. However, because most glomerular diseases in dogs and cats occur secondary to a NIN process, it is likely that early detection and effective treatment of the NIN process can reduce, or in some cases, eliminate, glomerular damage.

Prognosis

The prognosis for dogs with glomerular disease is variable and best based on a combination of the severity of dysfunction (i.e., the magnitude of proteinuria and presence or absence of azotemia), the presence or absence of hypertension or thromboembolism, the response to therapy, and the assessment of renal histology. Clinical experience suggests the disease is progressive in many cases, although the rate of progression is highly variable. In some animals, progression may be slow enough that they can lead relatively normal lives.

As is the case in people, it is likely that the natural progression of disease in dogs and cats will vary among the different types of glomerular disease. Well-controlled, prospective clinical trials evaluating the efficacy of additional treatment regimes (e.g., aldosterone antagonists and angiotensin receptor blockers; immunosuppressive treatment of specific histologic subtypes of glomerular disease) will undoubtedly provide valuable information and increase our ability to treat this disease. A major factor confounding interpretation of treatment efficacy studies is the variable biologic behavior of different types of glomerular disease. In human patients, for example, proliferative GN and MPGN have a poor prognosis as compared with MN (Bohle et al. 1992). Until results of such trials become available, if an underlying disease process cannot be identified and corrected, ACEIs, early renal failure diets, and low-dose aspirin are recommended.

Controversies

Despite widespread use of immunosuppressive agents in people with glomerular disease and an increasing frequency of use in dogs with glomerular disease, there has not been a controlled study supporting the efficacy of immunosuppressive agents in dogs with these diseases. There is evidence that corticosteroids can exacerbate proteinuria. However, definitive statements about the use of corticosteroids or other immunosuppressive drugs cannot be made until results of controlled studies of these agents in the specific glomerular diseases are available.

The relationship between proteinuria and progressive nephron loss in dogs is controversial. In dogs with chronic kidney disease, heavy proteinuria, as defined as UPC > 1, was associated with greater risk of uremic crisis and death (Jacob et al. 2005). Likewise, cats with chronic kidney disease and a UPC of > 0.4 had a shortened survival time (Syme et al. 2006). These studies provide indirect evidence that proteinuria is associated with progression of renal damage. Although one can then presume that heavy and persistent proteinuria associated with glomerular diseases may also be associated with tubular damage and progressive renal failure, this has not been proven in the dog as it has in people and rodents.

References

Bohle, A., et al. (1992). The long-term prognosis of the primary glomerulonephritides. *Path Res Pract* **188**: 908–924.

Brown, S.A., et al. (1993). Long-term effects of antihypertensive regimens on renal hemodynamics and proteinuria. *Kidney Int* **43**: 1210–1218.

Brown, S.A., et al. (1998). Beneficial effects of chronic administration of dietary n-3 polyunsaturated fatty acids in dogs with renal insufficiency. *J Lab Clin Med* **131**: 447–455.

Burkholder, W.J., et al. (2004). Diet modulates proteinuria in heterozygous female dogs with x-linked hereditary nephropathy. *J Vet Intern Med* **18**: 165–175.

Center, S.A., et al. (1987). Clinicopathologic, renal immunofluorescent, and light microscopic features of GN in the dog: 41 cases (1975–1985). *J Am Vet Med Assoc* **190**: 81–90.

Clark, W.F., et al. (1976). The platelet as a mediator of tissue damage in immune complex GN. *Clin Nephrol* **6**: 287–289.

Cook, A.K. and Cowgill, L.D. (1996). Clinical and pathologic features of protein-losing glomerular disease in the dog: A review of 137 cases. *J Am Anim Hosp Assoc* **32**: 313–322.

Cowgill, L.D. (1991). Clinical significance, diagnosis and management of systemic hypertension in dogs and cats. In: *Managing Renal Disease and Hypertension*. Hill's Pet Products and Harmon Smith Inc, pp. 35–44.

DiBartola, S.P., et al. (1989). Clinicopathologic findings in dogs with renal amyloidosis: 59 cases (1976–1986). *J Am Vet Med Assoc* **195**: 358–364.

Epstein, M. (2001). Aldosterone as a mediator of progressive renal disease: pathogenic and clinical implications. *Am J Kidney Dis* **37**: 677–688.

Grauer, G.F., et al. (1989). Experimental *Dirofilaria immitis-associated* GN induced in part by in situ formation of immune complexes in the glomerular capillary wall. *J Parasitol* **75**: 585–593.

Grauer, G.F., et al. (1992a). Effects of a thromboxane synthetase inhibitor on established immune complex GN in dogs. *Am J Vet Res* **53**: 808–813.

Grauer, G.F., et al. (1992b). Comparison of the effects of low-dose aspirin and specific thromboxane synthetase inhibition on whole blood platelet aggregation ATP secretion in healthy dogs. *Am J Vet Res* **53**: 1631–1635.

Grauer, G.F., et al. (2000). Effects of enalapril vs placebo as a treatment for canine idiopathic glomerulonephritis. *J Vet Intern Med* **14**: 526–533.

Green, R.A. and Kabel, A.L. (1982). Hypercoagulable state in three dogs with nephrotic syndrome: role of acquired antithrombin III deficiency. *J Am Vet Med Assoc* **181**: 914–917.

Green, R.A., et al. (1985). Hypoalbuminemia-related platelet hypersensitivity in two dogs with nephrotic syndrome. *J Am Vet Med Assoc* **186**: 485–488.

Grodecki, K.M., et al. (1997). Treatment of X-linked hereditary nephritis in Samoyed dogs with angiotensin converting enzyme (ACE) inhibitor. *J Comp Path* **117**: 209–225.

Harris, K.P., et al. (1996). Proteinuria: a mediator of interstitial fibrosis? *Contrib Nephrol* **118**: 173–179.

Jacob, F., et al. (2005). Evaluation of the association between initial proteinuria and morbidity rate or death in dogs with naturally occurring chronic renal failure. *J Am Vet Med Assoc* **226**: 393–400.

Jaenke, R.S. and Allen, T.A. (1986). Membranous nephropathy in the dog. *Vet Pathol* **23**: 718–733.

Johnson, R.J. (1997). Cytokines, growth factors and renal injury: where do we go now? *Kidney Int* **52**: S2–S6.

Keilani, T., et al. (1993). Improvement of lipid abnormalities associated with proteinuria using fosinopril, an angiotensin-converting enzyme inhibitor. *Ann Intern Med* **118**: 246–254.

Koeman, J.P., et al. (1987). Proteinuria in the dog: a pathomorphological study of 51 proteinuric dogs. *Res Vet Sci* **43**: 367–378.

Lees, G.E., et al. (2002). Glomerular proteinuria is rapidly but reversibly increased by short-term prednisone administration in heterozygous (carrier) female dogs with x-linked hereditary nephropathy (abstract). *J Vet Intern Med* **16**: 352.

Lees, G.E., et al. (2005). Assessment and management of proteinuria in dogs and cats: 2004 ACVIM Forum consensus statement (small animal). *J Vet Intern Med* **19**: 377–385.

Lewis, R.J. (1976). Canine glomerulonephritis: results from a microscopic evaluation of fifty cases. *Can Vet J* **17**: 171–176.

Longhofer, S.L., et al. (1991). Effects of a thromboxane synthetase inhibitor on immune complex GN. *Am J Vet Res* **52**: 480–487.

MacDougall, D.F., et al. (1986). Canine chronic renal disease: prevalence and types of GN in the dog. *Kidney Int* **29**: 1144–1151.

Miyauchi, Y., et al. (1992). Glomerulopathy with IgA deposition in the dog. *J Vet Med Sci* **54**: 969–975.

Muller-Peddinghaus, R. and Trautwein, G. (1977). Spontaneous GN in dogs 1. Classification and Immunopathology. *Vet Pathol* **14**: 1–13.

Murray, M. and Wright, N.G. (1974). A Morphologic study of canine glomerulonephritis. *Lab Invest* **30**: 213–221.

Nash, A.S., et al. (1979). Membranous nephropathy in the cat: a clinical and pathological study. *Vet Rec* **105**: 71–77.

Reddi, A.S., et al. (1991). Enalapril improves albuminuria by preventing glomerular loss of heparan sulfate in diabetic rats. *Biochem Med Metab Biol* **45**: 119–131.

Remuzzi, G. (1995). Abnormal protein traffic through the glomerular barrier induces proximal tubular cell dysfunction and causes renal injury. *Curr Opin Nephrol Hypertens* **4**: 339–342.

Rouse, B.T. and Lewis R.J. (1975). Canine glomerulonephritis: prevalence in dogs submitted at random for euthanasia. *Can J Comp Med* **39**: 365–370.

Syme, H.M., et al. (2006). Survival of cats with naturally occurring chronic renal failure is related to severity of proteinuria. *J Vet Intern Med* **20**: 528–535.

Tang, S., et al. (1999). Apical proteins stimulate complement synthesis by cultured human proximal tubular epithelial cells. *J Am Soc Nephrol* **10**: 69–76.

Vaden, S.L., et al. (1995). The effects of cyclosporin versus standard care in dogs with naturally occurring glomerulonephritis. *J Vet Intern Med* **9**: 259–266.

Vilafranca, M., et al. (1994). Histological and immunohistological classification of canine glomerular disease. *J Vet Med* **41**: 599–610.

Wheeler, D.C., et al. (1989). Hyperlipidemia in nephrotic syndrome. *Am J Nephrol* **9**: S78–S84.

54

Amyloidosis

Joe Bartges and Jonathan Wall

Amyloidosis refers to a heterogeneous group of clinical disorders caused by extracellular deposition of insoluble abnormal amyloid fibrils derived from aggregation of misfolded, normally soluble, protein (DiBartola 1995; Nishi et al. 2008). Amyloid precursor proteins comprise a group of structurally and functionally diverse molecules; however, when incorporated into the fibril they adopt a characteristic beta-pleated sheet structural conformation. More than 25 different proteins form amyloid fibrils *in vivo*. Although the fibrils share a common structural configuration they are associated with clinically distinct conditions. It is the nature of the amyloid precursor protein that defines the disease, and dictates organ distribution of the pathology (Table 54.1). There is no clinical or pathological evidence of disease in absence of such deposits. In local amyloidosis, amyloid is restricted to a particular organ or tissue. In systemic amyloidosis, deposits are present in any or all viscera, connective tissue, and vascular walls. Amyloidosis can be spontaneous or arise as a complication of a preexisting disease that produces either an inherently amyloidogenic abnormal protein or greatly increased amounts of potentially amyloidogenic normal protein. Hereditary amyloidosis is caused by mutations in genes that result in the production of structurally destabilized proteins. These mutant proteins exhibit a greater propensity for unfolding relative to their wild-type counterpart, which renders them amyloidogenic (Pepys 2006). Amyloid deposition occurs with Alzheimer's disease and type 2 diabetes mellitus, but unlike amyloidosis it is not established that amyloid causes these diseases.

Etiopathogenesis

The pathogenesis of amyloid relies principally on the misfolding of the various amyloid fibril precursor proteins. As a result of high concentration of precursor proteins or due to the introduction of destabilizing amino acid substitutions, the precursor protein adopts a non-native pro-amyloid conformation which is an absolute requirement for fibril formation. All amyloid fibrils share a common core structure in which the subunit proteins are arranged in a stack of, often twisted, anti-parallel, beta-pleated sheets aligned with their long axes perpendicular to the fibril long axis. Proteins that form amyloid transiently populate partly unfolded intermediate molecular states that expose the beta-sheet domain, enabling them to interact with similar molecules in a highly ordered fashion. Propagation of the resulting low molecular weight aggregates into mature amyloid fibrils is a thermodynamically favorable, auto-catalytic process that relies on a sustained supply of the fibril precursor protein. In many cases, the precursor proteins isolated from tissue amyloid deposits are truncated indicating that partial proteolytic cleavage has occurred. It remains unclear whether this occurs before, during, or after formation of amyloid fibrils; however, loss of the C-terminal domain of the immunoglobulin light chain protein renders it highly fibrillogenic (Wall et al. 1999).

Amyloid deposits accumulate in the extracellular space, progressively disrupting normal tissue architecture, and consequently impairing organ function. They can also produce space-occupying effects at microscopic and macroscopic levels. Although amyloid is inert in that it does not stimulate a local or systemic inflammatory response, deposits may exert cytotoxic effects and possibly promote apoptosis. The rate of amyloid accumulation has a major impact on organ function, which can be preserved for long periods in the presence of a heavy but stable amyloid load. This may reflect adaptation to gradual

Nephrology and Urology of Small Animals. Edited by Joe Bartges and David J. Polzin. © 2011 Blackwell Publishing Ltd.

Table 54.1 Partial list of human amyloid precursor proteins and their disease

Amyloid	Precursor protein	Acquired (A) or hereditary (H)	Systemic (S) or localized (L)	Disorder and tissue involvement
AL	Immunoglobulin light chain	A	S and L forms	Primary AL and myeloma-associated
AA	(Apo)serum amyloid protein A	A, H	S	Secondary or reactive amyloidosis
ATTR	Tranthyretin	A, H	S	Familial or senile systemic
AApoAI	Apolipoprotein AI	A, H	S and L forms	Familial systemic and localized aortic and meniscus
$A\beta_2M$	β_2-microglobulin	A	S (L?)	Hemodialysis-associated (and joints?)
AIAPP	Islet amyloid polypeptide (amylin)	A	L	Islets of Langerhans and insulinomas
$A\beta$	$A\beta$ protein precursor ($A\beta$PP)	A, H	L	Alzheimer's disease and aging
APrP	Prion protein	A	L	Spongiform encephalopathies

Source: Adapted from Westermark et al. (2007).

amyloid accumulation or may relate to toxic properties of newly formed amyloid material.

Although many different amyloidogenic proteins have been described in human medicine, renal amyloidosis in dogs and cats is typically associated with systemic AA amyloidosis. The fibrils are composed of an N-terminal fragment of the acute-phase apolipoprotein serum amyloid A protein (sAA). There are four human sAA genes, five in mice, and atleast three genes in cats. Human sAA1.1, 1.2, 3, and 4 are located on chromosome 11 and in the mouse they are located on chromosome 7. Of the human genes, sAA4 is expressed constitutively, whereas sAA1.1 and 1.2 are acute phase reactants. In human beings and mice sAA1.1 is the major component of amyloid deposits, in mice it is the only isoform that forms amyloid. In mice, the AA protein extracted from amyloid contains 76 amino acids and has a molecular weight of 8.4 kd. In humans there is considerable heterogeneity in the fragmentation pattern of sAA in the amyloid deposits in which peptides ranging from 45 amino acids to almost full length have been identified. The sAA protein found in cats and dogs differs from that in mice and human beings, in that, it contains an 8 amino acid insertion between positions 66 and 67 (protein sequence numbering; Figure 54.1) (Kluve-Beckerman et al. 1989). Human sAA contains possible binding sites for laminin

and fibronectin at positions 28 (YIGSD) and 38 (RGN), respectively (amino acid numbering according to Figure 54.1; Kisilevsky and Tam 2002). Due to amino acid substitutions the laminin-binding site in mouse, cat, and dog sAA is more degenerate, but the fibronectin-reactive site remains conserved.

The amino acid sequence of sAA in amyloid isolated from a domestic cat with amyloidosis differed by 3 amino acids from AA amyloid occurring in Abyssinian cats (underlined residues in Figure 54.1). (Johnson et al. 1989) This suggested that the low incidence of AA observed in short-haired domestic cats, as compared to the Abyssinian and Siamese breeds, may be due to structural changes in the protein resulting from these 3 amino acid substitutions.

Human sAA protein contains 104 amino acids and has a molecular weight of ~12 kd, mouse, cat and dog sAA proteins are one amino acid shorter in length but share considerable sequence identity to the human form (Figure 54.1). sAA is one of several acute-phase proteins synthesized by the liver in response to cytokine (IL-6, IL-1β, and TNF-α) production by macrophages in response to tissue injury. (Benson 1982; DiBartola 1995; Ceron et al. 2005; Bayramli and Ulutas 2008; Tamamoto et al. 2008) Serum amyloid A protein is released from hepatocytes and binds to high-density lipoproteins

```
           1         11        21        31        41        51
MOUSE .GFFSFVHEAF QGAGDMWRAY TDMKEANWKN SDKYFHARGN YDAAQRGPGG VWAAEKISDG
HUMAN RSFFSFLGEAF DGARDMWRAY SDMREANYIG SDKYFHARGN YDAAKRGPGG VWAAEAISDA
DOG   .QWYSFVSEAA QGAWDMLRAY SDMREANYKN SDKYFHARGN YDAAQRGPGG AWAAKVISDA
CAT   .EWYSFLGEAA QGAWDMWRAY SDMREANYIG ADKYFHARGN YDAARRGPGG VWAAKVISDA


           61                 71         81        91        101
MOUSE REAFQE         FFGR GHEDTIADQE ANRHGRSGKD PNYYRPPGLP DKY
HUMAN RENIQR         FFGH GAEDSLADQA ANEWGRSGKD PNHFRPAGLP EKY
DOG   RENSQRITDLLRFGDSGH GAEDSKADQA ANEWGRSGKD PNHFRPAGLP DKY
CAT   RENSQRVTDFFRHGNSGH GAEDSKADQE ANEWGRSGKD PNHYRPEGLP DKY
```

Figure 54.1 Comparison of sAA protein amino acid sequences. The 8 amino acid insert in the cat and dog sAA protein is shown in italics. Amino acids that differ between the short-haired domestic cat and the Abyssinian and Siamese breeds are shown in bold.

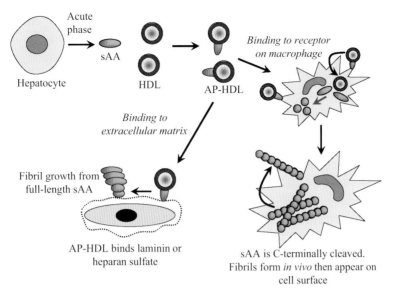

Figure 54.2 AA amyloidogenesis. Schematic representation of the formation of AA amyloid fibrils from hepatocyte-derived sAA protein. sAA produced in the liver in response to pro-inflammatory cytokines enters the circulation and is rapidly bound by high-density lipoprotein (HDL_3) displacing apolipopratin AI, to from acute-phase HDL (AP-HDL). AP-HDL can bind saturable receptors on the surface of macrophages where it is rapidly internalized into the endosome/lysomomal pathway. At low pH and in the presence of proteolytic enzymes, the HDL particle disassociates and the sAA is C-terminally truncated yielding amyloidogenic fragments which aggregate into fibrils within the cell. The fibrils eventually become extracellular and catalyze the formation of more amyloid. Alternatively, AP-HDL can bind to laminin or heparan sulfate proteoglycan molecules in the extracellular matrix of e.g., fibroblasts, which results in loss of the HDL particle and an increase in beta-sheet structure of the sAA. In this case full length sAA may form fibrils and act as a seed for further sequestration of sAA molecules.

displacing apolipoproteins A-I, A-II, or C, and circulates as a complex with high-density lipoproteins (Figure 54.2) (Benditt et al. 1982). Normal serum concentration of serum amyloid A protein is approximately 0.1 mg/dL, but its concentration can increase 100- to 1,000-fold after tissue injury. It begins to increase 2–4 hours after an inflammatory stimulus, peaks at 12–18 hours, and decreases to baseline by 36–48 hours if the stimulus is removed; when inflammation persists, sAA protein concentrations remain elevated (Benson et al. 1977). Serum amyloid A protein serves as precursor of AA amyloid in tissues.

The formation and deposition of AA amyloid has been shown to involve both cellular and extracellular components (Figure 54.2). In mice, the deposition of experimentally induced AA occurs initially in the perifollicular region of the spleen implicating an early role for macrophages. Indeed, transfer of monocytes from a mouse with amyloid to a suitably primed mouse in acute phase resulted in a rapid induction in amyloid deposition (Sponarova et al. 2008). The ability to seed AA amyloid *in vivo* is well established. Almost 30 years ago, it was shown that the soluble extract of a spleen containing AA amyloid, when injected IV, accelerated the deposition of AA in a primed mouse (Axelrad et al. 1982). The precise nature of this, so-called amyloid enhanc-

ing factor, remains unknown; however, pure synthetic amyloid fibrils possess amyloid enhancing capabilities (Johan et al. 1998) and it is highly likely that extracts of amyloid-laden tissues contain small fragments of fibrils that can act as a nidus for the propagation of the pathology (Lundmark et al. 2002). In vitro, when synthetic sAA apolipoprotein is added to macrophages in culture fibrils develop which possess the birefringent properties of amyloid when stained with Congo red. In the presence of amyloid enhancing factor fibril formation is accelerated and much more extensive (Kluve-Beckerman et al. 2002). This model system was used to demonstrate that sAA traffics through the endosome-lysosome compartments and is incompletely catabolized by proteases resulting in the formation of a truncated amyloid-forming protein. Fibrils form in intracellular compartments initially but then appear on the surface of the cells where they may act as amyloid enhancing factor and catalyze the progression of amyloid formation (Figure 54.2).

In addition to the importance of macrophages, extracellular matrix components, notably heparan sulfate (HS) proteoglycans are intimately involved in the formation of AA. Transgenic mice that lack significant amounts of tissue HS due to over-expression of heparanase do not develop AA amyloid (Li et al. 2005). Furthermore, preventing the interaction of the sAA with HS in vitro or *in vivo* reduces the deposition of AA amyloid (Kisilevsky et al. 2004). These observations led to the development and evaluation in mice and human beings, of anti-amyloid therapeutics that inhibit the interaction of sAA with HS glycosaminoglycans.

Amyloid is a complex matrix that includes, in addition to fibrils, many other molecules including serum amyloid P component (SAP), glycosaminoglycans, apolipoproteins, and fibronectin. Amyloid P component is identical to and derived from the normal circulating plasma protein, serum amyloid P component, a member of the pentraxin protein family that includes C-reactive protein. Serum amyloid P consists of 5 identical subunits, each with a molecular mass of approximately 25 kd, which are non-covalently associated in a pentameric disk-like ring. All amyloid deposits, irrespective of the nature of the precursor protein, contain significant amounts of SAP, which binds to the deposits in a calcium-dependent manner. Although not a proteinase inhibitor, its binding to amyloid fibrils in vitro protects them against proteolysis. In contrast to its normal rapid clearance from plasma, serum amyloid P persists for prolonged periods within amyloid deposits. The deposition of AA in mice is not dependent on the presence of SAP as knockout mice lacking the SAP protein still develop the pathology; however, ultrastructural studies of the fibrils indicated that they are morphologically different from those formed in vivo in the presence of SAP (Inoue et al. 2005).

Like SAP, glycosaminglycans are ubiquitously associated with amyloid deposits regardless of the chemical type of amyloid. As described above, they can sequester precursor proteins, mediate processing and folding of amyloidogenic proteins, induce beta-pleated sheet structure, and facilitate polymerization and deposition of amyloid fibrils (Shirahama 1989; Ohashi et al. 2002; Yamaguchi et al. 2003; Relini et al. 2008). Fibronectin binds to macrophages and serum amyloid A protein and may promote amyloidogenesis (Connolly et al. 1988; Westermark et al. 1991; Takahashi et al. 2002).

The pathogenesis of AA amyloidosis is not completely understood; however, the role of macrophages and HS proteoglycans is undeniable. AA amyloid is the most common amyloid in the animal kingdom, and due to its potential transmissibility via a rudimentary seeding mechanism, it represents a severe condition in both domestic and wild animal populations.

Amyloidosis in dogs and cats

Reactive amyloidosis occurs most commonly in dogs and cats, and is a familial disease in the Shar pei dog and Abyssinian cat; (Chew et al. 1982; Boyce et al. 1984; DiBartola et al. 1985; DiBartola et al. 1986; DiBartola et al.

1989a; Johnson et al. 1989; DiBartola et al. 1990; Loeven 1994; Clements et al. 1995; Van Der Linde-Sipman et al. 1997; Dubuis et al. 1998; Niewold et al. 1999; van Rossum et al. 2004; Flatland et al. 2007), however, it has been described in other breeds of dogs secondary to Ehrlichiosis (Luckschander et al. 2003), Hepatozoonosis (Macintire et al. 1997), Borreliosis (Dambach et al. 1997), monoclonal gammopathy (Brown 1996), polyarteritis in juvenile Beagles (Snyder et al. 1995), polyarthritis in an Akita (DiBartola 1995), Leishmania (Poli et al. 1991), dermatomyositis in a collie (Hargis et al. 1989), systemic lupus in a miniature Schnauzer (Grindem and Johnson 1984), cyclic hematopoiesis (Machado et al. 1978), and in related Beagles (Hargis et al. 1981; Bowles and Mosier 1992; Rha et al. 2000), walker hounds (DiBartola et al. 1989b), and Foxhounds (Mason and Day 1996), and in other breeds of cats including a European breed (Cavana et al. 2008), and Siamese (Godfrey and Day 1998; Niewold et al. 1999).

Most dogs and cats diagnosed with renal amyloidosis are older. Mean age of affected dogs was 9 years (Slauson et al. 1970; DiBartola et al. 1989b) with a range of 1–15 years; 91% were older than 5 years in a study of 44 cases. (Slauson et al. 1970) Mean age of affected cats is 7 years with range of 1–17 years; 65% are older than 5 years (Lucke and Hunt 1965; Nakamatsu et al. 1966; Clark and Seawright 1969; Crowell et al. 1972; Saegusa et al. 1979; Hartigan et al. 1980).

Diagnosis

In dogs and cats, renal amyloidosis usually results in progressive renal disease and associated clinical signs and laboratory changes. Although renal amyloidosis is usually a result of AA amyloidosis, most dogs and cats do not have a history or evidence of a predisposing chronic inflammatory cause (DiBartola 1995). Clinical signs of affected animals include anorexia, lethargy, weight loss, polyuria/polydipsia, vomiting, and occasionally diarrhea; nephrotic syndrome may be present. Thromboembolic disease and associated clinical signs (i.e., dyspnea with pulmonary thromboembolism, hindlimb paresis with iliac or femoral artery thromboembolism, etc.) may occur in as many as 40% of dogs, but occurs uncommonly in cats (Slauson and Gribble 1971). Physical examination findings are variable and usually related to presence of associated chronic renal failure, uremia, and/or nephrotic syndrome. Shar pei dogs may have an associated fever and hock swelling that precedes manifestation of renal amyloidosis.

Laboratory results are consistent with protein-losing nephropathy (hypoalbuminemia, proteinuria, and possibly hypercholesterolemia) and renal failure (non-regenerative, normocytic, normochromic anemia,

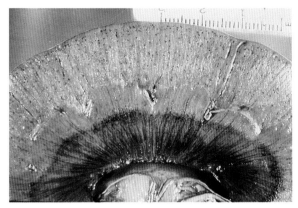

Figure 54.3 Cut surface of canine kidney stained with Lugol's iodine demonstrating amyloid deposition in glomeruli (pinpoint areas in cortex) and medullary insterstitium (streaking in medulla).

azotemia, hyperphosphatemia, metabolic acidosis, and hypocalcemia associated with hypoproteinemia). Cats are less likely to have large amount of proteinuria as amyloidosis is more likely to affect the renal medulla than the glomerulus. In addition to proteinuria, some animals have glucosuria with euglycemia and cylindruria (DiBartola 1995). Some animals may have a bacterial urinary tract infection. Imaging often reveals small kidneys in cats and variably-sized kidneys in dogs. Systemic arterial hypertension is often present with glomerular amyloidosis.

Diagnosis of renal amyloidosis is based on demonstration of amyloid deposition in kidneys. When Lugol's iodine is applied to the cut surface of a kidney affected with amyloidosis, amyloid appears as bluish-black material (Figure 54.3). On microscopic examination of renal tissue, amyloid appears as bluish infiltration with hematoxylin and eosin (Figure 54.4). Evaluation of sections stained with Congo red before and after permanganate

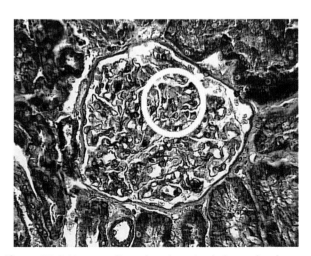

Figure 54.4 Hematoxylin and eosin-stained glomerulus demonstrating amyloid (blue staining, circle) in a dog.

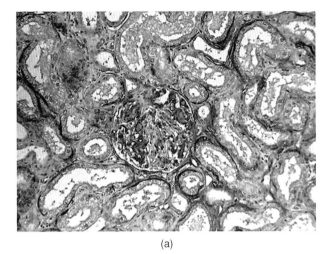

(a)

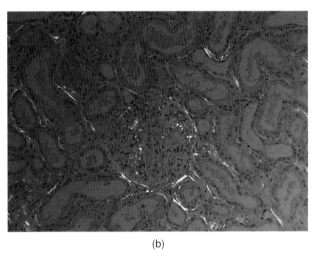

(b)

Figure 54.5 Detection of AA amyloid in a dog. (a) Immunohistochemical visualization of AA protein in amyloid using a mouse anti-AA monoclonal antibody. (b) Congo red stain of same glomerulus demonstrating apple green birefringence of amyloid coincident with the immunohistochemical stain.

oxidation allows a presumptive diagnosis of AA amyloidosis versus other types. Amyloid deposits appear green and birefringent when stained with Congo red and viewed under polarized light (Figure 54.5), and AA amyloid loses its Congo red affinity after permanganate oxidation (van Rijswijk and van Heusden 1979). An ancillary method, the Shtrasburg method, has been shown to confirm AA amyloidosis in dogs and cats as well (Shtrasburg et al. 2005). In dogs other than Shar pei dogs, amyloidosis is primarily a glomerular disease and can be diagnosed by a renal cortical biopsy. Early in the course of the disease, deposits are observed in the vascular pole of the glomerulus, in the glomerular capillary wall, and in the mesangium. When medullary amyloidosis occurs with glomerular involvement in Abyssinian and other domestic cats, renal cortical biopsies are negative for amyloidosis. Medullary amyloidosis without glomerular involvement occurs in at least 25% of Abyssinian cats and 33% of Shar pei dogs (DiBartola 1995). Renal papillary necrosis may be present and occurs from interference of blood flow by medullary amyloid deposits. Chronic tubule-interstitial disease indicative of chronic renal disease is often present. Other organs may be affected with amyloid deposition, but are not usually impaired functionally.

Treatment

Identify and treat any underlying inflammatory or neoplastic condition predisposing to amyloidosis. Treatment of acute or chronic renal failure should be instituted, if present. In Shar pei dogs with "fever-hock syndrome", analgesics to control the arthropathy and pyrexia is warranted. There is currently no specific treatment for AA amyloidosis, and prognosis is considered poor.

Dimethylsulfoxide (DMSO) may be beneficial because it may reduce concentrations of precursor serum amyloid A protein or by reducing interstitial inflammation and fibrosis (DiBartola 1995). Side-effects of DMSO treatment include nausea and a garlic-like odor. Intravenous DMSO can lead to transient hemoglobinuria due to hemolysis and perivascular inflammation and thrombosis, and when administered chronically can cause lens opacities (DiBartola 1995). When administered subcutaneously, dilute DMSO 1:4 with sterile water. Success of DMSO administration is controversial and only a few reports exist of improvement with DMSO therapy (Gruys et al. 1981; Spyridakis et al. 1986; DiBartola 1995). Colchicine may be beneficial in patients with amyloidosis before progression to renal failure. Colchicine impairs release of serum amyloid A protein from hepatocytes by binding to microtubules and preventing secretion and may interfere with amyloid enhancing factor production (Benson and Kleiner 1980; Brandwein et al. 1985; Zemer et al. 1986). It is thought that colchicine treatment will not reverse amyloid deposition; however, cases in human medicine do exist (Livneh et al. 1993; Kagan et al. 1999).

Newer treatments in human beings with AA amyloidosis (often associated with rheumatoid arthritis) include IL-1 receptor antagonism (Moser et al. 2009), anti-inflammatory drugs (Stankovic and Grateau 2008; Potysova et al. 2009), TNF-alpha blockers (Gottenberg et al. 2003; Mpofu et al. 2003; Drewe et al. 2004; Ravindran et al. 2004; Smith et al. 2004; Manenti et al. 2008), eprodisate (a compound that interferes with interactions between amyloidogenic proteins and glycosaminoglycans) (Dember et al. 2007), and chlorambucil (Tan et al. 1995). Whether these treatments would be effective in veterinary medicine is unknown.

References

Axelrad M.A., et al. (1982). Further characterization of amyloid-enhancing factor. *Lab Invest* **47**(2): 139–146.

Bayramli, G. and B. Ulutas (2008). Acute phase protein response in dogs with experimentally induced gastric mucosal injury. *Vet Clin Pathol* **37**(3): 312–316.

Benditt, E.P., et al. (1982). SAA, an apoprotein of HDL: its structure and function. *Ann N Y Acad Sci* **389**: 183–189.

Benson, M.D. (1982). In vitro synthesis of the acute phase reactant SAA by hepatocytes. *Ann N Y Acad Sci* **389**: 116–120.

Benson, M.D. and E. Kleiner (1980). Synthesis and secretion of serum amyloid protein A (SAA) by hepatocytes in mice treated with casein. *J Immunol* **124**(2): 495–499.

Benson, M.D., et al. (1977). Kinetics of serum amyloid protein A in casein-induced murine amyloidosis. *J Clin Invest* **59**(3): 412–417.

Bowles, M.H. and D.A. Mosier (1992). Renal amyloidosis in a family of beagles. *J Am Vet Med Assoc* **201**(4): 569–574.

Boyce, J.T., et al. (1984). Familial renal amyloidosis in Abyssinian cats. *Vet Pathol* **21**(1): 33–38.

Brandwein, S.R., et al. (1985). Effect of colchicine on experimental amyloidosis in two CBA/J mouse models. Chronic inflammatory stimulation and administration of amyloid-enhancing factor during acute inflammation. *Lab Invest* **52**(3): 319–325.

Brown, G. (1996). A monoclonal gammopathy-induced canine renal amyloidosis. *Can Vet J* **37**(2): 105.

Cavana, P., et al. (2008). Noncongophilic fibrillary glomerulonephritis in a cat. *Vet Pathol* **45**(3): 347–351.

Ceron, J.J., et al. (2005). Acute phase proteins in dogs and cats: current knowledge and future perspectives. *Vet Clin Pathol* **34**(2): 85–99.

Chew, D.J., et al. (1982). Renal amyloidosis in related Abyssinian cats. *J Am Vet Med Assoc* **181**(2): 139–142.

Clark, L. and A.A. Seawright (1969). Generalised amyloidosis in seven cats. *Pathol Vet* **6**(2): 117–134.

Clements, C.A., et al. (1995). Splenic vein thrombosis resulting in acute anemia: an unusual manifestation of nephrotic syndrome in a Chinese Shar Pei with reactive amyloidosis. *J Am Anim Hosp Assoc* **31**(5): 411–415.

Connolly, K.M., et al. (1988). Elevation of plasma fibronectin and serum amyloid P in autoimmune NZB, B/W, and MRL/1pr mice. *Exp Mol Pathol* **49**(3): 388–394.

Crowell, W.A., et al. (1972). Generalized amyloidosis in a cat. *J Am Vet Med Assoc* **161**(10): 1127–1133.

Dambach, D.M., et al. (1997). Morphologic, immunohistochemical, and ultrastructural characterization of a distinctive renal lesion in dogs putatively associated with Borrelia burgdorferi infection: 49 cases (1987–1992). *Vet Pathol* **34**(2): 85–96.

Dember, L.M., et al. (2007). Eprodisate for the treatment of renal disease in AA amyloidosis. *N Engl J Med* **356**(23): 2349–2360.

DiBartola, S.P. (1995). Renal amyloidosis. In: *Canine and Feline Nephrology and Urology*, edited by C.A. Osborne and D.R. Finco. Baltimore, MD: Williams & Wilkins, pp. 400–415.

DiBartola, S.P., et al. (1985). Isolation and characterization of amyloid protein AA in the Abyssinian cat. *Lab Invest* **52**(5): 485–489.

DiBartola, S.P., et al. (1986). Tissue distribution of amyloid deposits in Abyssinian cats with familial amyloidosis. *J Comp Pathol* **96**(4): 387–398.

DiBartola, S.P., et al. (1989a). Serum amyloid A protein concentration measured by radial immunodiffusion in Abyssinian and non-Abyssinian cats. *Am J Vet Res* **50**(8): 1414–1417.

DiBartola, S.P., et al. (1989b). Clinicopathologic findings in dogs with renal amyloidosis: 59 cases (1976–1986). *J Am Vet Med Assoc* **195**(3): 358–364.

DiBartola, S.P., et al. (1990). Familial renal amyloidosis in Chinese Shar Pei dogs. *J Am Vet Med Assoc* **197**(4): 483–487.

Drewe, E., et al. (2004). Treatment of renal amyloidosis with etanercept in tumour necrosis factor receptor-associated periodic syndrome. *Rheumatology (Oxford)* **43**(11): 1405–1408.

Dubuis, J.C., et al. (1998). Two cases of renal amyloidosis in the shar pei. *Schweiz Arch Tierheilkd* **140**(4): 156–160.

Flatland, B., et al. (2007). Liver aspirate from a Shar Pei dog. *Vet Clin Pathol* **36**(1): 105–108.

Godfrey, D.R. and M.J. Day (1998). Generalised amyloidosis in two Siamese cats: spontaneous liver haemorrhage and chronic renal failure. *J Small Anim Pract* **39**(9): 442–447.

Gottenberg, J.E., et al. (2003). Anti-tumor necrosis factor alpha therapy in fifteen patients with AA amyloidosis secondary to inflammatory arthritides: a followup report of tolerability and efficacy. *Arthritis Rheum* **48**(7): 2019–2024.

Grindem, C.B. and K.H. Johnson (1984). Amyloidosis in a case of canine systemic lupus erythematosus. *J Comp Pathol* **94**(4): 569–573.

Gruys, E., et al. (1981). Dubious effect of dimethylsulphoxide (DMSO) therapy on amyloid deposits and amyloidosis. *Vet Res Commun* **5**(1): 21–32.

Hargis, A.M., et al. (1989). Severe secondary amyloidosis in a dog with dermatomyositis. *J Comp Pathol* **100**(4): 427–433.

Hargis, A.M., et al. (1981). Relationship of hypothyroidism to diabetes mellitus, renal amyloidosis, and thrombosis in purebred beagles. *Am J Vet Res* **42**(6): 1077–1081.

Hartigan, P.J., et al. (1980). Generalized amyloidosis in the domestic cat. *Ir Vet J* **34**: 1–4.

Inoue S., et al. (2005) Formation of experimental murine AA amyloid fibrils in SAP-deficient mice: high resolution ultrastructural study. *Amyloid* **12**(3): 157–163.

Johan K., et al. (1998) Acceleration of amyloid protein A amyloidosis by amyloid-like synthetic fibrils. *Proc Natl Acad Sci U S A.* **95**(5): 2558–2563.

Johnson, K.H., et al. (1989). Amino acid sequence variations in protein AA of cats with high and low incidences of AA amyloidosis. *Comp Biochem Physiol B* **94**(4): 765–768.

Kagan, A., et al. (1999). Reversal of nephrotic syndrome due to AA amyloidosis in psoriatic patients on long-term colchicine treatment. Case report and review of the literature. *Nephron* **82**(4): 348–353.

Kisilevsky, R. and S.P. Tam (2002) Acute phase serum amyloid A, cholesterol metabolism, and cardiovascular disease. *Pediatr Pathol Mol Med* **21**(3): 291–305.

Kisilevsky, R., et al. (2004) Inhibition of amyloid A amyloidogenesis in vivo and in tissue culture by 4-deoxy analogues of peracetylated 2-acetamido-2-deoxy-alpha- and beta-d-glucose: implications for the treatment of various amyloidoses. *Am J Pathol* **164**(6): 2127–2137

Kluve-Beckerman, B., et al. (1989). Primary structures of dog and cat amyloid A proteins: comparison to human AA. *Comp Biochem Physiol B* **94**(1): 175–183.

Kluve-Beckerman B., et al. (2002) A pulse-chase study tracking the conversion of macrophage-endocytosed serum amyloid A into extracellular amyloid. *Arthritis Rheum.* **46**(7): 1905–1913

Li, J.P., et al. (2005) In vivo fragmentation of heparan sulfate by heparanase overexpression renders mice resistant to amyloid protein A amyloidosis. *Proc Natl Acad Sci U S A.* **102**(18): 6473–6477.

Livneh, A., et al. (1993). Colchicine in the treatment of AA and AL amyloidosis. *Semin Arthritis Rheum* **23**(3): 206–214.

Loeven, K.O. (1994). Hepatic amyloidosis in two Chinese Shar Pei dogs. *J Am Vet Med Assoc* **204**(8): 1212–1216.

Lucke, V.M. and V.M. Hunt (1965). Interstitial nephropathy and papillary necrosis in the domestic cat. *J Pathol Bacteriol* **89**: 723–728.

Luckschander, N., et al. (2003). Renal amyloidosis caused by Ehrlichia canis. *Schweiz Arch Tierheilkd* **145**(10): 482–485.

Lundmark, K., et al. (2002) Transmissibility of systemic amyloidosis by a prion-like mechanism. *Proc Natl Acad Sci U S A.* **99**(10): 6979–6984. Erratum in: (2003) *Proc Natl Acad Sci U S A.* **100**(6): 3543.

Machado, E.A., et al. (1978). The cyclic hematopoietic dog: a model for spontaneous secondary amyloidosis. A morphologic study. *Am J Pathol* **92**(1): 23–34.

Macintire, D.K., et al. (1997). Hepatozoonosis in dogs: 22 cases (1989–1994). *J Am Vet Med Assoc* **210**(7): 916–922.

Manenti, L., et al. (2008). Eprodisate in amyloid A amyloidosis: a novel therapeutic approach? *Expert Opin Pharmacother* **9**(12): 2175–2180.

Mason, N.J. and M.J. Day (1996). Renal amyloidosis in related English foxhounds. *J Small Anim Pract* **37**(6): 255–260.

Moser, C., et al. (2009). Successful treatment of familial Mediterranean fever with Anakinra and outcome after renal transplantation. *Nephrol Dial Transplant* **24**(2): 676–678.

Mpofu, S., et al. (2003). Cytostatic therapy for AA amyloidosis complicating psoriatic spondyloarthropathy. *Rheumatology (Oxford)* **42**(2): 362–366.

Nakamatsu, M., et al. (1966). Case of generalized amyloidosis in the cat. *Nippon Juigaku Zasshi* **28**(5): 259–265.

Niewold, T.A., et al. (1999). Familial amyloidosis in cats: Siamese and Abyssinian AA proteins differ in primary sequence and pattern of deposition. *Amyloid* **6**(3): 205–209.

Nishi, S., et al. (2008). New advances in renal amyloidosis. *Clin Exp Nephrol* **12**(2): 93–101.

Ohashi, K., et al. (2002). Affinity binding of glycosaminoglycans with beta(2)-microglobulin. *Nephron* **90**(2): 158–168.

Pepys, M.B. (2006). *Amyloidosis.* Annu Rev Med **57**: 223–241.

Poli, A., et al. (1991). Renal involvement in canine leishmaniasis. A light-microscopic, immunohistochemical and electron-microscopic study. *Nephron* **57**(4): 444–452.

Potysova, Z., et al. (2009). Renal AA amyloidosis: survey of epidemiologic and laboratory data from one nephrology centre. *Int Urol Nephrol* **41**(4): 941–945.

Ravindran, J., et al. (2004). Case report: response in proteinuria due to AA amyloidosis but not Felty's syndrome in a patient with rheumatoid arthritis treated with TNF-alpha blockade. *Rheumatology (Oxford)* **43**(5): 669–672.

Relini, A., et al. (2008). Heparin strongly enhances the formation of beta2-microglobulin amyloid fibrils in the presence of type I collagen. *J Biol Chem* **283**(8): 4912–4920.

Rha, J.Y., et al. (2000). Familial glomerulonephropathy in a litter of beagles. *J Am Vet Med Assoc* **216**(1): 46–50, 32.

Saegusa, S., et al. (1979). Concurrent feline immune-complex nephritis. Tubular antigen-positive and renal amyloidosis. *Arch Pathol Lab Med* **103**(9): 475–478.

Shirahama, T. (1989). Proteoglycans in amyloidogenesis. *Neurobiol Aging* **10**(5): 508–510; discussion 510–512.

Shtrasburg, S., et al. (2005). An ancillary tool for the diagnosis of amyloid A amyloidosis in a variety of domestic and wild animals. *Vet Pathol* **42**(2): 132–139.

Slauson, D.O. and D.H. Gribble (1971). Thrombosis complicating renal amyloidosis in dogs. *Vet Pathol* **8**(4): 352–363.

Slauson, D.O., et al. (1970). A clinicopathological study of renal amyloidosis in dogs. *J Comp Pathol* **80**(2): 335–343.

Smith, G.R., et al. (2004). Etanercept treatment of renal amyloidosis complicating rheumatoid arthritis. *Intern Med J* **34**(9–10): 570–572.

Snyder, P.W., et al. (1995). Pathologic features of naturally occurring juvenile polyarteritis in beagle dogs. *Vet Pathol* **32**(4): 337–345.

Sponarova, J., et al. (2008) AA-amyloidosis can be transferred by peripheral blood monocytes. *PLoS ONE* **3**(1): e3308.

Spyridakis, L., et al. (1986). Amyloidosis in a dog: treatment with dimethylsulfoxide. *J Am Vet Med Assoc* **189**(6): 690–691.

Stankovic, K. and G. Grateau (2008). Amyloidosis AA. *Nephrol Ther* **4**(4): 281–287.

Takahashi, N., et al. (2002). Establishment of a first-order kinetic model of light chain-associated amyloid fibril extension in vitro. *Biochim Biophys Acta* **1601**(1): 110–120.

Tamamoto, T., et al. (2008). Verification of measurement of the feline serum amyloid A (SAA) concentration by human SAA turbidimetric immunoassay and its clinical application. *J Vet Med Sci* **70**(11): 1247–1252.

Tan, S.Y., et al. (1995). Treatment of amyloidosis. *Am J Kidney Dis* **26**(2): 267–285.

Van Der Linde-Sipman, J.S., et al. (1997). Generalized AA-amyloidosis in Siamese and Oriental cats. *Vet Immunol Immunopathol* **56**(1–2): 1–10.

van Rijswijk, M.H. and C.W. van Heusden (1979). The potassium permanganate method. A reliable method for differentiating amyloid AA from other forms of amyloid in routine laboratory practice. *Am J Pathol* **97**(1): 43–58.

van Rossum, M., et al. (2004). Analysis of cDNA sequences of feline SAAs. *Amyloid* **11**(1): 38–43.

Wall, J., et al. (1999) Thermodynamic instability of human lambda 6 light chains: correlation with fibrillogenicity. *Biochemistry* **38**(42): 14101–14108.

Westermark, G.T., et al. (1991). Fibronectin and basement membrane components in renal amyloid deposits in patients with primary and secondary amyloidosis. *Clin Exp Immunol* **86**(1): 150–156.

Westermark, P., et al. (2007). A primer of amyloid nomenclature. *Amyloid* **14**(3): 179–183.

Yamaguchi, I., et al. (2003). Glycosaminoglycan and proteoglycan inhibit the depolymerization of beta2-microglobulin amyloid fibrils in vitro. *Kidney Int* **64**(3): 1080–1088.

Zemer, D., et al. (1986). Colchicine in the prevention and treatment of the amyloidosis of familial Mediterranean fever. *N Engl J Med* **314**(16): 1001–1005.

55

Disorders of renal tubules

Joe Bartges

Normal physiology

The nephron, the functional unit of the kidney, consists of a glomerular capillary network, a proximal convoluted tubule, the loop of Henle, a distal convoluted tubule, and a collecting duct. While renal function is often thought of in terms of azotemia, a reflection of glomerular function, tubular function is responsible for the final composition of urine through reabsorption and secretion of compounds (e.g., electrolytes, water). It is also involved in metabolism of hormones (e.g., erythropoietin, renin), and in maintaining systemic acid-base balance.

Tubulopathies can be classified as either isolated or complex defects, and as congenital or acquired (Bartges 1999). They may involve alteration in carbohydrate, nitrogen, electrolyte, mineral, fluid, and acid-based metabolism. There are several underlying principles of tubulopathies: (Chesney and Novello 1995) (1) Tubular disorders involve an abnormality of transport function. (2) Clinical and biochemical abnormalities reflect the site of tubular function. (3) Inherited tubular disorders involve loss of a transport protein or an error of metabolism. (4) Diseases that perturb energy production or structural integrity of tubular cells result in complex disorders. (5) Therapeutic principles are simple and involve replacement of the substance lost in urine or avoidance of the toxic substance. (6) Dose of replacement therapy relates to the altered site. If the altered site is responsible for bulk reabsorption, larger replacement doses will be required than at a site with less reclamation of a lost compound.

Isolated tubular disorders

Disorders of carbohydrate metabolism

Glucosuria

Glucosuria associated with euglycemia

Glucosuria with normal blood glucose concentrations is termed renal glucosuria. Renal glucosuria is uncommon, but has been reported in Scottish terriers, mixed breed dogs, as a familial disorder in Norwegian elkhounds, and in dogs with congenital renal disease such as Lhasa Apso/Shit Tzus. Renal glucosuria occurring with normal renal function (primary renal glucosuria) in human beings is due to a transport defect either in the brush border membrane or in the transtubular reabsorptive process for glucose. Two forms of this disorder have been described. Type A variant represents a reduction in both the renal threshold for glucose and maximal rate of glucose reabsorption ($Tm_{glucose}$). Type B glucosuria patients have a low renal threshold for glucose but a normal $Tm_{glucose}$. Dogs with primary glucosuria have polydipsia and polyuria due to osmotic diuresis induced by glucosuria. Glucosuria may predispose to bacterial or fungal urinary tract infections; therefore, signs of lower urinary tract disease may be present. However, dogs with renal glucosuria may also be asymptomatic. Diagnosis of renal glucosuria is based on documentation of persistent glucosuria without ketonuria and euglycemia; a normal serum fructosamine concentration may aid in confirming historical persistent euglycemia (Thoresen and Bredal 1999). There is no specific treatment. Hypoglycemia

Nephrology and Urology of Small Animals. Edited by Joe Bartges and David J. Polzin. © 2011 Blackwell Publishing Ltd.

does not occur, and restriction of dietary carbohydrate does not alter urinary glucose excretion. Appropriate antimicrobial therapy is indicated in animals that develop urinary tract infections.

Glucosuria associated with hyperglycemia

Any condition resulting in hyperglycemia may result in glucosuria if glomerular filtration of glucose exceeds $Tm_{glucose}$. The $Tm_{glucose}$ is exceeded when blood glucose concentrations exceed 180–220 mg/dL in dogs and 260–310 mg/dL in cats. Hyperglycemia and glucosuria may occur with diabetes mellitus, pancreatitis, hyperadrenocorticism, central nervous system lesions (variable), pheochromocytoma, and hyperprogesteronemia, or with administration of glucose containing solutions, glucocorticoids (rarely), adrenocorticotropic hormone, glucagon, progestational compounds, epinephrine, morphine, and phenothiazines.

Pentosuria

Pentosuria occurs in human beings because of overflow of pentoses (5 carbon cyclic sugars) from blood into urine (Chesney and Novello 1995). Pentosuria has not been described in dogs or cats either because it does not exist or because glucose oxidase impregnated test strips are used and so pentosuria is missed.

Disorders of nitrogen metabolism

Aminoaciduria

Amino acids are reabsorbed in the proximal tubule by several major shared transport systems: cyclic and neutral amino acids and glycine, dibasic amino acids, dicarboxylic amino acids, and beta-amino acids. Greater than 95% of filtered amino acids are reabsorbed by the proximal tubule. Aminoaciduria occurs due to one of several different defects. First, plasma concentration of an amino acid may be increased as a result of a metabolic defect, which increases the quantity filtered at the glomerulus. If tubular reabsorptive capacity for that amino acid is exceeded, overload aminoaciduria occurs. Second, there could be a defect in the proximal tubule brush border amino acid transport system. Because the amino acid transport systems found in the proximal tubule are in some cases the same as those in the intestine, transport defects may be found simultaneously in both tissues. Third, the proximal tubule cell may take up the amino acid but fail to metabolize it or fail to return it into the blood because of a defect in basolateral membrane transport. Lastly, aminoaciduria could arise from a more generalized defect, as in toxic nephropathies and Fanconi syndrome.

Cystinuria

Cystinuria is an inborn error of metabolism characterized by increased urinary excretion of cystine, which predisposes to cystine urolith formation. Normally, circulating cystine is filtered freely at the glomerulus, and 99–100% is actively reabsorbed in the proximal tubule. Decreased tubular reabsorption of cystine and, in some cases, other amino acids (lysine, glycine, ornithine, arginine) has been observed in dogs with cystine uroliths (McNamara et al. 1989; Hoppe et al. 1993). Aminoaciduria is associated with low or normal plasma levels of affected amino acids. Some affected dogs have a net secretion of cystine (Bovee and Segal 1984). Decreased tubular reabsorption of cystine and lysine may be due to a membrane transport defect. Jejunal mucosal uptake of cystine is not apparently reduced (Holtzapple et al. 1969).

Many breeds of dogs have been reported to develop cystine uroliths, but English bulldogs, Newfoundlands, and dachshunds appear to be predisposed (see Chapter 69) (Case et al. 1992; Lulich et al. 1995; Ling et al. 1998; Henthorn et al. 2000). Data contained in published pedigrees from inbred lines of dachshunds, basset hounds, and rottweilers suggest a sex-lined or autosomal recessive pattern of inheritance (Wallerstrom et al. 1992). Although cystine uroliths have been reported primarily in male dogs, they have been reported in female dogs also (Case et al. 1992; Lulich et al. 1995). Cystine uroliths appear to primarily affect young to middle-aged dogs (Case et al. 1992; Bartges et al. 1994).

Cystine uroliths have also been identified in cats (DiBartola et al. 1991; Osborne et al. 1996). In one cat, renal excretion of cystine, ornithine, lysine, and arginine were increased (DiBartola et al. 1991). Little information is available concerning cystinuria and cystine urolithiasis in cats.

Not all cystinuric dogs form uroliths; therefore, cystinuria is a predisposing rather than a primary cause of cystine urolith formation. Uroliths form, in part, because the solubility of cystine decreases in acidic urine, but it becomes more soluble in alkaline urine.

Treatment for cystine uroliths includes use of a low-protein diet, alkalinization therapy, and thiol-containing drugs such as 2-mercaptopropionylglycine (see Chapter 69) (Osborne et al. 1999; Hoppe and Denneberg 2001). Because cystine is an amino acid, consumption of a low-protein diet is associated with less cystine intake and excretion. Cystine is more soluble at a urine pH > 7.0; therefore, urinary alkalinization is of benefit in the dissolution and prevention of cystine uroliths (Barbey et al. 2000). Most low-protein diets are formulated to induce alkaluria. Thiol-containing drugs, such as D-penicillamine (15 mg/kg PO q12 hours) and

2-mercaptopropionylglycine (15–20 mg/kg PO q12 hours), decrease urinary cystine excretion by a thiol disulfide exchange reaction resulting in compounds that are more soluble than cystine (Lulich et al. 1995). Thiol-containing drugs may be used for dissolution and prevention of cystine uroliths. Use of 2-mercaptopropionylglycine (20 mg/kg PO q12 hours) was associated with preventing recurrence of cystine uroliths in 86% of dogs treated over a 14-year period (Hoppe and Denneberg 2001). Interestingly, in this study, urinary cystine levels decreased in dogs >5 years of age (Hoppe and Denneberg 2001).

Hypercarnitinuria

Carnitine is a nonessential sulfur-containing amino acid. Although carnitine is reabsorbed in the proximal renal tubule similar to other amino acids, it is less than that for other mammals (approximately 75% reabsorption in dogs compared with >90% in other mammals). Dilated cardiomyopathy has been associated with systemic carnitine deficiency (Keene et al. 1991). Recently, hypercarnitinuria has been reported to occur in cystinuric dogs in which dilated cardiomyopathy developed (Sanderson et al. 2001). Hypercarnitinuria likely represents a proximal renal tubular transport defect. Treatment for carnitine deficiency includes feeding a diet with adequate or increased carnitine content, or supplementation with L-Carnitine.

Other aminoacidurias

Other aminoacidurias have been observed to occur in human beings, but they have not been described in dogs or cats.

Uric aciduria

Uric acid is one of several biodegradation products of purine nucleotide metabolism. In most dogs and cats, allantoin is the major metabolic end product; it is the most soluble of the purine metabolic products excreted in urine (Bartges et al. 1992). However, in some breeds of dogs, such as Dalmatian coach hounds and English bulldogs, uric acid is the major purine metabolite that is excreted in urine (Bartges et al. 1994b). The ability of Dalmatians to oxidize uric acid to allantoin is intermediate between human beings and most non-Dalmatians dogs. Human beings have a serum uric acid concentration of 3–7 mg/dL, and excrete approximately 500–700 mg of uric acid in their urine per day. Most non-Dalmatians dogs have a serum uric acid concentration of less than 0.5 mg/dL, and excrete 10–60 mg of uric acid in their urine per day. Dalmatians have a serum uric acid concentration that is 2–4 times that of non-Dalmatians, and excrete more than 400–600 mg of uric acid in their urine per day (Sorenson and Ling 1993).

Studies of the fate of uric acid in Dalmatians have revealed unique hepatic and renal pathways of metabolism. Of these two metabolic sites, reciprocal allogenic renal and hepatic transplantations between Dalmatians and non-Dalmatians indicate that the hepatic mechanism is quantitatively the most significant. The liver of Dalmatians does not completely oxidize available uric acid, even though it contains a sufficient concentration of uricase. Compared to non-Dalmatians, Dalmatians convert uric acid to allantoin at a reduced rate. It has been hypothesized that their hepatic cellular membranes are partially impermeable to uric acid (Giesecke and Tiemeyer 1984).

The proximal renal tubules of Dalmatians reabsorb less uric acid than non-Dalmatians; a small amount is secreted by the distal tubules (Roch-Ramel and Peters 1978). In nonDalmatian dogs, 98–100% of the uric acid in glomerular filtrate is reabsorbed by the proximal tubules and returned to the liver for further metabolism.

The definitive mechanism of urate urolith formation in Dalmatian dogs remains unknown. Increased uric acid excretion is a risk factor rather than a primary cause. While all Dalmatians excrete relatively high quantities of uric acid in their urine, apparently, only a small percentage form urate uroliths. At one time, it was thought that urolith forming Dalmatians did not excrete greater quantities of uric acid in their urine than nonurolith forming Dalmatians. However, recent studies indicate that insensitive methods of measurement of urine uric acid concentration were responsible for this conclusion. When steps are taken to ensure that urine uric acid remains in solution, differences in urine uric acid concentrations between nonurolith forming Dalmatians and urolith forming Dalmatians may be expected.

Urate uroliths can be dissolved by feeding a low purine containing diet and administering a xanthine oxidase inhibitor, allopurinol (15 mg/kg PO q12 hours) (see Chapter 69) (Bartges et al. 1994a; Bartges et al. 1995; Bartges et al. 1999). Allopurinol impairs the conversion of xanthine to uric acid resulting in decreased concentrations of uric acid in blood and urine. However, increased concentrations of xanthine in blood and urine may result in xanthine urolith formation.

Xanthinuria

Xanthine is a product of purine metabolism and is converted to uric acid by the enzyme, xanthine oxidase (Bartges et al. 1992). Hereditary xanthinuria is a rarely recognized disorder of human beings characterized by a deficiency of xanthine oxidase. As a consequence, abnormal quantities of xanthine are excreted in urine as a major end product of purine metabolism. Because xanthine is the least soluble purine naturally excreted in urine, xanthinuria may be associated with urolith formation. In dogs, xanthinuria is usually associated with allopurinol administration. However, we have observed xanthine uroliths in a dog that did not receive allopurinol (unpublished data, Allen et al. 1998), and naturally occurring xanthine uroliths have been reported in three Cavalier King Charles spaniels (Kidder and Chivers 1968; Kucera et al. 1997; van Zuilen et al. 1997) and a Dachshund (see Chapter 69) (Flegel et al. 1998). Naturally occurring xanthine uroliths have also been observed to occur in cats (Osborne et al. 1996; White et al. 1997; Tsuchida et al. 2007). The mechanism(s) responsible for hyperxanthinuria and xanthine urolith formation in these animals are not known, but hyperxanthinemia was present.

Disorders of mineral and electrolyte metabolism

Calcium

Hypercalciuria may have several causes, and increases risk of calcium stone formation particularly calcium oxalate (see Chapter 69). Hypercalciuria may occur due to hypercalcemia, decreased renal tubular reabsorption of calcium (renal leak hypercalciuria), increased mobilization of calcium from bone (resorptive hypercalciuria), or increased intestinal absorption of calcium (absorptive hypercalciuria). Absorptive hypercalciuria may be differentiated from renal leak hypercalciuria by measuring 24-hour urinary calcium excretion during a fed and fasted state. Calcium excretion decreases during food deprivation in dogs with absorptive hypercalciuria, but not in dogs with renal leak hypercalciuria. It is thought that Miniature Schnauzers, and perhaps other breeds, that form calcium oxalate uroliths have absorptive hypercalciuria (Lulich et al. 1991). Treatment involves dietary modification to minimize urinary calcium excretion including sodium restriction, protein restriction, and alkalinization. Hydrochlorothiazide has also been shown to decrease urinary calcium excretion in healthy dogs (Lulich and Osborne 1992) and dogs that have formed calcium oxalate uroliths (Lulich et al. 2001) and urinary saturation for calcium oxalate in healthy cats, (Hezel et al. 2007) but its long-term safety and efficacy in dogs and cats that have formed calcium oxalate uroliths is unknown (Lulich et al. 1995).

Phosphorous

Phosphate transport disorders resulting in hyperphosphaturia and skeletal disease have been identified in human beings (Chesney and Novello 1995); however, in animals, hyperphosphaturia usually occurs as part of a complex tubulopathy.

Magnesium

Renal tubular Mg^{2+} wasting has been observed in some human beings with hypomagnesemia. Tetany, weakness, nausea, and hypocalcemia because of impaired PTH secretion and action may occur. Treatment with aminoglycoside or cisplatin can cause renal Mg^{2+} and K^+ wasting, leading to hypomagnesemia and hypokalemia. Treatment of hypomagnesemia consists of oral supplementation with magnesium salts; magnesium oxide is tolerated best (see Chapter 63).

Sodium and potassium

Hyperaldosteronism

Increased aldosterone production and secretion stimulates tubular reabsorption of Na^+ and excretion of K^+ and H^+, resulting in hypokalemia and metabolic alkalosis (see Chapters 61 and 62). Hyperaldosteronism may occur as a result of an adrenal tumor or hyperplasia (primary aldosteronism, Conn's syndrome), hyper-reninism due to a tumor of the juxtaglomerular apparatus or renovascular hypertension, from Bartter's syndrome (characterized by hyper-reninemia, metabolic acidosis, increased secretion of vasodilatory prostaglandins, and normal systemic arterial blood pressure) or from exogenous mineralocorticoid administration. Hyperaldosteronism has been observed in dogs, (Breitschwerdt et al. 1983; Rijnberk et al. 2001a; Johnson et al. 2006) and in cats (Ahn 1994; Flood et al. 1999; MacKay et al. 1999; Rijnberk et al. 2001b; Ash et al. 2005; DeClue et al. 2005; Gunn-Moore 2005; Rose et al. 2007). Treatment involves removal of the tumor if possible, K^+ supplementation, and administration of K^+ sparing diuretics (spironolactone or triamterene).

Hypoaldosteronism

Hypoaldosteronism due to decreased aldosterone production or decreased responsiveness to aldosterone has been observed in human beings (see Chapters 61 and 62). Hyperkalemia and metabolic acidosis occur; hypertension may be present. This occurs primarily as part of generalized hypoadrenocorticism; however, it has been reported in a dog with hyper-reninemic hypoaldosteronism (Lobetti 1998).

Renal tubular potassium secretion defect

Children with this syndrome have decreased renal tubular secretion of K^+, metabolic acidosis, short stature, urinary tract infections, calcium oxalate urolithiasis, and hypertension and weakness. The primary defect appears to be decreased secretion of K^+ with secondary impairment of proximal tubule bicarbonate (HCO_3^-) reabsorption. Chlorothiazide administration, HCO_3^- supplementation, and dietary Na^+ restriction are used to treat this disorder.

Disorders of vitamin metabolism

Methylmalonic aciduria associated with vitamin B12 deficiency

Methylmalonic aciduria has been observed in Giant Schnauzers, (Fyfe et al. 1991) two juvenile Border Collies, (Morgan and McConnell 1999; Battersby et al. 2005) a juvenile Beagle, (Fordyce et al. 2000), and a juvenile Labrador retriever (Podell et al. 1996) with intestinal malabsorption of vitamin B12 (cobalamin). Vitamin B12 deficiency occurs because of absent intrinsic factor-B12 receptors in the ileum. The trait appears to be autosomal recessive in nature. Affected puppies exhibit inappetence and failure to thrive between 6 and 12 weeks of age. Megaloblastic anemia occurs. Treatment involves parenteral administration of vitamin B12.

Malonic aciduria

A family of Maltese dogs with malonic aciduria but not methylmalonic aciduria has been described (O'Brien et al. 1999). Dogs presented at 3 years of age with episodes of seizures and stupor with hypoglycemia, acidosis, and ketonuria.

Disorders of water metabolism

Nephrogenic diabetes insipidus

Nephrogenic diabetes insipidus (nDI) is the term used to describe any disorder in which there is a structural or functional defect in the ability of the kidneys to respond to antidiuretic hormones (ADH) (see Chapter 42). Antidiuretic hormones induce increased water permeability in the distal tubule and collecting ducts by binding to a peritubular membrane receptor, resulting in activation of specific adenylate cyclases to form cyclic AMP. This compound leads to phosphorylation of other proteins that alter microtubular structures and permit augmented water permeability. Numerous drugs (e.g., furosemide, glucocorticoids, methoxyflurane), toxins (e.g., *E. coli* endotoxin), and conditions (e.g., hypokalemia, hypercalcemia, medullary cystic disease, interstitial nephritis, bacterial pyelonephritis, fungal pyelonephritis, cancer) can result in nDI (Cohen and Post 1999; Newman et al. 2003).

Congential nDI is a rare disorder associated with a deficiency of ADH receptors in the distal nephron (Lage

1973; Breitschwerdt et al. 1981; Court and Watson 1983; Takemura 1998; Greco 2001). Affected animals present at a young age for severe polyuria and polydipsia. Urine is hyposthenuric (urine specific gravity 1.001–1.005; urine osmolality less than 200 mOsm/kg), and does not increase above isosthenuric range during water deprivation. Animals do not respond to exogenous ADH. Treatment consists of massive amounts of water or dietary Na^+ restriction and use of thiazide diuretics (chlorothiazide, 10–20 mg/lb q12 hours) or hydrochlorothiazide (1–2 mg/lb q12 hours) (DiBartola 1995). Thiazide diuretic administration results in mild dehydration, enhanced proximal renal tubular reabsorption of Na^+, decreased delivery of tubular fluid to the distal nephron, and reduced urine output. Thiazides have been reported to reduce urine output by 20–30% in dogs with congenital nDI. Inhibitors of prostaglandin synthesis (ibuprofen, indomethacin, or aspirin) have been reported to reduce urine volume, increase urine osmolality, and reduce delivery of solute to the distal tubule in human beings. Reduction of dietary Na^+ and protein may reduce the amount of solute that must be excreted in urine, and may further reduce obligatory water loss and polyuria.

Central diabetes insipidus

Central diabetes insipidus occurs when there is a decrease or lack of ADH production or release. This can occur from decreased production by the hypothalamus (Green and Farrow 1974; Rogers et al. 1977; Feldman 1979; Browley 1980; Edwards et al. 1983; Post et al. 1989; Harb et al. 1996; Ramsey et al. 1999), destruction of the hypothalamus or pituitary gland, where it is stored in vesicles and released (Barr 1985; Davenport et al. 1986; Ferguson and Biery 1988; Authement et al. 1989; Goossens et al. 1995; Schwedes 1999; Smith and Elwood 2004; Aroch et al. 2005; Campbell and Bredhauer 2005; Hanson et al. 2005; Mellanby et al. 2005; Campbell and Bredhauer 2008; Nielsen et al. 2008). Urine is hyposthenuric (urine-specific gravity 1.001–1.005; urine osmolality less than 200 mOsm/kg), and does not increase above isosthenuric range during water deprivation. Animals respond to exogenous ADH. Treatment consists of providing ADH (1–4 drops of intranasal formulation in conjunctival sac q12–24 hours; 2–5 mcg of intranasal formulation SQ q12–24 hours; 0.1 mg or 0.2 mg tablet PO q8–12 hours). Water should be available at all times.

Disorders of acid-base metabolism

Renal tubular acidosis

Renal tubular acidosis is a rare group of disorders that lead to metabolic acidosis (see Chapter 66). There are two types described: decreased HCO_3^- reabsorption (proximal renal tubular acidosis, pRTA, type II), and defective acid excretion (distal renal tubular acidosis, dRTA, type I). Distal RTA associated with development of hyperkalemia resulting from hypoaldosteronism or aldosterone resistance has been termed Type IV RTA, but represents a type of dRTA.

The kidney maintains normal systemic acid-base balance by conserving HCO_3^- and excreting organic acids. Processes that are crucial in maintaining acid-base balance includes proximal reclamation of filtered HCO_3^-, proximal synthesis and medullary recycling of ammonium ion (NH_4^+), and distal secretion of hydrogen ion (H^+). Distal H^+ secretion occurs in the outer medullary and cortical collecting ducts and the inner medullary collecting duct. For each secreted H^+, a "new" HCO_3^- ion is transferred to the circulation via a Cl^-/HCO_3^- exchanger across the basolateral membrane. The most important transporter for apical secretion of H^+ is believed to be an electrogenic H^+-ATPase pump. Once secreted into the tubular lumen, passive back diffusion of H^+ does not occur under physiological conditions (Smulders et al. 1996).

Free H^+ can be excreted in urine only to a limited degree. They are bound either to filtered buffers to be excreted as titratable acid or to NH_3 to form NH_4^+. Net acid excretion (NAE) by the kidney is given by the equation:

$$NAE = (titratable\ acid + NH_4^+) - urinary\ loss\ of\ HCO_3^-.$$

In this equation, the contribution of buffer-bound H^+ excretion is referred to as titratable acid because it is measured by the amount of NaOH required to titrate the urine pH of a 24-hour urine sample to 7.40. The most important buffer is phosphate. Titratable acid in healthy adult beagles varied from 0.05 to 6.0 mmol/kg per 24 hours depending on diet consumed (Bartges et al. 1996).

The NH_4^+ is generated primarily in the proximal renal tubular cells from metabolism of glutamine. This results in formation of NH_4^+ and alpha-ketoglutarate. Alpha-ketoglutarate can be further metabolized for production of HCO_3^-, which is transported to extracellular fluid. Ammonia is secreted into the tubular lumen, presumably by substituting for H^+ on an internal binding site of the apical membrane Na^+/H^+ exchanger. Greater than 50% of NH_4^+ is subsequently reabsorbed in the thick ascending limb of the loop of Henle by a combination of Na^+ – NH_4^+-$2Cl^-$ cotransport and voltage-driven diffusion. This process is referred to as medullary recycling. Active reabsorption of NH_4^+ in the thick ascending limb provides a single effect for countercurrent multiplication of NH_4^+ in the renal medulla. Depending on the pH in the renal interstitium, NH_4^+ partly dissociates into NH_3 and

H^+. Dissociated H^+ is probably secreted into the lumen of the loop of Henle or collecting duct, converting luminal HCO_3^- remaining after proximal HCO_3^- reabsorption to H_2CO_3. Accumulated medullary NH_3 diffuses to areas with a low NH_3 concentration, including the medullary collecting tubules. Here, NH_3 passively diffuses into the lumen, where it serves as a proton acceptor to form NH_4^+ again. The NH_4^+ is lipid insoluble; therefore it cannot diffuse out of the lumen ("ion trapping"), and is secreted in urine. Binding of H^+ by NH_3 in the distal tubular lumen is crucial to maintain a favorable gradient for H^+ secretion and to a lesser extent NH_3 diffusion. Urinary NH_4^+ excretion in healthy adult beagles consuming various diets was 0.45–4.0 mmol/kg per 24 hours, (Bartges et al. 1996) and in 8 healthy cats fed 4 struvite management diets, it was 2.0–40 mmol/kg (Bartges et al. 1998). This ability to alter NH_4^+ excretion allows the kidney to increase acid excretion (NAE).

Not all of NH_4^+ produced by the kidney is excreted in the urine. In steady state conditions, approximately 50% are shunted to renal veins. The role of disturbances in shunting of NH_4^+ in the development of renal tubular acidosis has not been evaluated.

Urinary loss of HCO_3^- is the final component of the NAE equation. Bicarbonate excretion in healthy adult beagles consuming various diets was 0.07–0.25 mmol/kg per 24 hours (Bartges et al. 1996). Increased loss of HCO_3^- can be a source of decreased NAE even when the mechanisms discussed are fully intact. Normally, 85–90% of filtered HCO_3^- is reabsorbed in the proximal renal tubule secondary to glutamine metabolism. Another 2–5% is reabsorbed in the loop of Henle. "New" HCO_3^- is added to blood in the process of distal H^+ secretion.

Distal renal tubular acidosis

In dRTA, urine cannot be maximally acidified because of impaired H^+ secretion (and thus HCO_3^- generation) in collecting ducts, and urine pH is typically >6.0 despite moderately to markedly decreased plasma HCO_3^- concentration (Polzin et al. 1986; Watson et al. 1986). Urinary tract infection by urease-producing bacteria must be ruled out before the diagnosis of dRTA can be made. Nephrolithiasis, nephrocalcinosis, bone demineralization, and urinary potassium wasting with hypokalemia occur uncommonly. When plasma HCO_3^- concentration is increased to normal by supplementation, urinary fractional excretion of HCO_3^- becomes normal (<5%).

Four mechanisms are potentially involved in the pathogenesis of dRTA: a defective or partially absent proton pump (secretory defect), an unfavorable electrical gradient for H^+ secretion (voltage defect), back diffusion of H^+ (permeability defect), and insufficient supply of NH_3 to the distal nephron (NH_3 defect) (Smulders et al. 1996). Type IV dRTA is associated with hyperkalemia and is due to aldosterone deficiency, aldosterone resistance, or use of aldosterone antagonists such as spironolactone. It probably represents a combination of a rate-limited secretory defect, caused by the absence of the direct stimulation by aldosterone of H^+-ATPase and, less importantly, a voltage defect resulting from decreased distal Na^+ reabsorption. Hyperkalemia further adds to these mechanisms by its deleterious effects on NH_4^+ production and transport. In type IV dRTA, the ability to lower urinary pH is usually maintained. The term incomplete dRTA is used for disorders of distal acidification that become symptomatic only under conditions of an increased acid load. The "incompleteness" of acidification may simply be less severe, or increased ammoniagenesis may occur to compensate for decreased distal H^+ secretion.

Diagnosis of dRTA may be made by an ammonium chloride challenge test during which urine pH is monitored using a pH meter before and at hourly intervals for 6 hours after oral administration of 110 mg/kg of ammonium chloride. Normal dogs can reduce their urine pH to 5.0 and cats to 5.5. The amount of HCO_3^- supplementation required to correct metabolic acidosis in human beings with dRTA is variable, but is usually less than that required in pRTA. Alkali supplementation usually ranges from 1–5 mEq/kg per day. A combination of K^+ and Na^+ citrate may be preferred over HCO_3^- as the alkali supplement.

Proximal renal tubular acidosis

Proximal RTA results from a disturbance in proximal reclamation of filtered HCO_3^- (Jamieson and Chandler 2001; Hostutler et al. 2004). Urinary fractional excretion of HCO_3^- is usually >15% when plasma HCO_3^- concentration is increased to normal with supplementation. Bicarbonaturia is absent and urine pH is appropriately low when metabolic acidosis is present and plasma HCO_3^- concentration is decreased because distal acidifying ability is functional. When plasma HCO_3^- concentration is decreased, the filtered load of HCO_3^- is reduced, and almost all of the filtered HCO_3^- is reabsorbed in the distal tubules, despite the presence of the proximal tubule defect. Thus, pRTA can be viewed as a "self-limiting" disorder in which plasma HCO_3^- stabilizes at a lower than normal concentration after the filtered load falls sufficiently that distal HCO_3^- reabsorption can maintain plasma HCO_3^- at a new but lower steady-state concentration. The metabolic acidosis

of pRTA results not only from proximal HCO_3^- loss, but also from decreased NH_4^+ excretion, caused by either decreased proximal NH_4^+ synthesis or excessive NH_4^+ shunting to renal veins (Smulders et al. 1996).

Other abnormalities of proximal tubular function may accompany impaired HCO_3^- reabsorption in pRTA including defects in glucose, phosphate, Na^+, K^+, uric acid, and amino acid reabsorption. This condition of proximal tubular defects is known as Fanconi syndrome. Serum K^+ concentration is usually normal at time of diagnosis, but alkali therapy may precipitate hypokalemia and aggravate urinary K^+ wasting presumably by increasing distal delivery of Na^+ and HCO_3^-.

Diagnosis of pRTA is made by finding a urine pH <6.0 and hyperchloremic metabolic acidosis, but a urine pH >6.0 and increased urinary fractional excretion of HCO_3^- (>15%) after plasma HCO_3^- concentration has been increased to normal by alkali administration. Correction of metabolic acidosis by alkali therapy is more difficult in pRTA than in dRTA because of the marked bicarbonaturia that occurs when plasma HCO_3^- concentration is increased to normal. Sodium bicarbonate dosages in excess of 11 mEq/kg per day may be required to correct plasma HCO_3^-, and such therapy may result in hypokalemia. Potassium citrate may be a preferred source of alkali. One 540-mg tablet of potassium citrate will provide 5 mEq of K^+ and 1.7 mEq of citrate, and its metabolism will yield 5 mEq of HCO_3^- (DiBartola 1995).

Renal tubular acidosis is rare in dogs and cats. Both pRTA and dRTA have been observed occasionally. Distal RTA has been reported in cats and a dog with pyelonephritis caused by *E. coli* (Watson et al. 1986; Jamieson and Chandler 2001). Clinical signs included polyuria, polydipsia, anorexia, lethargy, enlarged kidneys, and isosthenuria. Distal RTA and hepatic lipidosis were reported in another cat without bacterial UTI (Brown et al. 1986). It may also occur as a consequence of ischemia-induced acute renal failure (Winaver et al. 1986). Clinical features of proximal and distal RTA are characterized in Table 55.1.

Complex tubular disorders

Fanconi syndrome

Urinary hyperexcretion of amino acids, phosphate, glucose, HCO_3^-, Ca^{2+}, K^+, and other ions, and proteins of molecular weights under 50,000 daltons, in conjunction with RTA and ADH-resistant polyuria, defines the complex tubulopathy termed Fanconi syndrome (Chesney and Novello 1995). There are inherited and acquired forms of Fanconi syndrome. The pathogenesis

Table 55.1 Clinical features of proximal and distal renal tubular acidosis

	Proximal RTA	Distal RTA
Hypercalciuria	Yes	Yes
Hyperphosphaturia	Yes	Yes
Urinary citrate	Normal	Decreased
Bone disease	Less severe	More severe
Nephrocalcinosis	No	Possible
Nephrolithiasis	Not usually	Yes
Hypokalemia	Mild	Mild to severe
Potassium wasting	Worsened by alkali therapy	Improved by alkali therapy
Alkali required for treatment	>11 mEq/kg per day	<4 mEq/kg per day
Other defects of proximal tubular function[a]	Yes	No
Reduction in plasma HCO_3^-	Moderate	Variable (can be severe)
Fractional excretion of HCO_3^- with normal plasma HCO_3^- concentration	>15%	<15%
Urine pH during academia	<6.0	>6.0
Urine pH after ammonium chloride	<6.0	>6.0

Source: (DiBartola 1995).
[a]Decreased reabsorption of sodium, potassium, phosphate, uric acid, glucose, and amino acids.

of the syndrome regardless of its cause involves one of two basic mechanisms. The first is that renal tubular membranes become leaky, allowing less efficient reabsorption of solutes. The second hypothesis suggests that the intracellular metabolism of renal tubule cells fail to produce sufficient energy to support transport. Any substance that could be "toxic" and alter renal tubular metabolism, such as heavy metals (e.g., lead, copper, mercury, organomercurials, Lysol, and maleic acid) and drugs (e.g., gentamicin, cephalosporins, outdated tetracycline, cisplatin, and salicylate) could impair transport processes. Fanconi syndrome may also occur with malignancies (e.g., multiple myeloma), monoclonal gammopathies, hyperparathyroidism, K^+ depletion, amyloidosis, nephrotic syndrome, vitamin D deficiency, interstitial nephritis associated with antitubular basement membrane antibodies, or as a complication of renal transplantation.

Fanconi syndrome occurs as a familial disease in Basenji dogs. It is estimated that 10–30% of Basenji dogs in the United States are affected (Noonan and Kay 1990). Other dogs that have been reported with idiopathic Fanconi syndrome include Border Terriers (Darrigrand Haag et al. 1996), Norwegian elkhounds (Finco 1976), a Whippet (Mackenzie and Van Den Broek 1982), a Yorkshire terrier (McEwan and Macartney 1987), a Sheltie (Bovee et al. 1979), a mixed breed dog (Padrid 1988), a Labrador retriever (Hostutler et al. 2004), and a Greyhound (Abraham et al. 2006). Fanconi syndrome also has been reported in a dog with gentamicin-induced acute renal failure (Brown 1986), in a dog with primary hypoparathyroidism with concurrent hypovitaminosis D (Freeman et al. 1994), in a dog with possible ethylene gly-

col toxicosis (Settles and Schmidt 1994), in dogs experimentally given 4-pentenoate (Boulanger et al. 1993), or maleic acid (Pouliot et al. 1992), in dogs with copper hepatopathy (Appleman et al. 2008; Hill et al. 2008), and in a dog with suspected pyelonephritis (Jamieson and Chandler 2001). Imidocarb treatment of dogs experimentally infected with *Babesia canis* resulted in vacuolar-hydropic degeneration, necrosis, and detachment of renal tubular epithelial cells from the basement membrane in some dogs, which could result in Fanconi syndrome (Mathe et al., 2007).

Dogs with Fanconi syndrome have abnormal fractional reabsorption of many solutes (Bovee 1984). Reabsorption of glucose, phosphate, and amino acids is abnormal in all affected dogs. Aminoaciduria is generalized in most dogs, but occasionally is limited to cystinuria with minor defects in reabsorption of methionine, glycine, and some dibasic amino acids. Many dogs also have variably severe reabsorptive defects for HCO_3^-, Na^+, K^+, and uric acid. Defective reabsorption of Na^+ and phosphate in Basenji dogs is manifested at approximately 3 years of age, and defective reabsorption of glucose and amino acids is apparent at approximately 4 years of age (Bovee 1984). The renal tubular disorder in affected Basenji dogs may be due to a metabolic or membrane defect affecting sodium movement or to increased back leak or to cell-to-lumen flux of amino acids. Isolated brush border vesicles from affected Basenji dogs showed decreased sodium-dependent glucose uptake but no decrease in cystine uptake (McNamara et al. 1989). Defective urinary concentrating ability in dogs with Fanconi syndrome represents a form of nDI. This defect may precede

Table 55.2 Summary of the Gonto protocol for dogs with idiopathic Fanconi syndrome

1. Ensure that fresh water is freely available at all times.
2. Feed any high-quality, dry dog food; at least once a week, feed a high-protein, canned, mammal-based (e.g., beef or lamb) dog food (for dogs with renal failure, feed a low-protein dry or canned diet).
3. Administer a vitamin-mineral supplement[a] for dogs.
    a. For dogs without clinical signs, administer 1/2 tablet, PO, every 12 hours.
    b. For dogs with clinical signs, administer 1 tablet, PO, every 12 hours (a higher dosage may be needed in dogs with hypokalemia or hypocalcemia).
4. Administer a calcium, vitamin D, and phosphorus supplement[b] for dogs (do not use in dogs with renal failure).
    a. For dogs without clinical signs, administer 1/2 tablet, PO, every 12 hours.
    b. For dogs with clinical signs, administer 1 tablet, PO, every 12 hours (a higher dosage is recommended for dogs with persistent loss of muscle mass and any signs of myalgia after correction of blood gas and serum biochemical abnormalities).
5. In dogs with polyuria and polydipsia, administer a multi-vitamin/mineral supplement[c] for human beings.
    a. Administer 1 tablet, PO, every 7 days.
    b. For dogs with renal failure, administer 1 tablet, PO, every 48 hours.
6. Administer an amino acid supplement.[d]
    a. For dogs without clinical signs, administer 1 tablet (or equivalent amount of powder), PO, every 7 days.
    b. For dogs with severe muscle wasting, poor hair coat, or skin problems, increase dosage to as high as 1 tablet, PO, every 48 hours.
    c. For dogs with renal failure, do not exceed 1/2 tablet, PO, every 24 hours.
7. Administer intact sodium bicarbonate tablets on the basis of venous blood gas findings (venous blood pH and $PvCO_2$).
    a. The initial dosage should be determined on the basis of venous blood pH and $PvCO_2$ (see Table 55.3).
    b. The daily dosage should be divided and administered, PO, every 12 hours.
    c. Dosage modifications should be based on the results of follow-up venous blood gas analyses.
8. Administer potassium supplements[e,f] on the basis of serum potassium concentration in dogs with persistent hypokalemia (monitor serum potassium concentration weekly until concentration stabilizes at target concentration).
    a. For dogs with serum potassium concentration between 1.5 and 2.0 mEq/L, administer 15 mEq, PO, every 12 hours.
    b. For dogs with serum potassium concentration between 2.1 and 2.75 mEq/L, administer 10 mEq, PO, every 12 hours.
    c. For dogs with serum potassium concentration between 2.76 and 3.75 mEq/L, administer 5 mEq, PO, every 12 hours.

Initial treatment guidelines are for dogs weighing between 10 and 12.5 kg (22 and 27 lb). Dosages should be adjusted for dogs substantially larger or smaller than this. Follow-up serum biochemical testing and venous blood gas analyses should be performed 8–10 weeks after initiation of treatment, 6 months later, and annually thereafter if the dog's condition remains stable. In dogs with renal failure, follow-up serum biochemical testing, venous blood gas analyses, and physical examinations should be performed more frequently.

Source: (http://www.voyuz.net/voyuz.net/Fanconi_Protocol.html).
[a]Pet Tab Plus, Pfizer Animal Health, Exton, Pa.
[b]Pet Cal, Pfizer Animal Health, Exton, Pa.
[c]Centrum, Wyeth, Madison, NJ.
[d]Amino Fuel, Twinlab, Hauppauge, NY.
[e]Tumil-K, King Animal Health, Bristol, Tenn.
[f]Urocit-K, Mission Pharmacal, San Antonio, Tex.

development of glucosuria. Glomerular filtration rate is normal in some affected dogs and reduced in others.

Clinical findings include polyuria, polydipsia, weight loss, poor haircoat, dehydration, and muscular weakness. The disease usually is identifiable in adult dogs when there is glucosuria and low urine specific gravity with a normal blood glucose concentration. Proteinuria usually is mild. Metabolic acidosis is variable in severity and hyperchloremic in nature, as expected with decreased proximal tubular reabsorption of HCO_3^-. Hypokalemia

can occur with longstanding disease, and may contribute to muscular weakness in some dogs. Azotemia and hyperphosphatemia are observed in dogs with advanced disease and renal failure. Renal clearance studies to identify reabsorptive defects for electrolytes and amino acids are necessary to differentiate Fanconi syndrome from primary renal glucosuria. Growth disturbances, metabolic bone disease, and nephrocalcinosis are observed in affected human patients, but have not been observed in dogs with Fanconi syndrome. Hyperchromatic karyomegaly

Table 55.3 Abbreviated table for calculating recommended initial daily dose of sodium bicarbonate in dogs with idiopathic Fanconi syndrome

PvCO$_2$ (mmHg)	Venous blood pH											
	7.40	7.35	7.30	7.25	7.20	7.10	7.00	6.90	6.80	6.70	6.60	6.50
20	9,072	9,072	10,368	10,368	11,664	14,256	15,552	16,848	18,144	18,144	19,440	20,736
30	7,776	7,776	9,072	9,072	10,368	12,960	14,256	15,552	16,848	16,848	18,144	19,440
32	6,480	6,480	7,776	7,776	9,072	11,664	12,960	14,256	14,256	15,552	16,848	18,144
34	6,480	6,480	6,480	6,480	7,776	9,072	10,368	11,664	12,960	14,256	15,552	16,848
36	5,184	5,184	6,480	6,480	7,776	9,072	10,368	11,664	11,664	12,960	14,256	15,552
38	5,184	5,184	5,184	5,184	6,480	7,776	9,072	10,368	10,368	11,664	12,960	14,256
40	3,888	3,888	3,888	3,888	5,184	6,480	7,776	9,072	9,072	10,368	11,664	12,960
42	2,592	2,592	2,592	2,592	3,888	5,184	6,480	7,776	7,776	9,072	10,368	11,664
44	1,296	1,296	1,296	1,296	2,592	3,888	5,184	6,480	6,480	7,776	9,072	10,368

Recommended daily dose of sodium bicarbonate is given in milligrams; the daily dose should be divided and given PO every 12 hours.
Source: (http://www.voyuz.net/voyuz.net/Fanconi_Protocol.html).

of renal tubular cells is a distinctive renal lesion in affected Basenji dogs, but its significance is unknown.

Progression of the disease in affected Basenji dogs is variable, although one study reported no shortening of expected life span (Yearley et al. 2004). Development of the Fanconi syndrome in other breeds appears to progress fairly quickly although spontaneous remission has been reported to occur (Jamieson and Chandler 2001; Hostutler et al. 2004). Some dogs develop chronic renal failure within a few months of diagnosis, and others remain stable for several years. Rapid progression and death may result from acute renal failure and papillary necrosis or acute pyelonephritis.

Treatment of dogs with Fanconi syndrome is limited to control of metabolic acidosis, replacement of substances lost in urine, appropriate antibiotic therapy for urinary tract infections, and conservative medical management of chronic renal failure. It may be difficult to control acidosis even with high doses of alkali therapy. This is a consequence of the marked bicarbonaturia that occurs whenever plasma HCO$_3$$^-$ concentration is increased with replacement to within the normal plasma range. Potassium citrate therapy provides both alkalinization and K$^+$ supplementation. The clinician should strive to maintain a serum HCO$_3$$^-$ concentration or total carbon dioxide concentration above 12 mEq/L, and a serum K$^+$ concentration of 4–6 mEq/L. Supplementation with vitamins, minerals, and amino acids has been recommended in addition to aggressive bicarbonate therapy (so-called Gonto Protocol; http://www.voyuz.net/voyuz.net/Fanconi_Protocol.html); however, no studies exist that validate the effectiveness or safety of this protocol (Tables 55.2 and 55.3).

In one study, 57 of 58 dogs with Fanconi syndrome were managed using this protocol and median survival time was 5.25 years; renal failure occurred in 12 of 29 dogs (41%) that were dead at the time of the study (Yearley et al. 2004).

References

Abraham, L.A., et al. (2006). Transient renal tubulopathy in a racing Greyhound. *Aust Vet J* **84**(11): 398–401.

Ahn, A. (1994). Hyperaldosteronism in cats. *Semin Vet Med Surg Small Anim* **9**(3): 153–157.

Appleman, E.H., et al. (2008). Transient acquired Fanconi syndrome associated with copper storage hepatopathy in 3 dogs. *J Vet Intern Med* **22**(4): 1038–1042.

Aroch, I., et al. (2005). Central diabetes insipidus in five cats: clinical presentation, diagnosis and oral desmopressin therapy. *J Feline Med Surg* **7**(6): 333–339.

Ash, R.A., et al. (2005). Primary hyperaldosteronism in the cat: a series of 13 cases. *J Feline Med Surg* **7**(3): 173–182.

Authement, J.M., et al. (1989). Transient, traumatically induced, central diabetes insipidus in a dog. *J Am Vet Med Assoc* **194**(5): 683–685.

Barbey, F., et al. (2000). Medical treatment of cystinuria: critical reappraisal of long-term results. *J Urol* **163**(5): 1419–1423.

Barr, S.C. (1985). Pituitary tumour causing multiple endocrinopathies in a dog. *Aust Vet J* **62**(4): 127–129.

Bartges, J.W. (1999). Disorders of renal tubules. In: *Textbook of Veterinary Internal Medicine*, edited by E.C. Feldman and S.J. Ettinger. Philadelphia, PA: WB Saunders, pp. 96–99.

Bartges, J.W., et al. (1992). Canine xanthine uroliths: risk factor management. In: *Current Veterinary Therapy XI*, edited by R.W. Kirk and J.D. Bonagura. Philadelphia, PA: WB Saunders, pp. 900–905.

Bartges, J.W., (1994a). *An Algorithmic Approach to Canine Urate Uroliths*. 12th Annual Veterinary Medical Forum of the American College of Veterinary Internal Medicine, San Francisco, Omnipress.

Bartges, J.W., et al. (1994b). Prevalence of cystine and urate uroliths in bulldogs and urate uroliths in Dalmatians. *J Am Vet Med Assoc* **204**(12): 1914–1918.

Bartges, J.W., et al. (1995). Influence of allopurinol and two diets on 24-hour urinary excretions of uric acid, xanthine, and ammonia by healthy dogs. *Am J Vet Res* **56**(5): 595–599.

Bartges, J.W., et al. (1996). Influence of four diets on uric acid metabolism and endogenous acid production in healthy Beagles. *Am J Vet Res* **57**(3): 324–328.

Bartges, J.W., et al. (1998). *Comparison of Struvite Activity Product Ratios and Relative Supersaurations in Urine Collected from Healthy Cats Consuming Four Struvite Management Diets.* Ralston Purina Nutrition Symposium, St. Louis, MO.

Bartges, J.W., et al. (1999). Canine urate urolithiasis. Etiopathogenesis, diagnosis, and management. *Vet Clin North Am Small Anim Pract* **29**(1): 161–191, xii-xiii.

Battersby, I.A., et al. (2005). Hyperammonaemic encephalopathy secondary to selective cobalamin deficiency in a juvenile Border collie. *J Small Anim Pract* **46**(7): 339–344.

Boulanger, Y., et al. (1993). Heterogeneous metabolism and toxicity of 4-pentenoate along the dog nephron. *Ren Physiol Biochem* **16**(4): 182–202.

Bovee, K.C. (1984). Genetic and metabolic diseases of the kidney. In: *Canine Nephrology*, edited by K.C. Bovee. Philadelphia, PA: Harwal Publishing Company, pp. 339–354.

Bovee, K.C., et al. (1979). Characterization of renal defects in dogs with a syndrome similar to the Fanconi syndrome in man. *J Am Vet Med Assoc* **174**(10): 1094–1099.

Bovee, K.C. and S. Segal (1984). Renal tubule reabsorption of amino acids after lysine loading of cystinuric dogs. *Metabolism* **33**(7): 602–607.

Breitschwerdt, E.B., et al. (1981). Nephrogenic diabetes insipidus in three dogs. *J Am Vet Med Assoc* **179**(3): 235–238.

Breitschwerdt, E.B., et al. (1983). Multiple endocrine abnormalities in Basenji dogs with renal tubular dysfunction. *J Am Vet Med Assoc* **182**(12): 1348–1353.

Browley, J. (1980). Diabetes insipidus in a dog. *Mod Vet Pract* **61**(11): 934–936.

Brown, S.A. (1986). Fanconi syndrome and acute renal failure associated with gentamicin therapy in a dog. *J Am Anim Hosp Assoc* **22**: 635.

Brown, S.A., et al. (1986). Distal renal tubular acidosis and hepatic lipidosis in a cat. *J Am Vet Med Assoc* **189**(10): 1350–1352.

Campbell, F.E. and B. Bredhauer (2005). Trauma-induced central diabetes insipidus in a cat. *Aust Vet J* **83**(12): 732–735.

Campbell, F.E. and B. Bredhauer (2008). Trauma-induced central diabetes insipidus in a cat. *Aust Vet J* **86**(3): 102–105.

Case, L.C., et al. (1992). Cystine-containing urinary calculi in dogs: 102 cases (1981–1989). *J Am Vet Med Assoc* **201**(1): 129–133.

Chesney, R.W. and A.C. Novello (1995). Defects of renal tubular transport. In: *Textbook of Nephrology*, edited by S.G. Massry and R.J. Glassock, 1st edition. Baltimore, MD: Williams & Wilkins, pp. 513–529.

Cohen, M. and G.S. Post (1999). Nephrogenic diabetes insipidus in a dog with intestinal leiomyosarcoma. *J Am Vet Med Assoc* **215**(12): 1818–1820, 1806.

Court, M.H. and A.D. Watson (1983). Idiopathic neurogenic diabetes insipidus in a cat. *Aust Vet J* **60**(8): 245–247.

Darrigrand Haag, R.A., et al. (1996). Congenital Fanconi syndrome associated with renal dysplasia in 2 Border Terriers. *J Vet Intern Med* **10**(6): 412–419.

Davenport, D.J., et al. (1986). Diabetes insipidus associated with metastatic pancreatic carcinoma in a dog. *J Am Vet Med Assoc* **189**(2): 204–205.

DeClue, A.E., et al. (2005). Hyperaldosteronism and hyperprogesteronism in a cat with an adrenal cortical carcinoma. *J Vet Intern Med* **19**(3): 355–358.

DiBartola, S.P. (1995). Renal tubular disorders. In: *Textbook of Veterinary Internal Medicine*, edited by S.J. Ettinger and E.C. Feldman, 2nd edition. Philadelphia, PA: WB Saunders, pp. 1801–1804.

DiBartola, S.P., et al. (1991). Cystinuria in a cat. *J Am Vet Med Assoc* **198**(1): 102–104.

Edwards, D.F., et al. (1983). Hypernatremic, hypertonic dehydration in a dog with diabetes insipidus and gastric dilation-volvulus. *J Am Vet Med Assoc* **182**(9): 973–977.

Feldman, E.C. (1979). Central diabetes insipidus in a dog. *Mod Vet Pract* **60**(8): 615–619.

Ferguson, D.C. and D.N. Biery (1988). Diabetes insipidus and hyperadrenocorticism associated with high plasma adrenocorticotropin concentration and a hypothalamic/pituitary mass in a dog. *J Am Vet Med Assoc* **193**(7): 835–839.

Finco, D.R. (1976). Familial renal disease in Norwegian elkhound dogs: physiologic and biochemical examinations. *Am J Vet Res* **37**: 87–91.

Flegel, T., et al. (1998). Xanthine urolithiasis in a dachshund. *Vet Rec* **143**(15): 420–423.

Flood, S.M., et al. (1999). Primary hyperaldosteronism in two cats. *J Am Anim Hosp Assoc* **35**(5): 411–416.

Fordyce, H.H., et al. (2000). Persistent cobalamin deficiency causing failure to thrive in a juvenile beagle. *J Small Anim Pract* **41**(9): 407–410.

Freeman, L.M., et al. (1994). Fanconi's syndrome in a dog with primary hypoparathyroidism. *J Vet Intern Med* **8**(5): 349–354.

Fyfe, J.C., (1991). Inherited selective intestinal cobalamin malabsorption and cobalamin deficiency in dogs. *Pediatr Res* **29**(1): 24–31.

Giesecke, D. and W. Tiemeyer (1984). Defect of uric acid uptake in Dalmatian dog liver. *Experientia* **40**: 1415–1416.

Goossens, M.M., et al. (1995). Central diabetes insipidus in a dog with a pro-opiomelanocortin-producing pituitary tumor not causing hyperadrenocorticism. *J Vet Intern Med* **9**(5): 361–365.

Greco, D.S. (2001). Diagnosis and treatment of juvenile endocrine disorders in puppies and kittens. *Vet Clin North Am Small Anim Pract* **31**(2): 401–409, viii.

Green, R.A. and C.S. Farrow (1974). Diabetes insipidus in a cat. *J Am Vet Med Assoc* **164**(5): 524–526.

Gunn-Moore, D. (2005). Feline endocrinopathies. *Vet Clin North Am Small Anim Pract* **35**(1): 171–210, vii.

Hanson, J.M., et al. (2005). Efficacy of transsphenoidal hypophysectomy in treatment of dogs with pituitary-dependent hyperadrenocorticism. *J Vet Intern Med* **19**(5): 687–694.

Harb, M.F., et al. (1996). Central diabetes insipidus in dogs: 20 cases (1986–1995). *J Am Vet Med Assoc* **209**(11): 1884–1888.

Henthorn, P.S., et al. (2000). Canine cystinuria: polymorphism in the canine SLC3A1 gene and identification of a nonsense mutation in cystinuric Newfoundland dogs. *Hum Genet* **107**(4): 295–303.

Hezel, A., et al. (2007). Influence of hydrochlorothiazide on urinary calcium oxalate relative supersaturation in healthy young adult female domestic shorthaired cats. *Vet Ther* **8**(4): 247–254.

Hill, T.L., et al. (2008). Concurrent hepatic copper toxicosis and Fanconi's syndrome in a dog. *J Vet Intern Med* **22**(1): 219–222.

Holtzapple, P.G., et al. (1969). Amino acid uptake by kidney and jejunal tissue from dogs with cystine stones. *Science* **166**: 1525–1527.

Hoppe, A. and T. Denneberg., (2001). Cystinuria in the dog: clinical studies during 14 years of medical treatment. *J Vet Intern Med* **15**(4): 361–367.

Hoppe, A., et al. (1993). Urinary excretion of amino acids in normal and cystinuric dogs. *Br Vet J* **149**(3): 253–268.

Hostutler, R.A., et al. (2004). Transient proximal renal tubular acidosis and Fanconi syndrome in a dog. *J Am Vet Med Assoc* **224**(10): 1611–1614, 1605.

Jamieson, P.M. and M.L. Chandler., (2001). Transient renal tubulopathy in a Labrador retriever. *J Small Anim Pract* **42**(11): 546–549.

Johnson, K.D., et al. (2006). Primary hyperaldosteronism in a dog with concurrent lymphoma. *J Vet Med A Physiol Pathol Clin Med* **53**(9): 467–470.

Keene, B.W., et al. (1991). Myocardial L-carnitine deficiency in a family of dogs with dilated cardiomyopathy. *J Amer Vet Med Assoc* **198**(4): 647–650.

Kidder, D.E. and P.R. Chivers (1968). Xanthine calculi in a dog. *Vet Rec* **83**: 228–229.

Kucera, J., et al. (1997). Bilateral xanthine nephrolithiasis in a dog. *J Small Anim Pract* **38**(7): 302–305.

Lage, A.L. (1973). Nephrogenic diabetes insipidus in a dog. *J Am Vet Med Assoc* **163**(3): 251–253.

Ling, G.V., et al. (1998). Urolithiasis in dogs. II: Breed prevalence, and interrelations of breed, sex, age, and mineral composition. *Am J Vet Res* **59**(5): 630–642.

Lobetti, R.G. (1998). Hyperreninaemic hypoaldosteronism in a dog. *J S Afr Vet Assoc* **69**(1): 33–35.

Lulich, J.P. and C.A. Osborne (1992). Effects of chlorothiazide on urinary excretion of calcium in clinically normal dogs. *Am J Vet Res* **53**(12): 2328–2332.

Lulich, J.P., et al. (1991). Evaluation of urine and serum metabolites in miniature schnauzers with calcium oxalate urolithiasis. *Am J Vet Res* **52**(10): 1583–1590.

Lulich, J.P., et al. (1995). Canine lower urinary tract disorders. In: *Textbook of Veterinary Internal Medicine*, edited by S.J. Ettinger and E.C. Feldman, 2nd edition. Philadelphia, PA: WB Saunders, pp. 1833–1861.

Lulich, J.P., et al. (2001). Effects of hydrochlorothiazide and diet in dogs with calcium oxalate urolithiasis. *J Am Vet Med Assoc* **218**(10): 1583–1586.

MacKay, A.D., et al. (1999). Successful surgical treatment of a cat with primary aldosteronism. *J Feline Med Surg* **1**(2): 117–122.

Mackenzie, C.P. and A. Van Den Broek (1982). The Fanconi syndrome in a Whippet. *J Small Anim Pract* **23**: 469–474.

Mathe, A., et al. (2007). Histological and ultrastructural studies of renal lesions in Babesia canis infected dogs treated with imidocarb. *Acta Vet Hung* **55**(4): 511–523.

McEwan, N.A. and L. Macartney (1987). Fanconi's syndrome in a Yorkshire terrier. *J Small Anim Pract* **28**: 737–742.

McNamara, P.D., et al. (1989). Cystinuria in dogs: comparison of the cystinuric component of the Fanconi syndrome in Basenji dogs to isolated cystinuria. *Metabolism* **38**(1): 8–15.

Mellanby, R.J., et al. (2005). Secondary hypothyroidism following head trauma in a cat. *J Feline Med Surg* **7**(2): 135–139.

Morgan, L.W. and J. McConnell (1999). Cobalamin deficiency associated with erythroblastic anemia and methylmalonic aciduria in a border collie. *J Am Anim Hosp Assoc* **35**(5): 392–395.

Newman, S.J., et al. (2003). Cryptococcal pyelonephritis in a dog. *J Am Vet Med Assoc* **222**(2): 180–183, 174.

Nielsen, L., et al. (2008). Central diabetes insipidus associated with primary focal B cell lymphoma in a dog. *Vet Rec* **162**(4): 124–126.

Noonan, C.H. and J.M. Kay (1990). Prevalence and geographic distribution of Fanconi syndrome in Basenjis in the United States. *J Am Vet Med Assoc* **197**(3): 345–349.

O'Brien, D.P., et al. (1999). Malonic aciduria in Maltese dogs: normal methylmalonic acid concentrations and malonyl-CoA decarboxylase activity in fibroblasts. *J Inherit Metab Dis* **22**(8): 883–890.

Osborne, C.A., et al. (1996). Diagnosis, medical treatment, and prognosis of feline urolithiasis. *Vet Clin North Am Small Anim Pract* **26**(3): 589–627.

Osborne, C.A., et al. (1999). Canine cystine urolithiasis. Cause, detection, treatment, and prevention. *Vet Clin North Am Small Anim Pract* **29**(1): 193–211, xiii.

Padrid, P. (1988). Fanconi syndrome in a mixed breed dog. *Modern Vet Pract* **69**: 162–165.

Podell, M., et al. (1996). Methylmalonic and malonic aciduria in a dog with progressive encephalomyelopathy. *Metab Brain Dis* **11**(3): 239–247.

Polzin, D.J., et al. (1986). Canine distal renal tubular acidosis and urolithiasis. *Vet Clin North Am Small Anim Pract* **16**(2): 241–250.

Post, K., et al. (1989). Congenital central diabetes insipidus in two sibling Afghan hound pups. *J Am Vet Med Assoc* **194**(8): 1086–1088.

Pouliot, J.F., et al. (1992). Brush border membrane proteins in experimental Fanconi's syndrome induced by 4-pentenoate and maleate. *Can J Physiol Pharmacol* **70**(9): 1247–1253.

Ramsey, I.K., et al. (1999). Concurrent central diabetes insipidus and panhypopituitarism in a German shepherd dog. *J Small Anim Pract* **40**(6): 271–274.

Rijnberk, A., et al. (2001a). Aldosteronoma in a dog with polyuria as the leading symptom. *Domest Anim Endocrinol* **20**(3): 227–240.

Rijnberk, A., et al. (2001b). Hyperaldosteronism in a cat with metastasised adrenocortical tumour. *Vet Q* **23**(1): 38–43.

Roch-Ramel, F. and G. Peters (1978). Urinary excretion of uric acid in nonhuman mammalian species. In: *Uric acid, Handbook of Experimental Pharmacology*, edited by W.N. Kelley and I.M. Weiner, Volume 51. Berlin: Springer-Verlag, pp. 211–255.

Rogers, W.A., et al. (1977). Partial deficiency of antidiuretic hormone in a cat. *J Am Vet Med Assoc* **170**(5): 545–547.

Rose, S.A., et al. (2007). Adrenalectomy and caval thrombectomy in a cat with primary hyperaldosteronism. *J Am Anim Hosp Assoc* **43**(4): 209–214.

Sanderson, S.L., et al. (2001). Evaluation of urinary carnitine and taurine excretion in 5 cystinuric dogs with carnitine and taurine deficiency. *J Vet Intern Med* **15**(2): 94–100.

Schwedes, C.S. (1999). Transient diabetes insipidus in a dog with acromegaly. *J Small Anim Pract* **40**(8): 392–396.

Settles, E.L. and D. Schmidt (1994). Fanconi syndrome in a Labrador retriever. *J Vet Intern Med* **8**(6): 390–393.

Smith, J.R. and C.M. Elwood (2004). Traumatic partial hypopituitarism in a cat. *J Small Anim Pract* **45**(8): 405–409.

Smulders, Y.M., et al. (1996). Renal tubular acidosis: pathophysiology and diagnosis. *Arch Intern Med* **156**: 1629–1636.

Sorenson, J.L. and G.V. Ling (1993). Metabolic and genetic aspects of urate urolithiasis in Dalmatians. *J Am Vet Med Assoc* **203**(6): 857–862.

Takemura, N. (1998). Successful long-term treatment of congenital nephrogenic diabetes insipidus in a dog. *J Small Anim Pract* **39**(12): 592–594.

Thoresen, S.I. and W.P. Bredal (1999). Serum fructosamine measurement: a new diagnostic approach to renal glucosuria in dogs. *Res Vet Sci* **67**(3): 267–271.

Tsuchida, S., et al. (2007). Xanthine urolithiasis in a cat: a case report and evaluation of a candidate gene for xanthine dehydrogenase. *J Feline Med Surg* **9**(6): 503–508.

van Zuilen, C.D., et al. (1997). Xanthinuria in a family of Cavalier King Charles spaniels. *Vet Q* **19**(4): 172–174.

Wallerstrom, B.I., et al. (1992). Cystine calculi in the dog: an epidemiological retrospective study. *J Small Anim Pract* **33**: 78–84.

Watson, A.D., et al. (1986). Distal renal tubular acidosis in a cat with pyelonephritis. *Vet Rec* **119**(3): 65–8.

White, R.N., et al. (1997). Naturally occurring xanthine urolithiasis in a domestic shorthair cat. *J Small Anim Pract* **38**(7): 299–301.

Winaver, J., et al. (1986). Impaired renal acidification following acute renal ischemia in the dog. *Kidney Int* **30**(6): 906–913.

Yearley, J.H., et al. (2004). Survival time, lifespan, and quality of life in dogs with idiopathic Fanconi syndrome. *J Am Vet Med Assoc* **225**(3): 377–383.

56

Congenital kidney diseases

George E. Lees

Introduction

Congenital kidney diseases are, by definition, present at birth. Inherited disorders are congenital in any case (the gene abnormality is present at birth), even when the structural and functional consequences of the defect only occur later in life. However, congenital conditions are not necessarily inherited. This is because normal organ development can be disrupted during gestation and the early neonatal period in a variety of ways that are not due to any genetic abnormality. Nevertheless, the most important congenital kidney diseases are conditions that are known to be genetic or are suspected to be inherited because of a familial or breed-associated pattern of disease occurrence. This information is important mainly due to the health implications for related animals and impact on breeding decisions.

Hereditary renal diseases have been recognized in several breeds or kindreds of dogs and cats (Lees 1996; DiBartola 2005), and more examples of such conditions are likely to be identified as kidney diseases having a familial pattern of occurrence are investigated thoroughly. The number and diversity of familial renal diseases that have been described in dogs are greater than those described in cats, but polycystic kidney disease in cats is likely the single most common inherited nephropathy that occurs in these two companion animal species worldwide. The main categories of familial nephropathies are renal dysplasia, primary glomerulopathies, polycystic kidney disease, amyloidosis, glomerulonephritis, and a miscellany of other diseases that are notable for occurrence in a particular breed (Table 56.1). The specific pathogenesis and underlying gene defect have been determined for only a few of these diseases; however, progress in this field is accelerating rapidly because of advancing technology and increasing availability of genetic information regarding these species.

Most familial renal diseases are progressive and ultimately fatal, but the rate of progression often varies considerably among individuals with the same disorder. Therapeutic efforts generally are focused on combating complications (e.g., hypertension, urinary tract infection) as they arise and using conventional strategies for the medical management of chronic renal failure to minimize disease progression and uremia.

Clinical findings

Chronic renal failure is the clinical syndrome produced by most of the congenital kidney diseases that require veterinary care, and it often develops while the animals are adolescents or young adults. In dogs with renal dysplasia and some primary glomerulopathies, onset of renal failure usually occurs at 3 months to 3 years of age, with peak occurrence at about 1 year of age. However, many familial nephropathies often produce renal failure later in life. For polycystic kidney disease, some primary glomerulopathies, amyloidosis, and glomerulonephritis, onset of renal failure is often at 3–7 years of age, depending on the condition.

Reduced appetite or anorexia, stunted growth or weight loss, polyuria and polydipsia, and vomiting are the most common clinical signs reported by the owners of dogs and cats with renal failure due to a familial nephropathy. Other signs that are often reported include poor hair coat, halitosis, and diarrhea. Hematuria, dysuria, and abdominal pain are the clinical signs associated with renal telangiectasia in Pembroke Welsh Corgi dogs, and hematuria also occurs in German Shepherd dogs with multifocal renal cystadenocarcinoma (see Chapters 57 and 79).

Nephrology and Urology of Small Animals. Edited by Joe Bartges and David J. Polzin. © 2011 Blackwell Publishing Ltd.

Table 56.1 Familial nephropathies in dogs and cats listed within disease categories by breeds reported to be affected and giving the mode of inheritance, if known

---

Dogs
  Renal dysplasia
    Lhasa Apso
    Shih Tzu
    Standard Poodle
    Soft-Coated Wheaten Terrier
    Chow Chow
    Alaskan Malamute
    Miniature Schnauzer
    Dutch Kooiker (Dutch Decoy) Dog
  Primary glomerulopathies
    Samoyed kindred and Navasota kindred (X-linked)
    English Cocker Spaniel (autosomal recessive)
    Bull Terrier (autosomal dominant)
    Dalmatian (autosomal dominant)
    Doberman Pinscher
    Bullmastiff
    Newfoundland
    Rottweiler
    Pembroke Welsh Corgi
    Beagle
  Polycystic kidney disease
    Bull Terrier (autosomal dominant)
    Carin Terrier and West Highland White Terrier (autosomal recessive)
  Amyloidosis
    Shar Pei
    English Foxhound
    Beagle
  Immune-mediated glomerulonephritis
    Soft-Coated Wheaten Terrier
    Bernese Mountain Dog (autosomal recessive, suspected)
    Brittany Spaniel (autosomal recessive)
  Miscellaneous
    Boxer – reflux nephropathy with segmental hypoplasia
    Basenji – Fanconi syndrome
    German Shepherd – multifocal cystadenocarcinoma (autosomal dominant)
    Pembroke Welsh Corgi – telangiectasia
Cats
  Polycystic kidney disease
    Persian (autosomal dominant)
  Amyloidosis
    Abyssinian (autosomal dominant with incomplete penetrance, suspected)
    Siamese and Oriental

Physical examination findings often include thin body condition, dehydration, mucous membrane pallor, uremic breath odor, and oral ulceration. Fibrous osteodystrophy or rubber jaw is occasionally observed, mainly in dogs that develop renal failure before 6 months of age. The kidneys of animals, especially cats, with polycystic kidney disease are often palpably enlarged. Otherwise, the kidneys usually are normal or reduced in size. Dogs with severe renal dysplasia often have especially small kidneys.

Laboratory testing most often reveals the expected abnormalities associated with chronic renal failure, namely impaired urine concentrating ability, azotemia, hyperphosphatemia, and nonregenerative anemia. These findings usually reflect the severity of the animal's renal failure independent of its cause. Urinalysis findings, however, frequently help discriminate among the common causes of juvenile or familial nephropathy. Dogs with primary glomerulopathies and familial glomerulonephritis consistently have persistent renal proteinuria (see Chapters 8 and 53) that emerges early in the course of disease and typically is of high magnitude (UPC $\geq$ 2). Dogs with renal dysplasia and dogs and cats with polycystic kidney disease usually exhibit little or no proteinuria, while proteinuria is an inconsistent finding that depends on the extent of glomerular involvement in dogs and cats with familial amyloidosis. Renal glucosuria is a consistent feature of the Fanconi syndrome in Basenji dogs but is occasionally observed in dogs with renal dysplasia or primary glomerulopathies. Hematuria is the cardinal feature of telangiectasia in Pembroke Welsh Corgi dogs, which may develop anemia due to blood loss in the urine. Bacterial urinary tract infection also sometimes develops as a secondary complication in dogs and cats with juvenile or familial nephropathies.

Diagnostic renal imaging is most helpful for animals with polycystic kidney disease in which a definitive diagnosis can be made by finding multiple cysts distributed in both kidneys using ultrasonography. In dogs with renal dysplasia, ultrasound can demonstrate abnormal size, shape, and sonic architecture of the kidneys, but it cannot distinguish renal dysplasia from other possible causes of small, fibrotic end-stage kidneys in affected dogs.

Diagnosis

For specific nephropathies known or suspected to be inherited in particular breeds, diagnosis of the condition generally rests on recognition of the expected clinical features, exclusion of other conditions that might produce similar signs, and ultimately upon identification of characteristic renal lesions. The exclusion of other disorders (especially those that are potentially treatable) is an important step because a variety of acquired diseases may occur in the same breeds and age-groups of animals that might have familial nephropathies. Careful interpretation of the results obtained from a thorough clinical investigation (i.e., history, physical examination, blood pressure determination, complete urinalysis, urine culture, and appropriate diagnostic imaging) is often adequate for presumptive diagnosis of familial nephropathy. Even when the diagnosis remains uncertain, however, such an investigation is generally sufficient to properly guide the animal's medical care. Nonetheless, definitive diagnosis of many familial nephropathies ultimately rests upon detection of characteristic lesions in kidney specimens obtained at necropsy or by biopsy (see Chapters 23 and 24). Light microscopic examinations are sufficient for many disorders, but especially for glomerular diseases, transmission electron microscopic and immunopathologic studies are often needed as well. Prior planning is generally needed to assure that specimens that will be suitable for these specialized evaluations are obtained when the tissue is collected because special materials and procedures are required. Centers that perform such studies should be contacted for guidance.

In breeds or families known to be at risk for certain familial nephropathies, apparently healthy animals can be screened with tests to enable early identification of affected individuals. The foremost examples of such screening are the use of ultrasonography to identify polycystic kidney disease and urinalyses to detect persistent renal proteinuria in animals that are at risk for glomerular disorders.

When a juvenile nephropathy is identified, questions about inheritance of the condition frequently arise. For breeds in which the specific nephropathy that has been diagnosed is known to be inherited, genetic counseling can be provided. In most other circumstances, heritability of the condition remains unknown unless or until studies of related animals show a familial pattern of disease occurrence.

Specific disorders

Renal dysplasia

Renal dysplasia is defined as disorganized development of renal parenchyma that is due to abnormal differentiation. For definitive diagnosis of this category of conditions, microscopic observation of structures in the kidney that are inappropriate for the stage of development of the animal is required. The presence of immature glomeruli and tubules usually within radial bands adjacent to more normally developed tissue (i.e., asynchronous differentiation of nephrons) is the most consistent feature (Picut and Lewis 1987b). Other findings indicative of renal dysplasia include persistent immature mesenchyme, persistent metanephric ducts, atypical tubular epithelial proliferation, and (albeit rare in dogs) dysontogenic metaplasia.

Secondary changes that are commonly observed include, compensatory hypertrophy and hyperplasia of glomerular tufts and tubules, interstitial fibrosis, tubulointerstitial nephritis, pyelonephritis, dystrophic mineralization, cystic glomerular atrophy, microcystic tubules, retention cysts, and glomerular lipidosis.

Renal dysplasia is most extensively reported and presumed to be familial in Lhasa Apso and Shih Tzu dogs (O'Brien et al. 1982; Picut and Lewis 1987b). Other breeds in which published reports have suggested that renal dysplasia occurs in a familial pattern include the Soft-Coated Wheaton Terrier (Eriksen and Gröndalen 1984; Nash et al. 1984), Standard Poodle (DiBartola et al. 1983), Alaskan Malamute (Vilafranca and Ferrer 1994), Golden Retriever (Kerlin and Van Winkle 1995; de Morais et al. 1996), Chow Chow (Brown et al. 1990), Miniature Schnauzer (Morton et al. 1990), and the Dutch Kooiker (Dutch Decoy) Dog (Schulze et al. 1998). Additionally, juvenile nephropathies with microscopic features of renal dysplasia have been reported in one or more unrelated dogs of so many different breeds that it seems likely that the disorder occurs at least sporadically in all breeds. The causes and pathogenesis of canine renal dysplasia are unknown. Renal dysplasia is widely accepted to be the same disease entity in both Lhasa Apso and Shih Tzu dogs, but whether the other familial or sporadic forms of renal dysplasia are fundamentally the same disease or different diseases having similar adverse effects on development of the kidneys in affected dogs is uncertain. To date, evidence documenting the validity of genetic testing for renal dysplasia has not been published for any breed.

Primary glomerulopathies

A number of primary glomerulopathies, including several of the most well characterized inherited renal diseases of dogs, have been described. Conditions in which an abnormality of the type IV collagen in the glomerular basement membrane (GBM) is known or suspected to cause the disease lead this category. All basement membranes contain collagen IV, but in the GBM, a special collagen network containing the $\alpha3$, $\alpha4$, and $\alpha5$ chains of type IV collagen is crucial for long-term maintenance of normal structure and function of the glomerular capillary wall. When this $\alpha3$-$\alpha4$-$\alpha5$(IV) network is not formed properly, distinctive ultrastructural changes that can be identified only by transmission electron microscopy develop in the GBM and initiate progressive renal disease leading to chronic renal failure. These conditions are analogous to the nephropathy that occurs in human Alport syndrome, which is a genetically and clinically heterogeneous group of diseases because the functional integrity of the GBM α3-α4-α5(IV) network can be disrupted in diverse ways. In dogs, as in people, mode of inheritance can be X-linked, autosomal recessive, or autosomal dominant.

X-linked hereditary nephropathies caused by mutations in the gene (*COL4A5*) encoding the α5(IV) collagen chain have been described in two canine families (Jansen et al. 1984; Jansen et al. 1987; Lees et al. 1999). In the Samoyed kindred, which was described first, a single nucleotide substitution in exon 35 (of 51) converts a glycine codon to a stop codon (Zheng et al. 1994). In the Navasota kindred, a 10-bp deletion in exon 9 creates a frame-shift and a stop codon in exon 10 (Cox et al. 2003). Thus, although unique within each kindred, both mutations cause *COL4A5* to encode truncated α5 chains incapable of combining with α3 and α4 chains to form α3-α4-α5 heterotrimers, which are required for assembly of the normal collagen IV network in the GBM. Consequently, the molecular, pathologic and clinical expressions of renal disease in both kindreds are similar. In affected males, GBM expression of collagen IV α5 chains, as well as that of α3 and α4 chains is totally absent as indicated by immunostaining with chain-specific antibodies (Harvey et al. 1998; Lees et al. 1999). Focal GBM splitting can be detected by electron microscopy beginning at about one month of age (Harvey et al. 1998). These changes subsequently progress in extent and severity, eventually producing the global and severe GBM thickening and multilaminar splitting that is the characteristic structural feature of this nephropathy. Persistent proteinuria, which is the first clinical manifestation of the disease, begins at 3–6 months of age, and renal function subsequently deteriorates progressively usually causing azotemia by 6–9 months of age and death from renal failure by 9–15 months of age (Jansen et al. 1987; Lees et al. 1999). The light microscopic features of the nephropathy are nonspecific, having the morphologic features of a membranoproliferative glomerulonephropathy accompanied by secondary changes in the tubulointerstitium. Carrier females have mosaic expression of the α3-α4-α5(IV) network in their GBM. They develop persistent proteinuria at about the same age as their affected brothers, but their nephropathy rarely progresses to renal failure until they are older than 5 years of age (Baumal et al. 1991).

An autosomal recessive hereditary glomerulopathy that is due to a mutation in the *COL4A4* gene occurs in English Cocker Spaniels (Lees et al. 1997; Davidson et al. 2007). In this breed, a single nucleotide substitution (A to T) in exon 3 (of 47) in *COL4A4* creates a premature stop codon that prevents proper synthesis of α4 chains. Without α4 chains, α3 and α5 chains are unable to form α3-α4-α5 heterotrimers, as required for the normal collagen IV network in the GBM. Immunos-

taining of kidneys from affected dogs shows absence of the normal α3-α4-α5(IV) network in their GBM, but expression of α5 chains is present in basement membranes (including the GBM) where they are co-expressed with α6 chains (Lees et al. 1998b). Except that males and females are affected equally, the inherited nephropathy in English Cocker Spaniels is clinically and pathologically similar to the X-linked disorders. Persistent proteinuria develops at 5–8 months of age, and renal function subsequently declines progressively leading to death from renal failure at 10–27 months of age (Lees et al. 1998a, 1998b). Definitive diagnosis of the condition once depended on transmission electron microscopy to demonstrate the characteristic multilaminar splitting and thickening of the GBM, or immunostaining to demonstrate the distinctively abnormal pattern of type IV collagen α-chain expression in renal basement membranes. However, a genetic test for the mutated *COL4A4* allele is currently available commercially worldwide and proper use of this test should eradicate this disease in the English Cocker Spaniel breed in the near future (Davidson et al. 2007).

Autosomal dominant inherited glomerulopathies have been described in Bull Terriers and Dalmatians, mainly from Australia (Robinson et al. 1989; Hood et al. 1991, 1995, 2000, 2002a, 2002b). The nephropathy in Bull Terriers has been studied more than the one in Dalmatians, but the two conditions are reported to have similar clinical and pathologic features. These disorders are characterized by ultrastructural abnormalities in the GBM that can be definitively diagnosed only by electron microscopy (Hood et al. 1995, 2000, 2002b). The GBM changes are similar to those that characterize the X-linked and autosomal recessive conditions described above. In contrast, however, immunostaining of kidney from affected Bull Terriers and Dalmatians shows a normal pattern of type IV collagen α-chain expression in their basement membranes (Hood et al. 2000, 2002b). These findings are consistent with possible existence of a functionally defective α3-α4-α5 network due to mutations in *COL4A3* or *COL4A4*, such as have been reported in the rare human forms of Alport syndrome that have autosomal dominant inheritance. However, gene defects that cause these nephropathies in Bull Terriers and Dalmatians have not been identified, and a few autosomal dominant human diseases with some features resembling Alport syndrome are caused by mutations in other genes (*MYH9, LMX1*). Clinical expression of canine autosomal dominant glomerulopathy is somewhat variable. All affected dogs have proteinuria (defined as UPC $\geq$ 0.3 by the investigators who studied these disorders), but the onset of renal failure occurs at 11 months to 8 years of age in Bull Terriers (Robinson et al. 1989) and at

8 months to 7 years of age in Dalmatians (Hood et al. 2002b). As is the case for the glomerulopathies described above, progression of these nephropathies to renal failure is associated with extensive secondary tubulointerstitial changes (Hood et al. 2002a, 2002b).

Other breeds in which a renal disease having the clinicopathologic features of a primary glomerulopathy has been described in related dogs include the Doberman Pinscher (Wilcock and Patterson 1979; Chew et al. 1983; Picut and Lewis 1987a), Bullmastiff (Casal et al. 2004), Beagle (Rha et al. 2000), Rottweiller (Cook et al. 1993; Wakamatsu et al. 2007), Pembroke Welsh Corgi (McKay et al. 2004), and Newfoundland (Koeman et al. 1994). The causes and pathogenesis of these conditions are uncertain, although the glomerular lesions sometimes have been examined at the ultrastructural as well as light microscopic levels.

Polycystic kidney disease

Autosomal dominant polycystic kidney disease is prevalent in Persian and Persian-cross cats, affecting approximately 38% of Persian cats worldwide (Beck and Lavelle 2001; Barrs et al. 2001; Cannon et al. 2001; Barthez et al. 2003). Recently, a single mutation in the feline *PKD1* gene has been incriminated as the cause of this disorder in many if not all affected cats (Lyons et al. 2004). A stop mutation caused by a single nucleotide transversion in exon 29 (of 46) was found in the heterozygous state in each of 48 affected cats (41 Persians and one cat each of seven other breeds) from the United States. Because the mutation is likely to be identical by descent within the breed, a DNA test is now possible to identify Persian and Persian-cross cats that have, or will develop, polycystic kidney disease, although the expectation that this single mutation causes the disease worldwide remains to be verified by further studies. In affected cats, multiple cysts form in both kidneys and occasionally in the liver. Renal cysts arise from tubules and occur in both the cortex and medulla (Eaton et al. 1997). They form early in life and gradually become more numerous and larger in size as the cat ages. Detection of multiple cysts distributed in both kidneys using ultrasonography is diagnostic. Cysts sometimes can be detected in kittens as young as 6–8 weeks of age; however, because the number and size of cysts increase with time, sensitivity of ultrasound as a diagnostic test for polycystic kidney disease increased from 75% at 16 weeks of age to 91% at 36 weeks of age in one study (Biller et al. 1996). Cyst growth eventually causes renomegaly, which can be an incidental finding during physical examination of seemingly healthy cats, and renal failure ensues later in adult life (at 3–10, average 7, years of age).

Autosomal dominant polycystic kidney disease also has been described in Bull Terriers, mainly in Australia (Burrows et al. 1994; O'Leary et al. 1999). Affected dogs are identified by ultrasonography when multiple (≥ 3) cysts distributed in both kidneys are detected in dogs with a family history of the disease. The gene mutation that causes this disease has not been identified (O'Leary et al. 2003), but dogs at risk for the disease can be screened with ultrasonography prior to breeding to minimize production of additional affected animals (O'Leary et al. 1999). Bull Terriers with polycystic kidney disease that develop renal failure do so as adults, and hepatic cysts have not been described in affected dogs. However, some Bull Terriers have renal lesions consistent with concurrent existence of both polycystic kidney disease and the hereditary GBM nephropathy (O'Leary et al. 2002).

Autosomal recessive polycystic kidney and liver disease has been described in the Carin Terrier and the West Highland White Terrier (McKenna and Carpenter 1980; McAloose et al. 1998). Affected puppies become clinically ill before two months of age and have marked enlargement of their livers and kidneys caused by the presence of numerous cysts in both organs.

Amyloidosis

Familial forms of reactive systemic amyloidosis with predilection for renal involvement occur in both dogs and cats (see Chapter 54). In dogs, familial renal amyloidosis has been described in Shar Peis most often (DiBartola et al. 1990; Rivas et al. 1993), but also in Beagles (Bowles and Mosier 1992) and English Foxhounds (Mason and Day 1996). In cats, this condition occurs mainly in Abyssinians (Chew et al. 1982; Boyce et al. 1984; DiBartola et al. 1986), but also has been reported in the Siamese and Oriental (a color variant of Siamese) breeds (Zuber 1993; Godfrey and Day 1998).

In Shar Pei dogs, familial amyloidosis usually causes renal failure in dogs that are 1–6 (average, 4) years of age (DiBartola et al. 1990). Some dogs have a history of previous episodes of high fever and joint swelling, and this disease in Shar Pei dogs may be analogous to familial Mediterranean fever in humans (May et al. 1992; Rivas et al. 1992). Some evidence suggests that amyloidosis in Shar Pei dogs is inherited in an autosomal recessive fashion (Rivas et al. 1993). Affected Shar Peis invariably have moderate to severe medullary interstitial amyloid deposits, but only two-thirds have glomerular deposits. Proteinuria and other elements of the nephrotic syndrome, which reflect the severity of glomerular involvement, occur in some dogs. Amyloid frequently is also deposited in many other organs. Severe amyloid deposition in the liver may cause hepatomegaly, jaundice, or hepatic rupture (Loeven 1994a, 1994b).

In Abyssinian cats, familial amyloidosis probably is inherited as an autosomal dominant trait with variable penetrance (DiBartola 2005). Renal amyloid deposits first appear between 9 and 24 months of age mainly in the medullary interstitium. Glomerular deposits are usually mild but occasionally can be severe, so proteinuria is a variable feature of renal amyloidosis in cats. Affected cats usually develop chronic renal failure at 1–5 (average, 3) years of age, but cats with mild deposits can live to be much older. Additionally, cats with severe medullary involvement sometimes develop papillary necrosis. Amyloid deposits are often also found in other organs, but in Abyssinian cats, extra-renal amyloid deposition usually is of little clinical consequence. In Siamese and Oriental cats with familial amyloidosis, however, severe amyloid deposition occurs predominantly in the liver and mainly causes intra-abdominal hemorrhage from hepatic rupture (Zuber 1993; Godfrey and Day 1998). Nonetheless, amyloid deposition also occurs in the kidneys and leads to renal failure in some affected cats. Amino acid sequences of amyloid AA proteins isolated from Siamese cats are slightly different from those of AA proteins from Abyssinian cats, possibly accounting for the difference in predominant site of amyloid deposition between the two breeds (Niewold et al. 1999).

Immune-mediated glomerulonephritis

A familial disorder that causes protein-losing enteropathy, protein-losing nephropathy, or both has been described in Soft-Coated Wheaten Terriers (Littman et al. 2000). Although pathogenesis of the disorder is incompletely understood, evidence suggests that food hypersensitivity and altered intestinal permeability develop first and that immune complex glomerulonephritis develops subsequently (Vaden et al. 2000a, 2000b). The mode of inheritance has not been defined, but the disorder is common among Soft-Coated Wheaten Terriers, particularly in the United States where the condition is estimated to affect as many as 10–15% of the dogs of this breed. Females are affected slightly more often than males, and the average age when renal disease is diagnosed in affected dogs is 6 years of age. Clinical signs associated with the nephropathy include polyuria, polydipsia, vomiting, and weight loss. Laboratory findings include proteinuria, hypoalbuminemia, and hypercholesterolemia, often associated with abnormalities attributable to renal failure (azotemia, hyperphosphatemia, and non-regenerative anemia). The disease is complicated by thromboembolism in about 12% of cases, and hypertension occurs occasionally (Littman

et al. 2000). By light microscopy, renal lesions are those of a membranous to membranoproliferative glomerulonephritis progressing to glomerular sclerosis accompanied by periglomerular fibrosis and secondary tubulointerstitial changes. Evidence of mesangial deposition of immunoglobulin A (IgA), IgM, and complement has been found in glomeruli of affected dogs using immunofluorescent labeling and electron microscopy (Afrouzian et al. 2001).

Membranoproliferative glomerulonephritis also has been described in 2- to 7-year-old Bernese Mountain Dogs (Minkus et al. 1994; Reusch et al. 1994). Pedigree analysis suggested autosomal recessive inheritance of the disorder. Laboratory findings were those of renal failure accompanied by marked proteinuria, hypoalbuminemia, and hypercholesterolemia. Glomerular ultrastructural lesions resembled those of human membranoproliferative glomerulonephritis type I with electron-dense immune deposits mainly in subendothelial locations and reduplication of the GBM. Immunolabeling consistently demonstrated glomerular IgM and complement deposition, with labeling for IgA or IgG detected only occasionally. Most of the affected dogs had high serum titers against *Borrelia burgdorferi*, but the organism could not be detected immunohistochemically in the tissues of affected dogs. Membranoproliferative glomerulonephritis also has been reported in Brittany Spaniels with a genetically determined deficiency of the third component of complement (Cork et al. 1991).

Miscellaneous conditions

The clinical and pathologic features of kidney disease in young (≤5 years of age) Boxer dogs have been described in reports from the United Kingdom and Norway (Chandler et al. 2007; Kolbjornsen et al. 2008). Clinically, the condition is characterized by the usual features of chronic renal failure; namely, impaired urine concentrating ability, azotemia, hyperphosphatemia, and anemia. Most dogs also exhibit mild to moderate proteinuria, and diagnostic imaging often reveals small, irregularly shaped kidneys with hyperechoic cortices and decreased corticomedullary differentiation. The condition occurs in both sexes, but affected dogs are more often females than males. Of note, urinary incontinence is reported in about half of affected dogs (including in both females and males), and bacterial urinary tract infections are found in nearly one-third of affected dogs (Chandler et al. 2007). Detailed histologic evaluation of kidneys from 7 young Boxers with end-stage kidney disease revealed a distinctive pattern of changes that was interpreted to be most likely the result of chronic atrophic non-obstructive pyelonephritis due to vesico-ureteral reflux (i.e., reflux nephropathy) and segmental renal hypoplasia attributable to the occurrence of some reflux-mediated injury to the kidney during development of the organ (i.e., during gestation and up to 3 weeks of age) (Kolbjornsen et al. 2008).

An inherited form of Fanconi syndrome, which is caused by generalized impairment of the reabsorptive functions of proximal renal tubules and results in excessive urinary losses of multiple solutes and water, occurs in Basenjis (see Chapter 55) (Bovee et al. 1979; Noonan and Kay 1990). Most affected dogs are 4–7 years of age when onset of the disease occurs, but substantial diversity in the spectrum and severity of reabsorptive defects exists among affected dogs. Polyuria, polydipsia, renal glucosuria, mild proteinuria, and aminoaciduria are consistent findings. Some dogs maintain normal serum biochemical profiles, but others may develop various derangements, most notably hyperchloremic metabolic acidosis or hypokalemia. Treatment generally is focused on minimizing the systemic effects of urinary losses of important solutes by supplementing their intake. A medical management protocol that espouses an aggressive approach to bicarbonate treatment as well as routine supplementation of amino acids, vitamins, and minerals has been promulgated (Gonto et al. 2003) and is widely used but has not been directly compared with any other management protocol. Some affected dogs develop renal failure, but a recent study found that the expected lifespan for affected dogs was similar to that for unaffected dogs and that affected dogs generally had a good or excellent quality of life as judged by their owners (Yearley et al. 2004). Notably, most of the dogs in the study were managed using the aggressive protocol. In addition, owner tolerance of polydipsia and polyuria is likely to be an important factor that influences life expectancy of dogs with Fanconi syndrome. Sporadic cases of persistent Fanconi syndrome also have been described in dogs of a number of other breeds, but evidence of familial occurrence of the condition in breeds other than the Basenji has not been reported.

Hereditary multifocal renal cystadenocarcinoma and nodular dermatofibrosis is a canine cancer syndrome originally described in German Shepherd dogs (see Chapters 57 and 79). The condition is inherited as an autosomal dominant trait, and a mutation in the canine *BHD* gene recently has been incriminated as the cause of the disorder (Lingaas et al. 2003). The disease is characterized by development of bilateral, multifocal tumors in the kidneys, numerous firm nodules in the skin and subcutis, and uterine leiomyomas. Affected dogs usually are diagnosed at 5–11 (average, 8) years of age when they are examined because of the skin lesions or a variety of nonspecific signs (Moe and Lium 1997).

Pembroke Welsh Corgis with telangiectasia have episodes of gross hematuria beginning at 2–8 years of age (Moore and Thornton 1983). Signs of abdominal distress or dysuria may occur as well. Several months often elapse between episodes, but urinary bleeding can be sufficiently severe to cause anemia or formation of blood clots in the urine. Affected dogs may develop nephrocalcinosis or calculi, and hydronephrosis may develop if a calculus or blood clot obstructs the ureter.

References

Afrouzian, M., et al. (2001). Immune complex mediated proliferative and sclerosing glomerulonephritis in Soft Coated Wheaten Terriers (SCWT): Is this an animal model of IgA nephropathy or IgM mesangial nephropathy? (abstract). *J Am Soc Nephrol* **12**: 670A.

Barrs, V.R., et al. (2001). Prevalence of autosomal dominant polycystic kidney disease in Persian cats and related-breeds in Sydney and Brisbane. *Aust Vet J* **79**: 257–259.

Barthez, P.Y., et al. (2003). Prevalence of polycystic kidney disease in Persian and Persian related cats in France. *J Feline Med Surg* **5**: 345–347.

Baumal, R., et al. (1991). Renal disease in carrier female dogs with X-linked hereditary nephritis; implications for female patients with this disease. *Am J Pathol* **139**: 751–764.

Beck, C. and R.B. Lavelle (2001). Feline polycystic kidney disease in Persian and other cats: a prospective study using ultrasonography. *Aust Vet J* **79**: 181–184.

Biller, D.S., et al. (1996). Inheritance of polycystic kidney disease in Persian cats. *J Hered* **87**: 1–5.

Bovee, K.C., et al. (1979). Characterization of renal defects in dogs with a syndrome similar to the Fanconi syndrome in man. *J Am Vet Med Assoc* **174**: 1094–1099.

Bowles, M.H. and D.A. Mosier (1992). Renal amyloidosis in a family of beagles. *J Am Vet Med Assoc* **201**: 569–574.

Boyce, J.T., et al. (1984). Familial renal amyloidosis in Abyssinian cats. *Vet Pathol* **21**: 33–38.

Brown, C.A., et al. (1990). Suspected familial renal disease in chow chows. *J Am Vet Med Assoc* **196**: 1279–1284.

Burrows, A.K., et al. (1994). Familial polycystic kidney disease in bull terriers. *J Small Anim Pract* **35**: 364–369.

Cannon, M.J., et al. (2001). Prevalence of polycystic kidney disease in Persian cats in the United Kingdom. *Vet Rec* **149**: 409–411.

Casal, M.L., et al. (2004). Familial glomerulonephropathy in the Bullmastiff. *Vet Pathol* **41**: 319–332.

Chandler, M.L., et al. (2007). Juvenile nephropathy in 37 boxer dogs. *J Small Anim Pract* **48**: 690–694.

Chew, D.J., et al. (1982). Renal amyloidosis in related Abyssinian cats. *J Am Vet Med Assoc* **181**: 139–142.

Chew, D.J., et al. (1983). Juvenile renal disease in Doberman Pinscher dogs. *J Am Vet Med Assoc* **182**: 481–485.

Cook, S.M., et al. (1993). Renal failure attributable to atrophic glomerulopathy in four related Rottweilers. *J Am Vet Med Assoc* **202**: 107–109.

Cork, L.C., et al. (1991). Membranoproliferative glomerulonephritis in dogs with a genetically determined deficiency of the third component of complement. *Clin Immunol Immunopathol* **60**: 455–470.

Cox, M.L., et al. (2003). Genetic cause of X-linked Alport syndrome in a family of domestic dogs. *Mamm Genome* **14**: 396–403.

Davidson, A.G., et al. (2007). Genetic cause of autosomal recessive hereditary nephropathy in the English cocker spaniel. *J Vet Intern Med* **21**: 394–401.

de Morais, H.S., et al. (1996). Juvenile renal disease in golden retrievers: 12 cases (1984–1994). *J Am Vet Med Assoc* **209**: 792–797.

DiBartola, S.P. (2005). Familial renal disease in dogs and cats. In: *Textbook of Veterinary Internal Medicine*, edited by S.J. Ettinger, and E.C. Feldman, 6th edition. St. Louis, MO: Elsevier Saunders, pp. 1819–1824.

DiBartola, S.P., et al. (1983). Juvenile renal disease in related Standard Poodles. *J Am Vet Med Assoc* **183**: 693–696.

DiBartola, S.P., et al. (1986). Tissue distribution of amyloid deposits in Abyssinian cats with familial amyloidosis. *J Comp Pathol* **96**: 387–398.

DiBartola, S.P., et al. (1990). Familial renal amyloidosis in Chinese shar pei dogs. *J Am Vet Med Assoc* **197**: 483–487.

Eaton, K.A., et al. (1997). Autosomal dominant polycystic kidney disease in Persian and Persian-cross cats. *Vet Pathol* **34**: 117–126.

Eriksen, K. and J. Gröndalen (1984). Familial renal disease in soft-coated Wheaten terriers. *J Small Anim Pract* **25**: 489–500.

Godfrey, D.R. and M.J. Day (1998). Generalised amyloidosis in two Siamese cats: spontaneous liver hemorrhage and chronic renal failure. *J Small Anim Pract* **39**: 442–447.

Gonto, S. (2003). *Fanconi Disease Management Protocol for Veterinarians*. Available at: www.basenjicompanions.org/health/images/Protocol2003.html (accessed October 24, 2008).

Harvey, S.J., et al. (1998). Role of distinct type IV collagen networks in glomerular development and function. *Kidney Int* **54**: 1857–1866.

Hood, J.C., et al. (1991). Proteinuria as an indicator of early renal disease in Bull terriers with hereditary nephritis. *J Small Anim Pract* **32**: 241–248.

Hood, J.C., et al. (1995). Bull terrier hereditary nephritis: a model for autosomal dominant Alport syndrome. *Kidney Int* **47**: 758–765.

Hood, J.C., et al. (2000). Ultrastructural appearance of renal and other basement membranes in the Bull terrier model of autosomal dominant hereditary nephritis. *Am J Kidney Dis* **36**: 378–391.

Hood, J.C., et al. (2002a). Correlation of histopathological features and renal impairment in autosomal dominant Alport syndrome in Bull terriers. *Nephrol Dial Transpl* **17**: 1897–1908.

Hood, J.C., et al. (2002b). A novel model of autosomal dominant Alport syndrome in Dalmatian dogs. *Nephrol Dial Transpl* **17**: 2094–2098.

Jansen, B., et al. (1984). Animal model of human disease: hereditary nephritis in Samoyed dogs. *Am J Pathol* **116**: 175–178.

Jansen, B., et al. (1987). Samoyed hereditary glomerulopathy: serial, clinical and laboratory (urine, serum biochemistry and hematology) studies. *Can J Vet Res* **51**: 387–393.

Kerlin, R.L. and T.J. Van Winkle (1995). Renal dysplasia in golden retrievers. *Vet Pathol* **32**: 327–329.

Koeman, J.P., et al. (1994). Proteinuria associated with glomerulosclerosis and glomerular collagen formation in three Newfoundland dog littermates. *Vet Pathol* **31**: 188–193.

Kolbjornsen, O., et al. (2008). End-stage kidney disease probably due to *reflux nephropathy with segmental hypoplasia (Ask-Upmark kidney)* in young Boxer dogs in Norway. A retrospective study. *Vet Pathol* **45**: 467–474.

Lees, G.E. (1996). Congenital renal diseases. *Vet Clin N Am-Small* **26**: 1379–1399.

Lees, G.E., et al. (1997). Glomerular ultrastructural findings similar to hereditary nephritis in 4 English cocker spaniels. *J Vet Intern Med* **11**: 80–85.

Lees, G.E., et al. (1998a). Early diagnosis of familial nephropathy in English cocker spaniels. *J Am Anim Hosp Assoc* **34**: 189–195.

Lees, G.E., et al. (1998b). A model of autosomal recessive Alport syndrome in English cocker spaniel dogs. *Kidney Int* **54**: 706–719.

Lees, G.E., et al. (1999). New form of X-linked dominant hereditary nephritis in dogs. *Am J Vet Res* **60**: 373–383.

Lingaas, F., et al. (2003). A mutation in the canine BHD gene is associated with hereditary multifocal renal cystadenocarcinoma and nodular dermatofibrosis in the German Shepherd dog. *Hum Mol Genet* **12**: 3043–3053.

Littman, M.P., et al. (2000). Familial protein-losing enteropathy and protein-losing nephropathy in Soft Coated Wheaten Terriers: 222 cases (1983–1997). *J Vet Intern Med* **14**: 68–80.

Loeven, K.O. (1994a). Hepatic amyloidosis in two Chinese Shar Pei dogs. *J Am Vet Med Assoc* **204**: 1212–1216.

Loeven, K.O. (1994b). Spontaneous hepatic rupture secondary to amyloidosis in a Chinese Shar Pei. *J Am Anim Hosp Assoc* **30**: 577–579.

Lyons, L.A., et al. (2004). Feline polycystic kidney disease mutation identified in PKD1. *J Am Soc Nephrol* **15**: 2548–2555.

Mason, N.J. and M.J. Day (1996). Renal amyloidosis in related English foxhounds. *J Small Anim Pract* **37**: 255–260.

May, C., et al. (1992). Chinese Shar Pei fever syndrome: a preliminary report. *Vet Rec* **131**: 586–587.

McAloose, D., et al. (1998). Polycystic kidney and liver disease in two related West Highland White Terrier litters. *Vet Pathol* **35**: 77–81.

McKay, L.W., et al. (2004). Juvenile nephropathy in two related Pembroke Welsh corgi puppies. *J Small Anim Pract* **45**: 568–571.

McKenna, S.C. and J.L. Carpenter (1980). Polycystic disease of the kidney and liver in the Cairn Terrier. *Vet Pathol* **17**: 436–442.

Minkus, G., et al. (1994). Familial nephropathy in Bernese mountain dogs. *Vet Pathol* **31**: 421–428.

Moe, L. and B. Lium (1997). Hereditary multifocal renal cystadenocarcinomas and nodular dermatofibrosis in 51 German shepherd dogs. *J Small Anim Pract* **38**: 498–505.

Moore, F.M. and G.W. Thornton (1983). Telangiectasia of Pembroke Welsh Corgi dogs. *Vet Pathol* **20**: 203–208.

Morton, L.D., et al. (1990). Juvenile renal disease in miniature schnauzer dogs. *Vet Pathol* **27**: 455–458.

Nash, A.S., et al. (1984). Progressive renal disease in soft-coated Wheaten terriers: possible familial nephropathy. *J Small Anim Pract* **25**: 479–487.

Niewold, T.A., et al. (1999). Familial amyloidosis in cats: Siamese and Abyssinian AA proteins differ in primary sequence and pattern of deposition. *Amyloid*. **6**: 205–209.

Noonan, C.H.B. and J.M. Kay (1990). Prevalence and geographic distribution of Fanconi syndrome in Basenjis in the United States. *J Am Vet Med Assoc* **197**: 345–349.

O'Brien, T.D., et al. (1982). Clinicopathologic manifestations of progressive renal disease in Lhasa Apso and Shih Tzu dogs. *J Am Vet Med Assoc* **180**: 658–664.

O'Leary, C.A., et al. (1999). Polycystic kidney disease in Bull Terriers: an autosomal dominant inherited disorder. *Aust Vet J* **77**: 361–366.

O'Leary, C.A., et al. (2002). Renal pathology of polycystic kidney disease and concurrent hereditary nephritis in Bull Terriers. *Aust Vet J* **80**: 353–361.

O'Leary, C.A., et al. (2003). No disease-associated mutations found in the coding sequence of the canine polycystic kidney disease gene 1 in Bull Terriers with polycystic kidney disease. *Anim Genet* **34**: 358–361.

Picut, C.A. and R.M. Lewis (1987a). Juvenile renal disease in the Doberman Pinscher: ultrastructural changes of the glomerular basement membrane. *J Comp Pathol* **97**: 587–596.

Picut, C.A. and R.M. Lewis (1987b). Microscopic features of canine renal dysplasia. *Vet Pathol* **24**: 156–163.

Reusch, C., et al. (1994). A new familial glomerulonephropathy in Bernese mountain dogs. *Vet Rec* **134**: 411–415.

Rha, J.Y., et al. (2000). Familial glomerulonephropathy in a litter of beagles. *J Am Vet Med Assoc* **216**: 46–50.

Rivas, A.L., et al. (1992). A canine febrile disorder associated with elevated interleukin-6. *Clin Immunol Immunopathol* **64**: 36–45.

Rivas, A.L., et al. (1993). Inheritance of renal amyloidosis in Chinese Shar-pei dogs. *J Hered* **84**: 438–442.

Robinson, W.F., et al. (1989). Chronic renal disease in bull terriers. *Aust Vet J* **66**: 193–195.

Schulze, C., et al. (1998). Renal dysplasia in three young adult Dutch kooiker dogs. *Vet Q* **20**: 146–148.

Vaden, S.L., et al. (2000a). Food hypersensitivity reactions in Soft Coated Wheaten Terriers with protein-losing enteropathy or protein-losing nephropathy or both: gastroscopic food sensitivity testing, dietary provocation, and fecal immunoglobulin E. *J Vet Intern Med* **14**: 60–67.

Vaden, S.L., et al. (2000b). Evaluation of intestinal permeability and gluten sensitivity in Soft-Coated Wheaten Terriers with familial protein-losing enteropathy, protein-losing nephropathy, or both. *Am J Vet Res* **61**: 518–524.

Vilafranca, M. and L. Ferrer (1994). Juvenile nephropathy in Alaskan Malamute littermates. *Vet Pathol* **31**: 375–377.

Wakamatsu, N., et al. (2007). Histologic and ultrastructural studies of juvenile onset renal disease in four Rottweiler dogs. *Vet Pathol* **44**: 96–100.

Wilcock, B.P. and J.M. Patterson (1979). Familial glomerulonephritis in Doberman pinscher dogs. *Can Vet J* **20**: 244–249.

Yearley, J.H., et al. (2004). Survival time, lifespan, and quality of life in dogs with idiopathic Fanconi syndrome. *J Am Vet Med Assoc* **225**: 377–383.

Zheng, K., et al. (1994). Canine X chromosome-linked hereditary nephritis: a genetic model for human X-linked hereditary nephritis resulting from a single base mutation in the gene encoding the alpha 5 chain of collagen type IV. *Proc Natl Acad Sci U S A* **91**: 3989–3993.

Zuber, R.M. (1993). Systemic amyloidosis in Oriental and Siamese cats. *Aust Vet Pract* **23**: 66–70.

57

Renal neoplasia

Carolyn Henry

Etiology and prevalence

Renal tumors may either be primary tumors or metastatic lesions from other primary sites. Of the metastatic renal tumors, lymphoma is one that may also present as a primary renal tumor, without evidence of lymphoma elsewhere in the body. As such, lymphoma will be included in the discussion of primary renal tumors that follows. Non-lymphoma primary renal neoplasia may be of mesothelial (sarcoma), epithelial (carcinoma), or mixed embryonal (nephroblastoma) origin. A list of reported canine and feline renal tumors is shown in Table 57.1. Of these, carcinomas are the most common primary renal tumors in dogs, accounting for approximately 60% of all cases. Sarcomas and nephroblastomas are less common, accounting for 34% and 6% of primary canine renal tumors, respectively, in one case series (Bryan 2006). In a report of 19 cats with primary non-lymphoma renal neoplasia, carcinomas were overwhelmingly represented with only one sarcoma, one nephroblastoma, and one adenoma (Henry 1999). Renal non-lymphoma neoplasia is relatively rare, accounting for less than 2% of all canine neoplasms (Baskin 1977; Sapierzynski 2006). Non-lymphoma primary neoplasia of the feline kidney is even less common, accounting for approximately 0.5% of all feline neoplasms (Henry 1999; Sapierzynski 2006). Overall, renal cell cancer is considered 4.5 times more likely in dogs than in cats (Meuten 2002). Older animals are most often affected, although nephroblastomas have been reported in young dogs and cats (Caywood 1980; Frimberger 1995). This is analogous to the juvenile onset of Wilms' tumor in people.

The cause of most primary renal neoplasia is unknown, although feline renal lymphoma may be associated with

FeLV (Mooney 1987). Dogs and cats with renal neoplasia are usually geriatric with the exceptions of FeLV-associated renal lymphoma and the aforementioned canine renal nephroblastoma (Bryan 2006). A male predominance has been reported for renal carcinomas in dogs, but this is not consistent across the literature (Hayes 1977; Klein 1988; Frimberger 1995; Meuten 2002). A male gender predisposition is also reported for all renal tumor types in cats, but small numbers of overall cases limit the ability to adequately assess this (Henry 1999; Meuten 2002; Sapierzynski 2006). The suspected male predisposition to renal cancer in dogs and cats is consistent with the male predominance reported for people (Meuten 2002; Linehan 2005).

Renal tumors may be unilateral or bilateral, although renal lymphoma in cats is usually bilateral (Mooney 1987). In a review of 82 dogs with non-lymphoma primary renal tumors, only carcinomas occurred bilaterally (Bryan 2006). Bilateral renal oncocytoma has been reported in a greyhound (Buergelt 2000). One other unique renal tumor that occurs bilaterally is the renal cystadenocarcinoma associated with nodular dermatofibrosis in German Shepherd dogs. (Moe 1997; Jonasdottir 2000) A mutation in the Birt-Hogg-Dube gene has been shown to be responsible for this syndrome. (Lingaas 2003) No other breed predispositions have been identified.

Clinical signs

In the early stage of disease, non-lymphoma primary renal tumors typically cause few clinical signs. Renal lymphoma may, on the other hand, be associated with clinical signs of illness or renal failure and renal cystadenocarcinoma of German Shepherd dogs may be first suspected due to presence of nodular skin lesions. Some of the clinical signs reported for dogs and cats

Nephrology and Urology of Small Animals. Edited by Joe Bartges and David J. Polzin. © 2011 Blackwell Publishing Ltd.

Table 57.1 Reported canine and feline primary renal tumors[a]

Epithelial	Mesenchymal	Others
Renal carcinoma	Spindle cell sarcoma	Lymphoma
Transitional cell carcinoma (Militerno 2003)	Osteosarcoma (Munday 2004)	Nephroblastoma
Transitional cell papilloma	Hemangiosarcoma (Ohler 1994; Locke 2006)	Giant cell tumor (Haziroglu 2005)
Tubular adenocarcinoma	Hemangioma (Peterson 1981; Eddlestone 1999)	Oncocytoma (Dempster 2000; Buergelt 2000)
Tubular and papillary adenocarcinoma	Renal sarcoma	
Renal adenocarcinoma	Leiomyosarcoma (Sato 2003)	
	Leiomyoma (Laluha 2006)	
Sarcomatoid renal adenocarcinoma (Britt 1985)	Malignant fibrous histiocytoma	
Renal tubular carcinoma	Fibroleiomyosarcoma	
Renal papillary carcinoma	Fibroma	
Clear cell renal carcinoma	Mixed mesenchymal tumor	
Papillary cystadenocarcinoma	Angiomyolipoma (Wang 2001)	
Renal Adenoma		

[a]Reported in Klein (1988), Henry (1999), or Bryan (2006) unless otherwise noted.

with primary renal tumors are listed in Table 57.2. Typical presenting complaints for symptomatic patients include lethargy, hematuria, palpable renomegaly, inappetance and weight loss (Klein 1988; Henry 1999; Bryan 2006). In advanced cases, patients may present in crisis, with acute collapse, hemoabdomen, ascites, or severe renal failure. Dogs with primary renal hemangiosarcoma (HSA) may present with hemoabdomen, but this occurs less frequently than with HSA of other visceral sites (Locke 2006). Overall, the course of renal HSA appears to be more insidious than that of HSA affecting other visceral sites, with a 60-day median duration of nonspecific clinical signs prior to diagnosis (Locke 2006). Dogs and cats with paraneoplastic polycythemia may be asymptomatic or may present with neurological signs including convulsions and seizures (Faissler 1998; Henry 1999).

Physical examination of affected patients may reveal pale mucous membranes, renomegaly, abdominal distension with a fluid wave, and flank pain. The latter is reportedly more common with renal sarcomas (Bryan 2006). Hemogram abnormalities tend to be non-specific, with the exception of polycythemia. However, most affected animals present with anemia, rather than with polycythemia (Klein 1988; Henry 1999; Bryan 2006). Serum biochemical analysis also tends to reveal nonspecific abnormalities. Fewer than 25% of affected dogs have serum biochemical changes (Bryan 2006). It has been reported that hypoalbuminemia is less common in dogs with renal sarcoma than with renal carcinoma or nephroblastoma (Bryan 2006). Proteinuria, hematuria, and pyuria may be detected on urinalysis, either associ-

ated with a secondary bacterial infection or due to the primary tumor (Frimberger 1995).

Diagnosis

Renal neoplasia is most often detected via radiographic or ultrasound imaging of the abdomen. Of these two methods, ultrasound is a more sensitive method of detection and permits evaluation of the renal architecture. Contrast radiographs (intravenous pyelogram) may improve the likelihood of detecting renal neoplasia, compared to plain film radiographs (Klein 1988; Bryan 2006). Advanced imaging with computed tomography or magnetic resonance imaging may be used to better define the size and extent of primary renal tumors and to facilitate surgical planning. See Table 57.3 for suggested diagnostic examinations. The Veterinary Bladder Tumor Antigen test (V-BTA, Alidex Inc., Redmond, WA) may have application for detecting intraluminal carcinomas of the kidney, although its use in this capacity is largely untested (Henry 2003).

Although lymphoma may arise primarily within the kidney, metastasis to or from other sites must be ruled out. In both feline and canine renal lymphoma, a tendency for metastasis to the central nervous system is reported (Mooney 1987; Batchelor 2006). Carcinomas can arise from the transitional urothelial lining or from the renal epithelium, resulting in simple carcinomas or adenocarcinomas with tubular or papillary differentiation. Clear cell renal carcinomas are characterized by clear-appearing cytoplasm caused by glycogen and lipid

Table 57.2 Characteristics of dogs with primary renal tumors

	Bryan (2006)	Klein (1988)
Carcinomas	60%	85%
Sarcomas	34%	11%
Nephroblastomas	6%	4%
MST carcinoma	16 months	8 months
MST sarcoma	9 months	NR
MST nephroblastoma	6 months	NR
Thoracic metastasis at diagnosis	16%	48%
Metastasis at death	77%	85%
Mean age at diagnosis	8.1 years	9.1 years
Bilateral disease	4%	32.4% Necropsied
Clinical signs		
Hematuria	32%	26%
Palpable abdominal mass	20%	41%
Inappetance	27%	50%
Pain	7%	15%
Weight loss	20%	39%
Hemogram abnormalities		
Anemia	33%	26%
Leukocytosis	20%	11%
Polycythemia	4.5%	2%
Serum biochemical abnormalities		
Elevated alkaline phosphatase	22%	15%
Elevated BUN	22%	26%
Elevated creatinine	20%	9%
Decreased albumin	19%	NR
Urinalysis abnormalities		
Hematuria	57%	33% gross 50% microscopic
Pyuria	53%	NR
Proteinuria	48%	61%
Isosthenuria	36%	NR

MST, median survival time.
Source: Adapted with permission from Henry and Higginbotham Small Animal Clinical Oncology, 2009, Elsevier.

content (Meuten 2002). These tumors tend to be a variant of simple or solid carcinoma.

Various paraneoplastic syndromes including fever, hypertrophic osteopathy, leukocytosis, polycythemia, hepatopathy, and hypoglycemia have been reported to occur with primary renal neoplasia (Lappin 1988; Henry 1999; Peeters 2001; Zini 2003; Battaglia 2005; Chiang 2006; Grillo 2007). Polycythemia may occur secondary to tumor production of erythropoietin, or because tumor-induced renal hypoxia causes the remaining normal tissue to over-produce erythropoietin (Peterson 1981). Hypertrophic osteopathy may occur both with primary nonmetastatic renal neoplasia and with renal malignancy that has metastasized to the thoracic cavity (Brodey 1958; Lucke 1976; Caywood 1980; Peeters 2001).

The metastatic rate for canine renal carcinomas has been reported to be as high as 48% at diagnosis, with 69% of all dogs having metastastic disease at death (Klein 1988; Bryan 2006). Sarcomas may arise from any of the mesenchymal cell populations within the kidney, and have a reported metastatic rate of 88% in dogs (Bryan 2006). The biologic behavior of canine nephroblastoma tends to be similar to that of carcinomas and sarcomas and the reported metastatic rate is 75% (Bryan 2006). Approximately two-thirds of all cats affected with primary renal neoplasia develop metastasis, with the exception of transitional cell carcinoma, for which the metastatic rate appears to be much higher (Henry 1999). Metastatic disease was identified in all 8 cats with renal TCC reported in the two largest feline renal tumor case series to date. (Carpenter 1987; Henry 1999) Benign renal tumors including hemangioma, adenoma, fibroma, and leiomyoma are occasionally reported in both species (Klein 1988; Mott 1996; Henry 1999). However, it is not uncommon for difficulty to arise in differentiating between benign (adenoma) and malignant (carcinoma) epithelial lesions on the basis of histological examination (Carpenter 1987; Henry 1999). Likewise, misdiagnosis of feline renal lymphoma as carcinoma has been reported in two case series (Carpenter 1987; Henry 1999). As such, it has been advised that a second opinion be routinely requested when a diagnosis of feline primary renal neoplasia is reported (Henry 1999).

Treatment

Therapy goals when treating primary renal neoplasia are dependent upon tumor type, location, and associated clinical signs and paraneoplastic syndromes. Acute therapy is often focused on stabilizing the patient prior to surgery by restoring blood volume, raising or lowering the hematocrit to a safe level, and minimizing azotemia. Surgical resection is the only therapy that has a demonstrated survival benefit for primary non-lymphoma renal tumors in dogs to date (Bryan 2006). Goals of surgery may include removal of the mass to halt hemorrhage, eliminate tumor cells in the body, and alleviate clinical signs and paraneoplastic syndromes. It is important to verify a lack of neoplastic disease in and adequate function of the remaining kidney if complete nephrectomy is recommended. Furthermore, ligation of the renal vein and removal of the entire ureter with the kidney is advised to minimize potential seeding or hematogenous spread of cancer cells (Fossum 2007). At the time of surgery, it is imperative that the opposite ureter be identified, so as to ensure that it is not unintentionally transected in the course of removing a large neoplasm (Fossum 2007). In one report, dogs undergoing surgery had a median

Table 57.3 Diagnostic Evaluation of Primary Renal Tumors

Diagnostic Evaluation of Primary Renal Tumors	
Test	Indications and/or results suggestive of renal neoplasia
CBC	Anemia, polycythemia
Chemistry profile	Azotemia, hypoproteinemia, hypoalbuminemia, elevated alkaline phosphatase
Urinalysis	Proteinuria, hematuria, pyuria, isosthenuria
Thoracic radiographs	Metastatic disease
Abdominal radiographs	Mid to dorsal abdominal mass, renomegaly, peritoneal effusion, retroperitoneal effusion
Abdominal ultrasound	Renal mass, metastatic disease (all organs possible)
Fine needle aspirate	May help differentiate carcinoma, sarcoma, lymphoma
Needle biopsy	May yield definitive diagnosis
Echocardiogram[a]	Rule out heart-based mass if hemangiosarcoma
V-BTA[a]	May be positive in renal TCC
Renal scintigraphy[a]	Confirm adequate renal function

Source: Adapted with permission from Henry and Higginbotham Small Animal Clinical Oncology, 2009, Elsevier.
[a]Additional/auxiliary tests.

survival time of 16 months compared to one month for those not treated surgically (Bryan 2006). Survival times exceeding four years have been reported for some dogs undergoing surgical resection of primary renal neoplasia (Lucke 1976; Bryan 2006).

Paraneoplastic syndromes often resolve within days to weeks of complete tumor excision. This is true not only for clinicopathologic abnormalities, but also for hypertrophic osteopathy when it is due to a nonmetastatic renal mass (Caywood 1980; Lappin 1988; Peeters 2001; Seaman 2003).

The only renal tumor for which chemotherapy is demonstrated to be of benefit is lymphoma (Mooney 1987; Batchelor 2006). The use of cytosine arabinoside as part of the chemotherapy protocol in dogs and cats with renal lymphoma is advocated in an effort to penetrate the CNS, given the likelihood of CNS metastasis associated with renal lymphoma in both species (Mooney 1987; Batchelor 2006). For non-lymphoma renal neoplasia, no chemotherapy provides a demonstrated survival benefit (Bryan 2006).

Prospective evaluation of protocols incorporating antimetabolites (i.e., gemcitabine and 5-FU), as are used in people with renal cancer, has not yet been reported in the veterinary literature (Linehan 2005). In one report of a dog with a surgically excised nephroblastoma, adjuvant vincristine and doxorubicin chemotherapy was administered (Seaman 2003). The dog was free of disease at the time of the report, more than 25 months after diagnosis. However, one can only speculate as to the impact of adjuvant chemotherapy in this case. Immunotherapy, another standard of care in human renal carcinomas, has not been adequately evaluated in dogs or cats (Linehan 2005).

Cyclooxygenase-2 expression has been demonstrated in two of three canine renal carcinomas in one report. (Khan 2001). However, a prospective evaluation of the efficacy of COX-2 inhibitors against renal carcinomas in dogs has not been done. The risk of impairing renal function with these agents would need to be weighed against the likelihood of inducing tumor remission.

Prognosis

Information regarding reported median survival times of dogs with various renal malignancies can be found in Table 57.2.

The prognosis for dogs with renal HSA is affected by whether or not hemoperitoneum is present at the time of diagnosis. While the median survival time for 14 dogs with hemangiosarcoma in one report was 278 days with a 1-year survival rate of 29%, those that presented with hemoperitoneum ($n = 2$) had a median survival time of only 62 days. Overall, the prognosis for renal HSA in dogs appears to be better than that seen with cardiac or splenic HSA. This may be due, in part, to the low metastatic rate at initial diagnosis (Locke 2006). There are too few reports of renal nephroblastoma to permit meaningful assessment of prognosis. Survival times in the dog have ranged from weeks to greater than two years, depending upon tumor stage and histopathology. The most favorable prognosis is afforded in cases with Stage I (confined to the kidney without disruption of the renal capsule or involvement of the renal sinus) disease that can be completely excised. Most reports of dogs treated for renal lymphoma indicate a poor outcome, with survival times of two months or less (Nelson 1983; Lascelles 2003; Snead 2005). However, there is one report of longer term survival (346 days) for a dog with bilateral renal lymphoma treated with vincristine, cyclophosphamide, cytosine arabinoside, and prednisolone (Batchelor 2006).

Case outcome data for cats with primary renal malignancy is scant in veterinary literature, but survival beyond one year is rarely reported. Cats with renal lymphoma have a wide range of survival times from days to more than six years (Mooney 1987). Low tumor stage and negative FeLV status are prognostic for better outcome with renal lymphoma.

References

Baskin, G.B. (1977). Primary renal tumors of the dog. *Vet Pathol* **14**(6): 591–605.

Batchelor, D.J. (2006). Long-term survival after combination chemotherapy for bilateral renal malignant lymphoma in a dog. *N Z Vet J* **54**(3): 147–150.

Battaglia, L. (2005). Hypoglycaemia as a paraneoplastic syndrome associated with renal adenocarcinoma in a dog. *Vet Res Commun* **29**: 671–675.

Britt, J.O. (1985). Sarcomatoid renal adenocarcinoma in a cat. *Vet Pathol* **22**(5): 514–515.

Brodey, R. (1958). Hypertrophic osteoarthropathy in a dog with pulmonary metastasis arising from a renal adenocarcinoma. *J Am Vet Med Assoc* **132**(6): 232–237.

Bryan, J.N. (2006). Primary renal neoplasia of dogs: a retrospective review of 82 cases. *J Vet Intern Med* **20**(5): 1155–1160.

Buergelt, C.D. (2000). Bilateral renal oncocytoma in a Greyhound dog. *Vet Path* **37**(2): 188–192.

Carpenter, J.L. (1987). Tumors and tumor-like lesions. In: *Disease of the Cat—Medicine and Surgery*, edited by J. Holzworth, 1st edition. Philadelphia, PA: WB Saunders, pp. 406–596.

Caywood, D.D. (1980). Hypertrophic osteoarthropathy associated with an atypical nephrolastoma in a dog. *J Am Anim Hosp Assoc* **16**(6): 855–865.

Chiang, Y-C. (2006). Hypertrophic osteopathy associated with disseminated metastasis of renal cell carcinoma in the dog: a case report. *J Vet Med Sci* **69**(2): 209–212.

Dempster, A.G. (2000). The histology and growth kinetics of canine renal oncocytoma. *J Comp Pathol* **123**(4): 294–298.

Eddlestone, S. (1999). Renal haemangioma in a dog. *J Small Anim Pract* **40**(3): 132–135.

Faissler, D. (1998). Convulsions in relation to polycythemia: literature review and case description. *Schweiz Arch Tierheilkd* **140**(3): 101–109.

Fossum, T.W. (2007). Surgery of the kidney and ureter. In: *Small Animal Surgery*, edited by T.W. Fossum, 3rd edition. St. Louis, MO: Mosby, Inc., pp. 635–662.

Frimberger, A.E. (1995). Treatment of nephroblastoma in a juvenile dog. *J Am Vet Med Assoc* **207**(5): 596–598.

Grillo, T.P. (2007). Hypertrophic osteopathy associated with renal pelvis transitional cell carcinoma in a dog. *Can Vet J* **48**: 745–747.

Hayes, H.M. Jr. (1977). Epidemiological features of canine renal neoplasms. *Cancer Res* **37**(8pt1): 2553–2556.

Haziroglu, R. (2005). Osteoclast-like giant cell tumor arising from the kidney in a dog. *Acta Veterinaria Hungarica* **53**(2): 225–230.

Henry, C.J. (1999). Primary renal tumors in cats: 19 cases (1992–1998). *J Feline Med Surg* **1**(3): 165–170.

Henry, C.J. (2003). Evaluation of a bladder tumor antigen test as a screening test for transitional cell carcinoma of the lower urinary tract in dogs. *Am J Vet Res* **64**(8): 1017–1020.

Jonasdottir, T.J. (2000). Genetic mapping of a naturally occurring hereditary renal cancer syndrome in dogs. *Proc Natl Acad Sci U S A* **97**(8): 4132–4137.

Khan, K.N.M. (2001). Expression of cyclooxygenase-2 in canine renal cell carcinoma. *Vet Pathol* **38**(1): 116–119.

Klein, M.K. (1988). Canine primary renal neoplasms: a retrospective review of 54 cases. *J Am Anim Hosp Assoc* **24**(4): 443–452.

Laluha, P. (2006). Leiomyoma of a kidney in a dog: a rare diagnosis. *Schweiz Arch Tierheilkd* **148**(6): 303–307.

Lappin, M.R. (1988). Hematuria and extreme neutrophilic leukocytosis in a dog with renal tubular carcinoma. *J Am Vet Med Assoc* **192**(9): 1289–1292.

Lascelles, B.D.X. (2003). Surgical treatment of right-sided renal lymphoma with invasion of the caudal vena cava. *J Small Anim Pract* **44**(3): 135–138.

Linehan, W.M. (2005). Cancer of the kidney. In: *Cancer Principles and Practice of Oncology*, edited by V.T. DeVita, Jr., S. Hellman, and S.A. Rosenberg, 7th edition. Philadelphia, PA: Lippincott, Williams and Wilkins, pp. 1139–1168.

Lingaas, F. (2003). A mutation in the canine BHD gene is associated with hereditary multifocal renal cystadenocarcinoma and nodular dermatofibrosis in the German Shepherd dog. *Hum Mol Gen* **12**(23): 3043–3053.

Locke, J.E. (2006). Comparative aspects and clinical outcomes of canine renal hemangiosarcoma. *J Vet Intern Med* **20**(4): 962–967.

Lucke, V.M. (1976). Renal carcinoma in the dog. *Vet Pathol* **13**(4): 264–276.

Meuten, D.J. (2002). Tumors of the urinary system. In: *Tumors in Domestic Animals*, edited by D.J. Meuten. Ames, IA: Iowa State Press, pp. 509–546.

Militerno, G. (2003). Transitional cell carcinoma of the renal pelvis in two dogs. *J Vet Med A* **50**: 457–459.

Moe, L. (1997). Hereditary multifocal renal cystadenocarcinoma and nodular dermatofibrosis in 51 German shepherd dogs. *J Small Anim Pract* **38**(11): 498–505.

Mooney, S.C. (1987). Renal lymphoma in cats: 28 cases (1977–1984). *J Am Vet Med Assoc* **191**(11): 1473–1477.

Mott, J.C. (1996). Nephron sparing by partial median nephrectomy for treatment of renal hemangioma in a dog. *J Am Vet Med Assoc* **208**(8): 1274–1276.

Munday, J.S. (2004). Renal osteosarcoma in a dog. *J Small Anim Pract* **45**(12): 618–622.

Nelson, R.W. (1983). Renal lymphosarcoma with inappropriate erythropoietin production in a dog. *J Am Vet Med Assoc* **182**(12): 1396–1397,

Ohler, C. (1994). Transient hemi-inattention in a dog with metastatic renal hemangiosarcoma. *J Am Anim Hosp Assoc* **30**: 207.

Peeters, D. (2001). Resolution of paraneoplastic leukocytosis and hypertrophic osteopathy after resection of a renal transitional cell carcinoma producing granulocyte-macrophage colony-stimulating factor in a young Bull Terrier. *J Vet Intern Med* **15**(4): 407–411.

Peterson, M.E. (1981). Inappropriate erythropoietin production from a renal carcinoma in a dog with polycythemia. *J Am Vet Med Assoc* **179**(10): 995–996.

Sapierzynski, R. (2006). Tumors of the urinary and genital systems in dogs and cats. Part I. Neoplasms of the kidney, urinary bladder and urethra. *Zycie Weterynaryjne* **81**(11): 739–743.

Sato, T. (2003). Leiomyosarcoma of the kidney in a dog. *J Vet Med A Physiol Pathol Clin Med* **50**(7): 366–369.

Seaman, R.L. (2003). Treatment of renal nephroblastoma in an adult dog. *J Am Anim Hosp Assoc* **39**(1): 76–79.

Snead, E.C. (2005). A case of bilateral renal lymphosarcoma with secondary polycythemia and paraneoplastic syndromes of hypogly-caemia and uvieitis in an English springer spaniel. *Vet Comp Oncol* **3**(3): 139–144.

Wang, F.I. (2001). Unilateral concurrence of pyelocaliceal diverticula and intracapsular angiomyolipoma in the kidney of a cat. *J Vet Diagn Invest* **13**(2): 167–169.

Zini, E. (2003). Sarcomatoid renal cell carcinoma with osteogenic differentiation and paraneoplastic hepatopathy in a dog, possi-bly related to human Stauffer's syndrome. *J Comp Pathol* **129**(4): 303–307.

58

Diseases of the ureter

Gilad Segev

Anatomy

The ureters are fibromuscular ducts carrying urine from the kidney to the urinary bladder (UB) by peristaltic activity transmitted from one muscle cell to the next (Osborne and Fletcher 1995). The ureters originate in the renal pelves and travel retroperitonealy along the aorta and vena cava, towards the UB. Near the pelvis, they join the lateral ligament of the bladder and insert into the dorsolateral aspect of the UB. The ureters cross the bladder wall obliquely and open into its neck in the trigon.

Vesicoureteral reflux

Vesicoureteral reflux is a retrograde urine movement from the UB to the ureters. It occurs when intravesicular pressure increases above intra-ureteral pressure. Normally, as the UB fills, the intravesicular pressure compresses the ureters, due to their oblique course through the bladder wall, thus preventing reflux (vesicoureteral valve). The length and diameter of the ureteral submucosal portion, its peristaltics, ureteral–UB pressure gradient, and detrusor muscle integrity are all factors that influence the vesicoureteral valve function. Vesicoureteral reflux is common in young animals and probably results from undeveloped ureterovesicular junction; however, it is often transient as the length of the ureteral submucosal portion increases during maturation (Christie 1973). Vesicoureteral reflux was documented in 10% of clinically normal adults dogs, more commonly in females, and was usually bilateral (Christie 1973). Reflux may be primary, or secondary to obstruction, ectopic ureters, infection, neuropathies, neoplasia, or iatrogenic ureteral or vesicular lesions. It may lead to renal damage if the refluxed urine is contaminated or in severe cases when

voiding pressure is transmitted to the renal pelvis. Reflux also predisposes to lower urinary tract infection (UTI) by urine recontamination and thus should be evaluated in cases of refractory UTI.

Diagnosis is based on various imaging techniques, using iodine-based contrast material infused into the UB. Radiographs are taken when the bladder is maximally distended, during voiding or after manual compression. Results should be interpreted with caution as reflux may occur in normal patients, depending on the type and depth of anesthesia and degree of bladder distention and compression (Christie 1973). Alternatively, reflux can be evaluated cystoscopically by filling the UB with dye and observing ureteral urine flow into the UB after dye was cleared from the bladder.

In young animals, treatment is not always indicated as the disorder is often self limiting. UTIs should be treated aggressively to prevent pyelonephritis, and urine should remain sterile as long as reflux is present. In adults, diagnostics are warranted to identify underlying ureteral or UB causes to facilitate therapy.

Ureterocele

Ureterocele is a cystic dilatation of the intravesicular sub-mucosal portion of the distal ureter (Tanagho 1972; McLoughlin and Bjorling 2003). Ureterocele is classified as orthotopic (simple), when it is entirely intravesicular, or ectopic. Ureteroceles, mostly congenital, were reported infrequently in dogs and as a single feline case report (McLoughlin et al. 1989; Stiffler et al. 2002; Eisele et al. 2005). It has also been reported as a complication of ectopic ureter correction in a dog (Martin et al. 1985). Like ectopic ureters, ureterocele is often concurrently present with other congenital abnormalities (McLoughlin and Bjorling 2003). Clinical signs include abdominal pain, lower urinary tract signs, and incontinence

Nephrology and Urology of Small Animals. Edited by Joe Bartges and David J. Polzin. © 2011 Blackwell Publishing Ltd.

(when ectopic). Complications associated with uretero- cele include UTI, ureteral obstruction (ipsilateral, con- tralateral or both), urethral obstruction, and secondary renal damage. Clinical signs are more likely in ectopic compared to orthotopic ureterocele; however, both can be asymptomatic.

Diagnosis is based on imaging techniques using ultra- sonography, CT, uroendoscopy, and contrast radiogra- phy, which can also demonstrate ureterocele patency (Lamb 1998; McLoughlin and Bjorling 2003). Uretero- celes may appear on as a "cobra head" sign in excretory urography or as a vesicular negative filling defect if the ipsilateral kidney function is impaired. Ultrasonograph- ically, simple ureterocele is a rounded thin-walled intra- vesicular hypoechoic structure. Ureteral communication can be demonstrated if the ureter is dilated (Lamb 1998).

Treatment aims include elimination of clinical signs, preservation of renal function, and prevention of vesi- coureteral reflux. Various surgical procedures have been described, including ureteronephrectomy, transurethral endoscopic incision, ureterocele omentalization, uretero- neocystostomy, and ureterocelectomy (Tattersall and Welsh 2006). Surgery must be individualized to the patient and is usually associated with a favorable outcome with complete elimination of clinical signs and improve- ment of hydronephrosis. If reflux is present, ureteroneo- cystostomy should be considered.

Ureteral obstruction

Ureteral obstruction (UO) may lead to a rapid build up of uremic toxins and progressive renal damage. The pres- ence of azotemia depends on the contralateral kidney function, the number of affected ureters, and the obstruc- tion severity. Although mostly acquired, congenital UO has been reported both in dogs and cats. UO can be clas- sified as intraluminal, intramural, and extramural. It can also be classified as acute or chronic, static or dynamic, partial or complete, and by its location. Intraluminal obstruction is the most common cause for UO in dogs and cats. It is usually caused by ureteral calculi; however, blood clots and inflammatory debris may also obstruct the ureter, particularly in cats. Intramural UO can result from a stricture, neoplasia (primary or metastasis), urete- rocele, fibroepithelial polyps, and proliferative ureteritis. Extramural UO results from retroperitoneal space occu- pying lesions, inadvertent ureteral ligation, or UB pathol- ogy. The incidence of feline UO has increased dramat- ically over the recent years and is a common etiology of acute uremia in cats (Kyles et al. 2005a). It typically results from ureteroliths, which are almost exclusively composed of calcium oxalate (Kyles et al. 2005a). UO is a challenging disorder often requiring highly sophisticated

diagnostic and therapeutic aids as well as unique surgical skills.

The pathophysiology of naturally occurring UO is not well documented. Most cats with UO present for medical care with advanced disease and both kidneys affected, although unilateral ureteroliths are more com- monly identified. (Kyles et al. 2005a) The severe azotemia present in most of these cats attests for a compromised contralateral kidney. The mechanical obstruction is aggravated by secondary local inflammation and spasm. Local ureteral damage (e.g., rupture and stricture) is a potential complication of UO, but increased intraureteral hydraulic pressure and decreased renal blood flow are more common consequences. The increased hydraulic pressure translates to increased pressure within renal tubules and Bowman's space and when high enough, may stop glomerular filtration altogether. If the contralat- eral renal function is preserved, clinical signs if present, are pain-related, and often overlooked, thus the episode may go unnoticed. If the obstruction is dynamic, it may resolve spontaneously. The degree and chronicity of UO are major factors determining the fate of the obstructed kidney. Prolonged and complete UO will result in renal fibrosis and/or hydronephrotic atrophy, however, if the obstruction resolves, these changes may not occur or may be incomplete. Thus, the affected kidney may have residual or normal function. Recurrent UO may lead to progressive renal damage.

If a complete UO does not resolve, renal fibrosis of the ipsilateral kidney and compensatory hypertrophy of the contralateral kidney occur. The end result is one small kidney and one large kidney–"big kidney-little kidney syndrome". Typically, patients are free of uremic signs at this steady state unless ureteral rupture has occurred, but may present pain related signs. Acute uremia man- ifests following obstruction of the hypertrophic kidney. Its severity depends on the degree of UO and the residual contralateral kidney function. If one ureter is completely obstructed, the severity of azotemia reflects the contralat- eral kidney function.

The clinical manifestation of UO can be acute or chronic and may result from uremia or from pain due to direct ureteral stimulation at the obstruction site and stretch of the collecting system and the renal capsule. Clinical signs are often nonspecific and include decreased appetite, lethargy, vomiting, hematuria and pain (Kyles et al. 2005a; Snyder et al. 2005). Interestingly, many azotemic cats with UO present a considerably better clin- ical demeanor compared to cats with similar levels of azotemia of other causes. Oliguria and anuria may be present; however, their absence does not rule out com- plete unilateral UO as urine may be produced by the contralateral kidney, even if the latter does not contribute substantially to overall GFR. Abdominal palpation may reveal abdominal pain (more common in dogs) and asymmetric kidneys, which is highly suggestive of UO. Typically, in cats with UO one kidney is small and irregular while the other is enlarged, firm and painful.

Common laboratory abnormalities of cats with ureteroliths included normocytic normochromic anemia (~50%), azotemia (80%), and hyperkalemia (35%) (Kyles et al. 2005a), whereas in dogs leukocytosis (50%) and azotemia (56%) are common (Snyder et al. 2005). Recent renal function data prior to the obstruction is extremely useful in azotemic patients when assessing the potential function of the obstructed kidney and the likelihood for successful outcome once ureteral patency has been restored. The relative contribution of each kidney and overall GFR are vital information that can guide therapy; however, these are difficult to assess as long as the obstruction is present. Urinalysis and urine sediment examination may demonstrate RBC, WBC, casts, crystals, and bacteria. Fifty percent of dogs and 8% of cats with ureteroliths have positive urine culture (Kyles et al. 2005a; Snyder et al. 2005). Only 6.5% of cats presented calcium oxalate crystaluria (Kyles et al. 2005a).

The diagnosis of UO is based on the history, clinical and clinicopathological signs and is confirmed by imaging techniques, often used in conjunction. The aim is to identify an obstruction and to assess the severity of secondary renal damage. Survey radiographs may demonstrate ureteroliths, as most are radio-opaque, with a reported sensitivity of ~80% (Kyles et al. 2005a; Snyder et al. 2005). Radiographs are extremely useful to follow ureteroliths' location and to determine if the obstruction is static or dynamic. Ultrasounography is a readily available non-invasive and useful tool to detect UO and to assess renal geometry and architecture. It had 77% and 100% sensitivity of detecting ureteroliths in cats and dogs, respectively (Kyles et al. 2005a; Snyder et al. 2005), but it is very equipment and operator-dependent. Typically, a shadowing hyperechoic structure consistent with an ureterolith is identified with a proximally torturous and dilated ureter. Hydronephrosis and dilatation of the collecting system may take days to develop, thus, their absence should not rule out UO. Dilatation progresses from proximally to distally, but may not necessarily reach the level of the obstruction. In cats with UO, typically one small kidney with chronic changes is observed while the other is enlarged with varying degree of hydronephrosis. Evaluation of chronic ipsilateral renal structural changes is essential, because if the obstructed kidney presents advanced chronic changes or marked hydronephrosis and marked parencymal loss the prognosis for renal function recovery once UO is relieved is poor. Combination of radiography and ultrasonography

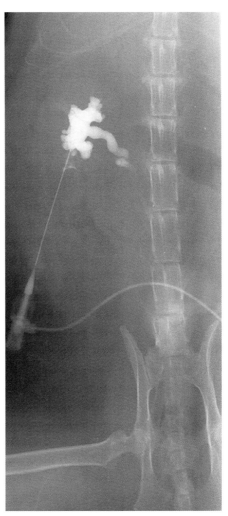

Figure 58.1 Ventrodorsal projection of ultrasonographic guided antegrade pyelography in a cat with ureteral obstruction. Note the dilated and tortuous ureter and the abrupt termination of the contrast enhancement in the distal part of the ureter, indicating the presence of an obstruction.

showed 90% sensitivity in identifying feline ureteroliths, emphasizing the importance of combining these tools. Intravenous urography can be used, but enhancement along the collecting system may not be sufficient due to decreased GFR (Lamb 1998). Alternatively, antegrade pyelography can be utilized if sufficient pelvic dilation is present (Figure 58.1) (Adin et al. 2003). Contrast CT is less invasive than antegrade pyelography and its high sensitivity allows use of a small contrast material amount, thereby decreasing potential nephrotoxicity.

Management of UO can be medical or surgical. The type and urgency of therapeutic intervention is determined by the nature of UO (i.e., static versus dynamic), its location, severity of uremia, presence of renal infection, and the risks associated with each procedure. When pain is the sole clinical manifestation, dynamic UO can be treated with analgesia and close monitoring to assure antegrade ureterolith movement. In human patients, distal ureteral ureteroliths <5 mm in diameter will resolve spontaneously in up to 98% of the patients (Segura et al. 1997); however, such guidelines do not exist in veterinary medicine. In uremic patients, therapy is first aimed at patient stabilization, and only secondarily at obstruction relief. Theoretically, fluid therapy will increase the hydraulic pressure on intraluminal obstructions and may promote antegrade movement; however, it should be exercised cautiously to prevent overhydration and circulatory failure. The same rationale may support the use of diuretics; however, this is not supported by evidence-based medicine. Other therapies, like glucagon, anti inflammatory drugs and ureteral muscle dilators, used in human patients, have not been evaluated extensively in dogs and cats. Extracorporeal wave lithotripsy has been successfully used in dogs to fragment ureteroliths, but the feline kidney is more sensitive to shock wave-induced injury. In severely azotemic patients, hemodialysis will allow patient stabilization prior to surgical intervention and will enable a longer period for dynamic intraluminal obstructions to spontaneously resolve. The risk for irreversible renal damage during this period, which depends on the degree and duration of the obstruction, should be considered. Studies assessing the renal response to feline UO are lacking. In dogs, complete ligation of the ureter for 4, 14, and 40 days resulted in 100%, 46%, and minimal renal function recovery, respectively, whereas partial ureteral ligation for 14, 28, and 60 days resulted in 100%, 31%, and 8%, repectively (Vaughan and Gillenwater 1971; Fink et al. 1980; Leahy et al. 1989). The period in which medical management can be attempted safely is yet to be determined; however, based on the limited available information, irreversible damage takes at least several days to occur even when the obstruction is complete.

Surgical intervention should be considered in cases of static UO (e.g., static ureterolith, stricture, or neoplasia), ureteral rupture and urine extravagation, severe infection of the obstructed kidney, and uncontrolled uremic signs or pain. Surgical options include nephrostomy tubes, ureterotomy, ureteroneocystostomy, nephrectomy, ureteral resection and anastamosis, and kidney transplantation (Kyles et al. 2005b). The type of surgery depends on the obstruction location, the surgeon's preference and the likelihood of regaining renal function. Nephrostomy tubes can be placed either surgically or percutaneously ultrasound-guided. These can be used in azotemic patients prior to surgery to restore GFR and urine drainage or in conjunction with medical management to allow a longer follow-up period for dynamic UOs. Complications are common and include urine leakage, poor drainage, and tube dislodgment (Kyles et al.

2005b). Ureterotomy is usually performed with intraluminal proximal obstructions. Ureterotomy or ureteroneocystostomy are performed with distal obstructions. The selected type of surgical procedure often depends on the surgeon's preference, as some perceive ureteroneocystostomy technically easier and with a lower complication rate. Ureteronephrectomy is considered when the obstruction cannot be eliminated or bypassed (e.g., proximal stricture, neoplasia) and with severe renal infection or damage (e.g., renal abscess). When an objective assessment of the relative contribution of each kidney to the overall GFR is not available, extreme caution should be exercised prior to nephrectomy. Presence of azotemia is evidence of significant impairment of the contralateral kidney; therefore, even minor contribution of each kidney may be crucial for a favorable outcome. As patients may develop future obstructions in the contralateral collecting system, the decision to perform nephrectomy, even in non-azotemic patients, should be cautiously considered. Thus, renal function (even partial) should be preserved whenever possible. Kidney transplantation should also be considered when other surgical and medical options have been exhausted. The risk of calculi formation in the allograft should be considered. In 5/19 cats that underwent transplantation, calculi were observed in the allograft, 120–665 days after surgery; (Aronson et al. 2006); nevertheless, renal transplantation is considered a viable option for feline UO.

The overall prognosis for non-azotemic patients is good (Kyles et al. 2005b; Snyder et al. 2005). One month survival rate for cats with UO was 75% (Kyles et al. 2005b). For these, survival rates at 6, 12, and 24 months were 91%, 92%, 88%, and 72%, 66%, 66% when managed surgically and medically, respectively (Kyles et al. 2005b). These results attest for the need for surgical intervention whenever indicated. Over half of the cats are expected to sustain CKD, and therefore, should be closely monitored. Moreover, the recurrence rate of UO in cats is as high as 40%, either ipsilaterally or contralaterally, with a median recurrence period of 12.5 months.

Ureteral injury and paraureteral urinoma

Ureteral injury can result from direct or indirect trauma, ureterolithiasis, and surgical iatrogenic. Urinary tract trauma mostly does not involve the ureters which are relatively protected by their location and flexibility. Nevertheless motor vehicle trauma is an important cause of urinary tract injuries and was the major cause for traumatic ureteral rupture (complete avulsions or partial tears) in a study of 10 animals (Weisse et al. 2002). Based on the small number of described cases, it is difficult to conclude whether any specific segment of the ureter is more prone to injury, as has been suggested in humans. Nevertheless, injuries have been described in both ureters at the ureteropelvic junction, midureter, and the ureterovesicular portion (Weisse et al. 2002). Ureteral injury has been reported as a complication of abdominal surgeries, mostly ovariohysterectomy, due to inadvertently incorporating the ureter in the ligature of the ovarian pedicle or cervical stump.

A ruptured ureter will result in retroperitoneal or peritoneal space urine accumulation depending on the rupture location and retroperitoneal integrity. Prolonged contact with urine will induce chemical peritonitis, and if infected, septic peritonitis as well. Urine may also be confined locally (see Urinoma). Patients often have a history of trauma or recent surgery. Clinical signs may resemble those of uremic patients, but are often related to concurrent injuries. In one study, only 2/10 patients presented signs related to the ureteral injury (e.g., anuria dysuria, hematuria) (Weisse et al. 2002). Thus, diagnosis is challenging and often delayed beyond the day of presentation.

Hematuria, is neither sensitive nor specific (Selcer 1982; Weisse et al. 2002). Radiography may reveal increased retroperitoneal space density and widening. Retroperitoneal fluids should be confirmed as urine before a diagnosis of ureteral rupture can be made. Contrast studies (radiography or CT) can aid in the diagnosis and demonstrate the urine extravagation site, thus, facilitating surgical and medical managenet (Lamb 1998; Weisse et al. 2002). Dilatation of the ipsilateral ureter and kidney may also be present (Thornhill and Cechner 1981; Selcer 1982). Ultrasonography may reveal retroperitoneal fluids, hydroureter, and hydronephrosis (Lamb 1998).

Initial treatment should concentrate on patient stabilization prior to surgical intervention. Concurrent injuries, shock, hyperkalemia and other complications should not be overlooked. Partial tears may heal spontaneously (Bjorling and Christie 1993). Surgical intervention, if needed, may include ureteral reanastomosis, ureteroneocystostomy, stenting across the defect, and ureteronephrectomy (Weisse et al. 2002). The choice of surgery depends on the location of the avulsion or tear. Post operative complications include dehiscence, urine extravasations and formation of stricture, fistula and urinoma. Animals that are successfully stabilized initially and do not develop acute renal failure have good outcome with surgical management (Weisse et al. 2002).

Urinoma is a potential complication of ureteral injury. It is also referred to as para-ureteral uriniferous pseudocyst or paraureteral pseudocyst. The extravagated urine stimulates a fibrous reaction, forming a capsule devoid of internal epithelial lining (pseudocyst) that engulfs the urine. Urinoma has been reported in both dogs and cats,

secondary to trauma, surgery, neoplasia, obstruction, and ureterolithiasis (Yeh et al. 1981; Schultze Kool et al. 1984; Tidwell et al. 1990; Moores et al. 2002; Worth and Tomlin 2004). They may cause UO, thus hydronephrosis and hydroureter may occur (Moores et al. 2002). The clinical signs are typically non specific and diagnosis is often delayed. Abdominal mass may be palpated if the urinoma is large. Abdominal ultrasonography demonstrates a hypoechoic mass and potentially dilatation of the collecting system and hydronephrosis. Analysis of aspirated fluid may confirm the presence of urine. If renal function is adequate contrast abdominal radiography or CT may demonstrate dilatation of the collecting system and potential ureteral–urinoma communication. Based on human experience, most obstructive urinomas can be successfully treated by ultrasound guided percutaneously drainage that relieve the obstruction, even if temporarily. Urinomas can be surgically resected thus alleviating an existing UO. When renal function is severely impaired, ureteronephrectomy is preformed (Moores et al. 2002).

Ectopic ureter

The ureter normally enters the dorsolateral caudal surface of the bladder and empties into the trigone after a short intramural course. Ectopic ureter results from termination of one or both ureters at a site other than the trigone as a result of an embryologic abnormality of the ureteral bud of the mesonephric duct. The degree of deviation of the ureteral bud from the normal position determines the location of the ectopic opening.

Vertebrates have one of three distinct excretory organs: the pronephros, mesonephros, or metanephros. Mammals and birds have developed metanephros. During development, the pronephros, mesonephros, and metanephros appear sequentially and parts of each are present in the developing embryo. In mammals, only the duct of the pronephros is retained as the mesonephric duct. The mesonephros is active in fetuses, but becomes vestigial in females and the mesonephric duct becomes the ductus deferens in males. The metanephric duct becomes the ureter and is derived from the distal mesonephric duct bud that lies close to the cloaca. The mesonephric and metanephric ducts share a common excretory duct and opening when the bladder forms. The metanephric duct grows towards the metanephros, which forms the kidney. As the bladder develops, the common duct is absorbed and the mesonephric and metanephric ducts acquire individual openings. As development continues, the mesonephric ducts displace caudally and open on a prominence on the dorsal urethral wall while the ureteral openings are in the bladder (Sutherland-Smith et al. 2004).

Ectopic ureters may be unilateral or bilateral and intramural or extramural. An extramural ectopic ureter bypasses insertion at the trigone and inserts distally in the urethra, vagina, or vestibule in females, or ductus deferens in males. An intramural ectopic ureter inserts at the trigone, but tunnels in the urethral wall to open distally. Variations of the intramural ectopic ureter include ureteral troughs, double ureteral openings, multiple fenestrated openings, and two intramural ureters opening in a single orifice (Stone and Mason 1990). Ectopic ureters may be associated with other congenital defects of the urogenital tract including agenesis, hypoplasia, or irregular shape of the kidneys; hydroureter; ureterocele; urachal remnants, pelvic bladder; vulvovaginal strictures; and persistent hymen (Mason et al 1990, McLoughlin and Chew 2000).

Young female dogs (median age of 10 months) are most commonly diagnosed with ectopic ureter; bilateral intramural ectopic ureters occur most commonly (Holt and Moore 1995; McLoughlin and Chew 2000). Males with ectopic ureter present later, with a median age of 24 months (Holt and Moore 1995), or they may be undiagnosed because they remain continent presumably due to the urethral length and external urethral sphincter. Breeds reported to be at greater risk for ectopic ureter include the Siberian husky, Labrador retriever, Golden retriever, Newfoundland, English bulldog, West Highland white terrier, fox terrier, Skye terrier, and miniature and toy poodles (McLoughlin and Chew 2000). A genetic basis may exist, but is unproven in most cases. Cats are rarely diagnosed with ectopic ureter.

Intermittent or continuous urinary incontinence since birth or weaning is the most frequently reported clinical sign in patients with ectopic ureter; however, most dogs void normally. Physical examination findings are often unremarkable, with the exception of moist or urine-stained hair in the perivulvar or preputial region. Urine scalding may cause secondary dermatitis, and owners may report frequent licking of the vulval or preputial area. Some dogs have vulvovaginitis, a vulvovaginal stricture, or a persistent hymen that can be detected digitally or with vaginoscopy. Dogs often have a history of bacterial urinary tract infections, which have been reported to occur in 64% of patients (Stone and Mason 1990). Some animals may respond partially or completely to pharmacologic management of urethral sphincter mechanism incompetence.

Survey radiography should be performed to assess size, shape, and location of kidneys and bladder. Excretory urography combined with pneumocystography (Figure 58.2) (McLoughlin and Chew 2000), abdominal ultrasonography (Lamb 1998), contrast urethrocystogra-

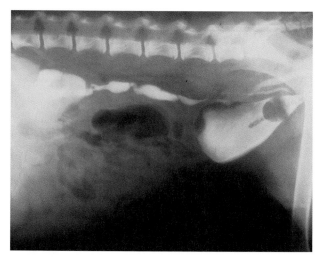

Figure 58.2 Excretory urogram and contrast cystogram demonstrating an extramural right ectopic ureter. The radiolucent defect in the bladder is the distal end of a foley catheter.

phy with vesicoureteral reflux, fluoroscopy, or contrast-enhanced computerized tomography may be used to diagnose ectopic ureter; however, urethrocystoscopy is more reliable especially when combined with other imaging modalities (Figure 58.3) (McLoughlin and Chew 2000). Dilation of the ectopic ureter is often, but not always, present.

While medical management may help control urinary incontinence, surgical correction or laser ablation is the preferred treatment. An extramural ectopic ureter is ligated at the distal end of the ureter at its attachment and reimplanted into the urinary bladder between the apex and the trigone (neoureterocystostomy). The bladder wall or urine from the renal pelvis should be collected at the

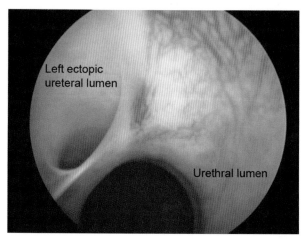

Figure 58.3 Cystoscopic image of an intramural left ectopic ureter in a 1.5 year old, female intact, Siberian Husky.

time of surgery and cultured because of the common occurrence of bacterial urinary tract infections.

Traditionally, intramural ectopic ureter is treated by ligation of the distal submucosal ureteral segment and creating a new ureteral opening in the trigone of the urinary bladder (neoureterostomy and urethral-trigonal reconstruction); however, incontinence persists commonly (44–67%) (McLaughlin and Miller 1991; McLoughlin and Chew 2000) because the intramural segment of ureter disrupts the functional anatomy of the internal urethral sphincter mechanism (McLoughlin and Chew 2000). In some of these cases medical treatment with drugs such as phenylpropanolamine or ephedrine sulfate may resolve or improve the incontinence. Transurethral laser ablation may also be used to correct intramural ectopic ureter (see Chapter 39). A rigid (in females) or flexible (in males) endoscope is inserted retrograde into the urethra; diagnostic urethrocystosopy is performed. A guide wire or catheter is inserted into the lumen of the ectopic ureter in order to protect the urethral wall. A laser fiber, diode (McCarthy 2006) or preferably Holmium:YAG (Berent and Mayhew 2007; Berent et al 2008), is inserted through the operating channel of the cystoscope and used to transect the free wall of the ectopic ureter until the opening is as close as possible to the normal anatomical location at the trigone. Following the procedure, dogs are more likely to be continent than with surgical correction (Berent and Mayhew 2007).

In patients where the kidney cannot be spared due to hydronephrosis or pyelonephritis, nephroureterectomy can be performed.

References

Adin, C.A., et al. (2003). Antegrade pyelography for suspected ureteral obstruction in cats: 11 cases (1995–2001). *J Am Vet Med Assoc* **222**(11): 1576–1581.

Aronson, L.R., et al. (2006). Renal transplantation in cats with calcium oxalate urolithiasis: 19 cases (1997–2004). *J Am Vet Med Assoc* **228**(5): 743–749.

Berent, A.C. and P.D. Mayhew (2007) Cystoscopic-guided laser ablation of intramural ureteral ectopia in 11 dogs (7 female, 4 males). *American College of Veterinary Surgeons: Scientific Abstracts*, 3.

Berent, A.C., et al. (2008) Use of cystoscopic-guided laser ablation for treatment of intramural ureteral ectopia in male dogs: four cases (2006–2007). *J Am Vet Med Assoc* **232**: 1026–1034.

Bjorling, D.E. and B.A. Christie (1993). Ureters. In: *Text Book of Small Animal Surgery*, edited by D. Slatter. Philadelphia, PA: WB Saunders, pp. 1443–1450.

Christie, B.A. (1973). Vesicoureteral reflux in dogs. *J Am Vet Med Assoc* **162**(9): 772–775.

Eisele, J.G., et al. (2005). Ectopic ureterocele in a cat. *J Am Anim Hosp Assoc* **41**(5): 332–335.

Fink, R.L., et al. (1980). Renal impairment and its reversibility following variable periods of complete ureteric obstruction. *Aust N Z J Surg* **50**(1): 77–83.

Holt, P.E. and A.H. Moore (1995) Canine ureteral ectopia: an analysis of 175 cases and comparison of surgical treatments. *Vet Rec* **136**: 345–349.

Kyles, A.E., et al. (2005a). Clinical, clinicopathologic, radiographic, and ultrasonographic abnormalities in cats with ureteral calculi: 163 cases (1984–2002). *J Am Vet Med Assoc* **226**(6): 932–936.

Kyles, A.E., et al. (2005b). Management and outcome of cats with ureteral calculi: 153 cases (1984–2002). *J Am Vet Med Assoc* **226**(6): 937–944.

Lamb, C.R. (1998). Ultrasonography of the ureters. *Vet Clin North Am Small Anim Pract* **28**(4): 823–848.

Leahy, A.L., et al. (1989). Renal injury and recovery in partial ureteric obstruction. *J Urol* **142**(1): 199–203.

Martin, R.A., et al. (1985). Bilateral ectopic ureters in a male dog. *J Am Anim Hosp Assoc* **21**: 80–84.

Mason, L.K. et al. (1990) Surgery of ectopic ureters: pre- and postoperative radiographic morphology. *J Am Anim Hosp Assoc* **26**: 73.

McCarthy, T. (September 1, 2006) Endoscopy brief: transurethral cystoscopy and diode laser incision to correct an ectopic ureter. *Veterinary Medicine Online* **101**(9): 558.

McLaughlin, R. and C.W. Miller (1991) Urinary incontinence after surgical repair of ureteral ectopia in dogs. *Vet Surg* **20**: 100–103.

McLoughlin, M.A. and D.E. Bjorling (2003). Ureters. In: *Text Book of Small Animal Surgery*, edited by D. Slatter, Volume **2**. Philadelphia, PA: WB Saunders, pp. 1619–1628.

McLoughlin, M.A. and D.J. Chew (2000) Diagnosis and surgical management of ectopic ureters. *Clin Tech Small Anim Pract* **15**: 17–24.

McLoughlin, M.A., et al. (1989). Canine ureteroceles: a case report and literature review. *J Am Anim Hosp Assoc* **25**: 699–706.

Moores, A.P., et al. (2002). Urinoma (para-ureteral pseudocyst) as a consequence of trauma in a cat. *J Small Anim Pract* **43**(5): 213–216.

Osborne, C.A. and T.F. Fletcher (1995). Applied anatomy of the urinary system with clincopathologic correlation. In: *Canine and Feline Nephrology and Urology*, edited by C.A. Osborne and D.R. Finco. New York: Williams & Wilkins, pp. 3–28.

Schultze Kool, L.J., et al. (1984). Retroperitoneal reabsorption of extravasated urine in renal transplant patients. *Radiology* **153**(3): 625–626.

Segura, J.W., et al. (1997). Ureteral Stones Clinical Guidelines Panel summary report on the management of ureteral calculi. The American Urological Association. *J Urol* **158**(5): 1915–1921.

Selcer, B.A. (1982). Urinary tract trauma associated with pelvic trauma. *J Am Anim Hosp Assoc* **18**: 785.

Snyder, D.M., et al. (2005). Diagnosis and surgical management of ureteral calculi in dogs: 16 cases (1990–2003). *N Z Vet J* **53**(1): 19–25.

Stiffler, K.S., et al. (2002). Intravesical ureterocele with concurrent renal dysfunction in a dog: a case report and proposed classification system. *J Am Anim Hosp Assoc* **38**(1): 33–39.

Stone, E.A. and L.K. Mason (1990) Surgery of ectopic ureters: types, method of correction, and postoperative results. *J Am Anim Hosp Assoc* **26**: 81–88.

Sutherland-Smith, J., et al. (2004). Ectopic ureters and ureteroceles in dogs: presentation, cause, and diagnosis. *Compend Contin Educ Pract Vet* **26**: 303–310.

Tanagho, E.A. (1972). Anatomy and management of ureteroceles. *J Urol* **107**(5): 729–736.

Tattersall, J.A. and E. Welsh (2006). Ectopic ureterocele in a male dog: a case report and review of surgical management. *J Am Anim Hosp Assoc* **42**(5): 395–400.

Thornhill, J.A. and P.E. Cechner (1981). Traumatic injuries to the kidney, ureter, bladder, and urethra. *Vet Clin North Am Small Anim Pract* **11**(1): 157–69.

Tidwell, A.S., et al. (1990). Urinoma, (para ureteral pseudocyst) in a dog. *Vet Radiol Ultrasound* **31**: 203–206.

Vaughan, E.D., Jr. and J.Y. Gillenwater (1971). Recovery following complete chronic unilateral ureteral occlusion: functional, radiographic and pathologic alterations. *J Urol* **106**(1): 27–35.

Weisse, C., et al. (2002). Traumatic rupture of the ureter: 10 cases. *J Am Anim Hosp Assoc* **38**(2): 188–192.

Worth, A.J. and S.C. Tomlin (2004). Post-traumatic paraureteral urinoma in a cat. *J Small Anim Pract* **45**(8): 413–416.

Yeh, E.L., et al. (1981). Ultrasound and radionuclide studies of urinary extravasation with hydronephrosis. *J Urol* **125**(5): 728–730.

59

Renal trauma

Patricia Sura

Renal trauma is diagnosed uncommonly in veterinary medicine (Thornhill and Cechner 1981; McLoughlin 2000), but is likely to receive wider attention with the increasing availability of advanced diagnostic imaging modalities. In humans, renal injuries represent the most common injuries to the urinary tract (McAninch 2000), occurring in approximately 10% of abdominal trauma cases (Shariat et al. 2007). In a study of 100 consecutive dogs with blunt pelvic trauma, 39 had concurrent urinary tract trauma (Selcer 1982). Superficial cortical lacerations, contusions, and other minor injuries represent 85% of all renal trauma cases (McAninch 2000). These injuries are likely to go unnoticed in most veterinary patients.

Anatomic location may be responsible for the protection afforded the kidneys from traumatic injury. The kidneys are sheltered by the ribs, spine, and thick epaxial musculature. They also have a degree of mobility permitted by their attachment to perirenal fat, which allows absorption of force and additional defense against damage (Thornhill and Cechner 1981; McLoughlin 2000).

The most common causes of renal injury in humans and animals are blunt trauma, falls from heights, and penetrating wounds (Thornhill and Cechner 1981; Santucci et al. 2004). Blunt trauma can either damage the kidney directly or lead to stretch injury and pedicle avulsion. Similarly, rapid deceleration from a fall can lead to pedicle injuries (Santucci et al. 2004). Injury occurs whenever the stress applied to the organ exceeds its ability to compensate and the chance of renal trauma increases with increasing impact velocity (Santucci et al. 2004).

Human renal injuries are classified as minor renal trauma (85%), major renal trauma (15%), and vascular injury (1%) (McAninch 2000). The American Asso-

ciation for the Surgery of Trauma (AAST) Organ Injury Scaling Committee was subsequently appointed to create a severity score by which renal injuries could be compared for the purpose of clinical research (Moore et al. 1989, 1995). The criteria for each score are detailed in Table 59.1. This information has been validated, and correlates well with the need for surgical repair, need for nephrectomy, and increased morbidity and mortality with increasing grades (Santucci et al. 2001; Kuan et al. 2006; Shariat et al. 2007). Predictive value of the grading system, along with the presence or absence of a perirenal hematoma and the need for a blood transfusion, was correct when used in an algorithm to determine whether surgery was required in 95% of patients (Santucci et al. 2001).

Thornhill and Cechner similarly divided veterinary renal injury into five descriptive categories (Thornhill and Cechner 1981). Bruising and ecchymosis is the most common, and typically resolves spontaneously. A hematoma arises when accumulation of blood occurs between the capsule and surrounding tissue. This accumulation of fluid may resorb, or result in a persistent cyst or abscess (Thornhill and Cechner 1981; McLoughlin 2000). Surgical drainage may be required in these cases. A fissure is an incomplete tear of the parenchyma extending through the capsule, resulting in a perinephric hematoma. In contrast, a laceration involves disruption of the retroperitoneum, resulting in blood and/or urine extravasation into the peritoneal space. Finally, rupture of the vascular pedicle may occur (Thornhill and Cechner 1981). This may result in death due to massive hemorrhage (McLoughlin 2000).

Clinical signs attributable to renal damage range from mild hematuria to an acute abdomen. Hemoperitoneum and uroperitoneum are also possible. Rapid loss of blood can contribute to hypovolemic shock and exsanguination, although mild to moderate parenchymal and

Nephrology and Urology of Small Animals. Edited by Joe Bartges and David J. Polzin. © 2011 Blackwell Publishing Ltd.

591

Table 59.1 American Association for the Surgery of Trauma grading scale for renal injuries

Grade[a]	Type	Description
I	Contusion	Microscopic or gross hematuria; urologic studies normal
	Hematoma	Subcapsular, nonexpanding without parenchymal laceration
II	Hematoma	Nonexpanding perirenal hematoma confined to renal retroperitoneum
	Laceration	<1.0 cm parenchymal depth of renal cortex without urinary extravasation
III	Laceration	>1.0 cm parenchymal depth of renal cortex without collecting system rupture or urinary extravasation
IV	Laceration	Parenchymal laceration extending through renal cortex, medulla, and collecting system
	Vascular	Main renal artery or vein injury with continued hemorrhage
V	Laceration	Completely shattered kidney
	Vascular	Avulsion of renal hilum, which devascularizes kidney

Source: With permission, Moore et al. (1989).
[a]Advance one grade for bilateral injuries up to grade III.

capsular bleeding is more common. In humans, 80–85% of renal hemorrhage resolves spontaneously (McAninch 2000). In addition, 76–87% of urine extravasation cases resolve without intervention (Santucci et al. 2004). While lacerations of the renal pelvis rarely respond to conservative management (Master and McAninch 2006), AAST grade IV and V renal lacerations with urine extravasation can heal remarkably well. In a study of 34 human patients with unilateral renal extravasation due to trauma, three (9%) required ureteral stenting to resolve the urine leakage, while the remaining 91% healed without further intervention (Alsikafi et al. 2006). Similarly in children, selective medical management of renal injury results in a 5–11% operation rate (Buckley and McAninch 2006). Ureteral stents or percutaneous nephrostomy tubes (Alsikafi and Rosenstein 2006) may be used as minimally invasive adjuncts to allow conservative healing of the kidney. In a report of uroperitoneum in 26 cats, only one cat had evidence of renal trauma and uroretroperitoneum necessitating nephrectomy (Aumann et al. 1998).

Hematuria in trauma patients suggests urinary tract injury. However, the degree of hematuria does not correlate with the amount of damage present (McAninch 2000; Santucci et al. 2004; Alsikafi and Rosenstein 2006) unless additional parameters are used in the evaluation. For example, in adult trauma patients with hematuria and systolic blood pressure <90, the chance of major renal injury is 62 times higher (12.5%) than if the blood pressure is >90 (0.2%) (Santucci et al. 2004).

Both veterinary and human trauma patients are typically triaged into hemodynamically stable and unstable groups, with treatment and further diagnostics planned accordingly. The best imaging modality to evaluate the hemodynamically stable human kidney is contrast enhanced computed tomography (McAninch 2000; Santucci et al. 2004; Alsikafi and Rosenstein 2006). This

modality can be used to confirm urinary extravasation, renal contusions, depth of lacerations, and pedicle injuries (Alsikafi and Rosenstein 2006). Its primary function is to determine whether surgical intervention is necessary (Santucci et al. 2004). The use of intravenous contrast material can provide a three-dimensional excretory urogram when evaluated with CT. This has replaced intravenous pyelogram as the most widely used examination for renal trauma in people (Al-Qudah and Santucci 2006; Alsikafi and Rosenstein 2006).

In veterinary patients, the use of CT is limited by the need for general anesthesia, limitation of scanners to secondary and tertiary referral centers, slow scan speed of non-helical machines, and expense (Herold et al. 2008). The trauma patient is typically stabilized, and surgery planned if there are penetrating wounds to the abdomen, additional surgical injuries present, or if intra-abdominal hemorrhage is uncontrollable (Herold et al. 2008). Widely available diagnostics, such as plain radiography, intravenous urography and abdominal ultrasonography are more typically employed.

In the hemodynamically stable animal, abdominal radiography is an appropriate non-invasive early diagnostic step. Loss of detail may be noted in the retroperitoneal space, as well as loss of renal margination, and space-occupying masses consistent with hematomas (Figure 59.1). Loss of retroperitoneal detail is a relatively non-specific finding. In a study of 100 dogs with pelvic trauma, 26 dogs had loss of retroperitoneal detail, with 43.5% (17) of those animals having concurrent urinary tract trauma (Selcer 1982). Excretory urography is indicated in these cases (Thornhill and Cechner 1981). Major causes of non-visualization of the kidney during excretory urography include pedicle avulsion, thrombosis, vascular spasm, and absence of the kidney (McAninch 2000). Excretory urography also is integral in documenting leakage of urine from the collecting system

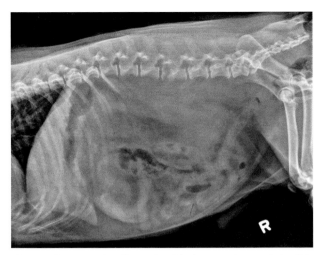

Figure 59.1 Lateral radiograph with decreased serosal detail in the retroperitoneal area with a large mass causing ventral displacement of the colon and small intestines, and cranial displacement of the stomach. This is consistent with a large renal hematoma, or shattered kidney with hemorrhage. There is also a displaced fracture of the fourth lumbar vertebra. Myelography confirmed spinal cord transection, and a necropsy was not performed. With permission, Federica Morandi, DVM, MS, DACVR, DECVDI.

(Figure 59.2). Abdominal ultrasonography may also be employed to evaluate renal parenchymal architecture.

Perhaps the most common use of ultrasonography in the trauma patient is the Focused Abdominal Sonography for Trauma (FAST) technique. FAST has been used in both adult and pediatric patients to assess severity of blunt trauma (Soudack et al. 2004; Helling et al. 2007). In

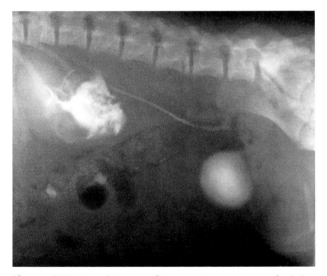

Figure 59.2 Lateral image of an excretory urogram depicting urine extravasation from the caudal pole of the left kidney, consistent with a laceration involving the collection system. Note the well-demarcated renal pelvis and continuity of the ureter. With permission, University of Tennessee Department of Radiology.

the human medical field, it has virtually eliminated diagnostic peritoneal lavage for the evaluation of the blunt trauma patient (Ollerton et al. 2006; Helling et al. 2007), and can segregate those patients requiring immediate surgery, further imaging, or simple observation. Specificity of this technique in the diagnosis of hemoperitoneum is 90–100% (Hoffman et al. 2009). FAST is not without limitations, in that parenchymal injuries, hollow viscus perforation, and retroperitoneal injuries may be missed with this technique. Renal injuries in people are 3.7 times more likely to be missed with FAST, but confirmed with ancillary testing such as CT or exploratory laparotomy (Hoffman et al. 2009). Veterinary application of this technique has been reported, with operators of various skill levels able to detect free abdominal fluid (Boysen et al. 2004). The use of this modality also allows focused abdominocentesis to collect fluid for analysis.

The blood supply to the canine kidneys is approximately 25% of total cardiac output (Brown 2003). Hemorrhage and rapid death is therefore possible from pedicle damage or severe lacerations to the parenchyma. Stabilization should consist of crystalloid and colloid support, with intense monitoring of hemodynamic parameters. Failure to respond to aggressive management is typically indicative of continued hemorrhage, and exploratory celiotomy is warranted. Absolute indications for surgery in humans are persistent, life-threatening blood loss, an expansile or pulsating renal hematoma, and renal pedicle avulsion (Santucci et al. 2004; Buckley and McAninch 2006).

A recent review of the management of hemoperitoneum in dogs recommended fluid resuscitation with crystalloids and colloids to a mean arterial pressure of 60 mmHg, with low normal resuscitation endpoints (Herold et al. 2008). This is performed to avoid clot disruption and rebleeding from a sudden increase in systolic pressure (Herold et al. 2008). In people, aggressive resuscitation is associated with an increased incidence of intraabdominal hemorrhage, compartment syndrome, and death (Balogh et al. 2003). A study in normal dogs revealed that isotonic crystalloids provide the most rapid increase in blood volume following infusion that rapidly declines due to redistribution. In contrast, colloid solutions provide a sustainable increase in blood volume, albeit at a lower magnitude (Silverstein et al. 2005). A combination of fluid types should be employed, with the goal of maintaining renal perfusion without creating an acute increase in systolic pressure.

Similarly, if a compression bandage is applied, sudden release of the abdominal counterpressure may release the tamponade effect and lead to immediate death (Herold et al. 2008). Vital parameters should be monitored every 5 minutes as pressure is released, and fluids administered as needed and compression reapplied if indicated (Vinayak and Krahwinkel 2004).

In general, vascular injuries of the kidney are rare. In humans, the renal artery is most commonly affected (60%), followed by the renal vein (30%) and combined injuries (10%) (Master and McAninch 2006). Suspect vascular injury is evaluated with an immediate arteriogram and computed tomography (McAninch 2000), or intraoperative one-shot intravenous pyelogram in unstable patients submitted to emergency celiotomy (Santucci et al. 2004). With this technique, a volume of contrast material is administered with fluoroscopic visualization in the operating room to evaluate renal perfusion, as well as to demonstrate some degree of contralateral kidney function. As salvage rates following vascular injury are reported to be 25–35% at best, nephrectomy is often pursued (Master and McAninch 2006). Confirmation of renal function has been described in the veterinary literature with cystotomy and visualization of the ureteral openings for urine production (Herold et al. 2008).

Due to the potential for exsanguination from renal hemorrhage, planned vascular control is used in the human field whenever celiotomy is planned for a hemorrhaging kidney. Occlusion times of <30 minutes (Master and McAninch 2006) are employed. In the dog, the aorta can be compressed digitally at the level of the celiac artery to quell intractable hemorrhage, and allow the use of atraumatic means (Rumel tourniquets or vascular clamps) to temporarily address the continuing hemorrhage and allow definitive repair (Burch et al. 1954; Herold et al. 2008). Canine renal vessels can be occluded for 30 minutes (Herold et al. 2008), and blood can be collected in a sterile container for autotransfusion if desired, provided that the presence of urine and gastrointestinal contents has been excluded (Vinayak and Krahwinkel 2004; Herold et al. 2008).

There is associated organ injury in 61–100% of renal trauma cases (Al-Qudah and Santucci 2006), with a high association of injuries necessitating operation in conjunction with AAST grade IV–V renal trauma in people (Buckley and McAninch 2006). Reconstructed human kidneys function at 2/3 normal on average (Master and McAninch 2006), and preservation of some renal function is possible in the majority of repaired renal lacerations (Santucci et al. 2004). Extrapolation is required, as this data is not available for companion animals, but renorrhaphy may be of benefit in the absence of pedicle injury to retain some degree of renal function, especially in animals with preexisting renal compromise.

Surgical principles of renorrhaphy include exposure of the entire kidney using vascular occlusion, sharp debridement of non-viable parenchyma, maintenance of accurate hemostasis, watertight closure of the collecting sys-

tem, reapproximation of parenchymal edges, use of an omental interposition flap, and providing a retroperitoneal drain (Master and McAninch 2006). Closed-suction drains are not appropriate, as they may increase leakage from the collecting system.

Trauma is the most common etiology leading to partial nephrectomy in humans (Master and McAninch 2006). The pelvis and diverticula are closed, and the intra-parenchymal vessels are ligated. Exposed parenchyma may be covered with capsule, transversus abdominis muscle, omentum, or a serosal patch (Master and McAninch 2006). In humans, 30% of a single functioning kidney is necessary to avoid dialysis (Master and McAninch 2006). Partial nephrectomy has been described in the veterinary literature, and adheres to the same principles as in humans (Rawlings et al. 2003).

Sequelae to renal damage include urinoma, renal abscess, hydronephrosis, renal vascular hypertension, and arteriovenous fistulae formation in humans (McAninch 2000; Buckley and McAninch 2006). Delayed hemorrhage may also be noted due to hematoma resorption and release of pressure from the offending vessel.

Urinomas occur in 1–7% of trauma patients, and can present as confined or free fluid (Al-Qudah and Santucci 2006). The condition may be asymptomatic, but fluid can dissect along fascial planes, causing flank pain and edema. Many resorb uneventfully, but percutaneous drainage or ureteral stents may be necessary for complete resolution (Al-Qudah and Santucci 2006). Of 34 conservatively managed people with renal lacerations, a single patient developed a urinoma. Other complications, such as hypertension or delayed hemorrhage did not occur (Alsikafi et al. 2006). The incidence of renal abscess due to contamination of the urinoma increases in frequency with coincident injury, metabolic disease states, and immunosuppression (Al-Qudah and Santucci 2006).

Urinomas have been reported in two cats, both of which were paraureteral and treated with nephrectomy (Moores et al. 2002; Worth and Tomlin 2004). Other interesting case reports have shown right kidney herniation through diaphragmatic defects in cats (Marolf 2002, Katic 2007), as well as a nephrocutaneous fistula secondary to blunt trauma in a dog (Lobetti and Irvine-Smith 2006). Penetrating injuries have also been demonstrated (Borthwick 1971; Lipson et al. 1972; Dorn and Stoloff 1975).

While hypertension can be induced in canine kidneys following sudden reduction in functioning mass (Finco 2004), post-traumatic pressure elevations have not been reported. In contrast, hypertension occurs in human renal trauma patients from renin overproduction, either due to arterial stenosis or occlusion, pressure on the kidney or AV fistulae (Al-Qudah and Santucci

2006). Prevalence of this phenomena has been reported in one study of 17,410 people as 0.57 per 1,000 (Chedid et al. 2006).

In conclusion, the diagnosis of renal trauma in veterinary patients is rare. Extrapolation of the human literature suggests that most cases of renal trauma can be managed conservatively, with close attention to patient status dictating the need and timing for surgery. If the principles of renorrhaphy are strictly followed, maintenance of some renal function may be anticipated, which could be of most significance in patients with preexisting renal compromise. Nephrectomy is warranted in cases of expanding, pulsatile renal hematomas, and renal pedicle avulsion.

References

Al-Qudah, H.S. and R.A. Santucci (2006). Complications of renal trauma. *Urol Clin North Am* **33**(1): 41–54.

Alsikafi, N.F. and D.I. Rosenstein (2006). Staging, evaluation and non-operative management of renal injuries. *Urol Clin North Am* **33**(1): 13–20.

Alsikafi, N.F., et al. (2006). Nonoperative management outcomes of isolated urinary extravasation following renal lacerations due to external trauma. *J Urol* **176**(6): 2494–2497.

Aumann, M., et al. (1998). Uroperitoneum in cats: 26 cases (1986–1995). *J Am Anim Hosp Assoc* **34**(4): 315–324.

Balogh, Z., et al. (2003). Supranormal trauma resuscitation causes more cases of abdominal compartment syndrome. *Arch Surg* **138**(6): 637–643

Borthwick, R. (1971). Foreign body in a cat's kidney. *J Small Anim Pract* **12**(11): 623–627.

Boysen, S.R., et al. (2004). Evaluation of a focused assessment with sonography for trauma protocol to detect free abdominal fluid in dogs involved in motor vehicle accidents. *J Am Vet Med Assoc* **225**(8): 1198–1204.

Brown, M.A. (2003). Physiology of the urinary tract. In: *Textbook of Small Animal Surgery*, edited by D. Slatter, 3rd edition. Philadelphia, PA: Elsevier Science.

Buckley, J.C. and J.W. McAninch (2006). The diagnosis, management, and outcomes of pediatric renal injuries. *Urol Clin North Am* **33**(1): 33–40.

Burch, B.H., et al. (1954). Temporary aortic occlusion in abdominal surgery. *Surgery* **35**(5): 684–689.

Chedid, A., et al. (2006). Blunt renal trauma-induced hypertension: prevalence, presentation and outcome. *Am J Hypertens* **19**(5): 500–504.

Dorn, A.S. and D. Stoloff (1975). Renal foreign body in a dog. *J Am Vet Med Assoc* **167**(8): 755–756.

Finco, D.R. (2004). Association of systemic hypertension with renal injury in dogs with induced renal failure. *J Vet Intern Med* **18**(3): 289–294.

Helling, T.S., et al. (2007). The utility of focused abdominal ultrasound in blunt abdominal trauma: a reappraisal. *Am J Surg* **194**(6): 728–733.

Herold, L.V., et al. (2008). Clinical evaluation and management of hemoperitoneum in dogs. *J Vet Emerg Crit Car* **18**(1): 40–53.

Hoffman, L., et al. (2009). Clinical predictors of injuries not identified by focused abdominal sonogram for trauma (FAST) examinations. *J Emerg Med* **36**(3): 271–279.

Katic, N., et al. (2007). Traumatic diaphragmatic rupture in a cat with partial kidney displacement into the thorax. *J Small Anim Pract* **48**(12): 705–708.

Kuan, J.K., et al. (2006). American Association for the Surgery of Trauma organ injury scale for kidney injuries predicts nephrectomy, dialysis and death in patients with blunt injury and nephrectomy for penetrating injuries. *J Trauma* **60**(2): 351–356.

Lipson, M.P., et al. (1972). Bullet lodged in kidney of a dog. *J Am Vet Med Assoc* **161**(3): 293.

Lobetti, R.G. and G.S. Irvine-Smith (2006). Nephro-cutaneous fistula in a dog. *J S Afr Vet Assoc* **77**(1): 40–41.

Marolf, A., et al. (2002). Radiographic diagnosis - right kidney herniation in a cat. *Vet Radiol Ultrasound* **43**(3): 237–240.

Master, V.A. and J.W. McAninch (2006). Operative management of renal injuries: parenchymal and vascular. *Urol Clin North Am* **33**(1): 21–32.

McAninch, J.W. (2000). Injuries to the genitourinary tract. In: *Smith's General Urology*, edited by E.A. Tanagho and J.W. McAninch, 15th edition. New York: McGraw-Hill.

McLoughlin, M.A. (2000). Surgical emergencies of the urinary tract. *Vet Clin N Am-Small Anim Pract* **30**(3): 581–601.

Moore, E.E., et al. (1989). Organ injury scaling: spleen, liver, and kidney. *J Trauma* **29**(12): 1664–1666.

Moore, E.E., et al. (1995). Organ injury scaling. *Surg Clin North Am* **75**(2): 293–303.

Moores, A.P., et al. (2002). Urinoma (para-ureteral pseudocyst) as a consequence of trauma in a cat. *J Small Anim Pract* **43**(5): 213–216.

Ollerton, J.E., et al. (2006). Prospective study to evaluate the influence of FAST on trauma patient management. *J Trauma* **60**(4): 785–791.

Rawlings, C.A., et al. (2003). Kidneys. In: *Textbook of Small Animal Surgery*, edited by D. Slatter, 3rd edition. Philadelphia, PA: Elsevier Science.

Santucci, R.A., et al. (2001). Validation of the American Association for the Surgery of Trauma organ injury severity scale for the kidney. *J Trauma* **50**(2): 195–200.

Santucci, R.A., et al. (2004). Consensus on genitourinary trauma. *BJU Int* **93**(7): 937–954.

Selcer, B.A. (1982). Urinary tract trauma associated with pelvic trauma. *J Am Anim Hosp Assoc* **18**(5): 785–793.

Shariat, S.F., et al. (2007). Evidence-based validation of the predictive value of the American Association for the Surgery of Trauma kidney injury scale. *J Trauma* **62**(4): 933–939.

Silverstein, D.C., et al. (2005). Assessment of changes in blood volume in response to resuscitative fluid administration in dogs. *J Vet Emerg Crit Car* **15**(3): 185–192.

Soudack, M., et al. (2004). Experience with focused abdominal sonography for trauma (FAST) in 313 pediatric patients. *J Clin Ultrasound* **32**(2): 53–61.

Thornhill, J.A. and P.E. Cechner (1981). Traumatic injuries to the kidney, ureter, bladder and urethra. *Vet Clin N Am-Small Anim Pract* **11**(1): 157–169.

Vinayak, A. and D.J. Krahwinkel (2004). Managing blunt-trauma induced hemoperitoneum in dogs and cats. *Comp Cont Educ Pract Vet* **26**(4): 276–291.

Worth, A.J. and S.C. Tomlin (2004). Post-traumatic paraureteral urinoma in a cat. *J Small Anim Pract* **45**(8): 413–416.

60

Renal and ureteral surgery

Karen Tobias

Compared with surgery of the lower urinary tract, renal and ureteral surgeries are often referred to specialty practices because of potential risk for severe intraoperative and postoperative complications. Some procedures, such as renal biopsy, can be relatively straightforward; however, preoperative and postoperative care can be challenging in patients with significant renal dysfunction or systemic illness.

Healing of the upper urinary tract

Healing of renal parenchyma is affected by the amount of vascular damage or necrosis present. When vascular injury is minimal, connective tissue and collagen rapidly repair renal parenchymal wounds. With parenchymal ischemia from compression, electrocoagulation, or vascular transection, inflammation, and infarction occur, delaying wound healing (Bellah 1989). Intraparenchymal hemorrhage increases the amount of fibrosis and renal damage, resulting in obliteration of local nephrons and dilation and obstruction of renal tubules in the area of the hematoma (Gerlaugh et al. 1960; Stone et al. 2002). Use of transparenchymal horizontal mattress sutures to stem hemorrhage, however, will cause parenchymal necrosis, fibrosis, scarring, and atrophy (Gahring et al. 1977). Healing is more rapid when intraparenchymal vessels are individually ligated.

Ureteral healing depends on the extent of damage and presence of urine leakage. Ureters that are crushed for up to 60 minutes will temporarily stenose at the site of injury (Brodsky et al. 1977). As long as local adventitia remains intact, renal function returns to normal within 3 months and radiographic evidence of ureteral stenosis resolves, although local aneurismal dilation of the ureter may persist. If local adventitia is lost, however, ureters may devascularize and 50% of affected ureters will develop persistent stricture (Brodsky et al. 1977).

The ureteral wall can regenerate completely when one-fourth of the diameter is present (Borkowski et al. 1979). With intraluminal stenting, re-epithelialization of a partially intact ureter is complete in 4–10 days. A fibrous bridge forms between the smooth muscle edges and eventually contracts to pull the smooth muscle together (Bellah 1989). The mural layer is completely regenerated in 4–6 weeks, although the regenerated muscular tissue is irregular and has fewer nerve fibers than normal ureteral musculature. When ureters are completely transected, the smooth muscle contracts and the mucosa retracts into a cuff. With splinting alone, the gap between transected ureteral ends is healed by development of a connective tissue tube that strictures after stent removal, resulting in ureteral obstruction (Huffman et al. 1956). Complete ureteral transections therefore require primary mucosa-to-mucosa repair. Because urine delays wound healing, stimulates fibrosis, and increases the risk of stricture, a leak-proof seal is ideal (Bellah 1989). Use of a continuous pattern for ureteral anastomosis provides a water-tight closure, results in smoother mucosal apposition, and is rapid; however, it may cause stricture because of a purse-string effect. Therefore, ureteroureteral or ureterocystic anastomosis is usually performed with an interrupted pattern (Bellah 1989; Mehl et al. 2005). Fine monofilament synthetic absorbable suture on a taper needle is most often used for ureteral repairs. Full-thickness sutures are completely covered by uroepithelium within 3 weeks. Ureteral peristalsis is diminished for 1–3 weeks after primary ureteral repair (Bellah 1989).

Complete ureteral obstruction can result in permanent renal damage, depending on the duration of the obstruction (Chapter 70). In healthy dogs, renal function will normalize if ureteral patency is restored within 7 days

Nephrology and Urology of Small Animals. Edited by Joe Bartges and David J. Polzin. © 2011 Blackwell Publishing Ltd.

after obstruction. Complete obstruction for more than 4 weeks results in total loss of function of the affected kidney (Wilson 1977). Placement of a catheter stent or nephrostomy tube for urinary diversion has been recommended to maintain renal function and prevent the deleterious effects of urine extravasation (Chapter 32). Ureteral catheter stents that divert urine from ureteral repair sites may improve ureteral regeneration and reduce scar tissue formation. Large catheters, however, delay re-epithelialization, inhibit peristalsis, incite fibrous tissue reaction, and increase the risk of infection and stricture. Therefore, routine stenting of ureters is not recommended. If urine diversion is required, a nephrostomy tube or periureteral drain can be placed (Bellah 1989). Nephrostomy tubes are also associated with a high complication rate (Kyles et al. 2005).

In most animals with extensive ureteral damage, nephroureterectomy is recommended, unless the contralateral kidney is dysfunctional. A variety of techniques have been used for ureteral reconstruction, including bladder flaps and tubes, intestinal conduits, free mucosal grafts, and replacement with synthetic materials. Of these, reconstruction with a full thickness pedicle bladder flap, such as a Baori flap, provides the best success.

Perioperative management

Surgery is recommended for patients with complete ureteral obstructions, unresponsive pyelonephritis, perinephric abscesses or cysts, unilateral renal neoplasia, severe ureteral or renal trauma, or congenital ureteral anomalies causing systemic illness or incontinence. Diagnostic tests, preoperative supportive care, and prognosis depend on the underlying condition.

Diagnostic tests

In general, complete blood count, biochemistry and coagulation panels, urinalysis (Chapter 7), urine culture (Chapter 9), and blood pressure measurements (Chapter 13) should be performed in any animal undergoing renal or ureteral surgery. Systolic blood pressure >180 mmHg is considered abnormal (Vaden et al. 2005). Risk of intra- or postoperative hemorrhage is increased in patients with azotemia, hypertension, or thrombocytopenia (Bigge et al. 2001). Buccal mucosal bleeding time is recommended in patients with uremia, which impairs platelet adhesion and aggregation (Bigge et al. 2001). A cross-match should be performed in any animal with coagulopathy or anemia or in which excessive bleeding is expected. Coagulation panels were reportedly abnormal in 39.8% of dogs and 51.9% of cats tested before renal biopsy (Vaden et al. 2005).

Abdominal radiographs (Chapter 15) and renal ultrasound (Chapter 16) are performed in most affected animals to evaluate renal and ureteral structure, identify urinary calculi, examine organs for primary or metastatic neoplasia, and obtain fluid or tissue samples. Bilateral renal involvement has been reported in 4–32% of dogs with primary renal tumors, primarily with neoplasia of renal tubular cell origin (Klein et al. 1988; Bryan et al. 2006). Abdominal metastases are noted in 54% of dogs with primary renal tumors, with the liver and ipsilateral adrenal gland most commonly affected (Klein et al. 1988). In cats with primary renal tumors, 36% have metastases to the abdominal cavity, including liver, adrenal gland, peritoneum, and mesentery (Henry et al. 1999). Abdominal ultrasound and radiographs should be repeated immediately before exploratory surgery in animals with ureteral calculi, since calculi may shift spontaneously into the bladder or renal pelvis (Dalby et al. 2006).

Thoracic radiographs should be performed in any animal in which neoplasia is suspected. Pulmonary metastases are noted on thoracic radiographs in 16–48% of dogs with primary renal tumors at the time of diagnosis; 77% have metastatic disease at the time of death (Klein et al. 1988; Bryan et al. 2006). In cats with nonlymphomatous primary renal tumors, pulmonary metastases are diagnosed preoperatively in 43% (Henry et al. 1999). Thoracic radiographs are also recommended in patients who are dyspneic or have undergone trauma. Hydrothorax and urothorax have been reported with perirenal cysts and diaphragmatic renal herniation, respectively (Rishniw et al. 1998; Störk et al. 2003).

Renal function should be evaluated by contrast studies (Chapter 15) or scintigraphy (Chapter 18), particularly if unilateral nephroureterectomy is being considered (Lanz and Waldron 2000). Systemic administration of contrast medium may exacerbate renal injury and result in hypotension or anaphylactic shock (Feeney et al. 1980). In patients with decreased renal function, diagnosis and localization of ureteral obstructions can be made with antegrade pyelography (ultrasound-guided percutaneous renal pelvis injection), although leakage of contrast material results in nondiagnostic studies in 28% of cats (Adin et al. 2003).

In patients with suspected ectopic ureters, cystoscopy (Chapter 19) is more accurate when compared to contrast radiography (Cannizzo et al. 2003). Cystoscopy permits identification of terminal ureteral openings and visualization of multiple ureteral fenestrations, troughs, and concurrent vestibular abnormalities. Additionally, many ectopic ureters can be corrected noninvasively with transcystoscopic laser ablation.

Preoperative care

When possible, uremia, blood pressure abnormalities, anemia, coagulopathies, and electrolyte imbalances should be corrected before anesthesia. Patients with hypoproteinemia will require oncotic support. An indwelling urinary catheter is placed to monitor urine production before and after surgery. Patients with erythrocytosis secondary to renal neoplasia may require phlebotomy (removal of 10–20 mL/kg of blood) and intravenous fluids to normalize packed cell volume and decrease the risk of intraoperative hemorrhage and postoperative thromboembolism (Nitsche 2004). Because complication rates are high after renal and ureteral surgery, medical management of nephric or ureteral calculi is usually attempted before considering surgery. Surgery is recommended for animals with complete obstruction, worsening azotemia, or unresponsive pyelonephritis (Kyles et al. 2005).

Maintenance of renal perfusion under anesthesia is critical; therefore, pre- and intraoperative hypotension should be corrected or prevented. Drugs that cause hypotension (e.g., acepromazine) or neprhotoxicity (e.g., aminoglycosides and nonsteroidal anti-inflammatory drugs) should be avoided. Animals with renal dysfunction are often premedicated with an anticholinergic drug and opioids and induced with intravenous propofol or an inhalant anesthetic delivered by mask. Anesthesia is maintained with isoflurane or sevoflurane, and blood pressure and urine output should be monitored during the procedure. Dopamine or dobutamine may be required intraoperatively in hypotensive animals. Epidural administration can reduce intraoperative anesthetic requirements and provide pre-emptive and postoperative analgesia.

The abdomen should be prepped from midthorax to pubis. If the incision is to be extended to the pubis or the urethra catheterized, the clip and prep should include the perivulvar or peripreputial region. Wide lateral preps are performed in patients that may require feeding tube or nephrostomy tube placement.

Besides standard surgical instruments and suction, fine needle holders, scissors, and thumb forceps should be available. For small ureters, 6–0 to 8–0 monofilament suture on a taper needle may be required. Magnification (ocular loupes or an operating microscope) is critical for ureteral surgery.

Postoperative care

Intravenous fluids are continued after surgery to maintain renal perfusion and prevent blood clot formation within the urinary tract (Figure 60.1). Postoperative anal-

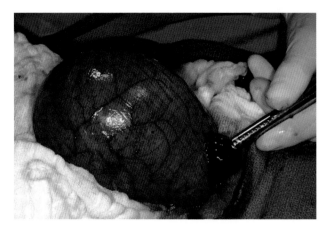

Figure 60.1 Ureteral and urethral obstruction from a large blood clot in the bladder.

gesia can be delivered by intermittent intravenous injections or a constant rate infusion of opioids. Animals should be monitored for anemia, oliguria or anuria, or evidence of urinary tract obstruction, and physical activity should be severely restricted for at least 24 hours. Depending on the surgery and the patient's condition, early postoperative follow-up may include serial red blood cell and platelet counts and biochemistry panels, blood pressure measurement, quantization of urine output, and reassessment of ureteral structure and function with ultrasonography or excretory urography.

Surgery of the kidneys

Renal biopsy

Introduction

Renal biopsies (Chapter 23) are primarily performed in animals with renal neoplasia (Chapter 57) or diseases of the renal cortex, such as protein-losing glomerulopathy (Chapter 53). They may also be recommended for patients with nephrotic syndrome without signs of systemic disease or acute, progressive renal failure (Chapter 49), for which the cause cannot be determined by less invasive means (Vaden et al. 2005). Because of the risk of complications, renal biopsies should only be performed when results are likely to alter patient management by providing an accurate diagnosis or facilitating prognostication (Vaden 2004). They are not necessary in patients with chronic or end stage renal disease or when owners are unwilling to pursue further therapy. Contraindications for renal biopsy include uncontrolled coagulopathy or hypertension, large or multiple renal cysts or abscesses, extensive pyeloneophritis, ureteral obstruction, and severe hydronephrosis (Rawlings et al. 2003; Vaden 2004, 2005).

In healthy adolescent dogs, serial renal biopsies with 18-gauge automatic biopsy needles do not significantly affect glomerular filtration rate (Groman et al. 2004).

A minimum of 5–10 glomeruli are needed for diagnosis of renal disease. A surgical approach is five times more likely to provide good-quality samples that only contain renal cortex because it allows adequate patient immobilization, complete visualization of the kidneys, and improved control of needle penetration and post-biopsy hemorrhage (Vaden et al. 2005). In animals with glomerular disease, samples should be of sufficient size so that portions can be submitted in formalin for light microscopy, in glutaraldelhyde or other appropriate fixatives for electron microscopy, and frozen for immunofluorescence (Vaden 2004).

Tissues may be obtained by parenchymal incision, or with a needle biopsy instrument through an open or laparoscopic approach. There is no difference in sample quality obtained by percutaneous or laparoscopic needle biopsy (Rawlings et al. 2003; Vaden et al. 2005). Disposable spring-loaded biopsy instruments are preferred over manually operated devices because they are easier to control and therefore more likely to provide good quality samples limited to the cortex (Vaden 2004). Needle sizes of 14- to 18-gauge have been recommended by various authors. In one study, samples obtained with 14-gauge double-spring-activated biopsy needles provided excellent quality specimens with large numbers of glomeruli, while samples obtained with 18-gauge biopsy needles often had few glomeruli and were crushed or fragmented (Rawlings et al. 2003). In another study, samples obtained with 16-gauge or 18-gauge needles were more likely to contain only cortex and less likely to contain medulla compared with samples obtained using a 14-gauge instrument (Vaden et al. 2005). Poor sampling techniques or insufficient sample size may result in incorrect diagnosis (Zatelli et al. 2003).

Techniques

Semi-automatic needle biopsy technique

Select a new 14- or 16-gauge biopsy needle with a 1.7–2.0 cm distal channel. Spring load the needle guide by pulling back on the handle. With some instruments, the needle guide can be retracted either 1 or 2 cm into the external gliding cannula. Depth of biopsy should be based on renal size and biopsy location. For generalized renal disease, select a biopsy site that will include only renal cortex, for example, across the cranial or caudal pole or longitudinally along the outer, convex surface of the kidney. Grasp the kidney with one hand to elevate it from the paralumbar fossa. If necessary, free it from its peritoneal attachments. Insert the tip of the guide into the parenchyma

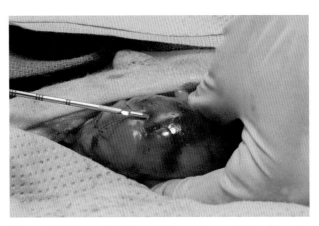

Figure 60.2 Insert the biopsy instrument parallel to the outer surface of the kidney so that it remains within the renal cortex.

to the level of the external gliding channel. Angle the needle so that it will travel within the outer fourth of the kidney (Figure 60.2). Keeping the instrument and kidney immobile, press on the end of the needle guide with your thumb to insert it into the renal cortex, then trigger the firing mechanism with your thumb to sever the parenchyma with the external channel. Remove the instrument from the kidney, and apply digital pressure to the resultant hole to control hemorrhage. If desired, take a second sample from a separate site or from the same site, angling in a different direction. If the biopsy site continues to bleed, close the capsule or overlying peritoneum with a simple interrupted or cruciate suture of 3–0 or 4–0 monofilament absorbable material on a taper needle. To expose the sampled tissue, spring-load the needle guide, then extend the needle guide from the external channel. Using a syringe and needle, spray the guide with a stream of sterile saline to gently dislodge the sample into a container.

Laparoscopic approach

Prep and drape the ventral and lateral abdominal surfaces. With the animal in dorsal recumbency, insert the primary trocar cannula (10 or 12 mm) on the midline, 3 cm caudal to the umbilicus, using an open technique. Place traction sutures on both sides of the linea alba to maintain a tight seal around the trocar cannula. With an insufflator, distend the peritoneal cavity with carbon dioxide. Insert the laparoscope through the cannula and attach the camera and light source. Place a second trocar cannula (5 mm) paramedian and caudal to the first cannula. Insert laparoscopic forceps through the 5 mm cannula to manipulate the viscera. Roll the dog slightly laterally to improve exposure of the kidney of interest. Stabilize the kidney with the laparoscopic forceps, then palpate the abdominal wall near the kidney. Make a small skin incision in the abdominal wall and insert a 16-cm long biopsy needle through the incision into the abdomen, visualizing the insertion with the laparosope. Position the biopsy needle tangential to the surface of the kidney and activate the spring mechanism. Examine the site for bleeding (Rawlings et al. 2003) (Chapter 21).

Wedge or core biopsy through an open approach

Although the kidney can be approached through a paracostal incision, a ventral midline celiotomy is more commonly performed. Elevate the kidney from the paralumbar fossa. Free the kidney from its peritoneal and sublumbar attachments if it is covered in fat or cannot be easily retracted from the abdomen, or if a focal lesion is present or the renal arteries are to be occluded with a tourniquet or vascular clamp. If an assistant is available, the renal arteries are palpated and digitally occluded between thumb and forefinger. If no assistant is available, reflect the kidney ventromedially; identify the renal artery and occlude it with a vascular clamp or Rumel tourniquet. The renal parenchyma will soften 30–60 seconds after arterial occlusion. Place a laparotomy pad dorsolateral to the kidney to keep it elevated. Limit continuous occlusion time to 20 minutes.

A sample can be obtained with a 4 mm skin punch biopsy or scalpel blade. With a no. 11 or 15 scalpel blade, make a crescent-shaped incision 5–10 mm long and about 5 mm deep into the renal cortex. The kidney will bleed readily at this time; if the artery is properly occluded, hemorrhage will be dark and flow continuously. If the artery is not occluded, hemorrhage will be bright red and pulsating. Connect the two ends of the incision with a straight cut, angling inward to sever remaining parenchymal attachments (Figure 60.3). Remove the sample by elevating it with the blade or gently lifting it by the cap-

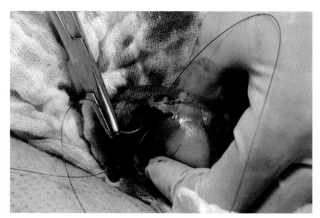
Figure 60.4 Take wide shallow bites of parenchyma and capsule to close the biopsy site.

sule or along one edge with fine thumb forceps, being careful not to crush the tissues.

If a skin punch biopsy is used, insert it through the capsule and into the parenchyma with a gentle twisting motion. Angle the biopsy punch as you withdraw it from the biopsy site to remove the sample. If the sample is not completely detached, use fine scissors to sever parenchymal attachments. In some cases, the sample will remain in the punch and can be removed by inserting saline or a stylet through the opposite end of the instrument.

Close the defect with simple interrupted or cruciate sutures of 3–0 or 4–0 absorbable monofilament material on a taper needle. Take wide bites, including parenchyma lateral to the incision (Figure 60.4). Follow the curve of the needle as you pass it through the tissues and do not lift up when passing the needle or tying the suture, as this will cut through the tissues and increase hemorrhage.

Complications

Complications are reported in 1–21.7% of animals undergoing surgical renal biopsies; rates are similar for wedge and needle techniques (Vaden et al. 2005). Complications are more likely to occur in animals with thrombocytopenia or prolonged clotting times (Bigge et al. 2001; Vaden et al. 2005). Other factors associated with complications include serum creatinine >5 mg/dL and patient age >4 years or weight less than 5 kg (Vaden 2004). Major complications are seen in 8.9% of animals, with severe hemorrhage being the most common. Uncontrolled systemic hypertension or administration of nonsteroidal anti-inflammatory drugs within the previous 5 days may increase the risk of hemorrhage (Vaden 2004). Other complications include hematuria, hydronephrosis secondary to renal pelvis or ureteral obstruction by blood clots, renal infarction, damage to renal vasculature, intrarenal arteriovenous fistula

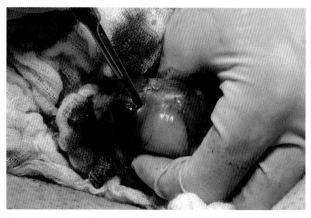
Figure 60.3 Make a semicircular incision in the renal parenchyma, then transect the biopsy specimen with a straight cut, angling inward.

formation, infection, cyst or intrarenal hematoma formation, and renal fibrosis (Bigge et al. 2001; Vaden 2004, 2005). Microscopic hematuria is expected in 20–70% of dogs and cats and generally resolves within 48–72 hours. Macroscopic hematuria is reported in 1–4% and usually resolves within 24 hours. Small perirenal hematomas may be seen in 10% of dogs and 17% of cats. Linear infarcts and parenchymal fibrosis and atrophy are common after biopsy, and retention cysts may develop along needle tracts. Effect on renal function is minimal in healthy animals (Vaden 2004, 2005). Death is reported in ≤3% of animals (Vaden 2004).

Repair of renal lacerations

Introduction

Capsular closure, with or without inclusion of superficial parenchyma, is used to control hemorrhage in animals with renal lacerations or incisions (Chapter 59). To reduce parenchymal engorgement and improve capsular apposition, the renal artery should be occluded digitally or with an atraumatic clamp before attempting repair. Bleeding from iatrogenic or traumatic renal lacerations that persists after placement of capsular or superficial parenchymal sutures may be controlled with sterile biodegradeable cyanoacrylate tissue adhesive. Sterile copolymer blends of ethyl and methoxypropyl cyanoacrylate are hydrolyzed and absorbed by the tissues within 60–90 days of application (Tobias et al. 2007). In patients with extensive trauma, nephroureterectomy may be required.

Suture closure

Once the parenchyma begins to soften after renal artery occlusion, appose the renal capsule with a simple interrupted, cruciate, mattress, or continuous pattern, using 3–0 or 4–0 absorbable monofilament suture on a taper needle. Although interrupted sutures take longer to place, they are usually more reliable in animals with thin capsules. Because the capsule tears easily, a superficial bite of parenchyma can be included with each suture. As with renal biopsy closure, follow the curve of the needle and do not lift up when taking tissue bites or tying knots. Apply digital pressure for 5 minutes to control continued hemorrhage (Bjorling and Petersen et al. 1990).

Cyanoacrylate capsular closure

As with the suture technique, temporarily occlude the renal arteries and, once the parenchyma becomes soft, hold the capsule edges in apposition with manual compression. Apply a thin layer of tissue adhesive over the laceration; do not allow the adhesive to enter the parenchy-

mal gap. Tissue adhesive will not adhere if applied too thickly or if the wound is bleeding vigorously. The adhesive dries within 60 seconds and induces histologic changes similar to suture (Tate et al. 2006; Tobias et al. 2007).

Nephrotomy

Introduction

The most common indication for nephrotomy is removal of renal calculi (Chapter 69). Because of potential complications, however, renal calculus removal is usually only performed in animals that have significant morbidity from infection, progressive renal dysfunction, or obstruction and that do not improve with medical management (Ross et al. 1999; Ross et al. 2007). Previous studies reported temporary postoperative decreases in glomerular filtration rate of 15–50% in normal dogs within 4 weeks after undergoing nephrotomy; however, renal perfusion in these dogs may have been affected by anesthetic protocol and intraoperative hypotension (Gahring et al. 1977; Fitzpatrick et al. 1980; Stone et al. 2002). Additionally, extensive compression of parenchyma with mattress sutures during nephrotomy closure can decrease perfusion (Gahring et al. 1977). Infusion of mannitol during total renal ischemia may reduce cell swelling and deterioration of renal function (Stone et al. 2002). With appropriate intraoperative support and surgical technique, unilateral nephrotomy has minimal effect on renal function in normal cats (Bolliger 2005). Effect in animals with preexisting renal dysfunction is unknown. Since nephrolithiasis is not associated with increased rates of mortality or disease progression in cats with mild or moderate chronic renal disease, medical management is recommended when renal function is stable (Ross et al. 2007).

Nephrotomy can be performed with a bisectional or intersegmental technique. In the bisectional technique, the kidney is divided along its longitudinal midline; thus, intraparenchymal vessels that cross the midline are severed. With the intersegmental technique, the parenchyma is divided along the vascular boundary between the two halves of the kidney, leaving major parenchymal vessels intact. In normal dogs, bisectional nephrotomy results in significantly greater intrarenal hemorrhage, cortical infarction, and cortical inflammation 8 days after surgery than intersegmental nephrotomy; however, neither technique decreases renal function (King 1974; Stone et al. 2002). In normal cats, bisectional nephrotomy with blunt parenchymal separation and no intraparenchymal vascular ligation has no significant effect on glomerular filtration rate, as long as hemorrhage and vascular disruption are minimal (King et al. 2006). Obstructive patterns may be seen on scintigraphy 48 hours after nephrotomy but usually resolve within 7 days.

Some authors recommend performing nephrotomies 4–6 weeks apart in animals with bilateral disease (Ross et al. 1999; Lanz and Waldron et al. 2000). The decision to perform bilateral versus unilateral staged nephrotomy depends on the patient's renal function, degree of obstruction, presence of severe pyelonephritis, and overall condition of the animal (Ross et al. 1999). If staged procedures are performed, renal function should be re-evaluated before performing the second surgery. Some authors recommend operating on the least affected kidney first since they feel it is less likely to be affected by anesthesia and surgery. Complete obstruction to urine outflow in patients with a concomitant urinary tract infection is a surgical emergency because of the risk of sepsis and acute renal failure (Ross et al. 1999).

Technique

Bisectional nephrotomy

Elevate the kidney from the paralumbar fossa and free it from its sublumbar attachments with sharp and blunt dissection. Often, the peritoneal attachments can be torn digitally. Small vessel from the peritoneum or sublumbar attachments may penetrate the renal capsule and will bleed when torn. Control hemorrhage with digital pressure or careful bipolar electrocautery. Occlude the renal artery(ies) with atraumatic vascular forceps, rumel tourniquet, or an assistant's fingers. Limit renal ischemic time to 20 minutes (Figure 60.5). If possible, occlude only the renal artery so that the renal parenchyma drains and becomes more pliable. Place a moistened laparotomy pad dorsolateral to the kidney to keep it elevated during the procedure.

Incise the renal capsule longitudinally along the midline of the convex surface of the kidney with a no.10 or no. 15 scalpel blade. Extend the incision over two-thirds of the kidney's length. Separate the renal parenchyma bluntly to the level of the pelvis with hemostatic forceps or the blunt end of a scalpel handle. Double ligate any blood vessels encountered during bisection with 4–0 or 5–0 absorbable suture material before transection.

Once the renal pelvis is exposed, remove calculi with forceps and submit for culture and quantitative analysis. Obtain a culture of the renal pelvis as well. Examine the pelvis for additional calculi, particularly within the recesses of the major calices. With a syringe, small catheter, or lacrimal cannula, flush the renal pelvis thoroughly with warm saline to remove any remaining mineral aggregates, clots, or debris. If desired, catheterize the ureter antegrade through the renal pelvis or retro-

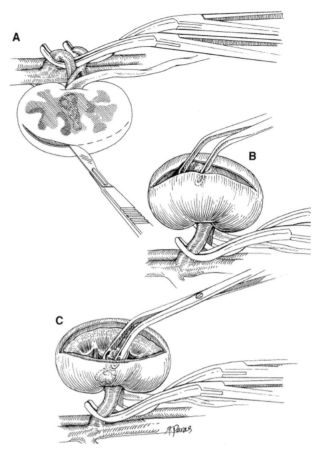

Figure 60.5 Nephrotomy (from Lanz and Waldron, 2000).

grade through a ventral cystotomy and gently flush to ensure patency. Close the nephrotomy site with 4–0 or 5–0 monofilament absorbable suture in a continuous or interrupted pattern, with suture bites placed through the renal capsule and a small amount of cortex (Lanz and Waldron et al. 2000; Stone et al. 2002). Release the vascular occlusion and examine the kidney for hemorrhage. Additional simple interrupted sutures are added when there is active hemorrhage; replacement of the bulldog clamp may be required to close the capsule if hemorrhage is significant (Lanz and Waldron 2000; King et al. 2006). Hemorrhage can also be reduced with direct pressure or by tacking omentum over the site (King et al. 2006). In some animals, bisectional nephrotomy can be closed by direct digital apposition and compression of the bisected renal parenchyma. Press the two halves together, then release the renal artery clamp. Maintain manual compression until hemostasis is achieved (Gahring et al. 1977).

Intersegmental nephrotomy

As with bisectional nephrotomy, elevate the kidney and free it from its peritoneal and sublumbar attachments.

Reflect the kidney ventromedially to expose its dorsal surface, and dissect the fat gently away from the renal pelvis to expose the dorsal and ventral branches of the renal artery. To determine the intersegmental boundary of vascular perfusion, place a vascular clamp on the dorsal branch of the renal artery, then administer 5 mL of indigo carmine into a peripheral vein. The portion of the kidney supplied by the ventral branch of the renal artery will be outlined by the dye. As with bisectional nephrotomy, temporarily occlude the renal arteries. Incise the renal capsule along the intersegmental plane, and bluntly separate the renal parenchyma (Stone et al. 2002).

Complications

Intrarenal hemorrhage is usually marked 1 day after nephrotomy. Persistent hemorrhage and vascular disruption may cause permanent parenchymal damage (Stone et al. 2002; King et al. 2006). Other potential complications include perirenal hemorrhage, persistent microscopic hematuria, and hydronephrosis secondary to blood clot obstruction (Stone et al. 2002; Bolliger et al. 2005; King et al. 2006). Perirenal hemorrhage may occur if sutures pull through the capsule and superficial cortex or if the parenchyma is not apposed sufficiently during the procedure. Postoperative urine leakage may occur in animals with hydronephrosis (Lanz and Waldron 2000). Renal pelvis hyperechogenicity secondary to mineralization is reported in 67% of cats after nephrotomy, and renal pelvis dilation is reported in 50%, although renal function may not be affected by either of these conditions (Bolliger et al. 2005). Although some authors recommend nephropexy to immobilize the kidney after nephrotomy (Lanz and Waldron 2000), reports of renal torsion have not been found in the literature.

Nephrostomy tube

Introduction

A nephrostomy tube provides temporary urine diversion from the renal pelvis and out the abdominal wall (Chapter 32). Nephrostomy tubes are primarily used in patients undergoing ureteral surgery when anastomotic leakage or obstructive swelling is expected (Bjorling and Petersen 1990). They have also been placed in animals that require stabilization before definitive surgery for ureteral obstruction (Nwadike et al. 2000) and for intrapelvic infusion of antimicrobials (Starkey and McLoughlin 1996). Types of tubes include flanged or pig-tail nephrostomy tubes and Foley or red rubber catheters. Kits are available for nonsurgical percutaneous insertion under ultrasound guidance. Because nephros-

tomy tubes are associated with a high rate of postoperative complications, routine placement after ureteral surgery is not recommended.

Technique

Clip, prep, and drape the ventral and lateral surfaces of the abdomen. Through a midline abdominal incision, perforate the peritoneum and abdominal musculature of the lateral abdominal wall near the kidney on the affected side, then incise the skin over the forceps. Insert a wire stylet into a 5 or 8 Fr catheter (e.g., red rubber or Foley). Pass the catheter through the abdominal wall incision into the abdomen, guiding it in with the forceps. Insert the catheter and stylet through the renal capsule and cortex and advance them into the renal pelvis. Holding the tube stable, remove the stylet carefully so that the catheter is retained in the renal pelvis.

If a proximal ureterotomy has been performed, a 20-gauge over-the-needle intravenous catheter can be advanced retrograde through the ureterotomy and renal pelvis and exited out through the renal cortex. Tie a length of suture material to a 5 Fr red rubber or Foley catheter and pass the suture through the over-the-needle catheter. Gradually withdraw the over-the-needle catheter and suture from the ureterotomy site, pulling the red rubber or Foley catheter gently through the renal cortex and pelvis and into the ureter. Cut the suture and gently retract the nephrostomy tube into the renal pelvis before securing the tube to the renal capsule and closing the ureterotomy.

To secure the tube, place a purse string suture of 4–0 absorbable monofilament through the capsule around the catheter and tighten gently. With two finger trap sutures, secure the catheter to the kidney capsule and then to the abdominal wall musculature. Tack the kidney to the body wall with mattress sutures of 4–0 absorbable monofilament, incorporating a small amount of renal cortex with each suture. With a fingertrap pattern, secure the nephrostomy catheter externally to the external abdominal musculature by taking deep bites through the skin and underlying muscle. Attach the catheter to a closed urinary collection system.

After the abdomen is closed, cover the exit wound with a sterile dressing to minimize risk of ascending infection. A restraint device (e.g., Elizabethan collar or side bars) should be placed on the animal to prevent premature removal. When the tube is no longer needed, the external finger trap sutures are removed; if a Foley catheter was used, the balloon is deflated, and the tube is removed with gentle continuous traction. The wound should seal within 2–3 days, unless the ureter is still obstructed (Bjorling and Petersen 1990).

Complications

Complications are seen in 46% of cats undergoing nephrostomy tube placement for ureteral obstruction and include uroperitoneum (25%), poor drainage, and dislodgement (Kyles et al. 2005). In cats undergoing ureteral surgery, mortality rates are higher for those that receive emergency nephrostomy tubes or dialysis catheters. Risk of dislodgement can be reduced by securing the catheter to the abdominal musculature instead of the skin alone. Leakage can be detected radiographically by injecting 1 mL of water soluble iodinated contrast material through the nephrostomy tube.

Pyelolithtomy

Introduction

Because damage to renal function is less likely, pyelolithotomy is preferred over nephrotomy for removal of calculi of the renal pelvis and proximal ureter, particularly when the renal pelvis is dilated (Chapters 58 and 69). With this technique, renal parenchyma is left intact, reducing the risk of intraparenchymal hematoma formation, and occlusion of the renal arteries is not required. Pyelolithotomy is difficult to perform when the renal pelvis is normal in size (Greenwood and Rawlings 1981).

Technique

Using blunt and sharp dissection, free the kidney from its sublumbar attachments and isolate it with moistened laparotomy pads. Reflect the kidney medially to expose its dorsal surface. Gently dissect overlying tissues from the renal pelvis, taking care not to damage branches of the renal vessels. With a no. 15 or no. 64 beaver blade, incise the renal pelvis and proximal ureter longitudinally (Figure 60.6). Extend the incision with fine scissors as needed. Remove large calculi with forceps and dislodge small calculi by flushing with a syringe with a catheter tip or attached lacrimal cannula. Submit the calculi for culture and quantitative analysis and obtain a fluid sample from the renal pelvis for culture. Flush the renal pelvis and proximal ureter gently and thoroughly with sterile saline to remove any debris or clots. If possible, catheterize the ureter antegrade and flush gently with sterile saline or perform a ventral cystotomy and catheterize and flush ureters retrograde to expel remaining calculi and verify ureteral patency (Greenwood and Rawlings 1981). If available, a small arthoscope can be inserted through the incision to examine the renal pelvis and proximal ureter for residual calculi. Alternatively, suture can be passed antegrade down the ureter to verify patency. Close the renal pelvis and proximal ureter

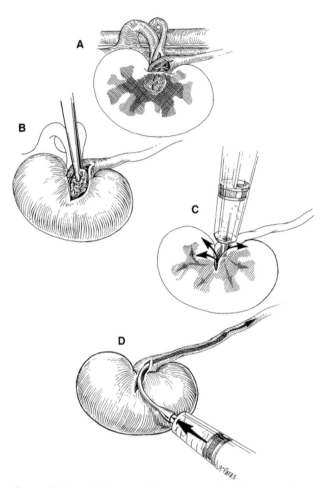

Figure 60.6 Pyelolithotomy (from Lanz and Waldron, 2000).

with 5–0 or 6–0 absorbable synthetic suture in a simple continuous pattern.

Complications

Leakage of urine may occur from the incision site if ureteral obstruction is present. Damage to renal vessels during dissection could further exacerbate renal dysfunction.

Perinephric cyst extirpation or omentalization

Introduction

A subcapsular perinephric pseudocyst is a serous fluid collection within a fibrous sac around one or both of the kidneys (Figure 60.7) (Chapter 56). The fibrous sac is often attached to the renal hilus or poles. Because perinephric pseudocysts lack an epithelial lining, they are not true cysts. Extravasated fluid may accumulate under or outside of the renal capsule; fluid is usually a transudate (Ochoa et al. 1999). Perinephric pseudocysts are bilateral in approximately 40–50% of cats (Ochoa et al.

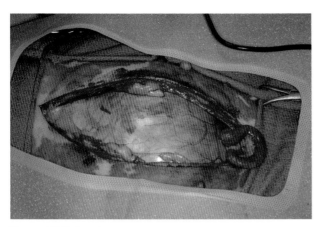

Figure 60.7 Renal cyst.

1999; Beck et al. 2000; Hill and Odesnik 2000; Inns 1997). Treatment may include ultrasound-guided drainage, capsulectomy, or nephroureterectomy (Ochoa et al. 1999). If fluid reoccurs after ultrasound-guided drainage, surgical removal of the capsule may be required. Survival times in cats treated with capsulectomy are longer than those that undergo unilateral nephrectomy (Beck et al. 2000). If the perinephric cyst becomes abscessed, nephroureterectomy is usually recommended unless function of the contralateral kidney is reduced. In that case, the abscess is surgically drained and omentalized.

Technique

Perform a ventral midline celiotomy and exploratory laparotomy. Identify the pseudocyst and, with metzenbaum scissors, dissect the lining away from the retroperitoneal fascia. Open and drain the cyst (Figure 60.8) and collect fluid for cytology, biochemical analysis, and culture. Resect the majority of the cyst wall, leaving at least 1 cm of capsular tissue along the renal attachment. Avoid dissection around the renal hilus (Beck et al. 2000). Insert

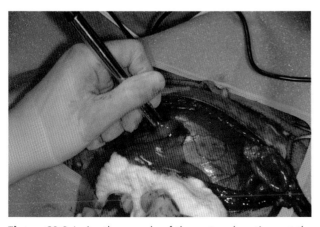

Figure 60.8 Incise the capsule of the cyst and suction out the contents.

the free end of the caudal omental fold into the remaining sac and tack it to the capsule remnants with interrupted, absorbable sutures (Hill and Odesnik et al. 2000; Inns 2007). If needed, extend the omentum by transecting its dorsal attachments near the greater curvature of the stomach, using cautery and ligation for hemostasis. For animals with bilateral pseudocysts, each corner of the extended omental sheet can then be advanced into the cyst cavity and tacked in place.

Complications

Although pseudocysts themselves are usually sterile, cats with perinephric pseudocysts often have urinary tract infections (Ochoa et al. 1999). Because perinephric pseudocysts are usually found in older cats with chronic renal failure, declining renal function is expected since pseudocyst resection does not prevent progression of renal disease. Ascites may develop in up to 25% of cats after surgery (Beck et al. 2000). If it does not gradually diminish or is compromising the patient, an echocardiogram and blood pressure measurements should be performed to determine whether cardiovascular dysfunction is present. Remnants of pseudocystic lining may continue to effuse after resection, and nephroureterectomy may be required to resolve the effusion (Rishniw et al. 1998).

Partial nephrectomy

Introduction

Partial nephrectomy has been recommended for animals with renal pole trauma in which persistent hemorrhage cannot be staunched by compression or capsular closure. In most instances, surgeons will perform a complete nephroureterectomy unless the contralateral kidney is also diseased.

Technique

Free the kidney from its peritoneal and sublumbar attachments with a combination of sharp and blunt dissection, and reflect it ventrally and medially to expose the renal vessels. Temporarily occlude the renal artery with an atraumatic vascular clamp, Rumel tourniquet, or an assistant's fingers, limiting continuous occlusion time to 20 minutes. Remove damaged, friable tissue with sharp transection, using a blade or scissors; leave the capsule intact, if possible. Remove renal artery occlusion temporarily to identify any intraparenchymal vessels that can be ligated, then reapply. Leave renal pelvis defects open, as with nephrotomy, and appose the overlying parenchyma, or close pelvis defects with 4–0 to 6–0 monofilament, rapidly absorbable suture in a continuous pattern (Bellah 1989; Bjorling and Petersen 1990).

If the renal capsule is present, appose it with 3–0 or 4–0 absorbable monofilament material in a continuous or interrupted pattern, taking superficial bites of renal parenchyma as needed. If the capsule is not intact, compress thick bleeding parenchymal tissue with multiple overlapping full thickness mattress sutures of 2–0 or 3–0 absorbable monofilament. Tighten the sutures firmly to appose and compress the parenchyma along the traumatized edge, then sharply transect the tissues beyond these sutures. Cover the exposed parenchyma with omentum, peritoneum, a seromuscular patch, or intestinal serosa (serosal patch), suturing it to the remaining capsule (Bjorling et al. 1990). If desired, place one or two transabdominal continuous suction drains near the kidney before closure to detect postoperative urine leakage. These can usually be removed 24–48 hours after surgery if no leakage is detective.

Complications

Renal dysfunction may progress in animals with severe renal trauma. Other potential complications include urine leakage and ureteral obstruction. Excretory urography can be performed several days after surgery to evaluate renal function and urine flow. In normal animals undergoing partial nephrectomy, use of peritoneal flaps to close capsular defects results in more renal atrophy than primary capsular apposition (Murphy and Best 1957).

Nephrectomy

Introduction

Indications for nephroureterectomy include unilateral primary renal or ureteral neoplasia (Figure 60.9) (Chap-

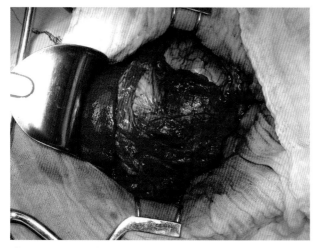

Figure 60.9 Renal carcinoma in a boxer dog. Note omental adhesions and extesive vascularity of the renal capsule.

ter 57), abscess, renal or ureteral trauma (Chapter 59), ectopic ureter (Chapter 58), acquired ureterovaginal fistula after ovariohysterectomy, benign idiopathic renal hemorrhage, or irreversible loss of function or severe pyelonephritis in animals with ureteral calculi (Chapter 58) (Holt et al. 1987; Bjorling and Petersen 1990; Lamb 1994; Lautzenhiser and Bjorling 2002; Weisse et al. 2002; Snyder et al. 2004; Bryan et al. 2006). Animals that undergo nephroureterectomy for ectopic ureters or ureteroceles also require ligation or resection of the distal ectopic tissue to reduce postoperative incontinence.

Structure and function of the contralateral kidney should be evaluated in all patients before considering nephrectomy. Unilateral nephroureterectomy is contraindicated in patients with bilateral renal disease, unless the kidney to be removed is expected to cause severe morbidity, such as with advanced pyelonephritis or abscess.

During surgery, renal arteries and veins in animals with hydronephrotic or nonfunctional kidneys may be difficult to detect. Extensive revascularization may be present, however, in neoplastic kidneys, requiring ligation of multiple peritoneal and sublumbar vessels.

After unilateral nephrectomy, the remaining kidney increases 10–15% in size because of cellular hypertrophy and, in young dogs, cellular hyperplasia. The rate of increase is rapid for the first 2–3 months, and then gradually slows. (Churchill et al. 1999) Compensatory hypertrophy is greatest in animals nephrectomized at <12 months of age (Urie et al. 2007). Creatinine increases slightly in normal dogs 2.5 years after unilateral nephrectomy (Urie et al. 2007).

Technique

Perform a midline celiotomy, starting at the xiphoid and extending caudally to the level of the bladder trigone. Expose the left or right kidney by medial retraction of the mesocolon or mesoduodenum, respectively. Free the kidney from its peritoneal and sublumbar attachments with sharp and blunt dissection or electrocautery (Figure 60.10). Often, a peritoneal incision can be extended by digital traction with index fingers. Ligate, hemoclip, or cauterize any peritoneal vessels that extend to the kidney (Figure 60.11). Reflect the kidney toward midline and expose the renal artery and vein near the aorta and caudal vena cava (Figure 60.12). Paired renal arteries may be present, particularly on the left side in the dog, while cats may have multiple renal veins. In intact animals that are not undergoing gonadectomy, expose the renal vessels between the hilus and any gonadal vessel tributaries. Separate the renal artery and vein, and triple ligate each, then transect the vessels between the two lateral most sutures.

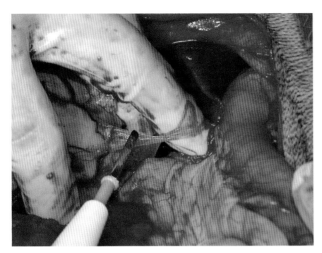

Figure 60.10 Divide the peritoneal attachments with blunt or sharp dissection or cautery.

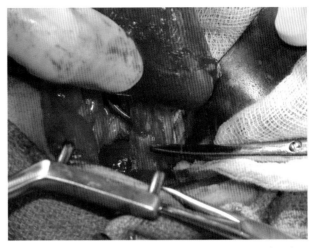

Figure 60.12 Identify the renal arteries and veins. In this dog, two renal arteries were present.

For added security, transfix vessels ≥4 mm in diameter. With sharp and blunt dissection, expose and elevate the ureter from the retroperitoneal space and follow it to its termination (Figure 60.13). Ligate the ureter near its termination with absorbable monofilament suture before transecting cranial to the ligature.

Complications

Although complications from the procedure itself are uncommon, animals may suffer morbidity from progression of renal dysfunction or metastatic disease after nephrectomy. Other potential complications include postoperative hemorrhage or, rarely, development of arteriovenous fistula from mass ligation of the renal artery and vein. Median survival after unilateral nephrec-

tomy in dogs with primary renal neoplasia is 16 months (range, 0–70 months) (Bryan et al. 2006). Dogs with renal hemangiosarcoma and hemoperitoneum have median survival of 62 days (Locke and Barber 2006). Postoperative chemotherapy does not significantly increase survival time (Bryan et al. 2006).

Surgery of the ureters

Ureteral catheterization

Introduction

Ureters are most commonly catheterized to verify patency in animals with ureteral calculi or to maintain patency during bladder or ureteral reconstruction (Greenwood and Rawlings 1981; Snyder et al. 2004). In animals with

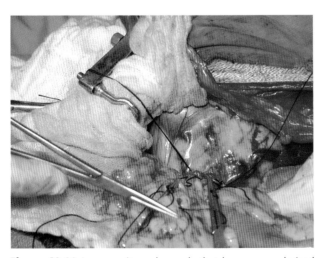

Figure 60.11 Large peritoneal vessels that have revascularized the renal parenchyma should be occluded with ligatures or staples.

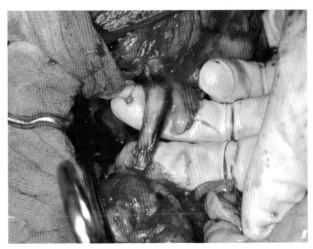

Figure 60.13 Follow the ureter to the bladder, and ligate and transect it close to its termination.

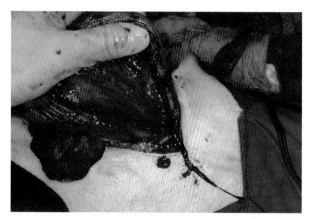

Figure 60.14 Idiopathic renal hematuria. A large clot extruded from the ureteral opening.

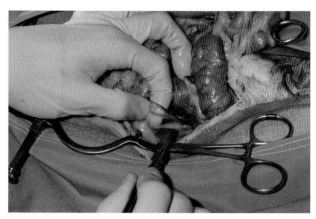

Figure 60.15 Midureteral calculus in a cat.

idiopathic renal hematuria (Figure 60.14), ureters are catheterized to collect samples from individual kidneys for microscopic analysis and culture (Holt et al. 1987). Normal cat ureters are usually too small to catheterize.

Technique

After performing a caudal midline celiotomy and exploratory, isolate the bladder with moistened laparotomy pads. Place a stay suture at the apex of the bladder to maintain traction. Perform a ventral midline cystotomy to expose the ureteral openings entering the dorsum of the bladder at the trigone. Suction the lumen gently to remove urine. Do not wipe bladder mucosa with sponges and avoid contact of mucosa with the suction tip, since mucosal swelling can easily interfere with visualization of the ureteral openings. Insert a 3.5 or 5 Fr red rubber catheter or close ended tomcat catheter cranially (about 5–10 mm) until resistance is felt at the S-bend of the ureter. Elevate the catheter and direct the tip dorsally and caudally until it passes through the S-bend, then advance the catheter cranially into the ureter. Palpate the vesicouretal junction and ureters dorsally to confirm placement. In animals with idiopathic renal hematuria, attach collection systems to each catheter to obtain individual urine samples.

Complications

Aggressive catheterization may cause obstruction from swelling. Ureteroliths may be inadvertently flushed into the renal pelvis.

Ureterotomy

Introduction

Ureterotomy is a technically demanding procedure that requires advanced training, specialized instruments, and

magnification. It is most frequently recommended for removal of calculi within the proximal third of the ureter, particularly when they are adhered to mucosa (Chapter 58) (Lanz and Waldron 2000; Hardie and Kyles 2004; Snyder et al. 2004).

Technique

After performing a ventral midline incision and exploratory laparotomy, identify the location of the ureteral calculus by palpation and visual inspection (Figure 60.15). Elevate the ureter from the paralumbar space, taking care to preserve the blood supply. Gently dissect periureteral fat from over the calculus. Using ocular magnification, make a longitudinal or transverse incision through the dilated portion of the ureter just proximal to the calculus, or directly over the calculus, with a #11, #15, or #64 blade (Figure 60.16) (Bellah 1989; Lanz and Waldron 2000; Hardie and Kyles 2004). Collect fluid from the ureterotomy side for culture and sensitivity. Extend the ureterotomy with a blade or fine scissors as needed. Avoid retrograde displacement of the calculus during

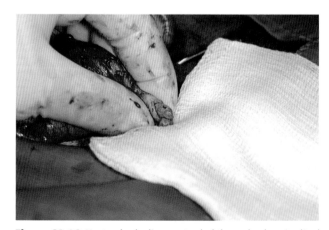

Figure 60.16 Ureteral calculi are extruded through a longitudinal ureterotomy.

ureteral manipulation (Dalby et al. 2006). Remove the calculus with fine forceps, and flush the ureteral ends with warm saline delivered through a lacrimal cannula. In dogs, perform a cystotomy, place a retrograde ureteral catheter, and flush the ureter to verify patency. Alternatively, insert a small arthroscope into the ureteral ends to check for residual calculi. In cats with small ureters, 5–0 polypropylene suture can be passed gently antegrade into the bladder or retrograde from the bladder to check patency. Submit the stone for quantitative analysis. Close the ureterotomy site with full thickness simple continuous or interrupted sutures of 5–0 to 8–0 absorbable material. Although longitudinal incisions can be closed transversely to increase ureteral diameter, this technique is unnecessary in dilated ureters and may cause obstruction of small ureters. If the ureteral mucosa or musculature is damaged extensively from the calculus, perform a ureteral resection and anastomosis (Lanz and Waldron 2000).

Complications

Potential complications include leakage, dehiscence, stricture, continued or progressive renal dysfunction, and recurrence of calculi (Snyder et al. 2004). In cats with ureteral calculi repaired by ureterotomy or ureteroneocystostomy, surgical complications were reported in 31% and perioperative mortality rate was 18% (Kyles et al. 2005). Uroperitoneum was reported in 16% of cats after ureterotomy; most of these cats required a second surgery to revise the ureterotomy closure (Kyles et al. 2005). Persistent obstruction is noted in 3% of cats undergoing ureterotomy for calculus removal.

Ureteral resection and anastomosis

Introduction

As with ureterotomy, ureteral resection and anastomosis is technically challenging. It is therefore performed uncommonly and use is usually limited to lesions of the proximal ureter. Indications may include ureteral stricture or damage from trauma or calculi (Chapters 58 and 59).

Technique

Perform a ventral midline celiotomy to expose the bladder, kidney, and ureter. Gently elevate the ureter from its sublumbar location, leaving as much periureteral tissue as possible to maintain blood supply. If desired, place stay sutures of 5–0 or 6–0 suture material in the periureteral tissues adjacent to the proposed sites of transection, leaving the maximum ureteral length to reduce anastomotic tension. Under magnification, transect the

ureters and remove any periureteral adipose tissue from the distal ends. Make a 3–4 mm longitudinal incision on opposite sides of each ureteral end to spatulate the tissue and increase the circumference of the anastomotic site. Place the spatulated ends opposite to one another, making sure that the ureters have not twisted. Appose the ends with full-thickness, simple, interrupted sutures of 6–0 to 8–0 absorbable monofilament material, placing the apical sutures first. Return the ureter to the sublumbar space and cover with omentum if desired. If postoperative obstruction is a concern, place a nephrostomy tube to temporarily divert urine for 2–7 days until swelling resolves and the mucosa is healed.

Complications

Ureteral obstruction from swelling or stricture is the most likely complication. Urine leakage or use of a ureteral stent will increase the risk of stricture formation.

Ureteroneocystostomy

Introduction

Transection of the ureter with reimplantation into the bladder is called ureteroneocystostomy. Indications for ureteroneocystostomy include renal transplantation (Chapter 31); reconstruction of ectopic, ruptured, avulsed, strictured, or inadvertently ligated ureters (Chapter 58); removal of ureteral calculi (Chapter 59); or resection of distal ureteral tumors (Chapter 57) (Lanz and Waldron 2000; McLoughlin and Chew 2000; Nwadike et al. 2000; Weisse et al. 2002; Reichle et al. 2003; Hardie and Kyles 2004; Steffey et al. 2004). Because the kidneys can be easily mobilized in many animals, ureteral reimplantation can be successfully performed when 3–4 cm of the proximal ureter remain. Animals with extensive ureteral resection will require renal descensus and nephropexy to reduce anastomotic tension.

Surgical prep for ureteral transplantation in animals with ectopic ureter should extend caudal to the pubis and include the perivulvar tissues in female dogs. During surgery, catheters that are passed antegrade through the ectopic distal ureteral segment may inadvertently exit from the vulva.

Ureteroneocystostomy is most commonly performed using an intravesicular approach, except in cats undergoing renal transplantation. In normal cats, creatinine concentrations and renal pelvis diameter tended to return to normal more quickly after undergoing interrupted extravesicular anastomosis (Mehl et al. 2005). In dogs with ectopic ureters, extravesicular reimplantation resulted in more complications than intravesicular anastomosis (Holt and Moore 1995). Use of a simple continuous pattern for extravesicular anastomosis increases postoperative mortality (Mehl et al. 2005). Ureters can be reimplanted at any location proximal to the trigone; short ureters are usually transplanted at the apex of the bladder to reduce anastomotic tension.

Some authors recommend formation of a short oblique submucosal tunnel (3:1 tunnel length to ureteral orifice diameter) during intravesicular ureteral implantation. In normal dogs, formation of a short oblique submucosal tunnel results in less fibrosis and ureteral dilation than a transverse pull through technique; however, vesicoureteral reflux is not seen in normal dogs with either technique (Waldron 1987).

If ectopic ureters or ureteroceles are present, the distal anomalous segment of the ureter must also be removed or ligated to reduce postoperative incontinence. Extramural ectopic ureters are ligated and transected as close to their termination as possible (Figure 60.17). The distal segment of an intramural ectopic ureter can be ligated from an extraluminal approach or dissected free via an intravesicular approach (see below). Resection of the intramural ectopic ureteral segment does not significantly improve outcome as compared with ligation of the ectopic remnant (Mayhew et al. 2006). Ureteroceles that occur external to the bladder ("ectopic") are resected and

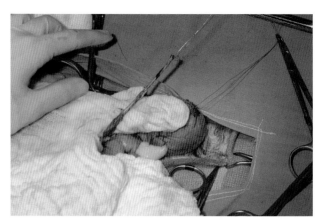

Figure 60.18 Stay suture through the ureteral end.

closed primarily. Orthotopic ureteroceles, which occur within the bladder lumen, can be partially resected and left open, as long as the ipsilateral ureteral stoma is in a normal position (McLoughlin and Chew 2000; Tattersall and Welsh 2006).

Technique: intravesicular ureteroneocystostomy

Perform a midline celiotomy, exposing the bladder and trigone. Extend the incision to the xiphoid for examination of the proximal ureter or kidney or to perform a renal descensus. Place a stay suture in the apex of the bladder for retraction to expose the proximal urethra. Place a second stay suture in the ureter 3–5 mm proximal to the proposed transection site before severing the ureter (Figure 60.18). If an intramural ectopic ureter is present, temporarily catheterize the distal ureteral segment. In all other animals, ligate the distal ureteral segment with 3–0 absorbable monofilament suture as close to its termination as possible.

Gently isolate the proximal ureteral end from surrounding fascia, sparing its arterial blood supply. Perform a ventral midline cystotomy. To facilitate manipulation of the tissues, place stay sutures intermittently along the incised edges of the bladder. If desired, excise a 4–5 mm ellipse of bladder mucosa at the proposed site of ureteroneocystostomy. Insert a fine-tipped mosquito hemostatic forceps from the lumen through the bladder wall. Grasp the ureteral stay suture with the forceps and pull the ureter through the bladder wall and into the bladder lumen (Figures 60.19 and 60.20). Verify that the ureter has not been twisted during placement. Remove any periureteral fat from around the distal end of the ureter and transect the ureteral tissue containing the stay suture. Using tenotomy or iris scissors, incise the ventral wall of the terminal ureteral end longitudinally for 2–5 mm to enlarge

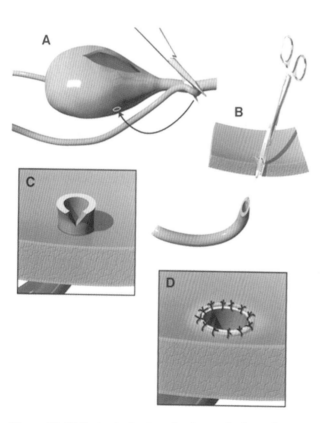

Figure 60.17 Ureteral reimplantation for repair of ectopic ureter (from McLoughlin and Chew, 2000).

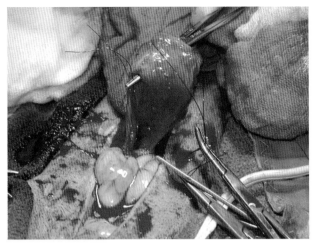

Figure 60.19 Insert a fine-tipped hemostat from the bladder lumen through the bladder wall and grasp the stay suture.

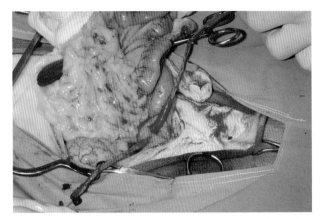

Figure 60.21 Cat with bilateral calculi of the proximal one-third of the ureter. Both ureters have been pulled through the bladder wall to the level of the calculi.

the opening (Figures 60.21 and 60.22). Appose ureteral mucosa to bladder mucosa with 5–8 simple interrupted sutures of 4–0 to 8–0 absorbable monofilament material on a taper needle, placing the first two sutures at the cranial and caudal ends of the new ureteral ostium (Figure 60.23) (Lanz and Waldron 2000; McLoughlin and Chew 2000). If possible, insert a red rubber catheter through the new ureteral opening and feed it several centimeters antegrade into the ureter. Place one or two simple interrupted sutures externally between the bladder serosa and ureteral muscle to further secure the ureter to the bladder (Figure 60.24).

If an ectopic ureteral segment is present, preplace several encircling sutures of 3–0 or 4–0 nonabsorbable or slowly absorbable monofilament material around the catheterized distal ectopic ureteral segment, starting and ending needle penetration externally on the serosal

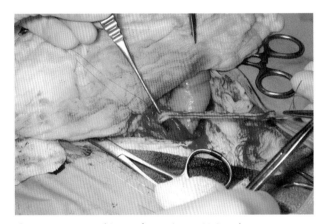

Figure 60.22 In this cat from Figure 60.21, the ureters were opened to the level of the calculi and the obstructions were removed. Handle only periurethral tissue with forceps.

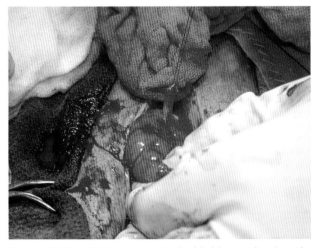

Figure 60.20 Pull the ureter into the bladder. In this dog, the bladder wall is everted to expose mucosa.

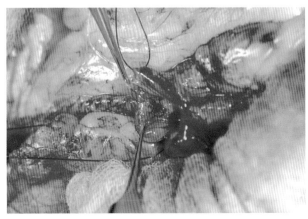

Figure 60.23 Neoureterostomy. The ureteral end was spatulated and sewn to bladder mucosa with interrupted sutures of fine absorbable monofilament.

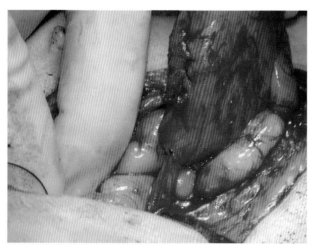

Figure 60.24 Two interrupted sutures were placed to secure the ureteral serosa to the bladder serosa.

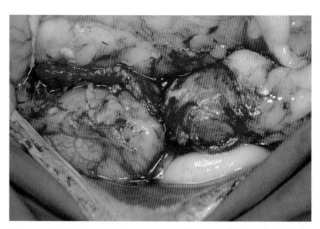

Figure 60.25 Cystonephropexy. In this cat, all but 2 cm of the proximal ureter were resected.

surface of the bladder. Remove the catheter and tie the sutures firmly to occlude the remaining ectopic intramural segment (Lanz and Waldron 2000; Taney et al. 2003).

Close the bladder with 3–0 or 4–0 monofilament suture in a simple continuous or inverting pattern. If desired, leave the retrograde ureteral catheter in place during closure of the cranial extent of the bladder to ensure ureteral patency; remove the catheter before completing the closure.

Technique: extravesicular ureteroneocystostomy

Make a 1 cm long, partial thickness incision through the apex of the bladder to expose the mucosa. Incise the distal end of the ureter longitudinally to spatulate the end. Make an incision through the bladder mucosa the same length as the spatulated ureter. Using 6–0 to 8–0 monofilament material on a taper needle, place a simple interrupted suture between the bladder and ureteral mucosa at the cranial and caudal ends of the incision. Insert a polypropylene suture into the ureteral lumen to ensure patency after the first two sutures are tied; remove this stenting suture before tying the final anastomotic suture. Appose the remaining cystic and ureteral mucosa along each side of the ureteroneocystostomy with a simple interrupted pattern (Mehl et al. 2005). Partially close the seromuscular bladder incision with 5–0 monofilament suture material, taking care not to obstruct the ureter (Hardie and Kyles 2004).

Technique: renal descensus

Mobilize the kidney by incising its peritoneal and fascial attachments. Pull the kidney caudally and medially

toward the bladder. Secure the caudal renal pole to the bladder (nephrocystopexy) with mattress sutures of 4–0 absorbable monofilament, taking bites of capsule and a small amount of renal cortex and including the bladder submucosa (Figure 60.25).

Alternatively, incise the peritoneum over the ipsilateral psoas muscle near the mobilized kidney. Pull the bladder cranial and tack it to the psoas muscle ("psoas hitch" or cystopexy) with 3–0 absorbable or nonabsorbable material. Pull the kidney caudally and tack it to the transversus abdominus and internal abdominal oblique muscles ("nephropexy"), using mattress sutures of 4–0 absorbable monofilament (Nwadike et al. 2000; Hardie and Kyles 2004).

Complications

Complications included hydroureter or hydronephrosis from temporary or permanent obstruction and uroabdomen from dehiscence or necrosis. Renal pelvic dilation, based on ultrasonography, is expected after ureteroneocystostomy because of postoperative swelling (Mehl et al. 2005). In normal dogs diagnosed with iatrogenic partial obstruction, based on results of scintigraphy, renal function gradually recovers 1–2 weeks after ureteroneocystostomy (Barthez et al. 2000). Hydroureter and hydronephrosis may occur with complete or partial obstruction of the ureter secondary to swelling, blood clots, or stricture formation. Hydroureter from edema or tissue trauma usually resolves in 4–6 weeks. If ureters are dilated before surgery, hydroureter will most likely be permanent. Of cats undergoing ureteroneocystostomy for ureteral calculi, 11% had persistent obstruction that required surgical revision and 15% developed uroabdomen because of distal ureteral necrosis or avulsion from the bladder (Kyles et al. 2005). In dogs with extravesicular reimplantation and anastomosis of the ectopic ureter, 8% required nephroureterectomy because of persistent hydronephrosis (Holt and Moore 1995).

In dogs with ectopic ureters, urinary incontinence persists in 44–67% (Lanz and Waldron 2000; Mcloughlin and Chew 2000). In cats with ectopic ureters, 92% are continent after ureteral transplantation and ligation of the distal ureteral segment (Holt and Gibbs 1992).

Neoureterostomy

Introduction

Intramural ectopic ureters (Chapter 58), which are the most common type of ectopic ureter, insert externally on the bladder at the normal site but continue to travel as submucosal tunnels or mucosal troughs through the trigone region. Submucosal ectopic segments may open at one or more sites along the urethra distal to the trigone or at the vestibule or vagina. In animals with intramural ectopic ureters, a new ureteral opening ("neoureterostomy") can be made by incising through the bladder mucosa into the ureter and apposing the mucosa of the two structures. Some authors recommend removal of any distal ectopic segments or troughs to improve urethral sphincter (McLoughlin and Chew 2000). Others prefer ligation of the distal ectopic segment. With the advent of cystoscopic-assisted laser ablation of distal intramural segments, surgical approach to this condition is becoming less common.

Technique

If the ectopic distal ureteral segment is to be removed, prep and drape female dogs to include the perivulvar region. Perform a ventral midline celiotomy, extending the incision caudally so that the bladder trigone can be visualized. Isolate the bladder and urethra with moistened sterile laparotomy pads. If necessary, place a stay suture in the apex of the bladder and retract it manually or secure it to Balfour retractors to facilitate bladder exposure.

Neoureterostomy with ligation of the ectopic segment

Perform a ventral midline cystotomy from the apex through the trigone. Examine and palpate the bladder to identify the intramural portion of the ureter. The ureter may appear as a small swelling and should feel like a tubular structure within the bladder submucosa. If the ureter is not evident, compress the urethra digitally to obstruct and dilate the ureter so that it can be palpated more easily. With a no. 15 scalpel blade or no. 64 beaver blade, make a 4–5 mm longitudinal incision through the dorsal bladder mucosa into the ureteral lumen at the cranial most

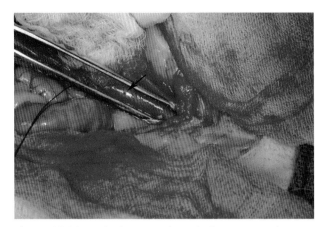

Figure 60.26 Urethral opening (arrow) of an intramural ectopic ureter.

extent of the intramural portion of the ureter. Catheterize the ureter antegrade and retrograde with two red rubber catheters. Suture the ureteral mucosa to the bladder mucosa with 4–0 to 6–0 absorbable monofilament material in a simple interrupted pattern. Preplace several sutures of 3–0 or 4–0 nonabsorbable material around the catheterized ectopic segment, with needle penetration starting and ending externally on the serosal surface of the bladder. Remove the catheter and tie the sutures firmly (Lanz and Waldron 2000; Taney et al. 2003). Close the bladder routinely.

Neoureterostomy with bladder neck reconstruction

Perform a ventral midline cystotomy and extend the incision through the ventral urethra to expose the ectopic opening (Figure 60.26). Catheterize the ureter retrograde through the ectopic opening with a red rubber tube (Figure 60.27). If the distal ureteral orifice cannot be identified, make an incision through the urethral mucosa

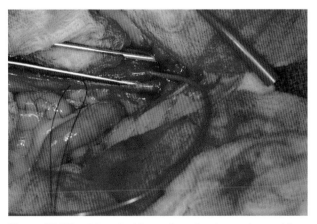

Figure 60.27 A 3 Fr red rubber catheter has been advanced from the ectopic opening retrograde into the intramural ectopic ureter.

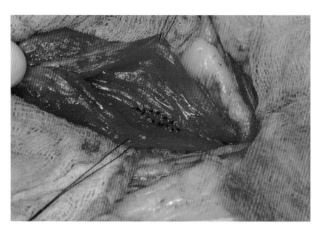

Figure 60.28 Final appearance after resection and closure of the intramural ectopic segment and neoureterostomy.

into the lumen of the distal ectopic submucosal ureter and catheterize the ectopic ureter retrograde from that point. With the catheter in place, dissect the ectopic ureter from the surrounding tissues with fine scissors, beginning distally. Include mucosa, submucosa, and some muscularis in the resection. Be careful to leave the dorsal urethral seromuscular layer intact. Continue dissection to the proximal most extent of the intramural ureter, just cranial to the trigone. Close the resulting urethral and bladder defect with 4–0 or 5–0 synthetic absorbable monofilament suture in a continuous or interrupted pattern; include underlying submucosa in urethral sutures (McLoughlin and Chew 2000). If hemorrhage is excessive during dissection, alternate dissection and closure as you continue proximally.

Transect the ureteral remnant 0.5 cm from where it passes transmurally through the bladder, then suture the ureteral mucosa of the new ureteral opening to the bladder mucosa with interrupted sutures of 5–0 or 6–0 absorbable monofilament (Figure 60.28). If a uterocele is present, partially resect the wall and close any urethral openings. If a ureteral trough is present, resect it and reconstruct the bladder as with submucosal tunnels.

If postoperative catheterization is desired, catheterize the bladder and urethra in female dogs before bladder and urethral closure by passing a red rubber catheter through the bladder lumen and into the urethra antegrade. Exit it out the vulva, and attach it to a balloon-tipped catheter with suture. Withdraw the red rubber catheter from the bladder lumen, guiding the balloon-tipped catheter through the urethra and into the bladder. Detach the red rubber catheter and discard it, then inflate the balloon-tipped catheter. Close the bladder and urethra with 4–0 absorbable monofilament suture in a simple continuous or interrupted pattern.

Complications

The most common complication of ectopic ureter repair is continued incontinence. In one study of dogs with ectopic ureters, 71% of dogs that underwent distal ureteral segment resection and bladder neck reconstruction and 50% that underwent distal segment ligation continued to have urinary incontinence. Recurrent urinary tract infections were reported in 15% and 29% of the resection and ligation groups, respectively (Mayhew et al. 2006). Causes of continued incontinence include sphincter mechanism incompetence, hypoplastic bladder, or recanalization of the ligated distal ureteral segment (Holt and Moore 1995; Mayhew et al. 2006). Culposuspension performed at the time of ectopic ureter repair may improve continence (Mouatt and Watt 2007).

Hydronephrosis and hydroureter may develop temporarily because of postoperative edema and inflammation. Stranguria is common after bladder neck reconstruction, and 14% of dogs will develop dysuria. Some animals may require temporary urethral catheterization until postoperative swelling resolves (McLoughlin and Chew 2000). Stricture formation is rare but may occur several weeks to months after surgery (Taney et al. 2003).

Bladder flap reconstruction of the ureter

Introduction

When ureteral length is extremely short because of trauma or extensive resection, the ureter can be reconstructed by formation of a full thickness tube using a pedicle flap from the bladder. The flap can be developed from a vascular portion of the dorsolateral or ventral bladder wall and will provide several centimeters of additional length. Renal descensus should be performed prior to flap development to determine the length of flap required to reach the proximal ureteral segment. Width of the flap should be based on bladder size but should be a minimum of 3 cm, depending on bladder thickness, to provide a tube 5–6 mm in diameter. Nephrocystopexy or nephropexy and psoas hitch are performed before or after ureteral anastomosis to reduce anastomotic tension.

Technique

Develop a single pedicle flap, based at the apex of the bladder, along the ventral or dorsolateral surface of the bladder, incorporating a major vessel if possible. The flap should be widest at its base to preserve blood supply. Length should be sufficient so that no tension will be present on the ureterovesicular anastomotic site after renal descensus. Place a stay suture in the end of the proximal ureteral segment. Pass a fine-tipped mosquito hemostat full thickness through the cranial end of the bladder flap, starting from the mucosa surface. Grasp the stay suture with the forceps and pull the ureter through the flap. Perform a ureteroneocystostomy as described above. Catheterize the new ureteral stoma and begin bladder closure by apposing the flap from side to side with 4–0 absorbable monofilament suture, starting cranially near the ureteroneocystostomy. Once the closure extends at least 1 cm caudal to the new ureteral stoma, remove the ureteral catheter. If desired, place a larger diameter red rubber catheter into the cranial end of the bladder tube and lay it along the length of the flap during closure; this will help to maintain bladder tube diameter as the tissues are apposed. Once tube closure is complete beyond the base of the flap, remove the catheter and close the rest of the bladder incision. If not yet performed, reduce tension on the site with a nephrocystopexy, or sublumbar nephropexy and cystopexy (psoas hitch).

Complications

Stenosis may occur at the ureteroneocystostomy (Gardiner et al. 1990). Vesicoureteral reflux may cause recurrent infection.

Ureterocolonic anastomosis

Considered a salvage procedure, ureterocolonic anastomosis has been performed in animals with urinary bladder or proximal urethral neoplasia. In normal dogs, ureterocolonic anastomosis maintains urinary continence but is fraught with complications, including azotemia, metabolic acidosis, hyperammonemia, neurologic disease, decreased glomerular filtration rate, ascending infection, and death. The procedure is therefore not recommended (Stone et al. 1988).

References

Adin, C.A., E.J. Herrgesell, et al. (2003). Antegrade pyelography for suspected ureteral obstruction in cats: 11 cases (1995–2001). *J Am Vet Med Assoc* **222**: 1576–1581.

Barthez, P.Y., D.D. Smeak, et al. (2000). Ureteral obstruction after ureteroneocystostomy in dogs assessed by technetium Tc 99 m diethylenetramine pentaacetic acid (DTPA) scintigraphy. *Vet Surg* **29**: 499–506.

Beck, J.A., C.R. Bellenger, et al. (2000). Perirenal pseudocysts in 26 cats. *Aust Vet J* **78**: 166–171.

Bellah, J.R. (1989). Wound healing in the urinary tract. *Sem Vet Med Surg Small Anim* **4**: 294–303.

Bigge, L.A., D.J. Brown, et al. (2001). Correlation between coagulation profile findings and bleeding complications after ultrasound-guided biopsies 434 cases (1993–1996). *J Am Anim Hosp Assoc* **37**: 228–233.

Bjorling, D.E. and S.W. Petersen (1990). Surgical techniques for urinary tract diversion and salvage in small animals. *Compend Contin Educ Pract Vet* **12**: 1699–1709.

Bolliger, C., R. Walshaw, et al. (2005). Evaluation of the effects of nephrotomy on renal function in clinically normal cats. *Am J Vet Res* **66**: 1400–1407.

Borkowski, A., K. Piechna, et al. (1979). Regeneration of the ureter and the renal pelvis in dogs from transversely transected and anastomosed strips of the ureteral wall. *Eur Urol* **5**: 352–358.

Brodsky, S.L., P.D. Ziminskind, et al. (1977). Effects of crush and devascularizing injuries to the proximal ureter: an experimental study. *Invest Urol* **14**: 361–365.

Bryan, J.N., C.J. Henry, et al. (2006). Primary renal neoplasia of dogs. *J Vet Intern Med* **20**: 1155–1160.

Cannizzo, K.L., M.A. McLoughlin, et al. (2003). Evaluation of transurethral cystoscopy and excretory urography for diagnosis of ectopic ureters in female dogs: 25 cases (1992–2000). *J Am Vet Med Assoc* **223**: 475–481.

Churchill, J.A., D.A. Feeney, et al. (1999). Effects of diet and aging on renal measurements in uninephrectomized geriatric bitches. *Vet Radiol Ultrasound* **40**: 233–240.

Dalby, A.M., L.G. Adams, et al. (2006). Spontaneous retrograde movement of ureteroliths in two dogs and five cats. *J Am Vet Med Assoc* **229**: 1118–1121.

Feeney, D.A., C.A. Osbourne, et al. (1980). Effect of multiple excretory urograms on glomerular filtration of normal dogs: a preliminary report. *Am J Vet Res* **41**: 960–963.

Fitzpatrick, J.M., M.S. Sleight, et al. (1980). Intrarenal access: effects on renal function and morphology. *Br J Urol* **52**: 409–414.

Gahring, D.R., D.T. Crowe, et al. (1977). Comparative renal function studies of nephrotomy closure with and without sutures in dogs. *J Am Vet Med Assoc* **171**: 537–541.

Gardiner, R.A., G.A. Mills, et al. (1990). Evaluation of a bladder advancement extension graft technique. *Br J Urol* **66**: 606–612.

Gerlaugh, R.L., W.E. DeMuth, et al. (1960). The healing of renal wounds. II. Surgical repair of contusions and lacerations. *J Urol* **83**: 529–534.

Greenwood, K.M. and C.A. Rawlings (1981). Removal of canine renal calculi by pyelolithotomy. *Vet Surg* **10**: 12–21.

Groman, R.P., A. Bahr, et al. (2004). Effects of serial ultrasound-guided renal biopsies on kidneys of healthy adolescent dogs. *Vet Radiol Ultrasound* **45**: 62–69.

Hardie, E.M. and A.E. Kyles (2004). Management of ureteral obstruction. *Vet Clin North Am Small Anim Pract* **34**: 989–1010.

Henry, C.J., S.E. Turnquist, et al. (1999). Primary renal tumors in cats: 19 cases (1992–1998). *J Feline Med Surg* **1**: 165–170.

Hill, T.P. and B.J. Odesnik (2000). Omentalisation of perinephric pseudocysts in a cat. *J Small Anim Pract* **41**: 115–118.

Holt, P.E. and C. Gibbs (1992). Congenital urinary incontinence in cats: a review of 19 cases. *Vet Rec* **120**: 437–442.

Holt, P.E., V.M. Lucke, et al. (1987). Idiopathic renal haemorrhage in the dog. *J Small Anim Pract* **28**: 253–263.

Holt, P.E. and A.H. Moore (1995). Canine ureteral ectopia: an analysis of 175 cases and comparison of surgical treatments. *Vet Rec* **136**: 345–349.

Huffman, W.L., J.F. McCorkle, et al. (1956). Ureteral regeneration following experimental segmental resection. *J Urol* **75**: 796–800.

Inns, J.H. (1997). Treatment of perinephric pseudocysts by omental drainage. *Aust Vet Pract* **27**: 174–177.

King, M.D., D.R. Waldron, et al. (2006). Effect of nephrotomy on renal function and morphology in normal cats. *Vet Surg* **35**: 749–758.

King, W.W. (1974). Renal wound healing. Histologic and histochemical sequences in the repair of intersegmental nephrotomies. *Inv Urol* **11**: 278–285.

Klein, M.K., G.C. Campbell, et al. (1988). Canine primary renal neoplasms: a retrospective review of 54 cases. *J Am Anim Hosp Assoc* **24**: 443–452.

Kyles, A.E., E.M. Hardie, et al. (2005). Management and outcome of cats with ureteral calculi: 153 cases (1984–2002). *J Am Vet Med Assoc* **226**: 937–944.

Lamb, C.R. (1994). Acquired ureterovaginal fistula secondary to ovariohysterectomy in a dog: diagnosis using ultrasound-guided nephropyelocentesis and antegrade ureterography. *Vet Radiol Ultrasound* **35**: 201–203.

Lanz, O.I. and D.R. Waldron (2000). Renal and ureteral surgery in dogs. *Clin Tech Small Anim Pract* **15**: 1–10.

Lautzenhiser, S.J. and D.E. Bjorling (2002). Urinary incontinence in a dog with an ectopic ureterocele. *J Am Anim Hosp Assoc* **38**: 29–32.

Locke, J.E. and L.G. Barber (2006). Comparative aspects and clinical outcomes of canine renal hemangiosarcoma. *J Vet Intern Med* **20**: 962–967.

Mayhew, P.D., K.C.L. Lee, et al. (2006). Comparison of two surgical techniques for management of intramural ureteral ectopia in dogs: 36 cases (1994–2004). *J Am Vet Med Assoc* **229**: 389–393.

McLoughlin, M.A. and D.J. Chew (2000). Diagnosis and surgical management of ectopic ureters. *Clin Tech Small Anim Pract* **15**: 17–24.

Mehl, M.L., A.E. Kyles, et al. (2005). Comparison of three ureteroneocystostomy techniques in cats. *Vet Surg* **34**: 114–119.

Mouatt, J.G. and P.R. Watt (2007). Ectopic ureter repair and colposuspension in seven bitches. *Aust Vet Pract* **31**: 160–167.

Murphy, J.J. and R. Best (1957). Healing of renal wounds. I. Partial nephrectomy. *J Urol* **78**: 504–510.

Nitsche, E.K. (2004). Erythrocytosis in dogs and cats: diagnosis and management. *Compend Contin Educ Pract Vet* **26**: 104–119.

Nwadike, B.S., et al. (2000). Use of bilateral temporary nephrostomy catheters for emergency treatment of bilateral ureter transection in a cat. *J Am Vet Med Assoc* **217**: 1862–1865.

Ochoa, V.B., S.P. DiBartola, et al. (1999). Perinephric pseudocysts in the cat: a retrospective study and review of the literature. *J Vet Intern Med* **13**: 47–55.

Rawlings, C.A., H. Diamond, et al. (2003). Diagnostic quality of percutaneous kidney biopsy specimens obtained with laparoscopy versus ultrasound guidance in dogs. *J Am Vet Med Assoc* **223**: 317–321.

Reichle, J.K., R.A. Person, et al. (2003). Ureteral fibroepithelial polyps in four dogs. *Vet Radiol Ultrasound* **44**: 433–437.

Rishniw, M., J. Weidman, et al. (1998). Hydrothorax secondary to a perinephric pseudocyst in a cat. *Vet Radiol Ultrasound* **39**: 193–196.

Ross, S.J., C.A. Osborne, et al. (2007). A case-control study of the effects of nephrolithiasis in cats with chronic kidney disease. *J Am Vet Med Assoc* **230**: 1854–1859.

Ross, S.J., C.A. Osborne, et al. (1999). Canine and feline nephrolithiasis. Epidemiology, detection, and management. *Vet Clin North Am Small Anim Pract* **29**: 231–250.

Snyder, D.M., M.A. Steffey, et al. (2004). Diagnosis and surgical management of ureteral calculi in dogs: 16 cases (1990–2003). *N Z Vet J* **53**: 19–25.

Starkey, R.J. and M.A. McLoughlin (1996). Treatment of renal aspergillosis in a dog using nephrostomy tubes. *J Vet Intern Med* **10**: 336–338.

Steffey, M., K.M. Rassnick, et al. (2004). Ureteral mast cell tumor in a dog. *J Am Anim Hosp Assoc* **40**: 82–85.

Stone, E.A., J.L. Robertson, et al. (2002). The effect of nephrotomy on renal function and morphology in dogs. *Vet Surg* **31**: 391–397.

Stone, E.A., M.C. Walter, et al. (1988). Ureterocolonic anastomosis in clinically normal dogs. *J Vet Res* **49**: 1147–1153.

Störk, C.K., A.J. Hamaide, et al. (2003). Hemiurothorax following diaphragmatic hernia and kidney prolapse in a cat. *J Feline Med Surg* **5**: 91–96.

Taney, K.G., K.W. Moore, et al. (2003). Bilateral ectopic ureters in a male dog with unilateral renal agenesis. *J Am Vet Med Assoc* **6**: 817–820.

Tate, P., B. Anneaux, et al. (2006). Evaluation of Tissumend II Sterile as a multipurpose absorbable tissue adhesive. *Int J Appl Res Vet Med* **4**: 74–85.

Tattersall, J.A. and E. Welsh (2006). Ectopic ureterocele in a male dog: a case report and review of surgical management. *J Am Anim Hosp Assoc* **42**: 395–400.

Tobias, K.M. (2007). Devices: Tissumend II sterile absorbable tissue adhesive. *Clinician's Brief* **5**: 47–48.

Urie, B.K., D.M. Tillson, et al. (2007). Evaluation of clinical status, renal function, and hematopoietic variables after unilateral nephrectomy in canine kidney donors. *J Am Vet Med Assoc* **230**: 1653–1656.

Vaden, S.L. (2004). Renal biopsy: methods and interpretation. *Vet Clin Small Anim* **34**: 887–908.

Vaden, S.L., J.F. Levine, et al. (2005). Renal biopsy: a retrospective study of methods and complications in 283 dogs and 65 cats. *J Vet Intern Med* **19**: 794–801.

Waldron, D.R., C.S. Hedlund, et al. (1987). Ureteroneocystostomy: a comparison of the submucosal tunnel and transverse pull through techniques. *J Am Anim Hosp Assoc* **23**: 285–290.

Weisse, C., L.R. Aronson, et al. (2002). Traumatic rupture of the ureter: 10 cases. *J Am Anim Hosp Assoc* **38**: 188–192.

Wilson, D.R. (1977). Renal function during and following obstruction. *Annu Rev Med* **28**: 329–339.

Zatelli, A., U. Bonfanti, et al. (2003). Echo-assisted percutaneous renal biopsy in dogs. A retrospective study of 229 cases. *Vet J* **166**: 257–264.

Section 6

Fluid, electrolyte, and acid–base disorders

61

Sodium disorders

David J. Polzin

Physiology of salt and water balance

The plasma sodium concentration is the ratio of plasma sodium to plasma water. Changes in the quantity of sodium or water could theoretically alter the sodium concentration, but most often disorders of plasma sodium reflect changes in water balance. The reason for this is that sodium and water are regulated largely independently to achieve different goals. As a consequence, the sodium concentration typically informs us more about the water content of the body than the sodium content.

Sodium is the principal cation in the extracellular fluid space (ECF). It remains in the extracellular space, and largely outside of the intracellular fluid space (ICF), because sodium is actively pumped from the ICF to the ECF in exchange for potassium ions by the Na-K-ATPase pump. The net effect of this is to maintain high concentration of sodium within the ECF and low concentrations in the ICF, whereas potassium exists in high concentrations within cells and low concentrations in the ECF. A slow ongoing leak of sodium into cells and potassium out of cells occurs, but the sodium–potassium pump maintains separation of these two ions into their appropriate fluid spaces.

In contrast to sodium and potassium, water freely moves to osmotic equilibrium across cell membranes between the ICF and ECF. Because water moves freely between ICF and ECF, the osmolality of both compartments is always the same, and the relative distribution of water between the ICF and ECF is determined by the relative number of osmotically active particles in each compartment. Sodium ions and their associated anions constitute the bulk of osmotically active particles normally found in the ECF.[1] Because sodium is the principal cation of the ECF and is largely restricted to the ECF, the *total body content* of sodium (an amount, not a concentration) determines the ECF volume.

The volume of the ECF is regulated by monitoring the "effective circulating volume" of the body and retaining or excreting sodium to maintain the appropriate volume. Sodium is not regulated to achieve sodium concentration, only volume, and there is no necessary correlation between the plasma sodium concentration and the ECF volume. "Effective circulating volume" refers to that part of the ECF that is in the arterial system and is effectively perfusing tissues (Rose 2001). It is essentially an unmeasurable entity that reflects tissue perfusion. The body measures effective circulating volume as the pressure perfusing arterial baroreceptors in the carotid sinus, atria, and glomerular afferent arterioles. When the baroreceptors detect an excess in ECF volume, they signal the kidneys to excrete sodium, whereas detection of volume contraction results in renal sodium retention (Chapter 2). This signaling system involves the renin–angiotensin system, sympathetic nervous system, atrial natriuretic peptide, pressure natriuresis, and antidiuretic hormone. Since water follows sodium, excretion of sodium contracts the ECF and retention of sodium expands the ECF. For the most part, sodium retention and contraction occurs in a largely isotonic fashion.

In contrast, plasma sodium concentration is measured by osmoreceptors in the hypothalamus that affect water intake (via thirst) and water excretion by the kidneys (via antidiuretic hormone—ADH). Water intake and water loss result in decreased and increased plasma osmolality, respectively. Since plasma sodium contributes the bulk of plasma osmolality, plasma sodium concentration changes in parallel with plasma osmolality. The body responds to a water load by suppressing ADH secretion, which decreases water reabsorption in the collecting tubules, thus facilitating the excretion of electrolyte-free

Nephrology and Urology of Small Animals. Edited by Joe Bartges and David J. Polzin. © 2011 Blackwell Publishing Ltd.

water. Dehydration promotes secretion of ADH, which leads to insertion of aquaporin 2 channels within the epithelium of the collecting tubules, thus facilitating reabsorption of water and excretion of concentrated urine. In this fashion, plasma osmolality is held within narrow limits with variation of as little as 1–2% in plasma osmolality initiating mechanisms that bring the plasma osmolality back to normal. However, in rare instances, ADH release can be stimulated by marked volume contraction of the ECF. In this setting, the need to maintain ECF volume to perfuse tissues over rides the usual control mechanisms based on osmolality (Chapter 42).

The total body content of sodium determines the ECF volume, whereas plasma osmolality and plasma sodium concentration reflect the ICF volume. In one construct, regulation of plasma osmolality is a means of monitoring and regulating cell volume. Intracellular osmoles are primarily composed of potassium salts of macromolecular ions that are restricted to the ICF. Since water moves to equilibrium and intracellular osmoles are largely fixed, reduction in plasma osmolality means water will move into cells (cells swell), while increased osmolality means water will move out of cells (cells shrink). Because there are roughly twice as many particles in the ICF as in the ECF, the ICF volume is approximately twice the size of the ECF. Movement of water in and out of cells with changes in osmolality is largely responsible for the clinical consequences of hyponatremia and hypernatremia.

Hyponatremia

Hyponatremia indicates an increase in water relative to sodium and is recognized as a serum sodium concentration below the normal range for a given laboratory (typically about <140 mmol/L in dogs and <149 mmol/L in cats). True hyponatremia is usually associated with a decrease in plasma osmolality. Two components are necessary for hyponatremia to develop: (1) a source of electrolyte-free water (EFW) and (2) ADH to prevent excretion of water. The most important defense against development of hyponatremia is renal excretion of EFW. Thus, hyponatremia almost always indicates a defect in water excretion.

Hyponatremia implies cell swelling as a consequence of a net movement of water into cells to achieve osmotic equilibrium. Exceptions to this rule include loss of certain potassium salts from the ICF or pseudohyponatremia (Halperin and Goldstein 1999). Loss of potassium salts from the ICF constitutes a reduction in total intracellular solute, which leads to movement of water out of cells. Pseudohyponatremia is a decrease in plasma sodium that occurs in association with a normal or increased effective plasma osmolality.[2] Hyperglycemia is an example of

pseudohyponatremia with an elevated effective plasma osmolality. Hyperglycemia draws water osmotically out of the ICF due to the osmotic effect of increased concentrations of glucose in the ECF. Mannitol and administration of intravenous immune globulins may produce the same effect (Rose 2001). Pseudohyponatremia with a normal effective plasma osmolality may occur with severe hyperlipidemia or hyperproteinemia. However, this error only occurs when plasma sodium concentration is measured using a flame photometer; it does not occur when the plasma sodium concentration is determined by ion selective electrode unless the plasma sample is diluted.

The clinical importance of recognizing that true hyponatremia (hypoosmotic hyponatremia) usually indicates cell swelling is that hyponatremia-induced swelling of the brain can lead to serious neurological compression injury because the brain is enclosed within a finite space. Acute hyponatremia is likely to result in brain swelling that, when severe, can lead to permanent neurological deficits or death. It has been suggested that a clinically significant acute shift in water requires about a 30–35 mOsm/L or more gradient between the plasma and brain tissue (Rose 2001). This represents a change in plasma sodium of approximately 15–18 meq/L (osmolality includes the sum of sodium ions and their associated anions). Neurological signs are most likely to develop when plasma sodium declines below 120 meq/L in dogs and 130 meq/L in cats (de Morais 2008). However, the rate of decline in osmolality may be as or more important than the actual plasma concentration.

The brain can adapt to cell swelling in chronic hyponatremia by moving solutes out of cells, thus reducing cell osmolality. Solutes removed from brain cells, called osmolytes, include sodium and potassium ions as well as organic solutes such as myoinositol and the amino acids glutamine, glutamate, and taurine. Removal of these solutes occurs over 1–3 days. Restoration of these solutes back into the brain cells as hyponatremia is corrected similarly takes several days to accomplish. This adaptation allows brain cells to maintain normal cell volume during hyponatremia, but places the cells at risk of cell contraction should hyponatremia be corrected too quickly.

The single most important decision to make in managing a patient with hyponatremia is to determine if the patient has acute or chronic hyponatremia. Acute hyponatremia is hyponatremia that has developed within the preceding 48 hours. The major risk associated with hyponatremia is brain swelling. It is important to accurately determine that the patient definitely has acute hyponatremia because it can be safely corrected rapidly, thus reducing the potential for persisting brain injury. However, as mentioned above, if the hyponatremia is corrected too quickly and the patient actually has chronic hyponatremia, osmotic demyelination syndrome[3] (ODS) may occur (see below). As a consequence, it is essential that the diagnosis of acute hyponatremia be definitively based on a demonstrated normal plasma sodium concentration no longer than 48 hours preceding the discovery of hyponatremia.

The ODS is a symmetrical demyelination commonly involving the base of the pons typically observed after therapy for hyponatremia, particularly if the hyponatremia is corrected too rapidly (Halperin and Goldstein 1999). Poor nutrition and hypokalemia are risk factors for development of ODS, probably because they delay restoration of intercellular osmolytes. Clinical signs of ODS vary widely but in its most severe form may include lethargy, weakness, ataxia, confusion, agitation, coma, and spastic or flaccid quadriparesis that develops days to a week after therapy. Diagnosis of ODS may be confirmed by MRI scanning. There is no known treatment.

Acute hyponatremia

When hyponatremia can be confirmed to have been present for less than 48 hours, hyponatremia is considered to be acute. Remember that acute discovery of a chronic condition does not make it an acute condition. Hyponatremia requires a source of water and the presence of ADH to prevent its excretion. Because the source for ADH in acute hyponatremia is usually obvious (Table 61.1), the principal diagnostic concern is to identify the source of electrolyte-free water. The principal risk to the patient is a rise in intracranial pressure and herniation of the brain secondary to brain swelling. The therapeutic principal is to rapidly correct the hyponatremia before it can cause brain injury.

Possible sources for water in patients with acute hyponatremia include administration of dextrose 5% in water, hypotonic saline, ingested water (including water-based enteral feeding supplements), water added to food for tube-feeding, and desalination of administered saline solutions. Desalination of administered saline solutions may occur when an excessive quantity of saline solution (e.g., normal saline) is administered intravenously to a patient, leading to overhydration and volume expansion. The physiologic response to overhydration is for the kidneys to excrete sodium. Normally, water would follow sodium into the urine; however, if ADH is present due to any of the conditions listed in Table 61.1, water may be retained as the sodium is excreted. The net effect would be to excrete the sodium load and retain water, thus producing hyponatremia. Desalination may also occur when isotonic saline is administered to a patient with the syndrome of inappropriate ADH secretion (SIADH—see

Table 61.1 Factors promoting antidiuretic hormone (vasopressin) release or activity

Physiologic stimuli
 Low "effective" circulating volume
 Pain
 Nausea
 Vomiting
 Anxiety
Absence of a physiologic stimulus
 Drugs that stimulate or augment ADH release
 Nicotine and Morphine (increase central ADH release)
 Some chemotherapeutic drugs (by causing nausea)
 Drugs that promote actions of ADH
 Oral hypoglycemics (e.g., chlorpropamide)
 Caffeine
 NSAIDs, aspirin
 Drugs that simulate ADH
 DDAVP
 Oxytocin
Endocrine causes:
 Adrenal insufficiency
 Hypothyroidism
Vasopressin-producing neoplasms
Vasopressin-producing granulomas
CNS or lung lesions (reset osmostat)
 Certain metabolic lesions (porphyria)

below) or when thiazide diuretics are administered to a patient with edema (diuretic causes salt loss, but ADH prevents excretion of water).

Acute hyponatremia that is mild (plasma sodium concentration has declined less than ~15 meq/L) and not associated with clinical signs can generally be managed by limiting the source of water. Water intake should be controlled until the cause for increased ADH abates. However, if acute hyponatremia is associated with clinical signs, more aggressive therapy is indicated and hyponatremia should be corrected quickly. Hypertonic saline may be administered until the neurological signs abate or plasma sodium concentration is close to 135 meq/L (Halperin and Goldstein 1999). When calculating the amount of sodium to administer, assume that the volume behaves as if the sodium is distributed throughout total body water:

$$\text{Dosage of sodium} = (\Delta_{Na^+}) \times TBW$$

Where (Δ_{Na^+}) is the desired increase in plasma sodium and TBW is total body water (~60% of body weight).

Hypertonic saline is recommended rather than isotonic saline because isotonic saline may be desalinated by the patient, thus worsening the hyponatremia.

Table 61.2 Causes for hypo-osmotic hyponatremia

Primary sodium loss
    Non-renal (gastrointestinal, edematous states, skin)
    Renal (renal failure, diuretics)
    Low aldosterone activity
Primary water gain
    Low cortisol levels
    Hypoalbuminemia
    Heart failure
    Hypothyroidism
    SIADH
    Primary polydipsia

Chronic hyponatremia

When hyponatremia has been present for more than 48 hours or is of undetermined duration, hyponatremia is considered to be chronic. Again, hyponatremia requires a source of water and the presence of ADH to prevent its excretion. The principal diagnostic concern with chronic hyponatremia is to identify why ADH is present (Table 61.1). Hypo-osmotic hyponatremia may result from losing sodium or from gaining water (Table 61.2). The principal risk to the patient is overaggressive therapy that lowers plasma sodium concentration too quickly, thus promoting ODS. The therapeutic principle is to slowly correct the hyponatremia to avoid inducing ODS.

In seeking a reason for ADH to be present, the first step is usually to establish whether the ECF is decreased. Determination of the patient's fluid status should be determined on the basis of the physical examination; it cannot be determined from the plasma sodium concentration. Hyponatremia can occur in patients who are volume contracted, volume expanded, or have a normal fluid volume. Patients who are volume contracted likely develop hyponatremia as a result of sodium loss. Hypovolemia may be detected as dry mucous membranes, increased skin turgor, tachycardia, increased hematocrit and total solids, and concentrated urine. Patients who have a normal to expanded ECF likely develop hyponatremia as a consequence of gaining water. Hypervolemia may be detected as gelatinous subcutaneous tissues, serous nasal discharge, chemosis, venous distension, peripheral edema, ascites, or pulmonary edema. However, since electrolyte-free water distributes throughout the total body water, the expansion of the ECF may be subclinical or very mild.

Sodium loss leading to ECF contraction usually occurs in an isotonic fashion. Hyponatremia then develops because the isotonic loss is replaced, at least in part, by electrolyte-free water (EFW). The EFW is retained despite hyponatremia because ADH release occurs as a consequence of volume contraction. In this setting, volume contraction may result from renal or non renal causes. When losses are of non-renal origin, urine sodium is usually low; however, reduced volume resulting from renal losses, gastric vomiting, or low aldosterone activity are likely to be associated with higher urine sodium excretion.

From a diagnostic standpoint, the amount of water taken in relative to the rate of excretion of EFW is an important factor in development of hyponatremia. It can be assessed by performing a tonicity balance: [Water In] > [EFW Out] = Hyponatremia. It is important to recognize that production of "concentrated" urine does not necessarily mean that sodium is being excreted. It is necessary to measure urine sodium to determine whether it is being retained or excreted. Low urine sodium is *usually* a good clinical marker for reduced effective circulating volume. The composition of urine must be compared to fluid/sodium intake to ascertain tonicity balance.

When hyponatremia results from a gain in body water, ECF volume is typically normal or expanded, but "effective" circulating volume may be normal or low. Conditions that may be associated with normal ECF volume, but decreased "effective" circulating volume include low cortisol levels, hypoalbuminemia, heart failure, and hypothyroidism. However, when "effective" circulating volume is normal, SIADH is the likely diagnosis.

SIADH is present when decreased effective circulating volume is not low and ADH release is not under the usual physiological control in a patient with hyponatremia. It can be produced by a variety of disorders including neurologic disorders, drugs, pulmonary disease, postoperative, severe nausea, ectopic ADH production (usually a neoplasm), or exogenous administration of ADH. SIADH is characterized by the following features: (1) hyponatremia and hypoosmolality; (2) urine osmolality that is inappropriately high (greater than 100 mOsm/L); (3) a urine sodium concentration that is not low despite hyponatremia (usually greater than ~40 meq/L in humans, unless the patient is volume depleted for some other reason); (4) normovolemia; (5) normal renal, adrenal, and thyroid function; and (6) normal acid–base and potassium balance (Rose 2001). Hyponatremia in patients with SIADH usually corrects with water restriction. The underlying cause for SIADH should be sought so that therapy for the primary disease may be provided.

Treatment of chronic hyponatremia involves raising the plasma sodium concentration at a safe rate and treating the underlying condition. The hyponatremia should be corrected slowly at a rate unlikely to induce ODS. Ideally, plasma sodium concentration should increase by no more than 8 meq/L/day. If the patient has moderate to severe malnutrition or hypokalemia, correction should be made more slowly. However, if the patient has severe neurological signs (e.g., seizure or coma) thought to be a consequence of hyponatremia itself, consider providing sufficient hypertonic sodium chloride solution to ameliorate the clinical signs (up to about 5 meq/L). This dosage of sodium is considered to be part of the increase allowable for the first day of therapy. The amount given over the 24-hour period appears more important than the rate of administration.

For patients with chronic hyponatremia resulting from sodium loss, the sodium deficit should be calculated as:

$$Na^+ \text{ deficit} = TBW \times Na^+ \text{ deficit per liter}$$

Where TBW is total body water ($\sim$60% of body weight), and the sodium deficit is the difference between the current plasma sodium concentration and the target sodium concentration. Total body sodium is used in this calculation because osmolality is the same in both the ECF and the ICF. The major indication for administering sodium chloride is to correct the volume deficit. This is usually done using normal saline. However, be aware that as the ECF volume deficit is corrected, the stimulus for ADH release may dissipate and water may be rapidly excreted causing a rapid reduction in plasma sodium. If this should happen, one option is to limit water diuresis by administration of ADH until the electrolyte and fluid deficits can be slowly and safely corrected.

Chronic hyponatremia resulting from water surplus may consist of (1) restricting water intake, (2) promoting water loss independent of ADH, and (3) reducing ADH levels. Water loss independent of ADH may be promoted by administering diuretics and replacing electrolytes (e.g., normal saline), but not water. Some causes for ADH release may be correctable, including: correcting volume depletion, providing colloid support for hypoalbuminemia, replacing hormones that are deficient (glucocorticoids, thyroid hormone), improve myocardial function, and withdraw drugs promoting ADH effects. In addition, ADH receptor antagonists (vapatans) can be used to selectively enhance renal EFW excretion; however, their safety, efficacy, and role in managing hyponatremia have not been established in dogs and cats (Francis and Tang 2004).

Hypernatremia

Hypernatremia reflects a relative increase in sodium compared to water and is recognized as a serum sodium concentration above the normal range for a given laboratory (typically about >150 mmol/L in dogs and >160 mmol/L

Table 61.3 Causes of hypernatremia

Pure water deficit
  Loss of electrolyte-free water without access with
    inadequate water consumption
  Diabetes insipidus
  Fever
  High environmental temperature
Dysfunctional thirst mechanism
  Primary hypodipsia
  Adipsia/hypodipsia with neurologic diseases
Hypotonic fluid loss
  Extrarenal loss
  Gastrointestinal
  Cutaneous
  Renal loss
  Third spacing (less likely)
Gain in sodium
  Salt poisoning
  Hypertonic fluid administration
  Hyperaldosteronism
  Hyperadrenocorticism (less likely)
Generation of intracellular osmoles
  Seizures
  Severe exertion

in cats). It may result from loss of EFW, loss of hypotonic fluids, or ingestion or administration of excessive quantities of sodium. Loss of EFW without the ability to replace water is by far the most common cause for severe hypernatremia in dogs and cats. Thirst is the primary defense against development of hypernatremia. It is such a powerful urge that hypernatremia will not develop if the thirst mechanism is intact and access to water is provided. Thirst is initiated when plasma sodium increases as little as 2 meq/L (Halperin and Goldstein 1999).

Successful management of hypernatremia requires recognition and treatment of the underlying disease (Table 61.3). Assessment of the ECF volume provides guidance as to the origin of hypernatremia. With pure water loss (EFW), the patient is hypovolemic, but because the reduction in volume is distributed throughout the TBW, patients may appear normally hydrated or only mildly dehydrated even with substantial loss of body water. In contrast, loss of hypotonic fluid (e.g., some gastrointestinal or urinary losses) typically results in overt signs of volume contraction or dehydration. In both of these instances, body weight will decrease. In the unusual instance where hypernatremia results from ingestion of excess sodium, recognition of an expanded ECF readily reveals the origin of the hypernatremia. Body weight typically increases in such patients. Transient hypernatremia may occur in association with severe exertion or seizures where metabolic generation of intracellular hyperosmolality may draw water from the ECF. In this setting, no change in body water or body weight occurs.

In the majority of hypernatremic patients, the ICF is contracted and patients are at risk of developing CNS hemorrhage subsequent to brain shrinkage. This is most likely to occur when hypernatremia is acute or severe (Halperin and Goldstein 1999). As mentioned above, significant changes in cell volume begin to occur with a gradient in excess of about 35 mOsm/L between the ECF and ICF. Clinical signs may include anorexia, lethargy, vomiting, muscular weakness, behavioral changes, disorientation, ataxia, seizures, coma, and death.

With chronic hypernatremia, brain cells generate intracellular osmoles, which limit the movement of water out of the cells. This effect is essentially the opposite of what occurs in hyponatremia in which the cell content of sodium, potassium, and organic solutes (glutamine, glutamate and inositol) is increased. As with hyponatremia, generation and elimination of these osmolytes requires several days. The clinical impact of this process is that correction of chronic hypernatremia must be done slowly to prevent brain swelling.

Current recommendation is to reduce the plasma sodium concentration slowly unless the patient is symptomatic for hypernatremia. Generally, plasma sodium should not be reduced more quickly than 12 meq/L/day.

When the patient is hypernatremic due to loss of water, the water deficit can be calculated by the formula:

Water Deficit = TBW × Lean Body Weight

$\times \{(\text{patient's plasma}[Na^+]/\text{normal plasma }[Na^+]) - 1\}$

Total body water may be reduced by the estimated volume depletion. When hypernatremia is due to loss of EFW alone, the water deficit is all that is required. It may be provided either orally or intravenously as 5% dextrose

in water depending on the condition of the patient. Continuing water loss should be mitigated if at all possible (e.g., by administration of ADH for diabetes insipidus). However, the water deficit does not account for any isosmotic fluid deficit that may be present with hypotonic fluid losses. The volume deficit that is present in addition to the water deficit may be replaced with isotonic fluid with due consideration as to how this will affect plasma sodium concentration. With severe hypernatremia, it may be necessary to provide fluid volume resuscitation using a solution similar to the patient's sodium concentration to avoid unintentionally rapid reduction in plasma sodium. Volume restoration of the ECF should be rapid if the patient is hypotensive. It may be necessary to measure ins and outs to assure that the net anticipated administration of free water is actually what the patient is receiving. The changes in plasma sodium should be carefully monitored during therapy.

Endnotes

1. Osmolalty of the ECF may be estimated by the formula: Calculated $P_{Osm} = (2 \times \text{plasma Na}) + ([glucose]/18) + ([BUN]/2.8)$.
2. Note that osmolality here refers to measured osmolality, not calculated osmolality.
3. ODS is sometimes called "pontine myelinosis."

References

de Morais, H. and S.P. DiBartola (2008). Hyponatremia: a quick reference. *Vet Clin Small Animal* **38**: 491–495.

Francis, G.S. and W.H.W. Tang (2004). Vasopressin receptor antagonists. *JAMA* **291**: 2017–2018.

Halperin, M.L. and M.B. Goldstein (1999). Fluid, electrolyte, and acid–base physiology. In: *A Problem-Based Approach*, 3rd ed. Philadelphia, PA: WB Saunders.

Rose, B.D. (2001). *Clinical Physiology of Acid–Base and Electrolyte Disorders*, 5th ed. New York: McGraw-Hill.

62

Potassium disorders

Andrea J. Sotirakopoulos and Sheri J. Ross

Normal potassium balance

Hypo- and hyperkalemia are among the most commonly recognized electrolyte abnormalities in both human and veterinary hospitalized patients. The significant morbidity and mortality associated with both hypo- and hyperkalemia underscore the need for prompt recognition and treatment. Potassium is the most abundant cation in the body; normal extracellular fluid (ECF) potassium concentration is approximately 4 mEq/L and the normal intracellular fluid (ICF) potassium concentration is approximately 140 mEq/L. Most of total body potassium (approximately 98%) is contained within cells, with muscle containing 60–70% (DiBartola and de Morais 2006). Only a small percentage (2%) of total body potassium is found in the extracellular compartment (Stanton and Giebisch 1992; Rose and Post 2001b). This differential distribution of potassium is the major determinant of the resting cell membrane potential. The resting membrane potential is maintained by the sodium-potassium-adenosinetriphosphatase (Na$^+$, K$^+$-ATPase) pump located within the plasma membrane of cells. This pump generates a net negative charge by exchanging three sodium ions (moving them out of the cell) for two potassium ions (into the cell) (Clausen and Everts 1989).

Small changes in distribution of potassium within the body may dramatically affect the resting membrane potential of nerve and muscle cells, including myocardial cells, with potentially fatal consequences. Control of potassium homeostasis is tightly regulated to match daily excretion with dietary intake. Regulation of total body potassium relies predominantly on the kidney. Over 90% of potassium excretion occurs through urine (Rose and Post 2001b), with the remaining 10% excreted in feces (Giebisch 1998). Extracellular potassium concentration may rise abruptly with increases in potassium intake as well as with processes or disease states that cause internal redistribution (Giebisch 1998). While the kidney is essential to chronic maintenance of total body potassium, more immediate control relies on a shift of potassium between intracellular and extracellular compartments (Giebisch 1998).

Internal distribution of potassium

Redistribution of potassium between intracellular and extracelluar fluid compartments provides protection from rapid changes in extracellular potassium concentration (Guyton and Hall 2006). This internal distribution of potassium is regulated by several factors including: serum concentrations of insulin and catecholamines, the presence of alkalosis or acidosis, cellular damage, and plasma tonicity (Giebisch 1998; Rose and Post 2001a).

Insulin and catecholamines (mainly epinephrine) promote uptake of potassium by extrarenal tissues such as skeletal muscle and liver (Vite and Gfeller 1994; Rose and Post 2001b). Following a meal, rising serum concentrations of glucose and potassium stimulate release of insulin and catecholamines. Epinephrine stimulated β_2-adrenergic receptors and insulin increase activity of the Na$^+$, K$^+$-ATPase pump, increasing cellular potassium uptake (Brown 1986).

The acid–base status of a patient may dramatically affect distribution of potassium between ICF and ECF. This interaction is complex and the magnitude of transcellular potassium shifts varies with both the severity and the underlying cause of the acid–base disturbance. In general, metabolic alkalosis causes movement of potassium from the ECF to the ICF (Vite and Gfeller 1994), while metabolic acidosis causes a shift in the opposite direction, resulting in loss of potassium from the cells (Vite and Gfeller 1994; Giebisch and Wagner 2007).

Nephrology and Urology of Small Animals. Edited by Joe Bartges and David J. Polzin. © 2011 Blackwell Publishing Ltd.

Sudden changes in plasma osmolality may also affect internal distribution of potassium. Serum hyperosmolality results in diffusion of intracellular water to extracellular compartments. This movement of water from cells creates solvent drag causing a net loss of potassium from cells. In contrast, serum hypoosmolality results in net movement of water into cells, resulting in a decreased ECF potassium concentration.

Regulation of potassium by the kidney

Potassium transport along the nephron

The kidneys are responsible for over 90% of total body potassium excretion and are critical in the maintenance of both short- and long-term potassium balance. Given their pivotal role in potassium balance, the kidneys must adjust potassium excretion quickly and with precision. Primary determinants of potassium excretion by the kidney are rates of (1) potassium filtration, (2) renal tubular potassium reabsorption, and (3) renal tubular potassium secretion (Guyton and Hall 2006). Within the nephron, approximately 66% of freely filtered potassium is reabsorbed along the proximal tubule. This reabsorption is mostly passive and driven by the positive tubule electrical potential and paracellular solvent drag (Giebisch and Wagner 2007).

Along the descending limb of the loop of Henle, a small amount of potassium is secreted into the tubule lumen from the medullary interstitium. Along the thick ascending limb of the loop of Henle, there is significant potassium reabsorption via the $Na^+, K^+ - 2Cl^-$ co-transporter. The summation of these events typically results in net reabsorption of potassium within the loop of Henle.

The distal nephron (late distal tubule and cortical collecting duct) is the most important site for net regulation of potassium excretion. Typically, dietary intake creates an excess of total body potassium resulting in net secretion into the tubule. However, potassium secretion may decrease or change to net reabsorption in states of potassium deficiency.

Potassium secretion in the distal nephron

Potassium secretion in the distal nephron is determined by the concentration gradient of potassium between tubular cells and tubular lumen, tubular flow rate, and transmembrane potential difference across the luminal membrane (DiBartola and de Morais 2006). Principal cells located in the late distal and cortical collecting tubules are responsible for secretion of potassium. Secretion of potassium into the tubular lumen requires both Na^+, K^+-ATPase pumps on basolateral membranes

and passive diffusion through potassium channels on luminal membranes. The basolateral Na^+, K^+-ATPase pump shifts potassium into the cell while moving sodium out of the cell into the interstitium (Giebisch 1998; Guyton and Hall 2006). Passive diffusion allows potassium to move from inside the cell into tubular fluid. The Na^+, K^+-ATPase pump creates the electrochemical gradient (high intracellular potassium concentration) facilitating secretion of potassium into the lumen via passive diffusion (Guyton and Hall 2006). Concentration of potassium in the extracellular fluid is a critical factor in regulation of potassium secretion. Rising potassium concentration in the ECF results in increased potassium secretion through increases in Na^+, K^+-ATPase pump activity, passive diffusion, and secretion of aldosterone (Guyton and Hall 2006).

Flow rate in the distal tubules also affects potassium secretion in that increases in tubular flow rate reduce intra-tubular potassium concentration, promoting further potassium secretion (DiBartola and de Morais 2006). Increases in distal tubular flow may be associated with diuretic therapy, increased sodium intake, and volume expansion. (Guyton and Hall 2006).

Secretion of potassium is also influenced by the amount of sodium and poorly reabsorbed anions delivered to the distal nephron. Sodium is usually reabsorbed, which increases the negativity of the luminal fluid and promotes diffusion of potassium out of cells. Likewise, poorly absorbed anions increase tubular negativity and promote potassium secretion.

Potassium deficiency is associated with increased activity and expression of H^+, K^+-ATPase pumps on the luminal membrane of α-intercalated cells of the collecting tubules. These cells promote reabsorption of potassium from the tubular lumen (Guyton and Hall 2006). Although important in management of mild hypokalemia, this response may be easily overwhelmed if potassium deficiency is severe or prolonged.

Control of potassium secretion: aldosterone

Aldosterone is primarily responsible for hormonal control of renal potassium excretion. Aldosterone is produced and secreted from zona glomerulosa cells of the adrenal cortex in response to many factors, including increases in serum potassium concentration and angiotensin II (produced in response to volume depletion). A potent feedback system is responsible for detecting an increase in ECF potassium concentration, which in turn stimulates aldosterone secretion. The resulting decrease in ECF potassium concentration ultimately reduces the amount of aldosterone secreted (Guyton and Hall 2006).

There are three major mechanisms by which aldosterone affects potassium regulation in the distal nephron. The first mechanism is by increasing intracellular potassium content by stimulating Na^+, K^+-ATPase pump activity. This increases the magnitude of the potassium concentration gradient across the apical membrane, resulting in an increased rate of potassium secretion into the luminal fluid. The second mechanism is by increasing permeability of potassium channels in the apical membrane, which increases the amount of potassium that may be excreted in a given time. The third mechanism is by increasing the rate of sodium uptake across the apical membrane. The resulting increase in the negativity of luminal fluid promotes the secretion of potassium (Giebisch and Wagner 2007).

Hypokalemia

Hypokalemia is defined as a serum potassium concentration below 3.6 mmol/L. Decreased serum potassium may cause hyperpolarization of cell membranes, thereby inhibiting the generation of action potentials by excitatory cells such as myocytes and neurons. Consequently, the predominant clinical signs associated with hypokalemia result from decreased nerve and muscle function. Polyuria and polydipsia occur commonly and result from a decrease in renal responsiveness to the action of ADH. In general, clinical signs depend on severity of hypokalemia, with mild hypokalemia (3–3.5 mmol/L) often being asymptomatic. Moderate hypokalemia (2.5–3.0 mmol/L) is usually accompanied by generalized muscle weakness and lethargy, while severe hypokalemia (<2.5 mmol/L) may be accompanied by significant muscle weakness and potentially even rhabdomyolysis. In cats, particularly those with chronic kidney disease, ventroflexion of the neck may be observed secondary to cervical muscle weakness. Extreme hypokalemia may cause ascending paralysis, culminating in respiratory failure and death.

Although uncommon, cardiac arrythmias may be observed due to delayed ventricular repolarization, especially in patients with preexisting heart disease. Electrocardiographic changes associated with hypokalemia are inconsistently observed, but include prolongation of QT intervals, ST segment deviations, and decrease in amplitude of T waves.

Causes of hypokalemia

Hypokalemia may result from decreased potassium intake, translocation of potassium from ECF to ICF, and/or increased gastrointestinal or renal losses of potassium (DiBartola and de Morais 2006) (Table 62.1).

Table 62.1 Causes of hypokalemia

Decreased potassium intake
   Severe malnutrition
   Iatrogenic (inadequate supplementation of parenteral fluids)

Altered transcellular potassium distribution
   Increased endogenous or exogenous insulin
   Catecholamine excess (stress, albuterol toxicity)
   Metabolic alkalosis
   Hypokalemic periodic paralysis (Burmese cats)

Increased potassium excretion
   Non-renal Excretion
   Vomiting
   Diarrhea
   Bentonite clay ingestion (cats-rare)
   Renal Excretion
   Diuretics (loop and thiazide)
   Post-obstructive diuresis
   Osmotic diuresis (uncontrolled diabetes)
   Primary aldosteronism
   Hyperadrenocorticism or exogenous glucocorticoids
   Renal tubular acidosis (Types 1 and 2)
   Hypomagnesemia

Decreased intake/iatrogenic hypokalemia

Decreased potassium intake is rarely the primary cause of hypokalemia in dogs and cats unless they are fed an atypical diet or have a chronic illness with prolonged anorexia (DiBartola and de Morais 2006). Iatrogenic dilutional hypokalemia may be observed in hospitalized patients receiving parenteral fluids with inadequate potassium supplementation to meet maintenance requirements. This is especially true in anorectic patients who do not receive timely nutritional support.

Translocation of potassium from ECF to ICF

Translocation of potassium from ECF to ICF may temporarily decrease plasma potassium concentration without altering total body potassium. In small animals, this redistribution has been reported with exogenous administration or endogenous release of insulin, catecholamine release, metabolic alkalosis, albuterol toxicity, and hypokalemic periodic paralysis (a hereditary disorder of Burmese cats). An increase in serum insulin concentration stimulates Na^+, K^+-ATPase pump activity and enhances cellular uptake of potassium (Ahee and Crowe 2000). Likewise, catecholamines may decrease serum potassium by stimulating the Na^+, K^+-ATPase pump, predominantly in skeletal muscle cells. Catecholamine release may increase during periods of stress associated with illness and hospitalization, contributing to hypokalemia. Metabolic alkalosis worsens hypokalemia due to movement of potassium into ICF in response to translocation of hydrogen ions out of the cell in an attempt to maintain the cellular electrical gradient (Langston 2008).

Albuterol is a β_2-adrenergic agonist commonly used as a bronchodilator. Overdoses of albuterol may cause significant hypokalemia and dysrhythmias (Vite and Gfeller 1994; McCown et al. 2008). Albuterol has been used in humans to treat hyperkalemia associated with renal disease (Murdock et al. 1991), hyperkalaemic familial periodic paralysis (Wang and Clausen 1976), and refractory hyperkalemia in hemodialysis patients (Allon et al. 1989; Allon and Copkney 1990).

Hypokalemic polymyopathy has been reported in Burmese cats between 2 and 12 months of age. This syndrome is characterized by recurrent episodes marked by hypokalemia, stiff gait, muscle weakness, ventroflexion of the neck, and increases in creatinine kinase concentration (Blaxter 1986; Mason 1988). Neither decreased potassium intake nor increased renal potassium excretion appear to be responsible for the pathogenesis of hypokalemia. A sudden and dramatic translocation of potassium from the ECF to the ICF seems to occur (Dickinson and LeCouteur 2004). Although the molecular basis for this polymyopathy in Burmese kittens has not been fully elucidated, a genetic basis similar to mutations in voltage-dependent ion channels seen in humans with hypokalemic periodic paralysis is suspected. (Elbaz et al. 1995; Vite 2002).

Increased loss of potassium

Typically, only a small amount of potassium is excreted in the feces; however, clinically significant losses of potassium may occur with protracted diarrhea. In dogs with intestinal obstruction, hypokalemia may be attributed to the loss of potassium through vomiting and fluid sequestration (Brown and Otto 2008). A modest amount of potassium may also be lost in vomitus of animals suffering from prolonged vomiting.

Although direct potassium losses from vomiting and diarrhea tend to be small, the ensuing volume depletion and metabolic alkalosis result in significant renal loss of potassium. Hypovolemia stimulates aldosterone release, thereby increasing sodium reabsorption and potassium excretion by principal cells of the collecting duct (Brown and Otto 2008). Metabolic alkalosis increases the amount of sodium bicarbonate delivered to the distal nephron, further enhancing secretion of potassium.

Hypokalemia has been reported in approximately 20–30% of cats with CKD (DiBartola et al. 1987; Elliot and Barber 1998) and is likely due to a combination of increased renal loses from polyuria and decreased intake

from chronic inappetance. Other conditions associated with significant urinary potassium losses include postobstructive diuresis following resolution of feline urethral obstruction (Bartges et al. 1996) and distal renal tubular acidosis (Soriano 2002; Dibartola and de Morais 2006).

A thorough medication history is important in all cases of hypokalemia as many medications promote hypokalemia. Certain diuretics, particularly furosemide, thiazide diuretics, and mannitol, can induce hypokalemia. Furosemide, a "loop diuretic," decreases reabsorption of sodium and chloride and increases excretion of potassium in the distal renal tubule (Plumb 2008). Exogenous mineralocorticoids such as fludrocortisone and DOCP cause a marked increase in potassium secretion in the distal nephron by mimicking effects of aldosterone. Very high doses of glucocorticoids or severe untreated Cushing's disease may produce some mineralocorticoid activity, but hypokalemia develops predominantly due to increased filtration and the resulting increase in sodium delivery to the distal nephron.

Primary hyperaldosteronism is caused by excessive aldosterone secretion from bilateral adrenal hyperplasia or an adrenal tumor; unilateral adrenal adenoma (or carcinoma), or in some cases, bilateral adrenal adenomas (Flood et al. 1999; Feldman and Nelson 2004a). In patients with primary hyperaldosteronism, there is a marked increase in sodium reabsorption and potassium secretion by the distal nephron. The marked increase in urinary potassium excretion may cause significant hypokalemia. These patients often present with volume-dependent hypertension, metabolic alkalosis, and marked hypokalemia.

Magnesium deficiency is often found concurrently with hypokalemia and may significantly inhibit therapeutic response to potassium supplementation. Combined magnesium and potassium deficiency may be observed in patients receiving loop or thiazide diuretics, or potentially nephrotoxic drugs such as aminoglycoside antibiotics, amphotericin B, or cisplatin. The mechanism of potassium loss secondary to magnesium deficiency is not entirely understood, but is believed to be associated with a decrease in magnesium-dependent inhibition of renal outer medullary potassium (ROMK) channels in the distal nephron. ROMK channels are responsible for the basal secretion of potassium in the distal tubule and cortical collecting ducts (Huang and Kuo 2007). Measurement of serum magnesium and correction of hypomagnesemia should be considered in patients with refractory hypokalemia (Kobrin and Goldfarb 1990).

Management of hypokalemia

The initial approach to the management of hypokalemia is the identification and correction, if possible, of the underlying disease process or contributing factors that resulted in the hypokalemia. A detailed history may help to identify possible etiologies (e.g., diuretic use). Therapeutic goals are to correct the potassium deficit and to minimize ongoing losses. It is imperative to recognize that correlation between serum potassium concentrations and total potassium deficit are poor. For example, initial serum potassium levels in patients with diabetic ketoacidosis may significantly underestimate total body potassium deficit. In this clinical scenario, serum potassium concentrations are artificially increased due to potassium translocation out of cells in response to insulin deficiency and metabolic acidosis. Given the inherent difficulties in accurately predicting the amount of potassium required to replenish total body deficit, frequent monitoring of serum potassium concentration is essential.

Initial management of moderate to severe hypokalemia usually requires parenteral administration of potassium, typically potassium chloride (or potassium phosphate) as an additive to 0.9% sodium chloride. Guidelines defining the amount of potassium chloride to add to parenteral fluids based on serum potassium concentration are provided in Table 62.2. To minimize the occurrence of cardiac arrhythmias, the rate of potassium administration should not exceed 0.5 mmol/kg/hr (DiBartola and de Morais 2001). Potassium chloride may also cause pain and potentially phlebitis if administered at concentrations exceeding 40 mmol/L via peripheral veins or greater than 60 mmol/L via central veins.

Oral potassium supplementation is preferable to parenteral supplementation for correction of mild to moderate hypokalemia and for control of ongoing potassium losses. Oral supplementation is safer than parenteral administration and is less likely to result in iatrogenic hyperkalemia. Potassium gluconate and potassium citrate are the most commonly used oral potassium sup-

plements. Although potassium chloride and potassium bicarbonate are available as oral formulations, they are associated with anorexia and vomiting and most pets find them unpalatable. Cats with hypokalemia and ongoing potassium loss secondary to CKD may be managed initially with oral potassium gluconate at 5–10 mEq/day divided into 2–3 doses. Once the potassium deficit has been replaced, the dose may be decreased to 2–4 mEq/day for maintenance (Langston 2008).

Hyperkalemia

Hyperkalemia is defined as serum potassium concentration greater than 5.0 mmol/L and can be classified as mild (5.0–6.0 mmol/L), moderate (6.0–8.0 mmol/L), or severe (>8.0 mmol/L) (Cowgill and Francey 2005). Clinical consequences of hyperkalemia are dependent upon the magnitude of increase in serum potassium and the rate at which the increase occurs. As with hypokalemia, clinical signs associated with hyperkalemia are generally related to impaired neuromuscular function. Elevated ECF concentrations of potassium decrease the electronegativity of the cellular membrane potential, leading to a partial depolarization of the cell. Initially, this change increases the excitability of the cell membrane, which explains the hyperesthesia and muscle twitching often observed in animals with moderate to severe hyperkalemia. With persistent hyperkalemia, cell membrane excitability is impaired due to delayed repolarization, leading to muscle weakness, paralysis, and impaired cardiac function.

Cardiotoxicity is the most clinically significant sequela of hyperkalemia, although the onset and severity does not seem to correlate well with serum potassium concentrations. Electrocardiographic (ECG) changes associated with hyperkalemia are documented in dogs and cats, and generally start to appear when serum potassium levels exceed 6.5–7.0 mmol/L (Ettinger et al. 1974; Tag and Day 2008). Initial ECG changes include increased amplitude ("tenting") of T waves, shortening of QT intervals, and flattening of P waves. Progression of hyperkalemia leads to prolongation of PR intervals and widening of the QRS complexes. Severe hyperkalemia dramatically decreases size of P waves due to diminishing conduction within the atria. Eventually, atrial conduction stops, P waves disappear, and significant bradycardia develops. As cardiac conduction continues to decrease, the QRS complex progressively widens and eventually merges with the T wave to form a sine wave, a harbinger of impending cardiac arrest (DiBartola and de Morais 2006) (Figure 62.1).

Causes of hyperkalemia

Although the following discussion addresses causes of hyperkalemia separately, it is important to realize that

Table 62.2 Guidelines for intravenous potassium supplementation in dogs and cats

Serum potassium concentration (mEq/L)	mEq KCl to add to 1 L fluid	Maximum fluid infusion rate[a] (mL/kg/hr)
<2.0	80	6
2.1–2.5	60	8
2.6–3.0	40	12
3.1–3.5	28	18
3.6–5.0	20	25

Source: Greene, R.W. and R.C. Scott (1975). Lower urinary tract disease. In: *Textbook of Veterinary Internal Medicine*, edited by S.J. Ettinger. Philadelphia: WB Saunders, p. 1572.
[a]Do not exceed 0.5 mEq/kg/h.

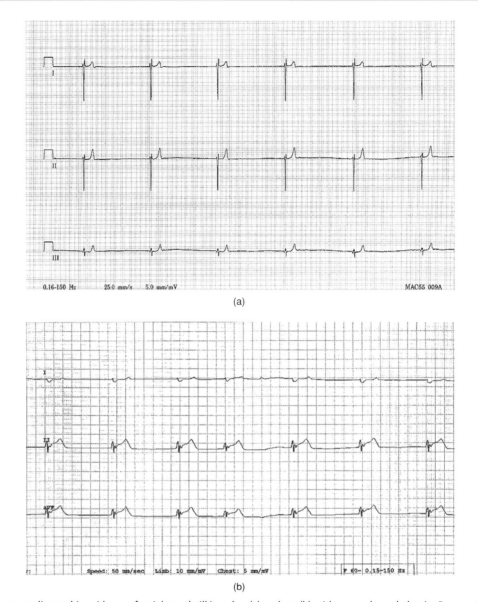

(a)

(b)

Figure 62.1 Electrocardiographic evidence of atrial standstill in a dog (a) and cat (b) with severe hyperkalemia. Progressive hyperkalemia may result in characteristic changes in the electrocardiogram (ECG); including tall, peaked T waves, and progressive flattening of the p wave as conduction through the artria is impaired. Eventually, conduction thought the atria ceases, resulting in atrial standstill (depicted above). Ventricular fibrillation may occur at any time during this progression. (ECGs courtesy of Drs. Sarah Miller and Joao Orvalho).

most patients who develop hyperkalemia have more than one contributing risk factor. Mechanistically, hyperkalemia may result from increased potassium intake, translocation of potassium from ICF to ECF, and/or decreased excretion (Table 62.3).

Increased intake

Increased oral intake of potassium is unlikely to result in significant hyperkalemia unless the patient has a concurrent defect in potassium excretion. Iatrogenic hyperkalemia resulting from overzealous potassium supplementation of intravenous fluids occurs more commonly. Inadequate dispersion of potassium chloride added to

parenteral fluids has also been associated with hyperkalemia. Inadequate mixing after addition of potassium chloride to a 1 L fluid bag could result in up to a 1,000-fold difference between maximum and minimum concentrations of potassium chloride in the fluid outflow (Thompson 1980).

Impaired distribution of potassium between the intracellular and extracellular spaces

Conditions causing a net shift of potassium from the intracellular space to the extracellular space may also result in hyperkalemia. This net shift occurs when potassium is prevented from entering cells or in situations

Table 62.3 Causes of hyperkalemia

Increased potassium intake
  Potassium supplements (enteral or parenteral)
  Certain herbal supplements (e.g., noni juice, alfalfa, dandelion)
  Stored packed red blood cells
  Penicillin G potassium (1.7 mEq/10^6U)

Altered transcellular potassium distribution
  Metabolic acidosis (mineral > organic acidosis)
  Insulin deficiency
  Hyperosmolality (diabetic ketoacidosis)
  Massive tissue damage (rhabdomyolysis, burns, trauma)

Decreased potassium excretion
  Chronic kidney disease, stage 4
  Acute kidney injury
  Decreased effective circulating volume (e.g., congestive heart failure)
  Mineralocorticoid deficiency
  Hypoadrenocorticism (Addison's disease)
  Hyporeninemic hypoaldosteronism (type IV renal tubular acidosis)
  Pseudohypoaldosteronism

Medications that impair K^+ excretion
  K^+-sparing diuretics (spironolactone, triamterene, amiloride)
  Trimethoprim, pentamidine
  Angiotensin-converting enzyme inhibitors and angiotensin receptor blockers
  Non-steroidal anti-inflammatory drugs
  Heparin
  Cyclosporin, tacrolimus

Pseudohyperkalemia
  Hemolysis (especially in Akitas)
  Thrombocytosis

where there is translocation/release of potassium from cells. Independently, these mechanisms do not usually result in significant hyperkalemia, but they may certainly exacerbate hyperkalemia from other causes.

Both insulin and β_2-adrenergic agonists stimulate cellular uptake of potassium and are potent determinants of transcellular potassium balance (Mandal 1997). Insulin deficiency and/or β_2-adrenergic blockade impair cellular uptake of potassium, resulting in increased serum potassium concentrations. In diabetic patients (insulin deficiency) this hyperkalemia is rarely recognized since hyperglycemia-driven osmotic diuresis causes overall potassium depletion. In these instances, serum potassium levels are misleading since they may underestimate total body deficit of potassium. Treatment of diabetic ketoacidosis (with insulin and intravenous fluid therapy) may

necessitate aggressive concurrent potassium supplementation in order to avoid dramatic hypokalemia.

An elevation in plasma osmolality may lead to increased serum potassium concentrations. Increased extracellular osmolality results in diffusion of water out of the cells. This movement of water carries potassium via a process known as solvent drag. Loss of intracellular water causes an apparent increase in intracellular potassium concentration, facilitating the movement of potassium out of the cell through channels in the cell membrane.

Acute metabolic acidosis

It is generally accepted that acidosis promotes hyperkalemia by shifting potassium from intracellular to extracellular compartments in exchange for intracellular buffering of hydrogen ions. However, the effects of metabolic acidosis on transcellular shifts of potassium are variable and depend on the cause and duration of the acidosis. A predictable increase in serum potassium concentration seems to only be associated with inorganic acidosis (e.g., HCl and NH_4Cl). Diabetic ketoacidosis and lactic acidosis, two of the most common causes of organic (nonmineral) metabolic acidosis, are not associated with significant increases in serum potassium, although a number of other factors related to the primary disease process could promote hyperkalemia. The mechanism(s) of this differing effect of mineral and organic acidemias on transmembrane movement of potassium appears to be related to the movement of organic anions into the cells without creating a gradient for hydrogen ions, thus obviating the efflux of intracellular potassium.

Increased potassium release from cells

Hyperkalemia resulting from intracellular potassium release may accompany any process, resulting in cell injury or death. Tissue damage, such as that seen with burns, rhabdomyolysis, snake and spider bites, and trauma, causes release of intracellular potassium from damaged cells (Gennari 2002). Except for cases with massive tissue destruction, the resulting hyperkalemia is not usually life-threatening; however, clinically significant hyperkalemia may occur in patients with concurrent kidney disease or other factors interfering with normal potassium excretion.

Although rare, acute tumor lysis syndrome may occur following treatment of certain malignancies with chemotherapy or radiation therapy and is characterized by severe hyperuricemia, hyperphosphatemia, hyperkalemia, hypocalcemia, and acute kidney injury. Following chemotherapy administration, synchronized cell death releases a significant amount of potassium and phosphate. Acute kidney injury, which may develop as a consequence of hyperuricemia, may exacerbate the hyperkalemia (Calia et al. 1996; Vickery and Thamm 2007).

Decreased renal potassium excretion

Normally, the kidneys are able to increase excretion of potassium as serum potassium concentration rises. Therefore, sustained hyperkalemia is almost always associated with some impairment of renal potassium elimination. Effective renal excretion of potassium is dependent on sufficient delivery of sodium and water to the distal nephron, aldosterone, and on a functional lower urinary tract. Thus, hyperkalemia may occur when one of these mechanisms is impaired due to kidney disease, decreased renal perfusion, a decrease in aldosterone, or urinary tract rent or obstruction.

Hyperkalemia is usually not a significant problem in chronic kidney disease until renal function has declined to less than 10% of normal. However, certain medications and excessive dietary intake may contribute to hyperkalemia at earlier stages. Hyperkalemia is the most common electrolyte abnormality encountered in anuric acute kidney injury and contributes significantly to morbidity and mortality in these patients.

Hypoaldosteronism

Hypoadrenocorticism (Addison's disease) is commonly associated with hyperkalemia due to a primary decrease in aldosterone production. Greater than 85% of adrenocortical cells must be lost before significant hyperkalemia develops (Feldman and Nelson 2004b). Hyporeninemic hypoaldosteronism (type IV renal tubular acidosis) is an important cause of hyperkalemia in human patients as it is often associated with diabetic nephropathy. Although this syndrome appears to be rare in veterinary medicine, it may be under-recognized as diagnostic tests are not readily available.

Primary gastrointestinal disease in dogs resulting from whipworm (trichuriasis) or salmonellosis has been associated with clinical signs and electrolyte abnormalities very similar to those seen with hypoadrenocorticism (DiBartola 1985). In these cases, significant sodium and bicarbonate-rich fluid are lost from the gastrointestinal tract, leading to an increase in thirst and subsequently to a dilutional hyponatremia. With continued losses of fluid and bicarbonate from the gastrointestinal tract, metabolic acidosis and hypovolemia develop. Hyponatremia and hypovolemia significantly decrease the amount of water and sodium in the distal tubule, leading to a marked decrease in potassium excretion (Graves et al. 1994). In addition, metabolic acidosis exacerbates hyperkalemia by shifting potassium extracellularly (Malik et al. 1990).

Medications

Hyperkalemia has been associated with the use of several medications, and this effect may be exacerbated in patients with concurrent kidney disease and in patients who receive an oral or parenteral potassium load. Many medications can directly or indirectly interfere with production of aldosterone, while other medications block effects of aldosterone at the receptor. Angiotensin converting enzyme (ACE) inhibitors decrease angiotensin II production, thereby decreasing aldosterone levels (Palmer 2004). Angiotensin receptor blockers increase potassium concentration but seem to have a slightly decreased propensity for this when compared with ACE inhibitors. Nonsteroidal anti-inflammatory drugs (NSAIDs) may contribute to hyperkalemia by indirectly decreasing aldosterone production. Prostaglandin inhibitors such as NSAIDs decrease renin production, which decreases production of aldosterone. Cyclosporin and tacrolimus have been associated with hyperkalemia via direct inhibition of the renin–angiotensin–aldosterone system and by direct effects on selective potassium and chloride channels in the distal tubule. When used in high doses, trimethoprim may also cause hyperkalemia by blocking sodium channels in the distal tubules, reducing sodium reabsorption and potassium excretion (Rubin et al. 1998). Although most diuretics increase urinary potassium excretion, causing hypokalemia, potassium-sparing diuretics such as spironolactone predispose to hyperkalemia. Spironolactone inhibits the effect of aldosterone by competitive inhibition of intracellular aldosterone receptors in the collecting duct. This decreases Na^+, K^+-ATPase activity and limits potassium excretion.

Miscellaneous

Hyperkalemia has been documented in several cases of pleural and peritoneal effusion (Zenger 1992; Bisset et al. 2001; Thompson and Carr 2002). Hyperkalemia can occur when there is third-space loss into body cavities and may be a result of an acquired defect in renal secretion of potassium. In these cases, relative hypovolemia and decreased glomerular filtration rate (GFR) lead to decrease in water and sodium delivery to the distal tubules, and to decreased secretion of potassium (Thompson and Carr 2002).

Urinary tract rent/obstruction

A common cause of severe hyperkalemia in veterinary medicine is urinary tract obstruction. In cats with acute urethral obstruction, life-threatening hyperkalemia may develop in under 48 hours. Once the obstruction has been relieved and the patient receives appropriate fluid therapy, hyperkalemia usually resolves rapidly. Acute ureteral obstruction (AUO) in cats is often associated with significant hyperkalemia and azotemia. Though calcium oxalate stones are usually the cause of feline AUO, nonmineralized obstructions (e.g., inspissated blood, sloughed renal tissue, ureteral strictures, etc.) are identified in approximately 30% of cases (Fischer 2006). In these cats, usually one ureter becomes obstructed and results in clinically subtle or silent disease. The associated kidney atrophies while the contralateral kidney hypertrophies, and laboratory values remain relatively unchanged until the hypertrophied kidney becomes obstructed, resulting in severe, acute, often life-threatening uremia and hyperkalemia. Often, the patient presents with life-threatening hyperkalemia, necessitating hemodialysis for stabilization prior to attempted surgical correction. Leakage of urine from the lower urinary tract (ureteral tear, ruptured bladder, etc.) may also result in significant postrenal azotemia and hyperkalemia. As with cases of urethral obstruction, hyperkalemia usually resolves rapidly once the underlying problem has been corrected.

Pseudohyperkalemia/spurious hyperkalemia

Pseudohyperkalemia or false elevations in measured serum potassium concentration may occur for several reasons. Generally, pseudohyperkalemia is attributed to potassium movement/leakage from cells during or after a blood draw (Rose and Post 2001b). Mechanical trauma during blood draw is the most common cause, especially in Akitas since they have high erythrocyte potassium content relative to their plasma and to that of other dogs (Degen 1987). Pseudohyperkalemia may also be observed in patients with marked elevations in platelet counts. Factitious hyperkalemia was documented in a group of 15 dogs with thrombocytosis (>600,000/uL) (Reimann et al. 1989). Serum potassium concentrations were higher than plasma concentrations in normal dogs and dogs with thrombocytosis due to release of potassium from platelets during clotting. In those dogs with thrombocytosis, the serum-plasma potassium difference was increased when the time between blood collection and separation of serum or plasma from cells was prolonged (Reimann et al. 1989).

Management of hyperkalemia

The initial step in the management of hyperkalemia is to determine if the hyperkalemia is life threatening and necessitates emergency management. If the patient has significant ECG changes, immediate intervention is required. Once any immediate danger has been addressed, management of hyperkalemia centers on diagnosing and correcting underlying cause(s).

In most cases, mild hyperkalemia (serum potassium concentration <6.0 mEq/L) rarely requires emergency treatment and resolves following replacement of any fluid deficits with potassium-free fluids such as normal saline. Fluid therapy results in hemodilution and causes an increase in both GFR and renal potassium excretion from improved renal blood flow (Cowgill and Francey 2005). If volume replacement and diuresis do not adequately reduce potassium, further medical management is indicated. Aggressive management of hyperkalemia should not be dictated by a specific serum potassium concentration, but rather clinical and ECG findings and the rapidity with which the hyperkalemia developed. In general, severe hyperkalemia (>8 mmol/L) is associated with cardiac conduction disturbances necessitating immediate intervention. The urgent management of hyperkalemia is usually based on one or more of the following approaches: opposing direct toxic effects of potassium on cellular membranes, promoting cellular uptake of potassium, and/or removing potassium from the body. The individual patient's response to therapies discussed below may vary, thus frequent measurements of serum potassium levels are recommended (Table 62.4).

Antagonism of cardiac effects: calcium

Intravenous calcium is the most rapid and effective way to antagonize myocardial toxic effects of hyperkalemia. Calcium directly antagonizes hyperkalemia-induced depolarization of the resting membrane potential by returning the membrane excitability toward normal. The membrane-stabilizing effect of calcium is independent of serum calcium concentration and has no direct effect on serum potassium concentration (Carvalhana et al. 2006). This protective effect is produced rapidly (within a few minutes), but the duration of action is short lived and lasts approximately 25–40 minutes. Calcium is usually administered as calcium gluconate available as a 10% solution. Initial dose for dogs and cats is 0.5–1.0 mL/kg intravenously over 15–20 minutes (Cowgill and Francey 2005). More rapid administration may cause worsening of bradycardia and potentiate ventricular arrhythmias. Continuous ECG and blood pressure monitoring should be performed throughout the infusion. Use of calcium chloride solutions is not recommended since they are acidifying and may cause significant tissue irritation with extravasation (Cowgill and Francey 2005). Because calcium gluconate has no direct effects on serum potassium concentration, it should be used for its cardiotoxic protective effects alone to give the

Table 62.4 Therapeutic options for the management of hyperkalemia[a]

Intervention	Change in serum [K$^+$]	Onset	Duration
Emergency management of severe hyperkalemia			
Correct dehydration	Decrease—dilutional	Immediate	20–30 min
Use K$^+$ free fluids (0.9% NaCl)			
Sodium bicarbonate (if acidosis present)	Decrease—translocation	10 min	1–2 h
Sufficient to correct acidosis			
If bicarbonate status unknown, 1–2 mEq/kg IV			
Dextrose ± Insulin	Decrease—translocation	10–20 min	2–3 h
1–2 mL/kg of 50% dextrose (diluted to 25%) IV OR			
Regular insulin 0.5–1.0 U/kg + 1–2 g dextrose/unit insulin			
Calcium gluconate	None	Immediate	15–30 min
0.5–1.0 mL/kg of 10% calcium gluconate IV over 10 min			
Loop diuretics	Decrease—excretion	1 h	Permanent
Only effective if non-oliguric			
Furosemide 2–4 mg/kg			
hydrochlorothiazide 2–4 mg/kg			
Sodium polystyrene sulfonate (Kayexalate®)	Variable	4–6 h	Permanent
Oral 2 g/kg in suspension (20 g in 100 mL of 20% sorbitol)			
Retention enema (50 g in 100 mL tap water)			
Dialytic management	Variable	10–15 min	Permanent
Long-term management of hyperkalemia			
Dietary K$^+$ restriction			
Discontinue medications that promote hyperkalemia			
Angiotensin-converting enzyme inhibitors			
Angiotensin receptor blockers			
Potassium sparing diuretics			
β-blockers			
NSAIDs			
Increase K$^+$ excretion			
Loop or thiazide diuretics if normal renal function			
Fludrocortisone if hypoaldosterone present			
Chronic sodium polystyrene sulfonate therapy			

[a]Therapy is tailored to the individual patient.

clinician sufficient time to institute other therapies that will actually decrease serum potassium concentrations and to diagnose the underlying disorder.

Redistribution of K$^+$ into cells

Sodium bicarbonate

In cases of severe hyperkalemia, a temporary reduction in serum potassium concentration may be achieved by administering medications promoting cellular uptake of potassium. Sodium bicarbonate increases extracellular pH and is associated with translocation of extracellular potassium into cells in exchange for hydrogen ions (Gennari 2002). Ideally, the dosage of sodium bicarbonate should be based on the calculated bicarbonate deficit; however, if measured serum bicarbonate concentrations are unavailable, sodium bicarbonate may be adminis-

tered at 1–2 mEq/kg intravenously over 15–20 minutes. Beneficial effects usually begin within 10 minutes and may persist for 1–2 hours (Clark and Brown 1995). If preexisting hypocalcemia is present (especially common in patients with ethylene glycol intoxication) sodium bicarbonate must be given cautiously as it may lower ionized blood calcium concentration and precipitate a hypocalcemic crisis. Sodium bicarbonate should not be used in animals that are overhydrated, hypernatremic, have metabolic alkalosis, or have respiratory compromise (impaired ability to exhale carbon dioxide).

Insulin and glucose

Infusions of regular insulin and glucose stimulate the Na$^+$, K$^+$-ATPase pump, shifting potassium from ECF to ICF in exchange for sodium and decreasing serum potassium concentration (Clark and Francey 1995; Ahee and Crowe 2000). Administration of glucose alone will stimulate release of endogenous insulin and reduce serum potassium. Typically, 1–2 mL/kg of 50% dextrose is diluted and given intravenously. Treatment with insulin and glucose may cause a greater reduction in potassium, but the patient's serum glucose must be carefully monitored, since resultant hypoglycemia is quite common. The typical treatment protocol is 0.5–1.0 U/kg of regular insulin with 2 g of dextrose for each unit of insulin administered. The potassium-lowering effect of insulin/glucose combination occurs as early as 10 minutes after administration and may persist for up to 6 hours (Allon 1996).

Catecholamines

As with insulin, catecholamines increase activity of the Na^+, K^+-ATPase pump promoting cellular uptake of potassium. The hypokalemiac effects are additive to those of insulin and independent of other factors such as pH and aldosterone. Administration of a β_2-agonist, (such as albuterol) via a metered-dose inhaler is often used as an adjunctive therapy for human patients with hyperkalemia. β_2-agonists are not recommended as monotherapy because their efficacy may be unpredictable, particularly in patients with concurrent kidney disease (Halperin and Kamel 1998).

Removal of potassium

The treatment strategies discussed above are temporary and do not result in reduction of total body stores of potassium. Therefore, once the patient has been stabilized, treatment is focused on removal of potassium from the body to ensure that significant hyperkalemia does not recur.

Diuretics/diuresis

Loop and thiazide diuretics are useful in treatment of chronic hyperkalemia, since they increase sodium and urine flow in the distal tubules thereby promoting kaliuresis (Carvalhana et al. 2006). A similar effect may be obtained in hospitalized patients with parenteral fluid administration. Although this is an effective strategy for elimination of potassium, use of diuretics/diuresis is limited by the patient's kidney function and ability to maintain adequate hydration and electrolyte balance.

Cation exchange resins

Sodium polystyrene sulfonate (SPS) resin (Kayxalate®) is a cation exchange resin that exchanges sodium for potassium. The majority of the resin's adsorption of potassium occurs in the colon, thus SPS may be administered orally or by enema. Suggested dose is 2 g/kg divided into 3–4 doses, as a suspension in 20% sorbitol (Cowgill and Francey 2005). This translates into rather large volumes that may complicate administration, especially in a noncooperative patient that does not have a enteral feeding tube. Despite addition of sorbitol, constipation remains a significant side effect. The propensity for constipation is increased with concurrent administration of aluminum hydroxide. SPS is not appropriate for treatment of acute severe hyperkalemia because of the delay in onset of action (Alfonzo et al. 2006).

Dialysis

Removal of potassium by hemodialysis or other renal replacement therapies is the most effective and rapid method of removing potassium from the body. Dialysis should be considered in severe or refractory cases of hyperkalemia, particularly when underlying kidney disease is suspected. Conventional hemodialysis lowers serum potassium concentrations more rapidly than peritoneal dialysis or continuous renal replacement therapies. The amount of potassium removed is determined by the concentration of potassium in the dialysate, duration of dialysis treatment, volume of blood dialyzed, characteristics of the dialyzer, and amount of ultrafiltration performed (Blumberg et al. 1997).

Long-term management of hyperkalemia

Long-term management of hyperkalemia requires that the underlying cause be identified and corrected. In some patients, the underlying cause may be obvious, such as the inability to excrete potassium observed with feline urethral obstructions. However, some animals may have several contributing factors and it is important to carefully consider all potential risk factors for hyperkalemia when prescribing medications and making dietary recommendations. For example, animals with kidney disease and/or heart disease may be on ACE inhibitors, in which case high potassium diets and other medications that predispose to hyperkalemia (e.g., NSAIDs or spironolactone) should be avoided or used only with careful monitoring. Important strategies for long-term management of hyperkalemia include avoiding medications that may predispose to hyperkalemia, carefully monitoring dietary potassium intake, and optimizing potassium excretion by both the kidneys and gastrointestinal tract.

References

Ahee, P. and A.V. Crowe (2000). The management of hyperkalaemia in the emergency department. *J Accid Emerg Med* **17**(3): 188–191.

Alfonzo, A., C. Isles, et al. (2006). Potassium disorders—clinical spectrum and emergency management. *Resuscitation* **70**(1): 10–25.

Allon, M. (1996). Effect of bicarbonate adminstration on plasma potassium in dialysis patients: interactions with insulin and albuterol. *Am J Kidney Dis* **28**: 508–514.

Allon, M. and C. Copkney (1990). Albuterol and insulin for treatment of hyperkalemia in hemodialysis patients. *Kidney Int* **38**(5): 869–872.

Allon, M., R. Dunlay, et al. (1989). Nebulized albuterol for acute hyperkalemia in patients on hemodialysis. *Ann Intern Med* **110**(6): 426–429.

Bartges, J., D.R. Finco, et al. (1996). Pathophysiology of urethral obstruction. *Vet Clin North Am Small Anim Pract* **26**(2): 255–264.

Bissett Sally, A., M. Lamb, et al. (2001). Hyponatremia and hyperkalemia associated with peritoneal effusion in four cats. *J Am Vet Med Assoc* **218**(10): 1590–1592.

Blaxter, A., P. Lievesley, et al. (1986). Periodic muscle weakness in Burmese kittens. *Vet Rec* **118**(22): 619–620.

Blumberg, A., H. Roser, et al. (1997). Plasma potassium in patients with terminal renal failure during and after haemodialysis; relationship with dialytic potassium removal and total body potassium. *Nephrol Dial Transplant* **12**: 1629–1634.

Brown, A.J. and C.M. Otto (2008). Fluid therapy in vomiting and diarrhea. *Vet Clin North Am Small Anim Pract* **38**(3): 653–675.

Brown, R.S. (1986). Extrarenal potassium homeostasis. *Kidney Int* **30**(1): 116.

Calia, C., A.E. Hohenhaus, et al. (1996). Acute tumor lyisis syndrome in a cat with lymphoma. *J Vet Intern Med* **10**(6): 409–411.

Carvalhana, V., L. Burry, et al. (2006). Management of severe hyperkalemia without hemodialysis: case report and literature review. *J Crit Care* **21**(4): 316–321.

Clark, B. and R.S. Brown (1995). Potassium homeostasis and hyperkalemic syndromes. *Endocrinol Metab Clin North Am* **24**(3): 573–591.

Clausen, T. and M.E. Everts (1989). Regulation of the Na,K-pump in skeletal muscle. *Kidney Int* **35**(1): 1–13.

Cowgill, L.D. and T. Francey (2005). Acute uremia. In: *Textbook of Veterinary Internal Medicine*, edited by S.J. Ettinger and E.C. Feldman, 6th edition. St. Louis: Saunders Elsevier, pp. 1731–1751.

Degen, M. (1987). Pseudohyperkalemia in Akitas. *J Am Vet Med Assoc* **190**(5): 541–543.

DiBartola, S.P. (1985). Clinicopathologic findings resembling hypoadrenocorticism in dogs with primary gastrointestinal disease. *J Am Vet Med Assoc* **187**(1): 60–63.

DiBartola, S.P. (2001). Management of hypokalaemia and hyperkalaemia. *J Feline Med Surg* **3**: 181–183.

DiBartola, S.P. and H.A. de Morais (2006). Disorders of potassium: hypokalemia and hyperkalemia. In: *Fluid, Electrolyte, and Acid–Base Disorders in Small Animal Practice*, edited by S.P. DiBartola, 3rd edition. St. Louis, MO: Saunders Elsevier, pp. 91–121.

DiBartola, S.P., H.C. Rutgers, et al. (1987). Clinicopathologic findings associated with chronic renal disease in cats: 74 cases (1973–1984). *J Am Vet Med Assoc* **190**(9): 1196–1202.

Dickinson, P.J. and R.A. LeCouteur (2004). Feline neuromuscular disorders. *Vet Clin North Am Small Anim Pract* **34**(6): 1307–1359.

Elbaz, A., J. Vale-Santos, et al. (1995). Hypokalemic periodic paralysis and the dihydropyridine receptor (CACNLIA3): genotype/phenotype correlations for two predominant mutations and evidence for the absence of a founder effect in 16 Caucasian families. *Am J Hum Genet* **56**(2): 374–380.

Elliot, J. and P.J. Barber (1998). Feline chronic renal failure: clinical findings in 80 cases diagnosed between 1992 and 1995. *J Small Anim Pract* **39**(2): 78–85.

Ettinger, P.O., T.J. Regan, et al. (1974). Hyperkalemia, cardiac conduction and the electrocardiogram. *Am Heart J* **88**(3): 360–369.

Feldman, E.C. and R.W. Nelson (2004a). Hyperadrenocorticism in cats (Cushing's syndrome). In: *Canine and Feline Endocrinology and Reproduction*, 3rd edition. St. Louis, MO: Elsevier Saunders, pp. 358–393.

Feldman, E.C. and R.W. Nelson (2004b). Hypoadrenocorticism (Addison's Disease). In: *Canine and Feline Endocrinology and Reproduction*, 3rd edition. St. Louis: Elsevier Saunders, pp. 394–439.

Fischer, J.R. (2006). Acute ureteral obstruction. In: *Consultations in Feline Internal Medicine*, edited by R. John, Vol. 5. St. Louis: Elsevier-Saunders, pp. 379–386.

Flood, S.M., J.F. Randolph, et al. (1999). Primary hyperaldosteroinism in two cats. *J Am Anim Hosp Assoc* **35**(5): 411–416.

Gennari, J.F. (2002). Disorders of potassium homeostasis hypokalemia and hyperkalemia. *Crit Care Clin* **18**(2): 273–288.

Giebisch, G. (1998). Renal potassium transport: mechanisms and regulation. *Am J Physiol* **274**(5): 817–833.

Giebisch, G. and R.C. Wagner (2007). Renal and extrarenal regulation of potassium. *Kidney Int* **72**: 397–410.

Graves, T.K., W.D. Schall, et al. (1994). Basal and ACTH-stimulated plasma aldosterone concentrations are normal or increased in dogs with trichuriasis-associated pseudohypoadrenocorticism. *J Vet Intern Med* **8**(4): 287–289.

Guyton, A.C. and J.E. Hall (2006). Textbook of Medical Physiology, 11th edition. Philidelphia, PA: Elsevier Saunders.

Halperin, M.L. and K.S. Kamel (1998). Potassium. *Lancet* **352**: 135–140.

Huang, C.L. and E. Kuo (2007). Mechanism of hypokalemia in magnesium deficiency. *J Am Soc Nephrol* **18**: 2649–2652.

Kobrin, S.M. and S. Goldfarb (1990). Magnesium deficiency. *Semin Nephrol* **10**(6): 525–535.

Langston, C. (2008). Managing fluid and electrolyte disorders in renal failure. *Vet Clin North Am Small Anim Pract* **38**(3): 677–697.

Malik, R., G.B. Hunt, et al. (1990). Severe whipworm infection in the dog. *J Small Anim Pract* **31**(4): 185–188.

Mandal, A. (1997). Hypokalemia and hyperkalemia. *Med Clin North Am* **81**(3): 611–639.

Mason, K. (1988). A hereditary disease in Burmese cats manifested as an episodic weakness with head nodding and neck ventroflexion. *J Am Anim Hosp Assoc* **24**: 147–151.

McCown, J.L., E.S. Lechner, et al. (2008). Suspected albuterol toxicosis in a dog. *J Am Vet Med Assoc* **232**(8): 1168–1171.

Murdock, I.A., R. Dos Anjos, et al. (1991). Treatment of hyperkalaemia with intravenous Salbutamol. *Arch Dis Child* **66**(4): 527–528.

Palmer, B.F. (2004). Managing hyperkalemia caused by inhibitors of the renin-angiotensin-aldosterone system. *N Engl J Med* **351**: 585–592.

Plumb, D.C. (2008). *Veterinary Drug Handbook*, 6th edition. Ames IA: Blackwell Publishing, pp. 413–415.

Reimann, K.A., G.G. Knowlen, et al. (1989). Factitious hyperkalemia in dogs with thrombocytosis. *J Vet Intern Med* **3**(1): 47–52.

Rose, B.D. and T.W. Post (2001a). Hypovolemic states. In: *Clinical Physiology of Acid-Base and Electrolyte Disorders*, edited by B.D. Rose and T.W. Post, 5th edition. New York: McGraw-Hill, pp. 415–446.

Rose, B.D. and T.W. Post (2001b). Introduction to disorders of potassium balance. In: *Clinical Physiology of Acid-Base and Electrolyte Disorders*, edited by B.D. Rose and T.W. Post, 5th edition. New York: McGraw-Hill, pp. 822–835.

Rubin, S.I., et al. (1998). Trimethoprim-induced exacerbation of hyperkalemia in a dog with hypoadrenocorticism. *J Vet Intern Med* **12**(3): 186–188.

Soriano, J.R. (2002). Renal tubular acidosis: the clinical entity. *J Am Soc Nephrol* **13**(8): 2160–2170.

Stanton, B.A. and G. Giebisch (1992). Renal potassium transport. *Am Phsyiol Soc* **8**(19): 813–874.

Tag, T.L. and T.K. Day (2008). Electrocariographic assessment of hyperkalemia in dogs and cats. *J Vet Emerg Crit Care* **18**(1): 61–67.

Thompson, M.D. and A.P. Carr (2002). Hyponatremia and hyperkalemia associated with chylous pleural and peritoneal effusion in a cat. *Can Vet J* **43**(8): 610–613.

Thompson, W.L. (1980). Incomplete mixing of drugs in intravenous infusions. *Crit Care Med* **8**(11): 603–607.

Vickery, K.R. and D.H. Thamm (2007). Successful treatment of acute tumor lysis syndrome in a Dog with multicentric lymphoma. *J Vet Intern Med* **21**(6): 1401–1404.

Vite, C.H. (2002). Myotonia and disorders of altered muscle cell membrane excitability. *Vet Clin North Am Small Anim Pract* **32**(1): 169–187.

Vite, C.H. and R.W. Gfeller (1994). Suspected Albuterol intoxication in a Dog. *J Vet Emerg Crit Care* **4**(1): 7–13.

Wang, P. and T. Clausen (1976). Treatment of attacks in hyperkalaemic familial periodic paralysis by inhalation of salbutamol. *Lancet* **301**: 221–223.

Zenger, E. (1992). Persistent hyperkalemia associated with nonchylous pleural effusion in a dog. *J Am Anim Hosp Assoc* **28**(5): 411–413.

63

Magnesium disorders

Elizabeth Rozanski

Magnesium is classically considered "the forgotten ion" in clinical practice due to relative inability to measure total body magnesium status, its primary role as an intracellular cation, and its less frequently highlighted role in normal physiology. Approximately 99% of total body magnesium is found intracellularly and similar to the more widely appreciated cation, calcium (Ca^{++}), serum magnesium is found in three fractions: protein-bound, complexed with anions (e.g., phosphate, bicarbonate), and ionized that is the active form (Schenck 2005a). As with calcium, magnesium balance is regulated carefully by intestinal absorption, renal reabsorption/secretion, and exchange with bone. Magnesium has multiple roles in the normal animal (Khanna et al. 1998; Toll et al. 2002). It serves as a co-factor of ATP production and catalyzes numerous other reactions, including regulation of intracellular calcium. Magnesium is absorbed from the gastrointestinal tract, primarily the small bowel, and excessive magnesium is excreted by the kidneys.

Measurement

The focus of this chapter is on disease in small animals that have been associated with alterations in magnesium status, as well as a brief discussion on those conditions in people who have been ascribed to raised or lowered magnesium levels. Any discussion of abnormalities in magnesium requires discussion of method of measurement. The simplest method is total serum levels, which may be obtained from most routine chemistry analyzers; however, similar to ionized calcium, ionized magnesium levels may more accurately reflect actual biologically active level. Magnesium values have also been assayed from tissue samples; however, this is impractical in daily clinical practice and has more potential importance as a research tool (Bebchunk et al. 2000). Most publications to date have looked primarily at total magnesium in sick dogs and cats. As point of care testing has increased in availability, ionized magnesium values are commonly available, specifically though the Nova Critical Care Xpress (Waltham, MA), which is very popular in veterinary emergency and critical care medicine settings (Gilroy et al. 2005).

Despite challenges with interpretation, low and high magnesium levels have been associated with a variety of conditions in people and companion animals. Normal ranges for ionized and serum magnesium in dogs is reported as 1.03–1.36 mg/dL and 1.61–2.51 mg/dL and 1.05–1.42 mg/dL and 1.70–2.99 mg/dL in cats. To convert to mmol/L, mg/dL is divided by 2.433, giving normal ionized magnesium values of 0.43–0.56 mmol/L in dogs and 0.43–0.58 mmol/L in cats. Conditions associated with high and low values are shown in Table 63.1.

Hypermagnesemia

Magnesium excesses are typically cleared by the kidney, thus increases in magnesium are most common in diseases that result in decreased glomerular filtration rate (GFR), such as renal failure. Increased magnesium levels may result from iatrogenic magnesium overdosage, either by incorrect calculation or through use of large doses of antacids (e.g., Mylanta® and Maalox®) or some cathartics. There are multiple case reports of children and elderly people with profound symptomatic hypermagnesemia associated with excessive cathartic usage, and a single report of an apparent mechanical mixer malfunction resulting in severe signs mimicking sepsis in two infants receiving total parenteral nutrition (TPN) (Qurechi and Melanokos 1996; Ali Am Walentik et al. 2003). One

Nephrology and Urology of Small Animals. Edited by Joe Bartges and David J. Polzin. © 2011 Blackwell Publishing Ltd.

Table 63.1 Common conditions associated with alterations in magnesium levels

---

Raised magnesium levels
    Renal failure
    Reduction in glomerular filtration rate (independent of renal failure)
    Iatrogenic or inadvertent
Lowered magnesium levels
    Gastrointestinal losses
    Protein-losing enteropathy
    Renal loss
    Endocrine disorders
    Sepsis
    Eclampsia (milk fever) in dogs
    Re-feeding syndrome
    Large volume resuscitation with Mg^{2+} free fluids
    Massive transfusion
    Other electrolytes disorders

---

report of a dog and a cat receiving iatrogenic magnesium overdosage described severe clinical signs including hypotension and bradycardia in both (Jackson and Drobatz 2004). These patients had ionized magnesium levels of 7–9 times normal range, which would be consistent with a severe overdosage. Iatrogenic overdosage is potentially more common as the therapeutic dose (see section on hypomagnesemia) is typically published in meq per kilogram per day, rather than as many other drugs are listed per minute or per hour, which may be confusing (Jackson and Drobatz 2004). All calculations for magnesium infusions should be made carefully.

In people, combination of an angiotensin-converting enzyme inhibitor (ACEi) and spironolactone may result in clinically important hypermagnesemia. However, in a study in small breed dogs with naturally occurring mitral valve disease, while treatment with a combination of ACEi and spironolactone did result in an increase in serum magnesium levels, it was not clinically important (Thomason et al. 2007). This supports that the simultaneous use of these medications in dogs with congestive heart failure is unlikely to result in clinical hypermagnesemia and may be used together.

Increases in ionized magnesium concentration were reported in 35% of dogs in one recent study on 76 dogs with hypoadrenocorticism (Adler et al. 2007). These increases were not statistically associated with the creatinine or with venous pH, suggesting that neither acidosis nor azotemia was the cause. It was postulated that decreased aldosterone action might have played a role in elevated ionized Mg^{2+} concentrations (Adler et al. 2007).

Surgery and anesthesia have been documented to result in a mild increase in ionized Mg^{2+} after a variety of anesthetic protocols and surgical procedures, although changes were not clinically relevant as values remained within normal range (Brainard et al. 2007).

Excessive dietary magnesium, although not necessarily serum levels, have been associated with the formation of magnesium ammonium phosphate (struvite) uroliths and resulted in creation of magnesium-restricted diets for dissolution and prevention of struvite urolithiasis (Chapter 69) (Houston et al. 2004). Effects of these magnesium-restricted diets were evaluated in a group of cats with hypertrophic cardiomyopathy; however, no apparent effect was detected, despite the role of magnesium in some forms of cardiac disease (Freeman et al. 1997).

Clinical signs of spontaneous hypermagnesemia are usually silent in pets with renal disease being more clearly apparent in those animals with marked over dosage (Jackson and Drobatz 2004; Cortes and Moses 2007). Signs of magnesium elevation include depression, weakness, flaccid paralysis, and diminished reflexes (Cortes and Moses 2007). Hypotension is associated with decreased systemic vascular resistance due to magnesium's effect on calcium channels. EKG changes will occur predictably at increasing levels of magnesium, with initial signs including a mild tachycardia, progressing to a bradycardia associated with QRS prolongation and an increased P-Q interval. Untreated, severe hypermagnesemia will result in ventricular fibrillation or asystole and subsequent death (Qurechi and Melanokos 1996).

Treatment of hypermagnesemia depends upon the severity of elevation and clinical signs. Any supplemental magnesium should obviously be discontinued. Some crystalloid fluids continue magnesium, notably Normosol®-R, Normosol®-M, Plasma-lyte® 148 and Plasma-lyte® 56. Lactated Ringer's solution and 0.9% saline do not contain magnesium (Cortes and Moses 2007). Loop diuretics (e.g., furosemide) may be useful as would a saline-based diuresis. In an acute setting, intravenous calcium gluconate at 50–150 mg/kg slowly will antagonize effects of magnesium toxicity. In people, use of dialysis has been described, but this has not been reported in veterinary medicine (Qurechi and Melanokos 1996; Kraft et al. 2005). Chronic mild hypermagnesemia that accompanies chronic renal failure (Chapter 48) may be well tolerated and not require a specific therapy.

Hypomagnesemia

Hypomagnesemia is considered a more common disturbance than hypermagnesemia with reports of up to 50% of critically ill people affected. Surveys in critically ill dogs and cats support that a similar number of companion animal patients may be affected (Khanna et al. 1998;

Toll et al. 2002). Hypomagnesemia is most often a result of increased renal loss, decreased intestinal absorption, redistribution, or a combination of two or more of these. Furthermore, other aspects of illness may magnify preexisting hypomagnesemia, such as sepsis, blood transfusions (in association with citrate), or extensive fluid or insulin therapy. In cattle and sheep, profound hypomagnesaemia is associated with certain type of pasture grazing and may result in a potentially fatal syndrome termed grass tetany; this is not a problem in nonruminant species (Martens and Schweigel 2000).

Clinical signs of mild hypomagnesemia may be hard to appreciate or distinguish from illness in general. Severely affected animals may have profound weakness or neurological signs or arrhythmias. Cardiac arrhythmias are associated with hypomagnesemia in people and are occasionally postulated to occur in dogs. One case report in a dog with hypercalcemia of malignancy due to an anal sac adenocarcinoma, which had been treated preoperatively with pamidronate, calcitonin, and saline, developed severe arrhythmia under anesthesia thought in part to be associated with resultant severe hypomagnesemia (Kadar et al. 2004). Perhaps the most important aspect of hypomagnesemia is the accompanying other metabolic and electrolytes disturbances, such as hypokalemia, hypocalcemia, or hyponatremia. Hypokalemia in particular is often observed in conjunction with hypomagnesemia, and in diabetic patients in particular, it may be very hard to correct hypokalemia without also addressing hypomagnesemia as serum potassium seems resistant to even very high rates of supplementation without corresponding correction of the magnesium deficiency. One abstract, presented at the ACVIM Forum in 2005, documented that dogs and cats with hypoparathyroidism appeared to have either "subnormal or marginal circulating concentrations of magnesium," which was postulated to decrease the cell membrane receptor sensitivity to ionized calcium and potentially negatively affect parathyroid hormone production (Schenck 2005b). Finally, another report described clinical signs associated with hypocalcemia and hypomagnesemia in five Yorkshire terriers or terrier-mixes, associated with a severe protein-losing enteropathy (Kimmel et al. 2000). Thus, magnesium status should be closely assessed in any patient with either hypokalemia or hypocalcemia and supplementation considered.

Endocrine disorders may be also associated with low magnesium levels. Hyperthyroidism in cats has been associated with a linear decline in ionized magnesium levels. The significance of this finding is currently unclear, but certainly cats affected with severe hyperthyroidism should be considered at risk for hypomagnesemia (Gilroy et al. 2006). Cats with diabetes mellitus and diabetic

ketoacidosis had lower ionized magnesium concentrations, but again the significance of this is unclear (Norris et al. 1999). A similar study in dogs with naturally occurring diabetes mellitus was unable to document differences in ionized magnesium between dogs with diabetes mellitus, healthy dogs, and dogs with diabetic ketoacidosis (Fincham et al. 2004).

Cavalier King Charles spaniels (CKCS), which have a high incidence of mitral valve prolapse (MVP), were found to have low magnesium levels in one study, while another study identified seemingly two groups of CKCS, one with low platelets with normal aggregation and low magnesium and another group with normal platelet numbers with increased platelet aggregation and normal serum magnesium, suggesting that not all CKCS are affected. MVP in people is known to be associated with hypomagnesemia, although the significance of this finding remains unclear in both people and spaniels (Pedersen and Mow 1998; Olsen et al. 2001).

Lactation results in loss of magnesium, although this is rarely detected as significant in the healthy mother. One article evaluating 27 bitches with eclampsia identified hypomagnesemia in 12 (44%) affected bitches, with the conclusion that low magnesium levels are common and supplementation may be warranted in moderately to severely eclampsic dogs (Aroch et al. 1999).

Refeeding syndrome is a unique but uncommon cause of magnesium depletion. After reintroduction of nutrients, specifically carbohydrates, there is an obligatory surge in insulin release, resulting in conversion from a catabolic to an anabolic state, thus increasing cellular requirements for phosphorus, potassium, and magnesium, which can lead to whole body electrolyte depletion. This can be magnified by preexisting magnesium depletion due to lack of dietary intake. One case report described severe refeeding syndrome, including hypomagnesemia in cat that was inadvertently locked in a garage for 49 days (Armitage-Chan et al. 2006).

Treatment of hypomagnesemia should be based upon clinical judgment. Patients with other electrolyte disturbances, specifically hypokalemia or hypocalcemia should be treated as should any animal with other clinical signs of weakness. Magnesium may be supplemented as outlined in Table 63.2.

In human medicine, supplemental intravenous magnesium is widely used for a variety of indications, including pre-term labor, asthma, cardiovascular disease, and/or arrhythmia, brain injury/stroke, and as an adjuvant anesthetic agent (Touyz 2004; Gupta et al. 2006). In dogs and cats, ancillary uses have been less commonly reported. One study did conclude that addition of magnesium sulphate was dose-sparing for thiopental and halothane in healthy dogs while another study reported

Table 63.2 Guidelines for actively supplementing magnesium

Recall that some fluid types (e.g., Normosol® and Plasma-lyte®) contain magnesium

Intravenous supplementation using magnesium sulfate

The following doses are equivalent:
  0.75–1 meq/kg per day
  0.03–0.04 meq/kg/h
  0.0005–0.0006 meq/kg/min

Be vigilant against inadvertent overdosage

Magnesium sulfate is supplied most commonly as a 50% solution with a concentration of 4 meq/mL

Alternatively, magnesium chloride is also available in a 20% solution with 2 meq/L

an apparent response to magnesium therapy in a dog with torsades des pointes (Baty et al. 1994; Anagnostou et al. 2008). The ultimate role of magnesium therapy in companion animal remains to be determined, but the preponderance of evidence suggests that this role will be expanding.

References

Adler, J.A., K.J. Drobatz, et al. (2007). Abnormalities of serum electrolyte concentrations in dogs with hypoadrenocorticism. *J Vet Intern Med* **21**: 1168–1173.

Ali Am Walentik, C., G.J. Mantych, et al. (2003). Iatrogenic acute hypermagnesesemia after total parenteral nutrition infusion mimicking septic shock syndrome: two case reports. *Pediatrics* **112**: e70–e72.

Anagnostou, T.L., I. Savvas, et al. (2008). Thiopental and halothane dose-sparing effects of magnesium sulphate in dogs. *Vet Anaesth Analg* **35**: 93–99.

Armitage-Chan, E.A., T.E. O'Toole, et al. (2006). Management of prolonged food deprivations, hypothermia and re-feeding syndrome in a cat. *J Vet Emerg Crit Care* **16**: S34–S41.

Aroch, I., H. Srebro, et al. (1999). Serum electrolyte concentrations in bitches with eclampsia. *Vet Record* **145**: 318–320.

Baty, C., D.C. Sweet, et al. (1994). Torsades de pointes-like polymorphic ventricular tachycardia in a dog. *J Vet Intern Med* **8**: 439–442.

Bebchunk, T.N., J.G. Hauptman, et al. (2000). Intracellular magnesium concentrations in dogs with gastric dilatation-volvulus. *Am J Vet Res* **61**: 1415–1417.

Brainard, B.M., V.L. Campbell, et al. (2007). The effects of surgery and anesthesia on blood magnesium and calcium concentrations in canine and feline patients. *Vet Anaesth Analg* **34**: 89–98.

Cortes, Y.E. and L. Moses (2007). Magnesium disturbances in critically ill patients. *Comp Con Ed Pract Vet* **29**: 420–427.

Fincham, S.C., K.J. Drobatz, et al. (2004). Evaluation of plasma-ionized magnesium concentration in 122 dogs with diabetes mellitus: a retrospective study. *J Vet Inten Med* **18**: 612–617.

Freeman, L.M., D.J. Brown, et al. (1997). Magnesium status and the effect of magnesium supplementation in feline hypertrophic cardiomyopathy. *Can J Vet Res* **61**: 227–231.

Gilroy, C.V., S.A. Burton, et al. (2005). Validation of the NOVA CRT8 for the measurement of ionized magnesium in feline serum. *Vet Clin Path* **34**: 124–131.

Gilroy, C.V., B.S. Horney, et al. (2006). Evaluation of ionized and total serum magnesium concentrations in hyperthyroid cats. *Can J Vet Res* **70**: 137–142.

Gupta, K., V. Vohra, et al. (2006). The role of magnesium as an adjuvant during general anesthesia. *Anaesthesia* **61**: 1058–1063.

Houston, D.M., N.E. Rinkardt, et al. (2004). Evaluation of the efficacy of a commercial diet in the dissolution of feline struvite bladder uroliths. *Vet Ther* **5**: 187–201.

Jackson, C.B. and K.J. Drobatz (2004). Iatrogenic magnesium overdosage: 2 case reports. *Journal of Veterinary Emergency and Critical Care* **14**: 115–123.

Kadar, E., J.E. Rush, et al. (2004). Electrolyte disturbances and cardiac arrhythmias in a dog following pamidronate, calcitonin and furosemide administration for hypercalcemia of malignancy. *J Am Anim Hosp Assoc* **40**: 75–81.

Khanna, C., E.M. Lund, et al. (1998). Hypomagnesemia in 188 dogs: a hospital population-based prevalence study. *J Vet Intern Med* **12**: 304–309.

Kimmel, S.E., L.S. Waddell, et al. (2000). Hypomagnesemia and hypocalcemia associated with protein-losing enteropathy in Yorkshire terriers: five cases (1992–1998). *J Am Vet Med Assoc* **217**: 703–706.

Kraft, M.D., I.F. Braiche, et al. (2005). Treatment of electrolyte disorders in adult patients in the intensive care unit. *Am J Health-Syst Pharm* **62**: 1663–1682.

Martens, H. and M. Schweigel (2000). Pathophysiology of grass tetany and other hypomagnesemias. Implications for clinical management. *Vet Clin North Am Food Anim Pract* **16**: 339–368.

Norris, C.R., R.W. Nelson, et al. (1999). Serum total and ionized magnesium concentrations and urinary fractional excretion of magnesium in cats with diabetes mellitus and diabetic ketoacidosis. *J Am Vet Med Assoc* **215**: 1455–1459.

Olsen, L.H., A.T. Kristensen, et al. (2001). Increased platelet aggregation response in Cavalier King Charles Spaniels with mitral valve prolapse. *J Vet Intern Med* **15**: 209–216.

Pedersen, H.D. and T. Mow (1998). Hypomagnesemia and mitral valve prolapse in Cavalier King Charles spaniels. *Zentralbl Veterinarmed A* **45**: 607–614.

Qurechi, T. and T.K. Melanokos (1996). Acute hypermagnesemia after laxative use. *Ann Emerg Med* **28**: 552–555.

Schenck, P.A. (2005a). Fractionation of canine serum magnesium. *Vet Clin Path* **34**: 137–139.

Schenck, P.A. (2005b). *Serum Ionized Magnesium Concentrations in Dogs and Cats with Hypoparathyroidism.* ACVIM 2005 Abstract. Available at: www.vin.com (accessed May 19, 2008).

Thomason, J.D., J.E. Rockwell, et al. (2007). Influence of combined angiotensin-converting enzyme inhibitors and spironolactone on serum K^+, Mg^{2+}, and Na^+ concentrations in small dogs with degenerative mitral valve disease. *J Vet Cardiol* **9**: 103–108.

Toll, J., H. Erb, et al. (2002). Prevalence and incidence of serum magnesium abnormalities in hospitalized cats. *J Vet Intern Med* **16**: 217–221.

Touyz, R.M. (2004). Magnesium in clinical medicine. *Front Biosci* **9**: 1278–1293.

64

Calcium disorders

John M. Kruger and Carl A. Osborne

Hypercalcemia and hypocalcemia are frequent disorders of calcium metabolism in dogs and cats. In one study, abnormal concentrations of total calcium were detected in approximately 16% of all canine serum samples submitted for biochemical determinations (Chew and Meuten 1982). Since precise control of extracellular calcium concentration is essential to maintain homeostasis, perturbations in calcium concentration can profoundly disrupt cellular and organ function, resulting in severe renal, gastrointestinal, cardiovascular, and neurologic dysfunction (Rosol et al. 1995).

Causes of hypercalcemia

Overview

Hypercalcemia may result from a number of remarkably diverse causes and pathophysiologic mechanisms (Tables 64.1 and 64.2). Basic pathophysiologic factors that, alone or in combination, may contribute to hypercalcemia include increased bone resorption, increased intestinal calcium absorption, mobilization of calcium from mineralized tissues, enhanced renal tubular calcium resorption, decreased bone accretion, increased calcium retention due to diminished glomerular filtration, increased protein binding of calcium, or increased calcium complexing with plasma anions (such as citrate and phosphorus). Laboratory error may also cause fictitious hypercalcemia.

Hypercalcemia of malignancy

Nonparathyroid neoplasms, especially lymphomas, account for 40–65% of hypercalcemic dogs and 10–30%

of hypercalcemic cats with classifiable disease (Table 64.1) (Chew and Carothers 1989; Elliot et al. 1991; Uehlinger et al. 1998; Savary et al. 2000; Bolliger et al. 2002). Malignancy-associated hypercalcemia may be the result of (1) tumor-derived circulating factors, which stimulate generalized osteoclastic bone resorption (so-called humoral hypercalcemia of malignancy), (2) tumor-induced local osteolysis, or (3) humoral and local pathogenic factors acting independently or in combination (Rosol and Capen 1992; Lucas et al. 2007).

Humoral hypercalcemia of malignancy results from enhanced osteoclastic bone resorption mediated by a systemically acting tumor-derived peptide that resembles parathyroid hormone (PTH) in both structure and physiologic properties (Osborne and Stevens 1973; Meuten et al. 1981; Meuten et al. 1983; Weir et al. 1988a, 1988b; Rosol and Capen 1992; Rosol et al. 1992; Bolliger et al. 2002). Like PTH, PTH-related protein (PTHrp) enhances osteoclastic bone resorption, promotes distal renal tubular calcium reabsorption, inhibits proximal tubule phosphorus reabsorption, and stimulates renal 25-hydroxyvitamin D-1-alpha-hydroxylase activity (Rosol and Capen 1992). Observations in hypercalcemic dogs with T-cell lymphoma and anal sac apocrine cell adenocarcinoma and cats with lymphoma, bronchogenic carcinoma, and squamous cell carcinoma suggest that PTHrp is the primary mediator of hypercalcemia associated with these neoplasms (Meuten et al. 1981; Meuten et al. 1983; Weir et al. 1988a, 1988b; Rosol and Capen 1992; Rosol et al. 1992; Lucas et al. 2007). However, tumor production of prostaglandins, cytokines, and calcitriol may have pathogenic roles in some forms of humoral hypercalcemia of malignancy (Rosol and Capen 1992; Rosol et al. 1992).

Hypercalcemia of malignancy also may result from tumor-induced local osteolysis. Primary or metastatic skeletal neoplasms may resorb bone directly or, more

Nephrology and Urology of Small Animals. Edited by Joe Bartges and David J. Polzin. © 2011 Blackwell Publishing Ltd.

Table 64.1 Causes of hypercalcemia in dogs

Common
  Some malignant neoplasms
    Lymphosarcoma
    Anal sac apocrine gland adenocarcinoma
  Hypoadrenocorticism
  Chronic renal failure
  Primary hyperparathyroidism (adenoma, adenocarcinoma, hyperplasia)

Uncommon, sporadic, or rare
  Acute renal failure (diuresis phase; e.g., rhabdomyolysis, gentamicin, raisins/grapes)
  Blood transfusion
  Hemoconcentration
  Hyperadrenocorticism (resolution phase)
  Hyperproteinemia
  Hypertrophic osteodystrophy
  Hypervitaminosis D
    Antipsoriasis creams containing calcitriene
    Iatrogenic (administration of calcitriol or other vitamin D preparations)
    Rodenticide intoxication (cholecalciferol)
  Hypothermia
  Idiopathic
  Infectious/Inflammatory
    Bacterial (neonatal septicemia, septic osteomyelitis, endometritis)
    Chronic nodular panniculitis
    Fungal (blastomycosis, histoplasmosis, coccidioidomycosis)
    Granulomatous dermatitis
    Granulomatous lymphadenitis
    Schistosomiasis
  Laboratory error (lipemia, hemolysis)
  Mammary hyperplasia
  Other neoplasms
    Acanthomatous ameloblastoma
    Carcinomas (skin, lung, nose, stomach, liver, pancreas, mammary gland, thyroid, adrenal medulla, testis, ovaries, undifferentiated)
    Hepatoblastoma
    Leukemia
    Malignant histiocytosis
    Malignant melanoma
    Metastatic bone neoplasms
    Multiple endocrine neoplasia
    Multiple myeloma
    Myeloproliferative disease
    Sarcomas (muscle, bone, adipose tissue, undifferentiated)
    Seminoma
    Thymoma

Table 64.2 Causes of hypercalcemia in cats

Common
  Chronic renal failure
  Idiopathic
  Some malignant neoplasms
    Lymphosarcoma
    Squamous cell carcinoma

Uncommon, sporadic, or rare
  Hyperproteinemia
  Hyperthyroidism
  Hypervitaminosis D
    Antipsoriasis creams containing calcitriene
  Iatrogenic (administration of calcitriol, or other vitamin D preparations)
    Plants (*Cestrum diurnum*)
    Rodenticide intoxication (cholecalciferol)
  Hypoadrenocorticism
  Hypothermia
  Infectious/Inflammatory
    Bacterial (nocardia, actinomyces)
    Chronic pancreatitis
    Feline infectious peritonitis
    Fungal (blastomycosis, histoplasmosis, cryptococcosis)
    Injection site granuloma
    Toxoplasmosis
  Laboratory error (lipemia, hemolysis)
  Liver disease (lipidosis, biliary hyperplasia/fibrosis)
  Obstructive uropathy
  Other neoplasms
    Carcinomas (skin, lung, thyroid, kidney, undifferentiated)
    Leukemia
    Metastatic bone neoplasms (squamous cell carcinoma)
    Multiple myeloma
    Myelodysplasia
    Myelofibrosis
    Myeloproliferative disease
    Sarcomas (bone, undifferentiated)
  Primary hyperparathyroidism (adenoma, adenocarcinoma, hyperplasia)

likely, stimulate osteoclastic bone resorption via tumor secretion of prostaglandins or other cytokines (Rosol and Capen 1992; Lucas et al. 2007). Although tumor-induced local osteolysis is a common cause of hypercalcemia in humans, it is infrequently recognized as a cause of hypercalcemia in dogs and cats (MacEwen and Siegel 1977; Chew and Carothers 1989; Elliot et al. 1991).

Hypoadrenocorticism

Hypoadrenocorticism may also be associated with hypercalcemia in dogs (Table 64.1) (Chew and Meuten 1982; Elliot et al. 1991; Uehlinger et al. 1998). Increased total calcium has been reported to occur in approximately 28–45% of dogs with spontaneous hypoadrenocorticism (Willard et al. 1982; Peterson et al. 1996; Uehlinger et al. 1998; Feldman and Nelson 2004a). Hypercalcemia has rarely been reported in cats with spontaneous hypoadrenocorticism; however, hypercalcemia has been observed in 25% of bilaterally adrenalectomized cats (Baumann and Kurland 1929; Peterson et al. 1989; Savary et al. 2000; Smith et al. 2002). The cause(s) of hypercalcemia of hypoadrenocorticism is most likely multifactorial. It may be attributable to one or a combination of the following: (1) increased calcium retention due to diminished glomerular filtration, (2) enhanced renal calcium reabsorption secondary to volume contraction, (3) hemoconcentration, acidosis, increased protein binding of calcium, (4) increased calcium complexing with plasma anions (such as citric acid and phosphorus), and (5) increased bone resorption (Walser et al. 1963; Muls et al. 1982; Montoli et al. 1992; Diamond and Thornley 1994; Adler et al. 1985). Plasma concentrations of protein-bound and complexed calcium were elevated in hypercalcemic adrenalectomized dogs, whereas plasma ionized calcium concentrations were usually within normal range (Walser et al. 1963). However, increased ionized calcium concentrations have been observed in some dogs and cats with hypoadrenocorticism (Walser et al. 1963; Smith et al. 2002; Adler et al. 1985).

Chronic renal failure

Chronic renal failure (CRF) in humans, dogs, and cats is commonly associated with renal secondary hyperparathyroidism that is characterized by normal to decreased calcium concentrations, hyperphosphatemia, increased plasma concentrations of PTH, decreased plasma concentrations of calcitriol and phosphatonin (fibroblast growth factor 23), and parathyroid hyperplasia (Chapter 48) (Polzin et al. 2005; Moe and Sprague 2008). However, a paradoxical irreversible form of hypercalcemia (so-called *tertiary hyperparathyroidism*) may be encountered in patients with long-standing renal secondary hyperparathyroidism. Increased serum total calcium concentrations have been observed in 14–22% of dogs and 10–21% of cats with CRF (DiBartola et al. 1987; Chew and Nagode 1990; Lulich et al. 1992; Barber and Elliot 1998; Gerber et al. 2003; Schenck and Chew 2005). Increased ionized calcium concentrations have been observed in 6–9% of dogs and in 6% of cats with CRF (Chew and Nagode 1990; Barber and Elliot 1998; Schenck and Chew 2005).

Autonomous hypersecretion of PTH by the parathyroid gland apparently plays a central role in the pathogenesis of tertiary hyperparathyroidism (Parfitt 1997).

Activation of parathyroid cell calcium-sensing receptors (CSR) and vitamin D receptors (VDR) normally suppress PTH synthesis and secretion and parathyroid tissue proliferation (Chen and Goodman 2004; Dusso et al. 2005). In some cases of humans with advanced CRF, the combined effects of hyperphosphatemia, decreased calcitriol levels, and decreased expression of CSRs and VDRs promote autonomous polyclonal, oligoclonal, or monoclonal parathyroid gland expansion and autonomous hypersecretion of PTH (Parfitt 1997; Llach and Velasquez Forereo 2001; Grzela et al. 2006; Lauter and Arnold 2008). PTH-mediated increases in osteoclastic bone resorption and resultant increases in ionized and total calcium concentrations in the face of hyperphosphatemia substantially increase the risk of nephrocalcinosis. Increased complexing of calcium with anions, hemoconcentration, and acidosis may also contribute to the pathogenesis of hypercalcemia of CRF, especially in patients with elevations in total calcium without concurrent increases of ionized calcium concentrations.

Primary hyperparathyroidism

Primary hyperparathyroidism is characterized by excessive uncontrolled production of PTH by hyperplastic or neoplastic parathyroid glands and is an uncommon cause of hypercalcemia in dogs and cats (Table 64.1) (Elliot et al. 1991; Savary et al. 2000; Feldman and Nelson 2004a). Solitary functional adenomas of the parathyroid gland have been the most commonly recognized cause of primary hyperparathyroidism in these species (Feldman and Nelson 2004a). Excess PTH enhances osteoclastic bone resorption, promotes renal tubular calcium reabsorption and phosphorus excretion, and stimulates 1-alpha-hydroxylase conversion of 25-hydroxyvitamin D_3 to calcitriol. Calcitriol increases intestinal calcium and phosphorus absorption and further enhances PTH-mediated osteoclastic bone resorption. In nonazotemic patients, the net effect of excess PTH is increased serum total and ionized calcium concentrations with normal to decreased serum phosphorus concentrations (Weir et al. 1986; Feldman and Nelson 2004a).

Hypervitaminosis D

Hypervitaminosis D is an uncommon cause of hypercalcemia in dogs and cats. It is usually associated with excess dietary or therapeutic vitamin D supplementation for treatment of hypoparathyroidism, or from accidental ingestion of cholecalciferol-containing rodenticides or human antipsoriasis creams containing the calcitriol analogue calcipotriene (calcipotriol) (Berger and Feldman 1987; Gunther et al. 1988; Hare et al. 2000; Schenck et al. 2006). Cholecalciferol undergoes rapid unregulated hepatic hydroxylation to form 25-hydroxyvitamin D_3 (Dusso et al. 2005). Although 25-dihydroxyvitamin D_3 has minimal biologic activity at physiologic concentrations, high plasma concentrations are capable of exerting direct effects on target tissues (Dzanis and Kallfelz 1988). Because active metabolites of vitamin D stimulate intestinal calcium and phosphorus transport, mobilize calcium from bone, and promote renal tubular reabsorption of calcium and phosphorus, excess vitamin D results in hypercalcemia, hyperphosphatemia, and dystrophic calcification of soft tissue (Spangler et al. 1979; Gunther et al. 1988; Rumbeiha et al. 1999, 2000; Dusso et al. 2005).

Infectious and inflammatory disorders

Hypercalcemia has been infrequently associated with chronic infections or inflammatory disorders in dogs and cats, including fungal, bacterial, viral, and parasitic infections and granulomatous dermatitis, panniculitis, and lymphadenitis (Tables 64.1 and 64.2). However, the reported prevalence of blastomycosis-associated hypercalcemia varies from 4–14% of affected dogs and up to 25% of affected cats (Dow et al. 1986; Arceneaux et al. 1998; Gilor et al. 2006; Crews et al. 2007). Studies in humans have revealed that inappropriate endogenous overproduction of calcitriol by activated macrophages is involved in the pathogenesis of hypercalcemia of chronic granulomatous disease (Sharma 2000). An increased serum calcitriol concentration has been observed in a dog with granulomatous lymphadenitis (Mellanby et al. 2006). However, concentrations of vitamin D metabolites apparently have not been reported in hypercalcemic dogs or cats with blastomycosis or other chronic inflammatory disorders.

Idiopathic hypercalcemia

Idiopathic disease is one of the most common causes of hypercalcemia in cats (Savary et al. 2000). They may develop a condition characterized by mildly to moderately increased total calcium, moderately to severely increased ionized calcium; normophosphatemia, low to normal concentrations of PTH, nondetectable PTHrp, and normal concentrations of 25-hydroxyvitamin D and calcitriol; and normal parathyroid gland morphology (McClain et al. 1999; Midkiff et al. 2000; Schenck et al. 2004). It has been reported in male and female cats of all ages. Longhaired cats may be disproportionally affected (Midkiff et al. 2000; Schenck et al. 2004). Urolithiasis (Chapter 69) has been observed in approximately 15–35% of cats with idiopathic hypercalcemia (Midkiff et al. 2000; Schenck et al. 2004). Although the majority of affected cats consumed acidifying diets, controlled studies evaluating whether diet is a risk factor in the patho-

genesis of idiopathic hypercalcemia are needed (McClain et al. 1999; Midkiff et al. 2000). Idiopathic hypercalcemia has been uncommonly encountered in dogs (Elliot et al. 1991; Uehlinger et al. 1998).

Miscellaneous causes of hypercalcemia

Hypercalcemia occasionally has been associated with a number of additional pathologic and nonpathologic disorders of dogs and cats (Tables 64.1 and 64.2). These causes represent a diverse group of disorders for which exact pathologic mechanisms responsible for hypercalcemia have yet to be defined.

Consequences of hypercalcemia

The severity of clinical signs will be influenced by the rate of increase in serum calcium concentration, the magnitude and duration of hypercalcemia, and the nature of the underlying disease. Of the many organ systems affected by hypercalcemia, the kidneys are particularly susceptible. Hypercalcemia-induced alterations in renal function and morphology are linked to many (if not all) of the clinical manifestations observed in hypercalcemic patients.

Alterations in renal function

Impaired urine concentrating ability leading to polyuria and compensatory polydipsia is an early clinical manifestation of hypercalcemia in dogs. Urine specific gravity values of hypercalcemic patients are consistently less than 1.030 and usually less than 1.020 (Kruger et al. 1996). Although polyuria is less commonly recognized in hypercalcemic cats compared to hypercalcemic dogs, approximately 66% of cats with primary hyperparathyroidism had urine specific gravities of less than 1.020 (Kallet et al. 1991; Marquez et al. 1995; Savary et al. 2000; Feldman and Nelson 2004a). A principal cause of hypercalcemia-induced polyuria appears to be the kidney's inability to respond to the antidiuretic hormone arginine–vasopressin (AVP), resulting in an acquired form of nephrogenic diabetes insipidus. AVP-elicited translocation of aquaporin-2 (APQ2) water channels into the apical membranes of collecting duct cells is the final rate-limiting step necessary for increased water reabsorption by the renal tubules (Nejsum 2005). Studies in rodent models have demonstrated that hypercalcemia is consistently associated with decreased collecting duct water permeability and urine osmolality, increased urine production and water intake, and decreased AQP2 protein expression and apical membrane localization (Levi et al. 1983; Earm et al. 1998; Sands et al. 1998; Wang et al. 2002, 2004). It has been proposed that these effects are mediated by calcium-induced activation of CSR on the apical surfaces of collecting duct cells and subsequent reduction in intracellular cAMP concentrations, activation of protein kinase C, stabilization of cell cytoskeleton, and decreased AQP2 expression and trafficking (Sands et al. 1997; Procino et al. 2004). Diminished collecting duct responsiveness to AVP is further compounded by reduced medullary tonicity and disruption of medullary osmotic gradients. Reduced medullary solute accumulation is likely related to decreased sodium reabsorption resulting from calcium-sensor receptor-mediated downregulation of major renal sodium transporters in the thick ascending limbs of the loops of Henle (Levi et al. 1983; Jesus Ferreira et al. 1998; Wang et al. 2004). Concurrent increases in renal medullary blood flow and subsequent medullary washout likely are additional contributing factors in disruption of medullary osmotic gradients (Brunette et al. 1974). Impaired ability to maximally concentrate urine may be further compounded by renal parenchymal injury due to hypercalcemia-induced calcification of tubular epithelium, interstitial tissues, and blood vessels (Kruger et al. 1996).

Elevations in serum calcium are frequently accompanied by variable reductions in GFR and variable increases in serum urea nitrogen and serum creatinine concentrations (Weller and Hoffman 1992; Kruger et al. 1996). Reductions in GFR and azotemia may result from prerenal factors, intrinsic renal factors, or combinations of both. Hypercalcemia may directly alter renal hemodynamics and glomerular filtration. Studies in several species have demonstrated that moderate to severe hypercalcemia consistently reduced GFR and renal blood flow as a result of renal vasoconstriction and a decrease in the glomerular ultrafiltration coefficient (Epstein et al. 1959; Chomdej et al. 1977; Humes et al. 1978; Levi et al. 1983; Zawada et al. 1986; Wang et al. 2004). Renal hemodynamic changes associated with hypercalcemia are potentially reversible; correction of hypercalcemia results in rapid restoration of GFR (Lins 1978; Sutton and Dirks 1986). However, if hypercalcemia is persistent and severe, sustained renal vasoconstriction and nephrocalcinosis may lead to progressive intrinsic renal tubular injury and intrinsic primary renal failure. In this case, the reversibility of intra-renal azotemia ultimately depends on the degree of renal tubular cell and tubular basement membrane damage (Osborne et al. 1969).

Other renal tubular defects associated with hypercalcemic disorders in humans include metabolic acidosis; metabolic alkalosis; hypercalciuria; aminoaciduria; glucosuria; and renal sodium, potassium, magnesium, and phosphorus wasting (Sutton and Dirks 1986). In general, renal tubular defects have not been well characterized in hypercalcemic disorders of dogs and cats (Kruger et al. 1996).

Alterations in renal morphology

Gross renal morphologic changes are evident with chronic or severe hypercalcemia. Kidneys may be normal to large in size, pale in color, speckled or mottled in appearance, and may have a finely granular or pitted surface texture (Barr et al. 1989). Gross evidence of renal mineralization may be observed as a distinctive white gritty band located adjacent to the cortical medullary junction (Kruger et al. 1996).

Microscopic changes associated with acute or mild hypercalcemia are characterized by variable calcification, degeneration, and necrosis of tubular epithelium as well as formation of obstructing intertubular casts in the ascending loops of Henle, distal tubules, and collecting ducts (Epstein et al. 1959; Carone et al. 1960; Spangler et al. 1979). Calcification of renal parenchyma is mild and randomly distributed, affecting primarily tubular epithelium and their basement membranes (Kruger et al. 1996). With severe or chronic hypercalcemia, the extent of tubular degeneration, necrosis, and obstruction as well as renal parenchymal calcification is proportionately greater. Renal calcification is widespread, involving cortical and medullary tubular epithelium and basement membranes, interstitial tissues, periglomerular capillary basement membranes, blood vessel walls, and Bowman's capsule (Carone et al. 1960; Spangler et al. 1979; Weller et al. 1982; Barr et al. 1989; Kruger et al. 1996). Nephrocalcinosis may be concurrently associated with fibrosis and infiltration of interstitial tissues with mononuclear cells. Glomerular lesions are usually characterized by mild degeneration.

Urolithiasis

Hypercalciuria predisposes patients to formation of uroliths composed of calcium phosphate or calcium oxalate (Chapter 69) (Klausner et al. 1986; Lulich et al. 2004). In one series of 168 dogs, calcium-containing uroliths were reported in 32% of patients with primary hyperparathyroidism (Feldman and Nelson 2004a). Similarly, calcium oxalate urolithiasis has been occasionally reported in cats with primary hyperparathyroidism (Marquez et al. 1995). Although urolithiasis is rarely recognized in association with other hypercalcemic disorders in dogs, radiopaque uroliths were identified in 35% of 20 cats with idiopathic hypercalcemia (Midkiff et al. 2000).

Urinary tract infections

Bacterial urinary tract infections (Chapter 71) have been observed in approximately 32% of dogs with primary hyperparathyroidism (Feldman and Nelson 2004a).

Several hypercalcemia-induced abnormalities of the urinary tract, including renal insufficiency, formation of dilute urine, and concurrent urolithiasis, represent risk factors for bacterial urinary tract infections in dogs with primary hyperparathyroidism (Osborne et al. 1979).

Diagnostic considerations for hypercalcemia

Depending on the reference laboratory, hypercalcemia is defined as a fasting total calcium concentration of greater than 12.0 mg/dL (3.8 mmol/L) in dogs and 11.0 mg/dL (2.75 mmol/L) in cats or an ionized calcium concentration greater than 6.0 mg/dL (1.5 mmol/L) in dogs and 5.7 mg/dL (1.4 mmol/L) in cats (Schenck et al. 2006). Since total calcium concentrations may not be directly proportional to ionized calcium concentration, ionized calcium determinations should be included in diagnostic evaluations whenever possible as they provide useful information for differentiating causes of hypercalcemia in dogs and cats (Schenck and Chew 2002, 2005; Lulich et al. 2004).

Identification of the cause or causes of hypercalcemia in dogs and cats and subsequent formulation of specific therapeutic plans depend on careful assessment of the history, physical examination findings, and results of hematologic, biochemical, endocrinologic, radiographic, ultrasonic, and histocytologic evaluations. Using the combined results of these routine evaluations, most disease processes that cause hypercalcemia in dogs and cats can be identified or at least localized to a specific anatomic region or organ system. Patients in whom a cause for hypercalcemia is not obvious from initial evaluations currently pose a diagnostic challenge. Disorders in these patients can often be differentiated using results of assays for ionized calcium and calcium regulating hormones, including serum intact molecule immunoreactive PTH, serum intact molecule or N-terminal immunoreactive PTHrP, 25-hydroxyvitamin D_3, and 1,25-dihydroxyvitamin D_3 (Table 64.3) (Kruger et al. 1996; Schenck et al. 2006).

Treatment strategies for hypercalcemia

Initiation of therapy directed toward the specific cause is the only consistently effective means of elimination or long-term control of hypercalcemia. However, symptomatic and supportive therapy is often required in patients with acute severe hypercalcemia. Symptomatic

Table 64.3 Laboratory abnormalities characteristic of common causes of hypercalcemia and hypocalcemia in dogs and cats

Cause	TCa	iCa	PO$_4$	Intact iPTH	PTHrP	25-OH Vit D	1,25(OH)$_2$ Vit D	SUN or SCr	Na$^+$/K$^+$ Ratio
HYPERCALCEMIA									
Hypercalcemia of malignancy	↑	↑	N,↓[†]	↓	↑,N	N	↓,N,↑	N[†]	N
Hypoadrenocorticism	↑	N,↑	N,↑	↓,N	N	N	N	↑	↓
Chronic renal failure (tertiary hyperparathyroidism)	↑	↑	↑	↑	N	N,↓	N,↓	↑	N**
Vitamin D intoxication (cholecalciferol)	↑	↑	N,↑	↓	N	↑	N,↑	N[†]	N
Primary hyperparathyroidism	↑	↑	N,↓[†]	N,↑	N	N	N,↑	N[†]	N
Feline idiopathic	↑	↑	N,↑	N,↓	N	↓,N,↑	↓,N,↑	N[†]	N
HYPOCALCEMIA									
Hypoalbuminemia	↓	N,↓	N	N,↑	N	N	N,↑	N	N
Chronic renal failure (secondary hyperparathyroidism)	N,↑,↓	N,↓	↑,N	↑	N	N,↓	N,↓	↑	N**
Obstructive uropathy	N,↓	N,↓	↑	N,↑	N	N	Unk	↑	↑
Eclampsia	↓	↓	↓	↑,N	N	N	N,↓	N	N
Ethylene glycol toxicity	↓	↓	↑,N	↑	N	N	N,↑	N[†]	N
Primary hypoparathyroidism	↓	↓	↑,N	↓,N	N	N	N,↓	N	N

Key: TCa = serum total calcium; iCa = serum ionized calcium; PO$_4$ = serum inorganic phosphorous; Intact iPTH = Intact molecule immunoreactive parathyroid hormone; PTHrP = immunoreactive parathyroid hormone related peptide; 25-OH Vit D = 25-hydroxyvitamin D; 1,25(OH)$_2$ Vit D = 1,25 dihydroxy vitamin D; SUN = blood urea nitrogen; SCr = serum creatinine; Na$^+$ = serum sodium; K$^+$ = serum potassium; N = normal; Unk = unknown.

[†]Values may be increased with reductions in GFR.

**Values may be decreased in oliguric renal failure.

and supportive therapies temporarily reduce elevated serum calcium concentrations and often ameliorate cardiac, neurologic, and renal toxicity. Short-term control of hypercalcemia provides additional time for formulation and initiation of specific diagnostic and therapeutic plans. Premature, overzealous, or inappropriate symptomatic therapy, however, may interfere with identification of specific causes and possibly expose patients to needless treatments with potentially life-threatening complications. The speed with which symptomatic therapy is initiated and the specific therapeutic agents are used depends on (1) pathogenesis; (2) duration, magnitude, and rate progression of hypercalcemia; (3) severity of associated clinical signs; (4) concomitant metabolic, endocrine, hematologic, cardiovascular, or renal abnormalities; (5) risk of progressive end-organ injury due to persistent hypercalcemia; and (6) availability of appropriate laboratory tests to monitor patient response in a timely fashion.

Regardless of the severity of hypercalcemia, extracellular fluid volume expansion is an essential component of the therapeutic regimen. Because sodium-dependent co-transport of calcium in proximal tubules accounts for approximately 70% of renal calcium reabsorption, restoration of extracellular fluid volume decreases proximal tubular sodium reabsorption and effectively promotes renal calcium excretion (Sutton and Dirks 1986). Dehydration should be corrected immediately by vigorous replacement therapy with 0.9% sodium chloride solution or other types of electrolyte solutions suited to patient needs (Table 64.4). Excessive fluid administration should be avoided in patients with pathologic oliguria, hypertension, congestive heart failure, or other edematous disorders, and in patients with preexisting hypokalemia or hypomagnesemia.

Patients with moderate to severe or rapidly progressing hypercalcemia often require additional therapy to promote further renal calcium excretion (Table 64.4). Furosemide and other loop diuretics promote renal calcium excretion and enhance the calciuric effects of fluid therapy by inhibiting calcium reabsorption in the thick ascending limb of the loops of Henle (Ong et al. 1974; Adin et al. 2003). Because use of diuretics in volume-contracted patients exacerbates hypercalcemia by accelerating fluid and electrolyte losses, correction of fluid and electrolyte deficits are essential prerequisites to furosemide therapy. Unlike furosemide, thiazide diuretics and the potassium-sparing diuretic amiloride may decrease renal excretion of calcium and are therefore contraindicated (Costanzo 1985).

In patients with severe or rapidly progressing hypercalcemia associated with increased bone resorption, agents that inhibit bone resorption are indicated. Glu-cocorticoids inhibit osteoclast-mediated bone resorption, decrease intestinal calcium absorption, and promote renal calcium excretion (Collins et al. 1963; Kim et al. 2007). In addition, glucocorticoids may be directly cytotoxic to steroid-sensitive neoplasms. Glucocorticoid responsive causes of hypercalcemia have been reported to include lymphoma, multiple myeloma, thymoma, hypervitaminosis D, granulomatous disease, hypoadrenocorticism, and feline idiopathic hypercalcemia (Schenck et al. 2006). Because glucocorticoids may substantially alter lymphoid morphology and may exacerbate infection-induced granulomatous disease, a definitive diagnosis should be established before glucocorticoid administration.

The naturally occurring polypeptide hormone calcitonin inhibits osteoclast-mediated bone resorption and enhances urinary calcium excretion (Cochran et al. 1970). Calcitonin is used in human patients because of the rapid onset of action, high degree of efficacy, and few contraindications or adverse effects (Wisneski 1990). However, the effects of the hormone are transient, with most patients becoming refractory to the drug in 2–4 days. Nevertheless, calcitonin seems to provide invaluable short-term adjunctive therapy in patients with severe hypercalcemia, especially when combined with a bisphosphonate (Sekine and Takami 1998). Experience with calcitonin in veterinary patients has been limited primarily to dogs with severe hypervitaminosis D (Table 64.4) (Dougherty et al. 1990; Garlock et al. 1991). Calcitonin has also been used in combination therapy for hypercalcemia associated with granulomatous disease in a cat (Mealey et al. 1999).

Bisphosphonates are synthetic pyrophosphate analogues with a high affinity for bone hydroxyapatite (Fan 2007). These agents are potent inhibitors of osteoclast-mediated bone resorption that act by disrupting osteoclast intracellular metabolism and by promoting osteoclast apoptosis. Bisphosphonates have been used to manage a variety of hypercalcemic disorders in humans, dogs, and cats (Wellington and Goa 2003; Schenck et al. 2006; Fan 2007). Newer second- and third-generation aminobisphosphonates, such as pamidronate, ibandronate, and zoledronate, are more effective and are associated with fewer adverse effects than earlier bisphosphonates (Wellington and Goa 2003; Fan 2007). Because of poor oral absorption, bisphosphonates are most effective when administered parenterally (Fan 2007). In veterinary patients, intravenous pamidronate has been used for management of hypercalcemia associated with malignancy, cholecalciferol and calcipotriene toxicity, feline nocardiosis, and feline idiopathic hypercalcemia (Table 64.4) (Rumbeiha et al. 1999, 2000; Pesillo et al. 2002; Kadar et al. 2004; Fan et al. 2005; Hostutler et al. 2005).

Table 64.4 Therapeutic agents for symptomatic management of hypercalcemia

Therapeutic agent	Dosage and route of administration	Onset of action[a]	Indications	Contraindications	Possible adverse effects
0.9% sodium chloride or other fluid that best suits patient needs	Hydration deficit plus 40–60 mL/kg IV infusion over 24 h	Rapid	Mild to severe hypercalcemia	Congestive heart failure, generalized edema, hypertension	Volume overload, hypokalemia, hypomagnesemia, hypernatremia
Furosemide	2–4 mg/kg IV, SC q 8–12 h; or 0.66 mg/kg bolus followed by CRI of 0.66 mg/kg/h	Immediate	Moderate to severe hypercalcemia	Dehydration, hypovolemia	Volume depletion, hypokalemia, hypomagnesemia, hypochloremic alkalosis, hypercalciuria
Prednisolone	1–2.2 mg/kg PO, SC, IV q 12 h	Rapid to delayed	Moderate to severe hypercalcemia due to steroid-responsive malignancy, hypervitaminosis D, granulomatous disease, hypoadrenocorticism, feline idiopathic hypercalcemia	Infectious disease, pancreatitis, hepatic insufficiency, renal failure, ulcerative colitis	Generalized catabolism, immunosuppression, pancreatitis, gastrointestinal ulceration, hepatopathy, myopathy, osteoporosis, others
Calcitonin	4–7 IU/kg SC q 6–8 h	Rapid	Mild to severe hypercalcemia when other therapy is ineffective or contraindicated	Hypersensitivity to calcitonin	Vomiting
Pamidronate	1–2 mg/kg IV infusion over 2 h q21–28 days	Rapid to delayed	Moderate to severe hypercalcemia due to malignancy, hypervitaminosis D, granulomatous disease, feline idiopathic hypercalcemia when other therapy is ineffective or contraindicated	Hypersensitivity to bisphosphonates	Vomiting, cardiac arrhythmia, renal failure, hypocalcemia, hypophosphatemia, hypomagnesemia
Sodium bicarbonate	1 mEq/kg IV every 10 to 15 min; maximum total dose of 4 mEq/kg	Immediate	Life-threatening hypercalcemic crisis	Alkalosis, congestive heart failure	Alkalosis, hypokalemia, paradoxical CSF acidosis, hypernatremia, ECF hyperosmolality, intracranial hemorrhage, coma, cardiac dysrhythmias
Sodium EDTA	25–75 mg/kg/h	Immediate	Life-threatening hypercalcemic crisis	Renal failure	Acute renal failure, hypocalcemia
Peritoneal dialysis	Low calcium or calcium-free dialysate IP	Rapid	Moderate to severe hypercalcemia with concurrent oliguric or anuric renal failure	Recent abdominal surgery, PKD, abdominal neoplasia	Peritonitis
Hemodialysis	Low calcium or calcium-free dialysate	Rapid	Moderate to severe hypercalcemia with concurrent oliguric or anuric renal failure	Few	Hypotension, hemorrhage, seizures, thromboembolism, sepsis

Key: CRI, constant rate infusion; CSF, cerebral spinal fluid; ECF, extracellular fluid; PKD, polycystic kidney disease; ND, not determined; D5W, 5% dextrose in water.

[a]Approximate time to beneficial therapeutic effect; maximum effect may occur later; immediate = <2 hours; rapid = 3–12 hours; delayed = >24 hours.

In a series of 7 dogs and 2 cats with hypercalcemia due to a variety of causes, pamidronate infusion resulted in a 15–64% decrease in serum total calcium concentration that persisted for 11 days to 9 weeks (median 8.5 weeks) (Hostutler et al. 2005). Interestingly, pamidronate has been used to manage renal tertiary hyperparathyroidism in hypercalcemic human patients with end-stage renal disease (Torregrosa et al. 2003). However, use of aminobisphosphonates for management of hypercalcemia in dogs and cats with end-stage renal disease has not been reported. Although veterinary experience with other aminobisphosphonates is limited, in humans, zoledronate has the advantages of increased potency, shorter infusion time, more rapid response, and longer duration of action compared to pamidronate (Wellington and Goa 2003; Fan et al. 2005).

Therapeutic agents that alter the relative concentration of ionized calcium or promote extrarenal calcium excretion are usually reserved for emergency short-term management of hypercalcemic crises (i.e., severe hypercalcemia resulting in life-threatening cardiac dysfunction and/or neurologic dysfunction). In this situation, immediate attempts should be made to reduce plasma ionized calcium with intravenous sodium bicarbonate or sodium EDTA (Table 64.4) (Kruger et al. 1996; Schenck et al. 2006). Both agents rapidly reduce plasma calcium concentration, but have short durations of effect (<2 hours) (Parfitt and Kleerekoper 1980; Meuten 1984; Chew et al. 1989). Because sodium bicarbonate and sodium EDTA may be associated with significant adverse effects, patients treated with these agents should be continuously monitored and should be switched to less hazardous forms of therapy as quickly as possible. Peritoneal (Chapter 30), pleural, or hemodialysis (Chapter 28) with low calcium dialysates are potentially useful for symptomatic therapy of a hypercalcemic crisis, especially if concomitant renal failure has limited other therapeutic options (Heyburn et al. 1980; Cowgill 1995).

Recently developed pharmaceutical agents that have potential roles in symptomatic treatment of hypercalcemia in dogs and cats include somatostatin congeners, nonhypercalcemic calcitriol analogues, calcimimetics, and osteoclast antiresorptive agents. Somatostatin congeners (e.g., lanreotide and octreotide) and noncalcemic calcitriol analogs (e.g., paricalcitol and doxercalciferol) are two classes of agents that may be useful for symptomatic treatment of dogs with hypercalcemia caused by PTHrp-producing neoplasms. These agents prevent excessive bone resorption by inhibiting tumor production of PTHrp (Anthony et al. 1995; Yu et al. 1995). Cinacalcet is a type II calcimimetic agent that functions as an allosteric modulator of the calcium-sensing receptor on the surface of the parathyroid cell (Ureña and Frazão 2003). By altering receptor conformation, cinacalcet enhances receptor sensitivity to extracellular calcium ions and thus inhibits PTH synthesis and secretion by parathyroid cells. The ability of cinacalcet to lower plasma PTH levels without exacerbating phosphate retention or increasing serum calcium concentrations has resulted in the use of this agent to successfully treat primary, secondary, and tertiary hyperparathyroidism and functional parathyroid carcinomas in humans (Wüthrich et al. 2007). Human recombinant osteoprotegerin is a novel investigational bone antiresorptive agent that functions as a decoy receptor for ligands that normally bind to receptors on osteoclasts and their precursors to promote osteoclast differentiation, activation, and survival. In rodent models, the speed and duration of reversal of humoral hypercalcemia of malignancy was significantly greater with osteoprotegerin than with high-dose pamidronate or zoledronate (Morony et al. 2005). Other therapeutic agents that have been used for control of hypercalcemia include mithramycin (plicamycin), gallium nitrate, and intravenous phosphate. However, use of these agents in human and veterinary medicine is limited or no longer recommended due to cost, adverse effects, or difficulty of administration (Kruger et al. 1996; Lucas et al. 2007; Pollak et al. 2008).

Causes of hypocalcemia

Overview

Hypocalcemia may result from a number of diverse causes and is commonly observed with urinary tract disorders (e.g., acute and CRF, nephrotic syndrome, and urethral obstruction (Table 64.5). However, hypocalcemia per se rarely induces significant functional or structural abnormalities of the urinary system. A notable exception to this generalization is CRF. Basic pathophysiologic factors that, alone or in combination, may contribute to hypocalcemia include decreased protein binding of calcium, decreased bone resorption, decreased intestinal calcium absorption, enhanced urinary calcium excretion, increased bone accretion, or increased calcium precipitation with plasma anions (such as citric acid, phosphorous, or oxalic acid).

Hypoalbuminemia

Hypoalbuminemia accounts for over half of patients with hypocalcemia and is frequently encountered in dogs and cats with protein-losing glomerular diseases that are frequently associated with severe proteinuria resulting in hypoalbuminemia and associated manifestations (e.g., nephrotic syndrome; Chapters 44 and 53) (Chew and Meuten 1982). Reductions in serum albumin

Table 64.5 Causes of hypocalcemia in dog and cats

Common
 Acute pancreatitis
 Acute renal failure
 Chronic renal failure (secondary renal hyperparathyroidism)
 Hypoalbuminemia
 Idiopathic
 Obstructive uropathy
 Puerperal tetany (eclampsia)

Uncommon, sporadic, or rare
 Cardiopulmonary resuscitation (CPR)
 Diabetes mellitus
 Gastrointestinal disease (e.g., gastroenteritis, gastric torsion)
 Ethylene glycol
 Hemorrhage
 Hyperthyroidism
 Hypoadrenocorticism
 Hypomagnesemia
 Hypoparathyroidism
  Atrophy (hypercalcemia-induced)
  Canine distemper virus
  Idiopathic (parathyroiditis)
  Infarction
  Postoperative (e.g., thyroidectomy, neck surgery)
 Hypovitaminosis D (rickets)
 Iatrogenic
  Acute rapid calcium-free fluid administration
  Bisphosphonate administration
  Blood or plasma transfusion (citrate anticoagulated blood products)
  Calcitonin administration
  Enrofloxacin administration
  Mithramycin administration
  Phosphate administration (oral or intravenous)
  Phosphate-containing enemas
  Sodium bicarbonate infusion
 Infectious/inflammatory (e.g., peritonitis, pyometra)
 Intestinal malabsorption (e.g., intestinal lymphangiectasia, protein losing enteropathy)
 Laboratory error
  EDTA contamination
  Gadolinium-based angiographic contrast agents
  Sample mishandling
 Liver disease
 Nutritional secondary hyperparathyroidism
 Rhabdomyolysis
 Renal transplantation
 Snake envenomation (*Vipera xanthina palestinae*)
 Soft tissue trauma
 Tumor lysis syndrome

concentrations decrease the protein-bound fraction of circulating calcium, resulting in mild decreases in serum total calcium concentrations. Since ionized calcium concentrations are usually unaffected, hypocalcemia due to hypoalbuminemia is rarely associated with clinical signs.

Chronic renal failure

CRF is a common cause of hypocalcemia in dogs (Chapter 48) (Chew and Meuten 1982). Decreases in total calcium have been observed in 10–23% of dogs and 8–15% of cats with CRF; whereas ionized hypocalcemia has been observed in 29–56% of affected dogs and 10–26% of affected cats (DiBartola et al. 1987; Chew and Nagode 1990; Lulich et al. 1992; Barber and Elliot 1998; Schenck and Chew 2002, 2005; Gerber et al. 2003; Schenck et al. 2006). Hypocalcemia is often a consequence of multiple biochemical and endocrinologic disturbances associated with advancing CRF (Chapter 48). In early stages of CRF, serum calcium and phosphorus concentrations are usually within normal ranges as a result of compensatory alterations in the metabolism and regulation of calcitriol, PTH, and phosphatonins (Polzin et al. 2005; Moe and Sprague 2008). As renal function deteriorates, however, the effects of phosphorus retention and diminished renal calcitriol synthesis predominate and overt hypocalcemia may develop due to increased calcium-phosphate complexing, reduced calcitriol-mediated intestinal calcium absorption, and increased skeletal resistance to the calcemic actions of PTH. The combination of low calcitriol, hypocalcemia, hyperphosphatemia, and elevated phosphatonin concentrations collectively serve to stimulate excess PTH secretion and progression of renal secondary hyperparathyroidism. Excess PTH may promote nephrocalcinosis and consequent progressive loss of renal function (Nagode et al. 1996).

Acute renal failure

Hypocalcemia may be observed in some dogs and cats with acute intrinsic renal failure (Chapter 49) (Vaden et al. 1997; Worwag and Langston 2008). In one study, decreased total calcium was observed in approximately 25% of 99 dogs with acute renal failure, and hypocalcemia was associated with a diminished likelihood of survival (Vaden et al. 1997). In patients with acute renal failure, hypocalcemia may be the direct result of the primary disease process (e.g., ethylene glycol intoxication, acute pancreatitis, or glomerulonephropathy/nephrotic syndrome) and/or the consequence of acute hyperphosphatemia resulting from abrupt severe deterioration of renal function. Hypocalcemia has been observed in approximately 50% of dogs and cats with ethylene glycol intoxication (Thrall et al. 1984; Connally et al. 1996).

After ingestion, ethylene glycol is rapidly metabolized to glycoaldehyde, glycolate, glyoxalate, and finally oxalic acid (Parry and Wallach 1974). The formation of calcium oxalate monohydrate (and to a lesser degree calcium oxalate dihydrate) results in hypocalcemia. Hypocalcemia may be evident prior to the development of azotemia as a result of initial complexing with oxalates, but it is more commonly associated with later stages of intoxication when acute intrinsic renal failure develops as a result of renal proximal tubular degeneration, necrosis, and intraluminal deposition of calcium oxalate crystals (Kersting and Nielsen 1966; Thrall et al. 1984; Grauer et al. 1987; Connally et al. 1996). Hypocalcemia at this later stage is most likely the result of acute hyperphosphatemia and subsequent increased calcium complexing, inhibition of the calcemic effects of PTH, impaired calcitriol synthesis, and diminished intestinal calcium absorption (Herbert et al. 1966; Tanaka and DeLuca 1973; Bover et al. 1999; Pollak et al. 2008).

Urethral obstruction

Urethral obstruction is a common life-threatening condition in cats and dogs that is often associated with azotemia, hyperphosphatemia, hyperkalemia, and acidosis (Chapters 70 and 77). Decreases in total and ionized calcium have been observed in cats with experimentally induced and naturally occurring urethral obstruction. In studies of naturally occurring disease, ionized hypocalcemia was detected in 34–74% of obstructed cats, whereas decreases in total calcium concentrations were detected in only 20–27% of affected cats (Drobatz and Hughes 1997; Lee and Drobatz 2003; Drobatz et al. 2005). Although significant decreases in ionized calcium were observed in dogs with experimentally induced bilateral ureteral obstruction, calcium disturbances have yet to be fully characterized in dogs with naturally occurring urethral obstruction (Tuma and Mallette 1983). Hypocalcemia in obstructed cats is rarely associated with clinical signs. However, hypocalcemia may contribute to cardiac and neurologic dysfunction in severely affected cats. Studies of cats with obstructive uropathy suggest that the mechanism of obstruction-induced hypocalcemia is not related to decreased PTH secretion or hypomagnesemia (Drobatz and Hughes 1997; Drobatz et al. 2005). Most likely, it involves the effects of acute hyperphosphatemia.

Consequences of hypocalcemia

Clinical manifestations of hypocalcemia are similar regardless of cause; however, the severity of signs may vary considerably depending on the magnitude, rate of decline, and duration of ionized hypocalcemia, and the presence of other concomitant electrolyte or acid–base disorders. Clinical signs are often not evident until total calcium concentrations fall below 6–7 mg/dL and ionized calcium concentrations of 0.7–0.8 mm/L (Feldman and Nelson 2004b). When present, signs of hypocalcemia are predominantly neurologic and neuromuscular (seizures, tetany, muscle tremors, fasciculations, and cramping, lameness, stiff gait, ataxia), but may also include signs related to the cardiovascular (bradycardia, tachycardia, hypotension), gastrointestinal (anorexia, vomiting, diarrhea, weight loss), respiratory (panting), ophthalmic (cataracts), and urinary (polyuria and polydipsia) systems (Feldman and Nelson 2004b; Schenck et al. 2006).

Diagnostic considerations for hypocalcemia

Depending on the reference laboratory, hypocalcemia is defined as a fasting total calcium concentration of less than 8.0 mg/dL (2.0 mmol/L) in dogs and 7.0 mg/dL (1.75 mmol/L) in cats or an ionized calcium concentration of less than 5.0 mg/dL (1.25 mmol/L) in dogs and 4.5 mg/dL (1.1 mmol/L) in cats (Schenck et al. 2006). Identification of the cause or causes of hypocalcemia in dogs and cats and subsequent formulation of specific therapeutic plans depend on careful assessment of the history and physical examination findings, and results of hematologic, biochemical, endocrinologic, radiographic, ultrasonic, and histocytologic evaluations. Using the combined results of these routine evaluations, most disease processes that cause hypocalcemia in dogs and cats can be identified. Patients in which a cause for hypocalcemia is not obvious from initial evaluations can often be differentiated using results of assays for calcium-regulating hormones, including ionized calcium, serum intact molecule immunoreactive PTH, 25-hydroxyvitamin D_3, and 1,25-dihydroxyvitamin D_3 (Table 64.3) (Schenck et al. 2006).

Treatment strategies for hypocalcemia

Treatment of hypocalcemia depends on the magnitude and rate of decline in serum calcium, the nature and severity of clinical signs, and the likelihood of progressive decreases in calcium concentrations. In general, therapeutic goals should be designed to raise serum calcium concentrations sufficiently to alleviate clinical signs, while avoiding the risks of overzealous treatment. Normalization of calcium concentrations into standard reference ranges is neither necessary nor desirable because excessive treatment may delay functional recovery of atrophied parathyroid glands and may increase the risk of hypercalcemia, hyperphosphatemia, soft-tissue mineralization, and urolithiasis. Animals with hypocalcemia due to hypoalbuminemia will not require specific therapy, assuming that ionized calcium concentrations are normal. Emergency treatment of severe hypocalcemia or hypocalcemia associated with severe clinical signs (e.g., seizures, tetany, cardiac dysfunction) entails parenteral 10% calcium gluconate administered intravenously slowly over 10–20 minutes to effect at a dose of 0.5–1.5 mL/kg (Schenck et al. 2006). The initial bolus can be followed by a continuous IV infusion of calcium until oral medications provide control of serum calcium concentrations. Although uncommon, our experiences and those of others suggest that subcutaneous administration of diluted preparations of calcium gluconate may be associated with severe dermatologic reactions in dogs and cats (Ruopp 2001; Schaer et al. 2001; Schenck et al. 2006).

Long-term management of chronic hypocalcemic disorders depends on the underlying cause. Treatment of overt hypocalcemia associated with CRF entails control of hyperphosphatemia, administration of calcitriol (2.5 to 5.0 ng/kg q24 h), and cautious use of oral calcium supplementation (Chapter 48) (Polzin et al. 2009). Because calcitriol may promote hypercalcemia, serum total and ionized calcium, phosphorous, and PTH concentrations should be monitored closely in patients with CRF receiving calcitriol therapy. Long-term management of hypocalcemia caused by primary hypoparathyroidism consists of oral administration of vitamin D preparations (e.g., ergocalciferol, dihydrotachysterol, or calcitriol) and calcium supplementation. Once vitamin D compounds reach their maximal effect, calcium supplements can often be discontinued (Feldman and Nelson 2004b). Hypercalcemia, hypercalciuria, nephrocalcinosis, and renal insufficiency are potential complications of long-term therapy for primary hyperparathyroidism (Kruger et al. 1996). Recent human studies have shown that synthetic human recombinant PTH maintains serum calcium concentrations without concurrent hypercalciuria (Winer et al. 2003). However, the safety and efficacy of human recombinant PTH for long-term management of hypoparathyroidism has not been evaluated in dogs and cats.

References

Adin, D.B., A.W. Taylor, et al. (2003). Intermittent bolus ingestion versus continuous infusion of furosemide in normal adult greyhound dogs. *J Vet Intern Med* **17**: 632–636.

Adler, A.J., N. Feran, et al. (1985). Effect of inorganic phosphate on serum ionized calcium concentration in vitro: a reassessment of the "trade-off hypothesis." *Kidney Int* **28**: 932–935.

Anthony, L.B., M.E. May, et al. (1995). Case report: lanreotide in the management of hypercalcemia of malignancy. *Am J Med Sci* **309**: 312.

Arceneaux, K.A., J. Taboada, et al. (1998). Blastomycosis in dogs: 115 cases (1989–1995). *J Am Vet Med Assoc* **213**: 658–664.

Barber, P.J. and J. Elliot (1998). Feline chronic renal failure: calcium homeostasis in 80 cases diagnosed between 1992 and 1995. *J Small Anim Prac* **39**: 108–116.

Barr, F.J., M.W. Patteson, et al. (1989). Hypercalcemic nephropathy in three dogs: sonographic appearance. *Vet Radiol* **30**: 169–173.

Baumann, E.J. and S. Kurland (1929). Changes in the inorganic constituents of blood in suprarenalectomized cats and rabbits. *J Biol Chem* **71**: 281–302.

Berger, B. and E.C. Feldman (1987). Primary hyperparathyroidism in dogs: 21 cases (1976–1986). *J Am Vet Med Assoc* **191**: 350–356.

Bolliger, A.P., P.A. Graham, et al. (2002). Detection of parathyroid hormone-related protein in cats with humoral hypercalcemia of malignancy. *Vet Clin Pathol* **31**: 3–8.

Bover, J., A. Jara, et al. (1999). Dynamics of skeletal resistance to parathyroid hormone in the rat: effect if renal failure and dietary phosphorous. *Bone* **25**: 279–285.

Brunette, M.G., J. Vary, et al. (1974). Hyposthenuria in hypercalcemia: the possible role of intrarenal blood flow redistribution. *Pflügers Arch* **350**: 9–23.

Carone, F.A., F.H. Epstein, et al. (1960). The effects upon the kidney of transient hypercalcemia induced by parathyroid extract. *Am J Path* **30**: 77–103.

Chen, R.A. and W.G. Goodman (2004). Role of calcium-sensing receptor in parathyroid gland physiology. *Am J Physiol Renal Physiol* **286**: F1005–F1011.

Chew, D.J. and M. Carothers (1989). Hypercalcemia. *Vet Clin North Am Small Anim Prac* **19**: 265–287.

Chew, D.J., M. Leonard, et al. (1989). Effect of sodium bicarbonate infusions on ionized calcium and total calcium in serum of clinically normal cats. *Am J Vet Res* **50**: 145–150.

Chew, D.J. and D.J. Meuten (1982). Disorders of calcium and phosphorus. *Vet Clin North Am Small Anim Prac* **12**: 411–438.

Chew, D.J. and L.A. Nagode (1990). Renal secondary hyperparathyroidism. In: *Proceedings of the 4th Annual Meeting of the Society for Comparative Endocrinology*, pp. 17–26.

Chomdej, P., P.D. Bell, et al. (1977). Renal hemodynamic and autoregulatory responses to acute hypercalcemia. *Am J Physiol* **232**: F490–F497.

Cochran, M., M. Peacock, et al. (1970). Renal effects of calcitonin. *Br Med J* **1**: 135–137.

Collins, E.J., E.R. Garrett, et al. (1963). Effect of adrenal steroids on radio-calcium metabolism in dogs. *Metabolism* **11**: 716–726.

Connally, H.E., M.A. Thrall, et al. (1996). Safety and efficacy of 4-methylpyrazole for treatment of suspected or confirmed ethylene glycol intoxication in dogs: 107 cases (1983–1995). *J Am Vet Med Assoc* **209**: 1880–1883.

Costanzo, L.S. (1985). Localization of diuretic action in microperfused rat distal tubules: Ca and Na transport. *Am J Physiol* **248**: F527–F535.

Cowgill, L.D. (1995). Application of peritoneal dialysis and hemodialysis in the management of renal failure. In: *Canine and Feline Nephrology and Urology*, edited by D.R. Finco and C.A. Osborne, 2nd edition. Baltimore, MD: Williams and Wilkins, pp. 573–596.

Crews, L.J., L.C. Sharkey, et al. (2007). Evaluation of total and ionized calcium status in dogs with blastomycosis: 38 cases (1997–2006). *J Am Vet Med Assoc* **231**: 1545–1549.

Diamond, T. and S. Thornley (1994). Addisonian crisis and hypercalcemia. *Aust NZ J Med* **24**: 316.

DiBartola, S.P., H.E. Rutgers, et al. (1987). Clinicopathologic findings associated with chronic renal disease in cats: 74 cases (1973–1984). *J Am Vet Med Assoc* **190**: 1196–1202.

Dougherty, S.A., S.A. Center, et al. (1990). Salmon calcitonin as adjunct treatment for vitamin D toxicosis in a dog. *J Am Vet Med Assoc* **196**: 1269–1272.

Dow, S.W., A.M. Legendre, et al. (1986). Hypercalcemia associated with blastomycosis in dogs. *J Am Vet Med Assoc* **188**: 706–709.

Drobatz, K.J. and D. Hughes (1997). Concentrations of ionized calcium in plasma of cats with urethral obstruction. *J Am Vet Med Assoc* **211**: 1392–1395.

Drobatz, K.J., C. Ward, et al. (2005). Serum concentrations of parathyroid hormone and 25-OH vitamin D3 in cats with urethral obstruction. *J Vet Emerg Crit Care* **15**: 170–184.

Dusso, A.S., A.J. Brown, et al. (2005). Vitamin D. *Am J Physiol Renal Physiol* **289**: F8–F28.

Dzanis, D.A. and F.A. Kallfelz (1988). Recent knowledge of vitamin D toxicity in dogs. *Proc Am Coll Vet Intern Med Forum* **6**: 289–291.

Earm, J.-H., B.M. Christensen, et al. (1998). Decreased aquaporin-2 expression and apical plasma membrane delivery in kidney collecting ducts of polyuric hypercalcemic rats. *J Am Soc Nephrol* **9**: 2181–2193.

Elliot, J., J.M. Dobson, et al. (1991). Hypercalcemia in the dog: a study of 40 cases. *J Small Anim Prac* **32**: 564–571.

Epstein, F.H., D. Beck, et al. (1959). Changes in renal concentrating ability produced by parathyroid extract. *J Clin Invest* **38**: 1214–1221.

Fan, T.M. (2007). The role of bisphosphonates in the management of patients that have cancer. *Vet Clin North Am Small Anim Prac* **37**: 1091–1110.

Fan, T.M., L.-P. de Lorimier, et al. (2005). Evaluation of intravenous pamidronate administration in 33 cancer-bearing dogs with primary or secondary bone involvement. *J Vet Intern Med* **19**: 74–80.

Feldman, E.C. and R.W. Nelson (2004a). Hypercalcemia and primary hyperparathyroidism. In: *Canine and Feline Endocrinology and Reproduction*, 3rd edition. Philadelphia, PA: WB Saunders, pp. 661–715.

Feldman, E.C. and R.W. Nelson (2004b). Hypocalcemia and primary hypoparathyroidism. In: *Canine and Feline Endocrinology and Reproduction*, 3rd edition. Philadelphia, PA: WB Saunders, pp. 716–742.

Garlock, S.M., M.E. Matz, et al. (1991). Vitamin D$_3$ rodenticide toxicity in a dog. *J Am Anim Hosp Assoc* **27**: 356–360.

Gerber, B., M. Hassig, et al. (2003). Serum concentrations of 1,25-dihydroxycholecalciferol and 25-hydroxycholecalciferol in clinically normal dogs and dogs with acute and chronic renal failure. *Am J Vet Res* **64**: 1161–1166.

Gilor, C., T.K. Graves, et al. (2006). Clinical aspects of natural infection with blastomycoses dermatitidis in acts: 8 cases (1991–2005). *J Am Vet Med Assoc* **229**: 96–99.

Grauer, G.F., M.A.H. Thrall, et al. (1987). Comparison of the effects of ethanol and 4-methylpyrzole on the pharmacokinetics and toxicity of ethylene glycol in the dog. *Toxicol Lett* **35**: 307–314.

Grzela, T., W. Chudzinski, et al. (2006). The calcium-sensing receptor and vitamin D receptor expression in tertiary hyperparathyroidism. *Int J Mol Med* **17**: 779–783.

Gunther, R., L.J. Felice, et al. (1988). Toxicity of a vitamin D$_3$ rodenticide to dogs. *J Am Vet Med Assoc* **193**: 211–214.

Hare, W.R., C.E. Dobbs, et al. (2000). Calcipotriene poisoning in dogs. *Vet Med* **95**: 770–778.

Herbert, L.A., J. Lenmann Jr, et al. (1966). Studies of the mechanism by which phosphate infusion lowers serum calcium concentration. *J Clin Invest* **45**: 1886–1894.

Heyburn, P.J., P.L. Shelby, et al. (1980). Peritoneal dialysis in the management of severe hypercalcemia. *Br Med J* **280**: 525–526.

Hostutler, R.A., D.J. Chew, et al. (2005). Uses and effectiveness of pamidronate disodium for treatment of dogs and cats with hypercalcemia. *J Vet Intern Med* **19**: 29–33.

Humes, H.D., J.L. Troy, et al. (1978). Influence of calcium on the determinants of glomerular ultrafiltration. *J Clin Invest* **61**: 32–40.

Jesus Ferreira, M.C., C. Helies-Toussaint, et al. (1998). Co-expression of a Ca^{2+}-inhibitable adenyl cyclase and of a Ca^{2+}-sensing receptor in the cortical thick ascending limb cell of the rat kidney. *J Biol Chem* **273**: 15192–15202.

Kadar, E., J.E. Rush, et al. (2004). Electrolyte disturbances and cardiac arrhythmias in a dog following pamidronate, calcitonin, and furosemide administration for hypercalcemia of malignancy. *J Am Anim Hosp Assoc* **40**: 75–81.

Kallet, A.J., K.P. Richter, et al. (1991). Primary hyperparathyroidism in cats: seven cases (1984–1989). *J Am Vet Med Assoc* **199**: 1767–1711.

Kersting, E.J. and S.W. Nielsen (1966). Experimental ethylene glycol poisoning in the dog. *Am J Vet Res* **27**: 574–582.

Kim, H.-J., H. Zhao, et al. (2007). Glucocorticoids and the osteoclast. *Ann NY Acad Sci* **1116**: 335–339.

Klausner, J.S., F.R. Fernandez, et al. (1986). Canine primary hyperparathyroidism and its association with urolithiasis. *Vet Clin North Am Small Anim Prac* **16**: 227–239.

Kruger, J.M., C.A. Osborne, et al. (1996). Hypecalcemia and renal failure: etiology, pathophysisology, diagnosis, and treatment. *Vet Clin North Am Small Anim Prac* **26**: 1417–1445.

Lauter, K.B. and A. Arnold (2008). Mutational analysis of CDKN1B, a candidate tumor-suppressor gene, in refractory secondary/tertiary hyperparathyroidism. *Kidney Int* **73**: 1137–1140.

Lee, J.A. and K.J. Drobatz (2003). Characterization of the clinical characteristics, electrolyte, acid-base, and renal parameters in male cats with urethral obstruction. *J Vet Emerg Crit Care* **13**: 277–233.

Levi, M., M.A. Ellis, et al. (1983). Control of renal hemodynamics and glomerular filtration rate in chronic hypercalcemia. *J Clin Invest* **71**: 1624–1632.

Lins, L.E. (1978). Reversible renal failure caused by hypercalcemia. *Acta Med Scand* **203**: 309–314.

Llach, F. and F. Velasquez Foreeo (2001). Secondary hyperparathyroidism in chronic renal failure: pathogenic and clinical aspects. *Am J Kidney Dis* **38**(supple 5): S20–S33.

Lucas, P., H. Lascote, et al. (2007). Treating paraneoplastic hypercalcemia in dogs and cats. *Vet Med* **102**: 314–331.

Lulich, J.P., C.A. Osborne, et al. (2004). Effects of diet on urine composition of cats with calcium oxalate urolithiasis. *J Am Anim Hosp Assoc* **40**: 185–191.

Lulich, J.P., C.A. Osborne, et al. (1992). Feline renal failure: questions, answers, questions. *Compend Contin Edu Prac Vet* **14**: 127–152.

MacEwen, E.G. and S.D. Siegel (1977). Hypercalcemia: a paraneoplastic disease. *Vet Clin North Am Small Anim Prac* **7**: 187–194.

Marquez, G.A., J.S. Klausner, et al. (1995). Calcium oxalate urolithiasis in a cat with a functional parathyroid adenocarcinoma. *J Am Vet Med Assoc* **206**: 817–819.

McClain, H.M., J.A. Barsanti, et al. (1999). Hypercalcemia and calcium oxalate urolithiasis in cats: a report of fine cases. *J Am Anim Hosp Assoc* **35**: 297–301.

Mealey, K.L., M.D. Willard, et al. (1999). Hypercalcemia associated with granulomatous disease in a cat. *J Am Vet Med Assoc* **215**: 959–962.

Mellanby, R.J., P. Mellor, et al. (2006). Hypercalcemia associated with granulomatous lymphadenitis and elevated 1,25 dihydroxyvitamin D concentration in a dog. *J Small Anim Prac* **47**: 207–212.

Meuten, D.J. (1984). Hypercalcemia. *Vet Clin North Am Small Anim Prac* **14**: 891–910.

Meuten, D.J., B.J. Cooper, et al. (1981). Hypercalcemia associated with an adenocarcinoma derived from the apocrine glands of the anal sac. *Vet Pathol* **18**: 454–471.

Meuten, D.J., G.J. Kociba, et al. (1983). Hypercalcemia in dogs with lymphosarcoma: biochemical, ultrastructural and histomorphometric investigations. *Lab Invest* **40**: 553–562.

Midkiff, A.M., D.J. Chew, et al. (2000). Idiopathic hypercalcemia in cats. *J Vet Intern Med* **14**: 619–626.

Moe, S.M. and S.M. Sprague (2008). Mineral bone disorders in chronic kidney disease. In: *The Kidney*, edited by B.M. Brenner and S.A. Levine, 8th edition. Vol. 2. Philadelphia, PA: Saunders Elsevier, pp. 1784–1813.

Montoli, A., G. Colussi, et al. (1992). Hypercalcemia in Addison's disease: calciotropic hormone profile and bone histology. *J Intern Med* **232**: 535–540.

Morony, S., K. Warmington, et al. (2005). The inhibition of RANKL causes greater suppression of bone resorption and hypercalcemia compared with bisphosphonates in two models of humoral hypercalcemia if malignancy. *Endocrinology* **146**: 3235–3243.

Muls, E., R. Bouillon, et al. (1982). Etiology of hypercalcemia in a patient with Addison's disease. *Calcif Tissue Int* **34**: 523–526.

Nagode, L., D. Chew, et al. (1996). Benefits of calcitriol therapy and serum phosphorus control in dogs and cats with chronic renal failure: both are essential to prevent or suppress toxic hyperparathyroidism. *Vet Clin North Am Small Anim Prac* **26**: 1293–1330.

Nejsum, L.N. (2005). The renal plumbing system: aquaporin water channels. *Cell Mol Life Sci* **62**: 1692–1706.

Ong, S.C., R.J. Shalhoub, et al. (1974). Effect of furosemide on experimental hypercalcemia in dogs. *Proc Soc Exp Biol Med* **145**: 227–233.

Osborne, C.A., J.S. Klausner, et al. (1979). Urinary tract infections: normal and abnormal host defense mechanisms. *Vet Clin North Am Small Anim Prac* **9**: 587–609.

Osborne, C.A., D.G. Low, et al. (1969). Reversible versus irreversible renal disease in the dog. *J Am Vet Med Assoc* **155**: 2062–2078.

Osborne, C.A. and J.B. Stevens (1973). Pseudohyperparathyroidism in the Dog. *J Am Vet Med Assoc* **162**: 125–135.

Parfitt, A.M. (1997). The hyperparathyroidism of chronic renal failure: a disorder of growth. *Kidney Int* **52**: 3–9.

Parfitt, A.M. and M. Kleerekoper (1980). Clinical disorders of calcium, phosphorous and magnesium metabolism. In: *Clinical Disorders of Fluid and Electrolyte Metabolism*, edited by M.H. Maxwell and C.R. Kleeman. New York: McGraw-Hill, pp. 947–1151.

Parry, M.F. and R. Wallach (1974). Ethylene glycol poisoning. *Am J Med* **57**: 143–150.

Pesillo, S.A., S.A. Khan, et al. (2002). Calcipotriene toxicosis in a dog successfully treated with pamidronate disodium. *J Vet Emerg Crit Care* **12**: 177–181.

Peterson, M.E., D.S. Greco, et al. (1989). Primary hypoadrenocorticism in ten cats. *J Vet Intern Med* **3**: 55–58.

Peterson, M.E., P.P. Kintzner, et al. (1996). Pretreatment clinical and laboratory findings in dogs with hypoadrenocorticism: 225 cases (1979–1993). *J Am Vet Med Assoc* **208**: 85–91.

Pollak, M.R., A.S.L. Yu, et al. (2008). Disorders of calcium, magnesium, and phosphate balance. In: *The Kidney*, edited by B.M. Brenner and S.A. Levine, 8th edition. Vol. 2. Philadelphia, PA: Saunders Elsevier, pp. 588–611.

Polzin, D.J., C.A. Osborne, et al. (2005). Chronic kidney disease. In: *Textbook of Veterinary Internal Medicine*, edited S.J. Ettinger and E.C. Feldman, 6th edition. St. Louis: Saunders Elsevier, pp. 1756–1785.

Polzin, D.J., S. Ross, et al. (2009). Calcitriol. In: *Kirk's Current Therapy XIV*, edited by J.D. Bonagura and D.C. Twedt. St. Louis: Saunders Elsevier, pp. 892–895.

Procino, G., M. Carmosino, et al. (2004). Extracellular calcium antagonizes forskolin-induced aquaporin 2 trafficking in collecting ducts cells. *Kidney Int* **66**: 2245–2255.

Rosol, T.J. and C.C. Capen (1992). Biology of disease: mechanisms of cancer-induced hypercalcemia. *Lab Invest* **67**: 680–702.

Rosol, T.J., D.J. Chew, et al. (1995). Pathophysiology of calcium metabolism. *Vet Clin Pathol* **24**: 49–63.

Rosol, T.J., L.A. Nagode, et al. (1992). Parathyroid hormone (PTH)-related protein, PTH, and 1,25-dihydroxyvitamin D in dogs with cancer-associated hypercalcemia. *Endocrinology* **131**: 1157–1164.

Rumbeiha, W.K., S.F. Fitzgerald, et al. (2000). Use of pamidronate disodium to reduce cholecalciferol-induced toxicosis in dogs. *Am J Vet Res* **61**: 9–13.

Rumbeiha, W.K., J.M. Kruger, et al. (1999). Use of pamidronate to reverse vitamin D_3-induced toxicosis in dogs. *Am J Vet Res* **60**: 1092–1097.

Ruopp, J.L. (2001). Primary hypoparathyroidism in a cat complicated by suspect iatrogenic calcinosis cutis. *J Amer Anim Hosp Assoc* **27**: 370–373.

Sands, J.M., F.X. Flores, et al. (1998). Vasopressin-elicited water and urea permeabilities are altered in IMCD in hypercalcemic rats. *Am J Physiol* **274**: F978–F985.

Sands, J.M., M. Naruse, et al. (1997). Apical extracellular calcium/polyvalent cation-sensing receptor regulates vasopressin-elicited water permeability in rat kidney inner medullary collecting duct. *J Clin Invest* **99**: 1399–1405.

Savary, K.C.M., G.S. Price, et al. (2000). Hypercalcemia in cats: a retrospective study of 71 cases (1991–1997). *J Vet Intern Med* **14**: 184–189.

Schaer, M., P.E. Ginn, et al. (2001). Severe calcinosis cutis associated with treatment of hypoparathyroidism in a dog. *J Am Anim Hosp Assoc* **27**: 364–369.

Schenck, P.A. and D.J. Chew (2002). Diagnostic discordance of total calcium and adjusted total calcium in predicting ionized calcium concentration in cats with chronic renal failure and other diseases. In: *Proceedings of the 10th Congress of the International Society of Animal Clinical Biochemistry*, Gainesville, FL.

Schenck, P.A. and D.J. Chew (2005). Prediction of serum ionized calcium concentration by serum total calcium measurement in dogs. *Am J Vet Res* **66**: 1330–1336.

Schenck, P.A., D.J. Chew, et al. (2006). Disorders of calcium: hypercalcemia and hypocalcemia. In: *Fluid, Electrolyte, and Acid-Base Disorders in Small Animal Practice*, edited by S.P. Dibartola, 3rd edition. St. Louis, MO: Saunders Elsevier, pp. 122–194.

Schenck, P.A., D.J. Chew, et al. (2004). Calcium metabolic hormones in feline idiopathic hypercalcemia. *J Vet Intern Med* **18**: 442.

Sekine, M. and H. Takami (1998). Combination of calcitonin and pamidronate for emergency treatment of malignant hypercalcemia. *Oncol Rep* **5**: 197–199.

Sharma, O.P. (2000). Hypercalcemia in granulomatous disorders: a clinical review. *Curr Opin Pulm Med* **6**: 442–447.

Smith, S.A., L.C. Freeman, et al. (2002). Hypercalcemia due to iatrogenic secondary hypoadrenocorticism and diabetes mellitus in a cat. *J Am Anim Hosp Assoc* **38**: 41–44.

Spangler, W.L., et al. (1979). Vitamin-D intoxication and the pathogenesis of vitamin D nephropathy in the dog. *Am J Vet Res* **40**: 73–83.

Sutton, R.A.L. and J.H. Dirks (1986). Calcium and magnesium: renal handling and disorders of metabolism. In: *The Kidney*, edited by B.M. Brenner and F.C. Rector, 3rd edition. Philadelphia, PA: WB Saunders, pp. 551–618.

Tanaka, Y. and H.F. DeLuca (1973). The control of 25-hydroxyvitatmin D metabolism by inorganic phosphorous. *Arch Biochem Biophys* **154**: 566–574.

Thrall, M.A., G.F. Grauer, et al. (1984). Clinicipathologic findings in dogs and cats with ethylene glycol intoxication. *J Am Vet Med Assoc* **184**: 37–41.

Torregrosa, J.-V., A. Moreno, et al. (2003). Usefulness of pamidronate in severe secondary hyperparathyroidism in patients undergoing hemodialysis. *Kidney Int* **63**(suppl. 85): S88–S90.

Tuma, S.N. and L.E. Mallette (1983). Hypercalcemia after nephrectomy in the dog: role of the kidneys and parathyroid glands. *J Lab Clin Med* **102**: 213–219.

Uehlinger, P., T. Glaus, et al. (1998). Hypercalcemia in dogs—retrospective study of 46 cases. *Schweiz Arch Tierheilkd* **140**: 188–197.

Ureña, P. and J.M. Frazão (2003). Calcimimetic agents: review and perspectives. *Kidney Int* **63**(suppl. 85): S91–S96.

Vaden, S.L., J. Levine, et al. (1997). A retrospective case-control of acute renal failure in 99 dogs. *J Vet Intern Med* **11**: 58–64.

Walser, M., B.H.B. Robinson, et al. (1963). The hypercalcemia of adrenal insufficiency. *J Clin Invest* **42**: 456–465.

Wang, W., C. Li, et al. (2002). AQP3, p-AQP2, and AQP2 expression is reduced in polyuric rats with hypercalcemia: prevention with cAMP-PDE inhibitors. *Am J Renal Physiol* **283**: F1313–F1325.

Wang, W., C. Li, et al. (2004). Reduced expression of renal Na^+ transporters in rats with PTH-induced hypercalcemia. *Am J Renal Physiol* **286**: F534–F545.

Weir, E.C., W.J. Burtis, et al. (1988a). Isolation of 16,000-Dalton parathyroid hormone-like proteins from two animal tumors causing humoral hypercalcemia of malignancy. *Endocrinology* **123**: 2744–2751.

Weir, E.C., R.W. Norrdin, et al. (1986). Primary hyperparathyroidism in a dog: biochemical, bone histomorphometric, and pathologic findings. *J Am Vet Assoc* **189**: 1471–1474.

Weir, E.C., R.W. Norrdin, et al. (1988b). Humoral hypercalcemia of malignancy in canine lymphosarcoma. *Endocrinology* **122**: 602–608.

Weller, R.E. and W.E. Hoffman (1992). Renal function in dogs with lymphosarcoma and associated hypercalcemia. *J Small Anim Prac* **33**: 61–66.

Weller, R.E., C.A. Holmberg, et al. (1982). Canine lymphosarcoma and hypercalcemia: clinical laboratory and pathologic evaluation of twenty-four cases. *J Small Anim Prac* **23**: 649–658.

Wellington, K. and K.L. Goa (2003). Zoledronic acid: a review of its use in the management of bone metastases and hypercalcemia of malignancy. *Drugs* **63**: 417–437.

Willard, M.D., W.D. Schall, et al. (1982). Canine hypoadrenocorticism: report of 37 cases and review of 39 previously reported cases. *J Am Vet Med Assoc* **180**: 59–62.

Winer, K.K., C.W. Ko, et al. (2003). Long-term treatment of hypoparathyroidism: a randomized controlled study comparing parathyroid hormone-(1–34) versus calcitriol and calcium. *J Clin Endocrinol Metab* **88**: 4214–4220.

Wisneski, L.A. (1990). Salmon calcitonin in the acute management of hypercalcemia. *Calcif Tissue Int* **46**: S26–S30.

Worwag, S. and C.E. Langston (2008). Acute intrinsic renal failure in cats: 32 cases (1997–2004). *J Am Vet Med Assoc* **232**: 728–732.

Wüthrich, R.P., D. Martin, et al. (2007). The role of calcimimetics in the treatment if hyperthyroidism. *Euro J Clin Invest* **37**: 915–922.

Yu, J., V. Papavasiliou, et al. (1995). Vitamin D analogs: new therapeutic agents for the treatment of squamous cancer and its associated hypercalcemia. *Anticancer Drugs* **6**: 101–108.

Zawada, E.T., et al. (1986). Systemic and renal vascular responses to dietary calcium and vitamin D. *Hypertension* **8**: 975–982.

65

Phosphorus disorders

David. J Polzin

Phosphorus is critical for many physiologic functions, including skeletal development, mineral metabolism, cell membrane phospholipid content and function, cell signaling, platelet aggregation, and energy transfer through mitochondrial function (Moe and Sprague 2008). Phosphate also plays an important role as a urinary buffer, facilitating excretion of hydrogen ions and as an intracellular buffer minimizing shifts in internal acid–base status.

Phosphorus appears in multiple forms in the body. Approximately 85% of body phosphorus occurs in the form of hydroxyapatite $[(Ca)_{10}(PO_4)_6(OH)_2]$ in bone, while 14% is found intracellularly in soft tissues and only 1% is contained within extracellular fluid (ECF) (Costanzo 2006; DiBartola and Willard 2006; Moe and Sprague 2008). Phosphate is the principal intracellular anion where it occurs largely in organic forms, but it can be readily converted to the inorganic form. Within cells it occurs with lipids (phospholipids), as part of the lipid bilayer of the cell membrane, with nucleic acids in DNA and RNA, as adenosine triphosphate (ATP) and diphosphate (ADP), providing the energy currency of cells, and as cyclic adenosine monophosphate (cAMP), an intracellular second messenger for many polypeptide hormones. Translocation into and out of ECF from the intracellular fluid (ICF) space occurs and can rapidly affect ECF concentrations.

In the ECF, 70% of phosphorous is organic (largely phosphate contained within phospholipids) and 30% is in the inorganic form. Approximately 15% of the inorganic portion is protein-bound with the remaining 85% either complexed to sodium, calcium, or magnesium or freely circulating as various forms of phosphate anions.

The freely circulating inorganic fraction is the portion measured and reported by clinical laboratories. In the ECF at a pH of 7.4, phosphate anions occur primarily in two forms: the divalent or alkaline form, monohydrogen phosphate (HPO_4^{2-}), and the monovalent or acid form, dihydrogen phosphate ($H_2PO_4^-$). At blood pH 7.4, the ratio of $[HPO_4^{2-}]$:$[H_2PO_4^-]$ is 4:1, yielding an average valence of 1.8 for phosphate in the ECF. The balance between the various forms of orthophosphate (an inorganic form of phosphate) is governed by the following set of equilibrium equations:

$$H_3PO_4 \leftrightarrow H_2PO_4^{1-} + H^+ \leftrightarrow HPO_4^{2-} + H^+ \leftrightarrow PO_4^{3+} + H^+$$
$$\text{pKa 2.0} \qquad \text{pKa 6.8} \qquad \text{pKa 12.4}$$

The normal ranges for serum phosphorus concentration are 2.5–5.5. mg/dL in dogs and 2.5–6.0 mg/dL in cats (Bates 2008). Serum phosphorus concentrations are slightly greater than plasma concentrations due to release of phosphorus from platelets and other cells during clotting (Schropp and Kovacic 2007). Values are typically greater in young animals compared to adults and may be influenced by dietary phosphorus intake. The effect of age is less pronounced in cats compared to dogs (Jacobs et al. 2000). Serum levels of phosphorus are not as tightly regulated as serum calcium, and they may vary by as much as 50% over the course of a day. Because dietary intake of phosphorus is the principal cause for the variation in serum phosphorus concentrations, serum phosphorus should be measured after at least a 12-hour fast.

Phosphorus balance

Three organs are involved in phosphorus homeostasis: the intestines, the kidneys, and the skeleton. The principal hormones responsible for modulating serum phosphorus levels are vitamin D (primarily calcitriol) and parathyroid hormone (PTH). However, more recently, there is

Nephrology and Urology of Small Animals. Edited by Joe Bartges and David J. Polzin. © 2011 Blackwell Publishing Ltd.

evidence for a role of circulating factors known as phosphatonins in regulation of serum phosphorus concentrations (Moe and Sprague 2008). Phosphatonins are hormones that regulate phosphorus excretion. Three phosphatonins identified include secreted frizzled-related protein 4 (FRP4), matrix extracellular phosphoglycoprotein, and fibroblast growth factor 23 (FGF23). An important role has recently been recognized for FGF23 in chronic kidney disease (CKD).

Daily phosphorus balance is primarily determined by the relationship between dietary intake and renal excretion of phosphorus. Because phosphorus is primarily located in the ICF space, plasma levels may poorly reflect total body phosphorus. For example, in CKD, total body phosphorus retention precedes development of hyperphosphatemia. Principal factors influencing plasma levels include dietary intake, regulatory substances such as fibroblast growth factor-23 (FGF-23), PTH, and $1,25(OH)_2$ cholecalciferol, ECF volume, and renal function (Schropp and Kovacic 2007; Moe and Sprague 2008). Phosphorus may enter or exit the exchangeable pool by movement into and out of the skeletal pool of phosphorus under the influence of PTH and $1,25(OH)_2$ cholecalciferol.

Intestinal handling of phosphorus

Phosphorus is a common constituent of canine and feline diets, originating primarily from meat, poultry, fish, and bone as well as from supplements added to diets. Typical canine and feline maintenance diets contain approximately 0.8–1.6% phosphorus on a dry matter basis with calcium to phosphorus ratio of 1.2 to 2:1. This reflects a daily intake ranging from 0.5 to 3.0 g of phosphorus per day (DiBartola and Willard 2006).

Intestinal absorption of phosphorus is largely passive, although a small portion is actively regulated. Passive phosphorus-concentration-dependent absorption occurs in the jejunum and ileum. Duodenal absorption is regulated by $1,25(OH)_2$ cholecalciferol via a sodium-dependent active transport mechanism. Intestinal adsorption of phosphorus is hindered by complex formation within the lumen of the intestine; calcium, aluminum, and lanthanum will form insoluble complexes with phosphorus that will hinder its absorption. In patients with reduced kidney function, phosphorus absorption continues and complexing of intestinal phosphorus to prevent absorption is used to advantage to limit hyperphosphatemia in these patients.

Renal handling of phosphorus

The kidneys are largely responsible for day-to-day regulation of serum phosphorus concentration. Daily phosphorus intake is usually balanced by renal excretion of an equal amount of phosphorus in urine. PTH and FGF23 are the major hormonal regulators of renal phosphorus excretion, while dietary intake of phosphorus is the major nonhormonal regulator.

Phosphate not bound to protein (about 85%) is freely filtered across glomerular capillaries. Approximately 80–90% of filtered phosphorus is then reabsorbed, largely by the proximal renal tubules, which is the primary site of regulated renal reabsorption of phosphorus. Additional phosphate reabsorption may occur in the distal tubules. Regulated phosphorus reabsorption involves the sodium–phosphate cotransporter Npt2b (Moe and Sprague 2008). The Npt2b rests in the terminal web and can be rapidly moved to the brush border in the luminal membrane of the proximal tubule cells in the presence of acute or chronic phosphorus depletion. The cotransporter is withdrawn from the brush border and catabolized after a phosphorus load or in the presence of PTH. This transport process is saturable and exhibits a transport maximum (T_m). Factors increasing phosphorus excretion are primarily increased plasma phosphorus and PTH. PTH regulates reabsorption of phosphorus in the proximal tubules by inhibiting its cotransporter, thereby lowering the T_m for phosphate reabsorption. Thus, PTH is phosphaturic; however, hypophosphaturia that occurs with phosphorus depletion will override the hyperphosphaturia induced by PTH (Moe and Sprague 2008).

Excretion of 10–15% of the total filtered load is a high percentage when compared to other electrolytes such as sodium, chloride, or bicarbonate. However, this relatively large fractional excretion is physiologically important because unreabsorbed phosphate serves as a urinary buffer for hydrogen ion (Moe and Sprague 2008).

Hyperphosphatemia

Hyperphosphatemia is defined as a serum phosphorus concentration exceeding 5.5 mg/dL in adult dogs or 6.0 mg/dL in adult cats.[1] Small to moderate increases above these values may be normal in puppies (up to 10.8 mg/dL in puppies) and kittens less than 1 year of age (DiBartola and Willard 2006). Because red blood cells contain abundant amounts of phosphorus, hemolysis should be excluded as a possible cause for hyperphosphatemia. In general, hyperphosphatemia may be caused by impaired renal excretion, increased phosphorus load, or a shift of phosphorus from tissues into the ECF.

Hyperphosphatemia itself does not appear to cause any clinical signs. The clinical consequences of hyperphosphatemia are predominantly a consequence of the associated hypocalcemia (tetany, seizures, and decreased cardiac contractility). Generally, as serum phosphorus increases, serum calcium declines. In this setting, hypocalcemia results from multiple causes including decreased $1,25(OH)_2$ cholecalciferol synthesis leading to decreased intestinal absorption of calcium, and deposition of calcium phosphorus complexes in tissues. Tissues most likely to be mineralized include previously injured tissues and proton-secreting organs such as the stomach and kidneys. Ectopic calcification of tissues is most likely to occur when the calcium × phosphorus product (both expressed as mg/dL) exceeds 55 (Moe and Sprague 2008). Hyperphosphatemia in patients with CKD facilitates secondary hyperparathyroidism and renal osteodystrophy (Chapter 48).

Causes of hyperphosphatemia

The principal causes for hyperphosphatemia are listed in Table 65.1. By far, the most common cause for hyperphosphatemia is impaired renal excretion of phosphorus in patients with impaired kidney function. When glomerular filtration rate (GFR) declines, positive phosphorus balance ensues as a consequence of impaired renal phosphorus excretion. However, in CKD, the initial decline in GFR and phosphorus retention are associated with release of FGF-23 and suppression of $1,25(OH)_2$ cholecalciferol synthesis and later PTH release, which all promote phosphaturia by reducing renal tubular reabsorption of phosphorus (Gutierrez et al. 2005). Because of this phosphaturic response, development of overt hyperphosphatemia does not occur until later in the course of CKD when the capacity of these compensatory adap-

Table 65.1 Principal causes of hyperphosphatemia

Reduced renal phosphorus excretion
    Acute kidney failure
    Chronic kidney disease
    Uroabdomen
    Urinary obstruction
    Hypoparathyroidism
    Acromegaly
    Hyperthyroidism
Exogenous intake of phosphorus
    Intravenous administration of phosphorus-containing solutions
    Ingestion of phosphate enemas
    Vitamin D intoxication (cholecalciferol rodenticides, calcipotriene)
Cell injury
    Tumor cell lysis
    Tissue trauma
    Rhabdomyolysis
    Hemolysis

tations is exceeded, typically when GFR is reduced to about 20% or less of normal. In contrast, there is inadequate time for these adaptations to completely develop in acute renal failure (ARF). As a consequence, hyperphosphatemia occurs earlier in the course of ARF, and the magnitude of hyperphosphatemia is greater relative to reduction in GFR. Urinary obstruction and uroabdomen are also associated with hyperphosphatemia due to impaired or ineffective renal excretion.

Several endocrine disorders may also be associated with hyperphosphatemia due to reduced phosphorus excretion. Hyperphosphatemia develops in hypoparathyroidism, but the associated hypocalcemia is of greater clinical importance. Since PTH promotes renal phosphorus excretion, lack of PTH (or resistance to its action) results in hyperphosphatemia. Thyroxine and growth hormone increase renal tubular reabsorption of phosphorus. Hyperphosphatemia was observed in 21% of 131 hyperthyroid cats in one study, and mild hyperphosphatemia has been reported in some acromegalic cats and dogs (Peterson et al. 1983; Peterson 1988; DiBartola and Willard 2006).

Excess gastrointestinal intake of phosphorus in any form may promote hyperphosphatemia (Table 64.1). Excess vitamin D promotes hyperphosphatemia by increasing intestinal absorption of phosphorus as well as calcium. In addition, administration of phosphorus-containing enemas should be avoided in patients with reduced kidney function because of the risk of absorption of large quantities of phosphorus from the gut.

During chemotherapy of rapidly lysing cells, such as those of lymphomas, a marked increase in phosphorus release from cells can exceed renal excretory capacity. The ensuing hyperphosphatemia may be accompanied by hyperkalemia and can lead to hypocalcemia. In addition, phosphorus can also be released from cells during acute rhabdomyolysis, crush injuries, or tissue infarction. Concurrent impairment of renal function can markedly enhance the magnitude of hyperphosphatemia resulting from any of these causes.

Treatment of hyperphosphatemia

Treatment of hyperphosphatemia should be directed at the underlying cause. Renal function should be optimized by correcting any prerenal or postrenal conditions. If renal function is adequate, phosphaturia should be promoted. ECF volume expansion with saline reduces renal tubular phosphorus reabsorption; increasing urine pH with sodium bicarbonate may also promote this effect. Reducing dietary phosphorus and providing intestinal phosphate binders are useful in reducing hyperphosphatemia in patients with CKD, although the reductions in serum phosphorus concentrations occur gradually over weeks to months. In patients with severe impairment of kidney function, dialysis is the most effective means of acutely reducing hyperphosphatemia. Management of hyperphosphatemia in patients with CKD is discussed in Chapter 48.

Hypophosphatemia

Since only about 1% of body phosphorus is in the ECF, hypophosphatemia may or may not reflect a decrease in total body phosphorus content. In general, the adverse effects of hypophosphatemia are more severe when total body phosphate depletion accompanies hypophosphatemia. Clinical effects of hypophosphatemia are most apparent in the hematologic, neuromuscular, cardiovascular, and skeletal systems (DiBartola and Willard 2006; Moe and Sprague 2008). When serum phosphorus declines to about 1.0 mg/dL or less, hemolysis may result, most likely the consequence of reduced red blood cell ATP levels promoting increased erythrocyte fragility. This effect is most commonly seen during therapy for diabetic ketoacidosis. In addition, platelets may have reduced function and thrombocytopenia may occur. Neuromuscular signs may include weakness and pain associated with rhabdomyolysis and anorexia, nausea, or vomiting due to intestinal ileus. Respiratory paralysis leading to death has been reported in hypophosphatemic humans. Metabolic encephalopathy characterized by coma, seizure, confusion, and irritability may also develop. A reversible impairment of cardiac contractility may occur. Skeletal demineralization may develop as a consequence of long-term derangements in PTH and calcitriol levels.

Causes of hypophosphatemia

Hypophosphatemia may result from increased urinary loss, decreased intake or translocation of phosphorus from the ECF into cells (Table 65.2). Increased urinary loss of phosphorus most often occurs in association with increased levels of PTH or renal tubular defects that impair phosphorus reabsorption. Primary hyperparathyroidism is associated with a trend toward reduced serum phosphate concentrations, although overt hypophosphatemia is inconsistently present. Clinical effects of hyperparathyroidism are primarily attributable to hypercalcemia, not hypophosphatemia. In Fanconi syndrome, hypophosphatemia results from defective renal tubular phosphorus reabsorption. In eclampsia, hypocalcemia stimulates PTH release, thereby promoting phosphaturia and hypophosphatemia. In humans, hypophosphatemia due to phosphaturia has been reported in association

Table 65.2 Principal causes of hypophosphatemia

Enhanced renal excretion of phosphorus
Primary hyperparathyroidism
Renal tubular disorders (e.g., Fanconi syndrome)
Eclampsia
Translocation of phosphorus into cells
Treatment of diabetic ketoacidosis
Insulin administration
Total parenteral nutrition
Refeeding
Hypothermia
Respiratory alkalosis
Decreased intake of phosphorus
Dietary deficiency
Gastrointestinal disorders
Vitamin D deficiency
Phosphate binders

with mesenchymal tumors that produce FGF-23 or FRP4 (Moe and Sprague 2008).

The origin of hypophosphatemia in patients with diabetes may be multifactorial. Diabetic patients, and particularly those with ketoacidosis, may be phosphorus depleted as a consequence of increased urinary losses and inadequate dietary intake. In this setting, insulin administration, which promotes movement of phosphorus from the ECF intracellularly, may be associated with marked hypophosphatemia. Refeeding and total parenteral nutrition after poor intake or starvation may stimulate tissue growth with translocation of phosphorus into cells. Alkalosis, particularly prolonged respiratory alkalosis, can promote intracellular shift of phosphorus because of the associated intracellular acidosis.

Hypophosphatemia may also result from decreased phosphorus intake or impaired phosphorus absorption (malabsorption, phosphate binders). In addition, vitamin D deficiency may impair phosphorus absorption and release from bone, leading to hypophosphatemia.

Treatment of hypophosphatemia

Treatment of hypophosphatemia is best directed at correcting the underlying disorder or nutritional deficiency. When hypophosphatemia can be anticipated, monitoring and prophylactic administration of supplemental phosphorus should be considered. Development of severe hypophosphatemia usually indicates underlying total body phosphorus depletion.

Phosphorus supplementation is appropriate for patients with clinical signs and those likely to develop clinical consequences (e.g., hypophosphatemia-associated hemolysis with therapy for diabetic ketoacidosis).

In such individuals, intravenous administration of phosphorus is usually indicated. However, intravenous phosphorus administration must be used with caution because it may promote hypocalcemia, tetany, renal failure, or metastatic calcification, especially when the calcium phosphorus product exceeds 55 mg^2/dL^2 (DiBartole and Willard 2006; Moe and Sprague 2008). Because the reduction in urinary phosphorus excretion that develops in hypophosphatemia may persist during therapy, hyperphosphatemia may develop during replacement therapy. To minimize these potential complications, phosphorus should be administered in small amounts (0.01–0.06 mmol/kg/h) by constant rate infusion over hours to days with repeated monitoring of the patient's response and serum phosphorus concentrations (every 6–8 hours). Because administered phosphorus rapidly translocates into the intracellular space, predicting the total dose requirement for phosphorus is not reliable. The goal is to raise serum phosphorus concentration to 2.0 mg/dL or greater. Depending on the patient's electrolyte needs, phosphorus may be administered as sodium phosphate or potassium phosphate. In cats under treatment for diabetic ketoacidosis with hypophosphatemia and hypokalemia, a common practice is to manage developing hypophosphatemia by providing 50–75% of the patient's potassium needs as potassium chloride with the remainder as potassium phosphate.

If the serum phosphorus is greater than 1.5 mg/dL and unlikely to decline further, treatment is usually unnecessary. However, if the patient is likely to be whole body phosphorus depleted, consider providing oral phosphorus supplementation in the form of skim or low-fat milk or phosphorus-containing buffered laxative.

Endnote

1. Normal ranges for serum phosphorus vary from laboratory to laboratory.

References

Bates, J.A. (2008). Phosphorus: as quick reference. *Vet Clin North America, Small Animal* **38**: 471–475.

Costanzo, L.S. (2006). *Physiology*. Philadelphia, PA: Saunders, pp. 282–283.

DiBartola, S.P. and M.D. Willard (2006). Disorders of phosphorus: hypophosphatemia and hyperphosphatemia. In: *Fluid, Electrolyte, and Acid-Base Disorders in Small Animal Practice*, edited by S.P. DiBartola. St. Louis, MO: WB Saunders, pp. 195–209.

Gutierrez, O., T. Isakova, et al. (2005). Fibroblast growth factor-23 mitigates hyperphosphatemia but accentuates calcitriol deficiency in chronic kidney disease. *J Am Soc Nephrol* **16**: 2205–2215.

Jacobs, R.M., J.H. Lumsden et al. (2000). Canine and feline reference values. In: Current Veterinary Therapy XIII, Edited by J.D. Bonagura. Philadelphia, PA: WB Saunders, p. 1213.

Moe, S.M. and S.M. Sprague (2008). Mineral bone disorders in chronic kidney disease. In: *The Kidney*, edited by B.M. Brenner, 8th edition. Philadelphia, PA: WB Saunders, pp. 1784–1813.

Peterson, M.E. (1988). Endocrine disorders in cats: four emerging diseases. *Comp Cont Educ Pract Vet* **19**: 1353–1362.

Peterson, M.E., P.P. Kintzer, et al. (1983). Feline hyperthyroidism: pretreatment clinical and laboratory evaluation of 131 cases. *J Am Vet Med Assoc* **183**: 103–110.

Schropp, D.M. and J. Kovacic (2007). Phosphorus and phosphate metabolism in veterinary patients. *J Vet Emerg Crit Care* **17**: 127–134.

66

Metabolic acid–base disorders

Marie E. Kerl

Metabolic acid–base abnormalities occur commonly in small animal patients presented for a wide variety of conditions. Determining the appropriate therapeutic response depends upon the clinician's ability to correctly diagnose the acid–base disorder and to understand appropriate treatment. This chapter will review normal blood gas physiology as well as the pathophysiology and diagnosis of blood gas disorders, with a focus on metabolic blood gas abnormalities.

Acid–base disorders are caused by changes in hydrogen ion concentration in circulation. The main organ systems that control the acid–base balance include the liver, lungs, and kidneys. Hydrogen ions are nonvolatile acids produced by normal metabolism and are renally excreted. An acid consists of a hydrogen ion (H^+) donor and a base (A^-), which is a proton acceptor. When placed in solution, acids dissociate into H^+ (acid) and A^-. Acidosis occurs with a gain of hydrogen ions in solution, whereas alkalosis occurs with a reduction of hydrogen ions (Rose 1994a; DiBartola 2006a). Acid production comes from three principal sources on a daily basis: production of carbon dioxide (CO_2), production of organic acids such as lactate and ketones, and production of inorganic acids (sulfate and phosphate), which are bio-products of dietary protein and amino acid metabolism (Morris and Low 2008). The liver is responsible for acid production through carbohydrate and lipid oxidation (CO_2 produced), dietary protein and amino acid metabolism producing sulfate, phosphate, and ammonia, and production of lactate and ketones (Morris and Low 2008). A small amount of base is also lost each day in the gastrointestinal tract, which effectively increases the acid load in the body (DiBartola 2006a).

Carbon dioxide is a volatile acid that can combine with water in the presence of carbonic anhydrase to form carbonic acid (H_2CO_3). Although carbonic acid can be formed in the absence of carbonic anhydrase, the reaction proceeds exceedingly slowly (DiBartola 2006a). Carbonic anhydrase is present in abundance in the body, especially in red blood cells and renal tubular cells. Carbon dioxide is routinely formed at consistent amounts during normal carbohydrate and fat metabolism and is excreted via the lungs during alveolar ventilation. The two sources of acid (H^+ and CO_2) are interrelated, as is shown in the carbonic acid equation:

$$H^+ + HCO_3^- <-> H_2CO_3 <-> H_2O + CO_2$$

Any cell containing carbonic anhydrase is capable of this reaction, and the chemical reaction can shift either direction, depending on the availability of substrate (Rose 1994a, Rose 1994d).

By definition, pH is the negative log of the hydrogen ion concentration. An acid gain results in a decrease in blood pH (acidemia), whereas an acid loss results in an increased pH (alkalemia). Because of the logarithmic nature of the equation, larger changes in H^+ concentration are required to decrease the pH by similar units than are required to increase the pH in alkalosis (Morris and Low 2008). Acid can be gained systemically from reduced renal elimination of a metabolically produced compound, or from ingestion of an exogenous acid source. Changes in CO_2 influence the H^+ concentration, as evidenced by the carbonic acid equation. As CO_2 is eliminated by increasing alveolar ventilation, carbonic acid dissociates to form more CO_2, and H^+ and bicarbonate (HCO_3^-) combine in turn to form more carbonic acid. This effectively lowers the H^+ concentration and increases pH. Conversely, as CO_2 increases from ventilation impairment, pH decreases. Acid–base disorders that are caused primarily by changes in alveolar

Nephrology and Urology of Small Animals. Edited by Joe Bartges and David J. Polzin. © 2011 Blackwell Publishing Ltd.

ventilation include primary respiratory acidosis and respiratory alkalosis. Discussion of primary respiratory acid–base disorders is beyond the scope of this chapter. The reader is referred to several excellent references on this subject (Rose 1994e, Rose 1994f; Johnson and Autran de Morias 2006).

Buffers act to bind H^+ to prevent large fluctuations in pH. A variety of buffer systems exist in the body, including nonbicarbonate buffers (proteins and phosphates) and HCO_3^-, which is the primary extracellular buffer. Bicarbonate is an effective buffer because it exists in relatively large concentrations compared with other buffers, and it participates in the carbonic acid equation to produce CO_2 gas, which can be eliminated through ventilation. The HCO_3^- buffer system, therefore, is considered an open system that can continue to buffer as long as the respiratory system is functional. In disease states causing HCO_3^- to be lost excessively from the urinary or gastrointestinal system, CO_2 and H_2O combine to form carbonic acid, which dissociates to increase H^+ and cause acidemia (Rose 1994d). Under normal function, the kidneys provide a consistent source of bicarbonate through reabsorption of filtered bicarbonate and regeneration of bicarbonate in the renal tubular cells. The proximal tubule reabsorbs 90–95% of the filtered bicarbonate load, and the remaining tubular segments reabsorb the remaining 10–15% (DiBartola 2006b). Acid that is gained on a daily basis through normal metabolic function is renally excreted through several mechanisms. Filtered H^+ ions combine with bicarbonate in the tubules to become H_2O and CO_2 via the carbonic acid equation. The CO_2 produced by this mechanism is absorbed across the luminal membrane and participates in the carbonic acid equation intracellularly to produce HCO_3^-, which is then absorbed at the basolateral membrane. Hydrogen is also excreted via titration with filtered sodium phosphate in exchange for sodium, or through production of ammonium ions in the tubular lumen utilizing ammonia from tubular excretion, filtration, or local production from glutamate metabolism within the tubular cells. All of these mechanisms result in tubular cell production of bicarbonate, which is then absorbed via the renal interstitium. Tubular cell $HCO3^-$ reabsorption depends upon appropriate concentrations of sodium and chloride ions, which participate in ion exchange to maintain electroneutrality, and a functional sodium–potassium ATPase pump to sustain an appropriate electrochemical gradient within the cells. The deficiency of any of these ions can perpetuate an acid–base disorder (DiBartola 2006a).

Various models have been developed to diagnose acid–base abnormalities and to determine contributing factors. A traditional approach to acid–base abnormalities involves inspection of the pH, HCO_3^-, and CO_2 values of a blood gas analysis as they are related via the Henderson–Hasselbalch equation (pH $= 6.1 \times$ log $\{HCO_3^-/0.03PCO_2\}$) and supplementing with calculation of the anion gap to further characterize metabolic acidosis (Rose 1994a; Morris and Low 2008). Another model, the physiochemical approach, (Stewart's approach) applies physical chemistry principles of electroneutrality, conservation of mass, and dissociation of electrolytes to better quantify the source of an acid–base disturbance and identify the causative mechanisms (Stewart 1981). This approach relies on determining three factors: the strong ion difference (sodium, potassium, calcium, magnesium, chloride, and lactate), the PCO_2, and total weak acid concentration (albumin, phosphates) (Stewart 1981). Since $HCO3^-$ is a dependent variable, it is not considered in calculations of this method. The reader is referred to several excellent references for further explanation of this method of calculating acid–base abnormalities (de Morias 2006; Kellum and Kellum 2007).

According to the Henderson–Hasselbalch equation, pH can be characterized by changes in HCO_3^- and partial pressure of carbon dioxide (PCO_2). Because a predictable change in HCO_3^- occurs with gain or loss of H^+ ions, HCO_3^- can be used to correctly identify acid–base abnormalities arising from metabolic disorders. In metabolic acidosis, an H^+ increase shifts the carbonic acid equation to result in a decrease in HCO_3^-; in metabolic alkalosis, an H^+ decrease has the opposite effect on HCO_3^-. This equation can also be used to predict how compensatory mechanisms engage to lessen the degree of change in the pH. When metabolic acidosis develops, the respiratory system is stimulated to increase the respiratory rate to eliminate CO_2 from the lungs and create respiratory alkalosis. Likewise, with a primary respiratory disorder, the opposite metabolic disorder is generated. The respiratory system provides rapid compensation, changing within minutes of onset of a metabolic disorder. Metabolic compensation occurs more slowly, becoming maximally effective within days. With either system, compensatory mechanisms should slow down as the pH approaches a normal range, and compensation should never completely normalize the pH (DiBartola 2006a).

Base excess, which is expressed in milliequivalents per liter (mEq/L), is the amount of base above or below the normal buffer base, a value calculated by taking into account the expected change in HCO_3^- secondary to acute changes in PCO_2. The general rule of thumb is that the HCO_3^- concentration rises about 1–2 mEq/L for each acute 10 mmHg increase in $PaCO_2$ above 40 mmHg to a maximum increase of 4 mEq/L and that the HCO_3^-

concentration falls 1–2 mEq for each acute 10 mmHg decrease in $PaCO_2$ below 40, to a maximum decrease of 6 mEq/L (Malley 1990). Some authors refer to a negative base excess as a base deficit.

By convention, a simple acid–base disorder is limited to the primary disorder and the appropriate compensatory response. A mixed disorder is one in which at least two separate abnormalities occur simultaneously. The reader is referred to Chapter 67 for a discussion of mixed acid–base disorders. Normal values at sea level for venous blood gas interpretation are pH, 7.35–7.45; PCO_2, 40–45 mmHg; and HCO_3^-, 19–24 mEq/L. Base excess normally should be −5–5 mEq/L (Kerl 2005a). An animal with metabolic acidosis has a pH below normal and a HCO_3^- below normal, while an animal with metabolic alkalosis has a pH above normal and an elevated HCO_3^-.

Metabolic acidosis results from the failure of normal systems, which compensate for acid–base abnormalities, occurring either through acid gain or failure of bicarbonate buffering. The quantity of acid can increase from a gain of H^+ through ingestion of an acid into the body, increased production of an endogenous acid, or failure to eliminate an acid load by the renal tubular cells. Metabolic acidosis can also be caused by a loss of HCO_3^- buffering ability. Differentiating these two causes of metabolic acidosis is important for both diagnosis of the underlying disorder and for determining correct therapeutic intervention.

Dissociation of acid into the H^+ ion and the corresponding anion occurs in circulation. When acid accumulates, HCO_3^- combines with H^+ to buffer the acid load, while the anion remains in solution. Because electroneutrality must be maintained as anions accumulate following acid dissociation, some other circulating anion must decrease correspondingly. Anion gap (AG) is a system that is useful in the classification of disorders causing metabolic acidosis. AG represents the difference between the four cations and anions commonly measured on a serum biochemical profile. The equation is stated:

$$AG = (Na^+ + K^+) - (Cl^- + HCO_3^-)$$

Although ranges for AG can vary somewhat based upon the reference ranges of electrolytes for various laboratories, a reference value of 16 ± 4 is typical (Kerl 2005a). When metabolic acidosis exists with an increased AG, there has usually been a gain of an endogenous or exogenous organic acid. Causes of AG metabolic acidosis, which are commonly encountered in small animal practice, include ethylene glycol intoxication (glycolate and other metabolites of ethylene glycol), uremia (phosphates and sulfates), tissue hypoxia (lactate), diabetic ketoacidosis (ketone bodies), salicylate intoxication, and other unusual intoxications (e.g., drugs, alcohol) (Elliott et al.

2003a; Elliott et al. 2003b; Lee and Drobatz 2003; de Morais et al. 2008). Tissue hypoxia causes an increased AG metabolic acidosis from lactic acidosis; however, there are likely other anions produced as well. In people and animals with various causes of AG metabolic acidosis, a number of Kreb's cycle intermediaries have been identified, which include isocitrate, succinate, a-ketoglutarate, and malate, as well as D-lactate, which is not measured on handheld lactate monitors (Forni et al. 2006). There appears to be prognostic significance of elevations in some of these unmeasured anions for people affected with certain disease processes (Dondorp et al. 2004). Lactate measurement has become commonly available in veterinary practice through the use of handheld lactate monitors, which measure L-lactate (Karagiannis et al. 2006). Older classification schemes identified lactic acidosis as being associated either with diseases characterized by impaired tissue oxygen delivery or with diseases not causing tissue hypoxia; however, even in hypoxic diseases, lactate concentrations are most likely elevated from other causes (de Morais et al. 2008). If the source of production of lactic acid resolves with appropriate resuscitative therapy, the lactate will be metabolized into bicarbonate and metabolic acidosis will resolve (Karagiannis et al. 2006). If the underlying disease cannot be resolved and the lactic acidosis persists, the prognosis is poor (de Morais et al. 2008). D-lactic acidosis has been identified in certain animals with congenital or acquired metabolic defects that cause failure of normal lactate metabolism by mitochondrial oxidative function (Packer et al. 2005; Kelmer et al. 2007). These metabolic defects result in a severe AG acidosis. Handheld lactate monitors would not identify the lactate in these animals since they only measure L-lactate (Karagiannis et al. 2006).

Metabolic acidosis characterized by a normal AG is caused by loss of bicarbonate buffers or a failure to excrete H^+ ions, with a corresponding increase in chloride to maintain electroneutrality (Kerl 2005a). This is often referred to as a hyperchloremic metabolic acidosis; however, that name can be somewhat misleading since hyperchloremic metabolic acidosis can sometimes be identified in the face of serum chloride that is within a laboratory reference range (DiBartola 2006b). Evaluating the proportion of sodium to chloride can be helpful to identify an animal with hyperchloremic metabolic acidosis. A difference of 30–40 milliequivalents (mEq) normally exists when measured serum chloride is subtracted from measured serum sodium. If the difference is less than 30 mEq/L, there is an excess of chloride in proportion to sodium, which is consistent with relative hyperchloremia (DiBartola 2006b). Hyperchloremic metabolic acidosis occurs less commonly than increased AG metabolic acidosis and is caused by renal tubular acidosis or by severe diarrhea and resultant loss of intestinal bicarbonate (Riordan and Schaer 2005). Iatrogenic hyperchloremic metabolic acidosis can also occur with administration of an alkali-free chloride containing crystalloid solution, such as 0.9% sodium chloride (0.9% NaCl) for intravenous volume replacement (Rose 1994b).

Renal tubular acidosis (RTA) is classified as proximal or distal based upon the area of defect (Riordan and Schaer 2005). Proximal RTA is characterized by a failure of bicarbonate absorption in the proximal tubular segments. This disorder causes an elevated urine fractional excretion of HCO_3^- when serum HCO_3^- is normal. Proximal RTA results in a self-limiting acidosis since the more distal tubular segments can absorb bicarbonate as the filtered bicarbonate load falls with systemic metabolic acidosis, thus limiting the acidosis (Kerl 2005b). Proximal RTA is most commonly identified as a feature of proximal tubular defects resembling Fanconi's syndrome. Other tubular defects seen commonly with Fanconi's syndrome include failure of absorption of glucose, phosphate, sodium, potassium, uric acid, and amino acids. Fanconi's syndrome had been described most commonly in basenji dogs and is observed sporadically in other breeds. Distal RTA is characterized by a failure to acidify the urine due to the loss of hydrogen excretory capacity of the distal tubule (Kerl 2005b). The hallmark of distal RTA is a urine pH greater than 6.0 despite moderate to marked systemic acidosis. Presence of a urinary tract infection with urease-producing bacteria should be ruled out prior to diagnosing distal RTA since these bacterial infections will increase urine pH. Causes of distal RTA reported in the literature include pyelonephritis, amphotericin B, and administration of outdated tetracycline (Riordan and Schaer 2005). Further information on renal tubular and congenital diseases can be found in Chapters 55 and 56.

Abnormalities associated with metabolic acidosis include lethargy, mental dullness or obtundation, decreased cardiac output, decreased blood pressure, and decreased hepatic and renal blood flow (Rose 1994b; Kerl 2005a; Packer et al. 2005; DiBartola 2006a; Kelmer et al. 2007; Kovacic 2008). In a clinical setting, it is challenging to tell whether clinical signs are caused by the acidemia or the underlying cause of the acid–base disorder or both (Kerl 2005a). For animals presenting with acute illness or decompensation of a chronic illness, treatment should be directed at the underlying disease, and treatment of the metabolic acidosis may be included in the overall treatment plan. Unless the patient has some impairment of normal ventilatory ability, compensatory mechanisms cause an increase in the respiratory rate, which allows the animal to eliminate CO_2 generated by carbonic acid formation, mitigating acidosis (DiBartola 2006a).

Treatment should be aimed at correcting the underlying disorder. This might involve improving tissue perfusion with appropriate resuscitative measures, eliminating ingested toxin or correcting metabolic, renal, or gastrointestinal disease (Kerl 2005a; DiBartola 2006a; de Morais et al. 2008; Kovacic 2008). With severe metabolic acidosis (pH of <7.15 and HCO_3^- <12 mEq/L), intravenous sodium bicarbonate may be administered judiciously according to the following formula, which can be used to calculate bicarbonate deficit:

$$Bicarbonate\ dose = (0.3)\ (Body\ weight\ [kg])$$
$$(Base\ deficit)$$

Half of this dose should be administered slowly intravenously for more than 6 hours, and the acid–base status should be re-evaluated prior to continuation of therapy. Rapid correction of metabolic acidosis can cause a number of undesired side effects, including hyperosmolarity, hypernatremia, and hypokalemia. Hypocalcemic tetany may be caused by shifting of calcium from the ionized to the protein-bound form after bicarbonate administration (Kerl 2005a). Paradoxical central nervous system (CNS) acidosis occurs when CO_2 generated following bicarbonate administration crosses the blood–brain barrier and takes part in the carbonic acid equation, essentially fueling acid production in the CNS. Iatrogenic metabolic alkalosis can also occur after administration of bicarbonate.

Metabolic alkalosis is most commonly caused by loss of chloride in excess of extracellular fluid volume, which typically occurs as a result of upper gastrointestinal (GI) fluid loss or sequestration (Rose 1994c). Other causes of chloride wasting include diuretic administration. Rarely, metabolic alkalosis may be caused by overzealous administration of sodium bicarbonate or another organic anion or by hyperaldosteronism (aka., Conn's syndrome), which causes sodium retention in excess of chloride (Rose 1994c). The most common clinical problem associated with metabolic alkalosis in small animal practice is gastric outflow obstruction (Boag et al. 2005). Cats with severe hypokalemia can develop metabolic alkalosis due to gastric hypomotility and pooling of gastric fluid, effectively causing a "third-spacing" of chloride without obvious or frequent vomiting. This third-spacing of chloride-rich secretions will lead to metabolic alkalosis when extracellular fluid depletion occurs.

During gastric outflow obstruction, appropriate renal compensation prevents an acid–base disorder until extracellular fluid volume depletion occurs secondary to the vomiting. In addition to the chloride deficit, aldosterone is released with hypovolemia, increasing renal uptake of sodium. Normally, sodium is reabsorbed with bicarbonate or chloride or is exchanged for potassium. Because gastric fluid has high chloride and potassium concentrations, animals with gastric outflow obstruction become systemically depleted of these electrolytes so that renal reabsorption of sodium can only occur with concurrent bicarbonate uptake (Kerl 2005a; DiBartola 2006b; de Morais et al. 2008). When chloride depletion and extracellular volume depletion initiate metabolic alkalosis, replacement of the chloride deficit will correct the acid–base disorder. Rarely, chloride-resistant metabolic alkalosis occurs in small animals. Causes of chloride-resistant alkalosis include primary hyperaldosteronism in which an aldosterone-secreting tumor releases aldosterone autonomously. This causes excessive wasting of distal tubular H^+ and potassium. Hyperadrenocorticism in people with adrenal tumors is associated with chloride-resistant alkalosis; however, metabolic alkalosis is an uncommon finding in dogs with hyperadrenocorticism (DiBartola 2006b).

Clinical signs of metabolic alkalosis are dictated by the underlying disorder generating the acid–base abnormality. Muscle twitching and seizures have been reported in animals with metabolic alkalosis (DiBartola 2006b). Signs associated with concurrent potassium depletion may include weakness, cardiac arrhythmias, renal dysfunction, and gastrointestinal motility disturbances (DiBartola 2006b).

Treatment of metabolic alkalosis is directed at resolving the underlying cause. Intravenous 0.9% sodium chloride is the fluid of choice to replace volume deficits and normalize chloride concentrations since these patients are often chloride-depleted. Fluids should not contain buffer (e.g., not lactated Ringer's solution) (Kerl 2005a). Pyloric outflow obstruction is often addressed surgically, or by removal of an obstructing foreign body. In animals with profuse vomiting unassociated with obstruction, drug therapy to minimize gastric hydrochloric acid (HCl) excretion may be warranted (e.g., famotidine, omeprazole). Because animals with metabolic alkalosis often have concurrent hypokalemia, cautious intravenous potassium chloride supplementation is often indicated (Kerl 2005a).

References

Boag, A.K., R.J. Coe, et al. (2005). Acid-base and electrolyte abnormalities in dogs with gastrointestinal foreign bodies. *J Vet Intern Med* **19**(6): 816–821.

de Morias, H.A. (2006). Strong ion approach to acid-base disorders. In: *Fluid, Electrolyte, and Acid-Base Disorders in Small Animal Practice*, edited by S.P. DiBartola. St. Louis, MO: Elsevier.

de Morais, H.A., J.F. Bach, et al. (2008). Metabolic acid-base disorders in the critical care unit. *Vet Clin N Am—Small Animal Pract* **38**(3): 559–574.

DiBartola, S.P. (2006a). Introduction to acid-base disorders. In: *Fluid, Electrolyte and Acid-Base Disorders in Small Animal Practice*, edited by S.P. DiBartola. St. Louis, MO: WB Saunders.

DiBartola, S.P. (2006b). Metabolic acid-base disorders. In: *Fluid, Electrolyte and Acid-Base Disorders in Small Animal Practice*, edited by S.P. DiBartola. St. Louis, MO: WB Saunders.

Dondorp, A.M., T.T.H. Chau, et al. (2004). Unidentified acids of strong prognostic significance in severe malaria (see comment). *Crit Care Med* **32**(8): 1683–1688.

Elliott, J., H.M. Syme, et al. (2003). Acid-base balance of cats with chronic renal failure: effect of deterioration in renal function. *J Small Anim Pract* **44**(6): 261–268.

Elliott, J., H.M. Syme, et al. (2003). Assessment of acid-base status of cats with naturally occurring chronic renal failure. *J Small Anim Pract* **44**(2): 65–70.

Forni, L.G., W. McKinnon, et al. (2006). Unmeasured anions in metabolic acidosis: unravelling the mystery. *Crit Care (London, England)* **10**(4): 220.

Johnson, R.A. and H. Autran de Morias (2006). Respiratory acid-base disorders. In: *Fluid, Eelctrolyte and Acid Base Disorders in Small Animal Practice*, edited by S.P. DiBartola. St. Louis, MO: WB Saunders.

Karagiannis, M.H., A.N. Reniker, et al. (2006). Lactate measurement as an indicator of perfusion. *Compend Contin Educ Pract Vet* **28**(4): 287–298.

Kellum, J.A. and J.A. Kellum (2007). Disorders of acid-base balance. *Crit Care Med* **35**(11): 2630–2636.

Kelmer, E., G.D. Shelton, et al. (2007). Organic acidemia in a young cat associated with cobalamin deficiency. *J Vet Emerg Crit Care* **17**(3): 299–304.

Kerl, M.E. (2005a). Acid-base, oximetry, and blood gas emergencies. In: *Textbook of Veterinary Internal Medicine*, edited by S.J. Ettinger and E.C. Feldman. St. Louis, MO: Elsevier.

Kerl, M.E. (2005b). Renal tubular diseases. In: *Textbook of Veterinary Internal Medicine*, edited by S.J. Ettinger and E.C. Feldman. St. Louis, MO: Elsevier.

Kovacic, J.P. (2008). Acid-base disturbances. In: *Small Animal Critical Care Medicine*, edited by D.C. Silverstein and K. Hopper. St. Louis, MO: Suanders Elsevier.

Lee, J.A. and K.J. Drobatz (2003). Characterization of the clinical characteristics, electrolytes, acid-base, and renal parameters in male cats with urethral obstruction. *J Vet Emerg Crit Care* **13**(4): 227–233.

Malley, W.J. (1990). Hypoxia: assessment and intervention. In: *Clinical Blood Gases: Application and Noninvasive Alternatives*, edited by W.J. Malley. Philadelphia, PA: WB Saunders.

Morris, C.G. and J. Low (2008). Metabolic acidosis in the critically ill: part 1. Classification and pathophysiology. *Anaesthesia* **63**(3): 294–301.

Packer, R.A., L.A. Cohn, et al. (2005). D-lactic acidosis secondary to exocrine pancreatic insufficiency in a cat. *J Vet Intern Med* **19**(1): 106–110.

Riordan, L. and M. Schaer (2005). Renal tubular acidosis. *Compend Contin Educ Pract Vet* **22**(7): 513–528.

Rose, B.D. (1994a). Acid-base physiology. In: *Clinical Physiology of Acid-Base and Electrolyte Disorders*, edited by B.D. Rose. New York: McGraw-Hill.

Rose, B.D. (1994b). Metabolic acidosis. In: *Clinical Physiology of Acid-Base and Electrolyte Disorders*, edited by B.D. Rose. New York: McGraw-Hill.

Rose, B.D. (1994c). Metabolic alkalosis. In: *Clinical Physiology of Acid-Base and Eelctrolyte Disorders*, edited by B.D. Rose. New York: McGraw-Hill.

Rose, B.D. (1994d). Regulation of acid-base balance. In: *Clinical Physiology of Acid-Base and Electrolyte Disorders*, edited by B.D. Rose. New York: McGraw-Hill.

Rose, B.D. (1994e). Respiratory acidosis. In: *Clinical Physiology of Acid-Base and Electrolyte Disorders*, edited by B.D. Rose. New York: McGraw-Hill.

Rose, B.D. (1994f). Respiratory alkalosis. In: *Clinical Physiology of Acid-Base and Electolyte Disorders*, edited by B.D. Rose. New York: McGraw-Hill.

Stewart, P.A. (1981). *How to Understand Acid-Base: A Quantitative Acid-Base Primer for Biology and Medicine*. New York: Elsevier.

67

Mixed acid–base disorders

Mark J. Acierno

Mixed acid–base disorders arise when two or more primary acid–base disturbances (metabolic acidosis, metabolic alkalosis, respiratory acidosis, and respiratory alkalosis) occur simultaneously in the same patient. Although mixed acid–base disorders are often thought of as difficult to understand, nothing could be further from the truth. A brief review of nomenclature, physiology, and the development of systematic approach to critically ill patients (Table 67.1) is all that is required to correctly identify and treat affected patients.

Correct use of terminology is essential when evaluating acid–base disturbances. Acidosis, acidemia, alkalosis, and alkalemia are terms that are sometimes used incorrectly. Acidosis refers to the physiologic process that leads to the accumulation of acid in the blood (Rose and Post 2001a). The resulting decrease in pH is called acidemia (Rose and Post 2001a). Thus, diabetic ketoacdosis is the physiologic process that results in an acidemia. Alkalosis refers to physiologic processes that increase serum alkali (Rose and Post 2001a). The resulting increase in pH is called alkalemia.

Surprisingly, the first step in assessing a patient's acid–base status is to obtain a thorough history and physical examination. Often, the clinician will find evidence of a possible acid–base disorder before the first laboratory tests are submitted. A history that is compatible with renal failure, diabetes mellitus, Fanconi's syndrome, or another condition associated with a primary acid–base disorder should prompt the submission of a blood gas analysis. When history is unhelpful, compatible conditions, such as diabetes, are often detected on routine laboratory tests. Many conditions that present emergently, such as heat stroke, congestive heart failure, and laryngeal paralysis, are also known to cause acid–base imbalances. Lastly, suspicion of toxin exposures, such as ethylene glycol, ethanol, and salicylate acid (aspirin), is a clear indication for the clinician to perform a blood gas analysis.

In order for blood gas analysis to be useful, the results must be accurate. Although some handheld point-of-care analyzers have been shown to provide reliable results in companion animals (Verwaerde et al. 2002), other unvalidated systems are sometimes used. These units may or may not be accurate in cats and dogs. Errors can also be introduced in the processing of samples and in the transcription of results. Care must be taken when blood samples are collected or stored in anticoagulation tubes as a significant decreases in CO_2 and bicarbonate will occur if the proportion of blood to sodium heparin is incorrect (Bloom et al. 1985). In the absence of cage-side testing, failing to immediately separate red blood cells from plasma can artificially increase P_{CO_2} measurements, while exposing serum to room air can have the opposite effect (Gambino and Schreiber 1966). Within living systems, pH, P_{CO_2}, and bicarbonate are in equilibrium and adhere to the Henderson–Hasselbalch equation. Therefore, we can use this formula to verify the "believability" of the results:

$$pH = 6.1 + \log([HCO_3^-]/0.03 * P_{CO2})$$

(Rose and Post 2001b; Breen 2001)

After determining the need for blood gas analysis and verifying the results, the next step is to identify any primary acid–base disorder. The primary disorder can be determined by evaluating serum bicarbonate in relation to pH (Figure 67.1) (Kraut and Madias 2001).

Decreased serum bicarbonate can occur with either a metabolic acidosis or as the compensatory response to respiratory alkalosis; however, decreases in serum bicarbonate and pH can only occur if the primary disorder is a metabolic acidosis (Kraut and Madias 2001). Decreased

Nephrology and Urology of Small Animals. Edited by Joe Bartges and David J. Polzin. © 2011 Blackwell Publishing Ltd.

Table 67.1 Steps in determining the presence of a mixed acid–base imbalance

1. Does the patient have a condition associated with acid/base disturbance
   a. Perform blood–gas
   b. Verify results
2. Identify primary disturbance
   a. If pH is abnormal, at *least* one acid–base disturbance exists
   b. If pH is normal and P_{CO2} or bicarbonate are abnormal, then a mixed disorder exists
3. Calculate expected compensation
   a. If not appropriate, mixed acid–base disorder exists or insufficient time for compensation to occur
   b. Appropriate compensation does not rule-out mixed acid–base disorder
4. Calculate AG
   a. High gap confirms existence of metabolic acidosis
      i. Normal gap does not disprove a metabolic acidosis
   b. Limits differentials
5. Determine Cl^-/Na^+ ratio
   a. Is strong ionic difference contributing to a mixed metabolic disorder?
6. Use clinical information, AG, and Cl^-/Na^+ ratio to evaluate for mixed metabolic disorders

serum bicarbonate accompanied by an increased pH is indicative of a respiratory alkalosis. An increase in serum bicarbonate can occur with either a metabolic alkalosis or as the compensatory response to respiratory acidosis. Increases in both bicarbonate and pH indicate a metabolic alkalosis, while increased bicarbonate with a decreased pH are suggestive of a respiratory acidosis (Kraut and Madias 2001).

Once the presence of a primary acid–base disorder has been established, the next step is to determine if there are one or more additional disturbances (Table 67.2). In the presence of simple acid–base disorder, bicarbonate and p_{CO2} always move in the same direction. When bicarbonate and p_{CO2} move in different directions, more than one disorder must be present (Kraut and Madias 2001).

While acid–base disorders that result in a pH out of the normal range and incongruent movement of bicarbonate and p_{CO2} produce obvious indicators of a mixed acid–base disorder, many others are more subtle and difficult to detect. For example, one might assume that a pH in the physiologic range eliminates the possibility of an acid–base disorder; however, mixed acid–base disturbance can have either an additive effect or a neutralizing effect on pH. Two simultaneous conditions that move pH in the same direction, such as respiratory and metabolic acidosis, will generate a pH that is lower than either condition individually. However, two counterbalancing conditions, such as respiratory alkalosis and metabolic acidosis can produce a pH that is high, low, or in the normal range. The presence of an abnormal HCO_3^-, p_{CO2}, or movement of these two parameters in opposite directions in the presence of a pH that falls in the normal range is an important indication that the patient has a mixed

Table 67.2 Examples of mixed acid–base disturbances

Neutralizing effect on pH
   Respiratory alkalosis and metabolic acidosis
      Septic shock (Goodwin and Schaer 1989)
      Heat stroke (Schall 1980)
      Gastric dilatation-volvulus (Muir 1982)
      Liver disease (Cornelius and Rawlings 1981)
      Salicylate toxicity (Oehme 1986)
   Mixed metabolic acidosis and hypochloremic alkalosis
   (de Morais and Leiswitz 2005)
      Renal failure with vomiting
      Lactic acidosis with vomiting
      DKA with vomiting
      Bicarbonate administration (Robinson and Hardy 1988)

Additive effect on pH
   Respiratory acidosis and metabolic acidosis
      Cardiopulmonary arrest (Lippert et al. 1988)
      Pulmonary edema (Ware and Bonagura 1986)
      Gastric dilatation-volvulus (Muir 1982)
   Respiratory alkalosis metabolic alkalosis
      Heart failure and diuretic use (Adams and Polzin 1989)
      Gastric dilatation-volvulus (Adams and Polzin 1989)
      Canine Babesiosis (Leisewitz et al. 2001)
      Sepsis associated with Parvovirus
   Mixed metabolic disorders
   Hyperchloremic and high AG metabolic acidosis
      Renal failure (de Morais and Leiswitz 2005)
      Resolving DKA (de Morais and Leiswitz 2005)
      Severe Babesiosis (*B. canis rossi*) (Leisewitz et al. 2001)
   Mixed high anion gap metabolic acisosis
      Renal failure with DKA (de Morais and Leiswitz 2005)
      DKA with lactic acidosis (de Morais and Leiswitz 2005)

acid–base disorder in which neither disorder is dominant. In these cases, the primary acid–base disturbance can be determined using the rules above if we assume that a pH that is toward the alkaline part of the normal range is increased and a pH toward the acidic part of the normal range is low.

Other mixed acid–base disorders will masquerade as simple acid–base disturbances resulting in an abnormal pH with apparently appropriate changes in bicarbonate and p_{CO_2}. In these cases, careful evaluation of the normal pulmonary and renal compensatory mechanisms will reveal that secondary acid–base disturbances are lurking.

Physiology of pH buffering and pulmonary/renal compensation

Cellular machinery is exquisitely sensitive to H^+ concentration, and therefore, maintaining blood pH in a narrow range is essential for life. There are three interrelated physiologic systems that work to resist blood pH changes: buffers, the respiratory system, and the kidneys.

A buffer is a pair of molecules, an acid and its conjugate base, which can resist changes in the pH of a solution by releasing H^+ ions when pH increases (becomes more alkaline) and binding H^+ ions when pH decreases (more acidic) (Ganong 2007a). The blood buffering system is the first line of defense in maintaining a stable pH. While plasma proteins, phosphates, and hemoglobin all play a role in blood buffering, it is the carbonic acid/bicarbonate system that is of paramount importance (Rose and Post 2001a; Guyton and Hall 2006).

If we examine the reaction below, we see that bicarbonate, which is produced by the kidneys, binds with free H^+ to form carbonic acid. If more H^+ ions are added to the blood, more carbonic acid is formed and the equation is driven to the left. In the presence of carbonic anhydrase, CO_2 and water are formed. The lungs expel the CO_2 and H^+ ion is removed from the body (Ganong 2007c).

$$CO_2 + H_2O \Leftrightarrow H_2CO_3 \Leftrightarrow H^+ + HCO_3^-$$

When looking at this formula in the context of the body, it becomes apparent that if the amount of CO_2 in the body is decreased, as can occur with increased pulmonary ventilation, the equation is driven to the left. Thus, more H^+ combines with bicarbonate to form carbonic acid, which then dissociates into water and CO_2. The result is an increase in blood pH. On the other hand, if pulmonary ventilation is impaired, the clearance H^+ is slowed and the pH of the blood falls.

Although regulation of respiration is influenced by P_{CO_2} and H^+ receptors in the carotid and aortic bodies, it is H^+ receptors in the medulla that exert the greatest effect (Ganong 2007b). An increase in H^+ concentration increases ventilation, and the magnitude of response is directly proportionate to the increase. Therefore, metabolic acidosis stimulates respiration, causing a decrease in P_{CO_2} and a commensurate reduction in H^+. Metabolic alkalosis, with its decreased H^+ concentration, suppresses ventilation, increasing P_{CO_2}, and causes a rise in H^+ concentration.

Respiratory compensation is the name given to the mechanism by which changes in blood H^+ concentrations affects pulmonary ventilation. Although a critical part of the acid–base system, the respiratory compensation capacity is limited and cannot fully correct blood pH.

Although they lack the immediate impact of respiratory compensation, the kidneys also play an important role in the regulation of blood bicarbonate and H^+ concentrations. In the renal tubule, bicarbonate is reabsorbed in exchange for H^+ ions, and the rate is proportionate to arterial P_{CO_2} (Ganong 2007d). During respiratory acidosis, P_{CO_2} is high, and therefore, renal H^+ excretion and bicarbonate resorption are enhanced. This compensatory mechanism provides additional buffering capacity. In respiratory alkalosis, low P_{CO_2} inhibits H^+ excretion and bicarbonate resorption, allowing blood bicarbonate levels to decrease. This compensatory mechanism helps prevent large pH changes associated with acid–base abnormalities; however, this system is relatively slow and unable to respond in acute conditions.

Calculating the expected compensatory response associated with each of the simple acid–base disturbances is important in detecting the presence of a mixed acid–base imbalances and determining the secondary disorder. Mixed acid–base disorders are often uncovered when a compensatory response is greater or less than would normally be expected (Table 67.3). It should be noted that while renal and pulmonary compensation in acid–base disturbances have been documented in humans and dogs (de Morais and DiBartola 1991), studies suggest that cats may not be capable of the same compensatory responses (Ching et al. 1989; Lemieux et al. 1990). Therefore, the following formulas for calculating compensation should not be applied to cats.

Metabolic acidosis can be the result of renal or gastrointestinal loss of bicarbonate, failure of renal acid secretion, metabolic synthesis of organic acids (ketones, lactate), or ingestion of toxins and is the most common acid–base disorder detected in cats and dogs (Cornelius and Rawlings 1981). Biochemical changes associated with metabolic acidosis include a decreased pH, decreased bicarbonate, and a compensatory decrease in P_{CO_2}. Once maximal respiratory compensation has occurred, which can take up to 12 hours, the P_{CO_2} can be expected to

Table 67.3 Expected compensatory responses in simple acid/base disorders

Disturbance	Metabolic change	Compensation
Metabolic acidosis	Each 1 mEq/L ↓ HCO$_3$-	P$_{CO2}$ ↓ by 0.7 mmHg
Metabolic alkalosis	Each 1 mEq/L ↑ HCO$_3$-	P$_{CO2}$ ↑ by 0.7 mmHg
Resp. acidosis—acute	Each 1 mmHg ↑ P$_{CO2}$	HCO$_3$$^-$ ↑ by 0.15 mEq/L
Resp. acidosis—chronic	Each 1 mmHg ↑ P$_{CO2}$	HCO$_3$$^-$ ↑ by 0.35 mEq/L
Resp. alkalosis—acute	Each 1 mmHg ↓ P$_{CO2}$	HCO$_3$$^-$ ↓ by 0.25 mEq/L
Resp. alkalosis—chronic	Each 1 mmHg ↓ P$_{CO2}$	HCO$_3$$^-$ ↓ by 0.55 mEq/L

decrease approximately by 0.7 mmHg for each 1.0 mEq/L decrease in bicarbonate (de Morais and DiBartola 1991). The following formula can be used to determine the expected P$_{CO2}$.

$$\text{Expected P}_{CO2} = \text{normal P}_{CO2} - [(\text{normal HCO}_3 - \text{measured HCO}_3) * 0.7]$$

In humans, the maximal amount of compensation that can occur is 10 mmHg (Kraut and Madias 2001), although this value has not been determined in dogs. Patients with a metabolic acidosis and sufficient time for compensation should have a measured P$_{CO2}$ within 2 mmHg of the expected value (Adams and Polzin 1989). If measured P$_{CO2}$ is less, a concurrent respiratory alkalosis should be suspected. If measured P$_{CO2}$ is more than 2 mmHg above the expected P$_{CO2}$, then a concurrent respiratory acidosis should be suspected.

Metabolic alkalosis is characterized by increase in serum bicarbonate concentration, which occurs as a consequence of a loss of H$^+$ from the body or a gain in bicarbonate. Examples include vomiting, hyperadrenocorticism, and iatrogenic administration of alkalinizing agents. Biochemical changes associated with metabolic alkalosis include an increased pH, an increased HCO$_3$$^-$, and a compensatory increase in P$_{CO2}$. Once maximal respiratory compensation has occurred, which can take up to 12 hours, the P$_{CO2}$ can be expected to increase by approximately 0.7 mmHg for each 1.0 mEq/L increase in bicarbonate (Borkan et al. 1987; de Morais and DiBartola 1991). The following formula can be used to determine the compensated P$_{CO2}$:

$$\text{Expected P}_{CO2} = \text{normal P}_{CO2} + [(\text{measured HCO}_3 - \text{normal HCO}_3) * 0.7]$$

The degree that P$_{CO2}$ can increase is limited since hypoxemia will eventually stimulate ventilation. In humans, P$_{CO2}$ will only correct to 55 mmHg (Weinberger et al. 1989). Patients with a metabolic alkalosis and sufficient time for compensation should have a measured P$_{CO2}$ within 2 mmHg of the expected value. If measured P$_{CO2}$ is less, a concurrent respiratory alkalosis is likely. If measured P$_{CO2}$ is more than 2 mmHg above the expected

value, then a concurrent respiratory acidosis should be suspected.

Respiratory acidosis, caused by an increase in CO$_2$, is the result of hypoventilation (Ganong 2001) and divided into two phases: acute respiratory acidosis and chronic respiratory acidosis. The acute phase, which occurs within 15 minutes, has minimal effect on serum bicarbonate and is largely the result of non-bicarbonate buffers (de Morais and DiBartola 2000). The chronic phase takes up to 5 days and involves a renal compensatory increase in serum bicarbonate. In the acute phase, serum bicarbonate increases just 0.15 mEq/L for each 1 mmHg increase in P$_{CO2}$. Chronically, serum bicarbonate can be expected to increase 0.35 mEq/L for each 1 mmHg increase in P$_{CO2}$ (de Morais and DiBartola 1991). The following formulas can be used to determine the expected bicarbonate in both chronic and acute respiratory acidosis:

$$\text{Acute: Expected HCO}_3 = \text{normal HCO}_3 + (\text{measured P}_{CO2} - \text{normal P}_{CO2} * 0.15)$$

$$\text{Chronic: Expected HCO}_3 = \text{normal HCO}_3 + (\text{measured P}_{CO2} - \text{normal P}_{CO2} * 0.35)$$

When measured bicarbonate varies by more than 2 mEq/L from the expected, a mixed acid–base disorder should be suspected. Decreased bicarbonate measurements are associated with a concurrent metabolic acidosis, while increases are associated with a concurrent metabolic alkalosis.

Respiratory alkalosis is the result of hyperventilation and can be the result of hypoxemia, pulmonary disease, or stimulation of the central respiratory center. Biochemical changes include an increased pH, a decreased P$_{CO2}$, and a serum bicarbonate that decreases over time. Respiratory alkalosis is divided into two phases: acute and chronic. In the acute phase, the kidneys have had little time to react and serum bicarbonate decreases 0.25 mEq/L for each 1 mmHg decrease in P$_{CO2}$ (de Morais and DiBartola 1991). The chronic phase takes up to 5 days and renal compensatory mechanisms decrease serum bicarbonate 0.55 mEq/L for each 1 mmHg decrease in P$_{CO2}$ (Adams and Polzin 1989; de Morais and DiBartola 1991). The following formulas can be used to determine the expected bicarbonate in both chronic and acute respiratory alkalosis:

$$\text{Acute: Expected HCO}_3 = \text{normal HCO}_3$$
$$- [(\text{normal P}_{CO2} - \text{measured P}_{CO2} * 0.25)]$$

$$\text{Chronic: Expected HCO}_3 = \text{normal HCO}_3$$
$$- [(\text{normal P}_{CO2} - \text{measured P}_{CO2} * 0.55)]$$

When measured bicarbonate varies by more than 2 mEq/L from the expected, a concurrent mixed acid–base disorder should be suspected; however, it may be possible that equilibration has not yet occurred. Decreased bicarbonate measurements are associated with a concurrent metabolic acidosis while increases are associated with a concurrent metabolic alkalosis.

Mixed acid–base disorders involving two diseases that both cause a metabolic acidosis can be difficult to detect. Bicarbonate, pH, P_{CO2}, and metabolic compensation may seem consistent with a simple disorder. In most cases, these mixed disorders are diagnosed by the clinician using information obtained on the history, physical examination, and blood work. For example, a patient may have diabetic ketoacidosis, resulting in dehydration, decreased perfusion, and secondary lactic acidosis. In this example, a combination of routine blood work, urine analysis, and an inexpensive lactate meter would provide the clinician with sufficient information to diagnosis the two conditions. Other secondary conditions may be more difficult to detect. Therefore, in all cases in which a metabolic acidosis has been diagnosed, a combination of the anion gap and $Na+:Cl^-$ ratio should be performed.

Anion gap

Strictly speaking, there is no "anion gap"; total serum anions must equal serum cations, otherwise charges would not balance. Determining actual ion concentration would require measuring all serum cations (cationic proteins, calcium, magnesium, potassium, sodium) and all serum anions (anionic proteins, bicarbonate, chloride, phosphate, sulfate and organic ions). In reality, sodium and potassium are the only cations, and chloride and bicarbonate the only anions routinely measured. Therefore, if we replace the unmeasured anions with UA and unmeasured cations with UC, we would have the following equations:

$$Na^+ + K^+ + UC = Cl^- + HCO_3^- + UA$$
$$\text{Or}$$
$$(Na^+ + K^+) - (Cl^- + HCO_3^-) = UA - UC$$

Since the total unmeasured anions exceed the unmeasured cations, the anion gap is positive. Normal values for the dog have been reported in the range of 12–25 mEq/L (Polzin et al. 1982). Values for cats are likely to be similar.

Many substances in the body such as cationic amino acids and ammonium chloride are metabolized in the liver to hydrochloric acid (HCL). When the H^+ is titrated by bicarbonate, Cl^- remains and there is no change in the measured anions (HCO_3^- and Cl^-). Therefore, the anion gap is unaffected. In cases of acidosis caused by renal or gastrointestinal loss of bicarbonate, the associated cation, sodium, is also lost, resulting in no change in the anion gap. Over-production of organic acids (Emmett 2006), toxins or the loss of renal H^+ excreting ability as is seen in chronic renal failure (Kraut and Kurtz 2005) are usually associated with increases in the anion gap. Some find the mnemonic "KIL-U" an easy way to remember the causes of elevations in the ion gap: ketones, ingestion (ethylene glycol, ethanol, salicylates), lactate, uremia.

The utility of the anion gap is threefold. First, although the presence of a normal anion gap does not eliminate the possibility of a metabolic acidosis, finding an increase establishes its presence. Secondly, since only a limited number of conditions result in an increased anion gap, its calculation is useful in limiting the differential diagnosis (Kraut and Madias 2007). Lastly, the finding of a high anion gap in a patient with disease not normally associated with this finding (e.g., renal tubular acidosis) directs the clinician to look for another cause of the metabolic acidosis.

Caution must be exercised when applying the anion gap to patients with hypoalbuminemia or hypoproteinemia as albumin and serum proteins contribute significantly to the unmeasured anions (Hatherill et al. 2002; Kraut and Madias 2007). It has been estimated that a 1 g/dL decrease in serum albumin or protein concentration results in a 4.1 mEq/L or 2.5 mEq/L respective reductions in the anion gap (Constable and Stampfli 2005). Therefore, the following adjusted anion gap formulas can be used in patients with hypoalbuminemia and hypoproteinemia.

$$AG_{alb} = AG + 4.1 * (3.77 - [alb])$$
$$AG_{protein} = AG + 2.5 * (6.7 - [TP])$$

Chloride/sodium ratio

In the Stewart model of acid–base balance, pH is determined by P_{CO2}, weak acids (e.g., protein), and the strong ionic difference. Chloride is the most important strong anion, while sodium is the primary strong cation. As the strong ion difference falls (e.g., Cl^- increases), pH becomes increasingly acidic, while increases in the

Table 67.4 Cl⁻/Na⁺ ratio

Cl−/Na+ ratio	Normal AG	Increased AG
Decreased	Hyperchloremic acidosis	Hyperchloremic metabolic acidosis
Increased	Hypochloremic alkalosis	Hypochloremic metabolic alkalosis

strong ionic difference (e.g., Cl^- decreases) causes blood to become alkalotic. The contribution of electrolytes to acid–base balance can be estimated by the chloride/sodium ratio (Durward et al. 2001; Fletcher and Dhrampal 2003). While references ranges have not been established for companion animals, it has been suggested that values greater than 0.78 in dogs and 0.80 in cats are associated with hyperchloremic metabolic acidosis, while values less than 0.72 in dogs and 0.74 in cats are associated with hypochloremic alkalosis (Table 67.4) (de Morais and Leiswitz 2005). This information can be helpful when mixed metabolic disturbances are suspected (Table 67.2).

Treatment

The most important aspects in formulating a treatment plan are to evaluate the current pH, understand the underlying disturbances, and anticipate the effect of any treatments. In the case of counterbalancing disorders,

treating one disorder without addressing the other can have catastrophic effects (Adrogue 2006). Patients with disorders that have an additive effect on pH may require more intensive and aggressive intervention. The treatment of individual primary acid–base disorders is discussed in Chapter 66.

Conclusion

The clinician can use the systematic approach presented in this chapter to determine if a patient has a mixed acid–base disorder (Figure 67.1); however, no simple set of heuristics can determine the cause of the imbalance. Ultimately, it is the patient's history, physical examination, and blood work that provide the underlying causes of the mixed acid–base disturbance. Once these causes have been elucidated, a treatment plan can be formulated that takes into account potential side effects.

References

Adams, L. and D. Polzin (1989). Mixed acid base disorders. *Vet Clin N Am Small Anim Pract* **19**: 307–326.

Adrogue, H.J. (2006). Mixed acid-base disturbances. *J Nephrol* **19**(Suppl 9): S97–S103.

Bloom, S.A., V.J. Canzanello, et al. (1985). Spurious assessment of acid-base status due to dilutional effect of heparin. *Am J Med* **79**: 528–530.

Borkan, S., T.E. Northrup, et al. (1987). Renal response to metabolic alkalosis induced by isovolemic hemofiltration in the dog. *Kidney Int* **32**: 322–328.

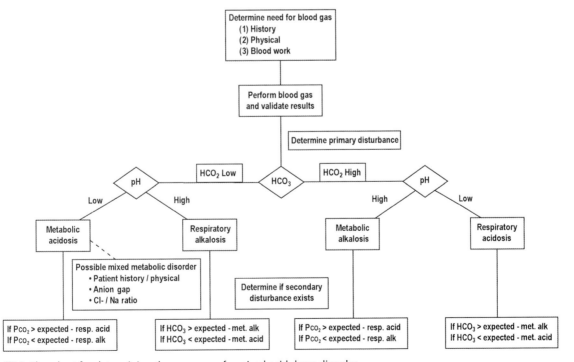

Figure 67.1 Flowchart for determining the presence of a mixed acid–base disorder.

Breen, P.H. (2001). Arterial blood gas and pH analysis. Clinical approach and interpretation. *Anesthesiol Clin N Am* **19**: 885–906.

Ching, S.V., M.J. Fettman, et al. (1989). The effect of chronic dietary acidification using ammonium chloride on acid-base and mineral metabolism in the adult cat. *J Nutr* **119**: 902–915.

Constable, P.D. and H.R. Stampfli (2005). Experimental determination of net protein charge and A(tot) and K(a) of nonvolatile buffers in canine plasma. *J Vet Intern Med* **19**: 507–514.

Cornelius, L.M. and C.A. Rawlings (1981). Arterial blood gas and acid-base values in dogs with various diseases and signs of disease. *J Am Vet Med Assoc* **178**: 992–995.

de Morais, H. and S. DiBartola (2000). Respiratory acid-base disorders. In: *Fluid Ther Small Anim Pract*, edited by S. DiBartola. Philadelphia, PA: WB Saunders, pp. 241–250.

de Morais, H. and S. DiBartola (1991). Ventilatory and metabolic compensation in dogs with acid-base disturbances. *J Vet Emerg Crit Care* **1**: 39–49.

de Morais, H.A. and A.L. Leiswitz (2005). Mixed acid base disorders. In: *Fluid, Electrolyte and Acid-Base Disorders in Small Animal Practice*, edited by S. DiBartola. Philadelphia, PA: WB Saunders, pp. 296–309.

Durward, A., S. Skellett, et al. (2001). The value of the chloride: sodium ratio in differentiating the aetiology of metabolic acidosis. *Intensive Care Med* **27**: 828–835.

Emmett, M. (2006). Anion-gap interpretation: the old and the new. *Nat Clin Pract Nephrol* **2**: 4–5.

Fletcher, S. and A. Dhrampal (2003). Acid-base balance and arterial blood gas analysis. *Surgery* **21**: 61–65.

Gambino, S.R. and H. Schreiber (1966). The measurement of CO_2 content with the autoanalyzer. A comparison with 3 standard methods and a description of a new method (alkalinization) for preventing loss of CO_2 from open cups. *Am J Clin Pathol* **45**: 406–411.

Ganong, W. (2001). Regulation of extracellular fluid compositiona and volume. In: *Review of Medical Physiology*. New York: Lange Medical Books, pp. 704–713.

Ganong, W. (2007a). The general and cellular basis of medical physiology. In: *Review of Medical Physiology*, edited by W. Ganong. Boston, MA: McGraw-Hill, pp. 1–50.

Ganong, W. (2007b). Regulation of respiration. In: *Review of Medical Physiology*. Boston, MA: McGraw-Hill, pp. 671–680.

Ganong, W. (2007c). Regulation of extracellular fluid compositiona and volume. In: *Review of Medical Physiology*. New York: Lange Medical Books, pp. 704–713.

Ganong, W. (2007d). *Regulation of Acid-Base*.

Goodwin, J.K. and M. Schaer (1989). Septic shock. *Vet Clin N Am Small Anim Pract* **19**: 1239–1258.

Guyton, A.C. and J.E. Hall (2006). Regulation of acid-base balance. In: *Textbook of Medical Physiology*. Philadelphia, PA: WB Saunders, pp. 383–401.

Hatherill, M., Z. Waggie, et al. (2002). Correction of the anion gap for albumin in order to detect occult tissue anions in shock. *Arch Dis Child* **87**: 526–529.

Kraut, J.A. and I. Kurtz (2005). Metabolic acidosis of CKD: diagnosis, clinical characteristics, and treatment. *Am J Kidney Dis* **45**: 978–993.

Kraut, J.A. and N.E. Madias (2001). Approach to patients with acid-base disorders. *Respir Care* **46**: 392–403.

Kraut, J.A. and N.E. Madias (2007). Serum anion gap: its uses and limitations in clinical medicine. *Clin J Am Soc Nephrol* **2**: 162–174.

Leisewitz, A.L., L.S. Jacobson, et al. (2001). The mixed acid-base disturbances of severe canine babesiosis. *J Vet Intern Med* **15**: 445–452.

Lemieux, G., C. Lemieux, et al. (1990). Metabolic characteristics of cat kidney: failure to adapt to metabolic acidosis. *Am J Physiol* **259**: R277–R281.

Lippert, A.C., A.T. Evans, et al. (1988). The effect of resuscitation technique and pre-arrest state of oxygenation on blood-gas values during cardiopulmonary resuscitation in dogs. *Vet Surg* **17**: 283–290.

Muir, W.W. (1982). Acid-base and electrolyte disturbances in dogs with gastric dilatation-volvulus. *J Am Vet Med Assoc* **181**: 229–231.

Oehme, F. (1986). Aspirin and acetaminophen. In: *Current Veterinary Therapy IX*, edited by R. Kirk. Philadelphia, PA: WB Saunders, pp. 188–190.

Polzin, D., J. Stevens, et al. (1982). Clinical evaluation of the anion gap in evaluation of acid-base disorders in dogs. *Compend Contin Educ Pract Vet* **4**: 102.

Robinson, E.P. and R.M. Hardy (1988). Clinical signs, diagnosis, and treatment of alkalemia in dogs: 20 cases (1982–1984). *J Am Vet Med Assoc* **192**: 943–949.

Rose, B.D. and T.W. Post (2001a). Acid base physiology. In: *Clinical Physiology of Acid-Base and Electrolyte Disorders*. New York: McGraw-Hill, pp. 299–324.

Rose, B.D. and T.W. Post (2001b). Regulation of acid-base balance. In: *Clinical Physiology of Acid-Base and Electrolyte Disorders*. New York: McGraw-Hill, pp. 325–371.

Schall, W. (1980). Heat stroke. In: *Current Veterinary Therapy VII*, edited by R. Kirk. Philadelphia, PA: WB Saunders, pp. 195–197.

Verwaerde, P., C. Malet, et al. (2002). The accuracy of the i-STAT portable analyser for measuring blood gases and pH in whole-blood samples from dogs. *Res Vet Sci* **73**: 71–75.

Ware, W. and J. Bonagura (1986). Pulmonary edema. In: *Canine and Feline Cardiology*, edited by P. Fox. New York: Churchill Livingstone, pp. 205–217.

Weinberger, S.E., R.M. Schwartzstein, et al. (1989). Hypercapnia. *N Engl J Med* **321**: 1223–1231.

Section 7

Systemic arterial hypertension

68

Systemic arterial hypertension

Scott Brown

The term systemic hypertension is held to be synonymous with sustained elevations of blood pressure (BP) and can generally be categorized into one of three types (Brown et al. 2007; Elliott and Watson 2009). *White-coat hypertension* is an elevation of BP caused by anxiety during the measurement process. *Secondary hypertension* is high BP concurrent with a clinical disease or condition known to cause hypertension or that is associated with administration of a therapeutic agent (e.g., parenteral fluids or drugs with vasoconstrictive or positive inotropic effects) that is known or suspected to cause an elevation of BP. Secondary hypertension may be associated with chronic kidney disease (CKD), hyperthyroidism, hyperadrenocorticism, diabetes mellitus, acute uremia, hyperaldosteronism, pheochromocytoma, and hypothyroidism. In cats, systemic hypertension is most commonly associated with CKD and hyperthyroidism, where prevalence rates approach 20–25% (Syme et al. 2002; Brown et al. 2007; Jepson et al. 2007). In dogs, CKD is also frequently associated with clinically important secondary hypertension.

A diagnosis of *idiopathic hypertension* is established when reliable BP measurements demonstrate a sustained BP elevation concurrent with normal hematology, biochemical panel, and urinalysis. While secondary hypertension remains the largest category of high BP in dogs and cats, idiopathic hypertension is more common than previously thought, accounting for approximately 18–20% of cases in cats (Maggio et al. 2000; Elliott et al. 2001). It is likely many of these animals have Stage I CKD, but this remains to be established. See Chapter 48 for explanation of the staging system for CKD proposed by the International Renal Interest Society (IRIS).

Isolated systolic or diastolic hypertension refers to occurrence of an elevated value for only systolic or only diastolic pressure. Such a finding may be artifactually produced by under- or over-estimation of the peak or trough of the BP curve by an indirect device. The presence of such an artifact should be considered whenever a very small (<20 mmHg) or large (>60 mmHg) pulse pressure is reported by an indirect device. True isolated hypertension of either type may represent white-coat, secondary, or idiopathic hypertension

Target-organ damage (TOD)

Systemic hypertension is problematic only because chronically sustained elevations of BP produce injury to tissues; the rationale for treatment of hypertension is to minimize or prevent this injury, which occurs in the kidney, eyes, brain, or cardiovascular system. Damage that results from the presence of sustained high BP is commonly referred to as end-organ or target-organ damage (TOD), and the presence of TOD is generally a strong indication favoring antihypertensive therapy.

In the kidney, TOD is generally manifest as an enhanced rate of decline of renal function, mortality, and/or proteinuria (Table 68.1) (Jacob et al. 2003; Brown et al. 2007; Syme et al. 2006; Jepson et al. 2007; Elliott and Watson 2009).

Magnitude of proteinuria should be assessed by measurement of urine protein/creatinine ratio or quantitative assessment of albuminuria as proteinuria is directly related to degree of elevation of BP and inversely related to efficacy of antihypertensive therapy in cats (Mathur et al. 2002; Jepson et al. 2007). Proteinuria is also related to degree of elevation of BP and to rate of decline of GFR in dogs (Finco 2004). Hypertension may be present in any stage of renal disease, as serum creatinine is not directly related to BP.

Nephrology and Urology of Small Animals. Edited by Joe Bartges and David J. Polzin. © 2011 Blackwell Publishing Ltd.

Table 68.1 Evidence of target organ damage (TOD) from systemic hypertension

Tissue	Hypertensive injury (TOD)	Clinical findings indicative of TOD	Diagnostic test(s) to identify TOD
Eye	Retinopathy	Acute onset of blindness Retinal detachment Intraocular hemorrhage Retinal vessel tortuosity or perivascular edema	Ophthalmic examination
Brain	Encephalopathy	Centrally localizing neurological signs (brain)	Neurological exam Magnetic resonance imaging or CT scan
Kidney	Progression of chronic kidney disease	Serial increases in serum creatinine concentration (decreases in GFR) Proteinuria	Serum creatinine and BUN Urinalysis with quantitative assessment of proteinuria GFR measurement
Heart and vessels	Left ventricular hypertrophy Cardiac failure	Left ventricular hypertrophy Gallop rhythm Arrhythmias Systolic murmur Evidence of cardiac failure Hemorrhage (e.g., epistaxis, stroke)	Auscultation Thoracic radiography Cardiac ultrasound Electrocardiogram

Ocular lesions are observed in many cats and dogs with hypertension, and while prevalence rates for ocular injury vary, it has been reported to be as high as 100% (Littman et al. 1988; Stiles et al. 1994; Maggio et al. 2000; Elliott et al. 2001). The syndrome is commonly termed hypertensive retinopathy and/or choroidopathy, and retinal detachment is the most commonly observed finding (Table 68.1). Acute onset of blindness from complete, bilateral exudative retinal detachment may be a presenting complaint in both species. Effective antihypertensive treatment can lead to retinal reattachment, but restoration of vision generally occurs in a minority of patients (Maggio et al. 2000).

Hypertensive encephalopathy (Bagley 2003) has been reported in dogs (Jacob et al. 2003) and cats (Littman 1994; Kyles et al. 1999; Maggio et al. 2000). Neurological signs have been reported to occur in nearly 1/2 of hypertensive cats (Littman 1994). This syndrome, in its early phases, is responsive to antihypertensive therapy (Brown et al. 2005). Observed clinical signs include lethargy, seizures, acute onset of altered mentation, altered behavior, disorientation, balance disturbances such as vestibular signs, head tilt, nystagmus, and focal neurological defects due to stroke-associated ischemia. Other CNS abnormalities, including hemorrhage and infarction are also observed in dogs and cats.

Cardiac changes present in hypertensive animals may include systolic murmurs and cardiac gallops and left ventricular hypertrophy (LVH) (Lesser et al. 1992). Although LVH may not be a risk factor for reduced sur-

vival time (Chetboul et al. 2003), effective antihypertensive therapy may reduce prevalence of LVH in affected cats (Snyder et al. 2001). Cardiac failure and other serious complications are infrequent but may occur. Animals with previously undiagnosed hypertension may unexpectedly develop signs of congestive heart failure after receiving fluid therapy. Epistaxis, presumably due to hypertension-induced vascular abnormalities, has been associated with systemic hypertension.

Selection of patients to screen for presence of hypertension

There are two clear indications for evaluating BP in a patient. First, BP should be measured in patients with clinical abnormalities consistent with TOD. A second indication for measurement of BP is presence of diseases or conditions casually associated with secondary hypertension as well as those being treated with pharmacological agents that may elevate BP. A thorough physical examination, including funduscopic evaluation, cardiac auscultation, and neurologic examination, should concurrently be performed in these at-risk populations to assess for TOD. While the positive relation between advancing age and prevalence of systemic hypertension is not as clear in animals as it is in people, conditions causing secondary hypertension are often more frequently observed in geriatric pets and it is prudent to routinely screen animals for the presence of these conditions (e.g.,

CKD and hyperthyroidism). At this time, there is no clear rationale for routine BP screening in animals that do not meet either of these criteria. In these patients, it would be expected that a higher proportion of elevated values are due to white-coat hypertension. If such screening is done, it should only be performed in older animals (e.g., ≥8 years of age) and results should be interpreted with an appreciation of the importance of excluding white-coat hypertension.

Measurement of systemic arterial BP

Diagnosis and management of hypertension in clinical patients should be based upon measurement of the patient's BP (Chapter 13). While it is critical for the veterinarian to fully appreciate the subtleties of BP measurement, it is generally preferred to have these measurements obtained by a skilled animal health technician who has been suitably trained. Acquiring expertise in the use of indirect BP measurement devices requires hours of training; experienced operators enhance the reliability of indirect measurement.

The BP may be affected by stress or anxiety associated with the measurement process (Brown et al. 2007). It is important for the measurement room to be quiet and that 5–10 minutes to be provided for the patient to acclimate to the room to reduce the likelihood of white-coat-effect hypertension (Belew et al. 1999). Many causes of measurement error will lead to an erroneously high value for BP. However, the minute-to-minute variability of BP, inconsistency of BP measuring devices, technical errors, transient dehydration, and parasympathetic overactivity all could lead to a falsely low value for BP.

The choice of device depends upon operator experience and preference. The cuff width should be 30–40% of the circumference at the chosen measurement site (Brown et al. 2007). Measurements may be taken on the antebrachium, brachium, tarsus, or tail. The position of the patient and cuff should be one that is well tolerated with the cuff at, or close to, the level of the right atrium. At least five consecutive, consistent indirect values should be obtained, the highest and lowest values discarded, and the remaining values averaged to produce the actual "measurement." Multiple measurements should be obtained, preferably separated by at least 24 hours, and these should always be accompanied by a thorough search for TOD and identification of conditions that may cause secondary hypertension.

A standard form for recording results of the BP measurement should be developed. The animal position and attitude, cuff size and site, and cuff site circumference (cm) should be carefully considered (ideally, these would also be noted in the animal record). All values obtained,

rationale for excluding values, the final (mean) result, and interpretation of the result by the veterinarian should be noted.

Treatment

The initial assessment of a patient suspected to have systemic hypertension should include recognizing conditions that may be contributing to an elevation of BP, identifying and characterizing TOD, and determining if there are any seemingly unrelated concurrent conditions that may complicate antihypertensive therapy. Because hypertension is often a silent, slowly progressive condition requiring vigilance and lifelong therapy, it is important to be absolutely certain about the diagnosis: a high BP measurement may represent idiopathic, secondary, or white-coat hypertension. Decisions to use antihypertensive drugs should be based on the integration of all clinically available information and a decision to treat, which may effectively mandate lifelong drug therapy and warrants periodic, judicious re-evaluation.

Use of BP staging to assess risk for future TOD

For treatment decisions, BP is categorized into stages on the basis of risk of developing subsequent TOD (Table 68.2).

While there are interbreed differences in BP in dogs and perhaps in cats, only the difference (20 mmHg higher values for each category) for Sight Hounds mandates separate categorization at this time (Cox et al. 1976; Bodey and Michell 1996). It is anticipated that publication of data in specific breeds of dogs and cats may justify further modification of this recommendation in the future.

In people, any reduction of BP that does not produce overt hypotension lowers the risk of TOD. Admittedly, this latter finding remains to be confirmed in dogs and cats, but the ACVIM Hypertension Consensus Panel

Table 68.2 Staging of blood pressure (BP; mmHg) in dogs and cats based on risk for future target-organ damage[a]

Systolic	Diastolic	Risk of future target organ damage	BP stage
<150	<95	None or minimal	N
150–159	95–99	Low	L
160–179	100–119	Moderate	M
≥180	≥120	High	H

[a]Where reliable measurements (see text) lead to different categories based on separate consideration of the patient's systolic and diastolic BP, the patient's BP stage should be taken as the higher risk.

(Brown et al. 2007) and IRIS (Elliott and Watson 2009) recommend that BP be categorized on the basis of risk of future TOD.

A BP below 150/95 mmHg, Stage N, should be interpreted as presenting minimal or no risk for TOD and antihypertensive therapy is not recommended. This level of BP also represents the treatment goal for antihypertensive therapy.

Decision to institute treatment

A decision to institute antihypertensive therapy should be based on reliable measurements of BP and proper staging. There are two exceptions: (1) patients with TOD consistent with hypertension that may rapidly progress (i.e., hypertensive retinopathy or encephalopathy) and (2) use of antihypertensive agents for another purpose, such as to reduce proteinuria in cats or dogs with CKD. In the first scenario, at least one reliable measurement should be obtained and withdrawal of medications should be considered after the initial crisis is resolved. In the second, it is preferred but not required to measure BP.

Some changes, such as LVH or hypertensive encephalopathy, may partially or wholly resolve with therapy. Antihypertensive therapy may reduce the incidence or delay the development of other abnormalities, such as hypertensive encephalopathy or choroidopathy. Antihypertensive therapy may slow disease progression in animals afflicted with CKD (Grauer et al. 2000; Brown et al. 2003). Most animals in this category, particularly those with TOD or secondary hypertension, are candidates for antihypertensive therapy. Others without TOD, particularly those with BP at the lower end of this range or those in which white-coat hypertension cannot be ruled out as the sole cause of the elevated BP, are generally not treated.

Some surveys of normal dogs and cats have reported values within or near the range of BP that comprise stage L. Further, it is likely that some animals in this category are exhibiting white-coat hypertension. The general consensus is that there is currently a paucity of data to support intervention when BP < 160/100 mmHg.

The rationale for treatment of patients in stage M is to limit future TOD, particularly in those animals with pre-existent TOD or secondary hypertension. While there is no general agreement, animals in stage M with idiopathic hypertension and no TOD are often not treated.

The rationale for treatment of patients with a high risk of TOD, stage H, is to limit the degree of TOD. While only extreme technical error or dramatic white-coat hypertension could produce such an elevated value for BP in a normal dog or cat, at least two measurement sessions should still be made to confirm the BP. The sole excep-

tion as noted above would be a patient in which rapidly progressive TOD, such as hypertensive retinopathy or encephalopathy, is already present. Animals in stage H with secondary or idiopathic hypertension are candidates to receive antihypertensive therapy and appropriate, disease-specific management of any conditions that might be causing secondary hypertension.

Antihypertensive therapy

As hypertension in dogs and cats is most often secondary (≥80% based on current data), antihypertensive drug therapy by itself is often not sufficient. Initial considerations should always include management of conditions likely to be causing secondary hypertension and treatment of TOD. Where possible, these considerations should be addressed with specific, targeted diagnostic and therapeutic regimens. Effective management of a condition causing secondary hypertension will lead to complete or partial resolution of the high BP in some, but not all, cases. Hypertension may remain or even worsen despite effective treatment of the primary condition (Ortega et al. 1996; Goy-Thollot et al. 2002; Brown et al. 2007).

Antihypertensive therapy must be individualized to the patient and its concurrent conditions. Regardless of the initial level of BP, the goal of therapy should be to maximally reduce the risk of TOD (Stage N: SBP < 150 and DBP < 95 mmHg). Certainly, a minimal goal of therapy is to achieve a reduction in stage of risk for TOD. Except in hypertensive crises (see below), this should be achieved with a gradual, persistent reduction of BP.

Although frequently recommended as an initial step in the pharmacological management of high BP, dietary salt restriction is controversial (Turner et al. 1990; Hansen et al. 1992; Greco et al. 1994; Buranakarl et al. 2004; Kirk et al. 2006), and available evidence suggests significant sodium restriction alone generally does not reduce BP and in fact activates the renin–angiotensin–aldosterone axis (Buranakarl et al. 2004) and may actually elevate BP in certain settings (Hansen et al. 1992; Greco et al. 1994). On the other hand, high salt intake may produce adverse consequences in some settings (Kirk et al. 2006), particularly in animals with CKD. Until more data are available, the selection of appropriate diet should be based on other patient-specific factors, such as underlying or concurrent diseases and palatability.

Once a decision is made to treat an animal with high BP, therapeutic intervention will almost always include a pharmacological agent. Angiotensin-converting enzyme inhibitors (ACEI) and calcium channel blockers (CCB) are the most widely used antihypertensive agents in

Table 68.3 Oral agents for routine antihypertensive therapy

Class	Drug (examples of trade name)	Usual oral dosage
Angiotensin converting enzyme inhibitor	Benazepril (Lotensin; Fortekor)	D: 0.5 mg/kg q 12–24 h C: 0.5 mg/kg q 12 h
	Enalapril (Vasotec; Enacard)	D: 0.5 mg/kg q 12–24 h C: 0.5 mg/kg q 24 h
Calcium channel blocker	Amlodipine (Norvasc)	D/C: 0.1–0.25 mg/kg q 24 h (up to 0.5 mg/kg in cats)
α_1 blocker	Prazosin (Minipress)	D: 0.5–2 mg/kg q 8–12 h C: 0.25–0.5 mg/cat q 24 h
	Phenoxybenazime (Dibenzyline)	D: 0.25 mg/kg q 8–12 hr or 0.5 mg/kg q 24 h C: 2.5 mg per cat q 8–12 hr or 0.5 mg/cat q 24 h
	Acepromazine (PromAce)	D/C: 0.5–2 mg/kg q8 h
Direct vasodilator	Hydralazine (Apresoline)	D: 0.5–2 mg/kg q 12 h (start at low end of range) C: 2.5 mg/cat q 12–24 h
Aldosterone antagonist	Spironolactone (Aldactone)	D/C: 1.0–2.0 mg/kg q 12 h
β Blocker	Propranolol (Inderal)	D: 0.2–1.0 mg/kg q 8 h (titrate to effect) C: 2.5–5 mg/cat q 8 h
	Atenolol (Tenormin)	D: 0.25–1.0 mg/kg q 12 h C: 6.25–12.5 mg/cat q 12 h
Thiazide diuretic	Hydrochlorothiazide (HydroDiuril)	D/C: 2–4 mg/kg q 12–24 h
Loop diuretic	Furosemide (Lasix)	D/C: 1–4 mg/kg q 8–24 h

D, dog; C, cat.

veterinary medicine. These agents produce renal vasodilation, which may be useful in hypertensive veterinary patients as they commonly have compromised kidney function.

Initial therapy is often ACEI in dogs and CCB in cats. The starting dose should be near the lower end of the recommended range (Table 68.3).

There is little rationale for starting at a lower dosage. If an antihypertensive agent of choice is only partially effective, the usual approach is to consider increasing the dosage or adding an additional drug. While not ideal, many veterinary patients with significant hypertension will require more than one agent. Combination therapy with ACEI and CCB at the lower end of the dosage range may be useful in cats where there is some evidence for a beneficial effect of ACEI in CKD (King et al. 2006) and an established antihypertensive efficacy for CCB (Elliott et al. 2001). Further, certain disease conditions may be best addressed with the addition of specific classes of agents to a CCB and/or ACEI, such as beta-blockers for hypertension-associated hyperthyroidism or alpha- and beta-blockers or surgical excision for pheochromocytomas, and aldosterone receptor blockers or surgical excision of adrenal tumors in animals with hypertension associated with hyperaldosteronism.

Client communication is important aspect of antihypertensive therapy. Before instituting therapy, the owner should appreciate that the goal of antihypertensive therapy is to prevent future adverse events, will not directly improve their pet's health, may be lifelong, and will require frequent re-evaluations.

Monitoring antihypertensive therapy

In general, hypertension is not an emergency, and 3–4 weeks should be allowed between dosage adjustments. There has been some concern about acute exacerbation of azotemia with ACEI, though this is an unusual complication and modest increases in serum creatinine concentration (<0.5 mg/dL) may occur and are generally tolerable. Nonetheless, a patient should be evaluated 3–14 days following any change in antihypertensive therapy. In unstable patients and those with IRIS stage III or IV CKD, this recheck should be conducted in a shorter timeframe, perhaps 3–7 days. Patients deemed to be hypertensive emergencies (see below) and hospitalized patients, particularly those receiving fluid therapy or pharmacological agents with cardiovascular effects, should be assessed daily. The purpose of these short-term assessment is to determine if there are any unexpected (e.g., new or worsening TOD) or adverse (e.g., marked worsening of azotemia or systemic hypotension) findings. A BP < 120/60 mmHg combined with clinical findings of weakness, syncope, and/or marked tachycardia indicates systemic hypotension and therapy should be adjusted accordingly.

Re-evaluation at 1–4 month intervals depending on stability (more frequent if BP or other conditions are unstable) and level of elevation (more frequent if BP remains > 180 mmHg) is appropriate. Follow-up evaluations, which are employed to assess efficacy of therapy and make adjustments if appropriate, should include measurement of BP, serum creatinine concentration, urinalysis with quantitative assessment of proteinuria, funduscopic examination, and other specific assessments depending on the individual circumstances (e.g., TOD, causes of secondary hypertension, and concurrent conditions) of the patient. A key predictive parameter for antihypertensive efficacy is the effect of therapy on the magnitude of proteinuria (Syme et al. 2006), and a benefit is predicted if the antihypertensive regimen used is antiproteinuric (e.g., reduces urine protein/creatinine by >50%). The frequency and nature of re-evaluations will vary depending on the BP risk stage, stability of BP, other aspects of the health of the patient, and frequency of dosage adjustment to antihypertensive therapy. Since signs of progression of TOD can be subtle, BP should be closely monitored over time in patients receiving antihypertensive therapy, even when hypertension is seemingly well-controlled.

Emergency treatment of hypertensive crises

Hypertension generally damages tissues by a slow, insidious process and is rarely an urgent situation. However, emergency antihypertensive therapy may be indicated when there is TOD likely to produce significant permanent abnormalities without rapid lowering of BP (i.e., hypertensive neurological and/or ocular injury) if the degree of BP elevation places the patient in the moderate or high risk category (i.e., systolic BP > 160 mmHg) (Elliott et al. 2001; Jacob et al. 2003). Animals with systolic BP of 140–159 mmHg that exhibit otherwise unexplained ocular or neurological damage that is potentially attributable to hypertensive, a short-term (3–7 day) trial of antihypertensive therapy can be cautiously employed. A decision to use antihypertensive therapy should be accompanied by identification and management of conditions that may complicate therapy, generally by causing secondary hypertension.

If a decision is made to treat an animal with high BP, therapeutic intervention will generally be with a parenteral agent such as hydralazine or an oral calcium channel blocker (Table 68.4) (Elliott et al. 2001).

If parenteral medications are used, continuous BP monitoring by arterial catheterization is recommended. Many clinicians prefer oral CCB, particularly in cats, because they generally decrease BP in severely hypertensive animals, regardless of primary disease. Amlodipine, for example, generally reduces BP by 25–50 mmHg in hypertensive cats within 4 hours of oral administration and poses limited risk of causing hypotension. If an oral CCB is used, it may be appropriate to send the animal home to reduce stress associated with hospitalization and re-evaluate in 24–72 hours.

Table 68.4 Agents for managing hypertensive crises (emergency therapy)

Class	Drug (examples of trade name)	Usual dosage and route of administration
Angiotensin-converting enzyme inhibitor	Enalaprilat (Vasotec IV)	0.2 mg/kg IV, repeated q1–2 h as needed (D/C)
Beta blocker	Esmolol (Brevibloc)	50–75 μg/kg/min IV by constant rate infusion (D)
Calcium channel blocker[a]	Amlodipine (Norvasc)	0.25–0.5 mg/kg orally q24 h (D/C)
Direct vasodilator[a]	Hydralazine (Apresoline)	0.2 mg/kg IV or IM, repeated q2 h as needed (D/C)
Direct vasodilator	Nitroprusside (Nipride, Nitropress)	1 μg/kg/min IV by constant rate infusion, with incremental increases of 1 μg/kg/min every 5 min, up to 10 μg/kg/min (D)
Mixed adrenergic blocker (primarily beta)	Labetalol (Trandate)	0.25 mg/kg IV over 2 min, repeated up to a total dose of 3.75 mg/kg in first hour followed by constant rate infusion of 25 μg/kg/min (D)

D, dog; C, cat.
[a] Most frequently employed agents.

References

Bagley, R.S. (2003). The brain as a target organ. In: *Essential Facts of Blood Pressure in Dogs and Cats*, edited by B. Egner, A. Carr, and S. Brown. Babenhausen, Germany: Vet Verlag, pp. 129–139.

Belew, A.M., T. Barlett, et al. (1999). Evaluation of the white-coat effect in cats. *J Vet Intern Med* **13**: 134–142.

Bodey, A.R. and A.R. Michell (1996). Epidemiological study of blood pressure in domestic dogs. *J Small Anim Pract* **37**: 116–125.

Brown, C.A., J.S. Munday, et al. (2005). Hypertensive encephalopathy in cats with reduced renal function. *Vet Pathol* **42**: 642–649.

Brown, S., C. Atkins, et al. (2007). Guidelines for the identification, evaluation, and management of systemic hypertension in dogs and cats. *J Vet Intern Med* **21**: 542–558.

Brown, S.A., D.R. Finco, et al. (2003). Evaluation of the effects of inhibition of angiotensin converting enzyme with enalapril in dogs with induced chronic renal insufficiency. *Am J Vet Res* **64**: 321–327.

Buranakarl, C., S. Mathur, et al. (2004). Effects of dietary sodium chloride intake on renal function and blood pressure in cats with normal and reduced renal function. *Am J Vet Res* **65**: 620–627.

Chetboul, V., H.P. Lefebvre, et al. (2003). Spontaneous feline hypertension: clinical and echocardiographic abnormalities, and survival rate. *J Vet Intern Med* **17**: 89–95.

Cox, R.H., L.H. Peterson, et al. (1976). Comparison of arterial hemodynamics in the mongrel dog and the racing greyhound. *Am J Physiol* **230**: 211–218.

Elliott, J., P.J. Barber, et al. (2001). Feline hypertension: clinical findings and response to antihypertensive treatment in 30 cases. *J Small Anim Pract* **42**: 122–129.

Elliott, J. and A.D.J. Watson (2009). Chronic kidney disease: staging and management. In: *Current Veterinary Therapy XIV*, edited by J.D. Bonagura and D.C. Twedt. St. Louis, MO: Elsevier Saunders, pp. 883–892.

Finco, D.R. (2004). Association of systemic hypertension with renal injury in dogs with induced renal failure. *J Vet Int Med* **18**: 289–294.

Goy-Thollot, I., D. Pechereau, et al. (2002). Investigation of the role of aldosterone in hypertension associated with spontaneous pituitary-dependent hyperadrenocorticism in dogs. *J Small Anim Pract* **43**: 489–492.

Grauer, G., D. Greco, et al. (2000). Effects of enalapril treatment versus placebo as a treatment for canine idiopathic glomerulonephritis. *J Vet Intern Med* **14**: 526–533.

Greco, D.S., G.E. Lees, et al. (1994). Effects of dietary sodium intake on blood pressure measurements in partially nephrectomized dogs. *Am J Vet Res* **55**: 160–165.

Hansen, B., S.P. DiBartola, et al. (1992). Clinical and metabolic findings in dogs with chronic renal failure fed two diets. *Am J Vet Res* **53**: 326–334.

Jacob, F., D.J. Polzin, et al. (2003). Association between initial systolic blood pressure and risk of developing a uremic crisis or of dying in dogs with chronic renal failure. *J Am Vet Med Assoc* **222**: 322–329.

Jepson, R.E., J. Elliott, et al. (2007). Effect of control of systolic blood pressure on survival in cats with systemic hypertension. *J Vet Intern Med* **21**: 402–409.

King, J.N., D.A. Gunn-Moore, et al. (2006). Tolerability and efficacy of benazepril in cats with chronic kidney disease. *J Vet Intern Med* **20**: 1054–1064.

Kirk, C.A., D.E. Jewell, et al. (2006). Effects of sodium chloride on selected parameters in cats. *Vet Ther* **7**: 333–346.

Kyles, A.E., C.R. Gregory, et al. (1999). Management of hypertension controls postoperative neurologic disorders after renal transplantation in cats. *Vet Surg* **28**: 436–441.

Lesser, M., P.R. Fox, et al. (1992). Assessment of hypertension in 40 cats with left ventricular hypertrophy by Doppler-shift sphygmomanometry. *J Small Anim Prac* **33**: 55–58.

Littman, M.P. (1994). Spontaneous systemic hypertension in 24 cats. *J Vet Intern Med* **8**: 79–86.

Littman, M.P., J.L. Robertson, et al. (1988). Spontaneous systemic hypertension in dogs: five cases (1981–1983). *J Am Vet Med Assoc* **193**: 486–494.

Maggio, F., T.C. DeFrancesco, et al. (2000). Ocular lesions associated with systemic hypertension in cats: 69 cases (1985–1998). *J Am Vet Med Assoc* **217**: 695–702.

Mathur, S., H. Syme, et al. (2002). Effects of the calcium channel antagonist amlodipine in cats with surgically induced hypertensive renal insufficiency. *Am J Vet Res* **63**: 833–839.

Ortega, T.M., E.C. Feldman, et al. (1996). Systemic arterial blood pressure and urine protein/creatinine ratio in dogs with hyperadrenocorticism. *J Am Vet Med Assoc* **209**: 1724–1729.

Snyder, P.S., D. Sadek, et al. (2001). Effect of amlodipine on echocardiographic variables in cats with systemic hypertension. *J Vet Intern Med* **15**: 52–56.

Stiles, J., D.J. Polzin, et al. (1994). The prevalence of retinopathy in cats with systemic hypertension and chronic renal failure or hyperthyroidism. *J Am Anim Hosp Assoc* **30**: 564–572.

Syme, H.M., P.J. Barer, et al. (2002). Prevalence of systolic hypertension in cats with chronic renal failure at initial evaluation. *J Am Vet Med Assoc* **220**: 1799–1804.

Syme, H.M., P.J. Markwell, et al. (2006). Survival of cats with naturally occurring chronic renal failure is related to severity of proteinuria. *J Vet Int Med* **20**: 528–535.

Turner, J.L., J.D. Brogdon, et al. (1990). Idiopathic hypertension in a cat with secondary hypertensive retinopathy associated with a high-salt diet. *J Am Anim Hosp Assoc* **26**: 647–651.

Section 8

Upper and lower urinary tract disorders

69

Canine and feline urolithiasis: diagnosis, treatment, and prevention

Jody P. Lulich, Carl A. Osborne, and Hasan Albasan

Urolithiasis is a general term referring to causes and effects of stones anywhere in the urinary tract. Urolithiasis should not be viewed conceptually as a single disease with a single cause but rather as sequelae of multiple interacting underlying abnormalities. Thus, the syndrome of urolithiasis may be defined as the occurrence of familial, congenital, and acquired pathophysiological factors that, in combination, progressively increase the risk of precipitation of excretory metabolites in urine to form stones (i.e., uroliths).

Anatomy of a stone

The term *urolith* is derived from the Greek word *uro* meaning urine and *lith* meaning stone. Unlike the gastrointestinal tract, solids that form in the urinary tract are abnormal because the urinary system is designed to dispose of the body's wastes in the form of a liquid. Under less than optimal conditions, some wastes, especially minerals, precipitate out of solution to form crystals. If these crystallized minerals are retained in the urinary system, they may grow and aggregate to form stones.

A crystal that forms within the urinary system may be viewed as a microlith; however, crystalluria (microlithura) is not synonymous with formation of macroliths (uroliths) and the clinical signs associated with them. Nor is crystalluria irrefutable evidence of a stone-forming tendency. In fact, crystalluria occurring in individuals with anatomically and functionally normal urinary tracts is often harmless and clinically unimportant. Identification of crystals in such individuals does

not justify therapy. On the other hand, detection of some types of abnormal crystals or aggregates of crystals commonly observed in healthy individuals may be of diagnostic, prognostic, and therapeutic significance (Lulich and Osborne 2009). For example, ammonium urate crystalluria may be indicative of portovascular disorders or primary hepatic disease.

A macroscopic urolith is primarily composed of one or more crystallized biogenic minerals in combination with relatively small quantities of organic matrix. Although one mineral usually predominates, composition of many uroliths is mixed. Combinations of minerals may be unevenly mixed throughout the urolith or they may be deposited in layers (laminations). Each urolith may contain a nidus, stone, shell, and surface crystals (Figure 69.1). The Minnesota Urolith Center uses the following terminology when reporting the results of urolith analysis (Lulich and Osborne 2009). We define the *nidus* or *nucleus* of a urolith as an area of obvious initiation of urolith growth. The term *stone* refers to the major body of the urolith. The term *shell* designates a layer of precipitated material that completely surrounds the body of the stone. The term *surface crystals* is used to describe an incomplete covering of the outermost surface of the urolith. In our studies, a urolith without a nidus or shell of different composition, which contains 70% or more of one type of mineral, is identified by that mineral. A urolith with less than 70% of one mineral is identified as a "*mixed*" urolith. A urolith with a nidus of one composition with one or more surrounding layers of different mineral composition from the nidus is called a "compound" urolith (Figure 69.1).

Nephrology and Urology of Small Animals. Edited by Joe Bartges and David J. Polzin. © 2011 Blackwell Publishing Ltd.

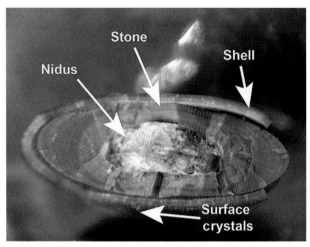

Figure 69.1 Anatomy of a compound urate stone with a nidus composed of struvite and a shell of calcium *oxalate monohydrate*.

Table 69.1 Comparing the ability survey radiography and ultrasonography to reveal urolith features

Urolith feature	Survey radiography	Ultrasonography
Radio-opacity	++++	−
Variations in Radio-opacity	+++	−
Shape	+++	+
Surface contour	+++	−
Diameter	+++	+++
Number	+ to +++	+ to ++
Location		
Kidney	+++	+++
Ureter	+++	+
Bladder	+++	++++
Urethra	+++	+

Urolith diagnosis

Uroliths represent one of the most common causes for lower urinary tract signs of disease (dysuria, inappropriate urination, hematuria, and pollakiuria). In contrast, clinical signs associated with upper tract uroliths are often silent, but should always be included in diagnostic differential lists for dogs and cats with kidney disease and persistent hematuria without signs of lower urinary tract disease.

Medical imaging is the cornerstone of urolith detection (Chapters 15, 16, and 17). The primary objective in performing radiographic or ultrasonographic evaluation is to verify urolith presence, location, number, size, density, and shape. In our experience survey radiography provides the most useful information for radio-opaque stones and the double contrast cystogram for radiolucent stones. Ultrasonography is a very sensitive method of detection, but does not provide sufficient information when urolith characteristics (size, shape, radio-opacity, number, etc.) are needed to select appropriate therapy (Table 69.1).

Knowledge of urolith composition is important because contemporary methods of management are primarily based on knowing this information. Several types of uroliths are commonly recognized in cats and dogs (Figures 69.2 and 69.3).

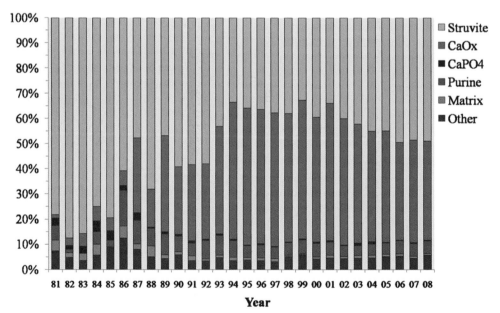

Figure 69.2 Changes in the prevalence of uroliths in cats between 1981 and 2009 (*n* = 106,194 submissions).

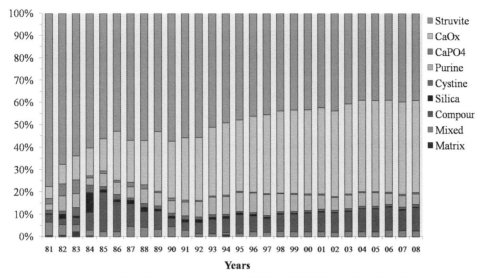

Figure 69.3 Changes in the prevalence of uroliths in dogs between 1981 and 2009 (*n* = 393,688 submissions).

When predicting mineral composition of uroliths, many factors are used (Tables 69.2–69.4) prior to determination by quantitative mineral analysis.

Although many use crystal identification as the primary method of predicting composition, crystalluria is not a consistent feature of urinalysis in dogs and cats with uroliths. For example, in one study of 30 cases of struvite urocystoliths in cats, struvite crystals were only detected in 17 patients (Osborne et al. 1990). Predicting mineral composition from survey radiographs offers many advantages because multiple pieces of information (e.g., radio-opacity, uniformity of radio-opacity,

Table 69.2

Mineral type			Predictors	
	Urine pH	Crystal appearance	Urine culture	Serum abnormalities
Magnesium ammonium phosphate	Neutral to alkaline	Four- to six-sided colorless prisms	Urease-producing bacteria *(Staphylococcus, Proteus, Enterococcus, Mycoplasma)*	None
Calcium oxalate	Acid to neutral	Dihydrate salt, colorless envelope, or octahedral shape; salt; small, monohydrate salt-spindles or dumbbell shape	Negative	Occasional hypercalcemia
Urate	Acid to neutral	Yellow-brown amorphous shapes or sphericals (ammonium urate)	Negative	Low-urea nitrogen and serum albumin in dogs with hepatic shunts
Calcium phosphate	Alkaline to neutral (brushite forms in acidic urine)	Amorphous, or long thin prisms	Negative	Occasional hypercalcemia
Cystine	Acid to neutral	Flat colorless, hexagonal plates	Negative	None
Silica	Acid to neutral	None observed	Negative	None

Table 69.3 Predicting mineral composition of canine uroliths based on radiographic appearance

Mineral	Radiographic opacity compared to soft tissue	Surface contour	Shape	Usual number	Approximate size
CaOx monohydrate	+++ to ++++	Smooth	Commonly round	20	2–7 mm
CaOx dihydrate	+++ to ++++	Rough	Rosette	>5, few large single	1–15 mm
Sterile MAP	++ to +++	Irregular, few smooth	Round to ovoid	1 to 3	5–15 mm
Infection MAP	+ to +++	Smooth to slightly rough	Round to faceted or pryamidal	>4 to many	4 to >20 mm
Urate	− to ++	Smooth	Round to oval	Few or too numerous to count	1–15 mm
CaP	+++ to ++++	Smooth	Round to cuboidal	Many, some few	2–6 mm
Cystine	− to +++	Smooth to bosselated	Round	Many to few	2–10 mm
Silica	++ to ++++	Smooth	Radiating spokes	One or many	2–10 mm
Xanthine	− to +	Smooth	Round to ovoid	Few to many	1–4 mm

CaOx, calcium oxalate; CaP, calcium phosphate; MAP, magnesium ammonium phosphate.

Table 69.4 Predicting mineral composition of feline uroliths based on radiographic appearance

Mineral	Radiographic opacity compared to soft tissue	Surface contour	Shape	Usual number	Approximate size
CaOx monohydrate	+++ to ++++	Smooth, but occasionally bosselated	Commonly round, but also rosette	>5	1–5 mm
CaOx dihydrate	+++ to ++++	Rough to smooth	Rosettes	>3	1–7 mm
Sterile MAP	++ to +++	Slightly rough	Round or discoid	Usually, 1–3, occassionally, many	3–10 mm
Infection MAP	+ to +++	Smooth to slightly rough	Round to faceted	Few to many	2 to >7 mm
Urate	− to ++	Smooth	Round to ovoid	Usually, 1, but up to 5	2–10 mm
CaP	+++ to ++++	Rough	Too rare to comment	Too rare to comment	1–4 mm
Cystine	− to +++	Rough	Round	Many, but some with few	1–4 mm
Silica	++ to ++++	Too rare to comment	Too rare to comment	Too rare to comment	1–4 mm
Xanthine	− to +	Smooth	Round to ovoid	1–3	1–5 mm

CaOx, calcium oxalate; CaP, calcium phosphate; MAP, magnesium ammonium phosphate.

shape, and surface contour) are processed from a single test (Tables 69.3 and 69.4). Although ultrasonography is gaining in popularity as a sensitive and safe method to detect uroliths, the information obtained should be considered complementary to survey radiology instead of a replacement. Small uroliths can also be retrieved from the urinary bladder for analysis without surgical intervention (Table 69.5) (Lulich and Osborne 1992). Urolith dissolution and prevention protocols devised on the basis of their quantitative mineral analysis typically provide the most consistent therapeutic results.

Clinical consequences of uroliths

Uroliths may spontaneously pass through various parts of the urinary tract, spontaneously dissolve, continue to grow, or become inactive (no growth occurs). Not all persistent uroliths are associated with clinical signs. In our experience, most inactive uroliths are not associated with urinary tract infection (UTI). Nonetheless, if uroliths remain in the urinary tract, dysuria, UTI, partial or total urinary obstruction, and polyp formation are potential sequelae.

UTI is common in dogs with urolithiasis. In most instances, UTI is the cause of struvite urolith formation in dogs and precedes stone formation. Once infection-induced struvite uroliths have formed, infected stones may contribute to the persistence and spread of infection to other portions of the urinary tract. In turn, presence of other urolith types is a risk factor for UTI. Factors contributing to increased risk of UTI include traumatic disruption of the mucosal lining of the urinary bladder, incomplete urine voiding, and sequestration of microorganisms in stones. Infections with urease-producing bacteria can result in deposition of magnesium ammonium phosphate on the surface of other urolith types, confounding diagnostic and management efforts to resolve the initial lithogenic events that are ultimately responsible for disease.

Polyp formation has been documented in several cases of dogs with urocystoliths. The events promoting polyp formation are unknown; however, it is logical to assume that chronic irritation to the urinary bladder mucosa and bacterial infection contributes to mucosal hyperplasia. Although, polyps have been routinely managed surgically, inflammatory polyps have also spontaneously regressed following eradication of uroliths and urinary infection.

Small uroliths located in the urinary bladder commonly pass into the urethra during the voiding phase of micturition. Uroliths whose diameter is slightly larger than the dilated proximal urethral lumen can become lodged in the urethra. Uroliths associated with complete and persistent obstruction affecting both kidneys results in uremia. Complete obstruction to urine outflow associated with UTI may result in rapid destruction of renal parenchyma and septicemia. If treatment is not provided, death can be expected to occur within 2–4 days.

Urolith management

Managing urolith removal

For decades, treatment of patients with uroliths has been the province of the surgeon; however, within the past 10 years, a variety of nonsurgical protocols have been developed to eradicate uroliths from the urinary tract (Table 69.5). The type of management selected will vary with the characteristics of the urolith (composition, size, contour, and location), the effects of the urolith on the patient, and the veterinarian's familiarity with available procedures (Tables 69.5–69.13).

Managing urethral obstruction

Once uroliths become lodged in the urethra, it is unlikely that they can be nonsurgically removed by antegrade voiding hydropropulsion. (Lulich et al. 1993) However, lithotripsy can be used to break the urethrolith into fragments small enough to pass through the urethra (Bevan and Lulich 2008; Lulich and Osborne 2009). To avoid urethral surgery when lithotripsy is not available, flushing urethroliths back into the bladder lumen by retrograde urohydropropulsion can, with a few exceptions, restore urethral patency (Osborne et al. 1999). The efficacy of this technique is dependent on dilating the portion of the urethral lumen containing urethroliths with fluid under pressure. To be consistently successful, one must be familiar with all aspects of the technique (Table 69.13).

Managing ureteral obstruction

Upper tract uroliths pose unique management problems in part because most are composed of calcium oxalate (Kyles et al. 2005; Lekcharoensuk et al. 2005). Medical protocols that will promote dissolution of calcium oxalate uroliths have not yet been developed. Difficulty in managing ureteroliths is magnified in cats because ureteral surgery is associated with significant risks, especially irreparable damage to the ureters and kidneys (Kyles et al. 2005). For these reasons, we recommend

Table 69.5 Methods of urolith removal

	Method	Suitable application	Considerations
Least invasive	Spontaneous voiding	Small (<3–5mm), asymptomatic urocystoliths with a relatively slow growth rate (i.e., calcium oxalate, calcium phosphate, uric acid) in female patients	Patients with uroliths larger than the urethral lumen may develop urethral obstruction Concomitant UTI should be eradicated
	Medical dissolution	Sterile struvite (Table 69.6), infection-induced struvite (Table 69.7), allopurinol-induced xanthine (Table 69.8), uric acid (Table 69.9), and cystine (Table 69.10) stones are amenable to medication dissolution.	Sterile struvite and allopurinol-induced xanthine uroliths dissolve within weeks Large infection-induced struvite stones may take 2–3 months to dissolve Stones in kidney require longer dissolution time than stones in the bladder Urethral obstruction is uncommon during dissolution of struvite stones for the following reasons: (1) Struvite uroliths commonly occur in females. (2) The wide urethra of females is less likely to obstruction. (3) Bacteria infection promoting dysuria, which may promote urolith movement into the urethral, is easily controlled with appropriate antimicobic administration.
Most invasive	Catheter retrieval (Table 69.11)	To retrieve small urocystoliths (<3 mm) for quantitative mineral analysis	Can be performed without anesthesia
	Voiding urohydropropulsion (VUH-Table 69.12)	To evacuate small to moderate size (<5–7 mm) urocystoliths of any composition	Not suitable for male cats unless they have a perineal urethrostomy Not suitable for patients with a urethral obstruction Not ideal for patients that have recently undergone bladder surgery Eradicate urinary infection prior to performing VUH.
	Stone basket retrieval	Urocystoliths smaller than (<5–7 mm) the distended diameter of the urethra	Performed during cystoscopy
	Urolith evacuators	Small urocystoliths or urolith fragments following lithotripsy in large female dogs	Most evacuators are designed to fit only the sheath of human cystoscopes. Can remove urolith fragments in large dogs too heavy to lift for voiding urohydropropulsion
	Intracorporeal lithotripsy	Urocystoliths in female dogs and cats and urethroliths in male dogs.	Performed during cystoscopy The flexibility of probes for laser lithotripsy permit fragmentation of urocystoliths in male dogs The urethra of the male cat will rarely accommodate cystoscopy equipment to perform lithotripsy Large hard uroliths (calcium oxalate monohydrate) in male dogs requires considerably longer times to fragment
	Extracorporeal shock wave lithotripsy (ESWL)	Ureteroliths and nephroliths in dogs	Uroliths in the renal pelvis are easier to fragment than ureteroliths The ability to perform ESWL without damaging feline kidney is controversial-newer generation lithotriptors may prove safer
Most invasive	Laparoscopic assisted cystotomy	Urocystoliths in dogs	Requires training in cystoscopy and laparoscopic surgery
	Cystotomy/ urethrotomy/ urethrostomy	Urocystoliths or uroliths lodged in the urethra	Consider retrograde urohydropropulsion of urethroliths prior to urethrotomy or urethrostomy Cystotomy—failure to remove all uroliths in 15–20% of cases
	Ureterotomy/ ureteroneocystotomy/ ureteroneoureterotomy	Clinically active ureteroliths	High degree of surgical skill required when performed on cats Surgery performed on dilated ureters has been associated with greater success than normal-sized ureters
	Pyelotomy/ nephrotomy	Nephroliths or ureteroliths flushed into the kidney	Some reduction in kidney function should be anticipated following surgery Difficult to locate some stones in renal pelvis

Table 69.6 Dissolution of sterile struvite uroliths

Diagnostic plan
  1. Perform appropriate diagnostic studies, including urinalysis (e.g., pH > 6.5, MAP crystalluria), diagnostic radiography (marginal to obvious radio-opaque urolith), and urine culture (infection-induced struvite uroliths are commonly caused by Staphyloccal species of bacteria), supporting the diagnosis of sterile MAP uroliths.
  2. Determine mineral composition of voided or retrieved uroliths. If unavailable, predict mineral composition by evaluating clinical data (Tables 69.2–69.4).

Therapeutic plan
  1. Consider mechanical removal (Table 69.5) if uroliths obstructing urine flow cannot be dislodged or if patients with a high risk of urine outflow obstruction cannot be monitored.
  2. Initiate therapy with a diet designed to dissolve magnesium ammonium phosphate uroliths (e.g., Hills Prescription diet s/d). No other food, supplements, or treats should be fed. Continue dietary therapy 1 month after radiographically detected dissolution (expected dissolution time = 3 to 5 weeks).

Plan to monitor efficacy of therapy
  1. Evaluate serial urinalyses. Urine pH should be acidic, urine specific gravity should be low (<1.015 in dog and <1.035 in cat (lower if using the canned food)), and struvite crystalluria should be absent.
  2. Continue calculolytic diet therapy for at least 1 month after survey radiographic disappearance of uroliths. The rationale is to provide therapy of adequate duration to dissolve small uroliths that cannot be detected by survey radiography (uroliths < 3 mm in diameter).
  3. If uroliths increase in size during dietary management or do not begin to decrease in size after approximately 2–4 weeks of appropriate medical management, alternative methods of removal should be considered. Difficulty in inducing complete dissolution of uroliths by creating urine that is undersaturated with calculogenic crystalloids should prompt consideration that (1) the wrong mineral component was diagnosed (larger (>0.5–0.7 mm) urate uroliths can mimic the radiographic appearance of struvite), (2) the nucleus of the urolith is of a different mineral composition than other portions of the urolith, or (3) the owner or the patient is not complying with medical recommendations.

Table 69.7 Recommendations for medical dissolution infection-induced struvite uroliths

Diagnostic plan
  1. Perform appropriate diagnostic studies, including urinalysis (e.g., pH > 6.5, MAP crystalluria), diagnostic radiography (radio-opaque urolith), and urine culture; infection (induced struvite uroliths are commonly caused by Staphylococcal species of bacteria).
  2. Determine mineral composition of voided or retrieved uroliths. If unavailable, predict mineral composition by evaluating clinical data (Tables 69.2–69.4).

Therapeutic plan
  1. Consider mechanical removal (Table 69.5) if uroliths obstructing urine flow cannot be dislodged or if patients with a high risk of urine outflow obstruction cannot be monitored.
  2. Eradicate urinary tract infection with appropriate antibiotics.
  Maintain antimicrobial therapy at the full dose during dissolution of uroliths and for approximately 1 month after dissolution (expected dissolution time = 2–3 months).
  3. Initiate therapy with a diet designed to dissolve struvite uroliths (e.g., Hills Prescription diet s/d). Other food, supplements, or treats should not be fed. Continue dietary therapy for approximately 1 month after radiographic confirmation dissolution.

Plan to monitor efficacy of therapy
  1. Evaluate serial urinalyses. Urine pH should be acidic, urine specific gravity should be low (<1.015 in dog and <1.035 in cat (lower if using the canned food)), and MAP crystalluria should be absent.
  2. Perform urine cultures to determine whether bacteria have been eradicated.
  3. Perform radiography monthly to assess urolith number, size, and position.
  4. If uroliths increase in size during therapy or do not begin to decrease in size after approximately 4–8 weeks of appropriate medical management, alternative management strategies (e.g., lithotripsy, cystotomy) can be considered. Difficulty in inducing complete dissolution of uroliths by creating urine that is undersaturated with the calculogenic crystalloids should prompt consideration that (1) the wrong mineral component was diagnosed, (2) the nidus of the urolith is of different mineral composition than outer portions of the urolith, or (3) the owner or the patient is not complying with medical recommendations, and (4) there is a persistent urinary tract infection.

Table 69.8 Recommendations for medical dissolution of allopurinol-induced xanthine uroliths

Diagnostic plan
  1. Perform appropriate diagnostic studies, including urinalysis (e.g., amorphous crystalluria), diagnostic radiography (marginally radio-opaque urolith requiring contrast cystourethrography and/or ultasonography),and a history of allopurinol administration, supporting the diagnosis of xanthine uroliths.
  2. If possible, verify mineral composition of voided or retrieved uroliths (Table 69.11).

Therapeutic plan
  1. Consider mechanical removal (Table 69.5) if uroliths obstructing urine flow cannot be dislodged or if patients with a high risk of urine outflow obstruction cannot be monitored.
  2. Discontinue allopurinol administration.
  3. Initiate therapy with a calculolytic diet with low quantities of purines that promotes urine alkalization (e.g., Prescription Diet Canine canned u/d for dogs or diets to manage patients with liver or kidney failure in cats). Other food or mineral supplements should not be fed.

Plan to monitor efficacy of therapy
  1. Evaluate serial urinalyses. Urine pH should be alkaline, urine specific gravity should be low (<1.015 in dog and <1.035 in cat (lower if using the canned food)), and crystalluria should be absent.
  2. Perform radiography monthly to assess urolith number, size, and position (expected dissolution time $= 1–2$ months). If uroliths grow during medical management or do not begin to dissolve in 4 weeks, alternative methods for urolith removal should be considered (Table 69.5).

managing cats with renal failure and ureteroliths by initially using noninvasive medical protocols designed to restore fluid volume, correct electrolyte and acid–base imbalances associated with uremia, and promote migration of ureterolith into the urinary bladder.

In concept, surgical removal of uroliths that obstruct a ureter should decrease the magnitude of renal dysfunction. However, determining when the benefits of ureteral surgery outweigh, the risks is often difficult. The timing of surgical intervention depends on the severity and

Table 69.9 Recommendations for medical dissolution of urate uroliths in dogs

Diagnostic plan
  1. Perform appropriate diagnostic studies, including urinalysis (amorphous crystalluria) and diagnostic radiography (marginally radio-opaque urolith ogten requiring contrast cystourethrography or ultasonography), supporting the diagnosis of urate uroliths. In breeds other than Dalmatians or English Bull dogs, consider liver function tests (provocative serum concentrations of bile acids and liver size). Decreased liver function is uncommonly associated with urate uroliths in cats.
  2. Determine mineral composition of voided or retrieved uroliths (Table 69.11). If unavailable, predict mineral composition by evaluating clinical data (Tables 69.2–69.4).

Therapeutic plan
  1. Consider mechanical removal (Table 69.5) if uroliths obstructing urine flow cannot be dislodged or if patients with a high risk of urine outflow obstruction cannot be monitored.
  2. Initiate therapy with a low purine calculolytic diet (Prescription Diet Canine u/d, l/d, or d/d; urate dissolution in cats is less predictable). Other food supplements should not be fed to the patient.
  3. Initiate therapy with allopurinol at a dosage of 15 mg/kg q l2 h PO (a lesser dose will be required in azotemic patients).
  4. If necessary, administer potassium citrate or sodium bicarbonate orally in order to eliminate aciduria. Strive for a urine pH of 7 or higher.

Plan to monitor efficacy of therapy
  1. Try to minimize follow-up studies that require urinary catheterization, but if necessary, give appropriate peri-catheterization antimicrobial agents to prevent iatrogenic catheter-induced UTI.
  2. Evaluate serial urinalyses. Urine pH should be greater than 7, specific gravity should be less than 1.020, and urate crystals should be absent.
  3. Perform serial radiography at monthly intervals to evaluate reductions in urolith number a size.
  4. Continue calculolytic diet and allopurinol for approximately 1 month after disappearance of uroliths as detected by medical imaging.

Table 69.10 Recommendations for medical dissolution of cystine uroliths

Diagnostic plan
    1. Perform appropriate diagnostic studies, including urinalysis (cystine crystalluria) and diagnostic radiography (marginally radio-opaque urolith requiring contrast cystourethrography or ultasonography), supporting a diagnosis of cystine uroliths.
    2. Determine mineral composition of voided or retrieved uroliths (Table 69.11). If unavailable, predict mineral composition by evaluating clinical data (Tables 69.2–69.4).

Therapeutic plan
    1. Consider mechanical removal (Table 69.5) if uroliths obstructing urine flow cannot be dislodged or if patients with a high risk of urine outflow obstruction cannot be monitored.
    2. Initiate therapy with calculolytic diet (e.g., Prescription Diet Canine canned u/d). Other food or mineral supplements should not be fed.
    3. Initiate therapy with N-(2-mecrcaptopropionyl)-glycine (2-MPG), approximately 15 mg/kg q l2 h PO. Other Thiol-containing drugs (D-penicillamine, captopril, and bucillamine) are available to augment cystine dissolution; however, because of their unproven efficacy or increased toxicity, they require more careful monitoring.
    4. If necessary, administer potassium citrate orally (75 mg/kg q l2 h) to induce alkaluria. Titrate dose to achieve a pH of 7 or slightly greater.

Plan to monitor efficacy of therapy (4–6 week intervals)
    1. Try to minimize follow-up studies that require urinary catheterization, but if they are required, give appropriate peri-catheterization antimicrobial agents to prevent iatrogenic catheter-induced UTI.
    2. Evaluate serial urinalyses. Urine pH should be greater than 7, specific gravity should be less than 1.020, and crystals should be absent.
    3. Perform serial radiography at monthly intervals to evaluate reductions in urolith number a size.
    4. Continue calculolytic diet, 2-MPG, and alkalinizing therapy for approximately 1 month after disappearance of uroliths as detected by radiography.

Table 69.11 Catheter retrieval of uroliths

1. Sedation	For most dogs, sedation is unnecessary; however, sterile lubricant with topical anesthetics (e.g., lidocaine) can improve patient comfort. Transurethral catheterization of most cats requires sedation.
2. Catheter selection	Select the largest catheter that can be easily inserted into the urethra. We commonly use sterile, 8 Fr or larger catheters flexible in dogs. The distal tip is smoothly cut so that the catheter is open at the end.
3. Measure catheter insertion length	Determine the length of catheter that must be inserted so that the open end reaches the trigone. This distance is easily determined by measuring urethral length from a radiograph.
4. Place catheter transurethrally	The well lubricated, sterile catheter from #2 above is advanced through the urethra into the bladder lumen, and the patient is placed in lateral recumbency
5. Fill the urinary bladder	If the urinary bladder is not distended with urine, it should be moderately distended with sterile physiologic solutions (e.g., LRS, normal saline).
6. Agitate the bladder while removing fluid	While aspirating fluid from the bladder through the catheter into a syringe, vigorously and repeatedly agitate the bladder. The bladder is agitated by placing your hand (palm up) between the patient (in the area of the bladder) and table. Repeatedly flex and extend your fingers to move the animal's abdomen (i.e., urinary bladder) up and down. This maneuver will disperse uroliths throughout fluid in the bladder lumen. Small uroliths in the vicinity of the catheter tip are easily aspirated into the catheter along with the fluid.
7. Repeat steps 5 and 6	It may be necessary to repeat this sequence of steps several times before a sufficient quantity of uroliths are retrieved. Difficulty in aspirating fluid may be caused by poor catheter position (position catheter tip in trigone of bladder) or occlusion of the catheter lumen with uroliths (injecting fluid back through the catheter should clear catheter lumen). The greatest opportunity to remove uroliths occurs when the bladder is almost empty. Therefore, we instill no more than 60 mL of saline, and use a 60 mL syringe to remove bladder contents (i.e., stones).

Table 69.12 Performing voiding urohydropropulsion

1. Anesthetize the patient	The type of anesthesia selected may vary based on the likelihood of success and gender of the patient. Consider reversible short acting anesthetics for patients with very small uroliths that are easily removed. Patients likely to go to surgery/lithotripsy should be placed under inhalation anesthesia. Immediately prior to voiding, consider injecting a short-acting drug like propofol to insure urethral relaxation; it is very helpful in male dogs.
2. Attach a 3-way stopcock to the end of the urinary catheter	The three-way stopcock facilitates control of the volume of fluid entering the bladder and containment of fluid once the bladder is filled.
3. Fill the urinary bladder and remove the catheter	Sterile physiologic solutions (LRS, normal saline) are injected through a transurethral catheter to distend the bladder. If fluid is expelled prematurely around the catheter prior to adequate bladder filling, the vulva and/or urethra can be gently occluded using your thumb and first finger. Placement of additional fluid may not be needed.
4. Position the patient such that the spine is approximately vertical	Repositioning the patient allows uroliths to accumulate at the neck of the bladder, facilitating their expulsion. Anatomically, the urethra does not become vertical until the caudal spine is 20–25 degrees anterior of vertical, but this may not be clinically important.
5. Agitate the bladder	Agitating the urinary bladder left and right is performed to dislodge uroliths loosely adhered to the bladder mucosa.
6. Express the urinary bladder	Apply steady digital pressure to the urinary bladder to induce micturition. Compress the urinary bladder dorsally and cranially (toward the back and head of the patient). Movement of the urinary bladder caudally toward the pelvic canal may cause the urethra to kink, preventing maximal urethral dilation. Once voiding begins, the bladder is more vigorously compressed.
7. Repeat steps 2–6	The bladder is flushed repeatedly until no uroliths are expelled.
8. Medical imaging	Radiography provides an appropriate method of assessing successful expulsion of uroliths. To enhance detection of remaining small uroliths, consider double-contrast cystography (only the lateral view is needed).

rate of progression of renal dysfunction, the potential for reversing renal dysfunction, the potential for urolith migration through the ureter, the presence of infection or uncontrollable pain, and risks associated with surgery of the ureters. If a urolith obstructs a ureter in a patient with previously compensated renal failure and causes an abrupt decline in renal function associated with life-threatening hyperkalemia and/or acidemia that cannot be controlled by peritoneal dialysis or hemodialysis, surgical intervention should be considered.

Although placement of nephrostomy tubes to bypass obstructed ureters may be considered as a method of temporarily improving renal function, maintaining nephrostomy tube position, seal, and patency for longer than 24 hours is often technically difficult (Nwadike et al. 2000; Hardie and Kyles 2004). In addition to severe unresponsive azotemia, if infection and pain cannot be appropriately managed, surgical ureterolith removal should be considered. Because of the high risk of irreparable ureteral damage associated with ureterotomy, surgical removal of ureterolith removal is not recommended if (1) ureteroliths are migrating through the ureter, (2) azotemia is resolving, (3) the associated kidney is non-

functional, or (4) surgeons are unfamiliar with appropriate surgical techniques.

Urolith prevention

Prevention of recurrent uroliths reduces the need for repeat surgery and is therefore cost effective. In general, preventative strategies are designed to eliminate or control the underlying causes of various types of uroliths. When causes cannot be identified or corrected, preventative strategies encompass efforts to minimize risk factors associated with calculogenesis. These strategies commonly include dietary and pharmacologic considerations (Figures 69.4–69.10).

Selection of an appropriate diet to prevent calcium oxalate urolith recurrence is challenging

Results of experimental and clinical investigations have demonstrated the importance of dietary modifications in medical protocols to prevent urolith recurrence. However, selecting an appropriate diet to prevent CaOx

Table 69.13 Retrograde urohydropropulsion

1. Decompress urinary bladder	Urethroliths cannot be safely flushed back into a bladder overdistended with urine. To empty the bladder, use a 22g, 1.5-inch needle attached to IV extension tubing, three-way stopcock, and large volume syringe to remove urine. By using the intravenous extension tubing and 3-way stopcock, the urinary bladder will not have to be repunctured after emptying a full syringe of urine. Excessive digital pressure should not be applied to the bladder wall while the needle is in its lumen lest urine be forced around the needle into the peritoneal cavity. Attempting complete evacuation of the bladder lumen is undesirable because the sharp point of the needle may then damage the bladder wall. We recommend that 10–15 mL of urine remain in the bladder.
2. Lubricate around the urethroliths	Fill one 12 mL syringe with 5 mL of saline and another 12 mL syringe with 5mLs of sterile water-soluble lubricant. Attach these two syringes with a 3-way stopcock. Mix the contents of both syringes by emptying one syringe into the other several times. After inserting a urethral catheter, inject 3–8 mL of mixture to lubricate around uroliths. This step is not always necessary.
3. Insert catheter	Insert a lubricated large bore flexible catheter. The tip of the catheter should remain distal to urethroliths.
4. Occlude pelvic urethra	Insert a gloved index finger into the rectum and occlude the urethral lumen by compressing the urethra against the floor or side of the bony pelvis.
5. Occlude distal urethra	With a moistened gauze sponge, occlude the distal urethra by compressing the distal tip of penis around the catheter.
6. Forcefully flush fluid through catheter	Fill a large syringe (20–35 mL) with sterile isotonic solution (e.g., saline, LRS, etc.). The normal bladder holds approximately 1.5–2.5 mL per kg of the patient's weight. With the syringe attached to the catheter, turn it upside down, and place the top of the plunger against the tabletop. Hold the syringe by the barrel and forcefully push it down over the plunger with the goal of dilating the urethral lumen with saline.
7. Relieve occlusion of pelvic urethra	Once the urethra becomes dilated, digital pressure applied to the pelvic urethra (but not the penile urethra) should be rapidly released.
8. Continue Flushing	Continue flushing fluid through the catheter and urethral lumen to propel urethroliths into the urinary bladder. Use caution not to over-distend the bladder lumen with saline. If the technique is repeated, accumulation of saline in the bladder lumen necessitates repeating decompressive cystocentesis.
9. Medical Imaging	Radiography provides an appropriate method of assessing whether or not all of the uroliths have been flushed into the bladder lumen. Transurethral catheterization is not a reliable method of verifying that all uroliths have been flushed out of the urethra.

uroliths is challenging because (1) the exact mechanisms underlying calcium oxalate urolith formation are not completely understood, (2) results of epidemiological studies do not always match physiology response of diet characteristics, and (3) diet efficacy has not been evaluated using clinically relevant endpoints. The following sections highlight each of these concerns.

Mechanisms underlying calcium oxalate urolith formation are not completely understood

Although formation of CaOx uroliths is associated with a complex and incompletely understood sequence of events, it is accepted that initial crystal formation and subsequent crystal growth are at least partly a reflection of urine supersaturation (Chapter 12). However, unlike other stone types, the urinary concentrations of calculogenic minerals may not be the predominant driving force for CaOx urolith formation. For example, 68 proteins were recently identified in matrix of CaOx uroliths from humans (Canales et al. 2008). We have identified over 30 proteins in CaOx uroliths from dogs (unpublished results). The functional relationship of some of these proteins is unknown and be present because they inadvertently become enveloped in stones as they form. Nonetheless, several proteins (e.g., osteopontin, nephrocalcin, Tamm-Horsfall, bikunin, and α1-antitripsin) are known

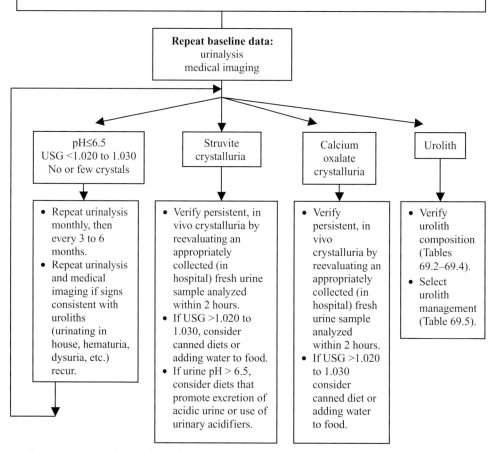

Medical:
- Metabolic risk factors promoting alkalemia (hypoxemia, chronic diuretic use, administration of antacids, chronic vomiting, and hyperaldosteronism) and subsequent alkaluria are rarely encountered. Sterile Struvite stones are commonly reported in cats and in English and American Cocker spaniel dogs.
- Reduction for some risk factors for Struvite urolith formation, including formation of acidic urine, may increase risk for calcium oxalate urolith formation.

Dietary:
- Diets restricted in phosphorus and magnesium that promote formation of acid urine (i.e., pH≤ 6.3), minimize formation of sterile Struvite uroliths.
- High moisture foods (i.e., canned formulations) are more effective because increased water consumption is associated with decreased urine concentrations of calculogenic minerals.

Pharmacological:
- Consider methionine or ammonium chloride to acidify the urine of patients consuming nonacidifying diets.
- Prolonged systemic over-acidification may result in metabolic acidosis, hypercalciuria, hypokalemia, and demineralization of bone.

Repeat baseline data:
urinalysis
medical imaging

pH≤6.5
USG <1.020 to 1.030
No or few crystals

Struvite
crystalluria

Calcium
oxalate
crystalluria

Urolith

- Repeat urinalysis monthly, then every 3 to 6 months.
- Repeat urinalysis and medical imaging if signs consistent with uroliths (urinating in house, hematuria, dysuria, etc.) recur.

- Verify persistent, in vivo crystalluria by reevaluating an appropriately collected (in hospital) fresh urine sample analyzed within 2 hours.
- If USG >1.020 to 1.030, consider canned diets or adding water to food.
- If urine pH > 6.5, consider diets that promote excretion of acidic urine or use of urinary acidifiers.

- Verify persistent, in vivo crystalluria by reevaluating an appropriately collected (in hospital) fresh urine sample analyzed within 2 hours.
- If USG >1.020 to 1.030 consider canned diet or adding water to food.

- Verify urolith composition (Tables 69.2–69.4).
- Select urolith management (Table 69.5).

Figure 69.4 Strategies to prevent sterile struvite urolith recurrence.

to influence crystal nucleation, growth, and aggregation. In experimentally induced hyperoxaluria, intratubular CaOx crystalluria was detected in osteoopontin and Tamm-Horsfall knockout mice, but did not occur in wild-type controls (Mo et al. 2007). These findings indicate the importance of other substances besides the concentrations of minerals in urine in the generation of CaOx uroliths.

Results of epidemiological studies do not always match physiology response of diet characteristics

Few studies have evaluated the risk of dietary ingredients on CaOx urolith formation. In these studies, the most influential dietary attributes have been urine acidifying potential and the quantities of calcium, protein,

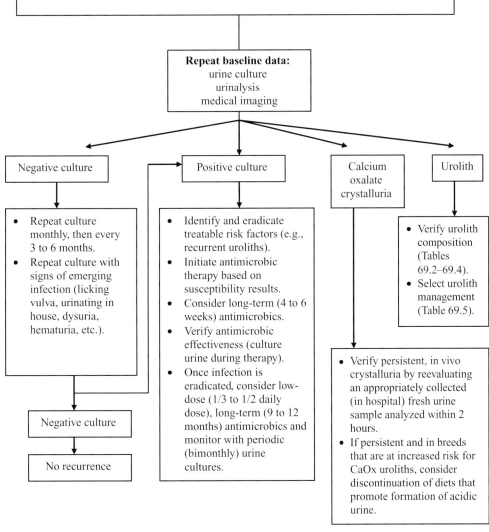

Medical:
- Eradication and prevention of urease-producing bacteria is essential to prevent urolith recurrence.
- If possible, correct structural (e.g., polypoid cystitis, congenital and acquired anomalies, perivulvar dermatitis, etc.) and functional (e.g., hyperadrenocortisim, diabetes mellitus, hypothyroidism, etc.) defects in host defenses predisposing to urinary tract infection.
- Avoid impairment of host defenses (e.g., corticosteroid administration, urinary catheterization, etc.).

Dietary:
- Diets restricted in phosphorus and magnesium that promote formation of acid urine may be helpful, but cannot be used as a substitute for good control of infection.

Pharmacological:
- Antimicrobic selection should be based on culture and susceptibility results.

Repeat baseline data:
urine culture
urinalysis
medical imaging

Negative culture
- Repeat culture monthly, then every 3 to 6 months.
- Repeat culture with signs of emerging infection (licking vulva, urinating in house, dysuria, hematuria, etc.).

Negative culture

No recurrence

Positive culture
- Identify and eradicate treatable risk factors (e.g., recurrent uroliths).
- Initiate antimicrobic therapy based on susceptibility results.
- Consider long-term (4 to 6 weeks) antimicrobics.
- Verify antimicrobic effectiveness (culture urine during therapy).
- Once infection is eradicated, consider low-dose (1/3 to 1/2 daily dose), long-term (9 to 12 months) antimicrobics and monitor with periodic (bimonthly) urine cultures.

Calcium oxalate crystalluria
- Verify persistent, in vivo crystalluria by reevaluating an appropriately collected (in hospital) fresh urine sample analyzed within 2 hours.
- If persistent and in breeds that are at increased risk for CaOx uroliths, consider discontinuation of diets that promote formation of acidic urine.

Urolith
- Verify urolith composition (Tables 69.2–69.4).
- Select urolith management (Table 69.5).

Figure 69.5 Strategies to prevent infection-induced struvite urolith recurrence.

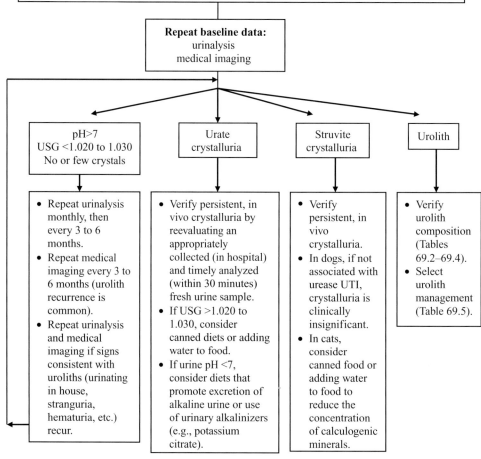

Medical:
- Canine breeds other than Dalmatians and Bulldogs commonly have portovascular anomalies. In these dogs, treatment of liver disease should complement treatment of uroliths.
- Impaired liver function is uncommonly documented in cats with urate uroliths.

Dietary:
- Provide reduced-protein (i.e., consistent with low purine) diets (Prescription diet u/d, l/d, d/d-egg) that promote diuresis and excretion of alkaline urine.
- High moisture foods (i.e., canned formulations) are more effective because increased water consumption is associated with decreased urine concentrations of calculogenic minerals.

Pharmacological:
- If dietary therapy alone is ineffective, consider long-term therapy with allopurinol (5 to 10 mg/kg/day). Higher doses of allopurinol, especially when given with higher protein foods, increase the risk of xanthine urolith formation.
- Consider potassium citrate if urine pH is not consistently ≥ 7.

Repeat baseline data:
urinalysis
medical imaging

pH>7
USG <1.020 to 1.030
No or few crystals

- Repeat urinalysis monthly, then every 3 to 6 months.
- Repeat medical imaging every 3 to 6 months (urolith recurrence is common).
- Repeat urinalysis and medical imaging if signs consistent with uroliths (urinating in house, stranguria, hematuria, etc.) recur.

Urate crystalluria

- Verify persistent, in vivo crystalluria by reevaluating an appropriately collected (in hospital) and timely analyzed (within 30 minutes) fresh urine sample.
- If USG >1.020 to 1.030, consider canned diets or adding water to food.
- If urine pH <7, consider diets that promote excretion of alkaline urine or use of urinary alkalinizers (e.g., potassium citrate).

Struvite crystalluria

- Verify persistent, in vivo crystalluria.
- In dogs, if not associated with urease UTI, crystalluria is clinically insignificant.
- In cats, consider canned food or adding water to food to reduce the concentration of calculogenic minerals.

Urolith

- Verify urolith composition (Tables 69.2–69.4).
- Select urolith management (Table 69.5).

Figure 69.6 Strategies to prevent urate urolith recurrence.

and sodium (Table 69.14) (Lekcharoensuk et al. 2002a, 2002b). Of the many dietary attributes evaluated, only two are consistently corroborated by results of experimental studies; diets formulated to promote more acidic urine and diets with low moisture content (i.e., kibble) increase the risk of CaOx formation. Therefore, canned diets designed to promote formation of neutral or alkaline urine should be considered to minimize CaOx urolith recurrence.

Diet efficacy has not been evaluated using clinically relevant endpoints

Ideally, studies to prevent CaOx urolith formation should be performed in dogs with a history of forming calcium oxalate stones. In addition, investigators and clients should be masked as to which dogs are randomly assigned the therapeutic food and the control food. Moreover, studies should reliable endpoints of urolith

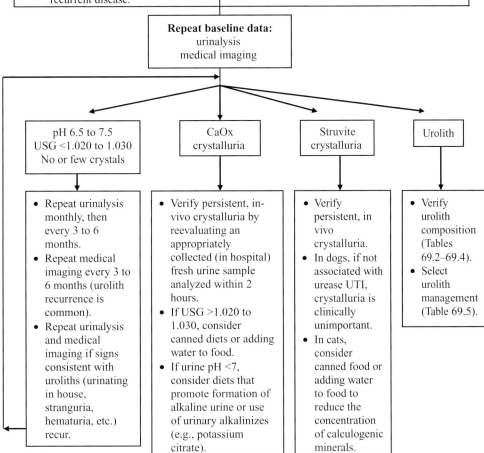

Medical:
- Hypercalcemia is uncommon, if detected, its cause should investigated and controlled.
- Hypercalciuria, a risk factor of CaOx urolithiasis has been associated with hyperadrenocorticism, exogenous glucocorticoid administration, and metabolic acidosis.

Dietary:
- Avoid calcium supplements and foods containing high quantities of oxalate (e.g., chocolate, peanuts, etc.)
- Provide reduced-protein diets (Prescription diet u/d, g/d) that promote diuresis and formation of alkaline urine.
- High moisture foods (i.e., canned formulations) are more effective because increased water consumption is associated with decreased urine concentrations of calculogenic minerals.

Pharmacological:
- Consider potassium citrate if urine pH is not consistently less than 7.
- Consider vitamin B6 (2 to 4 mg q 24 to 48 hours) in patients consuming primarily human food or diets of insufficient B6 content.
- Consider thiazide diuretics (hydrochlorothizide 2 mg/kg q12 hours) in dogs with highly recurrent disease.

Repeat baseline data:
urinalysis
medical imaging

pH 6.5 to 7.5
USG <1.020 to 1.030
No or few crystals
- Repeat urinalysis monthly, then every 3 to 6 months.
- Repeat medical imaging every 3 to 6 months (urolith recurrence is common).
- Repeat urinalysis and medical imaging if signs consistent with uroliths (urinating in house, stranguria, hematuria, etc.) recur.

CaOx crystalluria
- Verify persistent, in-vivo crystalluria by reevaluating an appropriately collected (in hospital) fresh urine sample analyzed within 2 hours.
- If USG >1.020 to 1.030, consider canned diets or adding water to food.
- If urine pH <7, consider diets that promote formation of alkaline urine or use of urinary alkalinizes (e.g., potassium citrate).

Struvite crystalluria
- Verify persistent, in vivo crystalluria.
- In dogs, if not associated with urease UTI, crystalluria is clinically unimportant.
- In cats, consider canned food or adding water to food to reduce the concentration of calculogenic minerals.

Urolith
- Verify urolith composition (Tables 69.2–69.4).
- Select urolith management (Table 69.5).

Figure 69.7 Strategies to prevent calcium oxalate urolith recurrence.

recurrence (i.e., medical imaging). We are not aware of any published studies meeting these basic criteria. So, how can veterinarians make recommendations? The two most commonly prescribed diets to prevent CaOx urolith recurrence in dogs are Prescription Diet u/d® and Urinary SO 14™. How do these diets compare (Table 69.15)?

New modalities to manage calcium oxalate prevention

Bisphosphonates to reduce urinary calcium excretion

Bisphosphonates are synthetic inorganic pyrophosphates that have a high affinity for binding divalent ions such as calcium. They are important pharmacologically because

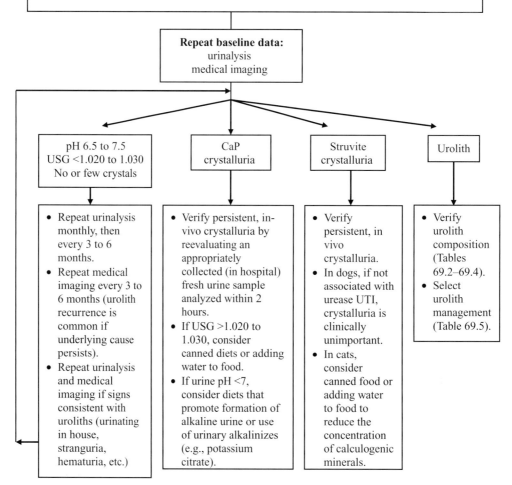

Medical:
- Hypercalcemia is not uncommon, if detected (ionized Ca), its cause should investigated and corrected.
- Hypercalciuria, a risk factor of CaP urolithiasis has been associated with hyperadrenocorticism, exogenous glucocorticoid administration, and metabolic acidosis.

Dietary:
- Avoid calcium supplements and vitamin D.
- Provide diets (prescription diet u/d) that promote diuresis and formation of alkaline urine.
- High moisture foods (i.e., canned formulations) are more effective because increased water consumption is associated with decreased urine concentrations of calculogenic minerals.

Pharmacological:
- Consider potassium citrate if urine pH is not consistently less than 7.
- Consider bisphosphonates (see New modalities to look for in the future).

Repeat baseline data:
urinalysis
medical imaging

**pH 6.5 to 7.5
USG <1.020 to 1.030
No or few crystals**
- Repeat urinalysis monthly, then every 3 to 6 months.
- Repeat medical imaging every 3 to 6 months (urolith recurrence is common if underlying cause persists).
- Repeat urinalysis and medical imaging if signs consistent with uroliths (urinating in house, stranguria, hematuria, etc.)

CaP crystalluria
- Verify persistent, in-vivo crystalluria by reevaluating an appropriately collected (in hospital) fresh urine sample analyzed within 2 hours.
- If USG >1.020 to 1.030, consider canned diets or adding water to food.
- If urine pH <7, consider diets that promote formation of alkaline urine or use of urinary alkalinizes (e.g., potassium citrate).

Struvite crystalluria
- Verify persistent, in vivo crystalluria.
- In dogs, if not associated with urease UTI, crystalluria is clinically unimportant.
- In cats, consider canned food or adding water to food to reduce the concentration of calculogenic minerals.

Urolith
- Verify urolith composition (Tables 69.2–69.4).
- Select urolith management (Table 69.5).

Figure 69.8 Strategies to prevent calcium phosphate urolith recurrence. With the exception of Brushite, calcium phosphates tend to be less soluble in alkaline urine. Whether patients will benefit from less-acid urine is unknown because acidification enhances urine calcium excretion. Calcium phosphate carbonate stones usually result from infections with bacteria elaborating urease. Therefore, calcium carbonate is a common component of struvite stones. Manage similar to infection-induced struvite stones by encouraging appropriate antimicrobic use and control of UTI and avoid dietary therapy promoting formation of acidic urine.

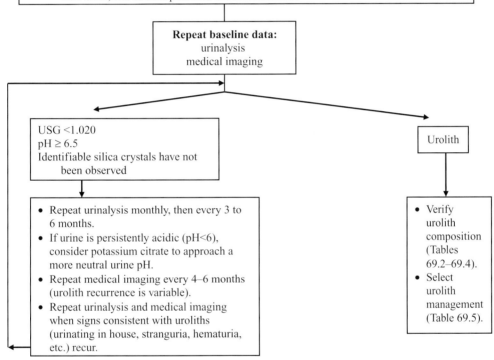

Figure 69.9 Strategies to prevent silica urolith recurrence.

these compounds stabilize bone minimizing calcium release in blood (Hostutleer et al. 2005) and excretion in urine (Basok et al. 2008) and are water soluble and renally excreted to bind calcium in urine.

Probiotics to reduce urinary oxalate excretion

Oxalobacter formigenes is an obligate anaerobic bacterium that resides in the intestine of most vertebrates and relies exclusively on the metabolism of oxalate as its sole source of energy. Human patients administered *Oxalobacter formigenes,* as enteric coated capsules reduced their urinary oxalate levels by 39–92% (Hoppe et al. 2006). Other intestinal bacteria (e.g., *Lactobacillus acidophilus*) also metabolize intestinal oxalate mini-

mizing its intestinal absorption and subsequent urinary excretion.

Preventing compound uroliths

Compound uroliths comprised approximately 8% of the uroliths submitted to the Minnesota Urolith Center (Figure 69.3). Compound uroliths form because factors initially promoting precipitation of one type of mineral have been superseded by factors promoting precipitation of a different mineral. Because risk factors that predispose to precipitation of different minerals in compound uroliths are often complex, designing effective medical protocols to manage them can be a unique challenge. In the absence of clinical evidence to the contrary, we

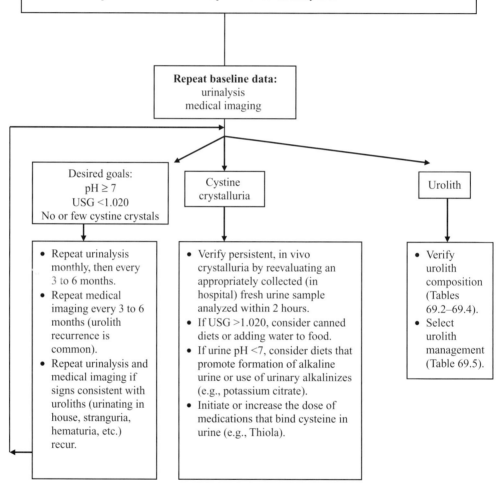

Medical:
- Urine nitroprusside test is a screening test for cystinuria.
- Genetic tests in Newfoundlands and Labrador retrievers are available to confirm genetic error in metabolism (Medical Genetics laboratory at the University of Pennsylvania).

Dietary:
- Provide reduced-protein diets that promote diuresis and formation of alkaline urine.
- High-moisture foods (i.e., canned formulations) are more effective because increased water consumption is associated with decreased urine concentrations of calculogenic minerals.

Pharmacological:
- If diet alone is ineffective, consider *n*-(2-mercaptoropionyl)-glycine (i.e., 2-MPG, also called Thiola™) at 10 to 30 mg/kg per day to maintain a urine cystine concentration below 200 mg/L.
- Consider potassium citrate if urine pH is not consistently ≥ 7.

Repeat baseline data:
urinalysis
medical imaging

Desired goals:
pH ≥ 7
USG <1.020
No or few cystine crystals

Cystine crystalluria

Urolith

- Repeat urinalysis monthly, then every 3 to 6 months.
- Repeat medical imaging every 3 to 6 months (urolith recurrence is common).
- Repeat urinalysis and medical imaging if signs consistent with uroliths (urinating in house, stranguria, hematuria, etc.) recur.

- Verify persistent, in vivo crystalluria by reevaluating an appropriately collected (in hospital) fresh urine sample analyzed within 2 hours.
- If USG >1.020, consider canned diets or adding water to food.
- If urine pH <7, consider diets that promote formation of alkaline urine or use of urinary alkalinizes (e.g., potassium citrate).
- Initiate or increase the dose of medications that bind cysteine in urine (e.g., Thiola).

- Verify urolith composition (Tables 69.2–69.4).
- Select urolith management (Table 69.5).

Figure 69.10 Strategies to prevent cystine urolith recurrence.

recommend prevention protocols principally designed to minimize recurrence of minerals that comprised the nucleus, rather than the outer layers (Lulich and Osborne 2000).

Logic suggests that the initial core (i.e., nidus) contributed to the formation of outer layers. Therefore, minimizing risk factors for precipitation of minerals found in the core minimize precipitation of minerals found in the outer layers. Because excessive concentration of minerals in urine is a prerequisite for urolith formation, it follows that increased water intake would logically lead to reduction in urine concentration of all lithogenic minerals, irrespective of their location or type and thus minimize recurrence. Formation of large volumes of less concentrated urine also decreases the risk of urolithiasis by increasing the frequency of

Table 69.14 Evaluation of dietary risk factors for calcium oxalate formation in dogs

Dietary component	Epidemiologic result	Comments	Conclusion
Urine acidifying potential	Diets promoting urine pH values less than 6.6 had the highest association with calcium oxalate formation in dogs consuming dry formulations of food (Lekcharoensuk 2002).	Acidic urine was also the most important risk factor for calcium oxalate urolith formation in cats (Kirk 1995; Lekcharoensuk 2001). Urine pH values greater than 6.5 were associated with decreased risk. This is physiologically plausible because in dogs alkalosis reduced urine calcium excretion (Marone 1983).	To reduce calcium oxalate, urolith recurrence select diets promoting alkalosis and urine pH values greater than 6.5.
Protein	Lower protein diets (1.9–5.8 g/100 kcal) were associated with increased risk. Higher protein diets (>6.25 g/100 kcal) were associated with fewer stones. Lekcharoensuk 2002)	Epidemiological studies do not demonstrate cause and effect but associations to investigate further. In contrast to the studies by Lekarchoensuk and colleagues, hypercalciuia from increased animal protein consumption (>77 g/day) increased the risk of calcium oxalate stones in man compared to the lowest intake (<50 g/day) (Curhan 1993). Several mechanisms are responsible for the hypercalciuria: (1) dietary protein increases glomerular filtration and thus the filtered load of calcium, (2) decreased renal fractional reabsorption of calcium is attributed to protein's acid load or due to the hyperinsulinemic effects of protein.	Until experimental studies evaluating different protein contents are performed in dogs with calcium oxalate stones, we recommend that protein be minimized to prevent calcium oxalate recurrence. The exact quantity has not been determined.
Calcium	Ironically, epidemiologic studies indicate that diets with lower quantities of calcium (<2.2 mg/kcal) are a risk factor for urolith formation.	In an experimental study in dogs, diets with the lowest calcium (1.8 mg/kcal) and oxalate (0.1 mg/kcal) were associated with the lowest relative supersaturation (RSS) for CaOx (Stevenson 2003). Diets with high caicium (7.5 mg/kcal) and low oxalate resulted in the highest CaOx RSS.	To reduce urolith recurrence diets should have lower quantities of calcium and oxalate

micturition and thus the frequency that crystals would be voided.

The most common compound urolith identified at the Minnesota Urolith Center contains a nidus of CaOx and outer layers of struvite. Unlike uroliths predominantly composed of CaOx, which occur more often in males, the majority of compound uroliths with a calcium oxalate core and outer layers of struvite occurred more commonly in female dogs. The paradox in managing patients forming uroliths with CaOx and struvite is that attempts to minimize risk factors for struvite formation (such as reducing urine pH, magnesium, and phosphorus) increase the risk for CaOx urolith forma-

tion. In this situation, we recommend that emphasis be placed on minimizing recurrence of CaOx uroliths, since CaOx was the nidus and cannot be dissolved medically. In contrast, struvite uroliths can often be dissolved by medical protocols. For uroliths containing a core of CaOx surrounded by a shell of infection-induced struvite, it is logical to assume that the initial episode of CaOx uroliths predisposed the patient to infection-induced struvite uroliths. Therefore, preventative management should include efforts to eradicate or control recurrent UTI's. Our preventative therapy would be identical even if the location of the minerals were reversed, a struvite nidus with outer layers of calcium oxalate.

Table 69.15 Comparing the dietary characteristic of diets commonly used to prevent CaOx urolith recurrence

	Prescription diet u/d		Urinary SO 14	
	Canned	Dry	Canned	Dry
Protein g/100 kcal	2.9	2.6	3.7	4.0
Fat g/100 kcal	5.8	4.7	5.9	4.0
Carbohydrate g/100 kcal	12.2	14.5	7.9	13.0
Calcium g/100 kcal	0.076	0.077	0.2	0.19
Phosphorus g/100 kcal	0.038	0.035	0.17	0.15
Sodium g/100 kcal	0.061	0.052	0.29	0.33
Potassium g/100 kcal	0.098	0.125	0.16	0.23
Magnesium g/100 kcal	0.011	0.011	0.012	0.016
Urine pH	7.1–7.7		5.5–6.0	
Urine Ca mmol/L	1.22 ± 0.18[a]		1.29 ± 0.90[b]	
Urine Ox mmol/L	0.744 ± 0.014[a]		0.91 ± 0.78[b]	
CaOx RSS	ND		7.76 ± 7.1[b]	

[a]This study was performed in 8 client-owned dogs with calcium oxalate urolithiasis. Dogs were fed the urolith prevention diet for 2 weeks at which time 24-hour urine samples were collected in metabolism cages. This study was performed at the University of Minnesota (Lulich, J.P., et al. (2001). J Am Vet Med Assoc **218**: 1583–1586).

[b]This study was performed in 13 client-owned dogs with calcium oxalate urolithiasis. Dogs were fed the urolith prevention diet for 1 month before daily voluntarily voided urine was collected by owners. This study was performed by the Waltham Centre for Pet Nutrition (Stevenson, A.E., et. al. (2004). Vet Therapeut **5**: 218–231).

References

Basok EK, A. Basaran, et al. (2008). Are new-generation bisphosphonates effective for the inhibition of calcium oxalate stone formation in a rat model? *Urologia Internationalis* **81**: 325–329.

Bevan, J.M. and J.P. Lulich (2008). *Comparison of Laser Lithotripsy and Cystotomy for the Management of Canine Urolithiasis*. Accepted for publication in *JAVMA*.

Canales, B.K., L. Anderson, et al. (2008). *J Endourol* **22**: 1161–1168.

Hardie, E.M. and A.E. Kyles (2004). Management of ureteral obstruction. *Vet Clin North America* **34**: 989–1010.

Hoppe, B., B. Beck, et al. (2006). Oxalobacter formigenes: a potential tool for the treatment of primary hyperoxaluria type 1. *Kidney Int* **70**: 1305–1311.

Hostutleer, R.A., D.J. Chew, et al. (2005). Uses and effectivnessof pamidronate disodium for treatment of dogs and cats with hypercalcemia. *J Vet Intern Med* **19**: 29–33.

Kyles, A.E., E.M. Hardie, et al. (2005). Management and outcome of cats with ureteral calculi: 153 cases (1984–2002). *JAVMA* **226**: 937–944.

Lekcharoensuk, C., C.A. Osborne, et al. (2005). Evaluation of trends in the frequency of calcium oxalate uroliths in the upper urinary tract of cats. *J Am Anim Hosp Assoc* **41**: 39–46.

Lekcharoensuk, C., C.A. Osborne, et al. (2002a). Associations between dietary factors in canned foods and formation of calcium oxalate uroliths in dogs. *Am J Vet Res* **63**: 163–169.

Lekcharoensuk, C., C.A. Osborne, et al. (2002b) Associations between dry dietary factors and canine calcium oxalate uroliths. *Am J Vet Res* **63**: 330–337.

Lulich, J.P., C.A. Osborne, et al. (2008). *Efficacy and Safety of Laser Lithotripsy to Remove Urocystoliths and Urethroliths in Dogs: 100 Consecutive Cases*. Accepted for publication *JAVMA*.

Lulich, J.P., C.A. Osborne (1992). Catheter-assisted retrieval of urocystoliths from dogs and cats. *Am J Vet Med Assoc* **201**: 111–113.

Lulich, J.P. and C.A. Osborne (2000). Compound uroliths: treatment and prevention. In: *Current Veterinary Therapy*, edited by J.D. Bonagura. Vol. **13**. Philadelphia PA: WB Saunders, pp. 874–877.

Lulich, J.P. and C.A. Osborne (2009). Changing paradigms in the diagnosis of urolithiasis. *Vet Clin North Am, Small Anim Pract* **39**: 79–91.

Lulich, J.P., C.A. Osborne, et al. (1993). Nonsurgical removal of urocystoliths by voiding urohydropulsion. *Am J Vet Med Assoc* **203**: 660–663.

Mo, L., L. Liaw, et al. (2007). Renal calcinosis and stone formation in mice lacking osteopontin, tamm-horsfall protein, or both. *Am J Physiol* **293**: F1935–F1943.

Nwadike, B.S., L.P. Wilson, et al. (2000). Use of temporary nephrosotomy catheters for emergency treatment of bilateral ureter transection in a cat. *J Am Vet Med Assoc* **217**: 1862–1865.

Osborne, C.A., J.P. Lulich, et.al. (1990). Medical dissolution of feline struvite urocystoliths. *JAVMA* **196**: 1053–1063

Osborne, C.A., J.P. Lulich, et al. (1999). Canine retrograde urohydropropulsion: 25 years of experience. *Vet Clin N Am: Small Anim Pract* (Editors: C.A. Osborne, J.P. Lulich, Bartges) **29**(1): 267–281.

70

Pathophysiology of urinary obstruction

Joe Bartges

Obstructive uropathy refers to abnormalities in structure or function of the urinary tract caused by impairment of normal flow of urine, resulting in local and systemic effects (Klahr and Harris 1992; Bartges and Finco 1996). Impairment of flow through the ureter or urethra due to physical obstruction results in characteristic clinical signs.

Pathophysiology

Acute urethral obstruction mimics ureteral obstruction in many aspects, including pathophysiological changes that occur in kidneys. Acute urethral obstruction may be induced and maintained by different causes, affecting the urethra at one or more sites. Irrespective of cause(s) of urethral obstruction, predictable clinical and biochemical abnormalities develop. Obstruction to urine flow results in increased pressure in the bladder and urethra proximal to site(s) of obstruction. Local pressure due to uroliths or matrix-crystalline plugs damage urethral mucosa. As intravesical pressure increases, damage occurs to urothelium and detrusor muscle. Nerves located in the bladder wall also are damaged, and inflammatory cells infiltrate. As back pressure persists and increases, ureters and kidneys are affected.

Most studies in animals have involved unilateral or bilateral ureteral obstruction rather than urethral obstruction (Klahr 1991; Klahr and Harris 1992); however, pathophysiologic changes associated with persistent urethral obstruction probably mimics bilateral ureteral obstruction induced in these models. With urethral obstruction, ureteral pressure increases, and this is transmitted to Bowman's space. As ureteral pressure increases,

there is a period during which renal blood flow increases because of decreased afferent arteriolar resistance mediated by release of vasodilatory prostaglandins (Allen and Vaughan 1978). During this hyperemic phase, glomerular filtration rate is decreased, but afferent arteriolar dilation increases intraglomerular pressure to counter increased pressure in Bowman's space (Yarger and Schocken 1980; Klahr and Harris 1992). After 24 hours, glomerular filtration rate decreases further due to two major vasoconstricting agents, thromboxane A_2 and angiotensin II, and possibly due to decreased endothelium-derived relaxing factor (Klahr 1991; Klahr and Harris 1992). Thromboxane A_2 is produced by infiltrating cells (blood monocytes and T lymphocytes) and possibly mesangial cells (Harris and Schreiner 1989; Yanagisawa and Morrissey 1990). During the obstructive period, angiotensin II may decrease glomerular filtration rate via mesangial cell contraction and may decrease the glomerular ultrafiltration coefficient. Although infusion of angiotensin II into normal animals increases net filtration pressure presumably because of greater efferent arteriolar constriction, blockage of angiotensin II formation after relief of obstruction increases glomerular filtration rate (Yarger and Schocken 1980). This increase in glomerular filtration rate may be due to a greater filtering surface area because angiotensin II causes mesangial cell contraction and subsequently reduces total glomerular capillary area available for filtration (Ausiello and Kreisberg 1980). Vasodilatory prostaglandins, such as prostaglandin E_2 and prostacyclin, which are produced in increased amounts by the obstructed kidney, may prevent further decrements in glomerular filtration rate by antagonizing vasoconstrictive effects of thromboxane A_2 and/or angiotensin II.

Leukocytes influx shortly after onset of acute ureteral obstruction (Schreiner and Unanue 1984). Leukocytes form distinctive rings around tubular cells particularly

Nephrology and Urology of Small Animals. Edited by Joe Bartges and David J. Polzin. © 2011 Blackwell Publishing Ltd.

in distal tubules (Schreiner and Harris 1988). Normal kidneys have a small number of resident macrophages in the renal cortex, mainly in glomeruli (Schreiner and Unanue 1984); however, normal medulla is completely devoid of resident leukocytes. In obstruction, mononuclear cells, primarily macrophages, are present in the medulla to the same extent as the cortex. This leukocyte invasion is associated with a relative depletion of resident macrophages from glomeruli. The second most abundant leukocyte is T-lymphocytes of the cytotoxic suppresser cell subclass. After relief of obstruction, macrophage and T-lymphocyte infiltrate decreases over days. Neutrophils are not normally present in the infiltrate.

Decreased glomerular filtration rate and renal blood flow result in azotemia and hyperphosphatemia. Although brief periods of obstruction result in minimal damage to kidneys, prolonged periods of obstruction are harmful. Recovery of glomerular filtration rate following relief of obstruction decreases as time of obstruction increases.

The degree and nature of tubular effects and their recovery depends on degree and duration of obstruction. With complete outflow obstruction, anuria ensues, resulting in potential for marked abnormalities in water, electrolyte, and acid–base balance. The major sites of abnormal function are located in the distal nephron. Tubular abnormalities include a concentrating defect, altered reabsorption of solutes and water, and impaired excretion of hydrogen and potassium. Once obstruction is relieved, renal function may reflect programmed homeostatic responses or aberrant consequences of renal injury. Sodium, potassium, phosphate, magnesium, and proton retention occur during obstruction; normal renal response is to enhance urinary excretion by increasing fractional excretion of retained substances. Water balance may be positive; polyuria ensues to correct water excess. Tubular damage during obstruction may compromise renal tubular function once obstruction is reversed.

Water reabsorption is impaired with obstruction. In fact, polyuria may exacerbate pressure associated with obstruction. Following relief of obstruction, an impaired ability to concentrate urine persists. The term postobstructive diuresis has been used to describe profuse polyuria that sometimes occurs after relief of obstruction. Initial diuresis with relief of obstruction may be attributed partially to homeostatic efforts for resolution of positive water and electrolyte balance and to diuresis associated with renal excretion of urea and other solutes. A defect in water homeostasis may persist because dehydrated patients cannot conserve water once obstruction is removed (Finco and Cornelius 1977). Renal ability to concentrate urine is impaired markedly, whereas ability to dilute urine is affected to a lesser degree.

Impaired concentrating ability may be due to increased medullary blood flow and washout of medullary hypertonic gradient and impaired response of medullary collecting ducts to antidiuretic hormone; atrial natriuretic peptide may also play a role. Thus, the concentrating defect in obstructive uropathy is presumably the result of decreased removal of solute from the thick ascending limb of the loop of Henle, decreased total number of juxtamedullary nephrons, washout of solutes from the medulla due to increased medullary blood flow, and decreased hydro-osmotic response of the cortical collecting duct to antidiuretic hormone (Saphasan and Sorrasuchart 1984).

Normal acid–base status is maintained by a combination of tubular reabsorption of filtered bicarbonate and excretion of hydrogen ion with ammonia and buffers primarily phosphates. Renal excretion of hydrogen ions effectively regenerates bicarbonate lost via the gastrointestinal tract or urinary tract or through respiratory buffering of metabolic acids. With urethral obstruction, retention of metabolic acids, consumption of bicarbonate to stabilize plasma and compartmental pH, generation of lactate associated with hypovolemia and hypoxia, and decreased conservation of bicarbonate in obstructive and postobstructive periods result in metabolic acidemia. Acidemia has significant direct and indirect effects. Direct effects include decreased myocardial contractility, stroke volume, and cardiac output; excitable membrane alterations leading to dysrhythmias; central nervous system depression; and dysfunction of metabolic pathways. Indirect effects include alterations in transcellular potassium distribution, plasma protein binding, ionization of pharmacologic agents, oxygen transport, tissue catabolism, and increased parasympathetic activity. Acutely following relief of obstruction of more than 24 hours' duration, dogs have impaired distal tubular proton excretion (Thirakomen and Koslov 1976). Dogs with long-term ureteral obstruction studied after recovery were able to both acidify and alkalinize urine after ammonium chloride and bicarbonate loading suggesting partial recovery of proton secretory function (Kerr 1956).

Fractional excretion of potassium increases after relief of obstruction. Although initially this may be interpreted as a homeostatic response to hyperkalemia, some animals develop hypokalemia during the postobstructive period. This observation indicates that there is impairment of normal homeostatic mechanisms. Increased urinary potassium excretion may be caused by increased delivery of sodium to the distal tubule, where sodium–potassium exchange occurs during sodium reabsorption. Medullary collecting duct may be the major site of the defect in potassium homeostasis.

Pathology

Urethral swelling, hemorrhage, and epithelial denudation may be present at the site of and proximal to the obstruction. The urinary bladder may be distended, hemorrhagic, and the epithelium denuded. Also, the urinary bladder wall may be thickened due to edema. Light microscopic examination of urinary bladders from dogs with experimental urethral obstruction of 10 hours' duration showed focal to diffuse submucosal hemorrhages, perivascular inflammatory infiltration, necrosis of urothelium, and fibrosis of the lamina propria (Tammela and Auto-Harmainen 1991). Axonal degeneration and edema of Schwann cells were found by electron microscopy. Although disruption of tight junctions between detrusor muscle cells is thought to occur, this has not been a consistent finding in experimental models. It is possible that bladder distention leads to reduced blood flow, which results in hypoxia, disturbances in energy metabolism, disturbances in activity of Na-K-ATPase membrane pumps, and injury to nerves located in the bladder wall (Seki and Karim 1992). These changes result in transient or permanent dysfunction of the bladder. Rupture of the urinary bladder may occur with prolonged urethral obstruction, particularly if the disease process is present in the urinary bladder before acute urethral obstruction.

Mild hydroureter and hydronephrosis may or may not be noted with acute lower urinary tract obstruction. If the patient lives for a sufficient period, urethral obstruction may lead to progressive loss of renal parenchyma. Histologically, glomeruli are preserved more readily than tubular elements, leading to a preponderance of glomeruli in residual cortical tissue. Fibrosis and cellular infiltration also occur (Morsing and Persson 1991).

References

Allen, J.T., E.D. Vaughan, et al. (1978). The effect of indomethicin on renal blood flow and ureteral pressure in unilateral ureteral obstruction in awake dogs. *Invest Urol* **15**: 324–327.

Ausiello, D.A., J.I. Kreisberg, et al. (1980). Contraction of cultured rat gomerular cells of apparent mesangial origin after stimulation with angiotensin II and arginine vasopressin. *J Clin Invest* **65**: 754–760.

Bartges, J.W., D.R. Finco, et al. (1996). Pathophysiology of urethral obstruction. *Vet Clin North Am Small Anim Pract* **26**(2): 255–264.

Finco, D.R. and L.M. Cornelius (1977). Characterization and treatment of water, electrolyte, and acid-base imbalances of induced urethral obstruction in the cat. *Am J Vet Res* **38**(6): 823–830.

Harris, K.P., G.F. Schreiner, et al. (1989). Effect of leukocyte depletion on the function of the postobstructed kidney in the rat. *Kidney Int* **36**(2): 210–215.

Kerr, W.S. (1956). Effects of complete ureteral obstruction in dogs on kidney function. *Am J Physiol* **184**: 521–526.

Klahr, S. (1991). New insights into the consequences and mechanisms of renal impairment in obstructive nephropathy [editorial]. *Am J Kidney Dis* **18**(6): 689–699.

Klahr, S. (1991). Pathophysiology of obstructive nephropathy: a 1991 update. *Semin Nephrol* **11**(2): 156–168.

Klahr, S. and K.P. Harris (1992). Obstuctive uropathy. In: *The Kidney*, edited by D.W. Seldin and G.G. Giebisch. New York: Raven Press.

Morsing, P. and A.E. Persson (1991). Tubuloglomerular feedback in obstructive uropathy. *Kidney Int Suppl* **32**(4): S110–S114.

Saphasan, S. and S. Sorrasuchart (1984). Factors inducing postobstructive diuresis in rats. *Nephron* **38**: 125–133.

Schreiner, G., K.P.G. Harris, et al. (1988). The immunological aspects of acute ureteral obstruction: immune cell infiltrate in the kidney. *Kidney Int* **34**: 487–493.

Schreiner, G. and E.R. Unanue (1984). Origin of the rat mesangial phagocyte and its expression of the leukocyte common antigen. *Lab Invest* **51**: 515–523.

Seki, N., O.M. Karim, et al. (1992). The effect of experimental urethral obstruction and its reversal on changes in passive electrical properties of detrusor muscle. *J Urol* **148**(6): 1957–1961.

Tammela, T., H. Auto-Harmainen, et al. (1991). Effect of prolonged experimental distention on the function and ultrastructure of the canine urinary bladder. *Ann Chrurgiae Gynaecolgiae* **80**: 301–306.

Thirakomen, K., N. Koslov, et al. (1976). Renal hydrogen ion excretion after release of unilateral ureteral obstruction. *Am J Physiol* **231**: 1233–1239.

Yanagisawa, H., J. Morrissey, et al. (1990). Role of angiotensin II in eicosanoid production in isolated glomeruli from rats with bilateral ureteral obstruction. *Am J Physiol* **258**: F85–F93.

Yarger, W.E., D.D. Schocken, et al. (1980). Obstructive nephropathy in the rat: possible roles for the renin-angiotensin system, prostaglandins, and thromboxanes in postobstructive renal function. *J Clin Invest* **65**: 400–412.

71

Urinary tract infection—bacterial

David Senior

Etiology

Urinary tract infection (UTI) can induce urethritis, prostatitis (in intact male dogs), cystitis, and pyelonephritis, and all of the urinary tract is at risk of colonization once UTI is established. Most UTI is caused by bacteria emanating from the gastrointestinal tract crossing the perineum and colonizing the external genitalia prior to retrograde invasion of the urethra and bladder against the flow of urine. A lesser number of lower UTIs go on to further ascend with colonization of the ureters and kidneys. Hematogenous renal infection, for example, from bacterial endocarditis, can induce septic infarcts and pyelonephritis although this is relatively uncommon.

In normal animals, the urinary tract proximal to the mid-urethra is a sterile environment and it remains resistant to infection even though it communicates directly with the external genitalia, an environment with a resident bacterial flora.

Development of UTI depends upon the balance between infectious agents and host resistance. Although UTI can occur when a very virulent organism invades a normal urinary tract, many times UTI develops when there is a disturbance of anatomical or functional host resistance factors that normally prevent microbial invasion. Common bacteria involved in UTI are shown in Table 71.1.

Pathogenesis

Development of UTI depends on a balance between virulent bacteria that tend to ascend the urinary tract and natural host defenses that tend to keep them out.

Nephrology and Urology of Small Animals. Edited by Joe Bartges and David J. Polzin. © 2011 Blackwell Publishing Ltd.

Host defense mechanisms

Host defense mechanisms purported to be important in protection against UTI are shown in Table 71.2.

Normal micturition

Diseases that impair the frequency or volume of micturition, or that permit residual urine to remain in the urinary bladder following micturition, predispose to infection. Urethral stricture secondary to fibrosis, hypertrophy, and tumors may interfere with normal urine outflow and provide sites for microbial colonization. Incomplete bladder emptying secondary to spinal lesions and acquired or congenital atonic bladder predispose to UTI.

Anatomical structures

A high-pressure zone in the urethra of female dogs may inhibit retrograde migration of bacteria toward the bladder. Symmetrical peristaltic contractions of the urethra identified in male dogs may have a similar effect. The oblique passage of the ureters through the bladder wall prevents vesicoureteral reflux when intravesicular pressure is high, for example, during voiding. Vulval involution is often associated with recurrent UTI (Figure 71.1). Congenital anomalies such as ectopic ureter bypass the normal anatomical defenses usually are associated with UTI.

Mucosal defense barriers

A thin surface layer of glycosaminoglycan (GAG) on the uroepithelium prevents bacterial attachment. Ovariectomized animals may be at greater risk of UTI due to impaired GAG production (Parsons 1982). Normal epithelial exfoliation of cells with bacteria attached may hamper bacterial colonization (Sobel and Kaye 1984). Urethral catheterization, passage of uroliths, neoplasia,

Table 71.1 Bacterial isolates in canine UTI

	Per cent of total isolates		
	a	b	c
E. coli	37.8	67	20.1
Staphylococcus spp.	14.5	21	9.6
Proteus mirabilis	12.4	3	15.4
Streptococcus spp.	10.7	6	10.6
Klebsiella pneumoniae	8.1	0	3.4
Pseudomonas aeruginosa	3.4	0	6.9
Enterobacter spp.	2.6	3	3.3
Number of isolates:	1,400	40	187

[a]Ling, G.V. et al. (1980a). *Vet Clin North Am* **9**: 617–630.
[b]Kivisto, A.K. et al. (1997). *J Sm Anim Pract* **18**: 707–712.
[c]Wooley, R.E. et al. (1976). *Mod Vet Pract* **57**: 535–538.

and chemical irritation (e.g., cyclophosphamide) can disrupt the normal mucosal barrier.

Antimicrobial properties of urine

Concentrated urine inhibits bacterial growth because of high concentrations of urea. Other organic acids derived from the diet also may inhibit bacterial growth. Dilute

Table 71.2 Local host defenses of the urinary tract

Normal micturition
   Adequate urine flow
   Frequent voiding
   Complete voiding
Anatomic structures
   Urethral high pressure zone
   Surface characteristics of urethral urothelium
   Urethral peristalsis
   Prostatic antibacterial fraction
   Length of urethra
   Ureterovesical flap valves and ureteral peristalsis
Mucosal defense barriers
   Antibody production
   Surface glycosaminoglycan layer
   Intrinsic mucosal antimicrobial properties
   Bacterial interference
   Exfoliation of cells
Antimicrobial properties of urine
   Extremes (high or low) of urine pH
   Hyperosmolality
   High concentration of urea
   Organic acids
Renal defenses
   Glomerular mesangial cells?
   Extensive blood supply and large blood flow

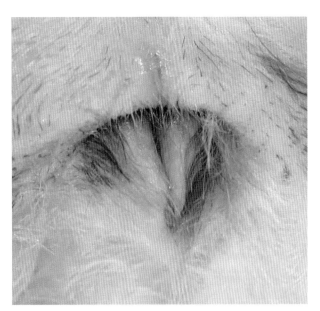

Figure 71.1 Vulval involution in a young female dog with recurrent urinary tract infection (Copyright David F. Senior BVSc., Louisiana State University, by permission).

urine associated with corticosteroid administration may predispose to infection. A high incidence (39%) of UTI has been reported in dogs with skin disease treated with corticosteroids (Ihrke et al. 1985). Urine contains a significant quantity of IgG and IgA, which may contribute to host defenses because bacteria coated by antibodies are less able to attach to the uroepithelium (Ling et al. 1985).

Bacterial virulence

Only a small proportion of the gastrointestinal flora can induce UTI (Parsons 1986). Motility, the ability to adhere to uroepithelial cells and efficient delivery of bacterial toxins to the mucosal wall may all be important virulence factors. Bacterial adherence is mediated by a variety of specific molecular configurations on or projecting from the surface of bacteria binding to receptors located on the uroepithelial cell wall (Senior et al. 1992). Bacterial urease production is an important virulence trait because urease causes devitalization of uroepitheial cells and smooth muscle paralysis, both of which facilitate bacterial invasion and persistence. Bacterial colicins inhibit the growth of other species of bacteria around them, which may be important in overcoming the protective effect of the normal flora of the external genitalia. Virulent bacteria produce aerophagin, hemolysins, and other substances that are capable of causing cell lysis with subsequent increased access to iron, an essential bacterial growth requirement.

The consequences of UTI are variable. In many cases, the signs of lower urinary tract inflammation are obvious and the condition responds readily to treatment. Chronic

UTI can persist undetected for a prolonged period in a commensal-like relationship with the host animal causing few if any detrimental effects. However, possible consequences of persistent UTI include struvite urolithiasis, chronic prostatitis, prostatic abscess formation, discospondylitis, and ascending renal infection with scarring, progressive loss of renal function, and chronic renal failure. Whether an infection will be benign or injurious cannot be predicted, so all cases of UTI should be treated vigorously.

Clinical signs

Typical signs of acute UTI are those of lower urinary tract inflammation. Animals with chronic UTI and animals with concurrent UTI and hyperadrenocorticism tend to be clinically silent.

When a UTI causes clinical signs, owners notice urgency, hematuria, dysuria, pollakiuria, and stranguria. Passage of urine can elicit a vocal pain response. Stranguria may continue after the bladder is empty. In lower UTI, the urine may appear progressively redder toward the end of urination. Urinary incontinence may develop. If the animal urinates in the house, hematuria and an ammonia-like odor to the urine may be noticed. When inflammation is confined to the urethra and external genitalia, the pain associated with urination can cause some animals to retain urine and not empty the bladder properly.

On physical examination, the patient may exhibit sensitivity to bladder palpation. If inflammation is severe, the bladder is usually small and the bladder wall may be thickened. Fever is seldom observed in lower UTI unless the inflammation is extreme. Chronic UTI can cause the bladder to become thickened due to edema, mucosal hyperplasia, and fibrosis. In animals with acute pyelonephritis, palpation of the kidneys can elicit a pain response.

Diagnosis

Differential diagnoses of lower urinary tract inflammation include UTI, urolithiasis (Figure 71.2), and lower urinary tract neoplasia (Figure 71.3). However, neoplasia is rare in dogs under 7 years of age. Urolithiasis and neoplasia are frequently accompanied by UTI.

The diagnosis of UTI is often made on clinical history and physical examination alone. Initial antimicrobial medications are prescribed on the basis of probable cause and past success. Urinalysis (Figure 71.4), urine culture, and antimicrobial sensitivity testing is recommended, particularly if previous treatment has been unsuccessful.

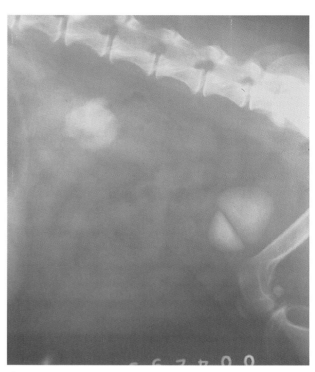

Figure 71.2 Radiographic appearance of bladder uroliths in a dog exhibiting signs of lower urinary tract inflammation (Copyright David F. Senior BVSc., Louisiana State University, by permission).

Method of collection alters interpretation of urinalysis and bacterial culture results. Urine samples for urinalysis and culture are best obtained by cystocentesis; voided samples are not suitable for this purpose. Collection of urine by cystocentesis can be facilitated with ultrasound guidance. Although catheterization can be used to collect

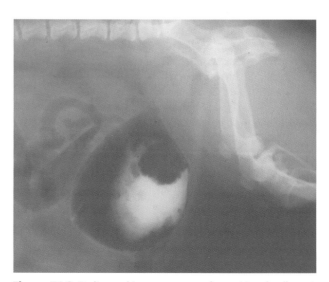

Figure 71.3 Radiographic appearance of transitional cell carcinoma of the bladder in a dog exhibiting signs of lower urinary tract inflammation (Copyright David F. Senior BVSc., Louisiana State University, by permission).

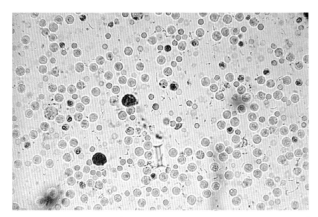

Figure 71.4 Typical inflammatory reaction seen in the urine sediment from a dog with acute bacterial cystitis. Red blood cells and white blood cells predominate (Copyright David F. Senior BVSc., Louisiana State University, by permission).

urine for urinalysis and culture, results obtained by cystocentesis are much easier to interpret (Comer and Ling 1981). Further, catheterization introduces bacteria into the urinary tract and traumatizes the urethral uroepithelium.

Typically with urinalysis of patients with UTI, the dipstick indicates increased proteinuria and hematuria and increased white blood cells, red blood cells, bacteria, and epithelial cells are observed in the urine sediment. With pyelonephritis, white blood cell casts and granular casts may be observed, but this is an inconsistent finding.

When pyuria is observed in the urine sediment in the absence of bacteriuria, urine culture should still be performed because positive cultures can be grown even when bacteria are not obvious on urine sediment. Absence of

abnormally high numbers of white blood cells and bacteria may not reliably rule out UTI if the urine specific gravity is low because of the dilution effect.

Bacterial culture should be performed as soon as possible after sample collection and certainly no longer than 4 hours. With cystocentesis samples, any bacterial growth is considered significant, but with catheterization, greater than 10^5 colonies per mL must be present to be considered significant. The most common bacterial isolates from canine UTI are shown in Table 71.1.

Antimicrobial sensitivity tests

Antimicrobial sensitivity tests on uropathogens are best performed using the minimum inhibitory concentration (MIC) method. Antimicrobial penetration into infected tissue of the bladder and urethra is dependent on the concentration of antimicrobial in urine, not plasma. The mean urinary concentration (MUC) achieved with standard dose regimens has been determined for most of the antimicrobial agents used to treat UTI. If an antimicrobial reaches an MUC of at least four times the in vitro MIC, treatment with that drug has a high chance of therapeutic success (Ling et al. 1984). Antimicrobial agents that cannot achieve four times the MIC are usually not effective. The MUC in dogs of commonly used antimicrobials when given at usual recommended doses is shown in Table 71.3. This data allows selection of appropriate drugs to treat UTI once MIC values for the isolated bacteria are known.

Recommended doses, dosing frequency, route of administration, and mean urinary concentration found

Table 71.3 Dosage and mean urinary concentration of the drugs commonly used to treat UTI[a] (Ling and Ruby 1983; Ling and Conzelman 1980b, 1980c, 1981; Rohrich et al. 1983; Sigel et al. 1981)

Agent	Dose	Route	Mean urine concentration ($\pm$ SD) µg/mL	MIC µg/mL
Ampicillin	25 mg/kg tid	P.O.	309 ($\pm$ 55)	77
Amoxicillin	11 mg/kg tid	P.O.	202 ($\pm$ 93)	50
Enrofloxacin	2.5 mg/kg bid	P.O.	40	10
Tetracycline	15 mg/kg tid	P.O.	138 ($\pm$ 65)	35
Chloramphenicol	33 mg/kg tid	P.O.	124 ($\pm$ 40)	31
Cephalexin	18 mg/kg tid	P.O.	500 (?)	125
Sulfisoxazole	22 mg/kg tid	P.O.	1,466 ($\pm$ 832)	366
Nitrofurantoin	5 mg/kg tid	P.O.	100 (?)	25
Trimethoprim-Sulfa	12 mg/kg bid	P.O.	246 ($\pm$ 150)	62
	2.2 mg/kg bid		55 ($\pm$ 19)	14
Kanamycin	6 mg/kg bid	S.Q.	530 ($\pm$ 151)	132
Gentamicin	1.5 mg/kg tid	S.Q.	107 ($\pm$ 33)	27
Amikacin	5 mg/kg tid	S.Q.	342 ($\pm$ 143)	85
Tobramycin	1 mg/kg tid	S.Q.	145 ($\pm$ 86)	36

[a] *Source*: Data courtesy of Dr. Gerald V. Ling, University of California, Davis.

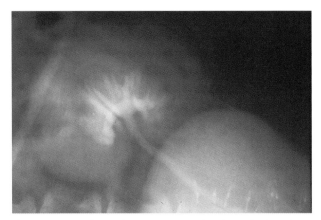

Figure 71.5 Radiographic appearance of pyelonephritis on intravenous pyelography. The diverticula of the renal collection system are thickened and distorted (Copyright David F. Senior BVSc., Louisiana State University, by permission).

in normal dogs is shown in Table 71.3. Note that dogs passing dilute urine may not achieve these levels.

The Kirby-Bauer disc-diffusion antimicrobial sensitivity test is based on antimicrobial concentrations achievable in plasma and tissue and is therefore applicable when prostatic and renal involvement is suspected.

Localization of infection

Differentiation between upper and lower UTI can be difficult. The presence of dilute urine, white blood cell casts in the urine sediment, irregular appearing diverticula and dilation of the renal pelvis on IVP, increased echogenicity of the renal pelvis on ultrasound, and peripheral leukocytosis are inconsistent indicators of renal infection. In advanced chronic pyelonephritis, the kidneys appear small and irregular, and the diverticula have irregular borders (Figure 71.5). Morphologic changes to the kidney on imaging do not prove that active renal infection is present at the time of the study. Bacterial culture on urine sampled directly from the renal pelvis by nephropyelocentesis can confirm renal involvement.

Upper UTI should always be considered a possibility, particularly if infection recurs after initial therapy. Repeat urinalysis and urine culture after treatment should be performed routinely. In intact male dogs with UTI, approximately 90% have concurrent colonization of the prostate.

Treatment

Choice of antimicrobial

Several bacteria commonly isolated from UTI in dogs and cats have predictable antimicrobial sensitivity provided they have not undergone recent antimicrobial treatment.

If cocci are observed in the urine sediment (*Staphylococcus intermedius*, *Streptococcus* spp., and *Enterococcus* spp.) or the urine is very alkaline and small rods in pairs are evident in the urine sediment (*Proteus mirabilis*), over 90% will be sensitive to ampicillin or amoxicillin. *S. intermedius* and *Proteus mirabilis* produce β-lactamase, so amoxicillin combined with the β-lactamase inhibitor clavulanic acid may be preferable. Both *S. intermedius* and *Proteus mirabilis* are powerful urease producers so extremely alkaline urine suggests their presence.

If rods are observed in the sediment of non-alkaline urine, the sensitivity of these bacteria is not predictable and urine culture and sensitivity must be performed. Antimicrobial sensitivity of *E. coli*, *Klebsiella* spp., and *Enterobacter* spp. are not predictable so sensitivity tests must be performed to determine appropriate treatment (Table 71.3). Fluoroquinolones are usually the best choice for *Pseudomonas aeruginosa* infections combining efficacy with low renal toxicity.

Duration of treatment

Treatment of UTI of the lower urinary tract should be continued for 14 days (Ling 1980; Ling 1984; Naber 1999). Treatment for 30 days is usually recommended for patients where prostatic or renal involvement is suspected.

With effective treatment, bacteria should not be detectable in the urine sediment by 3–5 days after initiation of treatment. Urine culture performed 10 days after cessation of treatment can document successful treatment or persistent or recurrent UTI.

Special considerations

Most oral antimicrobial agents should be given in three equally spaced doses daily to maintain effective concentration in the urine. Exceptions to this are the fluoroquinolones and potentiated sulfas, which can be given twice daily.

Provided antimicrobial sensitivity tests indicate that a drug is likely to be successful, adjunct treatment to acidify the urine is not necessary

Intact male dogs with UTI must always be treated assuming that the prostate is colonized. Antimicrobial selection should be based on prostatic penetration and treatment should be continued for 30 days. Acinar fluid in the canine prostate gland is acidic (pH 6.4) and antimicrobial agents penetrate the prostate from plasma, not from urine. Appropriate weak bases and/or lipid soluble antimicrobials include the fluoroquinolones (broad spectrum weak bases) (Dorfman et al. 1995), trimethoprim (a weak base), and doxycycline and chloramphenicol (lipid soluble). Penicillins and cephalosporins penetrate the prostate poorly and are inappropriate. Failure to clear infection from the prostate gland in a male dog with UTI sets the stage for recolonization by the same organism, establishment of chronic prostatitis, and formation of a prostatic abscess.

Although renal involvement in UTI is difficult to diagnose, the standard treatment regimen should be adjusted if pyelonephritis is suspected. Antimicrobial agents diffuse into renal tissue from plasma not from concentrated urine, so to be effective, drugs must achieve a plasma concentration of four times MIC. In addition, treatment for 30 days is warranted to ensure elimination of infection.

Treatment failure

Failure of an antimicrobial agent to sterilize the urine should alert the clinician to one or more of the following possibilities:

1. Inappropriate drug, dose, or duration of therapy. Owner compliance is important in this respect.
2. Failure of the antimicrobial agent to reach sufficient concentrations in urine despite appropriate drug administration. Intestinal malabsorption, impaired renal concentrating capacity, and development of antimicrobial resistance should be considered.
3. The presence of a nidus of infection that is capable of recolonizing the urinary tract once antimicrobial therapy is withdrawn. Pyelonephritis, prostatitis, neoplasia, persistent urachal remnant, and urolithiasis should be considered.
4. The presence of anatomical or functional abnormalities of the urinary tract that lower resistance to bacterial colonization. Many defects may be undetectable by available clinical diagnostic methods.

When UTI recurs after apparently effective treatment has been given for a reasonable period of time, underlying predisposing conditions should be sought. The external genitalia of female dogs should be examined for vulval involution. Urine retention after voiding should be determined by catheterization or ultrasound. In male dogs, prostatic involvement can be determined by ultrasonic examination with cytology and culture of prostatic aspirates. Imaging studies including ultrasound, plain, and contrast radiographic studies including IVP, double contrast cystography and retrograde and voiding urethrography, CT, and MRI combined with cystoscopy can rule out the presence of identifiable anatomical defects. Correction of anatomical and functional defects and underlying conditions often prevents recurrence of infection.

Prevention

When an animal suffers frequent recurrences of UTI despite adequate treatment and in the absence of detectable or correctable anatomic and functional disturbances, long-term management with antimicrobial agents may prevent additional recurrences. Patients should undergo initial treatment with an antimicrobial based on sensitivity results for 14 or 30 days, as required. Administration of an antimicrobial is then continued at 30–50% of the usual total daily dose given as a single dose at night before bedtime immediately after the animal voids. Treatment should be given for 6 months.

The long-term antimicrobial should be the same one used to treat the infection based on the last sensitivity test. Follow-up urine culture and sensitivity tests should be performed on a monthly basis to ensure that the patient remains free of infection. Resistant fecal and vaginal bacteria do not tend to develop with these low-dose regimens.

The orally administered urinary antiseptic methenamine mandalate has been suggested for prevention of UTI in patients with recurrent UTI. To be effective, this drug requires the formation of very acidic urine, which is difficult to achieve in dogs beyond 5 days. The efficacy of orally administered cranberry extract (available in capsule form), to prevent UTI in dogs, remains undocumented.

For follow-up urinalysis and bacterial culture, urine should always be collected by cystocentesis and never by catheterization. Catheterization predisposes animals to ascending infection.

Prognosis

The prognosis for successful treatment is good in patients that do not have major underlying predisposing causes that cannot be eliminated. For example, animals with unresectable bladder tumors are often prone to reinfection.

Caution

There is no evidence that canine and feline uropathogens are transferable across species and can cause UTI in humans. However, there is considerable evidence that treating a pet with an antimicrobial induces a change in the fecal flora of humans sharing the same household. The acquired resistance may be due to plasmid-mediated transfer of resistance from animal fecal flora to the fecal flora of closely associated humans (Schon et al. 1972; Levy et al. 1976). Patients with long-term refractory UTI with minimal clinical signs and no evidence of renal involvement may best be left untreated.

References

Biertuempfel, P.H., G.V. Ling, et al. (1981). Urinary tract infection resulting from catheterization in healthy adult dogs. *J Am Vet Med Assoc* **178**(9): 989–991.

Comer, K.M. and G.V. Ling (1981). Results of urinalysis and bacterial culture of canine urine obtained by antepubic cystocentesis, catheterization, and the midstream voided methods. *J Am Vet Med Assoc* **179**(9): 891–895.

Dorfman, M., J. Barsanti, et al. (1995). Enrofloxacin concentrations in dogs with normal prostate and dogs with chronic bacterial prostatitis. *Am J Vet Res* **56**(3): 386–390.

Ihrke, P.J., A.L. Norton, et al. (1985). Urinary tract infection associated with long-term corticosteroid administration in dogs with chronic skin diseases. *J Am Vet Med Assoc* **186**(1): 43–46.

Levy, S.B., G.B. FitzGerald, et al. (1976). Changes in intestinal flora of farm personnel after introduction of a tetracycline-supplemented feed on a farm. *N Engl J Med* **295**(11): 583–588.

Ling, G.V. (1980). Treatment of urinary tract infections. *Vet Clin North Am Small Anim Pract* **9**(4): 795–804.

Ling, G.V. (1984). Therapeutic strategies involving antimicrobial treatment of the canine urinary tract. *J Am Vet Med Assoc* **185**(10): 1162–1164.

Ling, G.V. and A.L. Ruby (1983). Cephalexin for oral treatment of canine urinary tract infection caused by Klebsiella pneumoniae. *J Am Vet Med Assoc* **182**(12): 1346–1347.

Ling, G.V., E.L. Biberstein, et al. (1980a). Bacterial pathogens associated with urinary tract infections. *Vet Clin North Am Small Anim Pract* **9**(4): 617–630.

Ling, G.V., G.M. Conzelman Jr, et al. (1980b). Urine concentrations of chloramphenicol, tetracycline, and sulfisoxazole after oral administration to healthy adult dogs. *Am J Vet Res* **41**(6): 950–952.

Ling, G.V., G.M. Conzelman Jr, et al. (1980c). Urine concentrations of five penicillins following oral administration to normal adult dogs. *Am J Vet Res* **41**(7): 1123–1125.

Ling, G.V., G.M. Conzelman Jr, et al. (1981). Urine concentrations of gentamicin, tobramycin, amikacin, and kanamycin after subcutaneous administration to healthy adult dogs. *Am J Vet Res.* **42**(10): 1792–1794.

Ling, G.V., P.J. Rohrich, et al. (1984). Canine urinary tract infections: a comparison of in vitro antimicrobial susceptibility test results and response to oral therapy with ampicillin or with trimethoprim-sulfa. *J Am Vet Med Assoc* **185**(3): 277–281.

Ling, G.V., J.M. Cullen, et al. (1985). Relationship of upper and lower urinary tract infection and bacterial invasion of uroepithelium to antibody-coated bacteria test results in female dogs. *Am J Vet Res* **46**(2): 499–504.

Naber, K.G. (1999). Short-term therapy of acute uncomplicated cystitis. *Curr Opin Urol* **9**(1): 57–64.

Parsons, C.L. (1982). Prevention of urinary tract infection by the exogenous glycosaminoglycan sodium pentosanpolysulfate. *J Urol* **127**(1): 167–169.

Parsons, C.L. (1986). Pathogenesis of urinary tract infections. Bacterial adherence, bladder defense mechanisms. *Urol Clin North Am* **13**(4): 563–568.

Rohrich, P.J., G.V. Ling, et al. (1983). In vitro susceptibilities of canine urinary bacteria to selected antimicrobial agents. *J Am Vet Med Assoc* **183**(8): 863–867.

Schon, E., V. Wagner, et al. (1972). Resistance of bacteria isolated from subjects with occupational chlortetracycline exposure. *Rev Czech Med* 1972 **18**(1): 1–12.

Senior, D.F., P. deMan, et al. (1992). Serotype, hemolysin production, and adherence characteristics of strains of *Escherichia coli* causing urinary tract infection in dogs. *Am J Vet Res* **53**(4): 494–498.

Sigel, C.W., G.V. Ling, et al. (1981). Pharmacokinetics of trimethoprim and sulfadiazine in the dog: urine concentrations after oral administration. *Am J Vet Res* **42**(6): 996–1001.

Sobel, J.D. and D. Kaye (1984). Host factors in the pathogenesis of urinary tract infections. *Am J Med* **76**(5A): 122–130.

72

Fungal urinary tract infection

Barrak Pressler

Fungal urinary tract infections are a rare cause of lower urinary tract disease in dogs and cats. Funguria may be due to primary (confined to the urinary tract and presumptively due to ascending infection) or secondary (systemic infections resulting in shedding of organisms into the urine) infections. Organisms of the genus *Candida* are most commonly identified. Regardless of the infecting species, fungal urinary tract infections often are challenging to treat because of the strong apparent association with concurrent immunosuppressive diseases or breaches in local immunity that oftentimes cannot be completely resolved.

Candida sp. urinary tract infections

Epidemiology

Candida spp. are normal inhabitants of the genital mucosa, upper respiratory tract, and gastrointestinal tract in people, dogs, and cats (Hazen and Howell 2007; Suchodolski 2008). Over 150 species have been described within the *Candida* genus (which now includes the historic genus *Torulopsis*), with *C. albicans* and *C. parapsillosis* being the most common species isolated from normal dogs (Hazen and Howell 2007; Suchodolski 2008). *Candida* spp. are yeast, as they reproduce by budding and are capable of fermenting carbohydrates; however, this is a morphologic rather than a true taxonomic classification. Yeasts most commonly have a budding, ovate appearance, but they will also occasionally appear filamentous, particularly in biofilms that form on mucosal and catheter surfaces or when tissue invasion has occurred (Bizerra 2008). As with bacterial urinary tract infection, can-

diduria presumptively occurs in dogs and cats following ascending infection to the lower urinary tract. *Candida* spp. are isolated from less than 1% of dogs and cats with urinary tract infections, and less than 2% of dogs with recurrent or resistant infections (Wooley and Blue 1976; Norris 2000; Ling 2001). The majority of infections in dogs, cats, and people are due to *C. albicans*, but several other species have been reported (Table 72.1) (Occhipinti 1994; Lundstrom and Sobel 2001; Pressler 2003; Jin and Lin 2005; Kauffman 2005).

Although bacterial urinary tract infections may occur in the absence of predisposing factors, in human and veterinary patients, candidal infections appear to be highly associated with breaches in local lower urinary tract defenses or systemic immunocompromise (Occhipinti 1994; Lundstrom and Sobel 2001; Wise 2001; Pressler 2003; Jin and Lin 2005; Kauffman 2005). Nosocomial infections in patients with indwelling urinary catheters are the most common cause of candiduria in people; approximately 10–15% of hospital-acquired urinary tract infections are due to *Candida* spp., versus less than 1% of out-patient populations (Lundstrom and Sobel 2001; Colodner 2008). Diabetes mellitus, recent antibiotic, chemotherapeutic, or steroid administration, female gender, and lower urinary tract disease are also highly associated with infection in people (Gubbins 1999; Lundstrom and Sobel 2001; Kauffman 2005). Antibiotics that have anti-anaerobe spectra of activity may particularly predispose to gastrointestinal candidal overgrowth, and thus candiduria (Kennedy and Volz 1985). Recent surgery, concurrent bacterial urinary tract infection, and intravenous catheterization may also be independent predictors of infection (Gubbins 1999; Lundstrom and Sobel 2001; Kauffman 2005).

Many of the risk factors associated with *Candida* spp. urinary tract infections in people appear to be associated with candiduria in dogs and cats as well (Pressler 2003;

Nephrology and Urology of Small Animals. Edited by Joe Bartges and David J. Polzin. © 2011 Blackwell Publishing Ltd.

Table 72.1 Species of fungi reported to cause primary urinary tract infections in dogs or cats

Aspergillus spp.
  A. fumigatus (Kirpatrick 1982)
  A. nidulans (Adamama-Moraitou 2001)
Candida spp.
  C. albicans (Fulton and Walker 1992; Brain 1993; Forward 2002; Kano 2002; Pressler 2003; Jin and Lin 2005)
  C. glabrata (Tan and Lim 1977; Pressler 2003; Toll 2003; Jin and Lin 2005)
  C. guilliermondii (Jin and Lin 2005)
  C. krusei (Pressler 2003; Jin and Lin 2005)
  C. parapsillosis (Kano 2002; Pressler 2003)
  C. rugosa (Pressler 2003)
  C. tropicalis (Pressler 2003; Jin and Lin 2005; Ozawa 2005)
Cryptococcus neoformans (Day and Holt 1994; Newman 2003; Jin and Lin 2005; Chapman and Kirk 2008)
Rhodotorula mucilaginosa (Jin and Lin 2005)
Trichosporone beigelii (Pressler 2003)

Jin and Lin 2005). Although systematic comparisons between animals with candiduria versus bacterial urinary tract infections have not been performed, patients with urinary tract stomata, diabetes mellitus, or lower urinary tract neoplasms such as transitional cell carcinoma appear to be predisposed to infection (Pressler 2003; Jin and Lin 2005). Approximately 17% of reported cases of candidal urinary tract infections have been in dogs or cats previously or simultaneously diagnosed with diabetes mellitus (Brain 1993; Forward 2002; Pressler 2003; Toll 2003; Jin and Lin 2005). However, the author's experience suggests that this is an underestimate of the true association between these two diseases, and as many as 30–40% of patients with *Candida* spp. urinary tract infection are diabetic. Although in-hospital urinary catheterization has not been reported in any cases of isolated candiduria, one dog with systemic candidiasis and diabetes mellitus developed infection following prolonged urethral catheterization (Heseltine 2003). In addition, many reported cases in dogs or cats have had concurrent lower urinary tract disease, with permanent stoma formation (urethrostomy or cystotomy tube placement) reported in approximately 40% of cases when the two largest veterinary retrospective studies are combined (Pressler 2003; Jin and Lin 2005). As expected, a variety of antibiotics, steroids, and chemotherapeutic agents have been commonly administered to affected animals within one month of diagnosis of *Candida* spp. infections (Pressler 2003; Jin and Lin 2005).

Clinical presentation and diagnosis

There are no historical or physical examination findings that allow differentiation of candiduria from other causes of lower urinary tract disease. Dogs and cats with candiduria may demonstrate typical signs of lower urinary tract disease (i.e., dysuria, pollakiuria, micro-, or macroscopic hematuria) or be asymptomatic (Pressler 2003; Jin and Lin 2005). On rare occasions, flocculent, white or yellow material may be grossly visible in urine from veterinary patients with candiduria. When this is observed, clinical suspicion for heavy biofilm formation or bezoar formation is increased. In the author's experience, patients with diabetes mellitus are more likely to have clinically silent infections, further stressing the need for routine urine cultures (Chapter 9) in patients with this disease. Likewise, dogs and cats with historically diagnosed but unsuccessfully treated *Candida* spp. urinary tract infections are often asymptomatic as well.

The most common reason *Candida* spp. urinary tract infections are first suspected is due to visualization of fungal elements on urine sediment examination. Although cutaneous *Candida* spp. are usually budding, organisms shed in urine may be budding or filamentous in appearance, reflecting shedding from the biofilm that often adheres to the bladder mucosa (Bizerra 2008). Finding fungal elements on routine urinalysis usually suggests that growth of *Candida* spp. is heavy. Alternatively, in patients where sediment examinations are performed to monitor for recurrence or response to therapy (i.e., times when number of organisms is expected to be low), urine cytospin preparations and/or modified Wright's staining of sediment may improve detection. Special stains of urine sediment such as Calcofluor white or lactophenol cotton blue are also occasionally used by clinical pathology or microbiology laboratories when fungal elements are suspected (Figure 72.1).

Identification of fungal elements should always be followed by urine culture to determine the infecting species. In some cases, the identification of *Candida* spp. first occurs by routine aerobic urine culture even though there was no clinical suspicion of funguria. Fortunately, *Candida* spp. readily grow on blood agar plates within 48 hours, and thus even when a specific fungal culture is not requested, most microbiology laboratories will identify candidal urinary tract infections. In those cases when candiduria is suspected or has been previously documented, a yeast or fungal culture should be requested. These cultures are performed on both blood and Sabouraud's media for 5–7 (yeast cultures) or 14 (fungal cultures) days, at both 37°C and ambient temperature. Sabouraud's media is not a better substrate than blood agar for fungal organism growth but is required for

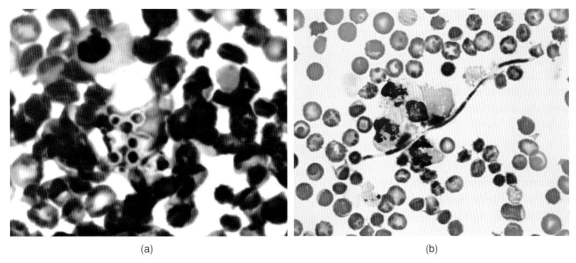

(a)   (b)

Figure 72.1 *Candida albicans* within urine sediment from a 5-year-old female spayed Labrador retriever being treated for multicentric lymphoma and acute-onset hematuria. Both budding (a) and filamentous (b) fungal elements are visible.

morphologic identification of genus and species based on growth characteristics. When fungal elements were not identified on initial urinalysis and the finding of candiduria on urine culture is unexpected, a second urine culture may be merited, particularly if the first sample was obtained via urinary catheter or mid-stream catch, or by cystocentesis in a patient with significant cutaneous disease. In the author's experience, dogs and cats may, in very rare circumstances, have transient candiduria.

Several other diagnostic tests have been used in experimental settings or have been investigated in people as more rapid methods for diagnosis of candiduria than standard fungal urine cultures. *Candida* spp.-specific polymerase chain reaction of urine samples has been reported in dogs and people; however, the ease of diagnosis by conventional diagnostic methods and the expense and specialized equipment required for PCR thus far makes this modality unappealing for routine use (Muncan and Wise 1996; Kano 2002; Ozawa 2005). In theory, PCR would be most useful in dogs and cats as a complement to culture in those cases where confirmation of successful treatment prior to cessation of antifungal therapy is desired. Serologic testing for *C. albicans* mannan protein antigen and antibodies has also been investigated in people. Unfortunately, correlation between the presence of antimannan antibodies and candiduria is extremely low, likely due to the ubiquitous nature of the organism and the high likelihood of previous exposure; the presence of circulating antigen in people is significantly associated with *Candida* spp. pyelonephritis, but not with candidal cystitis (Warnock 1976; Tokunaga 1993). Limited investigations of urine D-/L-arabinitol ratios in people suggest that this test is both sensitive and specific for detection of candiduria or can-

didal pyelonephritis, but this has not been investigated in dogs or cats (Tokunaga 1995; Hui 2004).

Treatment

Treatment of candiuria in people is recommended in all symptomatic patients, patients with systemic immunosuppressive diseases (and who are thus at risk of developing systemic candidiasis), and patients with noncorrectable risk factors. Patients with asymptomatic infections and no identifiable risk factors are initially recultured prior to treatment in order to confirm that candiduria is not transient; likewise, treatment is delayed in asymptomatic patients with correctable risk factors (such as indwelling urinary catheters) until these factors are removed and infection is found to persist. Unfortunately, because the most common risk factors in dogs and cats are not easily corrected (e.g., diabetes mellitus, permanent urinary tract stomata, and urinary tract neoplasia), withholding treatment in small animal veterinary patients is not recommended at this time. Ineffective treatment may lead to candidal pyelonephritis and/or fungemia.

Treatment of primary candiduria requires adequate excretion of active drug or metabolites into the urine. Of the antifungal agents widely used in veterinary medicine, only fluconazole and amphotericin B are excreted in significant amounts in active form by this route in people. Fluconazole is currently recommended as first-line therapy in people, dogs, and cats because it can be administered orally and has a high safety margin (Table 72.2) (Malani and Kauffman 2007). The majority of *C. albicans* isolates are sensitive to fluconazole, and thus routine antifungal sensitivity testing of this species does not appear

Table 72.2 Proposed treatment algorithm for fungal urinary tract infections

1. Identify and aggressively correct any concurrent breaks in local immunity or causes of systemic immunosuppression
2. Identify genus and species of infecting organism via urine fungal culture
    a. If *C. albicans*:
        i. Fluconazole, 5–10 mg/kg PO q12 h for 4–6 weeks
        ii. Repeat urine sediment examination and urine culture at 2–3 week intervals to confirm resolution of infection
        iii. Repeat urine sediment examination and urine culture 1 and 2 months after stopping therapy
    b. If non-*C. albicans*:
        i. Perform sensitivity testing of isolate against antifungal drugs to guide initial therapy
        ii. Consider penetration of drugs into urine when selecting therapy
3. If initial treatment with fluconazole fails to resolve infection, repeat antifungal drug sensitivity testing and consider:
    a. Intravesicular infusion of 1% clotrimazole (dogs; cats with permanent urinary tract stomata)
    b. Intravesicular infusion of amphotericin B (cats or dogs)
    c. Intravenous or subcutaneous amphotericin B (cats or dogs that have failed intravesicular therapy)
    d. Fluconazole at maximally recommended dose with addition of terbinafine (cats or dogs whose owners decline other treatment options)
    e. Benign neglect and regular monitoring for disease progression

necessary at the time of first diagnosis. However, other *Candida* spp., particularly *C. glabrata* and *C. krusei*, are more likely to be resistant to fluconazole, and sensitivity testing at first diagnosis is recommended to guide dose of fluconazole (as the MIC and break point may suggest that higher doses could be effective), or to determine if an alternative drug should be used (Rex 1995; Maenza 1996; Malani and Kauffman 2007).

Infections should always be considered "complicated" because of the association between candiduria and local or systemic immune system compromise. As such, treatment should be continued for a minimum of 4–6 weeks, with urine sediment examinations and/or cultures performed at 2–3 week intervals to confirm treatment efficacy. Frequency of resolution of infection in dogs and cats with fluconazole is unknown, but in the author's experience, it is approximately 50%; this is lower than reported success rates in people, likely because predisposing factors in veterinary patients are more difficult to control or resolve.

On the basis of personal experience and efficacy of alternative treatment options in people, the author's current treatment algorithm for animals with primary fungal urinary tract infections is presented in Table 72.2. For those patients who have persistent candidal urinary tract infections despite appropriate fluconazole therapy or who have recurrent infections, sensitivity testing of isolates should be performed. Several alternative treatment options have been reported by others and/or attempted by this author with varying degrees of success; none have been directly compared to fluconazole or each other to determine relative efficacy. Intravenous amphotericin B is primarily used for treatment of systemic candidiasis,

but single dose amphotericin B protocols (0.3–1.0 mg/kg) have also been reported for treatment of candiduria in people (Leu and Huang 1995; Fisher 2003). This author knows of successful treatment with multiple doses of amphotericin B in one dog with recurrent candiduria and urolithiasis, and treatment failure in one diabetic cat. Subcutaneous amphotericin B protocols have been reported for treatment of systemic cryptococcosis in dogs and cats and could potentially be used to treat candiduria as well (Malik 1996). Of other available antifungal drugs, oral itraconazole or ketoconazole do not result in high concentrations of active drug within urine. Nevertheless, in one retrospective study, a small number of patients had successful resolution of candiduria with these drugs (Pressler 2003). How well predisposing factors had been concurrently minimized or resolved in those patients is unknown. Newer parenteral triazole drugs (e.g., posaconazole, voriconazole) are not excreted into urine in active form and have not been used to treat candiduria to the author's knowledge; the same is true of terbinafine, which may be synergistic with some azole drugs but is not excreted into urine in active form (Humbert 1995; Barchiesi 1997; Malani and Kauffman 2007). Persistent or invasive candidal urinary tract infections in people have been treated with echinocandins (i.e., caspofungin, micafungin) despite poor urinary excretion of active drug, but the pharmacologic profiles, safety, and efficacy of these drugs in dogs or cats are unknown (Grooters and Taboada 2003; Bennett 2006; Lagrotteria 2007; Sobel 2007). It has been suggested that urine alkalinization may be a useful adjunctive therapy for candiduria in dogs and cats, as *Candida* spp. growth is inhibited at higher pH in vitro. This author has not appreciated improved resolution of infection in dogs and cats with alkalinization, and unfortunately, without concurrent dietary therapy, high doses of sodium bicarbonate are oftentimes required to reach target pH. Urine alkalinization is no longer favored in people in candiduria, and as a result this author does not manipulate urine pH as part of his standard protocol.

Intravesicular infusion of antifungal drugs has also been described. Advantages of this modality include direct instillation of large volumes of high concentration drugs, the ability to use drugs where safety (i.e., amphotericin B) would be limited by preexisting renal disease, and no need for owner administration of oral medications. Disadvantages include the need for repeat evaluations by veterinarians to perform drug instillation, difficulties associated with urinary catheterization (particularly in cats and female dogs), and risk of iatrogenic infection or bladder rupture. In people, the efficacy of intravesicular amphotericin B for long-term resolution of candiduria is equal to that of oral fluconazole, although amphotericin B may result in more rapid resolution of infection; nevertheless, because of the low power of these comparative studies and the difficulties associated with treatment, intravesicular drug administration is falling out of favor in people (Fan-Havard 1995; Leu and Huang 1995; Trinh 1995; Jacobs 1996; Wise 2001; Drew 2005). One cat with candiduria and a perineal urethrostomy treated by this author with a single dose of intravesicular amphotericin B failed to resolve candidal infection.

Alternatively, in dogs and cats, two case reports describe intravesicular infusion of 1% clotrimazole either transurethrally or via needle and syringe using ultrasound guidance (Forward 2002; Toll 2003). In addition, this author has treated approximately 20 cases of candiduria using a modified 1% clotrimazole protocol (Table 72.3). With a minimum of three infusions, the observed success rate for resolution of infection in patients who have failed fluconazole is approximately 50%. Successful resolution appears to be more likely in dogs and in nonobese animals. As previously discussed, resolution is likely correlated with successful identification and treatment of predisposing factors. Unfortunately, because 1%

clotrimazole is supplied in polyethylene glycol, it is highly viscous and very difficult to infuse through small diameter urinary catheters. As a result, administration of intravesicular clotrimazole in male cats has proven to be impractical in most cases (unless a larger catheter can be inserted through a perineal urethrostomy site).

Despite these various treatment options, approximately 25% of dogs and cats with candiduria appear to have persistent, asymptomatic infections despite at least two different treatment modalities. In these patients, the author only reattempts treatment when clinical signs recur, there is suspicion of ascending infection, or increased growth of *Candida* spp. is noted during periodic urine sediment examination. Studies are still required to determine whether this benign neglect approach is appropriate, and whether it can be attempted in all asymptomatic animals and not just those who have failed traditional therapy.

Noncandidal primary urinary tract infections

Although much rarer than *Candida* spp., other fungal organisms may also cause primary urinary tract infections in dogs or cats (Table 72.1). Unfortunately, too few cases have been reported to determine if predisposing factors, disease course, or optimal treatment differ from candiduria. In general, infection should be confirmed via a second urine culture, patients with confirmed infections should be evaluated for local or systemic causes of immunosuppression, and primary versus secondary funguria should be determined. Precise species identification of the infecting organism should always be performed. Of the common systemic mycoses, *Aspergillus* spp (Kirpatrick 1982; Adamama-Moraitou 2001) and *Cryptococcus neoformans* (Newman 2003; Chapman and Kirk 2008) rarely may cause primary infection of the lower and upper urinary tract in both dogs and cats. Despite these reports, if either agent is isolated from urine, clinicians should initially assume infection is systemic and determine other organ involvement before opting for oral fluconazole or localized intravesicular therapy.

Table 72.3 Intravesicular 1% clotrimazole protocol for treatment of fluconazole-resistant fungal urinary tract infections in dogs and cats

1. Catheterize and empty the bladder. Balloon catheters are preferred in dogs as they prevent premature voiding of drug in nonanesthetized patients; most cats will retain the infused drug if not allowed access to a litter box.
2. Infuse 7.5–10 mL/kg of 1% clotrimazole solution; volume should be determined by bladder palpation during infusion.
3. Infused fluid should be retained for a minimum of 15–30 minutes.
4. Repeat infusion q7 days for three treatments.
5. Repeat fungal urine culture 7 days after third treatment to determine whether additional infusions or alternative therapy should be considered.
6. Oral fluconazole therapy should be continued throughout the infusion protocol.

Susceptibility testing against various antifungal drugs is recommended for all non-*Candida* spp. urinary tract infections, as these atypical organisms are more likely to be resistant to one or more azole drugs. If organisms are resistant to fluconazole, then oral therapy with an alternative agent in conjunction with intravesicular infusion of clotrimazole or amphotericin B should likely be considered. Patients that fail this second line of therapy likely require intravenous or subcutaneous amphotericin B or newer antifungal agents.

Secondary funguria

Although rarer than primary urinary tract infections, *Candida* spp. and other typically nonpathogenic fungi may occasionally cause systemic infections in both dogs and cats. In most cases, the primary source of entry is unknown. Animals with systemic infection frequently have organisms identified on urine sediment examination or culture, and fungal hyphae within granulomata may be seen on histopathologic examination of kidneys (Gerding 1994; Clercx 1996; Heseltine 2003; Kuwamura 2006). Systemic clinical signs (e.g., fever) or hematologic or serum biochemical abnormalities in an animal with funguria should increase the suspicion of systemic infections.

The kidneys are a common site of involvement in dogs with systemic aspergillosis, and thus fungal hyphae are commonly identified in urine by routine sediment examination or culture (Wood 1978; Kabay 1985; Jang 1986; Kahler 1990; Dallman 1992; Robinson 2000). Cats with systemic *Aspergillus* spp. infection may also have renal involvement, albeit less frequently (Ossent 1987). Because of the higher frequency of systemic versus primary urinary tract aspergillosis in dogs, urinary aspergillosis should always prompt additional diagnostic testing to ensure that other organs are not involved. Systemic infections are usually treated with itraconazole and/or amphotericin B. Although the most commonly used azoles for aspergillosis have poor penetration into the urine, this is not a concern because urinary shedding in these cases is due to primary renal infection.

Dogs with systemic blastomycosis will on rare occasions also have organisms visible on routine urinalysis or concentrated urine sediment examination (Figure 72.2). Identification of *Blastomyces dermatitidis* within urine sediment may be more likely in intact male dogs with prostatic infection.

Anecdotally, presence of intact organisms within urine occurs almost exclusively in intact male dog with prostatic involvement. The blastomycosis serum or urine antigen test detects a surface antigen common to several fungal organisms rather than intact organisms. I have compared

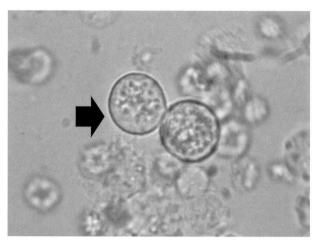

Figure 72.2 Blastomycoses (arrow), neutrophils, and epithelial cells on microscopic examination of unstained urine sediment (Magnification ×200).

the sensitivity of this test with urine sediment examination and fungal urine culture in dogs with confirmed systemic blastomycosis, and in all cases, urine cultures and sediment examinations failed to reveal organisms, whereas the antigen titer was supportive of infection (unpublished data). Therefore, although identification of *Blastomyces dermatitidis* organisms within urine is considered diagnostic for systemic infection, urine examination other than for the antigen test is not recommended for routine diagnostic evaluation of dogs with suspected infection.

Although localized nasal infection in cats is the most commonly encountered form of *Cryptococcus neoformans* infection, systemic infections are uncommonly encountered in cats and rarely in dogs. Identification of organisms within urine has been reported in cats with apparent localized nasal infection or those with obvious systemic involvement; however, systematic investigation of the frequency of urine shedding has not been performed (Gerds-Grogan and Dayrell-Hart 1997). Cats often have incidental lipiduria, and cryptococcal organisms may be difficult to differentiate from fat globules on routine, unstained urine sediment examination. Cryptococcal organisms are more uniform in size and found on a single focal plane as opposed to fat globules, which float throughout the sediment preparation and vary in size. Modified Wright's staining of suspected organisms also reveals internal structure that fat globules lack.

References

Adamama-Moraitou, K., C.G. Paitaki, et al. (2001). *Aspergillus* species cystitis in a cat. *J Feline Med Surg* **3**(1): 31–34.

Barchiesi, F., L. Fanconi Di Francesco, et al. (1997). In vitro activities of terbinafine in combination with fluconazole and itraconazole against isolates of *Candida albicans* with reduced susceptibility to azoles. *Antimicrobial Agents Chemother* **41**(8): 1812–1814.

Bennett, J. (2006). Echinocandins for candidemia in adults without neutropenia. *New Engl J Med* **355**(11): 1154–1159.

Bizerra, F., C.V. Nakamura, et al. (2008). Characteristics of biofilm formation by *Candida tropicalis* and antifungal resistance. *FEMS Yeast Res* **8**(3): 442–450.

Brain, P. (1993). Urinary tract candidiasis in a diabetic dog. *Aust Vet Pract* **23**: 88–91.

Chapman, T. and S. Kirk (2008). An isolated cryptococcal urinary tract infection in a cat. *J Am Anim Hosp Assoc* **44**(5): 262–265.

Clercx, C., K. McEntee, et al. (1996). Bronchopulmonary and disseminated granulomatous disease associated with *Aspergillus fumigatus* and *Candida* species infection in a golden retriever. *J Am Anim Hosp Assoc* **32**(2): 139–145.

Colodner, R., Y. Nuri, et al. (2008). Community-acquired and hospital-acquired candiduria: comparison of prevalence and clinical characteristics. *Eur J Clin Microbiol Infect Dis* **27**(4): 301–305.

Dallman, M., T.L. Dew, et al. (1992). Disseminated aspergillosis in a dog with diskospondylitis and neurologic deficits. *J Am Vet Med Assoc* **200**(4): 511–513.

Day, M. and P. Holt (1994). Unilateral fungal pyelonephritis in a dog. *Vet Pathol* **31**(2): 250–252.

Drew, R., R.R. Arthur, et al. (2005). Is it time to abandon the use of amphotericin B bladder irrigation? *Clin Infect Dis* **40**(10): 1465–1470.

Fan-Havard, P., C. O'Donovan, et al. (1995). Oral fluconazole versus amphotericin B bladder irrigation for treatment of candidal funguria. *Clin Infect Dis* **21**(4): 960–965.

Fisher, J., K. Woeltje, et al. (2003). Efficacy of a single intravenous dose of amphotericin B for *Candida* urinary tract infections: further favorable experience. *Clin Microbiol Infect* **9**(10): 1024–1027.

Forward, Z., A.M. Legendre, et al. (2002). Use of intermittent bladder infusion with clotrimazole for treatment of candiduria in a dog. *J Am Vet Med Assoc* **220**(10): 1496–1498.

Fulton, R., Jr. and R. Walker (1992). *Candida albicans* urocystitis in a cat. *J Am Vet Med Assoc* **200**(4): 524–526.

Gerding, P., L.D. Morton, et al. (1994). Ocular and disseminated candidiasis in an immunosuppressed cat. *J Am Vet Med Assoc* **204**(10): 1635–1638.

Gerds-Grogan, S. and B. Dayrell-Hart (1997). Feline cryptococcosis: a retrospective evaluation. *J Am Anim Hosp Assoc* **33**(2): 118–122.

Grooters, A. and J. Taboada (2003). Update on antifungal therapy. *Vet Clin North Am: Small Anim Pract* **33**(4): 749–758.

Gubbins, P., S.A. McConnell, et al. (1999). Current management of funguria. *Am J Health—System Pharm* **56**(19): 1929–1935.

Hazen, K. and S. Howell (2007). *Candida, Cryptococcus*, and other yeasts of medical importance. In: *Manual of Clinical Microbiology*, edited by P.R. Murray, 9th edition. Washington, DC: ASM Press.

Heseltine, J., D.L. Panciera, et al. (2003). Systemic candidiasis in a dog. *J Am Vet Med Assoc* **223**(6): 821–824.

Hui, M., S.W. Cheung, et al. (2004). Development and application of a rapid diagnostic method for invasive Candidiasis by the detection of D-/L-arabinitol using gas chromatography/mass spectrometry. *Diagnos Microbiol Infect Dis* **49**(2): 117–123.

Humbert, H., M.D. Cabiac, et al. (1995). Pharmacokinetics of terbinafine and of its five main metabolites in plasma and urine, following a single oral dose in healthy subjects. *Biopharm Drug Dispos* **16**(8): 685–694.

Jacobs, L., E.A. Skidmore, et al. (1996). Oral fluconazole compared with bladder irrigation with amphotericin B for treatment of fungal urinary tract infections in elderly patients. *Clin Infect Dis* **22**(1): 30–35.

Jang, S., T.E. Dorr, et al. (1986). *Aspergillus deflectus* infection in four dogs. *J Med Vet Mycol* **24**(2): 95–104.

Jin, Y. and D. Lin (2005). Fungal urinary tract infections in the dog and cat: a retrospective study (2001–2004). *J Am Anim Hosp Assoc* **41**(6): 373–381.

Kabay, M., W.F. Robinson, et al. (1985). The pathology of disseminated *Aspergillus terreus* infection in dogs. *Vet Pathol* **22**(6): 540–547.

Kahler, J., M.W. Leach, et al. (1990). Disseminated aspergillosis attributable to *Aspergillus deflectus* in a springer spaniel. *J Am Vet Med Assoc* **197**(7): 871–874.

Kano, R., Y. Hattori, et al. (2002). Detection and identification of the *Candida* species by 25 S ribosomal DNA analysis in the urine of candidal cystitis. *J Vet Med Sci* **64**(2): 115–117.

Kauffman, C. (2005). Candiduria. *Clin Infect Dis* **41**(Suppl 6): S371–S376.

Kennedy, M. and P. Volz (1985). Effect of various antibiotics on gastrointestinal colonization and dissemination by *Candida albicans*. Sabouraudia: *J Med Vet Mycol* **23**(4): 265–273.

Kirpatrick, R. (1982). Mycotic cystitis in a male cat. *Comp Cont Educ Small Anim Pract* **77**(9): 1365–1371.

Kuwamura, M., M. Ide, et al. (2006). Systemic candidiasis in a dog, developing spondylitis. *J Vet Med Sci* **68**(10): 1117–1119.

Lagrotteria, D., C. Rotstein, et al. (2007). Treatment of candiduria with micafungin: a case series. *Can J Infect Dis Med Microbiol* **18**(2): 149–150.

Leu, H.-S. and C.-T. Huang (1995). Clearance of funguria with short-course antifungal regimens: a prospective, randomized, controlled study. *Clin Infect Dis* **20**(5): 1152–1157.

Ling, G., C.R. Norris, et al. (2001). Interrelations of organism prevalence, specimen collection method, and host age, sex, and breed among 8,354 canine urinary tract infections (1969–1995). *J Vet Int Med* **15**(4): 341–347.

Lundstrom, T. and J. Sobel (2001). Nosocomial candiduria: a review. *Clin Infect Dis* **32**(11): 1602–1607.

Maenza, J., J.C. Keruly, et al. (1996). Risk factors for fluconazole-resistant candidiasis in human immunodeficiency virus-infected patients. *J Infect Dis* **173**(1): 219–225.

Malani, A. and C. Kauffman (2007). *Candida* urinary tract infections: treatment options. *Exp Rev Anti-Infect Ther* **5**(2): 277–284.

Malik, R., A.J. Craig, et al. (1996). Combination chemotherapy of canine and feline cryptococcosis using subcutaneously administered amphotericin B. *Aus Vet J* **73**(4): 124–128.

Muncan, P. and G. Wise (1996). Early identification of candiduria by polymerase chain reaction in high risk patients. *J Urol* **156**(1): 154–156.

Newman, S., C.E. Langston, et al. (2003). Cryptococcal pyelonephritis in a dog. *J Am Vet Med Assoc* **222**(2): 180–183.

Norris, C., B.J. Williams, et al. (2000). Recurrent and persistent urinary tract infections in dogs: 383 cases (1969–1995). *J Am Anim Hosp Assoc* **36**(6): 484–492.

Occhipinti, D., P.O. Gubbins, et al. (1994). Frequency, pathogenicity and microbiologic outcome of non-*Candida albicans* candiduria. *Eur J Clin Microbiol Infect Dis* **13**(6): 459–467.

Ossent, P. (1987). Systemic aspergillosis and mucormycosis in 23 cats. *Veterinary Record* **120**(14): 330–333.

Ozawa, H., K. Okabayashi, et al. (2005). Rapid identification of *Candida tropicalis* from canine cystitis. *Mycopathologia* **160**(2): 159–162.

Pressler, B., S.L. Vaden, et al. (2003). *Candida* spp. urinary tract infections in 13 dogs and seven cats: predisposing factors, treatment, and outcome. *J Am Anim Hosp Assoc* **39**(3): 263–270.

Rex, J., M.G. Rinaldi, et al. (1995). Resistance of *Candida* species to fluconazole. *Antimicrob Agents and Chemother* **39**(1): 1–8.

Robinson, W., M. Connole, et al. (2000). Systemic mycosis due to *Aspergillus deflectus* in a dog. *Aus Vet J* **78**(9): 600–602.

Sobel, J. (2007). Caspofungin in the treatment of symptomatic candiduria. *Clin Infect Dis* **44**(5): e46–e49.

Suchodolski, J., E.K. Morris, et al. (2008). Prevalence and identification of fungal DNA in the small intestine of healthy dogs and dogs with chronic enteropathies. *Vet Microbiol* **132**(3–4): 379–388.

Tan, R.J. and E.W. Lim (1977). Isolation of *Torulopsis glabrata* from a urine specimen of a Labrador bitch with urolithiasis. *Br Vet J* **133**(3): 324–325.

Tokunaga, S., M. Ohkawa, et al. (1993). Diagnostic value of determination of serum mannan concentrations in patients with candiduria. *Eur J Clin Microbiol Infect Dis* **12**(7): 542–545.

Tokunaga, S., M. Ohkawa, et al. (1995). D-arabinitol versus mannan antigen and candidal protein antigen as a serum marker for *Candida* pyelonephritis. *Eur J Clin Microbiol Infect Dis* **14**(2): 118–121.

Toll, J., C.M. Ashe, et al. (2003). Intravesicular administration of clotrimazole for treatment of candiduria in a cat with diabetes mellitus. *J Am Vet Med Assoc* **223**(8): 1156–1158.

Trinh, T., J. Simonian, et al. (1995). Continuous versus intermittent bladder irrigation of amphotericin B for the treatment of candiduria. *J Urol* **154**(6): 2032–2034.

Warnock, D., D.C. Speller, et al. (1976). Serological diagnosis of infection of the urinary tract by yeasts. *J Clin Pathol* **29**(9): 836–840.

Wise, G. (2001). Genitourinary fungal infections: a therapeutic conundrum. *Exp Opin Pharmacother* **2**(8): 1211–1226.

Wood, G.L., D.C. Hirsh, et al. (1978). Disseminated aspergillosis in a dog. *J Am Vet Med Assoc* **172**(6): 704–707.

Wooley, R. and J.L. Blue (1976). Bacterial isolations from canine and feline urine. *Mod Vet Pract* **57**(7): 535–538.

73

Viruses and urinary tract disease

John M. Kruger, Carl A. Osborne, Annabel G. Wise, Brian A. Scansen, and Roger K. Maes

For over a century, physicians have recognized a relationship between viral infections and urinary tract disease (Henoch 1884). Virus-induced disorders of the urinary system, especially those involving the kidneys, are now increasingly identified as major causes of morbidity and mortality in humans (Berns and Cohen 2007). Similarly, rapid advances in detection and localization of viruses in tissues and urine with contemporary molecular biologic methods have fostered a renewed interest in viral urinary tract infections (UTI) in companion animals.

As with all infectious diseases, clinical manifestations of viral UTIs are the cumulative result of the ability of a microorganism to establish infection and compromise host function and, conversely, the host's ability to resist or curtail infection (Murphy et al. 1999a). Because the virulence of a specific pathogen and the resistance of a given host may vary considerably, viral UTIs may be asymptomatic or may be associated with substantial morbidity and mortality. In general, viral pathogens may cause disease by (1) inducing cell injury or death, (2) altering cellular functions, (3) suppressing immune responses, or (4) stimulating systemic or organ-specific pathologic immune responses. It is noteworthy that virus-associated autoimmune diseases may occur in the absence of detectable viruses as a result of persistent nonreplicating viral components, virus-induced alterations in antigenic profiles of infected cells, or induction of antiviral antibodies capable of cross-reacting with self-proteins (Schattner and Rager-Zisman 1990).

Upper urinary tract disorders

Renal injury may be the direct result of virus-induced cytopathic effects on renal vascular, glomerular, tubular, and/or interstitial tissues, the secondary consequence of systemic infection and immune-mediated injury, or the result of both processes (Alpers and Kowalewska 2007; Faulhaber and Nelson 2007). Clinical manifestations of viral upper UTIs will be similar to other infectious and noninfectious causes of renal injury and may include varying combinations and degrees of proteinuria, hematuria, isosthenuria, and azotemia. A number of viral agents have been associated with human kidney diseases (Table 73.1). Likewise, several viruses have been associated with canine and feline kidney disorders (Table 73.1). Despite strong temporal associations between some viral infections and renal disease, a cause-and-effect relationship and specific mechanisms of renal injury have not been established in all cases.

Canine adenovirus

Canine adenovirus type 1 (CAV-1) is the cause of infectious canine hepatitis and is serologically and genetically distinct from canine adenovirus type 2 (CAV-2) (Wright 1976). CAV-1 is associated with systemic viremia, hepatitis, glomerulonephropathy, interstitial nephritis, and viruria, whereas CAV-2 is largely confined to the respiratory tract (Benetka et al. 2006). It is noteworthy that modified live CAV-1 vaccine strains may localize in renal tubular epithelium and have been associated with mild subclinical interstitial nephritis and persistent viruria (Appel et al. 1973). However, cross-reacting CAV-2 vaccine strains rarely, if ever, produce renal disease (Curtis et al. 1978).

After primary replication, CAV-1 rapidly disseminates to multiple tissues and body fluids. In the acute phase,

Nephrology and Urology of Small Animals. Edited by Joe Bartges and David J. Polzin. © 2011 Blackwell Publishing Ltd.

Table 73.1 Viruses associated with urinary tract disease

Host species	Virus	Associated conditions[a]	References
Human	Adenovirus types 11, 21	Hemorrhagic cystitis (children)	Mufson and Belshe 1976
	Coxsackievirus	Interstitial nephritis Glomerulonephritis	Burch and Colcolough 1969
	Cytomegalovirus	Interstitial nephritis[b] Hemorrhagic cystitis[b]	Platt et al. 1985; Spach et al. 1993
	Echovirus type 9	Glomerulonephritis	Yuceoglu et al. 1966
	Epstein-Barr virus	Interstitial nephritis Glomerulonephritis Renal leiomyoma[b]	Joh et al. 1998; Krishnan et al. 1999
	Erythrovirus B19	Hematuria[b] Cystitis[b] Glomerulonephritis[b]	Christensen et al. 2001
	Hantavirus	Tubulointerstitial nephritis Glomerulonephrititis	Miettinen et al. 2006
	Hepatitis virus types B, C	Glomerulonephritis Interstitial nephritis	Johnson and Couser 1990; Johnson et al. 1994
	Herpes simplex	Interstitial nephritis[b] Hemorrhagic cystitis	Silbert et al. 1990; McClanahan et al. 1994
	Herpes varicella-zoster	Hemorrhagic cystitis Glomerulonephritis	Meyer et al. 1959; Rossetti et al. 1996
	HIV	Collapsing focal glomerulosclerosis Interstitial nephritis Glomerulonephritis Hemorrhagic cystitis	Elem et al. 1991; D'Agati and Appel 1997
	Influenza A	Hemorrhagic cystitis Glomerulonephritis	Wilson and Smith 1972; Khakpour and Nik-Alchtar 1977
	Paramyxovirus (mumps)	Nephritis Hematuria	Utz et al. 1964; Hughes et al. 1966
	Polyomavirus BK	Tubulointerstitial nephritis[b] Ureteritis[b] Hemorrhagic cystitis[b]	Drachenberg et al. 2005
Canine	Canine adenovirus—1	Glomerulonephritis Interstitial nephritis Viruria	Wright 1976
	Canine herpesvirus	Hemorrhagic nephritis[c] Viruria	Carmichael 1970; Huxsoll and Hemelt 1970
	Canine distemper (paramyxovirus) virus	Urothelial swelling Viruria	Coffin and Liu 1957
Feline	Bovine herpesvirus-4	Hemorrhagic cystitis	Fabricant 1977
	Feline calicivirus	Hemorrhagic cystitis Viruria	Rich et al. 1971; Rice et al. 2002
	Feline immunodeficiency virus	Glomerulosclerosis Tubulointerstitial nephritis Amyloidosis	Poli et al. 1993; Poli et al. 1995
	Feline foamy virus	Hemorrhagic cystitis Glomerulonephritis	German et al. 2008
	Feline infectious peritonitis virus	Pyogranulomatous nephritis Interstitial nephritis Glomerulonephritis	Hayashi et al. 1982; Kipar et al. 2005
	Feline leukemia virus	Membranous glomerulonephritis Interstitial nephritis	Francis et al. 1980; Jakowski et al. 1980

[a]Cause-and-effect relationships have not been established in all cases.
[b]Disorder observed primarily in immunocompromised hosts.
[c]Disorder observed in neonatal puppies infected at less than 2 weeks of age.

the virus replicates in hepatocytes, vascular endothelium, lymphoid tissues, and circulating mononuclear cells and is associated with acute necrohemorrhagic hepatitis and generalized perivascular hemorrhage (Wright et al. 1973). Coincidental viral replication in glomerular capillary endothelial and mesangial cells results in a concurrent virus-induced glomerulonephropathy characterized by endothelial and mesangial cell degeneration and necrosis, disruption of visceral epithelial cells, proximal tubular epithelium degeneration, and proteinuria (Wright et al. 1973; Wright and Cornwell 1983). As virus neutralizing antibody titers rise at approximately 7–10 days post infection, subsequent mesangial and subendothelial deposition of circulating virus-antibody immune complexes induces a membranoproliferative glomerulonephritis (Wright et al. 1974; Wright and Cornwell 1983). By 10–14 days post infection, CAV-1 localizes in renal tubular epithelium where it is associated with focal interstitial nephritis, transient proteinuria, and a persistent viruria that may last for 6–9 months (Baker et al. 1954; Wright et al. 1981). At 30–40 days post infection, lesions of glomerulonephritis and interstitial nephritis and fibrosis are still evident but appear to be nonprogressive (Wright et al. 1981). Unlike the relationship of CAV-1 with chronic liver disease, however, persistent CAV-1 infection has not, as of yet, been associated with chronic progressive renal disease in dogs.

Canine herpesvirus

Canine herpesvirus (CHV) is a member of the alpha herpesvirus subfamily that causes severe, usually fatal, generalized systemic infections in seronegative neonatal puppies or immunocompromised animals; immunocompetent dogs exposed after 2 weeks of age develop only mild or inapparent upper respiratory tract or genital infections (Carmichael et al. 1965; Wright and Cornwell 1968; Appel et al. 1969; Carmichael 1970). Neonatal puppies less than 2 weeks of age are uniquely predisposed to CHV systemic infections because of their lower body temperature, inability to mount a febrile response, and poorly developed immune systems (Carmichael 1970; Huxsoll and Hemelt 1970). The hallmarks of generalized systemic infections in affected puppies are disseminated focal necrosis and hemorrhage in multiple organs, especially in the kidney, liver, lung, and spleen (Carmichael et al. 1965; Wright and Cornwell 1968). Grossly, kidneys are mottled in appearance due to multiple subcapsular cortical hemorrhages associated with wedge-shaped hemorrhagic lesions radiating outward from the medulla (Carmichael et al. 1965). Characteristic light microscopic renal lesions include fibrinoid necrosis of interlobular arteries, hemorrhage, glomerular degeneration, renal

tubular necrosis, interstitial nephritis, proteinuria, and hematuria (Carmichael et al. 1965; Wright and Cornwell 1968; Yamamura et al. 1992). The pathogenesis of CHV-induced nephropathy involves direct virus-induced cytolytic injury to the endothelium and smooth muscle of renal arteries, the renal tubular epithelium, and the connective tissues of the interstitium (Carmichael et al. 1965; Hashimoto et al. 1982; Yamamura et al. 1992; Schulze and Baumgärtner 1998). Renal infection is accompanied by CHV viruria in puppies with acute systemic disease (Huxsoll and Hemelt 1970). In dogs surviving acute infection, CHV is shed in nasal, oropharyngeal, and genitourinary secretions, and in feces for up to 2 weeks postinfection, the extent and duration of virus shedding in urine has not been determined (Karpas et al. 1968; Appel et al. 1969). After an appropriate host immune response, virus shedding ceases and CHV establishes lifelong latent infections of local ganglionic neurons and lymphoid tissues, including lumbosacral ganglia, the celiac plexus, and hypogastric lymph nodes (Burr et al. 1996; Schulze and Baumgärtner 1998; Miyoshi et al. 1999). Reactivation of latent CHV infections and subsequent genitourinary shedding of virus may be induced by stressful situations or by administration of systemic corticosteroids or other immunosuppressive agents (Okuda et al. 1993). However, the role of latent or recrudescent CHV infections in the development or progression of renal disease has not been determined.

Feline coronavirus

Feline infectious peritonitis (FIP) is a systemic, progressive, and ultimately fatal immunopathologic disease caused by a highly pathogenic feline coronavirus strain derived from a mutation of the more common and less pathogenic enteric strain of feline coronavirus (Hartmann 2005). The disease principally affects young cats less than 2 years of age (Rohrbach et al. 2001). Renal injury is common and is the direct result necrotizing pyogranulomatous vasculititis/nephritis associated with perivascular localization of activated coronavirus-infected monocyte/macrophages and coronavirus-specific immune complexes (Jacobse-Geels et al. 1982; Kipar et al. 2005). In addition, glomerulonephritis with or without concurrent vasculitis has been observed in cats with FIP. In one study of 85 naturally occurring cases of FIP, 71% of affected cats had light microscopic lesions of membranous, mesangioproliferative, or membranoproliferative glomerulonephritis (Hayashi et al. 1982). Identification of viral antigen–antibody complexes and complement in glomeruli of affected cats is consistent with immune-mediated glomerulonephritis occurring secondarily to systemic FIP infection.

Feline immunodeficiency virus

Feline immunodeficiency virus (FIV) is a member of the lentivirus subfamily of retroviruses that is similar to human immunodeficiency virus (HIV) in structure, biological properties, and clinical manifestations of infection (Bendinelli et al. 1995). Renal abnormalities have been reported in 8–24% of naturally infected FIV-positive cats from Japan, the United Kingdom, Australia, and New Zealand (Hopper et al. 1989; Ishida et al. 1989; Thomas et al. 1993). In studies of cats from a single endemically infected household in Italy, azotemia was observed in 50% and proteinuria in 95% of 21 FIV-positive cats (Poli et al. 1993; Poli et al. 1995). Abnormalities observed in naturally or experimentally infected FIV-positive cats include varying combinations and degrees of clinical signs consistent with renal failure, uremia, and the nephrotic syndrome, and laboratory findings of azotemia, hypoalbuminemia, and proteinuria (Thomas et al. 1993; Poli et al. 1993; Poli et al. 1995; Hofmann-Lehmann et al. 1997; Levy 2000). Renal lesions commonly observed in FIV-infected cats include mesangial thickening, segmental to diffuse glomerulosclerosis, tubular degeneration and/or necrosis, and interstitial mononuclear cell infiltrates; less common lesions include mesangial cell proliferation, glomerular or interstitial amyloid deposition, interstitial fibrosis, and microcystic tubular dilation (Matsumara et al. 1993; Poli et al. 1993; Dua et al. 1994; Bendinelli et al. 1995; Poli et al. 1995; Levy 2000).

HIV-associated nephropathy affects 3–10% of HIV-infected human patients and is clinically manifested by proteinuria and rapidly progressive renal failure (D'Agati and Appel 1997). Characteristic renal lesions include collapsing focal segmental glomerulosclerosis, podocyte hypertrophy and hyperplasia, tubular degeneration, microcystic tubular dilation, and interstitial inflammation and fibrosis (D'Agati and Appel 1997; Alpers and Kowalewska 2007). Recent studies suggest that HIV-associated nephropathy is a direct consequence of renal infection rather than a secondary consequence of systemic infection (Alpers and Kowalewska 2007). Similar light microscopic lesions and detection of anti-FIV IgG, infectious FIV, proviral DNA, and viral RNA in renal tissues of FIV-infected cats suggest that FIV-associated nephropathy may also involve direct viral injury to renal tissues (Poli et al. 1993; Poli et al. 1995). However, proof of this hypothesis requires further study.

Feline leukemia virus

Feline leukemia virus (FeLV) is a member of the oncornavirus subfamily of retroviruses that has been associated with membranous glomerulonephropathy, interstitial nephritis, proteinuria, nephrotic syndrome, and renal failure in chronically infected cats with or without concurrent lymphosarcoma or other myeloproliferative diseases (Cotter et al. 1975; Francis et al. 1980; Jakowski et al. 1980). Glomerulonephropathy was observed in 25–37% of necropsy specimens obtained from cats living in households with large populations of FeLV-infected cats (Francis et al. 1980; Jakowski et al. 1980). However, a substantially lower prevalence of glomerulonephropathy was observed in large necropsy-based surveys of FeLV-positive cats from the general population (Reinacher and Theilen 1987; Weijer and Daams 1976). In contrast to lentiviruses, FeLV-associated renal disease appears to occur secondarily to systemic infection and immune-mediated mechanisms of glomerular injury. Dysregulation of the immune system in chronically viremic cats is believed to induce formation of circulating immune complexes composed of viral antigens (whole virions, or solubilized proteins gp70, p27, or p15E) and antibodies that are deposited in glomeruli (Hardy 1982).

Feline foamy (syncytium-forming) virus

Feline foamy virus (FFV), formerly known as feline syncytium-forming virus, is a member of the spumavirus subfamily of retroviruses (Greene 2006). FFV infection is widespread in domestic and feral cat populations and is generally considered to be nonpathogenic. In a recent study, however, experimental FFV infection of SPF cats was associated with persistent viremia, anti-FFV IgG production, and microscopic lesions of mild glomerulonephritis characterized by increased cellularity of glomerular tufts and adhesions between the glomerular tuft and Bowman's capsule (German et al. 2008). Additional investigations are required to further characterize the pathologic features of FFV-induced renal disease in cats.

Lower urinary tract disorders

Viruses have long been implicated as causative agents in the etiopathogenesis of some forms of naturally occurring feline idiopathic cystitis (Chapter 75) (Fabricant 1977; Kruger et al. 1996). This hypothesis was supported by the isolation of a gamma herpesvirus (aka bovine herpesvirus type 4), retroviruses (aka FFV), and a calicivirus (aka feline calicivirus; FCV) from urine and tissues obtained from cats affected with lower urinary tract disease (Kruger et al. 1990). Similarly, a number of viral agents including adenoviruses, erythrovirus, herpes viruses, HIV, influenza, and polyomavirus have been associated with hemorrhagic cystitis and other lower urinary tract symptoms in humans (Table 73.1) (Sutcliffe et al. 2007). As of yet, viruses have not been implicated as causative agents in the pathogenesis of canine lower urinary tract disorders.

Clinical manifestations of viral lower UTIs are often indistinguishable from other infectious and noninfectious urinary tract diseases. Although the light microscopic features of acute viral UTIs have not been well characterized, urinary bladder lesions in cats with calicivirus-induced UTI consisted of urinary bladder mucosal petechial hemorrhages, urothelial ulceration, and submucosal edema and mononuclear inflammation (Kruger et al. 2007). These morphologic features are not unlike those observed in the urinary bladders of a limited number of cats with nonobstructive idiopathic cystitis (Lavelle et al. 2000; Reche and Hagiwara 2001; Specht et al. 2003). We emphasize, however, that these lesions can also be associated with any inflammatory process and are not pathognomonic for a diagnosis of viral UTI.

Feline calicivirus

Isolation of a feline calicivirus (FCV) from a Manx cat with spontaneous urethral obstruction in 1969, and subsequent experimental induction of obstructive uropathy in conventionally reared cats by urinary bladder inoculation supported a pathogenic role for FCV in some forms of feline lower urinary tract disease (Rich and Fabricant 1969; Rich et al. 1971). However, other investigators were unable to isolate FCV from urine obtained from cats with natural forms of feline lower urinary tract disease (Kruger et al. 1990). While these findings raised questions about the causative role of FCV, the inability to detect FCV may have been confounded by improper selection of cases (i.e., improper inclusion and exclusion criteria were used to select cats for study), the innately virucidal nature of feline urine, and use of insensitive or inappropriate virus detection methods (Scansen et al. 2004; Scansen et al. 2005).

Over the past two decades, there has been increasing evidence that FCV may have a causative role in the pathogenesis in at least some cases of feline idiopathic cystitis (Kruger et al. 1996; Rice et al. 2002; Kruger et al. 2007; Larson et al. 2007). In the 1980s, transmission electron microscopic examination of urethral matrix-crystalline plugs obtained from male cats with urethral obstruction revealed virus-like particles, similar in size (approximately 25–30 nm) and morphology to caliciviruses (Kruger et al. 1996). These calicivirus-like particles were observed in 38% of 92 urethral plugs obtained from male cats with urethral obstructive idiopathic cystitis. In the late 1990s, an improved virus isolation technique enabled isolation of two new FCV strains

(designated FCV-U1 and FCV-U2) from urine obtained from cats with idiopathic cystitis (Rice et al. 2002).

Subsequent development of a FCV p30 gene-based real-time reverse-transcriptase polymerase chain reaction (RT-PCR) assay optimized for feline urine allowed for large-scale epidemiologic and experimental studies investigating the causative role of FCV in idiopathic cystitis (Scansen et al. 2004, 2005). In a study characterizing lower urinary tract disease induced by FCV infection in specific-pathogen free (SPF) cats, FCV was detected by RT-PCR in urinary tract tissues from cats infected with either a urinary or respiratory strain of FCV (Kruger et al. 2007). Immunohistochemical staining confirmed localization of FCV antigens to the bladder urothelium. Light microscopy revealed that urinary bladder lesions were more severe and seen more frequently in cats infected with the urinary strain, whereas oral/respiratory tract lesions tended to be more severe and seen more frequently in cats infected with the respiratory strain. In a study investigating the prevalence of FCV urinary tract infection and FCV antibodies in cats with and without idiopathic cystitis (Larson et al. 2007), FCV RNA were detected by RT-PCR with similar frequency (approximately 6%) in urine from cats with idiopathic cystitis and cats with FCV-induced upper respiratory tract disease; viral nucleic acids were not detected in urine from asymptomatic vaccinated control cats. Mean FCV neutralizing antibody titers for cats with idiopathic cystitis and FCV-induced upper respiratory tract disease were significantly higher than the mean titer of asymptomatic vaccinated control cats. These observations confirmed FCV viruria in cats with and without respiratory signs and suggested increased exposure to FCV in cats with idiopathic cystitis.

Recent studies have identified the components of the functional receptor for FCV and include the junctional adhesion molecule 1 (JAM-1) and alpha 2,6-linked sialic acid (Makino et al. 2006; Stuart and Brown 2007). JAM-1 specifically localizes to the tight junctions of epithelial and endothelial cells and is involved in the regulation of tight junction integrity and permeability, as well as leukocyte–endothelial cell interactions (Ebnet et al. 2004). Sialic acids are negatively charged sugar molecules usually located at the ends of oligosaccharides attached to glycoproteins, glycolipids, and proteoglycans on the cell surface (Stuart and Brown 2007). It is likely that JAM-1 and sialic acid serve as serotype-independent tissue receptor components capable of mediating virus attachment, infection, and intracellular signaling (Barton et al. 2001; Makino et al. 2006; Stuart and Brown 2007). Since urothelial cell tight junctions and GAG layer are integral components of the urothelial barrier, it is plausible that FCV attachment, infection, and induction of cellular injury or death may alter the structural and/or functional integrity of the urothelium. Subsequent exposure of bladder wall tissues to urine constituents could result in sensory afferent nerve stimulation, mast cell activation, and/or induction of immune-mediated or neurogenic inflammatory responses (Elbadawi 1997; Birder 2005; Sant et al. 2007). Further studies are necessary to define the causative role of FCV in the pathogenesis of feline idiopathic cystitis.

Gamma herpesvirus (bovine herpesvirus-4)

In 1969, a cell-associated herpesvirus was isolated from pooled kidney organ explants from a litter of normal kittens, a kitten with upper respiratory disease, and a kitten with concurrent upper respiratory disease and urethral obstruction (Fabricant et al. 1971; Fabricant and Gillespie 1974). Subsequent antigenic and genomic analyses indicated that this herpesvirus was related to a group of gamma herpesviruses collectively referred to as bovine herpesvirus-4 (BHV-4) (Kruger et al. 1989). There is considerable evidence that BHV-4 can induce long-term viral UTIs in cats in a laboratory setting (Fabricant 1977; Kruger et al. 1990) and that BHV-4 infection is endemic in the feline population (Kruger et al. 2000). However, reproducible evidence that gamma herpesviruses cause naturally occurring symptomatic feline lower urinary tract disease is lacking.

Feline foamy (syncytium-forming) virus

In contrast to other viruses, FFV has been isolated from urine, urinary-tract tissues, and other tissues obtained from a large number of cats with lower urinary tract disease (Kruger et al. 1990). Additionally, FFV antibodies have been detected in serum samples obtained from cats with naturally occurring lower urinary tract disease (Shroyer and Shalaby 1978). FFV antibodies have also been detected in a large number of clinically normal cats (Pedersen et al. 1980). The relative ease and frequency with which FFV has been isolated from cats with lower urinary tract signs and the prevalence of FFV antibodies suggests a possible role in the pathogenesis of urinary tract disorders. However, it is difficult to assess the relative importance of FFV on the basis of available experimental and clinical evidence. Further investigations are necessary to determine the role, if any, of FFV virus in feline lower urinary tract disorders.

Diagnosis of viral UTI

Identification and localization of viruses within the urinary tract is an essential prerequisite to establishing a cause-and-effect relationship of viruses with urinary tract diseases. Since clinical signs, clinical laboratory data, and microscopic examination of tissues stained for routine light microscopy cannot reliably distinguish virus-induced disease from other urinary tract disorders, diagnosis of viral UTI should encompass specialized sampling, cultivation, and identification techniques suitable for each individual uropathogen. Exclusion of other known causes of upper or lower urinary tract disease should precede attempts to establish a diagnosis of viral UTI. Generally, diagnostic criteria for viral infections include (1) isolation and identification of viral agents; (2) direct demonstration of virus particles, viral antigens, or viral nucleic acids in tissues or body fluids; and/or (3) detection and quantitation of specific viral antibodies (Murphy et al. 1999b).

Virus isolation has historically been the diagnostic "gold standard" for diagnosis of viral UTI. However, virus isolation is time-consuming, expensive, and requires viable virus in the specimen and absence of substances that are toxic to cell culture or that inhibit viral replication. Molecular diagnostic methods, such as PCR or RT-PCR, circumvent many of the difficulties associated with conventional virus isolation methods and are increasingly being used for rapid detection of many viral agents (Murphy et al. 1999b). For example, a FCV p30 gene-based RT-PCR assay was found to be comparable to virus isolation in sensitivity and diagnostic range for detection of caliciviruses in urine and offered the advantages of reduced sample size, faster throughput, and better quantitation (Scansen et al. 2004).

Although PCR-based diagnostic assays are sensitive and rapid methods for virus detection, it is also recognized that urine is a particularly difficult substrate for amplification of nucleic acids (Scansen et al. 2005). In particular, RT-PCR assays are at risk for false-negative results due to RNA degradation by endogenous or exogenous RNases and/or the presence of endogenous RT-PCR inhibitors (Ballagi-Pordány and Belák 1996). In one study of routine submissions to a veterinary diagnostic laboratory, either partial or complete inhibition of RT-PCR was detected in approximately 20% of samples analyzed (Kleiboeker 2003). Preparation of nucleic acids for assay becomes a critical step that serves not only to concentrate and purify nucleic acids, but also to eliminate endogenous or exogenous enzymes that may damage nucleic acids (e.g., RNases) and to remove or inactivate PCR inhibitors. Studies on human and feline urine specimens indicate that the nucleic acid preparation method significantly influences the ability of PCR-based assays to detect viruses in urine and other complex biological specimens and emphasize the need to optimize methods of nucleic acid preparation for each viral assay and sample substrate (Demmler et al. 1988; Khan et al. 1991;

Behzadbehbahani et al. 1997; Echavarria et al. 1998; Biel et al. 2000; Scansen et al. 2005). In addition, incorporating an internal amplification control into the RT-PCR reaction allows for rapid detection of false-negative results caused by RT-PCR inhibitors and substantially increases the diagnostic reliability of RT-PCR assays (Ballagi-Pordány and Belák 1996; Kleiboeker 2003).

Treatment of viral UTI

The most effective treatment of viral UTIs lies in their prevention through use of appropriate immunization strategies and husbandry practices. Although interest in antiviral chemotherapeutics and biologic agents has grown considerably in recent years, antiviral agents available for clinical use are relatively few in number and are accompanied by only limited information regarding their safety and efficacy (Hartmann 2006). One exception is FCV. Parenteral administration of FCV-specific antiviral phosphorodiamidate morpholino oligomers effectively inhibited calicivirus replication, increased survival, decreased virus shedding, and hastened clinical recovery in kittens exposed to a severe virulent strain of FCV (Smith et al. 2008). Similarly, administration of anti-FCV mouse-cat chimeric monoclonal antibodies substantially reduced clinical signs in cats exposed to virulent FCV (Umehashi et al. 2002). However, antiviral agents have not been evaluated in cats with presumed FCV-induced lower urinary tract disease. In the absence of safe and effective antiviral agents, management of suspected virus-induced urinary tract disease in dogs and cats is limited to supportive and symptomatic care to alleviate clinical signs and minimize sequelae of infection.

References

Alpers, C.E. and J. Kowalewska (2007). Emerging paradigms in the renal pathology of viral diseases. *Clin J Am Soc Nephrol* **2**: S6–S12.

Appel, M., S.I. Bistner, et al. (1973). Pathogenicity of low-virulence strains of two canine adenoviruse types. *Am J Vet Res* **34**: 543–550.

Appel, M.J.G., M. Menegus, et al. (1969). Pathogenesis of canine herpesvirus in specific-pathogen-free dogs: 5-12-week-old pups. *Am J Vet Res* **30**: 2067–2073.

Baker, J.A., H.E. Jensen, et al. (1954). Canine infectious hepatitis—fox encephalitis. *J Am Vet Med Assoc* **124**: 214–216.

Ballagi-Pordány, A. and S. Belák (1996). The use of mimics as internal standards to avoid false negatives in diagnostic PCR. *Mol Cell Probes* **10**: 159–164.

Barton, E.S., J.C. Forrest, et al. (2001). Junction adhesion molecule is a receptor for reovirus. *Cell* **104**: 441–451.

Behzadbehbahani, A., P.E. Klapper, et al. (1997). Detection of BK virus in urine by polymerase chain reaction: a comparison of DNA extraction methods. *J Virol Methods* **67**: 161–166.

Bendinelli, M., M. Pistello, et al. (1995). Feline immunodeficiency virus: an interesting model for AIDS studies and an important cat pathogen. *Clin Microbiol Rev* **8**: 87–112.

Benetka, V., H. Weissenböck, et al. (2006). Canine adenovirus type 2 infection in four puppies with neurological signs. *Vet Rec* **158**: 91–94.

Berns, J.S. and A.H. Cohen (2007). Viruses and disease of the kidney. *Clin J Am Soc Nephrol* **2**: S1.

Biel, S.S., T.K. Held, et al. (2000). Rapid quantification and differentiation of human polyomavirus DNA in undiluted urine from patients after bone marrow transplantation. *J Clin Microbiol* **38**: 3689–3695.

Birder, L.A. (2005). More than just a barrier: urothelium as a drug target for urinary bladder pain. *Am J Physiol Renal Physiol* **289**: F489–F495.

Burch, G.E. and H.L. Colcolough (1969). Progressive coxsackie viral pancarditis and nephritis. *Annal Intern Med* **71**: 963–970.

Burr, P.D., M.E.M. Campbell, et al. (1996). Detection of canine herpesvirus 1 in a wide range of tissues using the polymerase chain reaction. *Vet Microbiol* **53**: 227–237.

Carmichael, L.E., R.A. Squire, et al. (1965). Clinical and pathologic features of a fatal viral disease of newborn pups. *Am J Vet Res* **26**: 803–814.

Carmichael, L.E. (1970). Herpesvirus canis: aspects of pathogenesis and immune response. *J Am Vet Med Assoc* **156**: 1714–1724.

Christensen, L.S., T.V. Madsen, et al. (2001). Persistent erythrovirus B19 urinary tract infection in an HIV-positive patient. *Clin Micro Infect* **7**: 507–509.

Coffin, D.L. and C. Liu (1957). Studies on canine distemper infection by means of fluorescein-labeled antibody. *Virol* **3**: 132–145.

Cotter, S.M., W.D. Hardy, et al. (1975). Association of feline leukemia virus with lymphosarcoma and other disorders in the cat. *J Am Vet med Assoc* **166**: 449–454.

Curtis, R., J.E. Jemmett, et al. (1978). The pathogenicity of an attenuated strain of canine adenovirus type 2 (CAV-2). *Vet Rec* **103**: 380–381.

D'Agati, V. and G.B. Appel (1997). HIV infection and the kidney. *J Am Soc Nephrol* **8**: 138–152.

Demmler, G.J., G.J. Buffone, et al. (1988). Detection of cytomegalovirus in urine from newborns by using polymerase chain reaction DNA amplification. *J Infect Dis* **158**: 1177–1184.

Drachenberg, C.B., H.H. Hirsch, et al. (2005). Polyomavirus disease in renal transplantation. Review of pathological findings and diagnostic methods. *Hum Pathol* **36**: 1245–1255.

Dua, N., G. Reubel, et al. (1994). An experimental study of primary feline immunodeficiency virus infection in cats and a historical comparison to acute simian and human immunodeficiency virus diseases. *Vet Immunol Immunopath* **43**: 337–355.

Ebnet, K., A. Suzuki, et al. (2004). Junctional adhesion molecules (JAMs): more molecules with dual functions? *J Cell Sci* **117**: 19–29.

Echavarria, M., M. Forman, et al. (1998). PCR method for detection of adenovirus in urine of healthy and human immunodeficiency virus-infected individuals. *J Clin Microbiol* **36**: 3323–3326.

Elbadawi, A. (1997). Interstitial cystitis: a critique of current concepts with a new proposal for pathologic diagnosis and pathogenesis. *Urology* **49**(Suppl. 5A): 14–40.

Elem, B., P.S. Patil, et al. (1991). Haematuria frequency syndrome in patients with positive HIV serology: observations in Zambia. *Brit J Urol* **67**: 146–149.

Fabricant, C.G. and J.H. Gillespie (1974). Identification and characterization of a second feline herpesvirus. *Infect Immun* **9**: 460–466.

Fabricant, C.G., J.M. King, et al. (1971). Isolation of a virus from a female cat with urolithiasis. *J Am Vet Med Assoc* **158**: 200–201.

Fabricant, C.G. (1977). Herpesvirus-induced urolithiasis in specific-pathogen-free male cats. *Am J Vet Res* **38**: 1837–1842.

Faulhaber, J.R. and P.J. Nelson (2007). Virus-induced cellular immune mechanisms of injury to the kidney. *Clin J Am Soc Nephrol* **2**: S2–S5.

Francis, D.P., M. Essex, et al. (1980). Increased risk for lymphoma and glomerulonephritis in a closed population of cats exposed to feline leukemia virus. *Am J Epidemiol* **111**: 337–346.

German, A.C., D.A. Harbour, et al. (2008). Is feline foamy virus really pathogenic. *Vet Immunol Immunopath* **123**: 114–118.

Greene, C.E. (2006). Feline foamy (syncytium-forming) virus infection. In: *Infectious Diseases of the Dog and Cat*, edited by C.E. Greene, 3rd edition. Philadelphia, PA: WB Saunders, pp. 154–155.

Hardy, W.D. Jr. (1982). Immunopathology induced by the feline leukemia virus. *Springer Semin Immunopathol* **5**: 75–106.

Hartmann, K. (2006). Antiviral and immunomodulary chemotherapy. In: *Infectious Diseases of the Dog and Cat*, edited by C.E. Greene, 3rd edition. Philadelphia, PA: WB Saunders, pp. 11–25.

Hartmann, K. (2005). Feline infectious peritonitis. *Vet Clin North Am Small Anim* **35**: 39–79.

Hashimoto, A., K. Hirai, et al. (1982). Experimental transplacental infection of pregnant dogs with canine herpesvirus. *Am J Vet Res* **43**: 844–850.

Hayashi, T., T. Ishida, et al. (1982). Glomerulonephritis with feline infectious peritonitis. *Jpn J Vet Sci* **44**: 909–916.

Henoch, E. (1884). Nephritis nach varicellen. *Berl Klin Wschr* **21**: 17.

Hofmann-Lehmann, R., E. Holznagel, et al. (1997). Parameters of disease progression in long-term experimental feline retrovirus (feline immunodeficiency virus and feline leukemia virus) infections: hematology, clinical chemistry, and lymphocyte subsets. *Clin Diag Lab Immunol* **4**: 33–42.

Hopper, C.D., A.H. Sparkes, et al. (1989). Clinincal and laboratory findings in cats infected with feline immunodeficiency virus. *Vet Rec* **125**: 341–436.

Hughes, W.T., A.J. Steigman, et al. (1966). Some implications of fatal nephritis associated with mumps. *Am J Dis Child* **111**: 297–301.

Huxsoll, D.L. and I.E. Hemelt (1970). Clinical observations of canine herpesvirus. *J Am Vet Med Assoc* **156**: 1706–1713.

Ishida, T., T. Washizu, et al. (1989). Feline immunodeficiency virus infection in cats of Japan. *J Am Vet Med Assoc* **194**: 221–225.

Jacobse-Geels, H.E.L., M.R. Daha, et al. (1982). Antibody, immune complexes, and complement activity fluctuates in kittens with experimentally induced feline infectious peritonitis. *Am J Vet Res* **43**: 666–670.

Jakowski, R.M., Essex, M. et al. (1980). Membranous glomerulonephritis in a household cluster of cats persistently viremic with feline leukemia virus. In: *Feline Leukemia Virus*, edited by W.D. Jr. Hardy, W. Essex, and A.J. McClelland. Amsterdam: Elsevier North Holland Inc., pp. 141–149.

Joh, K., Y. Kanetsuna, et al. (1998). Epstein-Barr virus genome-positive tubulointerstitial nephritis associated with immune complex-mediated glomerulonephritis in chronic active EB virus infection. *Virchows Arch* **432**: 567–573.

Johnson, R.J. and W.G. Couser (1990). Hepatitis B infection and renal disease: clinical, immunopathogenetic and therapeutic considerations. *Kidney Int* **37**: 663–676.

Johnson, R.J., R. Willson, et al. (1994). Renal manifestations of hepatitis C virus infection. *Kidney Int* **46**: 1255–1263.

Karpas, A., F.G. Garcia, et al. (1968). Experimental production of canine tracheobronchitis (kennel cough) with canine herpesvirus isolated from naturally infected dogs. *Am J Vet Res* **29**: 1251–1257.

Khakpour, M. and B. Nik-Alchtar (1977). Epidemics of hemorrhagic cystitis due to influenza A virus. *Postgrad Med J* **53**: 251–253.

Khan, G., H.O. Kangro, et al. (1991). Inhibitory effects of urine on the polymerase chain reaction for cytomegalovirus DNA. *J Clin Pathol* **44**: 360–365.

Kipar, A., H. May, et al. (2005). Morphologic features and development of granulomatous vasculitis in feline infectious peritonitis. *Vet Pathol* **42**: 321–330.

Kleiboeker, S.B. (2003). Applications of competitive RNA in diagnostic reverse transcription-PCR. *J Clin Microbiol* **41**: 2055–2061.

Krishnan, R., J.A. Freeman, et al. (1999). Epstein-Barr virus induced renal leimyoma. *J Urol* **161**: 212.

Kruger, J.M. and C.A. Osborne (1990). The role of viruses in feline lower urinary tract disease. *J Vet Int Med* **4**: 71–78.

Kruger, J.M., C.A. Osborne, et al. (1990). Herpesvirus induced urinary tract infection in SPF cats given methylprednisolone. *Am J Vet Res* **51**: 878–885.

Kruger, J.M., C.A. Osborne, et al. (1996). Viral infections of the feline urinary tract. *Vet Clin North Am Small Anim Prac* **26**: 281–296.

Kruger, J.M., C.A. Osborne, et al. (1989). Genetic and serologic analysis of feline cell-associated herpesvirus infection of the urinary tract in conventionally reared cats. *Am J Vet Res* **50**: 2023–2027.

Kruger, J.M., C.P. Pfent, et al. (2007). Feline calicivirus-induce urinary tract disease in specific-pathogen-free cats. *J Vet Intern Med* **21**: 684.

Kruger, J.M., P.J. Venta, et al. (2000). Prevalence of bovine herpesvirus 4 (BHV-4) infection in cats in central Michigan. *J Vet Intern Med* **14**: 593–597.

Larson, J., J.M. Kruger, et al. (2007). Epidemiology of feline calicivirus urinary tract infection in cats with idiopathic cystitis. *J Vet Intern Med* **21**: 684.

Lavelle, J.P., S.A. Meyers, et al. (2000). Urothelial pathophysiological changes in feline interstitial cystitis; a human model. *Am J Physiol Renal Physiol* **278**: F540–F553.

Levy, J.K. 2000. Feline immunodeficiency virus. In: *Current Veterinary Therapy XIII*, edited by J.D. Bonagura. Philadelphia, PA: WB Saunders, pp. 284–288.

Makino, A., M. Shimojima, et al. (2006). Junctional adhesion molecule 1 is a functional receptor for feline calicivirus. *J Virol* **80**: 4482–4490.

Matsumara, S., T. Ishida, et al. (1993). Pathologic features of acquired immunodeficiency-like syndrome in cats experimentally infected with feline immunodeficiency virus. *J Vet Med Sci* **55**: 387–394.

McClanahan, C., M.M. Grimes, et al. (1994). Hemorrhagic cystitis associated with herpes simplex virus. *J Urol* **151**: 152–153.

Meyer, R., H.P. Brown, et al. (1959). Herpes zoster involving the urinary bladder. *N Engl J Med* **260**: 1062–1065.

Miettinen, M.H., S.M. Mäkelä, et al. (2006). Ten-year prognosis of Puumala hantavirus-induced acute interstitial nephritis. *Kidney Int* **69**: 2043–2048.

Miyoshi, M., Y. Ishii, et al. (1999). Detection of canine herpesvirus DNA in the ganglionic neurons and the lymph node lymphocytes of latently infected dogs. *J Vet Med Sci* **61**: 375–379.

Mufson, M.A. and R.B. Belshe (1976). A review of adenoviruses in the etiology of acute hemorrhagic cystitis. *J Urol* **115**: 191–194.

Murphy, F.A., E.P.I. Gibbs, et al. (1999a). Determinants of viral virulence and host resistance/susceptibility. In: *Veterinary Virology*, 3rd edition. New York: Academic Press, pp. 111–125.

Murphy, F.A., E.P.I. Gibbs, et al. (1999b). Laboratory diagnosis of viral disease. In: *Veterinary Virology*, 3rd edition. New York: Academic Press, pp. 193–224.

Okuda, Y., A. Hashimoto, et al. (1993). Repeated canine herpesvirus (CHV) reactivation in dogs by an immunosuppressive drug. *Cornell Vet* **83**: 291–302.

Pedersen, N.C., R.R. Pool, et al. (1980). Feline chronic progressive polyarthritis. *Am J Vet Res* **41**: 522–535.

Platt, J.L., R.K. Sibley, et al. (1985). Interstitial nephritis associated with cytomegalovirus infection. *Kid Int* **28**: 550–552.

Poli, A., F. Abramo, et al. (1995). Renal involvement in feline immunodeficiency virus infection: p24 antigen detection, virus isolation and PCR analysis. *Vet Immunol Immunopathol* **46**: 13–20.

Poli, A., F. Abramo, et al. (1993). Renal involvement in feline immunodeficiency virus infection: a clinicopathologic study. *Nephron* **64**: 282–288.

Reche-Jr, A. and M.K. Hagiwara (2001). Histopathology and morphometry of urinary bladder of cats with idiopathic lower urinary tract disease. *Ciência Rural* **31**: 1045–1049.

Reinacher, M. and G. Theilen. (1987). Frequency and significance of feline leukemia virus infection in necropsied cats. *Am J Vet Res* **48**: 939–945.

Rice, C.C., J.M. Kruger, et al. (2002). Genetic characterization of 2 novel feline caliciviruses isolated from cats with idiopathic lower urinary tract disease. *J Vet Intern Med* **16**: 293–302.

Rich, L.J. and C.G. Fabricant (1969). Urethral obstruction in male cats: transmission studies. *Can J Comp Med* **33**: 164–165.

Rich, L.J., C.G. Fabricant, et al. (1971). Virus induced urolithiasis in male cats. *Cornell Vet* **61**: 542–553.

Rohrbach, B.W., A.M. Legendre, et al. (2001). Epidemiology of feline infectious peritonitis among cats examined at veterinary medical teaching hospitals. *J Am Vet Med Assoc* **218**: 1111–1115.

Rossetti, A., M. Tönz, et al. (1996). Acute glomerulonephritis with zoster. *Pediatr Infect Dis J* **15**: 643–644.

Sant, G.R., K. Kempuraj, et al. (2007). The mast cell in interstitial cystitis: role in pathophysiology and pathogenesis. *Urology* **69** (suppl. 4A): 34–40.

Scansen, B.A., J.M. Kruger, et al. (2005). In vitro comparison of RNA preparations methods for detection of feline calicivirus in urine of cats by use of a reverse transcriptase-polymerase chain reaction assay. *Am J Vet Res* **66**: 915–920.

Scansen, B.A., A.G. Wise, et al. (2004). Evaluation of a p30 gene-based real-time reverse transcriptase PCR assay for detection of feline calicivirus. *J Vet Internal Med* **18**: 135–138.

Schattner, A. and B. Rager-Zisman (1990). Virus induced autoimmunity. *Rev Infect Dis* **12**: 204–222.

Schulze, C. and W. Baumgärtner (1998). Nested polymerase chain reaction and in situ hybridization for diagnosis of canine herpesvirus infection in puppies. *Vet Pathol* **35**: 209–217.

Shroyer, E.L. and M.R. Shalaby (1978). Isolation of feline syncytia-forming virus from oropharyngeal swab samples and buffy coat cells. *Am J Vet Res* **39**: 555–560.

Silbert, P.L., L.R. Matz, et al. (1990). Herpes simplex virus interstitial nephritis in a renal allograft. *Clin Nephrol* **33**: 264–268.

Smith, A.W., P.L. Iversen, et al. (2008). Virus-specific antiviral treatment for controlling severe and fatal outbreaks of feline calicivirus infection. *Am J Vet Res* **69**: 23–32.

Spach, D.H., J.E. Bauwens, et al. (1993). Cytomegalovirus-induced hemorrhagic cystitis following bone marrow transplantation. *Clin Infect Dis* **16**: 142–144.

Specht, A.J., J.M. Kruger, et al. (2003). Light microscopic features of feline idiopathic cystitis. *J Vet Intern Med* **17**: 436.

Stuart, A.D. and T.D.K. Brown (2007). α2,6-Linked sialic acid acts as a receptor for feline calicivirus. *J Gen Virol* **88**: 177–186.

Sutcliffe, S., S. Rohrmann, et al. (2007). Viral infections and lower urinary tract symptoms in the third national health and nutrition examination survey. *J Urol* **178**: 2181–2185.

Thomas, J.B., W.F. Robinson, et al. (1993). Association of renal disease indicators with feline immunodeficiency infection. *J Am Anim Hosp Assoc* **29**: 320–326.

Umehashi, M., T. Imamura, et al. (2002). Post-exposure treatment of cats with mouse-cat chimeric antibodies against feline herpesvirus type 1 and feline calicivirus. *J Vet Med Sci* **64**: 1017–1021.

Utz, J.P., V.N. Houk, et al. (1964). Clinical and laboratory studies of mumps. *N Eng J Med* **270**: 1283–1286.

Weijer, K. and J.H. Daams (1976). The presence of leukaemia (lymphosacoma) and feline leukaemia virus (FeLV) in cats in The Netherlands. *J Small Anim Prac* **17**: 649–659.

Wilson, C.B. and R.C. Smith (1972). Goodpasture's syndrome associated with influenza A2 virus infection. *Ann Intern Med* **76**: 91–94.

Wright, N.G. (1976). Canine adenovirus: its role in renal and ocular disease: a review. *J Small Anim Pract* **17**: 25–33.

Wright, N.G. and H.J.C. Cornwell (1968). Experimental herpes virus infections in young puppies. *Res Vet Sci* **9**: 295–299.

Wright, N.G. and H.J.C. Cornwell (1983). Experimental canine adenovirus glomerulonephritis: histological, immunofluorescence and ultrastructural features of the early glomerular changes. *Br J Exp Path* **64**: 312–319.

Wright, N.G., W.I. Morrison, et al. (1974). Mesangial localization of immune complexes in experimental canine adenovirus glomerulonephritis. *Br J Exp Path* **55**: 458–465.

Wright, N.G., A.S. Nash, et al. (1981). Experimental canine adenovirus glomerulonephritis: persistence of glomerular lesions after oral challenge. *Br J Exp Path* **62**: 183–189.

Wright, N.G., H. Thompson, et al. (1973). Ultrastructure of the kidney and urinary excretion of renal antigens in experimental canine adenovirus infection. *Res Vet Sci* **14**: 376–380.

Yamamura, T., Y. Minato, et al. (1992). Electron microscopy of renal arterial lesions in a pup infected with canine herpesvirus. *Jap J Vet Sci* **54**: 779–780.

Yuceoglu, A.M., S. Berkovich, et al. (1966). Acute glomerulonephritis associated with Echo virus type 9 infection. *J Pediatr* **69**: 603–609.

74

Nematodes of the upper and lower urinary tract of dogs and cats

Carl A. Osborne, Jody P. Lulich, and Hasan Albasan

Parasitologists have classified literally thousands of nematodes. The name "Nematoda" is derived from a Greek term and is translated into English as "thread-like ones" (*nema*, "thread") and (*-ode*, "like").

Parasitism is characterized by an intimate relationship between two different species in which one (the parasite) uses the other (the host) as an environment from which it can derive life-sustaining nourishment. Life cycles of parasites may be classified as direct or indirect. Direct life cycles do not require an intermediate host. The definitive host is defined as the species in which the parasite reaches sexual maturity and produces progeny. Parasites with indirect life cycles such as *Dioctophyma renale* require one or more intermediate hosts to complete its life cycle. Morphological and physiological changes occur in the immature stage of the parasite while it lives in the intermediate host. Some life cycles are associated with paratenic hosts (aka transport hosts). The term "paratenic" describes an intermediate host that is not needed for the development of the parasite, but serves to maintain the parasite's life cycle. Parasites do not develop while living in paratenic hosts. Typically, the parasite does not feed on the paratenic host. Rather, the definitive host feeds on the paratenic host after the paratenic host has fed on the intermediate host containing the immature stage of the parasite. In this way, the paratenic host "transports" the underdeveloped parasite to the definitive host where it may resume growth toward sexual maturity. Terminal hosts (aka accidental hosts and dead-end hosts) are those in which the parasite does not

reach sexual maturity at a site in the body, which will allow them to propagate.

With expansive suburbanization, wild intermediate and paratenic hosts are living closer to man and domestic animals. Therefore, understanding of parasitic life cycles and host responses is essential to minimize risks of infections of man and domestic animals.

Dioctophyma renale

Taxonomy

Of the nematodes known to affect domestic animals and humans, few can rival the size and appearance of the giant kidney worm. The etymology of the Greek name "dioctophyma" is "di" = two; "octa" = 8; "phyma" = tubercles. It is based on the taxonomy of the cranial portion of this parasite (Karmanova 1968; Soulsby 1982).

Although adult female *D. renale* are one of the largest nematodes observed to infect domestic mammals, it apparently is not the largest nematode reported by others (Soulsby 1982; Bowman 1999). Review of the English literature indicates that the largest nematode species reported is *Placentonema gigantissima*. This nematode was discovered parasitizing the placenta of a Sperm Whale (*Physeter catodon*) (Gubanov 1951). It was 8.5 m in length with a diameter of 0.3 mm and contained 32 ovaries.

In dogs, adult female *D. renale* are significantly larger than males, reaching up to 100 cm in length and 1.2 cm in width (Karmanova 1968). In contrast, males are only 20–40 cm in length and 6 mm in width. In smaller hosts such as mink, adult females are smaller, reaching up to 60 cm in length (Maxie 1999; Mech and Tracy 2001). The larvae of *D. renale* range in length from 6 to 10 mm and

Nephrology and Urology of Small Animals. Edited by Joe Bartges and David J. Polzin. © 2011 Blackwell Publishing Ltd.

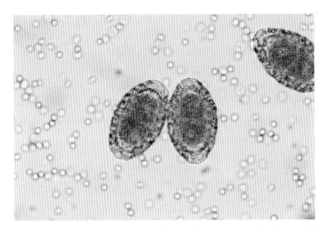

Figure 74.1 Dioctophyma renale ova (50× = original magnification; unstained).

in width from 0.1 to 0.2 mm. They are thread-like in appearance and are yellow to rust colored.

Adult male and female *D. renale* are typically blood (or vermillion) red in color when they are alive, but become brownish black after they die and degenerate. The term vermillion is derived from the Latin term "vermin" meaning worm. The characteristic red color may be associated with a hemoglobin-like blood pigment (erythrocruorin?).

The eggs are lemon-shaped and constant in size. They typically have a light tan or rust color with deep pits in their shells except at the poles that contain opercula. Eggs of *D. renale* measure 71–84 μm by 45–52 μm. Adult males have fleshy bell-shaped copulatory bursa that "dock" with the vulva of adult females located in the anterior portion of their body. A typical female *D. renale* has been estimated to produce approximately 18–20 million eggs in its lifetime (Figure 74.1).

The eggs may remain viable for up to 5 years. Desiccation and freezing temperatures are lethal to infective eggs of *D. renale* (Karmanova 1968). Although the lifespan of *D. renale* apparently has not been determined experimentally, there are estimates that some naturally occurring infections have lasted for 3–5 years (Karmanova 1968).

D. renale have a cuticle with three or more main outer layers consisting of collagen and other substances (Karmanova 1968). The outer layers are noncellular and are secreted by the epidermis. The cuticle apparently protects these nematodes as they invade various tissues of mammals. Longitudinal muscles obliquely arranged in bands line the body wall. Because their internal pressure is high, muscle contraction causes their body to flex rather than flatten. Contraction of these muscles allows the parasite to move by thrashing back and forth.

Free-living annelids (*Lumbriculus variegatus*) are essential intermediate hosts (Karmanova 1968). *Lum-*

briculus spp. (aka blackworms and mudworms) are phylogenically related to the earthworm (Karmanova 1968). Adult *L. variegates* are approximately 10 cm in length and 1.5 mm in diameter. They can be readily found in Europe, North America, and South America. They often inhabit shallow water of the edges of ponds, lakes, and marshes where they feed on decaying vegetation and microorganisms. *L. variegates* may also inhabit silt-sediments in deeper water. Any mammal that drinks water containing infected annelids has the potential of ingesting the infective third stage of *D. renale*.

Epidemiology

Dioctophyma renale is cosmopolitan in distribution (Karmanova 1968; Mace 1976a; Osbome et al. 1969). Cases of *D. renale* have been encountered in virtually every part of the world with a temperate climate. In North America, cases have been frequently encountered in Mississippi, Louisiana, Minnesota, Wisconsin, Michigan, and the central and eastern provinces of Canada (Osbome et al. 1969; Mech and Tracy 2001). The giant kidney worm has been reported in many species of animals, including dogs, mink, coyotes, jackals, raccoons, foxes, wolves, maned-wolves, beech martens, pine martens, otters, and weasels (Karmanova 1968; Osbome et al. 1969; Soulsby 1982). Isolated infections of seals, horses, and cows have been documented (Karmanova 1968; Soulsby 1982; Acha and Szyfres 1989; Mech and Tracy 2001; Hoffman et al. 2004). Humans are accidental hosts; there have been "believe it or not" case reports of adult *D. renale* passing through the urethra of women (Karmanova 1968). Because of the aquatic portion of its life cycle, water is an essential element of the habitat of *D. renale*. Therefore, it is not surprising that semiaquatic fish-eating mammals are the most common definitive hosts of *D. renale*. Fish and frogs often serve as paratenic hosts for this parasite. Mink are the most commonly infected mustelids and appear to be the principal definitive host in North America (Mace and Anderson 1975; Mace 1976b). Up to 50% of wild mink have been reported to be infected in some areas (Mech and Tracy 2001).

Life cycle

To complete the life cycle, both male and female parasites must be located in the same kidney of the host and the urinary tract must be patent. Fertile eggs are passed with urine voided by the host (Figure 74.2).

They embryonate in water and after 1–7 months produce first-stage larvae (Maxie 1999). The rate of their development is dependent on temperature of the water. The optimal temperature required for eggs to embryonate is between 25 and 30°C (Soulsby 1982). The eggs

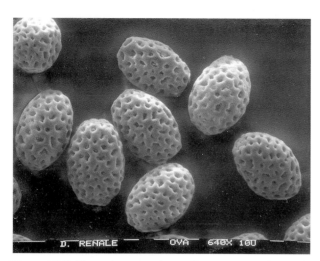

Figure 74.2 Dioctophyma renale ova (640× = original magnification. Scanning electron micrograph).

hatch only after being swallowed by the intermediate host, *Lumbriculus variegatus*. Contrary to earlier reports, this annelid apparently is the only intermediate host required to complete the life cycle (Karmanova 1968). A period of more than 100 days in *L. variegatus* is required for the second and third (infective) stage of the parasite to develop. The definitive host becomes infected by ingesting the infective larvae in annelids.

Paratenic hosts may also become a part of the life cycle. In the United States, frogs (*Rana climitans*) northern black bullheads (*Ictalurus nebulosus*) are paratenic hosts (Maxie 1999; Mech and Tracy 2001). In other countries, other species of fish (pike and pumpkin-seed fish) have been reported as paratenic hosts (Hoffman et al. 2004). Larvae encyst in the liver, mesentery, stomach wall, or abdominal muscles of paratenic hosts.

The definitive host becomes infected either by ingesting raw fish, frogs, other paratenic hosts, or by ingesting *L. variegates* (Karmanova 1968; Mace and Anderson 1975). After being swallowed by the definitive host, the infective larvae penetrate the walls of the stomach or intestines and migrate to the submucosa. Then, after approximately 5–7 days, they migrate to the liver and remain there for about 50 days. Migration to the right kidney and invasion of the renal pelvis follows (Karmanova 1968).

D. renale have been found more frequently in the right kidney than in the left (Karmanova 1968; Mace 1976a, 1976b; Soulsby 1982). The predilection for the right kidney has been attributed to the close anatomic relationship of the right kidney to the duodenum. According to some investigators, adult *D. renale* are found in the left renal pelvis when they penetrate the stomach at the greater curvature. Finding encysted *D. renale* around the liver is associated larval penetration at the lesser curvature of the stomach (Kommers et al. 1999). The time

required for infective larvae to become mature gravid females in the definitive host is 3.5–6 months. The entire life cycle requires approximately two years (Karmanova 1968; Mace and Anderson 1975; Soulsby 1982).

On occasion, *D. renale* have been encountered in the urinary bladder and/or ureter (Osbome et al. 1969; Nakagawa et al. 2007). The highest number of adults found in one dog is 34 (Monteiro et al. 2002).

The protein-rich fluid that surrounds adult worms in the renal pelves is almost entirely of host origin and likely is a rich source of nutrients that are absorbed across the body wall. We measured the urine protein/creatinine ratio of fluid surrounding a gravid adult female *D. renale* in the hydronephrotic right kidney of an adult dog and compared it to the UP/UC ratio of urine contained in the urinary bladder. The UP/UC ratio of the renal fluid was 301; the UP/UC ratio of urine aspirated from the bladder was 0.27. Other nematodes, such as the muscle dwelling *Trichinella spiralis*, also feed via transcuticular uptake of nutrients.

Pathophysiology

Kidney

Adult parasites have attained substantial size by the time they penetrate the kidney. The exact mechanisms involved with gaining access to the renal pelvis have not been reported. *D. renale* adults greater in length than renal dwelling adults have been found in the peritoneal cavity without any evidence of kidney penetration. Large adult parasites removed from the peritoneal cavity of one dog and transplanted to the same location in another dog have successfully penetrated the kidney of the recipient (Karmanova 1968). Entry of the parasite into the kidney probably results from the effects enzymes released by the parasite. Potent collagenases, hyaluronidases, and cysteine proteases released by nematodes can easily digest host tissues. Glands containing these enzymes may be located adjacent to the esophagus. Some infective larvae of nematodes also excrete large quantities of amines. Amines are strongly alkaline and very toxic. The parasite-derived amines may help infective larvae to penetrate tissue (Karmanova 1968).

Contrary to reports in the literature, available evidence does not support the theory that adult *D. renale* slowly devour the renal tissue of the host, reducing it to a hollow sack. The buccal cavity of the parasite is not used for the ingestion of intact renal tissues; solid particles have not been detected in the esophagus of *D. renale*. Although the exact mechanism(s) of destruction is not known for sure, it is apparent that obstruction caused by the growing adult parasite(s) and secondary hydronephrosis (or pyonephrosis) play a major role (Figures 74.3–74.5).

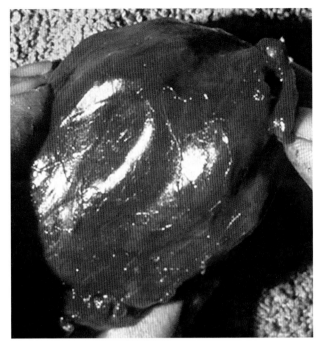

Figure 74.3 Photograph of the right kidney of a spayed female 14-month Golden retriever. The parasites have distorted the surface contour of the kidney.

Light microscopic examination of sections of kidneys from dogs with unilateral renal infection reveal changes typical of advanced hydronephrosis (i.e., obliteration of the majority of renal tubules surrounded by chronic inflammatory tissue and persistence of the structural architecture of many glomeruli). Ova of *D. renale* may be observed in the renal parenchyma adjacent to the

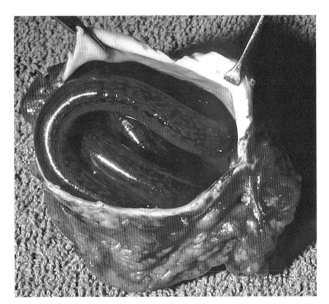

Figure 74.4 Photograph of an adult female and an adult male D. renale in the dilated renal pelvis of the right kidney.

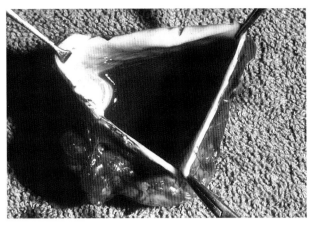

Figure 74.5 Photograph of the hydronephrotic right kidney with hemorrhagic modified transudate in the renal pelvis.

renal pelvis (Figure 74.6). The urothelium lining the renal pelvis is often hyperplastic in some areas and ulcerated in other areas.

In mink and dogs, bone has been reported in association with heteroplastic urothlelium (Osbome et al. 1969). The formation of mineralized bone is not unique to *D. renale* (Huggins 1931; Gruhn and Fisher 1960; Hall et al. 1972). Ostogenesis is likely related to the ability of some cells (such as transitional epithelium) to respond to growth factors such as bone morphogenic proteins. We have detected bone in hydronephrotic kidneys of cats that were not parasitized (Hall et al. 1972). Usually, only one kidney is affected with *D. renale*. The host maintains adequate renal function due to compensatory hypertrophy and hyperplasia of the remaining kidney. If both kidneys are parasitized, or if one kidney is parasitized and the opposite kidney has substantial comorbid dysfunction, varying stages of renal failure and uremia may occur.

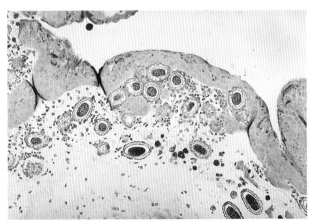

Figure 74.6 Photomicrograph of a section of a hydronephrotic right kidney of a dog. Numerous ova are present in the scarred renal tissue adjacent to hyperplastic urothelium.

Peritoneal cavity

In dogs, viable parasites located in the abdominal cavity or between lobes of the liver have frequently been reported as an incidental finding during ovariohysterectomies (Karmanova 1968). It is possible that, under certain conditions, the adult worms may remain in the peritoneal cavity for extended periods prior to penetration of a kidney. In a few cases, worms have been found in the peritoneal cavity while lesions indicative of partial kidney penetration by the parasite were present. However, adults and eggs of the parasite have been found in the peritoneal cavity without any detectable evidence of kidney penetration by the parasites (Karmanova 1968; Maxie 1999). Copulation of *D. renale* occurs in the kidney, and it has been suggested that mating can also occur in the peritoneal cavity. It is also possible that, after mating with females in the renal pelvis, male parasites exit the kidney into the peritoneal cavity (Karmanova 1968; Mace and Anderson 1975).

Eggs that are released by female worms pass through the urinary tract and are thought to provoke inflammation in the mucosa of the ureter and the bladder. The presence of eggs in the peritoneal cavity can also trigger the development of chronic peritonitis. Examination of the abdominal viscera from dogs with *D. renale* in the peritoneal cavity revealed hemorrhage, granulomatous inflammation, and fibrosis frequently involving the omentum, the surface of the liver, and less frequently the surface of the spleen (Karmanova 1968; Maxie 1999). In our experience, viable adult males (but not females) have been found in the peritoneal cavity of dogs without an associated inflammatory response. This suggests that females and/or their eggs stimulate a greater host inflammatory response than males.

Ascites may occur in dogs with *D. renale* in the peritoneal cavity. The fluid detected in the abdominal cavity is usually hemorrhagic. The quantity of ascitic fluid reported to be removed from dogs infected with *D. renale* ranged from approximately 20 mL to 3.2 L (Karmanova 1968).

Other sites

Adults and larvae of *D. renale* have been encountered in organs and tissues other than the kidneys, liver, and peritoneal cavity. *D. renale* has been reported in the urinary bladder, urethra, ureters, uterus, ovaries, mammary glands, stomach, abdominal wall, and thoracic cavity of dogs and other animals (Osbome et al. 1969). In terminal hosts (e.g., humans) *D. renale* has been reported in the subcutaneous tissue (Beaver and Theis 1979). Immature worms believed to be the infective third stage of *D. renale* have been reported in skin nodules of humans (Acha and Szyfres 1989). They have also been reported as large abdominal masses simulating neoplasms in man (Sun et al. 1986).

Clinical signs

The feeding of *L. variegatus* infected with *D. renale* to dogs typically induces vomiting due to effects of the parasite on the gastric mucosa (Karmanova 1968). Ingestion of uninfected annelids by dogs was not associated with vomiting. Microscopic examination of sections of stomach wall obtained from vomiting dogs infected with *D. renale* revealed submucosal hemorrhage adjacent to larvae (Karmanova 1968). Ferrets experimentally infected with *D. renale* via the ingestion of fish tissue containing the third stage of *D. renale* also vomited as a result of exposure to the parasite.

If only one kidney has been invaded with *D. renale* and the opposite kidney is normal, signs attributable to *D. renale* infestation are often absent. Hematuria observed by owners may be the first indication of an abnormality. Palpation of the abdomen may reveal an enlarged and/or misshaped hydronephrotic kidney.

If both kidneys are parasitized, clinical signs attributable to renal failure or uremia may occur. However, the host will die before extensive hydronephrosis of both kidneys has time to develop. The degree of renal dysfunction is influenced by (1) the number of parasites in the kidney, (2) the duration of infection, (3) the number of kidneys parasitized, and (4) and the presence of comorbid renal diseases.

Laboratory findings

When a gravid female worm is present in one or both kidneys that have a patent track to the exterior, microscopic examination of urine voided by the host usually reveals ova of *D. renale* (Ehrenford and Snodgrass 1955; Acha and Szyfres 1989). Pyuria, hematuria, and proteinuria with or without eggs are indicative of an inflammatory response. Renal function tests may reveal results typical of chronic renal failure when both kidneys are parasitized or when one only kidney contains parasites and the contralateral kidney is diseased.

Other tests

Radiography may reveal an enlarged hydronephrotic kidney. If intravenous urography is performed, it may be characterized by inability of the parasitized kidney to excrete the contrast agent. Ultrasonography may reveal that the affected kidney is hydronephrotic and contains excessive fluid (Soler et al. 2008). Ultrasound may also

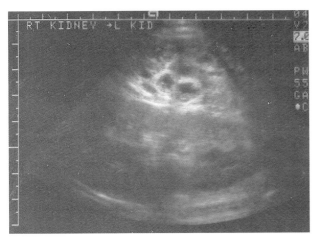

Figure 74.7 Transverse sonograph of the right kidney of a dog illustrating characteristic hyperechoic and hypoechoic pattern of D. renale

reveal characteristic hypoechoic loops associated with one or more of these parasites in the renal pelvis. Transverse plane sonographs of the affected kidney may reveal a thin hyperechoic rim that contains multiple circular structures of uniform diameter (Figure 74.7).

The outer layers of these structures are hyperechoic; the inner portions are hypoechoic. In the longitudinal plane, the structures appear as elongated hyperechoic bands alternating with elongated hypoechoic bands. If viable parasites are in the peritoneal cavity, sonography may reveal hyperechoic curvilinear bands in the region of the right caudal lobe of the liver and/or the cranial pole of the right kidney. Serially performed sonographs may reveal movement of the parasite(s) from one location to another. CT and MRI scans may also be used to detect *D. renale* in the renal pelvis of one or both kidneys, in the peritoneal cavity, or in varying positions between the lobes of the liver.

Diagnosis

If the gravid female parasite is located in the pelvis of a kidney that has a patent ureter, characteristic ova may be found by microscopic examination of urine sediment (Figures 74.1 and 74.2). When the worms are free in the peritoneal cavity, the diagnosis is usually made by ultrasonography, laparoscopy, computed tomography, and/or exploratory celiotomy. Parasites are often found between lobes of the liver.

Treatment

Nephrectomy is usually the treatment of choice when only one kidney is affected and the opposite kidney is

capable of sustaining homeostasis. In patients with parasites in both kidneys, nephrotomy and removal of the parasites may be indicated if sufficient functional tissue remains in both kidneys to maintain a reasonable quality of life. Unfortunately, by the time *D. renale* affecting both kidneys is recognized, the patients often have moderate to severe irreversible renal failure. Parasites that are incidental findings in the peritoneal cavity during celiotomy may be removed without further morbidity.

Pharmacologic treatment of adults and/or infective larvae discovered in any species has been virtually nonexistent. Review of the literature resulted in finding a report of a 44-year-old man with recurrent lumbar pain attributed to *D. renale* (Ignjatovic et al. 2003). According to the report, the patient had consumed undercooked fish or several months. The physicians stated that treatment consisting of two regimens of ivermectin resulted in a cure.

Prevention

Dogs and cats should not be fed raw fish or fish viscera, especially in areas where *D. renale* is known to exist. Likewise, they should not be given access to lake or pond water likely to contain infective stages of *D. renale*.

Although it is thought that infection with *D. renale* confers some protection against challenge exposure to the parasite, this empirical observation has not been documented by appropriate studies. However, less than 20% of the larvae that were orally administered to commercially reared mustelids were successful in reaching the kidneys (Mace and Anderson 1975).

Capillaria plica, Capillaria felis-cati

Taxonomy

The genus *Capillaria* contains many species that collectively parasitize all vertebrate classes (Butterworth and Beverly-Burton 1980). However, descriptions of the taxonomy of the genus *Capillaria* and various species of this genus are a mess. In 1819, Rudolphi first described nematodes found in the urinary bladder of wolves as *Trichosoma plica*, and this name was adopted by the scientific community. Sometime later, the name "Capillaria" was adopted. In 1951, Enzie reported *Capillaria felis-cati* from the urinary bladder of a domestic cat (Enzie 1951). However, Enzie's description of *C. felis-cati* was apparently based on the description of Freitus and Leent in 1936 (Butterworth and Beverly-Burton 1980). To add to the confusion, in 1982, the genus *Pearsonema* was adopted by some investigators instead of *Capillaria* (Moravec

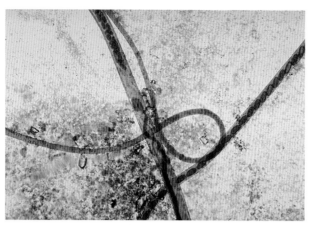

Figure 74.8 Photomicrograph of gravid Capllaria plica in the urine sediment of a dog (75× = original magnification. Unstained). Courtesy of Dr. David Senior, Louisiana State University.

1982; Waddell 1968a). Now, the genus names *Capillaria* and *Pearsonema* are used interchangeably. One of the problems in attempting to categorize species of these parasites to the genus *Capillaria* or to another new genus is that they all appear to be morphologically similar. In this chapter, we have used the name *Capillaria* and not *Pearsonema* as the genus name.

Capillaria aerophilia inhabits tissue (i.e., it is histozoic), whereas *C. plica* and *C. felis-cati* are lumen dwellers (i.e., they are coelozic). In contrast to *D. renale*, adult *C. plica* and *C. felis-cati* are small, fragile, thread-like yellowish parasites (Figure 74.8). Males are generally 16–53 mm long, whereas females are 17–53 mm long (Butterworth and Beverly-Burton 1980; Moravec 1982; Georgi and Georgi 1990).

The eggs have bipolar plugs, are colorless, and have a slightly pitted shell (Figure 74.9). They measure 63–68 by 24–27 μm (Butterworth and Beverly-Burton 1980; Georgi and Georgi 1990).

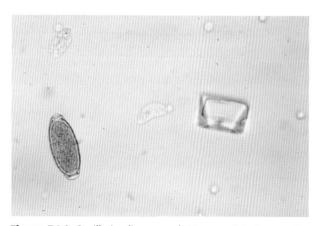

Figure 74.9 Capillaria plica ovum (160× = original magnification. Unstained).

Epidemiology

Capillaria plica is widely distributed throughout the world. It has been found in the urinary bladder, and less frequently in the ureters and renal pelves, of dogs, foxes, coyotes, raccoons, martens, mink badgers, otters, bobcats, skunks, weasels, and wolves. *Capillaria felis-cati* is found less commonly in the urinary bladder of cats. The two species of *Capillaria* have similar biologic properties and life cycles (Butterworth and Beverly-Burton 1980; Waddell 1968a; Moravec 1982).

Several species of wild animals appear to be the primary host. For example, 48% of 320 British wild red foxes were infected with *C. plica* (Beresford-Jones 1961). This parasite was also reported in 64% of 70 raccoons in western Kentucky (Cole and Shoop 1987). Although endemic infection rates as high as 59 and 72% have been reported in breeding kennels (Senior et al. 1980), infections with these parasites occur too infrequently in domestic dogs and cats housed indoors for these species to maintain the life cycle.

Life cycle

Although a direct life cycle has been proposed, there is strong evidence that earthworms are essential hosts for *C. plica* and *C. felis-cati* (Senior et al. 1980). According to the indirect life-cycle scenario, eggs containing a single cell are voided in the urine. First-stage larvae develop in approximately I month but apparently will not develop further unless they are ingested by an earthworm (*Lumbricus terrestris*). The definitive host becomes infected by eating earthworms that have first-stage larvae in their tissues. Infected larvae gain access to the lumen of the bladder via the circulatory system. Eggs first appear in the urine of the definitive host about 2 months after ingestion of infective larvae.

Direct transmission by feeding embryonated eggs to foxes failed to result infection, but ingestion of earthworms completed the life cycle (Beresford-Jones 1961). Ingestion of embryonated eggs by beagle puppies failed to cause infection, whereas ingestion of earthworms collected from yards of a kennel caused patent infection 61–68 days later (Senior et al. 1980). Eggs were not found in the urine voided by pups less than 8 months of age. Dogs selected for this study did not find earthworms palatable. Therefore, the investigators concluded that the dogs ingested them inadvertently or during grooming (Senior et al. 1980). Wild foxes and raccoons are more likely to eat earthworms than are domestic dogs and cats.

Pathophysiology

Adult worms weave the anterior portion of their bodies into the mucosa of the urinary bladder and at times into the mucosa of the ureters and renal pelvis. The macroscopic appearance of the kidney's renal pelves, ureters, urinary bladder, and urethra may be normal (Senior et al. 1980). However, light microscopy revealed submucosal edema of the urinary bladder in the vicinity of adult worms (Senior et al. 1980; Georgi and Georgi 1990). Desquamation of urothelial cells in the vicinity of the parasite also occurred. The submucosa contained dilated capillaries with margination of neutrophils along vessel walls. Focal areas of lymphocytes and plasma cells in the superficial mucosa were observed. There were relatively few eosinophils.

Clinical signs

Most dogs and cats with urinary capillariasis are asymptomatic; some become pollakiuric, polydipsic, and peri-uric (Waddell 1968a).

Laboratory findings

Urinalysis may reveal results (hematuria, proteinuria, and pyuria) typical of inflammation. Numerous clumps of transitional epithelial cells have also been observed in urine sediment (Senior et al. 1980). *C. plica* eggs are usually easy to identify, although at times they are difficult to find. Twenty-four-hour egg counts from eight infected dogs yielded mean counts ranging from approximately 600–25,000 (Senior et al. 1980). Egg counts from three infected dogs housed in cages for 84 days gradually diminished until eggs were undetectable. These observations were interpreted to indicate that infections with *Capillaria* species were self-limiting.

Diagnosis

A diagnosis is made by finding typical eggs via microscopic examination of urine sediment (Harris Lloyd 1981). Inability to detect parasite ova is not definitive evidence that the dog or cat is not infected. (e.g., absence of evidence is not always reliable evidence of absence).

Treatment

Urinary capillariasis is most often asymptomatic and may be self-limiting. Suggested treatments include (Waddell 1968b; Senior et al. 1980; Harris Lloyd 1981; Gillespie 1983; Kirkpatrick and Nelson 1987)

1. Several dogs appear to have been cured by single doses of ivermectin, 0.2 mg/kg, administered by subcutaneous injection.

2. Prolonged treatment with albendazole was effective in 85% of dogs infected with *C. plica*. The urine was negative for eggs 30 days after initiation of treatment. Oral doses of 50 mg/kg of albendazole were given twice daily for up to 30 days (Senior et al. 1980).

3. Mebendazole or albendazole (200 mg given orally twice per day) has been reported as the treatment of choice for human intestinal capillariasis (Bair et al. 2004).

Because evidence indicates that in the absence of reinfection, urinary capillariasis may be self-limiting, isolation of dog and cats from earthworms should be sufficient to eliminate a Capillaria bladder infection in less than 90 days (Waddell 1968a).

Prevention

Dogs and cats must be prevented from ingesting earthworms. Kennels and kennel yards should be surfaced with a material that prevents access of dogs (and cats) to earthworms.

References

Acha, P.N. and B. Szyfres (1989). *Zoonosis y Enfermedades Transmisibles Comunes al Hombre y a los Animales*, 2nd edition. Washington DC: Oranzacion Panamericano de la Salud, pp. 806–809.

Bair, M.J., K.P. Hwang, et al. (2004). Clinical features of human intestinal capillariasis in Taiwan. *World J Gastroenterol* **10**: 2391–2393.

Beaver, P.C. and J.H. Theis (1979). Diooctophymatid larval nematode in a subcutaneous nodule from man in California. *Am J Trop Med Hyg* **28**: 206–212.

Beresford-Jones, W.P. (1961). Observations on the helminths of British wild red foxes. *Vet Rec* **73**: 882–883.

Bowman, D.W., ed. (1999). *Bowman Georgis' Parasitology for Veterinarians*. Philadelpha, PA: WB Saunders.

Butterworth, E.W. and M. Beverly-Burton (1980). The taxonomy of capillaria spp. in carnivorous mammals from Ontario, Canada. *Systematic Parsitology* **1**: 211–236.

Cole, R.A. and W.L. Shoop (1987). Helminths of the raccoon (*Procyon lotor*) in western Kentucky. *J Parasitol* **73**: 762–768.

Ehrenford, F.A. and T.B. Snodgrass (1955). Incidence of canine dioctophymiasis (giant kidney worm infection) with a summary of cases in North America. *JAVMA* **126**: 415–417.

Enzie, F.D. (1951). Do whipworms occur in domestic cats in North America. *JAVMA* **119**: 210–213.

Georgi, J.R. and M.E. Georgi (1990). *Parasitology for Veterinarians*, 8th edition. Philadelphia, PA: WB Saunders, 206 p.

Gillespie, D. (1983). Successful treatment of canine *Capillaria plica* cystitis. *Vet Med/Small Anim Clin* **78**: 681.

Gruhn, J. and E.R. Fisher (1960). Heterotopic ossification and dystrophic calcification in infarcted rat kidney. *Arch Path* **69**: 90–100.

Gubanov, N.M. (1951). Giant nematoda from the placenta of Cetacea, *Placentonema gigantissima*. *Proc USSR Acad Sci* **77**: 1123–1125.

Hall, M.S., C.A. Osborne, et al. (1972). Hydronephrosis with heteroplastic bone formation in a cat. *JAVMA* **160**: 857–860.

Harris Lloyd, F. (1981). Feline bladderworm. *Vet Med/Small Anim Clin* **76**: 844.

Hoffman, V., T.J. Nolan, et al. (2004). First report of the giant kidney worm (*Dioctophyme renale*) in a harbor seal (*Phoca vitulina*). *J Parasitol* **90**: 659–660.

Huggins, C.B. (1931). Formation of bone under the influence of epithelium of the urinary tract. *Arch Surg* **22**: 377–408.

Ignjatovic, I., I. Stojkovic, et al. (2003). Infestation of the human kidney with *Dioctophyma renale*. *Urol Int* **70**: 70–73.

Karmanova, E.M. (1968). Biological peculiarities of nematodes of the order dioctophymidia. In: *Dioctophymidia of Animals and Man and Diseases Caused by Them. Fundamentals of Nematology*, Vol. **20**. Moscow: Nauka Publishers, pp. 24–121.

Kirkpatrick, C.E. and G.R. Nelson (1987). Ivermectin treatment of urinary capillariasis in a dog. *JAVMA* **191**: 701–702.

Kommers, D.G., M.R. Slha, et al. (1999). Dioctofimose em cães: 16 casos. *Ciência Rural* **29**: 517–522.

Mace, T.F. and R.C. Anderson (1975). Development of the giant kidney worm, *Dioctophyma renale* (Goeze, 1782) (Nematoda: Dioctophymatoidea). *Can J Zoo* **53**: 1552–1568.

Mace, T.F. (1976a). Bibliography of giant kidney worm *Dioctophyma renale*. *Wild Dis* **69**: 1–36.

Mace, T.F. (1976b) Lesions in mink (*Mustela vision*) infected with giant kidney worm. *J Wildl Dis* **12**: 88–92.

Maxie, M.G. (1999). *The Kidney*, 4th edition, Vol. **2**. In: *The Pathology of Domestic Animals*, edited by K.V.F. Jubb, P.C. Kennedy, and N. Palmer. San Diego: Academic Press, pp. 447–538.

Mech, L.D. and S.P. Tracy (2001). Prevalence of giant kidney worm (*Dioctophyma renale*) in wild mink (*Mustela vison*) in Minnesota. *Am Mid Nat* **145**: 206–209.

Monteiro, S.G., E.S.V. Sallis, et al. (2002). Infecção natural por trinta e quatro helmintos da espécie *Dioctophyma renale* (Goeze, 1782) em um cão. *Revista da Faculdade de Zootecnia, Veterinária e Agronomia Uruguaiana* **9**: 29–32.

Moravec, F. (1982). Proposal for a new systematic arrangement of nematodes of the family Capillariidae. *Folia Parasitol* **29**: 119–132.

Nakagawa, T.L.D.R., A.P.F. Rodrigues, et al. (2007). Giant kidney worm (*Dioctophyma renale*) infections in dogs from Northern Paraná, Brazil. *Vet Parasit* **145**: 366–370.

Osbome, C.A., J.B. Stevens, et al. (1969). *Dioctophyma renale* in the dog. *JAVMA* **155**: 605–620.

Senior, D.F., G.B. Solomon, et al. (1980). *Capillaria plica* infections in dogs. *JAVMA* **176**: 901–905.

Soler, M., L. Cardoso, et al. (2008). Imaging diagnosis—*Dioctophyma renale* in a dog. *Vet Rad Ultrasound* **49**: 307–308.

Soulsby, E.J.L. (1982). *Helminths, Arthropods, and Protozoa of Domesticated Animals*, 7th edition. Philadelphia, PA: Lea & Febiger, pp. 343–344.

Sun, T., A. Turnbull, et al. (1986). Giant kidney worm (*Dioctophyma renale*) infection mimicking retroperitoneal neoplasm. *Am J Surg Pathol* **10**: 508–512.

Waddell, A.H. (1968a). Further observations on *Capillaria feliscati* in the cat. *Australian Vet J* **44**: 33–34.

Waddell, A.H. (1968b). Anthelmintic treament for *Capillaria feliscati* in the cat. *Vet Rec* **82**: 598.

Section 9

Lower urinary tract disorders

75

Feline idiopathic cystitis

Jodi L. Westropp

Feline lower urinary tract disease (FLUTD) is an inclusive term used to describe any disorder affecting the urinary bladder or urethra of cats. Signs of LUTD in cats include variable combinations of pollakiuria, stranguria, periuria, dysuria, and hematuria. These lower urinary tract signs (LUTS) are not specific for any one particular disease; they can be seen in cats that have cystic calculi, bacterial urinary tract infections, neoplasia, or other mass lesions in the bladder. Overall, FLUTD has been reported in 4.6% of cats seen in private practices in the United States; a slightly higher prevalence was reported from Universities (F and Roudebush 2007). In approximately 2/3 of younger to middle-aged cats that present with these clinic signs, no definitive diagnosis can be made; therefore, this syndrome is called feline idiopathic cystitis (FIC) (Westropp and Buffington 2004). A synonym for this disease is idiopathic feline lower urinary tract disease (iFLUTD). Occasionally, clinicians will refer to this disease as interstitial cystitis (IC), because it is very similar to a disease that occurs in human beings. For consistency in this chapter, the term FIC will be used to refer to this idiopathic syndrome.

Signalment

FIC is generally seen in younger and middle-aged cats and is uncommonly diagnosed in cats greater than 10 years of age. Although it is reported in most studies that FIC occurs equally in both genders (Buffington et al. 1997a; Jones et al. 1997; Willeberg 1984), in one study, a male predisposition was suggested (Cameron et al. 2004). Although FIC can be obstructive or nonobstructive in its presentation, urethral obstruction is far more common

Nephrology and Urology of Small Animals. Edited by Joe Bartges and David J. Polzin. © 2011 Blackwell Publishing Ltd.

in male cats with no difference reported between intact and castrated males (Hostutler et al. 2005). In reported studies, excessive body weight, decreased activity, multiple cat households, and indoor housing have been associated with increased risk for FIC (Buffington 2002).

Pathophysiology
Histopathology

There are two forms of FIC, the nonulcerative and ulcerative form. Cats with FIC almost always present with the nonulcerative form; however, the "classic Hunner's ulcers" have been described rarely in cats (Clasper 1990). It is possible that the etiopathogenesis of these two forms of FIC are different. In humans with IC, those with Hunner's ulcers have more mononuclear cellular infiltrates in the perineural and perivascular areas of the bladder and can show urolthelial spongiosis and detachment (Peeker and Fall 2002). The nonulcerative subtype lacks the inflammatory cellular infiltrates. It has been shown in research on the bladder of cats with chronic FIC that histologic changes are generally nonspecific and may include an intact or damaged urothelium with sumbmucosal edema, dilation of submucosal blood vessels with marginated neutrophils, submucosal hemorrhage, and sometimes increased mast cell density (Buffington et al. 1997b). Histopathologic abnormalities are usually not specific for FIC. In an abstract, bladder histopathology in cats with FIC and urolithiasis was evaluated and a difference in the degree of lymphphocyte and mast cell infiltration as well as neovascularization was not shown, suggesting that these lesions are not pathognomonic for FIC (Specht et al. 2004). On the basis of the author's experience, no correlation between histology (and even cystoscopic) lesions and clinical signs appears to exist in cats.

Bladder abnormalities

Because cats with this disease present primarily for LUTS, a significant amount of research has been performed on the bladder. It has been shown in studies evaluating bladder permeability that there are marked increases in permeability after hydrodistention (Lavelle et al. 2000) and increased bladder permeability to sodium salicylate in cats with FIC (Gao et al. 1994). These findings may be mediated via the sympathetic nervous system. It has also been reported that cats with FIC excrete decreased amounts of both total urinary glycosaminoglycan (Buffington et al. 1996) (GAG) and a specific GAG (GP-51) (Press et al. 1995). GAG and GP-51 contribute to the surface mucus covering the urothelium and that is believed to inhibit bacterial adherence and urothelial injury from the noxious constituents of the urine.

It has been suggested that urothelial cells exhibit "neuronal-like" properties and activation by a variety of stimuli can evoke the release of various transmitters such as ATP and nitric oxide (Figure 75.1) (Birder 2006).

The urothelial cells themselves can be targets of these mediators and potentiate this inflammation. The bladder afferent neurons in cats with FIC exhibit an increased excitability to physical and chemical stimuli as compared to unaffected cats (Sculptoreanu et al. 2005). Sympathoneural–epithelial interactions appear to play an important role in permeability. Birder et al. (Birder et al. 2002) have shown that application of norepinephrine

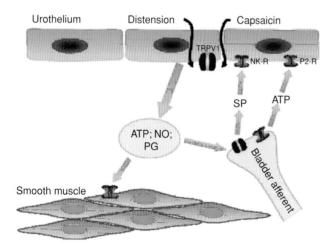

Figure 75.1 Schematic depicting possible interactions between bladder afferents, urothelial cells, and smooth muscle in the urinary bladder. Stimulation of receptors/channels on urothelial cells (e.g., ATP, distention, TRPV1) can release mediators (nitric oxide, NO; ATP; prostaglandin, PG) and target bladder nerves, altering afferent excitability. In turn, urothelial cells may be targets for transmitters released from bladder nerves. Pathology can damage urothelial cells, resulting in altered urothelial cells and neural function. Figure and description used with permission (Birder 2006).

(NE) to urinary bladder (UB) strips induces the release of nitric oxide from UB epithelium. Application of capsaicin results in the release of nitric oxide from epithelium as well as nervous tissue in the UB. In light of reports that nitric oxide may increase urothelial permeability (Jezernik et al. 2003; Oter et al. 2004), it is suggested by these results that some of the sympathetically mediated alterations in permeability may be mediated by NE via this mechanism.

In humans presenting with LUTS, urodynamics are often performed to rule out diseases, such as overactive bladder that could account for the clinical signs. Although these studies are not routinely performed in feline patients, in a recent publication, these procedures have been described and normal parameters have been established in a small group of healthy cats (Cohen et al. 2009). It has been shown in preliminary research evaluating urodyanmics in cats with FIC that there is no evidence of overactive bladder but occasional findings of decreased compliance have been noted (unpublished data).

Systemic abnormalities

Signs of FIC can wax and wane and appear to be exacerbated by stressful circumstances. A significant increase in tyrosine hydroxylase (TH) IR has been identified in the locus coeruleus (LC) (Reche and Buffington 1998) as well as in the paraventricular nucleus of the hypothalamus in cats with FIC (Welk and Buffington 2003). TH is the rate-limiting enzyme of catecholamine synthesis. Bladder distention stimulates neuronal activity in the LC, and the LC (Barrington's nucleus) is the origin of the descending excitatory pathway to the bladder (de Groat et al. 1993). Moreover, chronic stress can increase TH activity in the LC (Sands et al. 2000), with accompanying increases in autonomic outflow (Goldstein 1995). The LC contains the largest number of noradrenergic neurons and is the most important source of NE in the feline (and human) central nervous system. It is involved in such global brain functions as vigilance, arousal, and analgesia and appears to mediate visceral responses to stress (Valentino et al. 1999). The increased THIR observed in the LC of cats with FIC may provide a clue to the observation that clinical symptoms of FIC in cats and IC in humans follow a waxing and waning course and can be aggravated by environmental stressors (Buffington and Pacak 2001; Wesselmann 2001; Westropp et al. 2006).

In addition to increased LC activity, cats with FIC also have increased plasma NE concentrations (Buffington and Pacak 2001; Westropp et al. 2006). During stressful situations, elevated plasma and CSF catecholamine concentrations and their metabolites were found in FIC cats as compared to healthy cats. When evaluating catecholamine concentrations (CCE) in cats with FIC, we found that plasma DOPA, NE, and DHPG concentrations were significantly increased in FIC cats at all times during a moderate stress protocol ($p < 0.05$) as compared to healthy cats. Furthermore, as the healthy cats acclimated to the stress, their plasma catecholamine concentrations decreased, whereas in cats with FIC, even higher concentrations of plasma NE, epinephrine, and their metabolites were demonstrated (Westropp et al. 2006). The marked increment in (DOPA) suggests the possibility of a stress-induced increase in activity of TH, the rate-limiting step in CCE synthesis. In contrast, no effects on urine cortisol:creatinine were identified, suggesting an uncoupling of these two stress parameters.

Enhanced stimulus-induced local NE release from the bladder (Buffington et al. 2002) could lead to a functional desensitization of the central alpha-2 adrenoceptors (α2-AR) in cats with FIC (Westropp et al. 2007). In the brainstem (particularly the area of the LC), α-2 agonists inhibit NE release, whereas in the spinal cord, they inhibit transmission of nociceptive input to the brain (Stevens and Brenner 1996). To further test this hypothesis, we evaluated the functional sensitivity of the α2-AR in cats with FIC by evaluating their response to the selective α2-AR agonist, medetomidine. These studies were carried out under the same stress protocol we used to measure [CCE]. If the post-synaptic α2-ARs are normal, one would expect a decrease in heart rate and increase in pupil size after medetomidine administration. The decline in HR following medetomidine administration was significantly greater in healthy cats as compared to cats with FIC, although this difference was attenuated by day 35 ($p = 0.05$, Table 75.1).

The increase in pupil diameter following medetomidine administration was significantly greater in healthy cats as compared to FIC cats. We did not see any significant differences in post synaptic α2-AR function when evaluating sedation (Westropp 2005). It was revealed by

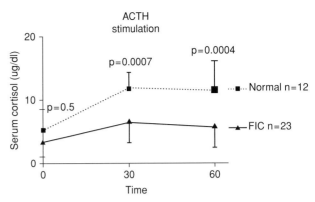

Figure 75.2 Mean serum cortisol response $\pm$ SD to 125 μg synthetic ACTH administered intramuscularly was significantly less in cats with FIC than in healthy cats (w2-way repeated measure ANOVA $p < 0.05$). Tukey–Kramer post hoc tests were used to compare groups at each time point.

electrical field stimulation studies of bladder strips from FIC cats that atipamezole, an α2-AR antagonist, did not alter the relaxing effect of NE, further suggesting that α2-ARs are downregulated in this disease (Buffington et al. 2002).

In addition to the sympathetic nervous system, abnormalities in the hypothalamic–pituitary–adrenal axis (HPA) have also been observed in cats with FIC. After a high dose (125 ug) of synthetic ACTH was administered, cats with FIC had significantly decreased serum cortisol responses as compared to healthy cats (Figure 75.2) (Westropp et al. 2003).

Although no obvious histological abnormalities were identified, the areas consisting of the zonae fasciculata and reticularis were significantly smaller in sections of glands from cats with FIC than in glands from healthy cats. Therefore, it appears that while the sympathoneural system is fully activated in this disorder, the HPA axis is not.

Viruses and FIC

The role of viruses has been and continues to be evaluated in cats that present with FIC (Fabricant et al. 1971; Kruger et al. 1991). Investigation of viruses as a causative agent of LUTS began in the 1960s. Virus-like particles (suspected to be calicivirus) were identified in the matrix of urethral plugs from some male cats with urinary obstruction (Osborne et al. 1996). The isolation of feline calicivirus, bovine herpesvirus 4 (strain FeCAHV), and feline syncytia-forming virus from cats with naturally occurring LUTS has also been reported (Kruger and Osborne 1990). Most recently, in the 40 cats that were evaluated, Rice et al. (2002) documented feline caliciviruses (FCVs) from 1 female cat with FIC and one

Table 75.1 Percent change in heart rate (HR) 10 minutes after 20 μg/kg of medetomidine was administered intramuscularly to cats on days 1, 3, 8, and 35. Healthy cats had a significantly greater decrease in HR after the alpha-2 agonist, medetomidine, was administered on all days compared to cats with feline idiopathic cystitis (FIC), except on day 35 ($p = 0.05$).

Percent change in HR after medetomidine administration	FIC (mean $\pm$ SD)	Healthy (mean $\pm$ SD)
Day 1	23% $\pm$ 15%*	34% $\pm$ 10%
Day 3	15% $\pm$ 14%*	37% $\pm$ 12%
Day 8	24% $\pm$ 9%*	32% $\pm$ 13%
Day 35	20% $\pm$ 10%	26% $\pm$ 16%

male cat with obstructive FIC. These viruses (FCV-U1 and FCV-U2, respectively) were genetically distinct from other known vaccine and field strains of FCV (Rice et al. 2002). In a published abstract, urinary shedding of the feline calcivirus was found in cats with FIC and suggests increased exposure to the feline calicivirus in FIC cats as compared to asymptomatic controls (Larson et al. 2007). The same group of researchers also inoculated specific pathogen-free cats with the urinary and respiratory FCV strains and found that both strains induced a similar spectrum of clinical and pathologic findings. What, if any, relationship viruses play in the etiopathogenesis in FIC remains unknown at this time (Kruger et al. 2007).

Obstructive FIC with urethral plugs

Urethral plugs are the most common cause of obstruction in male cats. In one series from the 1980s (Kruger et al. 1991), urethral plugs were the cause of obstruction in 60% of the cats, no cause was found in 30% of the cats, urolithiasis alone was documented in only 10% of the cases, and urolithiasis with bacterial urinary tract infection was observed in 2% of the cases. Occasionally, stricture and rarely neoplasia or a foreign body can cause the obstruction. Struvite urethroliths were the sole type reported in cats from the 1980s, but we have reported calcium oxalate urethroliths at the Gerald V. Ling Urinary Stone Analysis Laboratory (Cannon et al. 2007). It is the author's impression that urethral obstruction due to calcium oxalate urethroliths is more common in veterinary practice today than what has been previously reported in the literature. Furthermore, if calcium oxalate stones are noted in the urethra or bladder, they can be present in the upper urinary tract as well. On the basis of the examination of obstructed male cats with a urethroscope, idiopathic causes of obstruction also appear more common today.

It is unlikely for the urethra of female cats to become obstructed, but male cats have a narrow penile urethral lumen and are predisposed to obstruction with a urolith or urethral plug. The cause of the matrix formation in urethral plugs is currently unknown and is probably the outcome of several mechanisms. Many urethral plugs are composed of struvite with a proteinaceous matrix (Kruger et al. 1991), and this composition has not appeared to change over time. The cause(s) of urethral plugs is still unknown, but Osborne et al. have hypothesized that the concomitant occurrence of urinary tract infections and crystalluria may lead to the formation of matrix-crystalline plugs that obstruct various portions of the urethra, especially in male cats (Osborne et al. 1992). They hypothesized that Tamm-Horsfal mucoprotein (THP) is contained within urethral plugs. Once the THP coalesces with the crystals, white blood cells, and red blood cells, this coalescence can be surrounded by amorphous material and then obstruct the urethra.

In a small unpublished study, we found no evidence of THP in urethral plugs obtained from obstructed cats. However, the eletrophoretic pattern of the plugs resembled that of albumin and its degradation products, suggesting that the plug resulted from precipitated serum proteins. We hypothesize that vasodilatation and leakage of plasma proteins from the suburothelial capillary plexus ("bladder weeping") and secondary urethritis, which can be seen cystoscopically in cats with FIC, may trap crystals within the lumen of the male cat urethra, resulting in obstruction. It is likely that oozing of plasma proteins into urine during active inflammation increases the urinary pH that contributes to the precipitation of struvite crystals that participate in urethral plug formation. Although conventional wisdom indicates that urethral plugs form in the urethra, cystoscopic examination of the bladder has shown what appear to be plugs in the bladder. It is interesting that the mineral components of urethral plugs continue to be predominantly composed of struvite despite the apparent increase in the frequency of calcium oxalate urolithiasis. This may be due to the narrow range of "metabolic supersaturation" of struvite in urine. These, and other hypotheses, are not mutually exclusive, and plugs may form by different mechanisms depending on a variety of factors present at any particular instance.

For information on proper management of cats with urethral obstruction, refer to Chapters 36 and 77.

Summary

The pathophysiology of FIC likely involves complex interactions between a number of body systems. Abnormalities are not just localized to the bladder, but are present in the nervous, endocrine, and even cardiovascular systems (rush et al. 2002). It remains to be determined how these systems communicate and manifest as FIC in some cats but not in others. Environmental and behavioral stressors may also be associated with FIC. In order to better treat their patients, it is important for clinicians to understand that this syndrome is not just a "bladder disease" amenable to simple dietary or drug therapies.

Approach to the patient

Diagnostics

Because some 2/3 of cats with LUTS have FIC, and it appears that approximately 85% (Barsanti et al. 1982) of cats with FIC resolve their clinical signs in 2–3 days without treatment, it is debatable whether any diagnostics should be performed for a young cat with its first episode of LUTS. The basic tests are listed below and the clinician must decide based on the cat's signalment, history, and clinical signs, which tests will yield the most benefit for each individual patient.

Radiography and other imaging studies

Because FIC is a diagnosis of exclusion, diagnostics should be performed to rule out other causes of LUTS mentioned above. Urolithiasis can occur in approximately 12–15% (Buffington et al. 1997a) of cats with LUTS and an abdominal radiograph (Chapter 15) that includes the entire urinary tract should be performed. In those cats with recurrent episodes, a contrast cystogram and urethrogram (Chapter 15) can be helpful to better evaluate for the presence of nonradiopaque calculi and other lesions such as mass lesions, blood clots, and strictures. Contrast studies of the bladder and urethra in cats with FIC are usually unremarkable, though diffuse or asymmetrical thickening of the bladder wall is seen in about 15% of cases (Scrivani et al. 1997). In severe cases, extravasation of contrast material can be seen in the bladder wall. Contrast studies are especially indicated in elderly cats (>10 years of age) where FIC is not as likely. A contrast cystourethrogram is also beneficial for cases of obstructive FIC that do not respond to routine medical care and is necessary prior to performing a perineal urethrostomy in male cats. The clinician must be certain that no abnormalities are noted in the proximal urethra; if abnormalities are present, a perineal urethrostomy would be contraindicated. When performing any urinary contrast study, it is important that the descending colon is emptied prior to the procedure so that the entire urethra can be easily visualized.

An abdominal ultrasound (Chapter 16) should also be considered for cats that present for multiple episodes of FIC. It is a minimally invasive diagnostic that allows visualization of the bladder for abnormalities such as blood clots, polyps, neoplasia, and nonradioopaque stones such as cystine or ammonium urate. While ultrasound is a very useful diagnostic tool for this purpose, it is not the ideal diagnostic tool to evaluate the urethra. Radiography with or without contrast should always be performed to evaluate for stones or urethral plugs in that area.

Urinalysis and urine culture

A complete urinalysis (Chapter 7) should be performed at least once in cats that present with LUTS. Findings in cats with FIC are not specific and can include hematuria, and crystalluria, and even small amounts (5–10 WBC/hpf) of pyuria. The urine specific gravity is oftentimes very

concentrated, and if isosthenuria is present, diagnostics should be considered to evaluate the cat for underlying polyuric disorders.

As mentioned above, most cats that present with FLUTD are idiopathic and bacterial urinary tract infections are uncommon in younger, otherwise healthy cats. Less than 2% of young (<10 years of age) cats have been reported to have a true bacterial cystitis (Kruger et al. 1991; Buffington et al. 1997), and in another study, it was reported that 4.9% of cats presenting at a referral institution for LUTS had bacterial cystitis. However, a much higher percentage (22%) of cats with LUTS cultured positive by cystocentesis in a study evaluating cats from Norway (Eggertsdottir et al. 2007). Bacterial urinary tract infections also occur more often in cats that have had a perineal urethrostomy, repeated catheterizations, or have a concurrent disorder such as diabetes mellitus, chronic kidney disease, or hyperthyroidism (Bailiff et al. 2006; Mayer-Roenne et al. 2007). Quantitative urine culture (Chapter 9) should be performed in all cats with recurrent (>2) episodes, previous urethral obstructions, or catheterizations, as well in cats that have concurrent medical conditions.

Other diagnostics

Cystoscopy (Chapter 19) is available at many referral institutions and can be used to evaluate cats that have had repeated bouts of obstructive and nonobstructive FIC. Cats are placed under general anesthesia, and in females (and sometimes in males that have had a perineal urethrostomy), a rigid cystocscope (e.g., 25°, 2.8 mm (8.5 Fr) with 1.2 mm (3.6 Fr) biopsy channel Figure 75.3) can be introduced into the urethra and bladder with constant fluid insufflation to approximately 80 cm H_2O.

Care should be taken so as not to overdistend the bladder and cause trauma to the lower urinary tract. Cystoscopy in female cats usually provides excellent visualization of the urethra and bladder mucosa; small calculi,

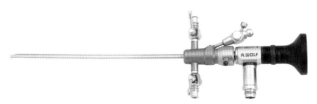

Figure 75.3 A typical rigid and flexible cystoscope that can be used for uroendoscopy in female and male cats, respectively. The flexible scope for male cats does provide good visualization of the urethra, but due to the small size, it is not ideal for imaging the bladder. A contrast cystogram can be helpful as an adjunct diagnostic if needed.

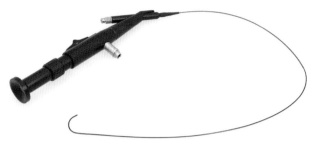

Figure 75.4 A typical rigid and flexible cystoscope that can be used for uroendoscopy in female and male cats respectively. The flexible scope for male cats does provide good visualization of the urethra, but due to the small size, it is not ideal for imaging the bladder. A contrast cystogram can be helpful as an adjunct diagnostic if needed.

a diverticulum, and masses can also be easily seen. Furthermore, if lesions are found, a small biopsy sample can be obtained through the scope. If one is having difficulty introducing the cystoscope through the urethra, the anesthesia depth should be reevaluated. A 1.1 mm flexible urethroscope is available for male cats, although due to the small size no operating channel for biopsies is possible (Figure 75.4).

This scope provides adequate visualization of the male cat urethra to evaluate for urethra plugs, strictures, urethral calculi, and foreign bodies. This scope does not provide sufficient visualization of the bladder to recommend its use on a routine basis; the author usually combines this test with a contrast cystogram in male cats.

Treatment of FIC

FIC can have a variable outcome. Clinical signs resolve spontaneously in as many as 85% of cats within 2–3 days, with or without treatment (Barsanti et al. 1982; Kruger et al. 2003; Westropp and Buffington 2004; Forrester and Roudebush 2007). As many as 50% of these cats will have another episode within 12 months and 39% recurred in a more recent study of cats consuming dry food (Markwell et al. 1999). It is not yet possible to predict which cats with FIC will relapse; some cats have multiple recurrences, while clinical signs never resolve in a small population of severely affected cats. In the author's experience, the most important consideration for a successful outcome is good communication with the owner. Oftentimes, after performing diagnostics on the cat and concluding that the disease is idiopathic, an appointment can be scheduled with only the owners present to thoroughly review the disease process, discuss short- and long-term treatment options, and be certain the owners have an understanding of this disease in their cat. No cure is currently available for FIC, and treatment options are aimed at keeping

the cat's clinical signs to a minimum and increasing the disease-free interval.

Treatment options for the acute episode

Antibiotics are rarely indicated for most cats that present for FLUTD and unless a cat has a documented bacterial urinary tract infection, empiric use of antibiotics is not warranted in cats with FIC. When a cat is diagnosed with FIC, analgesic therapy seems appropriate for the acute management of the disease. Providing analgesia with narcotics such as oral buprenorphine, butorphanol, or a fentanyl patch can be used depending on the severity of the pain. Nonsteroidal anti-inflammatory agents such as carprofen or meticam can also be used. However, this class of drugs should be used cautiously in obstructive FIC; the urethra should be patent and the azotemia should be resolved. Analgesic therapy can be provided for approximately 3–5 days, and if clinical signs have not significantly improved or resolved, further diagnostics should be performed. If the clinician is working with a case that has chronic FIC, analgesics can be dispensed for the cat with instructions for the owner to medicate the cat if clinical signs develop and then contact the veterinarian. Oftentimes, this treatment will be successful and the cat will not need to be evaluated at the veterinary hospital. If the clinician chooses to manage some cats in this manner, they must be confident that other differentials for FLUTD have been excluded and the cat has FIC. Breaking the chronic-pain–inflammation cycle may be important in the management of at least some cats with severe FIC.

Multimodal environmental modifications (MEMO)

On the basis of previous findings where catecholamines decreased after environemental modifications in research cats (Westropp 2005) MEMO therapy can be used to alter the cat's environment in hopes of reducing stress and decreasing the severity of the episodes and lengthening the intervals between the FIC episodes. This form of therapy was evaluated in client-owned cats with FIC implementing MEMO as the sole management strategy (Buffington et al. 2006). In an observational study, we evaluated 46 client-owned indoor-housed cats with FIC. In addition to their usual care, clients were offered recommendations for MEMO based on a detailed environmental history. Cases were followed for ten months by client contact to determine the effect of MEMO on LUTS and other signs. Significant ($p < 0.05$) reductions in LUTS, fearfulness, nervousness, signs referable to the respiratory tract, and a trend ($p < 0.1$) toward reduced aggressive behaviors were identified.

These results suggest that MEMO is a promising adjunctive therapy for indoor-housed cats with FIC.

Following a staged approach to therapy that begins with client education and MEMO seems beneficial in many cats with FIC. Establishing a technician-based program where a staff member follows these patients as often as necessary to be sure their cat's problems are explained thoroughly and that the clients gain enough understanding of the disease process to feel comfortable with managing their cat's disease can also be of great benefit. MEMO therapy involves obtaining a thorough environmental history including, but not limited to, the following topics:

1. Number of cats in the household
   a. Is inter-cat conflict an issue?
2. Number of other pets
3. Number of family members
4. Size and type of the household dwelling
5. Number of litter pans in the house
   a. How often are the cleaned?
   b. How often are they changed?
   c. Location in the house?
   d. Type of litter used?
   e. Depth of litter preferred by the cat?
6. Feeding
   a. Type of food (including brand, canned versus dry)?
   b. Location of bowls?
   c. Food preferences?
   d. Is competition for food present in the household?
7. Play/rest activity
   a. Preferred toys?
   b. Space in house available for play?
   c. Indoor/outdoor status?
   d. Preferred type of play?
   e. Resting/hiding areas preferred?
   f. Number of beds for the cat(s)?
8. Changes in household: This area includes topics such as construction, additions or subtractions to the home, and changes in the owner's lifestyle and regular routine.

These questions should be answered for every cat in the household. After the questionnaire has been discussed with the owner, a tailored MEMO therapeutic plan can be designed for each individual cat. Addressing only one or possibly two of the above categories at a time is recommended so as not to overwhelm the cat or the client with significant household changes. Because every cat seems to respond to their environment differently, no one recommendation can be made, but rather an individual plan is designed for each cat and owner. If more time is needed with the individual client, this plan can be discussed at an appointment with only the owner present. Considerations when tailoring a protocol should include the owner's commitment and attachment to the cat, the ability of the owner to implement the changes, and the cost of the changes suggested. For further suggestions as well as a good client resource, the reader is referred to the following website: www.indoorcat.org.

Dietary therapy

Some dietary modifications may reduce the risk of recurrence of clinical signs in affected cats. Efforts to acidify the urine using dry foods have no demonstrated value in treatment of cats with FIC. There is no known benefit to acidifying the urine or restricting magnesium in cats with FIC. No available evidence supports the idea that struvite crystalluria causes any damage to the underlying urothelium or worsens clinical signs of FIC. Struvite crystals can be incorporated in urethral plugs in obstructive FIC, and it seems prudent to recommend a higher moisture diet initially for all cats with this form of the disease. Increasing water intake may be beneficial for cats with FIC, and consumption of a canned food is one way to accomplish this. It has been reported that LUTS recurred in only 11% of affected cats during one year of feeding the canned formulation of a dietary product. Recurrence occurred in 39% of cats fed the dry formulation of the same food, suggesting that both constancy and consistency (i.e., increased water intake) may be important, but the reasons for this effect remain to be determined (Markwell et al. 1999). Increasing water intake will decrease the urine specific gravity and potentially decrease the concentration of noxious substances within the urine. Currently, only one commercial diet is marketed for FIC, but at this time no studies exist as to the efficacy of this diet in clinical cats.

Unfortunately, many cats will not readily consume a canned diet. It is not recommended to change a diet until the cat is home and feeling well so as not to induce a learned aversion to the recommended diet. The cat's regular food should still be provided and the preferred diet be placed next to the usual feeding bowl. If the cat eats the new diet readily, the old food can simply be removed over the next day or two. If the cat doesn't eat the new diet after an hour, the food should be removed until the next feeding and another attempt made at that time point, always providing fresh food for each new feeding. Once the new diet becomes familiar to the cat, it should start eating it readily. At that time, a decrease in the amount (about 25%) of the old diet can be done each day until the change is complete. If necessary, small quantities of the cat's favorite food such as meat or fish juice can be mixed with the new preferred food to increase the cat's interest in the diet. Meal feeding is generally an easier way to provide a change in a cat's diet and may provide more interaction with the owner and the cat which could be beneficial as well.

Pheromones

Pheromones are fatty acids that seem to transmit highly specific information between animals of the same species. Although the exact mechanisms of action are unknown, pheromones reportedly induce changes in both the limbic system and the hypothalamus that alter the emotional state of the animal (Pageat and Gaultier 2003). Feliway® (Abbott Laboratories, Abbott Park, IL), a synthetic analogue of this naturally occurring feline facial pheromone, was developed in an effort to decrease anxiety-related behaviors of cats. Treatment with this pheromone has been reported to reduce the amount of anxiety experienced by cats in unfamiliar circumstances, a response that may be helpful to these patients and their owners. Although a statistically significant difference was not found when Feliway® was compared to a placebo in cats with FIC, cats that had Feliway® used in the environment exhibited a trend for fewer bouts of cystitis and reduced negative behavioral traits (Gunn-Moore and Cameron 2004). Increased grooming and food intake in hospitalized cats (Griffith et al. 2000) also has been reported with the use of this pheromone. Feliway® is available in two forms. A spray can be used where the cat is urinating inappropriately as well as in cat carriers prior to transport. A room diffuser can be placed in a designated room that is modified to reduce stress and provide environmental enrichment for the cat. The diffuser is reported to cover approximately 650 square feet and last for approximately 1 month.

Pharmacologic therapy

Drug therapy with the tricyclic antidepressants (TCAs) may be helpful in chronic forms of FIC when MEMO, dietary, and phermonotherapy have not been successful to help manage clinical signs. Amitriptyline (Elavil®), and probably all TCA drugs, should not be used in the acute management of FIC (Kraijer et al. 2003) and may increase the risk of recurrence (Kruger et al. 2003). Amitriptyline, has been reported in uncontrolled trials to successfully decrease clinical signs of severe, recurrent FIC (Chew et al. 1998). It was shown in this series of cats with severe FIC that the clinical signs of some cats were reduced during amitriptyline treatment during a 12-month period. Amitriptyline (2.5–10 mg per cat SID) may provide analgesia by inhibition of NE reuptake at noradrenergic nerve terminals (Anderson 2001) and possibly due to inhibition of a wide range of nociceptive

neurons in the spinal trigeminal nucleus (Fromm et al. 1991). The author usually begins at the low end of the dose and recommends the medication be administered in the evening. The dosage can be slowly increased until the desired effects are achieved. If a favorable response is not achieved with this drug, it should be tapered slowly, over several weeks, and then discontinued. Side effects can include lethargy, weight gain, and urine retention because of the anticholinergic effects of this drug.

Clomipramine (Clomicalm®, veterinary label; and Anafranil®, human label) is also a tertiary amine like amitriptyline, but has more selectivity for blocking the reuptake of 5-HT. This drug has been shown to significantly decrease the number of episodes of urine spraying in cats (King et al. 2004). In that study, the initial dose used was 0.25–0.5 mg/kg orally once daily. Clomipramine has less anticholinergic properties as compared to amitriptylline; however, sedation is still a common side effect of this drug as well. Clomirpramine, in conjunction with environmental modification, has also been described to successfully decrease anxiety related and obsessive compulsive disorders in cats (Seksel and Lindeman 1998). The author has prescribed this in recurrent cases of FIC with anecdotal improvements in some patients. Other drugs such as fuoxetine (Prozac®) has been reported to help cats with inappropriate urinations with variable success rates (Pryor et al. 2001). Fluoxetine was used to help decrease the rate of urine marking after environmental alterations such as litter box hygiene and appropriate cleaning strategies.

As mentioned earlier, cats with FIC have decreased urinary GAG excretion. A defective GAG layer or damaged urothelium could permit hydrogen, calcium, potassium ions, or other constituents of urine to come into contact with sensory neurons innervating the urothelium. Because of this theory, GAG replacers such as pentosan polysulfate (Elmiron®) have been used to treat cats with FIC. In a placebo controlled study in which the effectiveness of oral glucosamine for the management of cats with FIC was evaluated, no significant differences were found between the two groups (Gunn-Moore and Shenoy 2004). However, the authors of this study did report a significant placebo effect, where both groups of cats improved significantly over the course of the study. One theory was that more positive interaction occurred with the cat, thereby decreasing stress.

Conclusion

FIC is a complex disease process that is not fully understood at this time. The clinician and client must understand that this disease is not limited to abnormalities related solely to the bladder. Because FIC can be a chronic, frustrating disease, excellent client communication in conjunction with MEMO therapy, analgesics, and possibly other pharmacologic agents can be of benefit in treating acute and chronic cases.

References

American Journal of Veterinary Research (in press).

Anderson, P. (2001). Amitriptyline. *Compend Contin Educ Pract Vet* 433–437.

Bailiff, N.L., R.W. Nelson, et al. (2006). Frequency and risk factors for urinary tract infection in cats with diabetes mellitus. *J Vet Intern Med* **20**: 850–855.

Barsanti, J.A., D.R. Finco, et al. (1982). Feline urologic syndrome: further investigation into therapy. *J Am Anim Hosp Assoc* **18**: 387–390.

Birder, L.A. (2006). Urinary bladder urothelium: molecular sensors of chemical/thermal/mechanical stimuli. *Vascul Pharmacol* **45**: 221–226.

Birder, L.A., M.L. Nealen, et al. (2002). Beta-adrenoceptor agonists stimulate endothelial nitric oxide synthase in rat urinary bladder urothelial cells. *J Neurosci* **22**: 8063–8070.

Buffington, C.A. (2002). External and internal influences on disease risk in cats. *J Am Vet Med Assoc* **220**: 994–1002.

Buffington, C.A. and K. Pacak (2001). Increased plasma norepinephrine concentration in cats with interstitial cystitis. *J Urol* **165**: 2051–2054.

Buffington, C.A., J.L. Blaisdell, et al. (1996). Decreased urine glycosaminoglycan excretion in cats with interstitial cystitis. *J Urol* **155**: 1801–1804.

Buffington, C.A., D.J. Chew, et al. (1997a). Clinical evaluation of cats with nonobstructive urinary tract diseases. *J Am Vet Med Assoc* **210**: 46–50.

Buffington, C.A.T., D.J. Chew, et al. (1997b). Animal model of human disease—feline interstitial cystitis. *Comp Pathol Bull* **29**: 3.

Buffington, C.A., B. Teng, et al. (2002). Norepinephrine content and adrenoceptor function in the bladder of cats with feline interstitial cystitis. *J Urol* **167**: 1876–1880.

Buffington, C.A., J.L. Westropp, et al. (2006). Clinical evaluation of multimodal environmental modification (MEMO) in the management of cats with idiopathic cystitis. *J Feline Med Surg* **8**: 261–268.

Cameron, M.E., R.A. Casey, et al. (2004). A study of environmental and behavioural factors that may be associated with feline idiopathic cystitis. *J Small Anim Pract* **45**: 144–147.

Cannon, A.B., J.L. Westropp, et al. (2007). Evaluation of trends in urolith composition in cats: 5,230 cases (1985–2004). *J Am Vet Med Assoc* **231**: 570–576.

Chew, D.J., C.A. Buffington, et al. (1998). Amitriptyline treatment for severe recurrent idiopathic cystitis in cats. *J Am Vet Med Assoc* **213**: 1282–1286.

Clasper, M. (1990). A case of interstitial cystitis and Hunner's ulcer in a domestic shorthaired cat. *N Z Vet J* **38**: 158–160.

Cohen, T.A., J.L. Westropp, et al. (2009). Evaluation of urodynamic procedures in female cats anesthetized with isoflurane or propofol. *Am J Vet Res* **70**(2): 290–296.

de Groat, W.C., A.M. Booth, et al. (1993). Neurophysiology of micturition and its modification in animal models of human disease. In: *Nervous Control of the Urogenital System*, edited by C.A. Maggi. Chur, Switzerland: Harwood Academic, pp. 227–290.

Eggertsdottir, A.V., H.S. Lund, et al. (2007). Bacteriuria in cats with feline lower urinary tract disease: a clinical study of 134 cases in Norway. *J Feline Med Surg* **9**: 458–465.

Fabricant, C.G., J.M. King, et al. (1971). Isolation of a virus from a female cat with urolithiasis. *J Am Vet Med Assoc* **158**: 200–201.

Forrester, D.S. and P. Roudebush (2007). Evidence-based management of feline lower urinary tract disease. *Vet Clin North Am Small Anim Pract* **37**: 533–558.

Fromm, G.H., M. Nakata, et al. (1991). Differential action of amitriptyline on neurons in the trigeminal nucleus. *Neurology* **41**: 1932–1936.

Gao, X., C.A. Buffington, et al. (1994). Effect of interstitial cystitis on drug absorption from urinary bladder. *J Pharmacol Exp Ther* **271**: 818–823.

Goldstein, D.S. (1995). *Catecholamines and Cardiovascular Disease*. New York: Oxford.

Griffith, C.A., E.S. Steigerwald, et al. (2000). Effects of a synthetic facial pheromone on behavior of cats. *J Am Vet Med Assoc* **217**: 1154–1156.

Gunn-Moore, D.A. and M.E. Cameron (2004). A pilot study using synthetic feline facial pheromone for the management of feline idiopathic cystitis. *J Feline Med Surg* **6**: 133–138.

Gunn-Moore, D.A. and C.M. Shenoy (2004). Oral glucosamine and the management of feline idiopathic cystitis. *J Feline Med Surg* **6**: 219–225.

Hostutler, R.A., D.J. Chew, et al. (2005). Recent concepts in feline lower urinary tract disease. *Vet Clin North Am Small Anim Pract* **35**: 147–170.

Jezernik, K., R. Romih, et al. (2003). Immunohistochemical detection of apoptosis, proliferation and inducible nitric oxide synthase in rat urothelium damaged by cyclophosphamide treatment. *Cell Biol Int* **27**: 863–869.

Jones, B., R.L. Sanson, et al. (1997). Elucidating the risk factors of feline urologic syndrome. *N Z Vet J* **45**: 100–108.

King, J.N., J. Steffan, et al. (2004). Determination of the dosage of clomipramine for the treatment of urine spraying in cats. *J Am Vet Med Assoc* **225**: 881–887.

Kraijer, M., J. Fink-Gremmels, et al. (2003). The short-term clinical efficacy of amitriptyline in the management of idiopathic feline lower urinary tract disease: a controlled clinical study. *J Feline Med Surg* **5**: 191–196.

Kruger, J.M., and C.A. Osborne (1990). The role of viruses in feline lower urinary tract disease. *J Vet Intern Med* **4**: 71–78.

Kruger, J.M., C.A. Osborne, et al. (1991). Clinical evaluation of cats with lower urinary tract disease. *J Am Vet Med Assoc* **199**: 211–216.

Kruger, J.M., Conway, T.S.et al. (2003). Randomized controlled trial of the efficacy of short-term amitriptyline administration for treatment of acute, nonobstructive, idiopathic lower urinary tract disease in cats. *J Am Vet Med Assoc* **222**: 749–758.

Kruger, J.M., C.P. Pfent, et al. (2007). *Feline Calicivirus-Induced Urinary Tract Disease in Specific-Pathogen-Free Cats*. Seattle, WA: ACVIM, pp. 648–649.

Larson, J., J.M. Kruger, et al. (2007). *Epidemiology of Feline Calicivirus Urinary Tract Infection in Cats with Idiopathic Cystitis*. Seattle, WA: ACVIM, 648 p.

Lavelle, J.P., S.A. Meyers, et al. (2000). Urothelial pathophysiological changes in feline interstitial cystitis: a human model. *Am J Physiol Renal Physiol* **278**: F540–F553.

Markwell, P.J., C.A. Buffington, et al. (1999). Clinical evaluation of commercially available urinary acidification diets in the management of idiopathic cystitis in cats. *J Am Vet Med Assoc* **214**: 361–365.

Mayer-Roenne, B., R.E. Goldstein, et al. (2007). Urinary tract infections in cats with hyperthyroidism, diabetes mellitus and chronic kidney disease. *J Feline Med Surg* **9**: 124–132.

Osborne, C.A., J.P. Kruger, et al. (1992). Feline matrix-crystalline urethral plugs-a unifying hypothesis of causes. *J Small Anim Pract* **33**: 172–177.

Osborne, C.A., J.P. Lulich, et al. (1996). Feline urolithiasis: etiology and pathophysiology. *Vet Clin North Am Small Anim Pract* **26**: 217–232.

Oter, S., A. Korkmaz, et al. (2004). Inducible nitric oxide synthase inhibition in cyclophosphamide-induced hemorrhagic cystitis in rats. *Urol Res* **32**: 185–189.

Pageat, P. and E. Gaultier (2003). Current research in canine and feline pheromones. *Vet Clin North Am Small Anim Pract* **33**: 187–211.

Peeker, R. and M. Fall (2002). Toward a precise definition of interstitial cystitis: further evidence of differences in classic and nonulcer disease. *J Urol* **167**: 2470–2472.

Press, S.M., R. Moldwin, et al. (1995). Decreased expression of GP-51 glycosaminoglycan in cats afflicted with feline interstitial cystitis. *J Urol* **153**: 288A.

Pryor, P.A., B.L. Hart, et al. (2001). Effects of a selective serotonin reuptake inhibitor on urine spraying behavior in cats. *J Am Vet Med Assoc* **219**: 1557–1561.

Reche, A.J. and C.A. Buffington (1998). Increased tyrosine hydroxylase immunoreactivity in the locus coeruleus of cats with interstitial cystitis. *J Urol* **159**: 1045.

Rice, C.C., J.M. Kruger, et al. (2002). Genetic characterization of 2 novel feline caliciviruses isolated from cats with idiopathic lower urinary tract disease. *J Vet Intern Med* **16**: 293–302.

Rush, J., L.M. Freeman, et al. (2002). Population and survival characerisitics of cats with hypertrophic cardiomyopathy: 260 cases (1990–1999). *JAVMA* **220**: 202–207.

Sands, S.A., R. Strong, et al. (2000). Effects of acute restraint stress on tyrosine hydroxylase mRNA expression in locus coeruleus of Wistar and Wistar-Kyoto rats. *Brain Res Mol Brain Res* **75**: 1–7.

Scrivani, P.V., D.J. Chew, et al. (1997). Results of retrograde urethrography in cats with idiopathic, nonobstructive lower urinary tract disease and their association with pathogenesis: 53 cases (1993–1995). *JAVMA* **211**: 741–748.

Sculptoreanu, A., W.C. de Groat, et al. (2005). Abnormal excitability in capsaicin-responsive DRG neurons from cats with feline interstitial cystitis. *Exp Neurol* **193**: 437–443.

Seksel, K. and M.J. Lindeman (1998). Use of clomipramine in the treatment of anxiety-related and obsessive-compulsive disorders in cats. *Aust Vet J* **76**: 317–321.

Specht, A., J.J. Kruger, et al. (2004). *Histochemical and Immunohistochemical Light Microscopic Features of Chronic Feline Idiopathic Aystitis*. Minneapolis, MN: ACVIM, p. 416.

Stevens, C.W. and G.M. Brenner (1996). Spinal administration of adrenergic agents produces analgesia in amphibians. *Eur J Pharmacol* **316**: 205–210.

Valentino, R.J., R.R. Miselis, et al. (1999). Pontine regulation of pelvic viscera: pharmacological target for pelvic visceral dysfunctions. *Trends Pharmacol Sci* **20**: 253–260.

Welk, K.A. and C.A. Buffington (2003). Effect of interstitial cystitis on central neuropeptide in receptor immunoreactivity in cats. In: *Department of Human Anatomy*. Columbus: The Ohio State University.

Wesselmann, U. (2001). Interstitial cystitis: a chronic visceral pain syndrome. *Urology* **57**: 102.

Westropp, J.L. (2005). Evaluation of the sympathetic nervous system and hypothalamic pituitary adrenal axis in cats with interstitial cystitis. In: *Department of Veterinary Clinical Sciences*. Columbus: The Ohio State University, p. 166.

Westropp, J.L., and C.A. Buffington (2004). Feline idiopathic cystitis: current understanding of pathophysiology and management. *Vet Clin N Am Small Anim* **34**: 1043.

Westropp, J.L., K. Welk, et al. (2003). Small adrenal glands in cats with feline interstitial cystitis. *J Urol* **170**(6): 2494–2497.

Westropp, J.L., P.H. Kass, et al. (2006). Evaluation of the effects of stress in cats with idiopathic cystitis. *Am J Vet Res* **67**: 731–736.

Westropp, J.L., C.A. Buffington, et al. (2007). In vivo evaluation of the alpha-2 adrenoceptors in cats with idiopathic cystitis. *Am J Vet Res* **68**(2): 203–207.

Willeberg, P. (1984). Epidemiology of naturally occurring feline urologic syndrome. *Vet Clin North Am Small Anim Pract* **14**: 455–469.

76

Micturition disorders

Julie Fischer and India F. Lane

Urinary incontinence

Introduction

Normal micturition consists of a *urine storage phase,* when the bladder slowly fills and relaxes while the urethra remains closed, and a *urine voiding phase,* when the bladder contracts and urine is expelled through a relaxed urethra. Appropriate urine storage and voiding depend on intricate and coordinated interaction of the nervous system, urinary bladder, and urethra. Disorders of urine storage usually manifest clinically as *urinary incontinence,* while disorders of voiding usually manifest as *urine retention.*

Neurophysiology of micturition

Key anatomic components of the lower urinary tract (LUT) include (1) *detrusor muscle,* the smooth muscle that forms the body and neck of the bladder; (2) the *internal urethral sphincter* (IUS) that is composed of smooth muscle of the urethrovesicular junction; (3) the *external urethral sphincter* (EUS) that includes striated muscle encircling portions of the urethra distal to the IUS (the position of the EUS varies somewhat by species and sex); and (4) the *ureterovesicular junction,* normally located proximal to the IUS, at the junction of the bladder body and neck. The urethral closure mechanism consisting of the bladder neck and smooth and striated urethral musculature is often termed the "outflow tract" or "outlet" (Figure 76.1).

Urothelial and suburothelial cell layers also contribute to neural control of micturition and to urinary response to irritating local mechanical or chemical stimuli.

The urine storage phase of micturition occurs chiefly under sympathetic (adrenergic) nervous control (Figure 76.2).

The hypogastric nerve (arising from spinal segments L_{1-4} in the dog, L_{2-5} in the cat) stimulates detrusor beta receptors, inducing smooth muscular relaxation and permitting filling under low pressure. In contrast, sympathetic stimulation of alpha-1 receptors of the bladder neck and urethral smooth muscle (IUS) induces smooth muscle contraction, closing the outlet and maintaining continence. Sympathetic input also modulates and minimizes parasympathetic-mediated contraction of the detrusor muscle, but some basal tone and low-intensity rhythmic activity does continue in the bladder during the storage phase. The pudendal nerve (arising from spinal segments S_{1-3}) supplies voluntary input to the striated urethral musculature (EUS). During the storage phase, this input stimulates nicotinic cholinergic receptors in the EUS, causing contracture and additional closure of the outlet when needed (e.g., during coughing or sneezing; to temporarily override an inappropriately timed urge to void).

Afferent information is transmitted from the bladder by the pelvic (filling sensation, need to void) and hypogastric (pain, overdistension) nerves, and from the bladder neck and urethra by the pudendal nerve. Messages regarding filling and contraction appear to flow through A-delta fibers, whereas C fibers transmit noxious stimuli. Signaling properties of the urothelium, and a suburothelial neural plexus most prominent in the bladder neck, also communicate sensory information locally, putatively by releasing ATP (Ferguson 1997). Collectively, the urothelium, subendothelial myofibroblasts, smooth muscle fibers, and associated afferent nerves represent the "stretch receptors" of the LUT.

As bladder filling progresses, information from these receptors is passed to higher centers, in particular to the

Nephrology and Urology of Small Animals. Edited by Joe Bartges and David J. Polzin. © 2011 Blackwell Publishing Ltd.

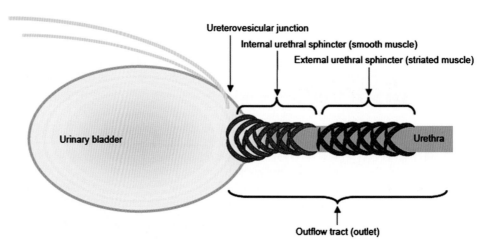

Figure 76.1 Basic anatomy of the lower urinary tract. (a) Urinary bladder, (b) ureterovesicular junction, (c) internal urethral sphincter (smooth muscle), (d) external urethral sphincter (striated muscle), (e) outflow tract (outlet), and (f) urethra.

hypothalamus and pontine micturtion centers. At a critical bladder volume, neurologic gates switch to maximize voiding capacity; however, voluntary (prefrontal and frontal cortex) release of inhibition is required for urethral relaxation and initiation of voiding.

The urine voiding phase of micturition occurs chiefly under parasympathetic (cholinergic) control. The pelvic nerve (arising from spinal segments S_{1-3}) stimulates muscarinic cholinergic receptors in the detrusor, causing contraction, which raises the intravesicular pressure. Simultaneously, sympathetic input to the outlet is inhibited at the level of the micturition center in the pons, allowing IUS and EUS relaxation. When intravesicular pressure exceeds outlet closure pressure, urine voiding occurs. After complete voiding, the system is "reset" for the filling stage to begin again. Numerous spinal and local interneu-

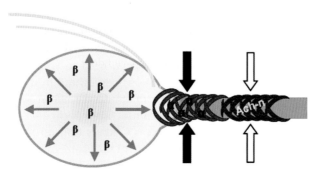

Figure 76.2 The urine storage phase of micturition. Sympathetic input to the beta receptors in the bladder stimulates detrusor relaxation; sympathetic input to the alpha receptors in the IUS stimulates smooth muscle contraction. Voluntary input to the nicotinic cholinergic EUS receptors stimulates striated muscle contraction. During the storage phase, outlet resistance must exceed intravesicular pressure to maintain continence. β, beta receptor; α, alpha receptor; Ach-n, nicotinic cholinergic receptor.

rons and interconnections preserve the "on–off" switching mechanism needed for coordinated bladder and outlet activity, both during storage and voiding phases. Figure 76.3 provides a schematic representation of the innervation of the LUT.

For more information, excellent reviews of applicable neurophysiology can be found in the references (Lane 2000a; Fowler et al. 2008).

Urinary incontinence

Urinary incontinence is defined as involuntary passage of urine through the urethra. Incontinence is most common in female dogs, but is also clinically recognized in male dogs and in cats. Urinary incontinence represents derangement in structure or function of one or more components of the storage mechanism: (1) anatomical abnormality of ureteral termination or urinary bladder or urethral development, (2) failure of the urinary bladder to sufficiently accommodate urine, or (3) failure of sufficiently functional urethral closure. Bladder and urethral dysfunction can be muscular (functional) or neurogenic in origin. Additionally, paradoxical or overflow incontinence is occasionally observed in animals with urine retention, when urinary bladder volume and pressure simply exceed outlet resistance, and spillover occurs. This section focuses on functional disorders of the bladder and urethra.

Urethral sphincter mechanism incompetence

Epidemiology

A weak urethral outlet mechanism is the most common cause of urinary incontinence in dogs (Table 76.1) and is

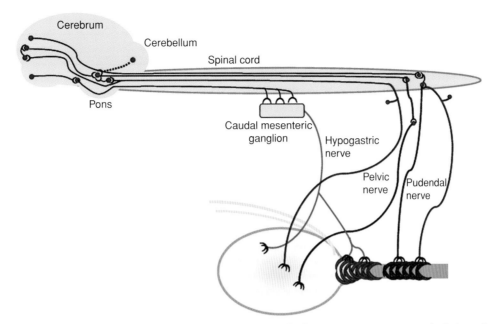

Figure 76.3 Schematic representation of central nervous system input to the lower urinary tract. Sympathetic input is supplied to the bladder and proximal urethra via the hypogastric nerve (grey); parasympathetic input is supplied via the afferent pelvic nerve (dark red) and sensation of stretch is relayed to higher centers via the afferent pelvic nerve (dark red). The afferent (dark red) and efferent (blue) branches of the pudendal nerve relay somatic input to and from the external urethral sphincter. Voiding is coordinated in the micturition center of the pons, with input from cerebrocortical centers.

termed *urethral incompetence* or *urethral sphincter mechanism incompetence.*

Young to middle-aged spayed female dogs are most often affected, usually developing incontinence within 3 years of ovariohysterectomy. Incidence of *spay-related incontinence or reproductive hormone responsive incontinence* may reach 20% of all spayed female dogs and is highest in large breed dogs (Thrusfield 1985; Arnold et al. 1989). Neutered males may be affected.

Urinary incontinence is particularly common in certain breeds of dogs, but is encountered in many mixed breed dogs as well. German shepherd dogs, Doberman pinschers, Labrador retrievers, old English sheepdogs, English springer spaniels, boxers, rottweilers, weimeraners, and Irish setters are overrepresented. Over 15% of Doberman owners reported urinary incontinence in a survey investigating causes of morbidity and mortality in the Netherlands (Bacon et al. 2002; Mandigers et al. 2006). Incontinence is notoriously difficult to control in this (and a few other) affected breeds. Doberman pinschers (27%) and boxers (16%) were the most common breed evaluated in Nickel et al.'s (1999) 77 refractory incontinence cases; Dobermans comprised 10 and 17% of dogs in two large series of colposuspension cases (Holt 1990; Marchevsky et al. 1999). The English springer spaniel, Labrador retriever, and German shepherd dog breeds were overrepresented in 100 dogs undergoing urethropexy (White 2001).

Pathophysiology

Although underlying causes of urethral incompetence are not known, multiple factors such as aging, decreased responsiveness of urethral receptors, abnormal urethral or bladder neck position, obesity, and vestibulovaginal anomalies may contribute. Decreased urethral closure pressure (Arnold et al. 1989) and subtle anatomical differences (Holt 1985a) have been documented in incontinent female dogs when compared to continent females. However, decreases in urethral pressure and changes in profile shape are also seen in healthy, continent dogs after ovariectomy (Reichler et al. 2004; Salomon et al. 2006), so a combination of factors likely influences the development of overt incontinence in spayed dogs.

Because of the strong association with spaying, veterinarians and pet owners are keenly interested in whether the timing of neutering influences development of urinary incontinence later in life. In a long-term (median 2 years) follow-up of early age and traditional age gonodectomy dogs, there was a very low incidence of urinary incontinence, which was not different between the two groups (Howe 2001). In a much larger group of dogs, incidence of urinary incontinence requiring treatment increased on a continuous scale with decreasing age at ovariectomy. Dogs ovariectomized younger than 3 months of age have a substantially increased risk of clinically significant incontinence (projected cumulative risk

Table 76.1 Characteristics of common disorders causing urinary incontinence

Disorder	Characteristics	Diagnostic methods
Acquired urethral sphincter mechanism incompetence (reproductive hormone responsive or "spay" incontinence)	Medium to large-breed adult dogs, usually female Prior ovariohysterectomy Intermittent urine leakage Resting urinary incontinence Otherwise normal	Response to treatment Urethral pressure profile
Urinary bladder storage dysfunction (detrusor instability, urge incontinence, overactive bladder)	Intermittent urinary incontinence Pollakiuria May appear behavioral or voluntary May be associated with excitement or activity	Response to treatment Cystometrography Cystourethrography
Ectopic ureter	Affected since birth Often continuous urine leakage	Contrast radiography/computed tomography Urethrocystoscopy Vaginourethrography Surgical exploration
Congenital urethral incompetence or hypoplasia	Severe or continuous urine leakage Juvenile animal Wide or short urethra in some cases Ectopic ureter not demonstrated	Cystourethrography Urethral pressure profile
Vaginal abnormality or urine pooling	Urine leakage at rest or when rising Urine leakage following voiding Recurrent or persistent vaginitis Vestibulovaginal stenosis/septum on digital examination	Vaginal examination and vaginoscopy Vaginourethrography
Prostatic disease (male dogs)	Intact or neutered Other signs of prostatic disease or concurrent dysuria Hind limb weakness/stiff, stilted gait	Abdominal radiographs Ultrasonography Contrast urethrography Prostatic brushing, aspirate, or biopsy
FeLV-associated urinary incontinence (cats)	Intermittent urine leakage Anisocoria	FeLV test

Table modified from Fischer and Lane (2007).

of 12.9% in the first 6 years of life) when compared with dogs ovariectomized after 3 months of age (projected cumulative risk of 5% in the first 6 years of life) (Spain et al. 2004). The optimal time for ovariohysterectomy is still debatable; there was no significant difference in relative risk for dogs neutered prior to versus after their first heat in a population of over 800 dogs reviewed in the United Kingdom (Thrusfield et al. 1998). In another population study, there was a lower incidence of urinary incontinence in dogs spayed before the first heat than in previous reports of dogs spayed after the first heat. However, the severity of incontinence appeared to be greater when it did occur in the former (earlier spay) group (Stocklin-Gautschi et al. 2001).

Recently, investigators have pinpointed structural and immunohistochemical changes associated with neuter-ing in dogs. When bladder and urethral segments from intact and neutered dogs were examined, both neutered male and neutered female dogs had a significantly higher percentage of collagen than muscle than did intact animals. Neutered females also had higher percentage of collagen in the proximal urethra than did neutered males. The authors speculated that excessive collagen deposition displacing or overwhelming muscular volume in the bladder and urethra could affect closure function (Ponglowhapan et al. 2008). Indeed, in another study, strips of urinary bladder smooth muscle from neutered males and females were less responsive than those from intact dogs (Coit 2008). Investigations of plasma and tissue concentrations of reproductive hormone receptors continue to both help elucidate and cloud the understanding of urinary incontinence in spayed dogs (Welle et al. 2006).

Urinary bladder dysfunction

Incontinence also results when the urinary bladder cannot store urine adequately (*detrusor instability, overactive bladder, bladder hypoaccomodation*). The definition of bladder overactivity includes the finding of involuntary bladder contractions at low bladder volumes, which is rarely documented in small animals. Despite the lack of documentation of classic diagnostic findings, bladder storage dysfunction may be more common than the literature suggests. Nickel et al. (1999) examined urodynamic studies in 77 incontinent dogs refractory to medical treatments and found that 15 dogs had urodynamic findings consistent with poor bladder storage function in addition to poor urethral function, and another 10 dogs had urodynamic abnormalities of bladder function alone. These dynamic findings appear to be consistent with increased collagen deposition in the bladders of spayed female dogs, as described earlier in this chapter.

Additionally, bladder storage function has been suspected in juvenile dogs and cats with congenital incontinence, especially those with ectopic ureters, or grossly hypoplastic bladders, or urethras. Reduced capacity and poor accommodation of urine (low compliance) was documented by cystometry in four of nine dogs with ectopic ureters in one study (Lane et al. 1995).

Diagnostic approach to urinary incontinence

History and urinary bladder size

The first step in diagnosis is to determine whether the problem is primarily with storing or with voiding urine (Table 76.2).

Disorders of storage are characterized by involuntary leakage of small amounts of urine with a small to normal urinary bladder size; a distended bladder should prompt an investigation for causes of urinary retention. Continuous leakage of urine is sometimes reported with anatomical disorders or with severe urethral incompetence. Affected animals usually appear healthy and void urine normally otherwise. The urinary bladder will be normal in size; the bladder may be easily expressed in relaxed dogs with severe urethral incompetence. The pattern of incontinence may offer clues as to the cause. Most dogs with urethral incompetence leak urine while resting or sleeping. Dogs with bladder dysfunction (also known as urge incontinence) are more likely to involuntarily void small amounts with activity or to exhibit pollakiuria in addition to incontinence. Severe or continuous incontinence is suggestive of anatomical abnormalities.

Neurological evaluation

In addition to the general physical examination, careful neurological assessment is indicated. Neurological impairment of bladder or urethral function is usually accompanied by other deficits. Mental alertness, proprioception, and gait are assessed broadly, with more specific attention devoted to anal tone, tail tone, and perineal sensation. Genitoanal reflexes are elicited by gently squeezing the base of the penis or the vulvar folds. An observable contraction ("wink") of the anal sphincter should be apparent if the pudendal nerve reflex arc (including sacral cord function) is intact (Figure 76.2). Deep palpation of the spine is indicated to detect pain or hyperesthesia, since disruption of any portion of the spinal cord can interrupt normal micturition reflexes. If any indication of neurogenic incontinence is detected, the diagnostic approach shifts to comprehensive assessment of brain and spinal cord.

Rectal/vaginal examination

Applying dorsal pressure during digital rectal examination may elicit subtle lumbosacral pain. Prostatic disorders, urethral masses or stones, perineal hernias, and weak anal sphincter tone also are picked up by digital rectal palpation. In female dogs, the urethra and urethral orifice are palpable on digital vaginal examination. Vaginal strictures or bands, particularly those occurring distal to the urethral orifice, may contribute to urine pooling or may occur concurrent with developmental abnormalities of the genitourinary tract, such as urethral incompetence or ectopic ureter.

Urinalysis and urine culture

A urinalysis and urine culture should be performed to identify infection or inflammation of the LUT. Urine specific gravity is a useful indicator of urine concentrating ability, and if the urine is poorly concentrated, evaluation of additional samples or investigation into polyuric disorders is indicated.

Additional diagnostic investigation (if needed)

In dogs that are otherwise healthy, neurologically normal, and free of urinary tract inflammation, urethral incompetence is the most likely diagnosis. A favorable response to pharmacologic treatments that increase urethral resistance should confirm the diagnosis.

Imaging

Further evaluation of the urogenital tract is justified in certain cases. Although radiographic imaging is of little

Table 76.2 Problem-specific historical questions and physical examination guidelines for patients with urinary incontinence or urinary retention

History (incontinence)
- When does leakage occur? Nocturnally/when resting or recumbent? Continuously? With excitation? Upon rising?
- How old was the patient when the problem began? In relation to neutering surgery?
- Is the leakage worsening, constant, or improving?
- Is the pet able to void normally?
- Is the pet conscious of the dribbling?
- Is the problem worse with a full bladder?
- Is urine volume increased in general?
- Are LUT signs present (pollakiuria, strangiuria, hematuria)?
- Any systemic signs of illness?
- What is estimated water consumption?
- Any history of prior urinary tract problems?
- Any recent abdominal, pelvic or urogenital surgery, or trauma?

History (urinary retention)
- How old was the patient when the problem began? In relation to neutering surgery?
- Any previous medical problems?
- What is estimated water consumption?
- Any history of prior urogenital disorders (e.g., urinary tract infections, urolithiasis, urethral obstructions)?
- Any systemic signs of illness?
- Any previous back surgery or trauma?
- Any recent abdominal, pelvic, or urogenital surgery, or trauma?
- How frequent are voiding attempts?
- Is any urine passed during voiding attempts?

Physical examination
- Is the bladder large or small?
- Is it firm or soft?
- Are the urethra and prostate/vagina normal on palpation?
- Is perineal/preputial urine staining/scald present?
- Is the neurologic examination normal?
  - Mentation and cranial nerves
  - Conscious proprioception, spinal reflexes, tail and anal tone, perineal reflexes, bulbourethral/vulvar reflex
  - Pupillary light reflexes
- Is bladder expressible?

Observed voiding
- Can the patient initiate and maintain a normal urine stream?
- What is the residual urine volume following voiding attempts?

Table modified from Fischer and Lane (2007).

use in the diagnosis of functional urethral incompetence, imaging should be pursued for incontinence (1) in male dogs or juvenile (<1 year) animals, (2) that closely follows ovariohysterectomy or other surgical procedure, (3) that is continuous or occurs in abnormal anatomic sites (e.g., urine leakage per rectum), or (4) that is accompanied by recurrent urinary tract infection, recurrent vaginitis, hematuria, crystalluria, or azotemia. Imaging is also recommended whenever surgical correction of incontinence is being considered, in order to rule out lesions or concurrent abnormalities that might affect surgical approach or outcome (Arnold 1992).

Although abdominal ultrasonography is useful for imaging of kidneys, bladder, and reproductive organs, visualization of urethra and vaginal conformation are not always possible. In order to fully evaluate the urinary tract, survey radiography, excretory urography, cystourethrography, or vaginourethrography may be chosen depending on the features of the individual patient. Usually, an excretory urogram in combination with contrast cystourethrography or vaginourethrography is completed. Computed tomography enhanced with contrast media is another excellent tool for delineating urologic structures.

Cystoscopy

Direct visualization of urogenital structures by vaginoscopy or cystoscopy is now considered essential in refractory cases (Chapter 19). Visualization of the vagina allows identification of strictures, bands, and evidence of urine pooling. In experienced hands, cystoscopic examination is a very sensitive tool for identification of ectopic ureteral terminations and also may be considered for further evaluation of suspected urethral or bladder neck lesions.

Functional studies—urodynamic procedures

More sophisticated functional studies can be pursued in complex scenarios or for patients that do not respond to appropriate trial therapy (Chapter 22). Although techniques vary, the studies basically offer a glimpse at the closure (or resistance) function of the urethra and the storage (compliance, capacity) and contractile function of the urinary bladder. The *urethral pressure profile* is measured by recording intraurethral pressure along the length of the urethra and documents the closure pressure of the urethral outlet. The *cystometrogram* is a recording of pressures within the urinary bladder as the bladder is filled with air, gas, or fluid medium. The filling slope and capacity of fluid infused can be used to estimate bladder compliance and capacity; involuntary, repeated, or early contractions can be documented. Both procedures are most useful when evaluating dogs or cats with refractory incontinence or multiple anatomical and functional abnormalities (Chapter 22).

Pharmacologic management of urinary incontinence

Management of decreased urethral resistance

Estrogen

Reproductive hormones are reasonably effective in improving continence in dogs with urethral incompetence. Estrogens such as diethylstilbesterol (DES), stilbesterol, estriol, and conjugated estrogens (Premarin) improve urethral resistance by increasing alpha-adrenergic receptor responsiveness and by improving urethral vascularity and other mucosal epithelial characteristics. Estrogen compounds are specifically useful in spayed females. While many estrogen products are readily available as hormone replacement treatment for women, the most reliable veterinary product, diethylstilbesterol (DES), is no longer commercially available due to the human health risks associated with the drug. DES is available from many veterinary compounding agencies; quality depends on the source. The effectiveness of most estrogen treatments is improved by using a "loading" phase, followed by a frequency of administration tailored to the individual patient and drug (Table 76.3).

A prolonged residual effect of estrogen administration can be seen in some dogs after a period of successful treatment, especially when DES or stilbesterol are employed. Administration can be stopped on a trial basis and restarted when incontinence returns (usually weeks to months).

Estrogens can also be used concurrently with phenylpropanolamine (PPA) and are theorized to be synergistic when combined therapy is used. In a small number of healthy Beagle dogs, however, urethral closure pressures increased after 7 days of estriol administration and did not increase further after addition of PPA to the treatment regimen (Hamaide et al. 2006). Estrogens are often chosen for dogs that do not tolerate alpha agonists, for those that are not completely continent on alpha agonists alone, and for clients who prefer the less frequent dosing regimen.

Veterinary practitioners have the most experience with DES or stilbesterol; treatment with these agents improves continence in 60–80% of treated dogs. Veterinarians in North America have less experience with other estrogen compounds, but recent studies confirm acceptable levels of effectiveness in female dogs. Response to estriol was studied in a large group ($n = 129$) of incontinent adult, spayed female dogs treated by practitioners in the Netherlands, Belgium, France, and Germany (Mandigers and Nell 2001). In an open-label trial, the dogs were given 2 mg estriol per day for a week, then the dose was reduced at weekly intervals to the minimal effective dose (typically 0.5–2.0 mg/dog given daily or every other day). Veterinarians classified 61% of the dogs as continent and 22% improved at day 42 of treatment, whereas owners reported an "excellent" response in 33% and a "good" or "adequate" response in 49%. Twelve dogs exhibited signs of estrus at the initial estriol dose, which resolved in all but one dog after dose reduction. No adverse hematologic effects were observed at day 42 in this study (Mandigers and Nell 2001). Dosing estriol every 2–3 days is supported by pharmacokinetic studies, in which plasma concentrations of the drug disappeared by 48 hours following the last dose (Hoeijmakers et al. 2003). Response to natural, conjugated estrogen (similar to Premarin) has been described in nine incontinent large breed dogs followed in a prospective manner. All dogs responded well to estrogen administration; daily administration was continued until two weeks of continence had been obtained. In seven of nine dogs in which dose information was reported, maintenance dosages ranged from 0.625 to 1.25 mg per dog, administered PO every 12–72 hours. In the remaining two dogs, administration every 4–7 days was

Table 76.3 Pharmacologic agents useful in the management of urinary incontinence

Agent	Classification	Recommended dosage	Possible adverse effects	Contraindications or comments
Diethylstilbesterol* (DES), stilbesterol*	Reproductive hormone	Dogs: 0.1–1.0 mg/dog PO q 24 h for 5–7 days, then weekly or as needed	Estrus Behavior change Myelosuppression Pyometra in intact female	Males Cats Pregnancy
Stilbesterol* (alternate regimen)	Reproductive hormone	Dogs: 0.04–0.06 mg/dog PO q 24 h for 7 days, reduced weekly to 0.01–0.02 mg/dog per day	As with DES	As with DES
Premarin*	Conjugated estrogen	Dogs: 0.02 mg/kg PO q 24 h for 5–7 days, then q 2–4 days or as needed	As with DES	As with DES
Estriol*	Reproductive hormone	Dogs: 0.5–1.0 mg/dog PO q 24 h for 5–7 days, then q 2–3 days as needed	As with DES	As with DES
Estriol* (alternate regimen)	Reproductive hormone	Dogs: 2.0 mg/dog PO q 24 h for 7 days, then reduce daily dose by 0.5 mg each week to establish minimal effective daily dose; then try every other day administration.	As with DES	As with DES
Testosterone cypionate	Reproductive hormone	Dogs: 2.2 mg/kg IM q 4–8 weeks	Behavior change Perianal adenoma Perineal hernias Prostatic disorders Aggression	Cardiac, renal, or hepatic disease
Testosterone propionate	Reproductive hormone	Dogs: 2.2 mg/kg IM q 2–3 days	As for testosterone cypionate	As for testosterone cypionate
Phenylpropanolamine (PPA)	Indirect alpha agonist	Dogs: 1.5 mg/kg PO q 8–12 hrs, or 12.5–75 mg PO q 8–12 h	Anxiety Aggression Anorexia Hypertension Tachycardia	Some cardiac disease Hypertension ± anxiety disorders
Ephedrine	Alpha agonist	Dogs: 1.2 mg/kg PO q 8 h	As with PPA	As with PPA
Pseudoephedrine	Alpha agonist	Dogs: 0.2–0.4 mg/kg (practically, 15–60 mg total dose per dog) PO q8–12 h	As with PP	As with PPA
Imipramine	Antimuscarinic, alpha/beta agonist	Dogs: 5–15 mg PO q 12 h	Sedation Dry mouth Urinary retention GI upset	Seizure disorders Use of other anticholinergic or CNS depressants, glaucoma, GI obstruction, renal or hepatic disease, cardiac arrythmias
Oxybutynin	Antimuscarinic	Cats and small dogs: 0.5–1.25 mg total per dose Larger dogs: 2.5–3.75 mg total per dose	As for imipramine	Glaucoma, GI obstruction, renal or hepatic disease, cardiac arrythmias, hypertension
Dicyclomine	Antimuscarinic	Dogs: 5–10 mg/dog PO q 8 h	As for imipramine	As for oxybutynin
Depot leuprolide	GnRH analog	Dogs: 11.25 mg/dog		May be redosed as needed May be used in combination with alpha agonists
Depot deslorelin	GnRH analog	Dogs: 5–10 mg/dog		May be redosed as needed As for leuprolide

Table modified from Fischer and Lane (2007).

effective. No hematologic effects of estrogen were observed in treated dogs for up to 49 months (Angioletti et al. 2004).

Possible adverse effects of estrogens include signs of estrus, hair loss, behavioral changes, and bone marrow suppression. Chronic, daily *estriolum* treatment was implicated in stump pyometra in an Irish Setter (Schotanus et al. 2008). Estrogenic side effects are most common during the loading dose of estriol and with higher doses of DES. Bone marrow suppression is unlikely in dogs treated with appropriate doses of the drugs listed here, but owners should be advised of this potentially fatal adverse effect. Estradiol cypionate (ECP), a repository preparation, should never be used for urinary incontinence in dogs because of the higher risk of bone marrow suppression. Estrogen administration should be avoided in male dogs due to resulting prostatic squamous metaplasia and in dogs with a history or breed predilection for immune-mediated disease, since estrogens are immunostimulatory. Estrogens are not very effective and poorly tolerated in cats, often inducing estrus-like behavior.

Alpha-adrenergic agents

Sympathomimetic drugs with alpha agonist effects, including PPA, phenylephrine, and pseudoephedrine, have been extremely effective in improving or controlling urinary incontinence. Excellent responses have been observed in most dogs treated with PPA, with 90% or greater responding in small studies (Richter and Ling 1985). Scott et al. (2002) reported results of PPA administration in a prospective, blinded, placebo-controlled study of 50 incontinent adult female dogs at various clinics in the United Kingdom that had been ovariohysterectomized at least 6 months prior to the study. Dogs were treated with either PPA (1 mg/kg q 8 hours in a syrup formulation) or placebo (sorbitol syrup only). Owner-reported frequency of unconscious urination and volume of urine loss were compared between the treated and control dogs at day 7 and 28 of treatment. By day 7, 55% PPA treated dogs were reported to have no unconscious urination as opposed to 26% of the dogs receiving placebo. By day 28, the percentage of continent PPA dogs rose to 85.7% while the number of continent placebo-treated dogs rose to 33.3%. Side effects were not significantly different between the two groups; however, occurrences of diarrhea and vomiting were reported in both groups. Gastrointestinal side effects are uncommon with PPA, but may be more likely with this formulation of the drug. While this study demonstrated a significantly better response to PPA than placebo, the placebo effect was unexpectedly high (Scott et al. 2002). This finding prob-

ably reflects the variable and intermittent nature of urinary incontinence in dogs; however, further study may be warranted regarding how owners view and report urine leakage during clinical trials. Owner observations differed from urodynamic findings in another study, where some owners reported good improvement after pseudoephedrine treatment without evidence of increase in closure measures (Byron et al. 2007). In this group of 9 female dogs, improvement in continence score, maximal urethral closure pressure, and functional area of the UPP was observed after PPA (1.5 mg/kg q 8 hours) administration (Byron et al. 2007). In another randomized, double-blinded study, female dogs responded well to 1.5 mg/kg q 12 hours; 21 of 24 dogs were continent and another 2 improved (Burgherr et al. 2007).

While most resources recommend administration of PPA two or three times per day for best effect, the dose is adjusted to the minimal amount needed to achieve continence. As with reproductive hormones, it is usually beneficial to start with the optimal dose until continence is achieved. However, a recent investigation in healthy intact Beagles challenges this assumption. Dogs were treated with PPA at once-, twice-, or three times daily intervals. Urodynamic changes (increased urethral pressure) were similar for all dosing frequencies, leading the authors to recommend once daily treatment for incontinent dogs (Carofiglio et al. 2006). Desensitization of receptors was suspected with TID administration. Responses in intact Beagles may not parallel those in incontinent spayed dogs; however, reduced frequency of administration may be effective in some dogs and may prevent development of tolerance during long-term treatment.

Ephedrine and pseudoephedrine are alternative alpha agonists with similar effects on urethral function. Their clinical use increases during periods when PPA is difficult to obtain. Nendick and Clark (1987) described pseudoephedrine (15–30 mg q 8–24 hours) as totally effective in 14/17 (82.4%) dogs in a retrospective study. Arnold found good results with ephedrine (1–2 mg/kg q 12 hours) in 28 of 38 (74%) female dogs, with some improvement noted in 37 of the 38 (Arnold 1992). However, in a series of nine female dogs studied in a crossover design, dogs exhibited significantly better improvement in continence and urodynamic variables during treatment with PPA than with pseudoephedrine (Byron et al. 2007). Clinical improvement was observed in only 6 of the 9 dogs during pseudoephedrine administration. Differences in response between the drugs may vary based on relative indirect and direct alpha-adrenergic activities of each; PPA appears to possess some direct activity while pseudoephedrine acts solely by indirect actions.

Adverse effects of alpha agonists include restlessness, tachycardia, anorexia, gastrointestinal side effects, aggression, and other behavioral changes. Adverse effects are usually dose-dependent and may vary among products. On the basis of human experience, the degree of adverse effects, cardiac effects, and development of tolerance have been expected to be higher with ephedrine compounds than with PPA. This expectation was confirmed in the dogs studied by Byron et al.; 5 of 9 dogs (56%) exhibited adverse behavioral effects including decreased appetite, increased panting, and lethargy. Although systemic hypertension is an important potential complication, significant changes in blood pressure have not been detected in prospective studies of incontinent dogs treated with PPA (Richter and Ling 1985; Byron et al. 2007). However, one older dog with borderline hypertension developed anesthesia-induced ventricular arrhythmias after a period of treatment with pseudoephedrine (Byron et al. 2007). Mild but significant increases in diastolic blood pressure were observed in healthy Beagles at 7 or 14 days after administration of PPA or ephedrine. Significant increases in systolic arterial pressure, to measurements above 220 mmHg, were observed in three healthy dogs treated with PPA twice daily in this study (Carofiglio et al. 2006). Caution is certainly advisable in high-risk patients; alpha agonists should not be administered in known hypertensive patients.

Like DES, PPA has been removed from commercial production for humans, but is produced by veterinary compounding pharmacies under an FDA compassionate use provision. Over-the-counter pseudoephedrine products are now semi-controlled by pharmacies in order to limit availability of the compound for methamphetamine production. Although PPA has been studied most often, all alpha agonists have a similar mechanism of action and approximate dose range (1.5 mg/kg PO q 8–24 hours) for the treatment of urethral incompetence. While most dogs will usually become continent or improve dramatically with either estrogen or alpha agonist administration, the two drugs can also be combined for synergistic effect in the same patient. Combination treatment allows estrogen to "prime" the urethral receptors for alpha agonist treatment. Starting doses are the same as for each drug when used individually, but the dose of both products can often be reduced slightly over time if the combination is effective.

GnRH analogs

Gonadotropin-releasing hormone (GnRH) analogs have recently been applied to the treatment of urinary incontinence. Reichler et al. (2003) reported experience with leuprolide, buserelin, and deslorelin, GnRH analogs that suppress sex hormone release. In theory, chronically unsuppressed FSH and LH release (due to lack of negative feedback) in ovariectomized dogs may contribute to urinary incontinence. Administration of GnRH analogs paradoxically results in reduced FSH and LH over time. In Reichler's series, the drugs appeared useful in 12 of 13 dogs with refractory incontinence, either alone or in combination with alpha agonists. In a more recent trial, 9 of 23 incontinent dogs treated with long-acting leuprolide were continent for prolonged periods (70–575 days); another 10 of the dogs had partial response. These 23 dogs, however, also responded to PPA, with 92% overall reduction in urine leakage (Reichler et al. 2006). The only urodynamic parameter that changed after depot leuprolide injection was cystometric threshold volume (an indicator of capacity and accommodation) (Reichler et al. 2006). There were no apparent adverse effects of GnRH treatment reported in this study, but long-term use of these drugs in dogs has not been evaluated. GnRH analogs may prove to be a valuable long-acting treatment that would alleviate the need for daily or weekly medication; however, availability and cost of GnRH analogs limit their use in the United States.

Management of urinary bladder overactivity

Antimuscarinic (anticholinergic) agents

Other pharmacologic agents that may be useful in unusual or refractory incontinence cases include anticholinergic (antimuscarinic) agents that enhance bladder storage. Anticholinergic agents are quite effective for *detrusor instability* (*overactive bladder* or *urge incontinence*) in which involuntary detrusor contractions occur, causing inappropriate leakage of urine. Most products also possess antispasmodic or analgesic activity, which facilitates response. True detrusor instability is rare in animals; oxybutynin and emepronium bromide have been effective in sporadic cases (Holt 1984; Lappin and Barsanti 1987).

Antimuscarinic agents can be considered on a trial basis in refractory incontinence, either alone or in combination with alpha agonists or reproductive hormones. Without urodynamic documentation of poor bladder storage function or detrusor instability, trial treatment can be considered in animals in which urge incontinence appears likely. These dogs or cats usually leak urine when active, either when walking, jumping, or moving; urine dribbling may appear behavioral since posturing may occur. Oxybutynin is most commonly recommended, and the author has limited experience using the new anticholineric, tolteridine. Other agents, including amitryptiline, imipramine, flavoxate, and dicyclomine, also have anticholinergic effects. Imipramine and amitryptiline, tricyclic antidepressants, may improve urine storage by several mechanisms, including anticholinergic, alpha-adrenergic and beta-adrenergic effects. Imipramine has not proven very effective in clinical application, however. Clients may be familiar with the heavily marketed product, tolterodine (Detrol, Pharmacia, & Upjohn), for overactive bladder in human patients. This antimuscarinic agent is touted for once-daily administration and reduced side effects when compared with other available agents. There are no published reports of the drug's use in small animals at this time. Side effects of antimuscarinic agents include dry mouth, blurred vision, urine retention, and gastrointestinal upset, and significantly limit tolerance of the drugs in people, but these compounds appear well tolerated by dogs. Ptyalism and gastrointestinal symptoms are possible in dogs and usually are remedied by dose reduction.

Agents with combined activities

Duloxetine, a serotonin and norepinephrine reuptake inhibitor, may improve striated muscle resistance as well as bladder capacity and has proven useful in women with stress incontinence (Norton et al. 2002; Van Kerrebroeck et al. 2004). The agent works by inhibition of serotonin and norepinephrine reuptake at the presynaptic neurons in the sacral spinal cord (Onuf's nucleus). In cats with experimentally induced irritated urinary bladder, a five-fold increase in bladder capacity and an eight-fold increase in urethral EMG activity were observed after duloxetine administration (Karl and Katofiase 1995). In women, a dose of 20–40 mg twice daily is effective in reducing incontinence by over 50% (Jost and Marsalek 2005) and is effective in women with severe clinical signs (Van Kerrebroeck et al. 2004). The most common adverse effect in women was nausea, which can be minimized by slow-dose escalation (Norton et al. 2002; Oelke et al. 2006). Experience is limited in small animals, where smooth muscle is the predominant contributor to urethral sphincter incompetence, but the drug could be useful as adjunct treatment in some cases.

Endoscopic and surgical management of urinary incontinence

Bulking agents, including cod-liver oil, Teflon, extracellular matrix, and collagen products, have been used to boost tissue resistance or size in the urethra and other tissues. Glutaraldehyde cross-linked bovine collagen currently is preferred for periurethral application in humans and dogs and does not migrate into other tissues. Collagen injection has been most commonly applied in female dogs refractory to PPA administration (Chapter 37). In

reported series 53–68% of dogs became continent after one or two injections. Most of the other dogs exhibited significant improvement after injection and with the postinjection addition of PPA treatment (Arnold et al. 1996; Barth et al. 2005; Byron et al. 2005). Mean duration of continence has been reported as 12 (Byron et al. 2005) to 17 months (Barth et al. 2005); excellent responses of greater than 30 months duration have been observed (Arnold). Transient adverse effects, including stranguria, hematuria, vaginitis, and urine retention, are possible. Repeated injection can be done when effectiveness wanes.

Surgical methods

Colposuspension is the most commonly described surgical procedure for incontinent female dogs (Chapter 82). In this procedure, the vagina is fixed to the ventral abdominal wall via sutures through the prepubic tendon, entrapping the urethra in a compressed and slightly cranial position (Gregory and Holt 1994). Other similar procedures fix the outer layers of the urethra (urethropexy), the prostate (Holt et al. 2005), or the deferent ducts (males) to the ventral abdominal wall. Initial results with these procedures have been promising, achieving short-term continence in 50–75% of patients (Holt 1990; Rawlings et al. 2001; White 2001). However, long-term continence is more elusive with this technique (Massat et al. 1993; Rawlings et al. 2001). In all of these groups, PPA or other medical treatments were often necessary to augment the response to surgery. With advances in endoscopic injection techniques and in patient selection for vulvoplasty, suspension procedures are rarely indicated today.

Vulvoplasty

Some incontinent dogs also have vaginal, vestibular, or vulvar conformational abnormalities. Many exhibit other LUT signs, including recurrent urinary tract and vaginal infections. Although it is not entirely clear how these conformational problems contribute to incontinence, urine retention in the vestibule and vagina may lead to urine pooling, episodic leakage, and recurrent urinary tract infection. Urine pooling is strongly suspected if urine dribbling occurs after voiding in female dogs. Vulvoplasty may improve urine drainage, decreasing vaginal irritation and decreasing urine leakage related to urine pooling (Crawford and Adams 2002; Hammel and Bjorling 2002). In a group of dogs with vestibulovaginal strictures reviewed by Hammel and Bjorling, 19 dogs had refractory urinary incontinence as part of their clinical presentation. Incontinence resolved with vulvoplasty alone in 6 dogs, and an additional 9 had improved response to PPA after surgery. The procedure appears to be a useful adjunct

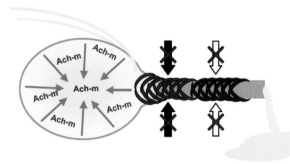

Figure 76.4 The urine voiding phase of micturition. Parasympathetic stimulation of muscarinic cholinergic receptors causes contraction of the detrusor muscle. Parasympathetic inhibition of sympathetic input to the IUS, and voluntary inhibition of EUS contraction causes passive relaxation of the outflow tract and causes intravesicular pressure to exceed outlet pressure, permitting urine voiding. Ach-m, muscarinic cholinergic receptor.

in the management of some dogs with urinary incontinence. Concurrent urethral incompetence, however, still may require medical treatment.

Urinary retention

During the storage phase of micturition, contraction of the bladder outlet combined with relaxation of the detrusor muscle permit low-pressure filling of the bladder with urine (Figure 76.2). Transition to the voiding phase entails relaxation of the bladder neck and proximal urethra, with simultaneous contraction of the detrusor (Figure 76.4).

Though the process of urine voiding may seem simple and straightforward, coordinated and complete voiding requires complex interaction among the components of the LUT, and the sympathetic, parasympathetic, and somatic nervous systems.

Etiologies of urinary retention

Incomplete voiding and consequent urinary retention result from inadequate urethral relaxation, inadequate detrusor contraction, or both. Etiologies and mechanisms of urinary retention are discussed below, and Table 76.4 presents characteristics of common causative disorders.

Inadequate detrusor contraction

Atony of the detrusor may be primary (neurogenic) or may be secondary (non-neurogenic) to chronically increased outlet resistance, whether mechanical or functional. Rarely, structural or mechanical detrusor abnormalities can cause functional failure. Chronic inflammation or infection of the bladder wall can, over time,

lead to replacement of smooth muscle with noncontractile fibrous tissue, leading to a noncompliant bladder with diminished contractility. Usually, however, detrusor fibrosis produces clinical signs associated with bladder noncompliance: decreased urine storage capacity and increased voiding frequency.

Neurogenic

Most voiding disorders due to inadequate detrusor contraction occur secondary to neurologic disease, most often spinal cord disease. Though lesions of the cerebral cortex or cerebellum have the potential to disrupt initiation or modulation of voiding, brain disease is more likely to cause clinical signs associated with storage dysfunction rather than with voiding dysfunction. Spinal cord lesions resulting in upper motor neuron or lower motor neuron clinical signs frequently also disrupt normal voiding function. See Figure 76.3 for a schematic representation of the innervation of the LUT.

Lower motor neuron disorders

Disruptions of the sacral spinal cord segments (cord segments S1-S3, located caudal to vertebra L5) or bilaterally of the pelvic nerve or pelvic plexus can result in varying degrees of detrusor atony and EUS hyporeflexia. On physical examination, patients with lower motor neuron disorders usually exhibit diminished or absent perineal reflexes and have distended bladders that are frequently easily expressible. Overflow incontinence is often seen when the bladder is full. Because the IUS derives innervation from the hypogastric nerve, IUS tone may be preserved in the presence of sacral lesions and can become fixed over time. Common causes of lower motor neuron disorders include cauda equina syndrome, sacroiliac luxation, intervertebral disk disease, sacrococcygeal separation or fracture ("tail-pull" injury), congenital malformation (e.g., in Manx cats), and neoplasia. Treatment for complete neurogenic detrusor atony and sphincter areflexia is generally unsuccessful, unless the underlying cause is correctable.

Parasympathomimetic agents such as bethanechol may be administered to help increase strength of detrusor contraction if partial innervation and function are present, but are ineffective and need not be administered if pelvic nerve function is absent. Patients can be managed at home with scrupulous bladder and nursing care, including aseptic urethral catheterization (preferred for male dogs) or manual bladder expression (for female dogs and cats) 3–4 times daily and frequent perineal cleaning to prevent urine scald. Patients should be monitored routinely for UTI and treated when infection is documented.

Table 76.4 Characteristics of common disorders causing urinary retention

Disorder	Characteristics	Diagnostics
Neurogenic causes		
Lesions of sacral spinal cord (lower motor neuron)	Distended, flaccid urinary bladder Bladder easily expressed Depressed genitoanal reflexes ± Lumbosacral pain Overflow incontinence possible	Neurologic examination Imaging (any or all of: radiograpy, myelography, epidurography, computed tomography, magnetic resonance imaging)
Lesions of suprasacral spinal cord (upper motor neuron)	Distended, firm urinary bladder Bladder not easily expressed Incomplete voiding possible Gait and proprioceptive deficits	Neurologic examination Imaging (any or all of: radiograpy, myelography, epidurography, computed tomography, magnetic resonance imaging)
Detrusor-urethral dyssynergia	Distended urinary bladder (may be firm or atonic) Bladder not easily expressed Incomplete voiding possible; stream may be initiated but not maintained Patient is otherwise normal	Observation, measurement of residual urine volume Urethral pressure profilometry ± cystometrography Response to alpha antagonists
Primary detrusor atony	Distended bladder Weak or absent urine stream Other signs of dysautonomia damage to hypogastric nerve	Observation, measurement of residual urine volume Response to treatment Cystometrography Dysautonomia testing
Non-neurogenic causes		
Anatomic urethral obstruction	Difficult urethral catheterization Dysuria and stranguria ± hematuria Caused by uroliths, neoplasia, blood clots, urethral plugs (cats)	Urethral catheterization Radiography/contrast cystourethrography Ultrasonography
Functional urinary obstruction	Distended bladder, difficult to express Easy urethral catheterization Voiding may be initiated, then interrupted Usually male dogs and cats Idiopathic or caused by urethral irritation or previous obstruction Rarely and transiently occurs following abdominal, pelvic, or pelvic limb surgery	Exclusion of anatomic or neurogenic causes Response to treatment with alpha antagonists Urethral pressure profile
Primary detrusor atony	Distended bladder Weak or absent urine stream Caused by overdistension from any cause of obstruction, muscle weakness, drugs	Observation, measurement of residual urine volume Response to treatment Cystometrography
Medications (e.g., opioids, anticholinergics/ antispasmodics, tricyclic antidepressants, calcium channel blockers)	Easy urethral catheterization Variable presentation otherwise	Medication history Exclusion of anatomic or functional obstruction Response to withdrawal of medication

Table modified from Fischer and Lane (2007).

Dysautonomia

Primary dysautonomia is a rare, idiopathic, neurodegenerative disorder of the sympathetic and parasympathetic (autonomic) nervous systems, caused by chromatolytic degeneration of neurons in the autonomic ganglia. Dysautonomia has been recognized in dogs and cats worldwide, as well as in horses and rabbits. In cats, dysautonomia has chiefly been reported in the United Kingdom and Scandinavia, but a recent retrospective described nine dysautonomic cats from Kansas and Missouri (Kidder 2008). In dogs, the large majority of reported cases have come from Kansas and Missouri (Longshore 1996; Harkin 2002).

Voiding dysfunction characterized by overflow incontinence from bladder atony and urethral sphincter areflexia may be the chief presenting complaint in the dysautonomic patient, but other signs of autonomic dysfunction (e.g., dilated, nonresponsive pupils; xerostomia; nictitans prolapse; absent anal sphincter tone; regurgitation and/or vomiting) are usually discovered in the patient history or on physical examination. Results of specific clinical and pharmacologic testing (described in Harkin 2002; Kidder 2008) confirm an antemortem diagnosis with a high degree of certainty. Dysautonomia most often produces polysystemic pathology with clinically devastating results; management is generally unrewarding if the gastrointestinal tract is affected (e.g., ileus, megaesophagus). If signs are largely confined to the urinary tract, however, satisfactory management may be possible with parasympathomimetic agents and bladder expression or intermittent catheterization.

Myogenic

Detrusor atony from overdistension

Sustained overdistension from any cause can contribute to loss of detrusor function. Detrusor smooth muscle fibers coordinate contraction via tight junctions, and excessive and/or prolonged stretch separates these tight junctions, disrupting neuromuscular transmission and resulting in weak, uncoordinated, or absent contractile effort (Kato et al. 1990; Ling 1995). Cats and dogs with more acute urinary obstruction and overdistension are presented for stranguria, anuria, or overflow incontinence and usually have large, flaccid bladders on physical examination (Animals with very acute obstruction usually have turgid, painful bladders; Chapter 77). The bladder will stay distended after voiding attempts, which are generally partial or weak. Perineal reflexes remain intact but detrusor contraction is diminished or absent. For such patients, maintenance of an indwelling urinary catheter (for 72 hours up to 14 days) with a closed collection system may be required to re-establish tight junctions and permit detrusor function to return. Chronic atony and urine distension may be more subtle in presentation.

Hospitalization, recumbency, orthopedic surgery, or other painful conditions that preclude normal posturing or voiding may lead to urinary retention. Retention is generally transient in these cases; short-term

indwelling or intermittent urethral catheterization suffices for management. Although parasympathomimetic agents may help improve the quality of detrusor contractions, these prokinetic agents must not be given without first definitively establishing a low-resistance outflow conduit, either with indwelling catheterization, by removal of an anatomic obstruction, or with pharmacologic agents that relax the urethral outlet (in the case of functional obstruction). Urethral relaxants alone are usually not sufficient to produce adequate urine flow in the initial stages of recovery, so indwelling catheterization is recommended during early management. Prognosis depends on the cause and reversibility of underlying conditions, but is generally good for recovery of detrusor function in acute cases. Chronicity diminishes the odds of full functional return.

Pharmacologic causes of urinary retention

Pharmacologic agents often contribute to urinary retention in humans, especially in conjunction with anesthesia, pain, or bladder overdistension. Urinary retention has been reported in dogs following systemic administration of agents from several classes of pharmacological agents, including tricyclic antidepressants, anticholinergic agents, opioids, and calcium channel blockers; intrathecal administration of morphine has also been implicated in cases of urinary retention (Richelson 1983; Drake et al. 1998; Herperger 1998; Kona-Boun 2003). Urinary effects of these agents are usually transient, but urinary catheterization may be required until normal voiding function resumes.

Inappropriate outlet resistance

Anatomic/mechanical obstruction

Mechanical disruption of bladder outflow occurs commonly in dogs and cats, due most frequently to urolithiasis, obstructive feline idiopathic cystitis, or neoplasia and may certainly interfere with normal voiding. Generally, though, these types of LUT diseases cause urinary obstruction, prior to development of bladder atony (Chapter 77).

Myogenic

Functional urinary obstruction

The term "functional obstruction" describes a condition in which amplified sympathetic nervous input increases urethral sphincter tone, thus inappropriately raising outlet pressure and restricting or precluding urine flow during voiding attempts. Functional obstruction may sometimes have a neurogenic component to its pathology or may result from direct irritation of the urethra. Anxiety produced by ineffectual voiding attempts may then further increase sympathetic stimulus. Functional obstruction due to spasm of the urethral musculature occurs commonly in cats following urethral instrumentation for relief of mechanical obstruction.

Management of functional obstruction includes treatment or prevention of bladder atony from overdistension with indwelling urethral catheterization if necessary and possible, while simultaneously decreasing IUS and/or EUS resistance as discussed in the section on upper motor neuron disorders (Lane et al. 2000). Anxiolytic therapy may be helpful to decrease stress and consequently sympathetic input to the LUT; commonly used anxiolytic medications are included in Table 76.5.

Prognosis is variable, but is favorable in cases of acute urethral irritation (e.g., cats with urethral spasm postobstruction).

Functional obstruction following relief of a mechanical obstruction in cats happens frequently, and thus merits specific discussion. Though many of these cats have just had an indwelling urinary catheter removed, resolution of the functional component of the obstruction may require replacement of an indwelling urinary catheter for a variable period of time (usually 1–3 additional days). Although no evidence-based measures exist to prevent the development of urethrospasm, the following suggestions may reduce the risk of functional obstruction due to urethral irritation and/or inflammation, following relief of mechanical urethral obstruction (Fischer 2003).

- Leave only soft, nonirritating catheters in the urethra. Less irritating catheter types include silicone, Teflon, and soft infant feeding-tubes. Polypropylene catheters (tom-cat catheters) cause irritation when left in contact with the urethral mucosa. They are also the catheters most likely to cause bladder trauma when left indwelling.
- Consider the use of urethral relaxant medication during and after the period of catheterization. Prazosin is a safe and effective urethral smooth muscle relaxant in cats; diazepam and dantrolene relax skeletal muscle (see Table 76.1).
- Consider the one-time use of a nonsteroidal anti-inflammatory such as ketoprofen at the time of catheterization. This may be contraindicated in animals with renal azotemia.
- Ensure patency of the indwelling catheter at all times. The bladder should be empty when the catheter is in place, and urine output and bladder size should be monitored to ensure this.
- Consider the use of anxiolytic and/or mildly tranquilizing medication during and immediately after

the period of indwelling catheterization. Diazepam (injectable), acepromazine, and amitriptyline are several options. These medications may reduce stress and straining, thus decreasing sympathetic input to the LUT.

Neurogenic

Upper motor neuron disorders

Upper motor neuron lesions result from spinal cord lesions between the sacral segments and the pontine micturition center and cause reflex detrusor contraction simultaneous with uninhibited sphincter contraction. Patients with upper motor neuron disorders often have overt paresis or paralysis of the hind limbs and usually cannot urinate voluntarily. On physical examination, the bladder is usually distended, turgid, and difficult or impossible to express early in the disease course. Manual bladder expression should be undertaken carefully, because aggressive attempts at expression can result in bladder rupture and because repeated expression may interfere with detrusor muscle recovery. Intermittent aseptic urethral catheterization several times daily is preferred, particularly in male dogs, to reduce risk of bladder trauma and ensure complete emptying.

After days to weeks, local spinal reflexes may resume and allow for some voiding activity. Involuntary bladder emptying is typically initiated when threshold capacity is reached; this phenomenon is termed an automatic or reflex bladder. When automatic bladder activity occurs, management with manual expression may be possible, since stimulation of detrusor contraction now should result in sphincter relaxation and enable partial to complete emptying. Automatic (or reflex) bladder function is rarely seen in dogs, however, and is usually partial when it does occur, so pharmacologic assistance is usually necessary. Urethral smooth muscle relaxants, such as the alpha-antagonists (e.g., prazosin, tamsulosin) and skeletal muscle relaxants (e.g., baclofen, diazepam, dantrolene), may facilitate complete bladder emptying by relaxing the IUS and EUS, respectively. Residual urine volume should be quantified periodically to assess efficacy of therapy.

Detrusor-urethral dyssynergia

In veterinary literature, *detrusor-urethral dyssynergia* has been classified as either a neurogenic or a myogenic disorder, because it may be caused by a partial lesion of the reticulospinal tract, a lesion cranial to the caudal mesenteric ganglion, or idiopathic in origin. In human patients, the term usually implies neurogenic dyssynergia, documented by specific neurologic and urodynamic

Table 76.5 Formulary of agents useful in the management of urinary retention

Category/agent	Mechanism	Recommended dosage	Possible adverse effects	Contraindications or comments
Urethral relaxants				
Acepromazine	Skeletal muscle relaxation via neuroleptic effect, smooth muscle relaxation via alpha-antagonism	Up to 0.1 mg/kg IV q 12–24 h (doses as low as 0.02 mg/kg IV may be effective) 1.1–2.2 mg/kg PO q 12–24 h	Hypotension Sedation Exacerbation of seizure disorder Disinhibition	Hypovolemia Cardiac disease Seizure disorder
Baclofen	Skeletal muscle relaxation	Dog: 1–2 mg/kg PO q 8 h Cat: not recommended	Weakness GI upset Pruritus	
Bethanechol	Parasympathomimetic	Dogs: 5–25 mg PO q 8 h Cats: 1.25–5 mg PO q 8 h	Ptyalism Vomiting Diarrhea	Outlet obstruction or high outlet resistance GI obstruction Atropine is antidotal
Cisapride	Prokinetic, may enhance acetylcholine release	Dogs 0.5 mg/kg PO q 8 h Cats: 1.25–5 mg/cat PO q 8–12 h	Diarrhea Possible abdominal pain	GI obstruction Reduce dose with hepatic insufficiency
Dantrolene	Skeletal muscle relaxation via direct effects	Dog: 1–5 mg/kg PO q 8–12 h Cat: 0.5–2.0 mg/kg PO q 8 h 1.0 mg/kg IV	Weakness Sedation GI upset Hepatotoxicity	Cardiac disease
Diazepam	Skeletal muscle relaxation via central effects (benzodiazepine)	Dog: 2–10 mg/dog PO q 8 h Cat: 1–2.5 mg/cat PO q 8 h or prn	Sedation Paradoxic excitation Idiopathic hepatic necrosis (with PO use in cats only) Polyphagia	Pregnancy Hepatic disease
Phenoxybenzamine	Smooth muscle relaxation via nonspecific alpha-antagonism	Dog: 0.25 mg/kg PO q 8–12 h or 2.5–20 mg/dog PO q 8–12 h Cat:1.25–7.5 mg/cat PO q 8–12 h	Hypotension Tachycardia GI upset	Cardiac disease Hypovolemia Glaucoma Renal failure Diabetes mellitus (type II)
Prazosin	Smooth muscle relaxation via α_1 antagonism	Dog: 1 mg/15 kg PO q 8–12 h Cat: 0.25–0.5 mg/cat PO q 12–24 h	Hypotension Mild sedation Ptyalism	Cardiac disease Renal failure
Terazosin	Smooth muscle relaxation via α_1 antagonism	Dog: 0.5–5.0 mg/dog q 12–24 h Cat: not determined	Hypotension Mild sedation Ptyalism	Cardiac disease Renal failure
Tamsulosin	Smooth muscle relaxation via selective α_{1A} antagonism	Dog	Hypotension with overdose	Do not use in cats
Anxiolytic agents				
Acepromazine	See above	See above	See above	See above
Alprazolam	Centrally acting anxiolytic benzodiazepine	Cat: 0.125–0.25 mg/cat PO q 12 h	As for diazepam, except idiopathic hepatic necrosis has not been documented.	May be a good alternative to diazepam if oral therapy is needed

(continued)

Table 76.5 continued

Category/agent	Mechanism	Recommended dosage	Possible adverse effects	Contraindications or comments
Amitriptyline	Tricyclic antidepressant, anxiolytic, alpha antagonist, antihistimine, analgesic, anticholinergic	Cat: 1–2 mg/kg per day PO or 2.5–10 mg/cat per day PO	Sedation Neutropenia, thrombocytopenia Urinary retention Weight gain	Do not use if bladder atony is suspected. Use cautiously and discontinue if worseing of urinary retention is suspected.
Diazapam	See above	See above	See above	See above

Table modified from Fischer and Lane (2007).

criteria. A dyssynergic state results when initiation of detrusor contraction is accompanied by simultaneous contraction of the urethral musculature (either the IUS, the EUS, or both), resulting in the urinary bladder contracting against markedly increased outlet pressure. Idiopathic dyssynergia, also considered a "functional urethral obstruction," is most commonly a disorder of male dogs and may be exacerbated by excitation or exertion (psychological, physical, or sexual), probably because of increased sympathetic input. Dyssynergic dogs will often initiate a urine stream that then is quickly attenuated and may repeat such behavior several times before abandoning attempts to void. Residual urine volume is greater than 10 mL.

Documentation of dyssynergia is difficult in clinical practice, because it requires simultaneous electromyographic assessment of detrusor and sphincter muscle activity during voiding. A clinical diagnosis can be made based on the signalment, physical examination findings, voiding pattern, and exclusion of mechanical obstruction. Urethral pressure profilometry may confirm increased outlet resistance and can help localize the region of abnormal resistance to the IUS, EUS, or both (Lane et al. 2000). Management of dyssynergia centers on decreasing IUS and/or EUS resistance (as discussed in the section on upper motor neuron disorders) and restoring detrusor function if necessary.

The diagnostic approach to urinary retention

Patient history and physical examination

The diagnostic approach to urinary retention is designed to (1) rule out neurological and obstructive disorders, (2) assess the status of the urinary bladder contractile force and urethral outlet resistance, and (3) investigate possible underlying etiologies. For urinary retention as for other micturition disorders, meticulous questioning and thoughtful observations provide the basis for diagnosis.

Specific historical questions related to urinary retention are listed in Table 76.2. Most animals with urinary retention have a distended bladder that is readily palpable on physical examination, and some will have historical or physical examination evidence of overflow incontinence. Digital rectal examination should include identification and careful palpation of the urethra (lying on ventral midline), the prostatic region, and possibly the trigone of the bladder (in a very small dog). Use of the free hand on the caudal abdomen to tip the bladder back into the pelvis will assist with palpation of the prostatic region and possibly the trigone. A digital vaginal examination should be performed in female dogs, and the urethral orifice should be identified. The region of the urethral orifice and ventral vaginal wall should be carefully palpated for thickening or irregularity. Critical assessment of neurologic status, particularly of the hind limb reflexes and reflexes testing the sacral arc (e.g., perineal, bulbospongiosus/vulvar), is specifically indicated in patients with urinary retention.

Observation of voiding behavior also is a key component of the initial assessment. Particular attention should be given to the patient's ability to initiate and maintain a urine stream. Patients with anatomic obstruction typically strain and produce little to no urine. Functionally obstructed animals may initiate a normal stream that is quickly attenuated or may posture to urinate for long periods of time without straining. Animals with bladder atony may slowly initiate a weak stream that can be augmented with manual abdominal compression. Some animals with more chronic atony will not attempt to void at all. Normal voiding results in an empty or nearly empty urinary bladder. If the bladder is easily palpable following voiding, manual expression should be gently attempted to assess contractile responsiveness and outlet resistance. Inability to manually express a distended bladder increases the likelihood of anatomic or functional outlet obstruction.

After observing voiding attempts, residual volume is quantified or estimated. Postvoiding bladder size can be estimated by palpation, radiography, or ultrasonography (Atalan et al. 1999). Urethral catheterization enables detection of mechanical urethral obstruction and permits acute bladder drainage as well as quantification of residual urine volume. In healthy animals, resistance to the passage of a urethral catheter is encountered at the urethral flexure in male cats and the distal os penis and pelvic brim of male dogs. Urethral catheters may easily pass by small uroliths, by some intraluminal soft tissue lesions, and through regions of extraluminal urethral compression; ability to catheterize the urethra does not fully rule out anatomic obstruction. Normal residual urine volume in dogs is 0.1–3.4 mL/kg (median 0.2 mL/kg) (Atalan et al. 1999). Serial measurement of residual urine volume provides objective assessment of response to therapy.

Clinicopathologic assessment

In general, urinary retention is not associated with any abnormalities on the biochemistry profile or the CBC. The urinalysis may show a variety of changes either associated with the underlying disease (e.g., neoplastic transitional cells in a dog with obstructive trigonal transitional cell carcinoma) or consequent to the fact of urinary retention itself (e.g., discoloration, increased number of sloughed epithelial cells). Bacterial urinary tract infection occurs commonly in dogs and cats with urinary retention, since complete voiding is an important host defense against bladder colonization. The postrenal azotemia and hyperkalemia frequently seen with mechanical urethral and ureteral obstruction are not generally seen with urinary retention.

Imaging

The possibility of mechanical urethral obstruction must be evaluated during the initial assessment of any animal with urinary retention; this is chiefly performed through urethral catheterization and imaging. Plain radiographs will rule out most obstructive stone disease when the uroliths are radio-opaque (e.g., calcium oxalate, struvite). Plain radiographs should also be scrutinized for the presence of soft-tissue masses (e.g., enlarged prostate), which could contribute to mechanical obstruction, and spinal changes (e.g., intervertebral disk disease, bony neoplasia), which could signal or explain a neurogenic component to the urinary retention.

Retrograde cystourethrography using iodine-based contrast will help demonstrate radiolucent stones as well as small stones near the os penis. Filling defects in the bladder or urethra may suggest the presence of radiolucent stones or of intraluminal masses. Use of air as negative contrast, following the iodine-based positive contrast, provides better evaluation of the bladder wall and trigone.

Ultrasound is an excellent modality for evaluation of the trigone, proximal urethra, and prostate or prostatic region, but the pubic bone precludes evaluation of the full length of the urethra. Moderate distension of the bladder with urine or saline aids ultrasonographic assessment, particularly of the bladder wall.

Urethrocystoscopy permits direct visualization and biopsy of urethral obstructions and has proven valuable for detection of lesions that do not manifest with conventional imaging studies. Advanced imaging of the spinal cord (e.g., myelography/epidurography, computed tomography, magnetic resonance imaging) may be necessary to confirm or localize subtle neurological lesions.

Urodynamic assessment

Urethral pressure profilometry and cystometrography are specialized urodynamic assessment methods of urinary bladder and resting urethral function. The availability of these procedures is limited to a handful of university and specialty hospitals, and their sensitivity for diagnosing dynamic disorders (e.g., detrusor-urethral dyssynergia) is limited in small animals. Fortunately, functional studies are rarely required for diagnosis and management of urinary retention. The principles and applications of urethral pressure profilometry and cystometrography are discussed in Chapter 22.

Management of urinary retention

Bladder management

Regardless of the cause or extent of detrusor hypofunction, preventing bladder overdistension and preventing urinary retention are critical to patient management. Bladder overdistension interferes with functional detrusor recovery (Kato et al. 1990; Bross et al. 1999), and urinary retention predisposes to bacterial UTI. In cats and in female dogs, maintenance of a soft indwelling urinary catheter attached to a closed collection system is strongly recommended if the bladder has been overdistended and/or detrusor injury is suspected (e.g., with pets with acute mechanical urethral obstruction). For male dogs, clean, intermittent urethral catheterization (q 4–8 hours as needed to keep the bladder from becoming large) is a straightforward and preferred method of bladder care, since it carries a lower risk of inducing ascending UTI than does an indwelling urinary catheter. Manual bladder expression rarely results in complete bladder emptying, may traumatize the bladder wall (especially in pets with increased outlet resistance), and may cause retrograde reflux of urine into the renal pelvis, resulting in mechanical upper urinary tract damage and/or ascending pyelonephritis. For cats and female dogs, manual expression may be necessary for chronic bladder management since repeated catheterization is clinically impractical and not feasible for owners; use of smooth and/or skeletal muscle relaxants to decrease outlet resistance is particularly important in these pets to minimize adverse effects of manual expression.

Urinary tract infection (UTI) can be both a predisposing factor to (less commonly) and a sequela of (very commonly) urinary retention. Urine obtained via cystocentesis should be submitted for bacterial culture and sensitivity and persistent UTI should be treated with an appropriate antimicrobial, preferably after catheterization is no longer required. Treatment with systemic antibiotics concomitant with indwelling urinary catheterization can predispose to resistant bacterial infection. Simple bacterial cystitis can be treated following the initial phase of management and preferably after normal voiding resumes. Immediate antimicrobial therapy is indicated in the face of clinical or clinicopathological evidence of systemic bacterial infection (fever, elevated white blood cell count, malaise, etc.). Periodic reculture of cystocentesis-sampled urine is warranted as long as abnormal voiding patterns persist.

Management of detrusor hypofunction

Bethanechol is a parasympathomimetic, direct cholinergic drug that theoretically stimulates or augments smooth muscle contraction. In cases of detrusor hypofunction, bethanechol has traditionally been used to help restore and enhance detrusor contraction, though for this drug to be effective the detrusor and pelvic nerves must be at least partially intact (Steers 1996). The oral form of bethanechol is relatively poorly absorbed, and the subcutaneous form should be used quite cautiously and in small doses (Lees and Moreau 1984). Given subcutaneously bethanechol can, at therapeutic doses, cause vomiting, salivation, and diarrhea, and if overdosed can cause cholinergic crisis resulting in cardiovascular collapse, bronchoconstriction, and death (Ling 1995). The parenteral form should therefore be used extremely cautiously (if at all, for urinary applications) and at the lowest effective dose. Bethanechol should never be given intramuscularly or intravenously. In cases of adverse reaction, atropine is antidotal. Neither oral nor subcutaneous bethanechol should be used alone in the face of increased outlet resistance; smooth and/or skeletal muscle relaxant therapy should be started first so the bladder is not contracting against a closed door, of sorts. Both cisapride and beta-blocking medications have been used in humans for the treatment of detrusor atony, and cisapride has been recommended for this use in dogs; though yet unproven, they may theoretically be effective in augmenting response to bethanechol in unresponsive patients (Coates 2004).

Management of inappropriate outlet resistance

Anatomic obstructions and underlying neurologic lesions must be corrected directly when possible. For neurogenic and functional disorders, however, outlet resistance can be reduced by pharmacologic therapy to enhance voiding. Nonselective α and selective α_1 adrenergic antagonists block sympathetic receptors in the α-innervated urinary smooth muscle fibers and result in IUS and bladder neck relaxation, with a resultant decrease in outlet resistance (Poirier 1988; Hashimoto et al. 1992; Brune 1996; Steers 1996). Veterinarians have traditionally used phenoxybenzamine, a nonselective, irreversible, or slowly reversible α-antagonist, to decrease outlet resistance in small animals (Poirier 1988; Breslin 1993; Steers 1996), but prazosin, an α_1-selective antagonist, is a potent, effective, and economical alternative to phenoxybenzamine and has rendered its use obsolete (Lepor 1990; Breslin 1993; Fischer 2003).

Because of its α_1 selectivity, use of prazosin in small animals may carry a lower incidence of side effects than use of phenoxybenzamine, as has been demonstrated in humans (Jønler et al. 1994). The most common side effect of prazosin use in humans is postural hypotension, particularly during initial dosing (Carruthers 1994; Jønler et al. 1994); intravenous prazosin dropped systolic and mean blood pressures to a greater degree than phenoxybenzamine in one study in dogs (Fischer 2003). Though oral prazosin doses that cause urethral relaxation often causes measurable blood pressure decreases in dogs and cats, clinical signs of hypotension are rare. Ideally, blood pressure is monitored during initial therapy with prazosin; the drug should be avoided in critically ill patients until volume depletion and hypotension are corrected. Prazosin capsules are available in 1, 2, and 5 mg sizes, and dogs can receive 1 mg/15 kg body weight PO q 8–12 hours (Fischer and Lane 2007). Cats can receive 0.25–0.5 mg per cat q 8–12 hours, so capsules must be divided (Lane 2000). If hypotension or depression occurs, the dose should be reduced or the administration frequency decreased. Administration of half the target prazosin dose for the first 24–48 hours of therapy may reduce the chance of a postural hypotensive episode, though this type of adverse effect occurs very infrequently in euvolemic animals (Carruthers 1994; Jønler et al. 1994; Steers 1996).

Tamsulosin is a newer antagonist that exhibits strong selectivity for the α_1 receptors in the urinary tract (α_{1A}) over the vascular α_1 receptors (α_{1B}). This selectivity results in the capacity for greater efficacy as a urethral smooth muscle relaxant with minimized risk of hypotension, and thus a greater margin of safety when used in dogs (Ohtake et al. 2006; Sato et al. 2007). The metabolism of tamsulosin is not precisely and consistently described, and some sources suggest that glucuronidation may be involved; because of this, *tamsulosin cannot currently be recommended for use in cats*. Silodosin is another commercially available α_1-antagonist that shows even greater α_{1A} receptor selectivity in canine tissues than does tamsulosin and may prove to be a useful therapy, but veterinary clinical data and experience with silodosin are lacking at this point (Tatemichi et al. 2006). In experimental studies in dogs, doses of 1–100 mcg/kg IV and PO have been used to evaluate tamsulosin's effect on urethral pressure and arterial blood pressure (Sudoh et al. 1996; Witte e al. 2002; Ohtake et al. 2006). Oral tamsulosin doses of 1–10 mcg/kg produced dose-dependent blockade of phenylephrine-induced urethral pressure increase in a clinically effective range (Witte et al. 2002); this author (JRF) has used 10 mcg/kg PO q day in dogs with presumptive urethral-sphincter dyssynergia with good clinical effect and without adverse effects. Some clinicians use smooth muscle antispasmodic agents (e.g., propantheline, oxybutynin) in a similar fashion to relax both bladder and urethra, but the urethral effects may be quite weak.

Skeletal muscle fibers (EUS) are arranged in specific portions of the urethra. Some dogs, and especially cats, with dysfunctional voiding will require additional relaxation of this striated muscle in order to sufficiently relax the urethral outlet. We commonly use diazepam for this purpose (Mawby 1990), though acepromazine, dantrolene, and aminopropazine can also serve as skeletal muscle relaxants (Moreau and Lappin 1989; Marks 1993; Streater-Knowlen et al. 1995; Steers 1996). Baclofen may be considered in dogs only. Acepromazine effectively reduces smooth and striated muscle tone after single doses; however, continued dosing may lead to significant sedation or hypotension. Dantrolene, baclofen, and aminopropazine are not commonly used in veterinary medicine but are mentioned here for completeness. Skeletal muscle relaxants may be a more important component of urethral relaxant therapy for cats than for dogs because of the higher relative proportion of skeletal muscle in the feline urethra compared to the canine urethra (Cullen 1983). Oral diazepam administration can cause idiosyncratic hepatic necrosis in cats; oral administration of diazepam, particularly long-term administration, should be done with caution in this species. Empirically, alprazolam, another benzodiazepine, appears to cause urethral relaxation in cats and also has anxiolytic/tranquilizing effects (Overall 1997), offering a promising alternative to diazepam when an oral benzodiazepine is needed for a feline patient. Methocarbamol, a centrally acting muscle relaxant, also causes generalized muscle relaxation through unknown mechanisms (possibly via generalized sedative effect) and is most often used for pets with metaldehyde poisoning or intervertebral disk disease. Though methocarbamol has not been specifically investigated for use in decreasing urethral outlet resistance, if other agents are not readily available or are contraindicated in a particular patient, it may be a reasonable choice. All skeletal muscle relaxants mentioned here can cause sedation, which may be profound at higher doses.

Duration of urethral relaxant therapy depends in part on the cause of increased outlet resistance. For example, a cat with urethrospasm and functional obstruction following the relief of an anatomical obstruction may only require a few days of urethral relaxants; the drug can then be gradually tapered and discontinued. Conversely, a dog with idiopathic functional urethral obstruction may well require lifelong therapy to maintain adequate voiding function. For many pets with increased outlet resistance due to spinal cord injury, urethral relaxants can be tapered and eventually discontinued as the pet's neurologic function returns. Administration is usually continued for several days after effective voiding is observed.

Summary

The clinical sign of urinary incontinence indicates derangement of the normal physical and/or physiological parameters governing the storage phase of micturition; animals leak urine due to inappropriately decreased outlet closure pressure, a noncompliant or overactive bladder, and/or anatomic abnormality that undermines normal continence mechanisms. The clinical sign of urinary retention indicates derangement of the normal physical and/or physiological parameters governing the voiding phase of micturition; animals retain urine due to inappropriately increased outlet pressure, inappropriately decreased detrusor contraction during voiding, and/or mechanical obstruction to urine outflow. Optimal management hinges on identification of the abnormal neurological and/or muscular activity, thus permitting targeted therapies. Prognosis depends on etiology, severity, and duration of the derangement, but urinary incontinence and urinary retention can be resolved or adequately treated in many veterinary patients.

References

Abdel-Azim, M., M. Sullivan, et al. (1991). Disorders of bladder function in spinal cord disease. *Neur Clin* **9**: 727.

Adin, C.A., J.P. Farese, et al. (2004). Urodynamic effects of a percutaneously controlled static hydraulic urethral sphincter in canine cadavers. *Am J Vet Res* **65**: 283–288.

Angioletti, A., I. DeFrancesco, et al. (2004). Urinary incontinence after spaying in the bitch: incidence and oestrogen-therapy. *Vet Res Comm* **28**: 153–155.

Arnold, S. (1992). Relationship of incontinence to neutering. In: *Current Veterinary Therapy XI: Small Animal Practice*, edited by R.W. Kirk. Phildelphia, PA: W.B. Saunders, pp. 875–877.

Arnold, S., P. Arnold, et al. (1989). Incontinentia urinae bei der kastrierten Huendin: Haeufigkeit und Rassedisposition. *Schweiz Arch Tierheilkd* **131**: 259–263.

Arnold, S., M. Hubler, et al. (1996). Treatment of urinary incontinence in bitches by endoscopic injection of glutaraldehyde cross-linked collagen. *J Small Anim Pract* **37**: 163–168.

Atalan, G., F.J. Barr, et al. (1999). Frequency of urination and ultrasonographic estimation of residual urine in normal and dysuric dogs. *Res Vet Sci* **68**: 295–299.

Bacon, N.J., O. Oni, et al. (2002). Treatment of urethral sphincter mechanism incompetence in 11 bitches with a sustained-release formulation of phenylpropanolamine hydrochloride. *Vet Rec* **151**: 373.

Barth, A., I.M. Reichler, et al. (2005). Evaluation of long-term effects of endoscopic injection of collagen into the urethral submucosa for treatment of urethral sphincter incompetence in female dogs: 40 cases (1993-2000). *J Am Vet Med Assoc* **226**, 73.

Breslin, D., D.W. Fields, et al. (1993). Medical management of benign prostatic hyperplasia: a canine model comparing the in vivo efficacy of α_1 adrenergic antagonists in the prostate. *J Urol* **149**: 395.

Bross, S., S. Schumacher, et al. (1999). Effects of acute urinary bladder overdistension on bladder response during sacral neurostimulation. *Eur Urol* **36**, 354–359.

Brune, M.E., S.P. Katwala, et al. (1996). Effects of selective and non-selective α_1-adrenoreceptors on intraurethral and arterial pressures in intact conscious dogs. *Pharmacology* **53**: 356.

Burgherr, T., I. Reichler, et al. (2007). Efficacy, tolerance and acceptability of Incontex in spayed bitches with urinary incontinence [German]. *Schweiz Arch Tierheikd* **149**: 307–313.

Byron, J.B., D.J. Chew, et al. (2005). Transurethral collagen implantation for treatment of canine urinary incontinence. ACVIM Forum, Abstract 120.

Byron, J.K., P.A. March, et al. (2007). Effect of phenylpropanolamine and pseudoephedrine on the urethral pressure profile and continence scores of incontinent female dogs. *J Vet Intern Med* **21**: 47–53.

Carofiglio, F., A.J. Hamaide, et al. (2006). Evaluation of the urodynamic and hemodynamic effects of orally administered phenylpropanolamine and ephedrine in female dogs. *Am J Vet Res* **67**: 723–730.

Carruthers, S.G. (1994). Adverse effects of a1-adrenergic blocking drugs. *Drug Safety* **11**(1): 12–20.

Coates, J. (2004). Neurogenic micturition disorders. ACVIM Forum, Minneapolis.

Coit, V.A., I.F. Gibson, et al. (2008). Neutering affects urinary bladder function by different mechanisms in male and female dogs. *Eur J Pharmacol* **14**: 153–158.

Crawford, J.T. and W.M. Adams (2002). Influence of vestibulobaginal stenosis, pelvic bladder, and recessed vulva on response to treatment for clinical signs of lower urinary tract disease in dogs: 38 cases (1990–1999). *J Am Vet Med Assoc* **221**: 995–999.

Cullen, W.C, T.F. Fletcher, et al. (1983). Morphometry of the female feline urethra. *J Urol* **129**: 190.

de Groat, W.C. (2008). Neuroanatomy and neurophysiology: innervation of the lower urinary tract. In: *Female Urology*, edited by R. Shlomo and R. Larissa. Philadelphia: Saunders.

Drake, M.J., P.M. Nixon, et al. (1998 Jul). Drug-induced bladder and urinary disorders. Incidence, prevention and management. *Drug Saf.* **19**(1): 45–55.

Espineira, M.M.D., F.W. Viehoff, et al. (1998). Idiopathic detrusor–urethral dyssynergia in dogs: a retrospective analysis of 22 cases. *J Small Anim Pract* **39**: 264–270.

Ferguson, D.R., I. Kennedy, et al. (1997). ATP is released from rabbit urinary bladder cells by hydrostatic pressure changes—a possible sensory mechanism? *J Physiol* **505**: 503–511.

Fischer, J.R. and I.F. Lane (2003). Medical treatment of voiding dysfunction in dogs and cats. *Vet Med* **98**(1): 67–73.

Fischer, J.R., I.F. Lane, et al. (2003). Urethral pressure profile and hemodynamic effects of phenoxybenzamine and prazosin in non-sedated male beagle dogs. *Can J Vet Res* **67**: 30–38.

Fischer, J.R. and I.F. Lane (2007). Incontinence and urinary retention. In: *BSAVA Manual of Canine and Feline Nephrology and Urology*, edited by J. Elliott and G. Grauer, 2nd edition. pp. 26–40.

Fowler, C.J., D. Griffiths, et al. (2008). The neural control of micturition. *Nat Rev Neurosci* **9**: 453–466.

Gregory, S.P. and P.E. Holt (1994). The immediate effect of colposuspension on resting and stressed urethral pressure profiles in anaesthetized incontinent bitches. *Vet Surg* **23**: 330.

Hamaide, A.J., J.G. Grand, et al. (2006). Urodynamic and morphologic changes in the lower portion of the urogenital tract after administration of estriol alone and in combination with phenylpropanolamine in sexually intact and spayed female dogs. *Am J Vet Res* **67**: 901–908.

Hammel, S.P., D.E. Bjorling (2002). Results of vulvoplasty for treatment of recessed vulva in dogs. *J Am Anim Hosp Assoc* **38**: 79–83.

Hashimoto, S., S. Kigashi, et al. (1992). Neurogenic responses of urethra isolated from the dog. *Eur J Pharmacol* **213**(1): 117.

Hoeijmakers, M., B. Janszen, et al. (2003). Pharmacokinetics of oestriol after repeated oral administration to dogs. *Res Vet Sci* **75**: 55–59.

Holt, P.E. (1984). Efficacy of emepronium bromide in the treatment of physiological incontinence in the bitch. *Vet Rec* **114**: 355f.

Holt, P.E. (1985a). Importance of urethral length, bladder neck position and vestibulovaginal stenosis in sphincter mechanism incompetence in the incontinent bitch. *Res Vet Sci* **39**: 364–372.

Holt, P.E. (1985b). Urinary incontinence in the bitch due to sphincter mechanism incompetence: prevalence in referred dogs and retrospective analysis of sixty cases. *J Small Anim Pract* **26**: 181–190.

Holt, P.E. (1990). Long-term evaluation of colposuspension in the treatment of urinary incontinence due to incompetence of the urethral sphincter mechanism in the bitch. *Vet Rec* **127**: 537–542.

Holt, P.E. and S.P. Gregory (1991). Can urethral pressure profilometry predict the response to colposuspension in the bitch. *Vet Rec* **128**: 281–282.

Holt, P.E., R.J. Coe, et al. (2005). Prostatopexy as a treatment for urethral sphincter mechanism incompetence in male dogs. *J Small Anim Pract* **46**: 567–570.

Hosgood, G. Urethral disease and obstructive uropathy. In: *Disease Mechanisms in Small Animal Surgery*, edited by M.J. Bojrab. Philadelphia: Lea & Febiger, 528 p.

Howe, L.M., M.R. Slater, et al. (2001). Long-term outcome of gonadectomy performed at an early age or traditional age in dogs. *J Am Vet Med Assoc* **218**: 217.

Jønler, M., M. Riehmann, et al. (1994). Benign prostatic hyperplasia. Current pharmacologic treatment. *Drugs* **47**(1): 66–81.

Jost, W.J. and P. Marsalek (2005). Duloxetine in the treatment of stress urinary incontinence. *Ther Clin Risk Mgmt* **1**: 259–264.

Karl, K.B. and M.A. Katofiase (1995). Effects of duloxetine, a combined serotonin and norepinephrinae reuptake inhibitor, on central neural control of lower urinary tract function in the chloralose-anesthetized female cat. *J Pharmacol Exp Ther* **274**: 1014–1024.

Kato, K., A.J. Wein, et al. (1990). Short-term functional effects of bladder outlet obstruction in the cat. *J Urol* **143**(5): 1020–1025.

Kobayashi, S., M. Endou, et al. (2003). The sympathomimetic actions of l-ephedrine and d-pseudoephedrine: direct receptor activation or norepinephrine release? *Anesth Anlg* **97**: 1239–1245.

Lane, I.F. (2000a). Diagnosis and management of urinary retention. *Vet Clin N Am Small Anim Pract* **30**: 25–57.

Lane, I.F. (2000b). Urinary obstruction and functional urinary retention. In: *Textbook of Veterinary Internal Medicine: Diseases of the Dog and Cat*, edited by S. Ettinger and E. Feldman, Vol. **1**. Philadelphia: WB Saunders, pp. 93–96.

Lane, I.F. (2000c). Use of anticholinergic agents in lower urinary tract disease. In: *Kirk's Current Veterinary Therapy XIII*, edited by J.D. Bonagura. Philadelphia, PA: Saunders, pp. 899–902.

Lane, I.F. (2003). Treating urinary incontinence. *Vet Med* **98**(1): 58f.

Lane, I.F., M.R. Lappin, et al. (1995). Evaluation of preoperative urodynamic measurements in nine dogs with ectopic ureters. *J Am Vet Med Assoc* **206**, 1348–1357.

Lane, I.F., J.R. Fischer, et al. (2000). Functional urethral obstruction in 3 dogs: clinical and urethral pressure profile findings. *J Vet Intern Med* **14**(1), 43–49.

Lappin, M.R. and J.A. Barsanti (1987). Urinary incontinence secondary to idiopathic detrusor instability: cystometrographic diagnosis and pharmacologic management in two dogs and a cat. *J Am Vet Med Assoc* **191**, 1439f.

Lees, G.E. and P.M. Moreau (1984). Management of hypotonic and atonic bladders in cats. *Vet Clin North Am (Small Anim Pract)* **14**, 641.

Lepor, H. (1990). Role of alpha adrenergic blockers in the treatment of benign prostatic hyperplasia. *Prostate* **3**(Suppl): 66.

Ling, G.V. (1995). *Lower Urinary Tract Diseases of Gogs and Cats: Diagnosis, Medical Management, Prevention*. St. Louis: Mosby-Year Book, Inc.

Mandigers, P.J.J. and T. Nell (2001). Treatment of bitches with acquired urinary incontinence with oestriol. *Vet Rec* **149**: 765–767.

Mandigers, P.J.J., T. Senders, et al. (2006). Morbidity and mortality in 928 dobermanns born in the Netherlands between 1993 and 1999. *Vet Rec* **158**: 226–229.

Marchevsky, A.M., G.A. Edwards, et al. (1999). Colposuspension in 60 bitches with incompetence of the urethral sphincter mechanism. *Aus Vet Pract* **29**: 2–7.

Marks, S.L., I.M. Straeter, et al. (1993). The effects of phenoxybenzamine and acepromazine maleate on urethral pressure profiles of anesthetized healthy male cats [abstract]. *J Vet Int Med* **7**: 122.

Massat, B.J., C.R. Gregory, et al. (1993). Cystourethropexy to correct refractory urinary incontinence due to urethral sphincter mechanism incompetence: preliminary results in ten bitches. *Vet Surg* **22**, 260–268.

Mawby, D.I., S.M. Meric, et al. (1990). Pharmacologic relaxation of the urethra in male cats: A study of the effects of phenoxybenzamine, diazepam, nifedipine, and xylazine. *Can J Vet Res* **55**: 28.

Moreau, P.M. (1982). Neurogenic disorders of micturition in the dog and cat. *Comp Cont Ed Pract Vet* **4**: 12.

Moreau, P.M. and M.R. Lappin (1989). Pharmacologic management of urinary incontinence. In: *Current Veterinary Therapy X: Small Animal Practice*, edited by R.W. Kirk. Philadelphia: WB Saunders, 1214 p.

Nendick, P.A. and W.T. Clark (1987). Medical therapy of urinary incontinence in ovariectomized bitches: a comparison of the effectiveness of diethylstilbestrol and pseudoephedrine. *Aus Vet J* **64**: 117–118.

Nickel, R.F., M.V. Vink-Noteboom, et al. (1999). Clinical and radiographic findings compared with urodynamic findings in neutered female dogs with refractory urinary incontinence. *Vet Rec* **145**: 11–15.

Norton, P.A., N.R. Zinner, et al. (2002). Duloxetine versus placebo in the treatment of stress urinary incontinence. *Am J Obstet Gynecol* **187**: 40–48.

O'Brien, D.P. (1990). Disorders of the urogenital system. *Sem Vet Med Surg (Small Anim)* **5**: 57–66.

Oelke, M., J.P. Roovers, et al. (2006 May). Safety and tolerability of duloxetine in women with stress urinary incontinence. *BJOG* **113**(Suppl 1): 22–26.

Ohtake, A., S. Sato, et al. (2006). Effects of tamsulosin on resting urethral pressure and arterial blood pressure in anaesthetized female dogs. *J Pharm Pharmacol* **58**(3): 345–350.

Oliver, J.E., Lorenz, M.D.et al. (1997). Disorders of micturition. In: *Handbook of Veterinary Neurology*, edited by J. Oliver, 3rd edition. Philadelphia: WB Saunders, 73 p.

Overall, K.L. (1997). *Clinical Behavioral Medicine for Small Animals*. St. Louis: Mosby-Year Book, Inc., 239 p.

Poirier, M., J.P. Riffaud, et al. (1988). Effects of five alpha-blockers on the hypogastric nerve stimulation of the canine lower urinary tract. *J Urol* **140**: 165.

Ponglowhapan, S., D.B. Church, et al. (2008). Differences in the proportion of collagen and muscle in the canine lower urinary tract with regard to gonadal status and gender. *Theriogenology* **70**: 1516–1524.

Rawlings, C., J.A. Barsanti, et al. (2001). Evaluation of colposuspension for treatment of incontinence in spayed female dogs. *J Am Vet Med Assoc* **219**, 770–775.

Reichler, I.M., M. Hubler, et al. (2003). The effect of GnRH analogs on urinary incontinence after ablation of the ovaries in dogs. *Theriogenology* **60**: 1207–1216.

Reichler, I.M., E. Pfeiffer, et al. (2004). Changes in plasma gonadotropin concentrations and urethral closure pressure in the bitch during the 12 months following ovariectomy. *Theriogenology* **62**: 1391–1402.

Reichler, I.M., E. Hung, et al. (2005). FSH and LH plasma levels in bitches with differences in risk for urinary incontinence. *Theriogenology* **63**: 2164.

Reichler, I.M., W. Jochle, et al. (2006). Effect of a long acting GnRH analogue or placebo on plasma LH/FSH, urethral pressure profiles and clinical signs of urinary incontinence due to Sphincter mechanism incompetence in bitches. *Theriogenology* **66**(5): 1227–1236.

Richelson, E. (1983 Jan). Antimuscarinic and other receptor-blocking properties of antidepressants. *Mayo Clin Proc* **58**(1): 40–46.

Richter, K.P. and G.V. Ling (1985). Clinical response and urethral pressure profile changes after phenylpropanolamine in dogs with primary sphincter incompetence. *J Am Vet Med Assoc* **187**: 605–611.

Sato, S., A. Ohtake, et al. (2007). Relationship between the functional effect of tamsulosin and its concentration in lower urinary tract tissues of dogs. *Biol Pharm Bull* **30**: 81–486.

Schotanus, B.A., J. deGier, et al. (2008). Estrolium treatment in the bitch: a risk for uterine infection? *Reprod Domest Anim* **43**: 176–180.

Scott, L., F. Leddy, et al. (2002). Evaluation of phenylpropanolamine in the treatment of urethral sphincter mechanism incompetence in the bitch. *J Small Anim Pract* **43**, 493–496.

Spain, C.V., J.M. Scarlett, et al. (2004 Feb 1). Long-term risks and benefits of early-age gonadectomy in dogs. *J Am Vet Med Assoc* **224**(3): 380–387.

Steers, W.D., D.M. Barret, et al. (1996). Voiding function and dysfunction: Diagnosis, classification, management. In: *Adult and Pediatric Urology*, edited by Gillenwater, 3rd edition. St. Louis: Mosby, 1220 p.

Stocklin-Gautschi, H.M., I.M. Reichler, et al. (2001). The relationship of urinary incontinence to early spaying in bitches. *J Repro Fert* **57**: 233–236.

Streater-Knowlen, I.M., S.L. Marks, et al. (1995). Urethral pressure response to smooth and skeletal muscle relaxants in anesthetized, adult male cats with naturally acquired urethral obstruction. *Am J Vet Res* **56**: 919.

Sudoh, K., H. Tanaka, et al. (1996). Effect of tamsulosin, a novel alpha 1-adrenoceptor antagonist, on urethral pressure profile in anaesthetized dogs. *J Auton Pharmacol* **16**(3): 147–154.

Tatemichi, S., Y. Tomiyama, et al. (2006). Uroselectivity in male dogs of Silodosin (KMD-3213): a novel drug for the obstructive component of benign prostatic hyperplasia. *Neurol Urodynam* **25**: 792–799.

Thrusfield, M.V. (1985). Association between urinary incontinence and spaying bitches. *Vet Rec* **116**: 695.

Thrusfield, M.V., P.E. Holt, et al. (1998 Dec). Acquired urinary incontinence in bitches: its incidence and relationship to neutering practices. *J Small Anim Pract* **39**(12): 559–566.

Van Kerrebroeck, P., P. Abrams, et al. (2004). Duloxetine versus placebo in the treatment of European and Canadian women with stress urinary incontinence. *B J Obstet Gynaecol* **111**: 249–257.

Welle, M.M., I.M. Riechler, et al. (2006). Immunohistochemical localization and quantitative assessment of GnRH-, FSH-, And LH-receptor mRNA expression in canine skin: a powerful tool to study the pathogenesis of side effects after spaying. *Histochem Cell Biol* **126**: 527–535.

White, R.N. (2001). Urethropexy for the management of urethral sphincter mechanism incompetence in the bitch. *J Small Anim Pract* **42**, 481–486.

White, R.A. and C.J. Pomeroy (1989). Phenylpropanolamine: an alpha-adrenergic agent for the management of urinary incontinence in the bitch associated with urethral sphincter mechanism incompetence. *Vet Rec* **125**, 478–480.

Witte, D.G., M.E. Brune, et al. (2002). Modeling of relationships between pharmacokinetics and blockade of agonist-induced elevation of intraurethral pressure and mean arterial pressure in conscious dogs treated with alpha(1)-adrenoceptor antagonists. *J Pharmacol Exp Ther* **300**(2): 495–504.

77

Urethral diseases

Joe Bartges

Urethral disease occurs commonly in dogs and cats, often in association with diseases of the urinary bladder. Clinical signs of urethral disease are associated with signs of lower urinary tract disease (e.g., pollakiuria, stranguria, periuria, hematuria, etc.) or to obstruction of urine flow. Physical examination should include palpation of the perineal region and rectal examination as the pelvic urethra is palpable through the rectal wall running dorsal to the pelvic bones. Common diseases affecting the urethra in dogs and cats include urethral obstruction and urinary incontinence due to urethral sphincter mechanism incompetency.

Hypospadias

Hypospadias is a congenital anomaly of the external genitalia in which there is fusion failure of the urogenital folds and incomplete development of the penile urethra (Figure 77.1) (Galanty et al. 2008).

Types include glandular, penile, scrotal, perineal, and anal according to site of the urethral opening. It can be classified as mild, moderate, or severe. In severe cases, lesions such as underdevelopment or absence of the penis, failure of fusion of the scrotum, and failure of the urethra to close in the perineal area may be seen. Other abnormalities associated with hypospadias include retained testicles, kidney agenesis, bone or anorectal defects, umbilical hernia, hydrocephalus, and urinary incontinence and ascending urinary tract infections (McFarland and Deniz 1961; Ader and Hobson 1978; Hayes and Wilson 1986). Chromosome analysis can be used to differentiate hypospadias from true hermaphroditism (Cassata et al. 2008). No corrective surgery is indicated with minimal

defects, moderate urethral defects can be treated with a two-layer closure, and major defects with excision of the external genitalia and urethrostomy (Vahlensieck 1973; Rawlings 1984; Burger et al. 1992; Pavletic 2007; Galanty et al. 2008).

Urethrorectal fistula

Urethrorectal fistula occurs because of failure of separation of the fetal cloaca into the anterior urethrovesical segment and posterior rectal segment by the urorectal septum resulting in a permanent communication between urethra and rectum. It has also been described as an acquired disease due to prostatic abscessation in a dog (Agut et al. 2006). Clinical signs are related to abnormal micturition occurring typically after weaning. Urine is observed to pass from the rectum, and cystitis, perineal dermatitis, hematuria, infection-induced struvite urolithiasis, and diarrhea may occur (Miller 1980). Diagnosis is made by direct visualization or contrast studies verifying the communication. Treatment involves surgical correction of the congenital defect (Whitney and Schrader 1988). With acquired urethrorectal fistula, conservative therapy utilizing an indwelling urinary catheter, antibiotics, and omentalization of the prostatic abscess has been described (Agut et al. 2006).

Urethritis

Urethritis refers to inflammation of the urethra. Inflammation may be primary in nature or secondary to other diseases, including trauma, urolithiasis (Figure 77.2), or neoplasia (Figure 77.3) (Polzin and Jeraj 1980; Olausson et al. 2005).

Oftentimes, urethritis occurs with cystitis usually bacterial in dogs or idiopathic in cats. Inflammation occurs due to breakdown of urothelial lining and may result in

Nephrology and Urology of Small Animals. Edited by Joe Bartges and David J. Polzin. © 2011 Blackwell Publishing Ltd.

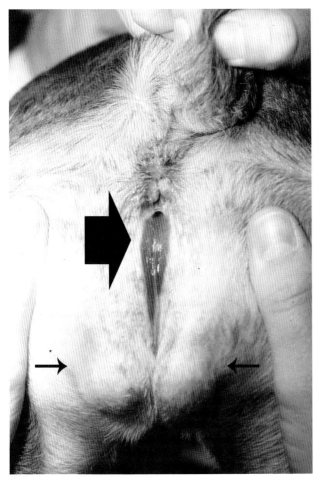

Figure 77.1 Hypospadias (large arrow) in a 5-month-old, intact male, English bulldog. Small arrows identify testicles.

ulceration and erosion. Proliferative urethritis may occur secondary to chronic bacterial infection or immune-mediated disease. Granulomatous (lymphoplasmacytic) urethritis is characterized by epithelial hyperplasia and infiltration with lymphocytes and plasma cells and is

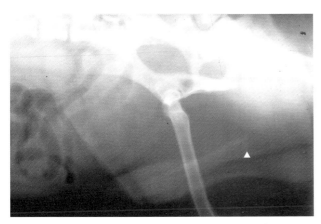

Figure 77.2 Lateral survey abdominal radiograph of a 4-year-old, intact male, English bulldog with urethral obstruction due to a cystine urolith (arrow); urocystoliths are also present.

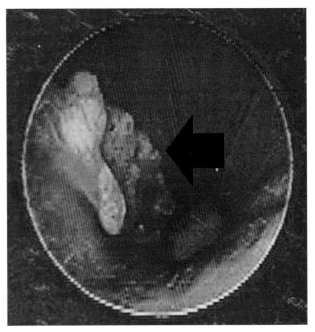

Figure 77.3 Cystoscopic view of urethral transitional cell carcinoma (arrow) in a 10-year-old, spayed female, mixed breed dog.

associated with chronic bacterial infection (Moroff et al. 1991). Clinical signs are consistent with lower urinary tract disease. Diagnosis is made by rectal palpation of the urethra, by contrast urethrography (Figure 77.4) or cystoscopy (Figure 77.5).

Biopsy of the urethra confirms the inflammatory nature. Treatment for urethritis includes antimicrobial therapy for the bacterial infection, and, possibly, anti-inflammatory therapy if granulomatous urethritis is present. Anti-inflammatory therapy with prednisone (1 mg/kg PO q 24 hours), cyclophosphamide (2.2 mg/kg PO q 24 hours for 4 days per week), or piroxicam

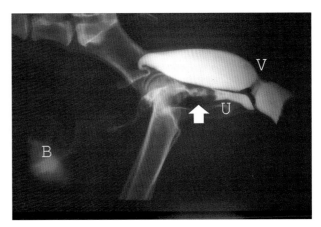

Figure 77.4 Lateral abdominal contrast vaginourethrocystography in a 4-year-old, spayed female, Chow-cross with granulomatous (lymphoplasmacytic) urethritis. V, vagina; U, urethra; B, bladder.

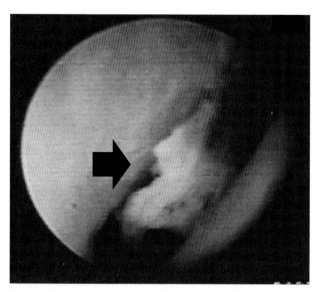

Figure 77.5 Cystoscopic view of granulomatous (lymphoplasmacytic) urethritis (arrow) in a 6-year-old, spayed female, Irish setter secondary to chronic bacterial cystitis due to *Escherichia coli*.

(0.3 mg/kg PO q 24 hours) may be tried. For proliferative urethritis, anti-inflammatory therapy as described or immunosuppressive therapy (azathioprine at 2 mg/kg PO q 24–48 hours or prednisone at 2 mg/kg PO q 24 hours) with concurrent antimicrobial therapy is recommended. If urethral obstruction is present, a cystostomy catheter (Chapter 32) may be required until regression of inflammatory infiltration and urethral obstruction (Salinardi et al. 2003).

Urethral prolapse

Urethral prolapse occurs when the distal urethra protrudes through the urethral orifice of the penis. It appears as a red or purple mass at the tip of the penis and occurs commonly in English bulldogs, but has been reported in other breeds (Kirsch et al. 2002; Ragni 2007). Clinical signs may not be present, or the dog may lick at the prepuce, have stranguria, or have bleeding from the prepuce. Diagnosis of urethral prolapse is made by visualization; it must be differentiated from neoplasia. If the prolapse is not causing problems, then treatment may not be required. Urethral prolapse is treated by attempting to manually reduce the prolapsed tissue; applying hypertonic saline may facilitate the attempt. A loose purse-string suture is then placed; however, recurrences are common. Surgical reduction or urethropexy is often the treatment of choice (Chapter 83) (Kirsch et al. 2002).

Neoplasia

Primary neoplasia of the urethra is uncommon in dogs and cats; however, extension of bladder or prostatic

neoplasia may occur (Chapter 79). Transitional cell carcinoma and squamous cell carcinoma occur most commonly, but other tumor types have been described (Tarvin et al. 1978; Szymanski et al. 1984; Batamuzi and Kristensen 1996; Caney et al. 1998; Davis and Holt 2003; Liptak et al. 2004; Mirkovic et al. 2004; Olausson et al. 2005; Takagi et al. 2005; Tucker and Smith 2008). Diagnosis is made by rectal palpation of the urethra, by contrast urethrography, or cystoscopy. Treatment involves surgical removal or laser ablation, if possible, and/or chemotherapy (Chapter 79); insertion of a urethral stent to relieve obstruction may also be done (Chapter 32) (Latal et al. 1994; Elwick et al. 2003; Weisse et al. 2006).

Urethral trauma

Urethral trauma may occur from blunt or penetrating injuries, especially from traumatic urinary catheterization (Figure 77.6) (Jones et al. 1981; Bjorling 1984; Hay and Rosin 1997; Anderson et al. 2006).

Blunt trauma due to vehicular trauma may cause urethral trauma due to pubic or os penis fractures. Iatrogenic trauma may occur with urinary catheterization especially when using a stiff polypropylene catheter. Clinical signs relate to the lower urinary tract. Additionally, urine may collect subcutaneously or intra-abdominally. Hematuria may be the only clinical sign. Diagnosis is made by contrast urethrography or cystoscopy. Treatment includes placement of an indwelling urinary catheter (Meige et al. 2008) and surgical correction or urinary diversion (Hay and Rosin 1997; Boothe 2000; Anderson et al. 2006). Urethrostomy may be necessary if the urethra is not salvageable.

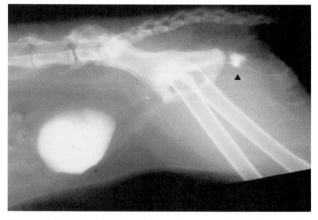

Figure 77.6 Lateral retrograde contrast urethrocystogram of a 3-year-old, castrated male, domestic shorthaired cat with urethral trauma and leakage of contrast (arrow) from catheterization to relieve a urethral obstruction.

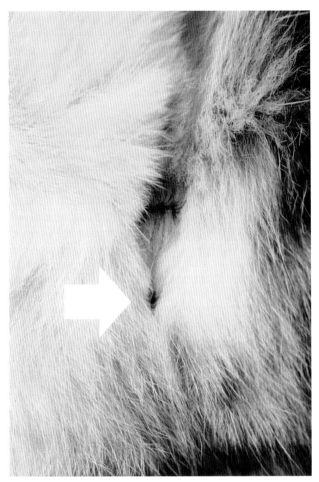

Figure 77.7 Urethral stricture at site of previous perineal urethrostomy in a 3-year-old, castrated male, domestic shorthaired cat.

Urethral stricture

Urethral stricture usually occurs secondary to urethral trauma, especially urinary catheterization in cats (Figure 77.6) (Corgozinho et al. 2007; Meige et al. 2008), or surgery (Figure 77.7) (Osborne et al. 1996; Phillips and Holt 2006).

Clinically, dogs and cats with urethral strictures have hematuria and stranguria or are unable to urinate. There is often a history of a traumatic or surgical event, although urethral stricture may occur secondary to a neoplastic process such as a transitional cell carcinoma. Diagnosis is made by visualization if the stricture is at the site of a previous urethrostomy procedure, by contrast urethrography, or cystoscopy. Treatment includes surgical correction, dilation of the strictured area, or insertion of a urethral stent (Latal et al. 1994; Smeak 2000; Bennett et al. 2005; Phillips and Holt 2006; Corgozinho et al. 2007; Wood et al. 2007).

Urethral sphincter mechanism incompetency (urinary incontinence)

Urethral sphincter mechanism incompetency is the most common cause of urinary incontinence in dogs occurring primarily in spayed female dogs (Chapters 76). Dogs typically present several years after ovariohysterectomy and clinical signs include unconsciously leaving a puddle of urine where the dog lays. While awake, urination is normal and incontinence is not present. Bacterial urinary tract infection occurs commonly with urinary incontinence and is not associated typically with active urine sediment, although it is associated with worsening of urinary incontinence. Medical treatment involves administration of estrogenic or alpha-agonist agents alone or in combination. In dogs that are medically unresponsive, surgical techniques and urethral bulking agents are available (Chapter 38 and 83).

Urethral obstruction

Obstructive uropathy refers to abnormalities in structure or function of the urinary tract caused by impairment of normal flow of urine, and the resulting local and systemic effects of that impairment (Klahr and Harris 1992; Bartges et al. 1996). Impairment of flow through the urethra either due to physical obstruction (Figures 77.2, 77.8–77.10) or due to detrusor or urethral dysfunction results in characteristic clinical signs.

Although there are many causes of urethral obstruction, urolithiasis is the most common cause in dogs and crystalline-matrix urethral plugs, and uroliths are the most common in cats and will be addressed in this chapter.

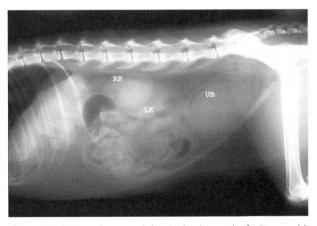

Figure 77.8 Lateral survey abdominal radiograph of a 7-year-old, castrated male, domestic shorthaired cat with urethral obstruction due to calcium oxalate uroliths. B, urinary bladder; RK, right kidney; LK, left kidney.

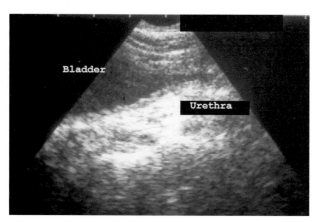

Figure 77.9 Abdominal ultrasound image of cat described in Figure 77.8. The bladder is distended and the wall appears thickened. The proximal urethra is dilated.

Clinical signs

Signs of obstructive uropathy vary considerably depending on degree of urine outflow impairment, duration of disease, and presence of secondary bacterial infection. Patients with urethral obstruction may or may not have preceding signs of lower urinary disease. They may only exhibit clinical signs localized to the lower urinary tract, such as dysuria, hematuria, pollakiuria, inability to pass urine, or pain, or they may exhibit polysystemic signs of uremia, such as vomiting, anorexia, and depression. Owners may mistake animals with urethral obstruction as being constipated or having abdominal or back pain.

Physical examination may reveal a physiologically normal-appearing animal or they may be depressed, in shock, or unconscious. A large painful bladder may be palpable. Bradycardia, hypothermia, pale mucous membranes with prolonged capillary refill time, hyperpnoea,

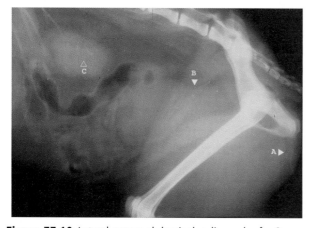

Figure 77.10 Lateral survey abdominal radiograph of a 9-year-old, castrated male, domestic shorthaired cat with calcium oxalate urethroliths causing obstruction, A, cystolith, B, and nephroliths, C.

and halitosis may be present. The tip of the penis may be dark purple and swollen. One or more uroliths may be palpated in the urethra. Rectal examination should be performed, when possible, to rule out a pelvic urethral urolith or obstruction from neoplasia or prostatic disease.

Blood samples for complete blood cell counts and serum biochemical analysis and a urine sample for analysis and possible culture should be collected. Cystocentesis may be performed successfully even with urethral obstruction if care is taken to insert the hypodermic needle gently and angling the tip towards the trigone while stabilizing the urinary bladder. When the patient is stable, survey abdominal radiography should be performed. Additional imaging such as ultrasonography, contrast urethrocystography, or urethrocystoscopy may be considered.

Clinical consequences

Clinical consequences of urethral obstruction are often, but not always, associated with signs of uremia. Partial or early outflow obstruction may not impair renal function sufficiently to cause uremia; however, clinical signs of uremia usually occur within 24 hours of complete urethral obstruction. As functional renal mass decreases or as intravesical, ureteral, and renal pressure increases, urine concentrating ability is lost. Increased tubular volume of urine and increased tubular pressure occur, resulting in azotemia and uremia. Early detection and removal of obstruction results in prompt disappearance of signs of uremia, although renal abnormalities may persist for a longer time. Also, urethral obstruction may lead to detrusor atony or urethral injury. Urethral and bladder mucosal damage, urinary tract infection, and urethral or bladder rupture may also occur.

Treatment

Emergency stabilization

Priorities of treating a patient with urethral obstruction depend on degree of obstruction and systemic responses to the obstruction. If the animal is extremely depressed, oxygen should be administered, intravenous catheter placed, and blood and urine samples obtained. Fluid therapy should be instituted with rate based on physiologic status of the patient. Estimate degree of dehydration and administer an isotonic replacement electrolyte solution over 6–12 hours if minimally dehydrated, over 4 hours if moderately dehydrated, and over 1–2 hours if shock is present. Rate of fluid therapy should be assessed and adjusted based on response to therapy including heart rate, electrocardiogram, respiratory rate, and thoracic auscultation. If bradyarrhythmia is present due to hyper-kalemia, it should be treated aggressively.

Hyperkalemia

Clinical and experimental studies have shown that obstructive uropathy alters sodium, potassium, magnesium, phosphorous, and calcium metabolism (Finco and Cornelius 1977; Burrows and Bovee 1978). Hyperkalemia is caused by acidemia, decreased renal excretion of potassium, and tissue catabolism. Alterations in P-R interval, S-T segment, and T waves on electrocardiograms are associated frequently with hyperkalemia. Dysrhythmias may also occur including third-degree heart block and ventricular arrhythmias. Varying degrees of neuromuscular weakness and flaccid paralysis occur as a result of impaired impulse transmission. Serum concentration of potassium approaching 10 mEq/L may be associated with bradycardia and cardiac arrest.

Immediate life-threatening arrhythmias due to hyperkalemia should be treated first. Treatment can include calcium gluconate (50–100 mg/kg IV over 2–3 minutes, monitor ECG) to counteract effect of hyperkalemia at the sino-atrial node, or measures to decrease serum potassium concentration (bicarbonate (1–2 mEq/kg IV)), 10% dextrose infusion (4–10 mL/kg IV), insulin (0.1–0.25 IU/kg IV q 2–4 hours), or dextrose and insulin infusion (0.5 IU/kg regular insulin + 4 mL of 50% dextrose/IU of insulin IV).

Fluids

Dehydration should be addressed immediately; intravenous fluid therapy with a replacement crystalloid is best. Rate of hydration depends on degree of shock present, but should be completed within 6–12 hours unless heart disease is present.

Metabolic acidosis

Metabolic acidosis is present in acute urethral obstruction; however, usually it is not severe enough (pH < 7.0) to warrant specific treatment.

Hypocalcemia

Ionized hypocalcemia may occur in cats with urethral obstruction and exacerbates the effects of hyperkalemia; it is treated with calcium gluconate if needed (Lee and Drobatz 2003).

Relieving urethral obstruction

Following stabilization, the patient is sedated or anesthetized, and urethral obstruction is relieved (Chapters

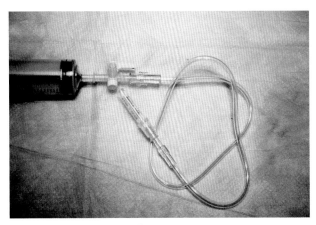

Figure 77.11 22 gauge, $1^1/_2$-inch hypodermic needle attached to an IV extension set and three-way stopcock for removing larger quantities of urine from the bladder by cystocentesis.

35 and 36). If the patient is severely depressed or unconscious, relieving the urethral obstruction may be possible without sedation or anesthesia. Many protocols are available to facilitate relief of urethral obstruction, including morphine (0.1–0.3 mg/kg IM), butorphanol (0.2–0.4 mg/kg IV or IM), propofol (2–4 mg/kg IV), short-acting barbiturate (5 mg/kg IV), isoflurane anesthesia administered by mask, and ketamine (2.5–5.0 mg/kg IV) mixed with diazepam (0.125–0.25 mg/kg IV) or midazaolam (0.125–0.25 mg/kg IV or IM) or acepromazaine (0.05–0.1 mg/kg IV).

Cystocentesis should be performed using a 22-gauge, $1^1/_2$-inch hypodermic needle or a 22-gauge over-the-needle catheter attached to an IV extension set and three-way stopcock (Figure 77.11) in order to decompress the urinary bladder and to collect diagnostic samples.

Stabilize the hypodermic needle or catheter in order to avoid further damage to the urinary bladder and uroabdomen. Urethral catheterization should be performed as soon as possible (Chapters 35 and 36). In male cats, a urethral crystalline-matrix plug may be dislodged by massaging the distal penis between the thumb and forefinger and applying gentle pressure to the bladder (Figure 77.12).

If the obstruction is not relieved, retrograde hydropropulsion should be performed (Chapter 35). An alternative treatment for urethroliths is lithotripsy (Chapter 34) (Davidson et al. 2004; Adams et al. 2008; Defarges and Dunn 2008; Lulich et al. 2009).

Indwelling urinary catheter

Decision for placing an indwelling urinary catheter is dependent upon ease or difficulty that the urethral obstruction was relieved, stream of urine obtained after relieving urethral obstruction, presence of a large amount

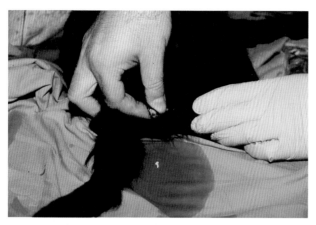

Figure 77.12 Urethral plug (small arrow) dislodged from a 5-year-old, castrated male, domestic shorthaired cat by massaging the penile urethra (large arrow) and applying gentle pressure on the urinary bladder.

of crystalline and/or gelatinous debris in urine after copious flushing of the urinary bladder, degree of bladder overdistention and likelihood of detrusor atony, degree of systemic illness of the patient, and cause of urethral obstruction. A closed system is used with an indwelling urinary catheter (Figure 77.13).

Administration of an alpha$_2$-receptor antagonist (prazosin or phenoxybenzamine) helps to decrease urethral spasm secondary to the catheter (Straeter-Knowlen et al. 1995; Fischer et al. 2003). Depending on cause of urethral obstruction, definitive treatment and appropriate preventative measures should be undertaken (Osborne et al. 1996). Antibiotics should not be administered while an indwelling urinary catheter is present. Although concomitant administration of antibiotics decreases incidence of bacterial urinary tract infections, when infections occur they exhibit a higher degree of antimicrobial resistance (Barsanti et al. 1985). In one study of induced sterile cystitis in cats with indwelling urinary catheters, some cats receiving amoxicillin developed bacterial cystitis and at necropsy had positive bacterial cultures from kidneys (Barsanti et al. 1992).

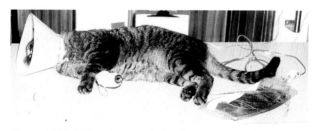

Figure 77.13 Closed system indwelling urinary catheter in a 6-year-old, castrated male, domestic shorthaired cat following relief of a urethral obstruction due to a presumed crystalline-matrix urethral plug.

Female dogs and cats

Occasionally, female dogs and cats present with urethral obstruction due to urolithiasis. They are managed as described previously. Urethroliths are often palpable on rectal examination and may be retropulsed into the urinary bladder using a combination of urethral catheterization and flushing and digital moving of the urolith per rectum.

Complications

Bacterial infection

Bacterial infection may be a complication of obstructive uropathy. Infection may be present before onset of acute urethral obstruction or be introduced as a consequence of procedures used to relieve obstruction. Alkaline urine associated with infection by urease-producing microorganisms may predispose to struvite crystalluria and urolithiasis or to struvite-matrix plug formation. Infection is difficult to eradicate while urinary stasis exists. Signs of lower urinary tract infection may persist after urethral obstruction is relieved. Outflow obstruction predisposes the upper tract to ascending bacterial infection due to vesicoureteral reflux.

Micturition dysfunction

After prolonged retention of urine, patients may have difficulty emptying their bladders. This may be due to decreased bladder elasticity, damage to nerves in the bladder wall, damage to contractile elements in the bladder wall, or to urethral edema or inflammation, resulting in urethral spasm (Tammela et al. 1991). Detrusor atony or urethral swelling or spasm may be transient or may persist for an unpredictable period depending on the underlying disease and the amount of irreversible damage caused by urethral obstruction and may impact on survival. Goal of treatment is to restore normal bladder and urethral function.

Postobstructive diuresis

Relief of urethral obstruction is accompanied by alterations in ability to modulate water and sodium balance. This postobstructive diuresis can affect hydration status and electrolyte balance. Degree of diuresis can be very profound and may require prolonged intravenous or subcutaneous administration of large amounts of fluids. Measuring urine output and body weight after relieving urethral obstruction aids in determining necessary fluid therapy to maintain hydration.

Intrinsic renal failure

Although postrenal azotemia occurs more commonly than renal azotemia with urethral obstruction, primary renal failure may occur. Many factors lead to renal failure including loss of renal parenchyma due to sustained increased intrarenal pressure, cytokine production by infiltrating leukocytes into renal parenchyma, electrolyte imbalances, fibrosis of damaged renal parenchyma, and renal ischemia due to dehydration associated with urethral obstruction and postobstructive diuresis (Saphasan and Sorrasuchart 1984). Treatment of urethral obstruction should be directed at correcting imbalances in homeostasis due to urethral obstruction.

Death

Obstructive uropathy that persists for more than 24 hours usually results in postrenal uremia. This occurs because increased back pressure induced by obstruction to outflow impairs glomerular filtration, renal blood flow, and tubular function (Kerr 1956). After obstruction of the urethra of normal cats, death occurred in 3–6 days (Finco and Cornelius 1977). Death may be a result of cardiopulmonary failure associated with fluid and electrolyte imbalances, particularly potassium, or development of acute oliguric/anuric renal failure. Damage to the mucosal surface of the urinary bladder and presence of bacterial urinary tract infection shorten survival times.

Prognosis

Prognosis for animals with urethral obstruction is dependent upon the cause of the obstruction, ease of relieving obstruction, and success of preventative therapy. In one study of 45 male cats with urethral obstruction, reobstruction due to uroliths or crystalline-matrix plugs occurred in approximately 1/3, clinical signs recurred in approximately 1/2, and euthanasia was performed in 1/5 (Gerber et al. 2008).

If obstruction cannot be relieved, is recurrent despite appropriate treatment, or if penile trauma occurs during attempted relief of urethral obstruction (Figure 77.5), surgical urinary diversion (scrotal urethrostomy or perineal urethrostomy) should be considered (Chapter 83) (Smeak 2000; Corgozinho et al. 2007). Complications of scrotal urethrostomy in dogs are typically hemorrhage at time of surgery or stricture at the site, whereas perineal urethrostomy in cats may be associated with stricture formation, urine leakage, and recurrent bacterial urinary tract infection (Scavelli 1989; Newton and Smeak 1996; Bass et al. 2005; Corgozinho et al. 2007). For urethral obstruction due to neoplasia, urethral stents or cystostomy catheters may be used (Salinardi et al. 2003).

References

Adams, L.G., A.C. Berent, et al. (2008). Use of laser lithotripsy for fragmentation of uroliths in dogs: 73 cases (2005–2006). *J Am Vet Med Assoc* **232**(11): 1680–1687.

Ader, P.L. and H.P. Hobson (1978). Hypospadia: a review of the veterinary literature and a report of three cases in the dog. *J Am Anim Hosp Assoc* **14**: 721–727.

Agut, A., X. Lucas, et al. (2006). A urethrorectal fistula due to prostatic abscess associated with urolithiasis in a dog. *Reprod Domest Anim* **41**(3): 247–250.

Anderson, R.B., L.R. Aronson, et al. (2006). Prognostic factors for successful outcome following urethral rupture in dogs and cats. *J Am Anim Hosp Assoc* **42**(2): 136–146.

Barsanti, J.A., J. Blue, et al. (1985). Urinary tract infection due to indwelling bladder catheters in dogs and cats. *J Am Vet Med Assoc* **187**(4): 384–388.

Barsanti, J.A., E.B. Shotts, et al. (1992). Effect of therapy on susceptibility to urinary tract infection in male cats with indwelling urethral catheters. *J Vet Intern Med* **6**(2): 64–70.

Bartges, J.W., D.R. Finco, et al. (1996). Pathophysiology of urethral obstruction. *Vet Clin North Am Small Anim Pract* **26**(2): 255–264.

Bass, M., J. Howard, et al. (2005). Retrospective study of indications for and outcome of perineal urethrostomy in cats. *J Small Anim Pract* **46**(5): 227–231.

Batamuzi, E.K. and F. Kristensen (1996). Urinary tract infection: the role of canine transmissible venereal tumour. *J Small Anim Pract* **37**(6): 276–279.

Bennett, S.L., G.E. Edwards, et al. (2005). Balloon dilation of a urethral stricture in a dog. *Aust Vet J* **83**(9): 552–554.

Bjorling, D.E. (1984). Traumatic injuries of the urogenital system. *Vet Clin North Am Small Anim Pract* **14**(1): 61–76.

Boothe, H.W. (2000). Managing traumatic urethral injuries. *Clin Tech Small Anim Pract* **15**(1): 35–39.

Burger, R.A., S.C. Muller, et al. (1992). The buccal mucosal graft for urethral reconstruction: a preliminary report. *J Urol* **147**(3): 662–664.

Burrows, C.F. and K.C. Bovee (1978). Characterization and treatment of acid-base and renal defects due to urethral obstruction in cats. *J Am Vet Med Assoc* **172**(7): 801–805.

Caney, S.M., P.E. Holt, et al. (1998). Prostatic carcinoma in two cats. *J Small Anim Pract* **39**(3): 140–143.

Cassata, R., A. Iannuzzi, et al. (2008). Clinical, cytogenetic and molecular evaluation in a dog with bilateral cryptorchidism and hypospadias. *Cytogenet Genome Res* **120**(1–2): 140–143.

Corgozinho, K.B., H.J. de Souza, et al. (2007). Catheter-induced urethral trauma in cats with urethral obstruction. *J Feline Med Surg* **9**(6): 481–486.

Davidson, E.B., J.W. Ritchey, et al. (2004). Laser lithotripsy for treatment of canine uroliths. *Vet Surg* **33**(1): 56–61.

Davis, G.J. and D. Holt (2003). Two chondrosarcomas in the urethra of a German shepherd dog. *J Small Anim Pract* **44**(4): 169–171.

Defarges, A. and M. Dunn (2008). Use of electrohydraulic lithotripsy in 28 dogs with bladder and urethral calculi. *J Vet Intern Med* **22**(6): 1267–1273.

Elwick, K.E., L.D. Melendez, et al. (2003). Neodymium: Yttrium-aluminum-Garnet (Nd:YAG) laser ablation of an obstructive urethral polyp in a dog. *J Am Anim Hosp Assoc* **39**(5): 506–508.

Finco, D.R. and L.M. Cornelius (1977). Characterization and treatment of water, electrolyte, and acid-base imbalances of induced urethral obstruction in the cat. *Am J Vet Res* **38**(6): 823–830.

Fischer, J.R., I.F. Lane, et al. (2003). Urethral pressure profile and hemodynamic effects of phenoxybenzamine and prazosin in non-sedated male beagle dogs. *Can J Vet Res* **67**(1): 30–38.

Galanty, M., P. Jurka, et al. (2008). Surgical treatment of hypospadias. Techniques and results in six dogs. *Pol J Vet Sci* **11**(3): 235–243.

Gerber, B., S. Eichenberger, et al. (2008). Guarded long-term prognosis in male cats with urethral obstruction. *J Feline Med Surg* **10**(1): 16–23.

Hay, C.W. and E. Rosin (1997). Repair of an intrapelvic urethral tear in a bitch caused by iatrogenic trauma. *Vet Rec* **140**(2): 48–49.

Hayes, H.M., Jr. and G.P. Wilson (1986). Hospital incidence of hypospadias in dogs in North America. *Vet Rec* **118**(22): 605–607.

Jones, G.H., W.T. Testerman, et al. (1981). Ruptured urethra caused by trauma in a dog. *Vet Med Small Anim Clin* **76**(5): 672–673.

Kerr, W.S. (1956). Effects of complete ureteral obstruction in dogs on kidney function. *Am J Physiol* **184**: 521–526.

Kirsch, J.A., J.G. Hauptman, et al. (2002). A urethropexy technique for surgical treatment of urethral prolapse in the male dog. *J Am Anim Hosp Assoc* **38**(4): 381–384.

Klahr, S. and K.P. Harris (1992). Obstuctive uropathy. In: *The Kidney*, edited by D.W. Seldin and G.G. Giebisch. New York: Raven Press.

Latal, D., J. Mraz, et al. (1994). Nitinol urethral stents: long-term results in dogs. *Urol Res* **22**(5): 295–300.

Lee, J.A. and K.J. Drobatz (2003). Characterization of the clinical characterstics, electrolytes, acid-base, and renal parameters in male cats with urethral obstruction. *J Vet Emerg Crit Care* **13**(4): 227–233.

Liptak, J.M., S.P. Brutscher, et al. (2004). Transurethral resection in the management of urethral and prostatic neoplasia in 6 dogs. *Vet Surg* **33**(5): 505–516.

Lulich, J.P., L.G. Adams, et al. (2009). Changing paradigms in the treatment of uroliths by lithotripsy. *Vet Clin North Am Small Anim Pract* **39**(1): 143–160.

McFarland, L.Z. and E. Deniz (1961). Unilateral renal agenesis with ipsilateral cryptorchidism and perineal hypospadias in a dog. *J Am Vet Med Assoc* **139**: 1099–1100.

Meige, F., S. Sarrau, et al. (2008). Management of traumatic urethral rupture in 11 cats using primary alignment with a urethral catheter. *Vet Comp Orthop Traumatol* **21**(1): 76–84.

Miller, C.F. (1980). Urethrorectal fistula with concurrent urolithiasis in a dog. *Vet Med Small Anim Clin* **75**(1): 73–76.

Mirkovic, T.K., C.L. Shmon, et al. (2004). Urinary obstruction secondary to an ossifying fibroma of the os penis in a dog. *J Am Anim Hosp Assoc* **40**(2): 152–156.

Moroff, S.D., B.A. Brown, et al. (1991). Infiltrative urethral disease in female dogs: 41 cases (1980–1987). *J Am Vet Med Assoc* **199**(2): 247–251.

Newton, J.D. and D.D. Smeak (1996). Simple continuous closure of canine scrotal urethrostomy: results in 20 cases. *J Am Anim Hosp Assoc* **32**(6): 531–534.

Olausson, A., S.M. Stieger, et al. (2005). A urinary bladder fibrosarcoma in a young dog. *Vet Radiol Ultrasound* **46**(2): 135–138.

Osborne, C.A., D.D. Caywood, et al. (1996). Feline perineal urethrostomy: a potential cause of feline lower urinary tract disease. *Vet Clin North Am Small Anim Pract* **26**(3): 535–549.

Osborne, C.A., J.M. Kruger, et al. (1996). Medical management of feline urethral obstruction. *Vet Clin North Am Small Anim Pract* **26**(3): 483–498.

Pavletic, M.M. (2007). Reconstruction of the urethra by use of an inverse tubed bipedicled flap in a dog with hypospadias. *J Am Vet Med Assoc* **231**(1): 71–73.

Phillips, H. and D.E. Holt (2006). Surgical revision of the urethral stoma following perineal urethrostomy in 11 cats (1998–2004). *J Am Anim Hosp Assoc* **42**(3): 218–222.

Polzin, D.J. and K. Jeraj (1980). Urethritis, cystitis, and ureteritis. *Vet Clin North Am Small Anim Pract* **9**(4): 661–678.

Ragni, R.A. (2007). Urethral prolapse in three male Yorkshire terriers. *J Small Anim Pract* **48**(3): 180.

Rawlings, C.A. (1984). Correction of congenital defects of the urogenital system. *Vet Clin North Am Small Anim Pract* **14**(1): 49–60.

Salinardi, B.J., S.L. Marks, et al. (2003). The use of a low-profile cystostomy tube to relieve urethral obstruction in a dog. *J Am Anim Hosp Assoc* **39**(4): 403–405.

Saphasan, S. and S. Sorrasuchart (1984). Factors inducing post-obstructive diuresis in rats. *Nephron* **38**: 125–133.

Scavelli, T.D. (1989). Complications associated with perineal urethrostomy in the cat. *Probl Vet Med* **1**(1): 111–119.

Smeak, D.D. (2000). Urethrotomy and urethrostomy in the dog. *Clin Tech Small Anim Pract* **15**(1): 25–34.

Straeter-Knowlen, I.M., S.L. Marks, et al. (1995). Urethral pressure response to smooth and skeletal muscle relaxants in anesthetized, adult male cats with naturally acquired urethral obstruction. *Am J Vet Res* **56**(7): 919–923.

Szymanski, C., R. Boyce, et al. (1984). Transitional cell carcinoma of the urethra metastatic to the eyes in a dog. *J Am Vet Med Assoc* **185**(9): 1003–1004.

Takagi, S., T. Kadosawa, et al. (2005). Urethral transitional cell carcinoma in a cat. *J Small Anim Pract* **46**(10): 504–506.

Tammela, T., H. Auto-Harmainen, et al. (1991). Effect of prolonged experimental distention on the function and ultrastructure of the canine urinary bladder. *Ann Chrurgiae Gynaecolgiae* **80**: 301–306.

Tarvin, G., A. Patnaik, et al. (1978). Primary urethral tumors in dogs. *J Am Vet Med Assoc* **172**(8): 931–933.

Tucker, A.R. and J.R. Smith (2008). Prostatic squamous metaplasia in a cat with interstitial cell neoplasia in a retained testis. *Vet Pathol* **45**(6): 905–909.

Vahlensieck, W. (1973). Hypospadias-repair with histoacrylic tissue adhesive and without indwelling catheter drainage. *Urol Res* **1**(1): 2–5.

Weisse, C., A. Berent, et al. (2006). Evaluation of palliative stenting for management of malignant urethral obstructions in dogs. *J Am Vet Med Assoc* **229**(2): 226–234.

Whitney, W.O. and L.A. Schrader (1988). Urethrorectal fistulectomy in a dog, using a perineal approach. *J Am Vet Med Assoc* **193**(5): 568–569.

Wood, M.W., S. Vaden, et al. (2007). Cystoscopic-guided balloon dilation of a urethral stricture in a female dog. *Can Vet J* **48**(7): 731–733.

78

Prostatic disease

Margaret Root Kustritz

Applied anatomy and physiology

The prostate is the only accessory sex organ of male dogs. Male cats have a prostate and bulbourethral glands. Diseases of the accessory sex organs of male cats are very uncommon and will not be discussed.

The prostate encircles the neck of the urinary bladder. Prostatic fluid empties into the prostatic urethra via a number of small duct openings, the seminis colliculus. Histologically, the prostate is made up of two major lobes with a fibrous median raphe. The large lobes are made up of lobules of secretory tissue separated by bands of nondistensible connective tissue. There is little smooth muscle tissue in the canine prostate.

The prostate increases in size and vascularity with increasing age in intact dogs. This is a normal phenomenon and is not necessarily always associated with disease.

Androgens are primary effectors of prostate growth and function (Shidaifat et al. 2007a). Testosterone is converted to dihydrotestosterone (DHT) via the enzyme 5-alpha-reductase. DHT has a higher binding affinity than testosterone and less readily dissociates from receptors, thereby exerting a greater effect than native testosterone (Grino et al. 1990). Castration causes discernible prostatic atrophy within days, with a 50% reduction in size by 3 weeks and a 70% reduction in size by 9 weeks after surgery (Barsanti 1997).

Prostatic fluid secretion is constitutive in intact male dogs, with volume of fluid produced not associated with frequency of breeding (Johnston et al. 2000). Prostatic fluid flows into the urinary bladder and into the urethra, creating the mucoid mass called smegma at the preputial orifice that is commonly seen in intact male dogs.

Nephrology and Urology of Small Animals. Edited by Joe Bartges and David J. Polzin. © 2011 Blackwell Publishing Ltd.

Prostate disease is common in aged, intact male dogs and can occur in castrated males. Overall prevalence of prostate disease in dogs in one study was reported as 75.6% in 500 dogs aged 1–21 years of age (Mukaratirwa and Chitura 2007). Conditions that will be discussed are benign prostatic hypertrophy/hyperplasia (BPH), prostatitis/prostatic abscesses, paraprostatic cysts, and prostatic neoplasia.

Diagnostic testing for prostatic disease

Physical examination

Rectal examination (Chapter 4) is part of examination of all male dogs with clinical signs of lower urinary tract disease. The prostate is palpable at the cranial aspect of the pubis; however, when enlarged, it may be located more cranially. By pushing dorsally and caudally on the caudal abdomen with the other hand, the prostate may be pushed to the cranial aspect of the pubis and may be palpable via rectal examination. When enlarged, the prostate may be identified by abdominal palpation.

Imaging of the prostate

In healthy intact male dogs, the prostate should be less than 70% of the distance between the sacral promontory and cranial aspect of the pubis on lateral survey abdominal radiography (Chapter 15). It should be round and smooth. A triangular-shaped fat pad is present between the cranioventral aspect of the prostate and the caudoventral aspect of the urinary bladder (Johnston and Feeney 1986). Ultrasonographically (Chapter 16), the prostate in a healthy intact male dog is round and smooth and has a diffuse inhomogeneous echotexture. Contrast may reflux into the prostate gland of a healthy intact male dog on retrograde contrast urethrocystography (Chapter 15); the prostatic urethral mucosa should be smooth and may be narrowed.

Cytologic examination of prostatic fluid and tissue

Urinalysis and urine culture

A complete urinalysis (Chapter 7) should be performed on all male dogs with signs of lower urinary tract disease. Microscopic examination of urine sediment may reveal hematuria, pyuria, or occasionally neoplastic cells. Aerobic bacteriologic culture of urine should also be performed (Chapter 9).

Ejaculate

Manual ejaculation is the most common method of semen collection used in dogs. Collect canine semen in a comfortable, quiet environment with nonslip flooring. Most male dogs will ejaculate in the absence of a teaser bitch; however, use of a teaser bitch facilitates collection. Dogs that are painful may resist ejaculation or be unable to ejaculate. Semen should be collected using a latex artifical vagina attached to a sterile, graduated plastic centrifuge tube because this best simulates natural service and the copulatory lock. The narrow end of the collecting cone is pulled over the sterile centrifuge tube. The top of the latex-collecting cone is folded over to form a final length such that the tip of the erect penis will be just above the centrifuge tube, minimizing contact of the ejaculate with the latex cone but not permitting the tip of the penis to be traumatized by the collecting tube. A small amount of water-soluble lubricant is placed around the top fold of the collecting cone, which facilitates removal later. Do not allow lubricant to come in contact with the ejaculate. If a teaser bitch is used, two people should be present: one to hold the teaser bitch and the other for the male. The handler of the bitch should kneel in front of her and keep her standing. The male dog is allowed to sniff at the bitch's hindquarters, and he may be allowed to mount her. Brisk and enthusiastic massage of the bulbous glandis through the prepuce of the male will also elicit erection. As soon as erection occurs, the hand manipulating the prepuce can be used to move the prepuce proximal to the bulbus glandis while the other hand introduces the collecting cone with attached centrifuge tube over the engorging penis. Ideally, the collecting cone is passed to just proximal to the bulbus glandis and a tight grip maintained at the area. Application of circumferential pressure proximal to the bulbus glandis simulates the pressure of the vulvar lips during the copulatory lock, and the pressure of the latex cone around the erect penis simulates intravaginal pressure. The male will thrust vigorously for several minutes, ejaculating the presperm and sperm-rich fractions of semen, on average 21 seconds after beginning manual stimulation (Johnston et al. 2001). Collected semen may be submitted for bacteriological culture (Chapter 9) and cytology (Chapter 26).

Prostatic massage

Prostatic massage is an alternative technique for collecting prostatic fluid from dogs where semen cannot be collected due to pain, inexperience, or temperament (Barsanti 1995). In cases of suspected prostatic neoplasia with invasion of the prostatic urethra, specimens from prostatic massage are more likely to contain neoplastic cells than an ejaculate (Barsanti and Finco 1984). After the dog is allowed to urinate, he is placed in lateral recumbency and a urinary catheter is passed transurethrally into the urinary bladder (Chapter 5). The bladder is emptied and the residual urine submitted for urinalysis (Chapter 7) and aerobic bacterial urine culture (Chapter 9) if not previously performed. Flush the bladder several times with sterile fluid. Retract the urinary catheter to a position just distal to the prostate as determined by rectal palpation. The prostate is massaged per rectum or per abdomen or both for 1–2 minutes. Inject 5–10 mL of sterile 0.9% saline slowly through the catheter while manually occluding the urethral orifice around the catheter to prevent reflux. Gently aspirate through the catheter while advancing the catheter into the urinary bladder in order to collect epithelial cells from the prostatic and proximal urethra and the fluid that was injected into the urinary bladder. The fluid is submitted for cytologic examination (Chapter 26) and for culture (Chapter 9).

Fine-needle aspiration

In cases where the prostate can be identified by abdominal palpation or using ultrasonographic guidance (Chapter 16), fine-needle aspiration of prostate tissue can be performed using a 22-gauge, 1 1/2–inch hypodermic needle and 6–12 mL syringe. Sedation rarely is necessary. The sample aspirated into the needle and/or syringe hub is then expelled onto microscopic slides and cytologic examination performed (Chapter 26). Care must be taken with cystic disease or abscessation as rupture of the cyst or abscess may occur.

Biopsy

Traumatic catheterization or brush biopsy

In cases where involvement of the prostatic urethra is suspected, a traumatic urinary catheter biopsy or urethral brush technique can be combined with prostatic massage (Barsanti 1995). Prostatic massage is performed as described previously except that after placing the urinary catheter in the prostatic urethra using guidance by rectal palpation, the urinary catheter is moved rapidly back and forth while applying negative pressure with a syringe and pushing ventrally on the prostate per rectum. Negative pressure is maintained as the catheter is then advanced into the urinary bladder for retrieval of infused sterile fluid. Alternatively, urinary catheter biopsy can be performed independently of prostatic massage. Place approximately 6 mL of sterile physiologic saline in a 12 mL syringe attached to the urinary catheter. The catheter is inserted into the urethra and guided to the level of the prostatic urethra by rectal palpation. Inject 4–5 mL of the sterile saline through the catheter and move the catheter briskly back and forth while applying negative pressure on the syringe. Fluid can be submitted for cytological examination (Chapter 26) and pieces of tissue can be submitted for histopathologic examination.

Endoscopic and fluoroscopic biopsy of prostatic urethra

In cases where prostatic urethral involvement is suspected, biopsy of the invading cancer through and in the uroepithelium can be obtained using endoscopy (Chapter 19) or fluoroscopic guidance (Chapter 25). Biopsy samples are examined histopathologically.

Tru-cut biopsy

Using ultrasonographic guidance, a Tru-cut biopsy sample may be obtained (Chapter 16). Sedation of the patient is recommended prior to sampling.

Surgical biopsy

Tru-cut or excisional biopsy of the prostate can be obtained through an open surgical approach (Chapter 83).

Prostatic diseases

Benign prostatic hypertrophy

Signalment

BPH consists of both hypertrophy and hyperplasia of secretory and connective tissues in the prostate. The condition occurs spontaneously only in dogs and men. This is an age-related change and is not recognized to be preneoplastic in dogs. There is histologic evidence of BPH in 16% of dogs by 2 years of age, with 50% having BPH by 4–5 years of age (Berry et al. 1986). No breed predisposition has been reported; be aware that normal Scottish Terriers have a prostate that is four times larger than that of other dogs with similar body weight (O'Shea 1962). BPH does not occur in castrated males.

Clinical signs

Many animals with BPH identified by rectal palpation or imaging of the prostate have no associated clinical signs. The most common clinical sign reported is dripping of bloody fluid from the urethra unassociated with urination (Krawiec and Heflin 1992; Read and Bryden 1995). This occurs because of development of intraparenchymal cysts and increasing vascularity of the prostate with increasing size (Barsanti 1997). The prostatic fluid secreted is blood-tinged and so more visible to the owner than the normal clear prostatic fluid that commonly runs through the postprostatic urethra.

A common clinical sign of BPH in men is dysuria or perceived inability to completely empty the bladder during micturition. This is caused by contraction of smooth muscle around the prostatic urethra decreasing urine outflow. This is an uncommon presenting complaint in dogs because of the relative paucity of smooth muscle within the canine prostate. However, because dogs do not exhibit signs of BPH with minimal prostatomegaly, clinical presentation for signs referable to increased size of the prostate is more common in dogs than in men. These signs include rectal tenesmus and defecation of ribbon-shaped stools (Krawiec and Heflin 1992).

Urinary tract signs are associated with BPH in 27% of cases, with hematuria that most commonly described (Krawiec and Heflin 1992). Systemic signs of disease are uncommon in dogs with uncomplicated BPH.

Diagnosis

Complete blood count (CBC) and chemistry profile results are within normal limits in dogs with uncomplicated BPH (Read and Bryden 1995). Hematuria is present on urinalysis. BPH most often is a rule-out diagnosis, after unsuccessful investigation for prostatitis or prostatic abscesses in intact or castrated males, and prostatic neoplasia in castrated or intact males. Significant prostatomegaly is present. Often, this can be identified by rectal palpation. In dogs with a pelvic prostate, the prostate is symmetrical as a ventral, bilaterally symmetrical mass. The prostate encircles the bladder neck and since the urinary bladder is freely movable from the pelvis into the abdomen, as the prostate increases in size with age, it may pull the urinary bladder forward and fall into the abdomen. If the prostate cannot be felt rectally or abdominally, you may try wheelbarrowing the dog up onto his back legs so the prostate falls back into the pelvis, or try pushing abdominal contents caudally with your free hand toward the gloved finger in the rectum. Digital rectal examination of the prostate as a diagnostic

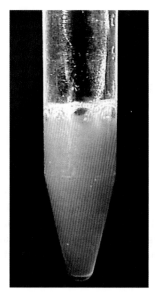

Figure 78.1 Ejaculated prostatic fluid from dog with prostate disease.

test has high specificity (75%) but low sensitivity (53%) (Mukaratirwa and Chitura 2007).

In dogs with BPH, the prostate is symmetrically enlarged and nonpainful. Prostatic fluid varies in color from tan to red (Figure 78.1). Prostatic fluid or tissue cultures are negative or nonsignificant (see "Prostatitis"). Abdominal ultrasonography reveals diffuse prostatomegaly with a homogeneous parenchyma (Figure 78.2). Very small cysts may be seen, scattered diffusely throughout the parenchyma.

In human medicine, assessment of various secretory proteins in serum, most notably prostate specific antigen (PSA), is used to diagnose prostate disease. Measurement of secretory proteins, including PSA and canine prostate

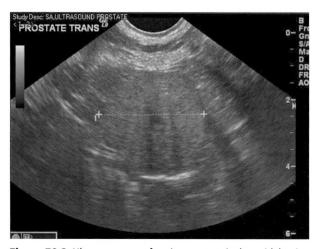

Figure 78.2 Ultrasonogram of canine prostate in dog with benign prostatic hypertrophy/hyperplasia (BPH).

specific esterase, has not been demonstrated to be clinically useful in dogs for diagnosis of prostate disease (Bell et al. 1995).

Treatment

The most effective treatment for BPH in dogs is castration (Rhodes 1996). After castration, secretory epithelial cells die and basal cells lose the capacity to differentiate into secretory cells (Shidaifat et al. 2004). Clinical signs of BPH resolve within 4 weeks (Read and Bryden 1995). No medical therapy has been demonstrated to be as effective as castration.

Medical therapies used historically involved use of estrogens or progestogens. Estrogen, either oral or injectable, is associated with squamous metaplasia of prostatic epithelium and subsequent increased predisposition to prostatitis (Merk et al. 1986). Progestogens, either oral (megestrol acetate 0.50 mg/kg once daily for 4–8 weeks) or injectable (medroxyprogesterone acetate 3 mg/kg subcutaneous every 10 months), have been demonstrated to resolve clinical signs of BPH without negatively impacting semen quality in dogs (Bamberg-Thalen and Linde-Forsberg 1993; Olson 1984). Side effects of progestogen therapy include increased appetite and possible hypothyroidism or diabetes mellitus (Bamberg-Thalen and Linde-Forsberg 1993).

The preferred medical therapy is use of the 5-alpha reductase inhibitor, finasteride (Iguer-Ouada and Verstegen 1997; Sirinarumitr et al. 2001). Because this drug inhibits transformation of testosterone to dihydrotestosterone but does not inhibit testosterone secretion, it decreases prostate size without affecting libido or spermatogenesis. The drug may be more effective in dogs with greater prostatomegaly (Jia et al. 2006). The recommended dose regimen is 5 mg once daily per os in dogs up to 50 kg of body weight for up to 4 months. Most dogs show significant reduction in prostatomegaly and clinical signs within 2–4 weeks after institution of therapy. No side effects have been reported (Iguer-Ouada and Verstegen 1997; Sirinarumitr et al. 2001; Sirinarumitr et al. 2002). Prostate enlargement will recur after the drug is withdrawn. Therapy with finasteride is recommended to control clinical signs of disease as a stopgap to permit the owners to achieve what they need to with that dog before castration is performed. This may include showing the dog in conformation, breeding to specific bitches, or semen collection for cryopreservation.

Experimental therapies for BPH described in dogs as research subjects for human medicine that are not yet available clinically in veterinary medicine include intraprostatic injection of botulinum toxin and thermal ablation via ultrasound (Chuang et al. 2006; Liu et al. 2006; Sasaki et al. 2006).

Prevention

Prostatomegaly is a normal consequence of age in dogs left intact. Dogs with no clinical signs of disease need not be treated at all. BPH is a predisposing cause of prostatitis; aged, intact males may benefit from regular evaluation for prostatitis by culture of prostatic fluid or tissue as described below. Herbal therapy with saw palmetto is not a useful preventative therapy in dogs (Barsanti et al. 2000). Castration is a highly effective therapy for clinical signs of BPH and a highly effective technique for prevention.

Prostatitis/prostatic abscesses

Signalment

Prostatitis is diffuse infection with associated inflammation of the prostate gland. Prostatic abscesses are accumulations of purulent fluid within a cystic space in a persistently infected prostate. The prostate is constantly exposed to microorganisms that are part of the normal flora in the distal urethra. Inherent protective mechanisms include retrograde flow of prostatic fluid and urine, the tight prostatic capsule, presence of local immune factors including IgA and antibacterial proteins, and persistent contractile activity emptying prostatic acini (Dorfman and Barsanti 1995; Barsanti 1997; Shafik et al. 2006). Development of prostatitis implies some underlying problem in the prostate leading to a breakdown of these protective mechanisms. Any dog with prostatitis should be evaluated for underlying BPH or prostatic neoplasia.

Clinical signs

Clinical presentation of dogs with prostatitis varies with duration of disease. Chronic prostatitis often is associated with the clinical presentation of the underlying disease (see BPH and prostatic neoplasia). Acute prostatitis is associated with demonstration of a pain response when the prostate is palpated and is more likely to be associated with systemic signs of disease including fever, lethargy, abdominal pain, and dyschezia (Krawiec and Heflin 1992; Dorfman and Barsanti 1995; Kawakami et al. 2006). Urinary tract signs associated with prostate infection include dysuria, urethral discharge, and hematuria (Krawiec and Heflin 1992; Dorfman and Barsanti 1995; Kawakami et al. 2006). Dogs with a prostatic abscess may present with virtually no clinical signs of disease or with rupture into the peritoneal cavity, with acute abdomen and signs of septic shock.

Diagnosis

Results of routine bloodwork are not well correlated with presence of disease in dogs with prostatitis (Barsanti et al. 1983). Similarly, cytology of ejaculated prostatic fluid is not well correlated with culture results and should not be used to determine whether or not cultures should be performed (Barsanti et al. 1983; Root Kustritz et al. 2005).

Ejaculated prostatic fluid is not sterile as it accumulates microorganisms from the distal urethra. However, collection of prostatic fluid by manual ejaculation is a noninvasive procedure and may be preferred in experienced, intact male dogs. All cultures should be quantitative; growth of more than 10,000 bacteria/mL of a single organism is significant. Fluid and cells can be collected by prostatic massage. In this technique, the sedated dog is placed in lateral recumbency and a urinary catheter passed. The urinary bladder is emptied and flushed with saline. The catheter is pulled back into the area of the prostatic urethra and a gloved finger in the rectum used to massage the prostate, showering cells and fluid into the prostatic urethra from where it is aspirated via the catheter. Finally, ultrasound can be used to guide collection of a fine-needle aspirate (FNA) sample directly from prostate tissue. Because there is no normal flora in the prostatic urethra or prostate tissue, any positive culture from these samples is considered significant. Culture results from ejaculated prostatic fluid were positively correlated with culture results from tissue collected by FNA in 80% of cases in one study (Barsanti et al. 1983).

In general, diagnostic findings by FNA are concordant with diagnosis by histopathology in canine prostate disease 75% of the time (Powe et al. 2004). FNA usually does not require sedation.

Bacterial prostatitis due to aerobic organisms is most common, with *E.coli, Staphylococcus* sp., *Klebsiella* sp., and *Proteus* sp. the most common organisms identified as causative (Krawiec and Heflin 1992). *Brucella canis* has been demonstrated experimentally as a cause of prostatitis in dogs (Dorfman and Barsanti 1995). Anaerobic organisms have been identified in some cases of canine prostatitis (Soki et al. 2002). Fungal prostatitis also is reported, most commonly secondary to systemic blastomycosis (Barsanti and Finco 1979; Krawiec and Heflin 1992).

Abdominal ultrasonography reveals findings associated with underlying disease (see BPH and prostatic neoplasia). Prostatic inflammation is associated with increased mottling of the parenchyma. This is a nonspecific finding on ultrasonography; culture should be performed for definitive diagnosis of prostatitis. Prostatic abscesses will be apparent as large, circular

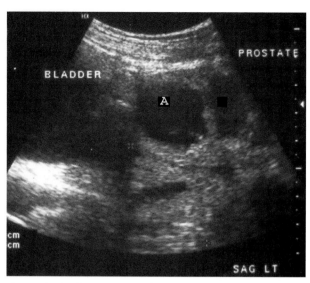

Figure 78.3 Ultrasonogram of canine prostate in dog with prostatic abscess (A).

hypo- to anechoic areas within the prostatic parenchyma (Figure 78.3).

Treatment

Appropriate antibiotic therapy should be based on culture and sensitivity. Culture of ejaculated prostatic fluid correctly permits diagnosis of prostatitis in about 60% of cases (Ling et al. 1983). Culture of prostatic tissue is reported to be 25% more accurate than culture of prostatic fluid (Barsanti et al. 1983). Although one may be hesitant to consider collecting a FNA sample from potentially infected tissue, there are no reports in the literature of adverse effects after collection of FNA samples from the prostate with ultrasound guidance in dogs (Root Kustritz 2006).

In dogs with acute prostatitis, there is significant disruption of the prostatic capsule, meaning that almost any antibiotic can penetrate prostatic tissue. In dogs with chronic prostatitis, only those antibiotics that are highly lipid soluble, not highly protein-bound, and ionize at the pH of prostatic tissue will penetrate and remain within the prostate (Dorfman and Barsanti 1995). Fibromuscular stroma separating the lobules within the canine prostate restrict flow of drugs within the tissue (Wientjes et al. 2005). Antibiotics that meet the appropriate criteria include fluoroquinolones, trimethoprim-sulfa combinations, and chloramphenicol. Because chloramphenicol is not routinely stocked in veterinary clinics, the former two classes of drug are most routinely used. Among fluoroquinolones, enrofloxacin and ciprofloxacin have been demonstrated to reach significantly high concentrations

in prostatic tissue (Martiarena and Llorente 1993; Dorfman et al. 1995; Albarellos et al. 2006).

Historically, many publications stressed necessity of measurement of prostatic fluid pH to determine which antibiotics would ionize and remain in tissue. However, it has been demonstrated that pH of prostatic fluid does not differ when comparing normal dogs to those with acute or chronic prostatitis (Barsanti et al. 1983; Threlfall and Chew 1999). Fluoroquinolones are zwitterions, ionizing at multiple pHs, and it has been demonstrated that enrofloxacin moves into the prostate equally well when comparing normal dogs to dogs with chronic bacterial prostatitis (Dorfman et al. 1995).

Initial antibiotic therapy should be instituted for 4–6 weeks. Owners should be made aware that long-term use of trimethoprim-sulfa combinations may be associated with side effects including keratoconjunctivitis sicca, hypothyroidism, and folic acid anemia (Rubin 1990; Torres et al. 1996). Repeat culture of prostatic fluid or tissue should be performed 1 week after antibiotic therapy is completed and, if clear, repeated again one month later. If the underlying cause of prostatitis is not addressed (for example, castrating the dog to control BPH), evaluation for prostatitis should be performed every 3–6 months.

Prostatic abscesses historically were treated surgically, with marsupialization or omentalization of the abscess cavity (Freitag et al. 2007). These procedures require great surgical expertise and are associated with significant side effects. More recently, ultrasound guided aspiration of abscesses has been described, with good long-term success. The regimen includes initial ultrasound-guided drainage with rechecks every 1–6 weeks and repeated drainage if necessary, and supportive antibiotic therapy and castration (Boland et al. 2003). In a study describing eight dogs with prostatic abscesses, the median number of drainage procedures was two, clinical signs resolved in all dogs and no side effects were noted, and there was no recurrence of disease within the follow-up period of up to 5 months (Boland et al. 2003). Another study described ultrasound-guided drainage of prostatic abscesses and subsequent filling of the abscess cavity with tea tree oil in six dogs; 67% of those dogs required two treatments, with complete resolution of clinical signs in all dogs by 6 weeks after initial diagnosis (Kawakami et al. 2006).

Prevention

Because prostatic infection occurs secondary to some other prostate disease, preventative strategies must be associated with prevention of those conditions, for example by use of castration to prevent development of BPH. It has been well demonstrated that castration hastens resolution and prevents recurrence of prostatitis in dogs

(Cowan et al. 1991). Prevention of prostatitis by periodic empirical therapy with antibiotics has not been described and is not recommended so as not to promote development of resistant bacteria.

Paraprostatic cysts

Signalment

Paraprostatic cysts are fluid-filled masses most commonly arising craniolateral or caudal to the prostate. They are hypothesized to be remnants of the embryonic Wolffian ducts (Girard and Despots 1995; Lisciandro 1995). Large and giant breed dogs appear to be over-represented.

Clinical signs

Clinical appearance of disease is not apparent until paraprostatic cysts are very large and impinge on neighboring structures. Clinical signs may include rectal tenesmus and lethargy, with up to 45% of dogs presenting with systemic signs of illness (Stowater and Lamb 1989; Krawiec and Heflin 1992). Urinary tract signs associated with paraprostatic cysts occur in 26% of cases and include stranguria and bloody urethral discharge (Stowater and Lamb 1989; Krawiec and Heflin 1992).

Diagnosis

Abdominal ultrasonography is the preferred technique for identification of paraprostatic cysts and for identification of these masses as separate from the urinary bladder. The cysts are visible as large anechoic structures that may be septate (Stowater and Lamb 1989) (Figure 78.4). Because these masses usually do not directly communicate with the prostatic parenchyma, prostate diagnostics usually are unremarkable (Marquez Black et al. 1998).

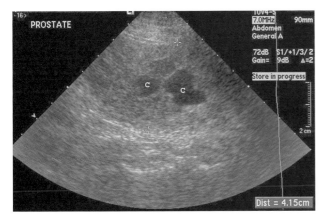

Figure 78.4 Ultrasonongram of canine prostate with associated cysts (C).

Treatment

Surgical excision is the preferred therapy. Surgery may be difficult if the cyst is large or has adhered to adjacent organs (White et al. 1987). Urinary incontinence is an occasional postoperative complication, reported in 9% of dogs in one small study (White et al. 1987).

Prostatic neoplasia

Signalment

Prostatic neoplasia in dogs usually is primary, with malignant adenocarcinoma by far the most common tumor type identified. Incidence of prostatic adenocarcinoma is 0.2–0.6% in dogs (Obradovich et al. 1987; Teske et al. 2002). Benign primary neoplasia of the prostate has not been reported in dogs. Secondary tumors that may localize in the prostate include transitional cell carcinoma, hemangiosarcoma, squamous-cell carcinoma, and lymphosarcoma (Barsanti 1997; Winter et al. 2006; Bryan et al. 2007).

Prostatic neoplasia with or without overlying prostatitis is the only prostate disease seen in castrated dogs. Several studies have demonstrated a 2–4 times increased risk for development of prostatic neoplasia in castrated dogs compared to those left intact (Bell et al. 1991; Teske et al. 2002; Sorenmo et al. 2003; Bryan et al. 2007). Among castrated dogs, Beagles, Bouvier des Flandres, Doberman Pinschers, English Springer Spaniels, German Shorthair Pointers, Scottish Terriers, Shetland Sheepdogs, and West Highland White Terriers are reported to be at increased risk (Teske et al. 2002; Bryan et al. 2007). Cause-and-effects have not been identified. Length of time from castration to diagnosis of prostatic neoplasia is variable and hormone changes identified after castration do not favor angiogenesis (Teske et al. 2002; Shidaifat et al. 2007b). Prostatic neoplasia in dogs is not androgen-dependent (Obradovich et al. 1987; Gallardo et al. 2007). Tumor behavior may be influenced by alterations in estrogen and progesterone receptors in neoplastic tissue compared to normal prostatic tissue or by oxidative stress (Aydin et al. 2006; Grieco et al. 2006; Gallardo et al. 2007). Any castrated dog with prostatomegaly should be considered to have prostatic neoplasia until proven otherwise.

Clinical signs

Prostatic adenocarcinoma most often has metastasized prior to diagnosis. Clinical signs may be referable to the prostate or to sites of metastasis and include anorexia, weight loss, dyschezia, and abdominal pain (Krawiec and Heflin 1992; Winter et al. 2006; Shidaifat et al. 2007b). Most common sites of metastasis are the liver, lungs, regional lymph nodes, vertebrae, spleen, colon or rectum,

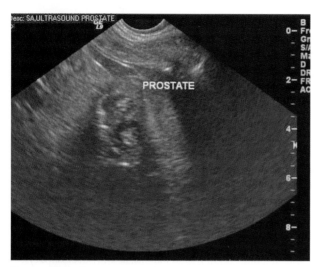

Figure 78.5 Ultrasonogram of canine prostate in dog with prostatic adenocarcinoma.

urethra, urinary bladder, and kidneys (Bell et al. 1991). Urinary tract signs may include stranguria, hematuria, and persistent urinary bladder distension (Krawiec and Heflin 1992; Winter et al. 2006).

Diagnosis

Systemic disease may be evidenced by changes on complete blood count including leukocytosis due to neutrophilia with a left shift, increased alkaline phosphatase (ALP) on chemistry profile, and pyuria and hematuria on urinalysis (Bell et al. 1991). Assessment for metastases by radiography should be performed but owners must be made aware that in 40% of cases with metastases to the lungs, they will not be visible on radiographs (Bell et al. 1991).

Because prognosis in cases with prostatic adenocarcinoma is grave, definitive diagnosis is of paramount importance. Abdominal ultrasonography may reveal the scattered hypoechogenicity of mineralization and a whorled appearance of the parenchyma (Figure 78.5) (Bell et al. 1991). However, these are nonspecific signs. Collection of a FNA or biopsy sample via ultrasound guidance is strongly recommended. Studies have demonstrated that FNA permits accurate diagnosis of prostatic neoplasia in 80% of cases and biopsy in 79–90% of cases (Bell et al. 1991; Nickel and Teske 1992). Biopsy requires sedation of the patient and is most commonly performed using a triggered core biopsy instrument (Tru-Cut, Travenol Laboratories Inc., Deerfield IL).

Treatment

There is no reported cure for prostatic adenocarcinoma in dogs. Total or subtotal prostatectomy is associated with significant decrease in quality of life due to development of urinary incontinence (Basinger et al. 1989; Goldschmid and Bellenger 1991). Prostatectomy using a laser, one-time injection of interleukin-2 and ongoing therapy with meloxicam has been demonstrated in one study to be associated with less postoperative urinary incontinence (L'Eplattenier et al. 2006). Adjunctive therapies, including chemotherapy and intraoperative radiation therapy, are not well described and may not address metastatic disease. Palliative therapy with anti-inflammatory agents has been described; in one study, it was demonstrated that dogs treated with a COX-2 inhibitor had decreased tumor proliferation and inhibition of tumor angiogenesis and had a significantly longer median survival time (Sorenmo et al. 2004). One recommended palliative therapy is piroxicam (0.3 mg/kg per os once daily).

Dogs with urethral obstruction due to prostatic neoplasia at present have few therapeutic options. Percutaneous drainage of the urinary bladder is obviously not a viable long-term solution. Human products that may be of benefit but are not yet clinically readily available in veterinary medicine include button-type urinary fistulas that attach the urinary bladder wall to the body wall and urethral stents (Yoon et al. 2006).

Prevention

Exact cause-and-effect relationship between castration and occurrence of prostatic neoplasia is not described. Although prostatic neoplasia is a high morbidity and mortality disorder, it is of low incidence. The decision regarding whether or not to castrate a dog as a means of prevention against development against prostatic neoplasia when aged must be made on a case-by-case basis.

References

Albarellos, G.A., L. Montoya, et al. (2006). Ciprofloxacin and norfloxacin pharmacokinetics and prostatic fluid penetration in dogs after multiple oral dosing. *Vet J* **172**: 334–339.

Aydin, A., Z. Arsova-Sarafinovska, et al. (2006). Oxidative stress and antioxidant status in non-metastatic prostate cancer and benign prostatic hyperplasia. *Clin Biochem* **39**: 176–179.

Bamberg-Thalen, B. and C. Linde-Forsberg (1993). Treatment of canine benign prostatic hyperplasia with medroxyprogesterone acetate. *J Am Anim Hosp Assoc* **29**: 221–226.

Barsanti, J.A. (1995). Collection and analysis of prostatic fluid and tissue. In: *Canine and Feline Nephrology and Urology*, edited by C.A. Osborne and D.R. Finco. Baltimore, MD: Williams & Wilkins, pp. 122–135.

Barsanti, J.A. (1997). Diseases of the prostate gland. Proceedings, Society for Theriogenology, Montreal Canada, pp. 72–80.

Barsanti, J.A. and D.R. Finco (1979). Canine bacterial prostatitis. *Vet Clin North Am* **9**: 679–700.

Barsanti, J.A. and D.R. Finco (1984). Evaluation of techniques for diagnosis of canine prostatic diseases. *J Am Vet Med Assoc* **185**: 198–200.

Barsanti, J.A., K.W. Prasse, et al. (1983). Evaluation of various techniques for diagnosis of chronic bacterial prostatitis in the dog. *J Am Vet Med Assoc* **183**: 219–224.

Barsanti, J.A., D.R. Finco, et al. (2000). Effects of an extract of *Serenoa repens* on dogs with hyperplasia of the prostate gland. *Am J Vet Res* **61**: 880–885.

Basinger, R.R., C.A. Rawlings, et al. (1989). Urodynamic alterations associated with clinical prostatic diseases and prostatic surgery in 23 dogs. *J Am Anim Hosp Assoc* **25**: 385–392.

Bell, F.W., J.S. Klausner, et al. (1991). Clinical and pathologic features of prostatic adenocarcinoma in sexually intact and castrated dogs: 31 cases (1970–1987). *J Am Vet Med Assoc* **199**: 1623–1630.

Bell, F.W., J.S. Klausner, et al. (1995). Evaluation of serum and seminal plasma markers in the diagnosis of canine prostate disorders. *J Vet Int Med* **9**: 149–153.

Berry, S.J., J.D. Strandberg, et al. (1986). Development of canine benign prostatic hyperplasia with age. *Prostate* **9**: 363–373.

Boland, L.E., R.J. Hardie, et al. (2003). Ultrasound-guided percutaneous drainage as the primary treatment for prostatic abscesses and cysts in dogs. *J Am Anim Hosp Assoc* **39**: 151–159.

Bryan, J.N., M.R. Keeler, et al. (2007). A population study of neutering status as a risk factor for canine prostate cancer. *Prostate* **67**: 1174–1181.

Chuang, Y.C., C.H. Tu, et al. (2006). Intraprostatic injection of botulinum toxin type-A relieves bladder outlet obstruction in human and induces prostate apoptosis in dogs. *BMC Urol* **6**: 12.

Cowan, L.A., J.A. Barsanti, et al. (1991). Effects of castration on chronic bacterial prostatitis in dogs. *J Am Vet Med Assoc* **199**: 346–350.

Dorfman, M., J. Barsanti, et al. (1995). Enrofloxacin concentrations in dogs with normal prostate and dogs with chronic bacterial prostatitis. *Am J Vet Res* **56**: 386–390.

Dorfman, M. and J.A. Barsanti (1995). CVT update: treatment of canine bacterial prostatitis. In: *Current Veterinary Therapy XII*, edited by J.D. Bonagura and R.W. Kirk. Philadelphia, PA: WB Saunders, pp. 1029–1032.

Freitag, T., R.M. Jerram, et al. (2007). Surgical management of common canine prostatic conditions. *Comp Cont Ed* **29**: 656–673.

Gallardo, F., T. Mogas, et al. (2007). Expression of androgen, oestrogen alpha and beta, and progesterone receptors in the canine prostate: differences between normal, inflamed, hyperplastic and neoplastic glands. *J Comp Path* **136**: 1–8.

Girard, C. and J. Despots (1995). Mineralized paraprostatic cyst in a dog. *Can Vet J* **36**: 573–574.

Goldschmid, S.E. and C.R. Bellenger (1991). Urinary incontinence after prostatectomy in dogs. *Vet Surg* **20**: 253–256.

Grieco, V., E. Riccardi, et al. (2006). The distribution of oestrogen receptors in normal, hyperplastic and neoplastic canine prostate, as demonstrated immunohistochemically. *J Comp Path* **135**: 11–16.

Grino, P.B., J.E. Griffin, et al. (1990). Testosterone at high concentrations interacts with the human androgen receptor similarly to dihydrotestosterone. *Endocrinology* **126**: 1165–1172.

Iguer-Ouada, M., and J.P. Verstegen (1997). Effect of finasteride (Proscar MSD) on seminal composition, prostate function and fertility in male dogs. *J Rep Fert* **51**: 139–149.

Jia, G., J.T. Heverhagen, et al. (2006). Pharmacokinetic parameters as a potential predictor of response to pharmacotherapy in benign prostatic hyperplasia: a preclinical trial using dynamic contrast-enhanced MRI. *Mag Res Imaging* **24**: 721–725.

Johnston, G.R. and D.A. Feeney (1986). Radiographic evaluation of the urinary tract in dogs and cats. In: *Contemporary Issues in Small Animal Practice (Nephrology and Urology)*, edited by E.B. Breitschwerdt. New York: Churchill Livingstone, pp. 203–273.

Johnston, S.D., K. Kamolpatana, et al. (2000). Prostatic disorders in the dog. *Anim Repro Sci* **60–61**: 405–415.

Johnston, S.D., M.V. Root Kustritz, et al. (2001). Semen collection, evaluation, and preservation. In: *Canine and Feline Theriogenology*, edited by S.D. Johnston, M.V. Root Kustritz, and P.N.S. Olson. Philadelphia, PA: WB Saunders, pp. 289–306.

Kawakami, E., M. Washizu, et al. (2006). Treatment of prostatic abscesses by aspiration of purulent matter and injection with tea tree oil into the cavities of dogs. *J Vet Med Sci* **68**: 1215–1217.

Krawiec, D.R. and D. Heflin. (1992). Study of prostatic disease in dogs: 177 cases (1981–1986). *J Am Vet Med Assoc* **200**: 1119–1122.

L'Eplattenier, H.F., S.A. VanNimwegen, et al. (2006). Partial prostatectomy using Nd:YAG laser for management of canine prostatic carcinoma. *Vet Surg* **35**: 406–411.

Ling, G.V., J.E. Branam, et al. (1983). Canine prostatic fluid: techniques of collection, quantitative bacterial culture, and interpretation of results. *J Am Vet Med Assoc* **183**: 201–206.

Lisciandro, G.R. (1995). What is your diagnosis? (Paraprostatic cyst in a dog). *J Am Vet Med Assoc* **206**: 171–172.

Liu, J.B., D.A. Merton, et al. (2006). Contrast-enhanced ultrasound for radio frequency ablation of canine prostates: initial results. *J Urol* **176**: 1654–1660.

Marquez Black, G., G.V. Ling, et al. (1998). Prevalence of prostatic cysts in adult, large breed dogs. *J Am Anim Hosp Assoc* **34**: 17–180.

Martiarena, B.M. and P. Llorente (1993). Ciprofloxacin as antibiotic treatment in bacterial prostatitis. *Rev Med Vet Buenos Aires* **74**: 130–136.

Merk, F.B., M.J. Warhol, et al. (1986). Multiple phenotypes of glandular cells in castrated dogs after individual or combined treatment with androgen and estrogen. Morphometric, ultrastructural, and cytochemical distinctions. *Lab Invest* **54**: 442–456.

Mukaratirwa, S. and T. Chitura (2007). Canine subclinical prostatic disease: histological prevalence and validity of digital rectal examination as a screening test. *J So Afr Vet Assoc* **78**: 66–68.

Nickel, R.F. and E. Teske (1992). Diagnosis of canine prostatic carcinoma. *Tidjschrift Voor Diergeneeskunde* **117** (Suppl 1): 32S.

O'Shea, J.D. (1962). Studies on the canine prostate gland. I. Factors influencing its size and weight. *J Comp Path* **72**: 321–331.

Obradovich, J., R. Walshaw, et al. (1987). The influence of castration on the development of prostatic carcinoma in the dog: 43 cases (1978–1985). *J Vet Int Med* **1**: 183–187.

Olson, P.N. (1984). Disorders of the canine prostate gland. Proceedings, Society for Theriogenology, Denver, CO, pp. 46–59.

Powe, J.R., P.J. Canfield, et al. (2004). Evaluation of the cytologic diagnosis of canine prostatic disorders. *Vet Clin Pathol* **33**: 150–154.

Read, R.A. and S. Bryden (1995). Urethral bleeding as a presenting sign of benign prostatic hyperplasia in the dog: a retrospective study (1979–1993). *J Am Anim Hosp Assoc* **31**: 261–267.

Rhodes, L. (1996). The role of dihydrotestosterone in prostate physiology: comparisons among rats, dogs and primates. *Proceedings, Society for Theriogenology*, Kansas City, MO, pp. 124–135.

Root Kustritz, M.V. (2006). Collection of tissue and culture samples from the canine reproductive tract. *Theriogenology* **66**: 567–574.

Root Kustritz, M.V., S.D. Johnston, et al. (2005). Relationship between inflammatory cytology of canine seminal fluid and significant aerobic bacterial, anaerobic bacterial or mycoplasma cultures of canine seminal fluid: 95 cases (1987–2000). *Theriogenology* **64**: 1333–1339.

Rubin, S.I. (1990). Managing dogs with bacterial prostatic disease. *Vet Med* **85**: 387–394.

Sasaki, K., T. Azuma, et al. (2006). Chronic effect of transrectal split-focus ultrasound ablation on canine prostatic tissue. *J Vet Med Sci* **68**: 839–845.

Shafik, A., A.A. Shafik, et al. (2006). Contractile activity of the prostate at ejaculation: an electrophysiologic study. *Urol* **67**: 793–796.

Shidaifat, F., M. Daradka, et al. (2004). Effect of androgen ablation on prostatic cell differentiation in dogs. *Endo Res* **30**: 327–334.

Shidaifat, F., B. Al-Trad, et al. (2007a). Testosterone effect on immature prostate gland development associated with suppression of transforming growth factor-beta. *Life Sci* **80**: 829–834.

Shidaifat, F., M. Gharaibeh, et al. (2007b). Effect of castration on extracellular matrix remodeling and angiogenesis of the prostate gland. *Endo J* **54**: 521–529.

Sirinarumitr, K., S.D. Johnston, et al. (2001). Effects of finasteride on size of the prostate gland and semen quality in dogs with benign prostatic hypertrophy. *J Am Vet Med Assoc* **218**: 1275–1280.

Sirinarumitr, K., T. Sirinarumitr, et al. (2002). Finasteride-induced prostatic involution by apoptosis in dogs with benign prostatic hypertrophy. *Am J Vet Res* **63**: 495–498.

Soki, J., E. Fodor, et al. (2002). Isolation and characterization of an imipenem-resistant *Bacteroides fragilis* strain from a prostate abscess in a dog. *Vet Micro* **84**: 187–190.

Sorenmo, K.U., M. Goldschmidt, et al. (2003). Immunohistochemical characterization of canine prostatic carcinoma and correlation with castration status and castration time. *Vet Comp Oncol* **1**: 48–56.

Sorenmo, K.U., M.H. Goldschmidt, et al. (2004). Evaluation of cyclooxygenase-1 and cyclooxygenase-2 expression and the effect of cyclooxygenase inhibitors in canine prostatic carcinoma. *Vet Comp Oncol* **2**: 13–23.

Stowater, J.L. and C.R. Lamb (1989). Ultrasonographic features of paraprostatic cysts in nine dogs. *Vet Rad* **30**: 232–239.

Teske, E., E.C. Naan, et al. (2002). Canine prostatic carcinoma: epidemiological evidence of an increased risk in castrated dogs. *Mol Cell Endo* **197**: 251–255.

Threlfall, W.R. and D.J. Chew (1999). Diagnosis and treatment of canine bacterial prostatitis. *Comp Cont Ed* **21**: 73–88.

Torres, S.M.F., P.J. McKeever, et al. (1996). Hypothyroidism in a dog associated with trimethoprim-sulphadiazine therapy. *Vet Derm* **7**: 105–108.

White, R.A.S., M.E. Herrtage, et al. (1987). The diagnosis and management of paraprostatic and prostatic retention cysts in the dog. *J Small Anim Prac* **28**: 551–574.

Wientjes, M.G., J.H. Zheng, et al. (2005). Intraprostatic chemotherapy: distribution and transport mechanisms. *Clin Cancer Res* **11**: 4204–4211.

Winter, M.D., J.E. Locke, et al. (2006). Imaging diagnosis—urinary obstruction secondary to prostatic lymphoma in a young dog. *Vet Rad Ultrasound* **47**: 597–601.

Yoon, C.J., H.Y. Song, et al. (2006). Covered retrievable prostatic urethral stents: feasibility study in a canine model. *J Vasc Interv Radiol* **17**: 1813–1819.

79

Neoplasia of the lower urinary tract

Jeffrey Phillips

Urinary system tumors include benign and malignant neoplasia of the kidney, bladder, urethra, and tumors that arise from accessory sexual glands in the male. Traditionally, these neoplasms have been treated with surgery only with prognosis dependent on tumor type, clinical stage, location, and surgical resectability. Unfortunately, in both human and veterinary oncology, effective surgical treatment of these tumors, especially those of the lower urinary system, can be quite difficult because of anatomic constraints. Thus, for nonresectable tumors, incompletely resected tumors, or tumors associated with significant metastatic risk, adjuvant treatments such as chemotherapy are important modalities. Addition of such treatments has provided modest improvements in survival and in some cases significant palliative benefits.

Tumors of the urinary bladder and urethra

Tumors of the urinary bladder and urethra are uncommon in dogs accounting for ~1% of all canine neoplasms (Osborne et al. 1968). One retrospective study evaluated medical records from 13 veterinary universities from 1964 to 1975 and identified only 114 cases of primary canine bladder malignancy (Hayes 1976). In cats, tumors of the lower urinary tract system are seen less frequently and are uniformly malignant (Osborne et al. 1968; Sapierzynski et al. 2007).

Signalment for dogs and cats is predictable with the majority of patients middle-aged to older. Breed predisposition for development of canine bladder tumors has been described in the Airedale terrier, Scottish terrier, Westhighland white terrier, Beagle, and Sheltie being significantly over-represented while German Shepherds and

Golden Retrievers are under-represented (Hayes 1976; Norris et al. 1992; Sapierzynski et al. 2007). Several reports suggest a gender predilection for these tumors in female dogs (Strafuss and Dean 1975; Hayes 1976); however, more recent reports fail to identify a gender preference (Norris et al. 1992; Sapierzynski et al. 2007). No breed or gender predilections have been described for development of feline lower urinary tract tumors.

The majority of canine lower urinary tract tumors are malignant (approximately 95%) although benign mesenchymal variants have been reported. Histologic tumor types seen in cats and dogs include transitional cell carcinoma (approximately 90% of cases), squamous cell carcinoma (approximately 1%), adeno- and undifferentiated carcinoma (approximately 1%), and a variety of mesenchymal tumors (approximately 7%) (Meuten 2002). Benign tumor types have only been reported in dogs and include fibroma and leiomyoma.

Secondary neoplasms involving the bladder have also been reported in cats and dogs. The most common secondary tumors involving the bladder are extensions of prostatic and urethral tumors although differentiation from a primary bladder origin with urethral extension is difficult. Other secondary bladder tumors include metastatic lesions from mesenchymal and, more commonly, epithelial tumors. Lymphoma involving primarily the urinary bladder has also been reported in cats and dogs although this comprises less than 1/3 of all secondary neoplasms of the bladder (Meuten 2002).

Clinical signs seen in dogs with bladder tumors are consist of lower urinary tract symptoms such as hematuria, pollakiuria, or dysuria (88%) and less frequently polyuria, polydipsia, and incontinence (Norris et al. 1992). Nonlower urinary tract signs include lameness due to bony metastases, abdominal pain, and lethargy (Norris et al. 1992). In cats, lower urinary tract symptoms include hematuria (76%), stranguria (40%), pollakiuria

Nephrology and Urology of Small Animals. Edited by Joe Bartges and David J. Polzin. © 2011 Blackwell Publishing Ltd.

(35%), urinary tract obstruction (14%), and inappropriate urination (14%) (Wilson et al. 2007).

Hematologic findings in dogs with primary bladder tumors include neutrophilia (20%) and anemia (8%). Serum chemistry abnormalities include elevated liver enzyme activity (45%), azotemia (13%), and hypercalcemia (5%) (Norris et al. 1992). In cats, no consistent hematologic changes have been described; however, at presentation up to 50% of cats have been reported to be azotemic (Wilson et al. 2007). Urinalysis results are typically abnormal in both dogs (93%) and cats (80%) with >50% of all patients exhibiting active urinary tract infections (Norris et al. 1992; Wilson et al. 2007). Paraneoplastic syndromes seen in patients with bladder tumors include hypercalcemia, hypertrophic osteopathy, hyperestrogenism, cachexia, immune-mediated thrombocytopenia and/or anemia, and polycythemia (Caywood et al. 1980; Norris et al. 1992). Further information on each of the specific subtypes of primary lower urinary tract tumors is presented in the following sections.

Epithelial tumors of the lower urinary tract

The majority of epithelial neoplasms of the lower urinary tract are considered malignant; however, benign conditions such as polypoid cystitis and fibroepithelial polyps have also been described (Martinez et al. 2003; Patrick et al. 2006). These benign conditions are characterized by inflammation, epithelial proliferation, and development of polypoid masses. Importantly, there is no evidence that these represent preneoplastic lesions (Martinez et al. 2003). Because these lesions are generally classified as inflammatory rather than neoplastic lesions, only malignant epithelial neoplasms will be discussed.

Transitional cell carcinoma

Transitional cell carcinoma is the most common tumor of the lower urinary tract in cats and dogs accounting for >90% of cases (Norris et al. 1992). Other tumor types include squamous cell carcinoma, adenocarcinoma, and undifferentiated carcinoma. Because there are no unique clinical features associated with the different epithelial malignancies, only transitional cell carcinoma is presented. Transitional cell carcinoma is locally invasive and has a moderate metastatic rate with >50% of dogs and >20% of cats exhibiting evidence of metastases at time of death (Norris et al. 1992; Wilson et al. 2007). Affected dogs and cats are middle-aged to older with a median age of onset of 10 years in dogs and 15 years in cats. In dogs, there is a well-recognized breed predilection with Shelties, Scottish terriers, and Westhighland white terriers (amongst other breeds) being significantly overrepresented (Norris et al. 1992). No breed preference has

been identified in cats. Female dogs were thought to be at increased risk for the development of these tumors historically, although more recent studies have failed to support this. In cats, no gender bias has been identified.

There are several proposed mechanisms that underlie development of canine bladder tumors. The high prevalence of these tumors in select breeds suggests a genetic basis at least in some breeds. Ongoing research at the National Cancer Institute is trying to identify a genetic variant associated with tumor development in these select breeds. Environmental factors have also been shown to be associated with canine bladder tumor development. In one study, topical insecticide exposure increased risk by up to 3.5/year (Glickman et al. 1989) although another study failed to identify a similar increased risk within Scottish terriers (Raghavan et al. 2004). A study examining risk associated with herbicide exposure and bladder tumor formation (in Scottish terriers) noted increased risk (odds ratio, 4.42) in exposed dogs. Furthermore, this risk was increased (odds ratio, 7.19) for dogs exposed to both herbicides and insectides (Glickman et al. 2004). Other genetic and/or environmental factors that may be associated with increased risk of bladder tumor formation include obesity, cyclophosphamide usage, and exposure to aromatic amines (Glickman et al. 1989); however, current veterinary literature fails to document these associations. To date, no risk factors have been identified in the cat.

Histology of canine and feline urothelial tumors is divided based on local growth pattern into flat lesions and papillary neoplasms (which project into the lumen) (Table 79.1; Patrick et al. 2006).

Flat lesions are considered reactive, dysplastic, carcinoma in situ, or overtly neoplastic and likely comprise <20% of lesions (Knapp et al. 2000a). Only overtly neoplastic lesions are truly invasive and there is some disagreement on their prevalence (Meuten 2002; Patrick et al. 2006). Papillary lesions comprise infiltrating (90%) and noninfiltrating (10%) variants (Knapp et al. 2000a). Noninfiltrating variants are uncommon and relatively low-grade malignancies, while infiltrative variants (flat and papillary) are the most common urothelial tumor and of high-grade malignancy.

Flat and papillary noninfiltrating lesions are locally extensive but do not invade the bladder wall stroma and are unlikely to metastasize. While these are traditionally considered either benign proliferations or low-grade malignancies, progression to more aggressive types commonly occurs, especially among patients with carcinoma in situ. Infiltrating lesions of papillary and nonpapillary forms are highly invasive locally and typically involve the lamina propria and/or the muscularis propria (Patrick et al. 2006). Typical location of lesions (regardless of

Table 79.1 Histologic variants and malignant potential of canine urothelial tumors (Meuten 2002; Patrick et al. 2006)

Type of lesion	Growth pattern	Malignant potential
Flat (nonpapillary)		
Dysplatic, reactive, etc.	Confined to mucosa	None
Carcinoma in situ	Confined to mucosa	May progress to overtly malignant
Infiltrative	Involve mucosa and deeper layers	Highly malignant
Papillary (luminal growth)		
Papilloma	Confined to mucosa	None
Noninfiltrative	Involve mucosa ± substantia propria	Metastases unlikely, may progress to more aggressive types
Infiltrative	Most common variant that involves mucosa and deeper layers	Highly malignant

histology) in cats and dogs is fairly predictable. The majority of canine patients develop tumors in the region of the trigone with up to 50% of male patients having prostatic involvement (Figure 79.1) (Hayes 1976).

In cats, more than half of patients develop tumors in the ventral aspect of the bladder (Wilson et al. 2007). Regardless of primary tumor location, many cats and dogs have or will develop other intravesicular disease sites. Furthermore, there is some support to the concept of "field cancerization" when assessing local extent of these tumors. This concept implies that the entire urothelial mucosa has been exposed to some inciting source of preneoplastic changes and is thus at risk of transforming into overtly neoplastic mucosa. While the true inciting source is unknown, this concept can be used to explain the multifocal growth patterns of most tumors (Figure 79.2).

With respect to systemic behavior, invasive lesions have high metastatic rates with up to 50% of dogs and at least 20% of cats exhibiting metastatic disease at the time of death (Norris et al. 1992; Wilson et al. 2007). Common metastatic sites in dogs include lungs (51%), sublumbar lymph nodes (48%), urethra and prostate (50%), and bony sites (10%) (Norris et al. 1992; Wilson et al. 2007). Staging tests recommended for patients with bladder tumors include complete blood cell counts, serum chemistry, urinalysis, urine culture, abdominal ultrasonography, and thoracic and abdominal radiography. Ancillary tests include double-contrast cystography, cystoscopy, urine sediment analysis, and tumor biopsy (Figure 79.3).

A presumptive diagnosis of transitional cell carcinoma can be obtained through a combination of signalment, imaging results, and cytologic or histologic tumor analysis. Cytologic diagnosis can be accomplished with urine sediment, traumatic catheterization, or percutaneous needle aspiration. Urine sediment analysis is the

preferred method of diagnosis and successfully identifies 30–50% of affected dogs (Chapters 7 and 26) (Norris et al. 1992). "Traumatic" urethral catheterization and/or prostatic/urethral washes can also be useful, diagnosing up to 90% of affected dogs (Norris et al. 1992). Percutaneous transabdominal aspiration cytology of bladder tumors, however, should be avoided due to risk (albeit low-risk of approximately 1–3%) of needle-tract tumor implantation (Nyland et al. 2002; Vignoli et al. 2007). Cystoscopic evaluation and tumor biopsy can be helpful in dogs with early-stage flat and/or noninfiltrating lesions (Chapter 19).

A noninvasive screening test that has proven useful in select cases is the veterinary bladder tumor antigen test. This test is a rapid latex agglutination dipstick test that detects the presence of "bladder tumor analytes" (Billet et al. 2002). While the sensitivity of this test is quite high for detection of bladder tumors (85–90%), specificity is quite low, especially in dogs with nonneoplastic lower urinary tract disease (35–41%) (Billet et al. 2002; Henry et al. 2003a). Because of low specificity, the test is most suited to rule out the presence of lower urinary tract neoplasia. In this setting, the negative predictive value can be as high as 99% (Henry et al. 2003a). Results of all clinical staging diagnostics are used to determine WHO tumor stage (Table 79.2).

Treatment options

Treatment of choice for any solid tumor of the bladder is surgical resection. This approach is complicated in veterinary patients by two factors; the majority of clinical patients present with extensive (nonresectable, stage III) disease, and the concept of "field cancerization" leads to high recurrence rates (up to 70% in humans). Those patients who truly have lower clinical stages (I and perhaps II) are potential candidates for local therapies. Local

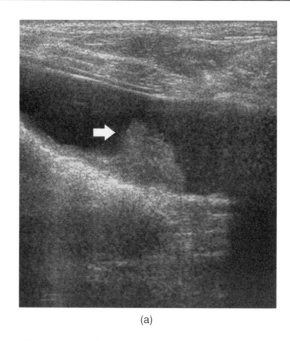

(a)

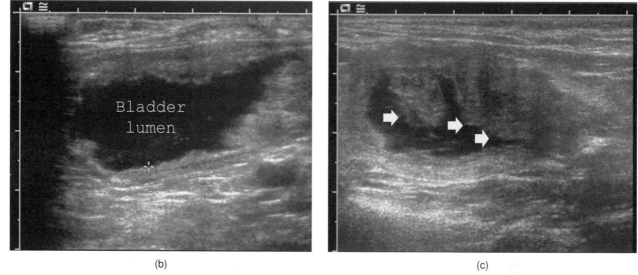

(b)   (c)

Figure 79.1 (a) Ultrasound image of a canine transitional cell carcinoma showing typical trigonal location of tumors, note papillary infiltrative growth (arrow). (b) Ultrasound image of a canine transitional cell carcinoma illustrating multifocal growth pattern (nonpapillary infiltrative). (c) Ultrasound image of a feline transitional cell carcinoma located in the ventral portion of the bladder (arrows).

therapeutic options include mucosal resection, photo-dynamic therapy, laser ablation, radiation therapy, and partial or complete cystectomy. The typical patients with advanced local and/or systemic disease are candidates for palliative techniques such as chemotherapy (systemic and intravesicular), NSAIDs, cystotomy tube placement, and urethral dissection or stent placement (Chapter 32).

Mucosal resection is a transurethral technique useful only for small and noninfiltrative lesions. This technique entails endoscopic visualization of the affected region followed by either electrosurgical or laser resection of the lesion (Chapters 19 and 39). While this approach is appli-

cable for humans, where more than 75% will present with early-stage disease, most veterinary patients have invasive tumors that cannot be resected using these techniques. Photodynamic therapy and carbon dioxide laser ablation have similar indications as mucosal resection and thus have only been used on an experimental basis in canine patients (Nseyo et al. 1993; Upton et al. 2006).

Several reports have described use of radiation therapy for the treatment of canine bladder tumors (Withrow et al. 1989; DeLuca et al. 1994; Poirier et al. 2004; Murphy et al. 2008). Single-dose intraoperative and multidose (fractionated) protocols have been used.

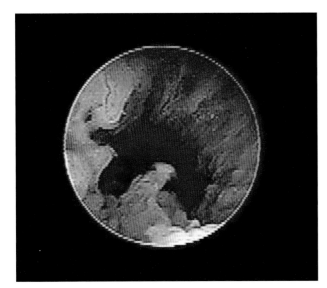

Figure 79.2 Cystoscopic image of a transitional cell carcinoma of the bladder.

Toxicities ranged from minimal (hematuria, pollakiuria, colitis) to severe signs, such as secondary tumor formation (rhabdomyosarcoma), bladder fibrosis, urethral stenosis, colonic perforation, and ureter stenosis. While toxicity increased with dosage, there was no clear relationship between protocol used, dose per treatment, and side effects. Newer approaches have attempted to minimize toxicity while maximizing tumor dosage. These methods involve techniques to maintain constant bladder (and thus tumor) position along with intertreatment target repositioning with CT guidance to maximize tumor and minimize normal tissue dosage (Murphy et al. 2008). Overall, clinical responses with radiation therapy

is less than 20% and efficacy for improving survival is unknown.

Surgical methods for treatment of bladder tumors include both partial and complete cystectomies. Unfortunately, the majority of veterinary patients will not be appropriate candidates for these methods due to advanced clinical stage and tumor location within the trigonal region. While the trigonal location of most canine tumors is not amenable to partial resections, other locations in patients with early stage disease may be considered. In a series of 11 canine patients, partial cystectomies (±chemotherapy) encompassing 40 and 70% of the bladder was performed (Stone et al. 1996). Local recurrence was documented or suspected in 9 dogs and median overall survival was 12 months.

Techniques for complete cystectomy and ureteral diversion have also been described. These include subtotal cystectomies with uretero-colonic anastomosis, regenerative urinary bladder augmentation using small intestinal submucosa, and other (nonpublished) methods to create a pseudo bladder from a hydronephrotic kidney (Pope et al. 1997; Stone et al. 1988). The uterero-colonic diversion approach, while successful in eliminating all gross tumor, is associated with severe metabolic complications such as hyperammonemia, metabolic acidosis, and azotemia. In one series of ten dogs treated with this approach, median survival was <2 months and 6/10 dogs died with evidence of metastatic disease (Stone et al. 1988).

Perhaps a more promising approach utilizes small intestinal submucosal grafts as a scaffold to allow bladder augmentation and regeneration. These grafts have been shown to allow for successful regeneration of 40–60% of the bladder in a period of 8–12 weeks following subtotal

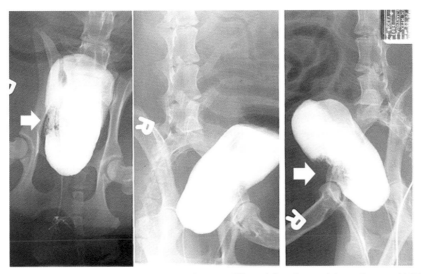

Figure 79.3 Double contrast cystogram demonstrating trigonal region filling defect (arrows) in an 8 year old SF Mixed breed dog with transitional cell carcinoma.

Table 79.2 Clinical stages (TNM) of canine and feline bladder tumors (Owen 1980)

T: Primary tumor	
Tis: Carcinoma in situ	T2: Tumour invading the bladder wall, with induration
T0: No evidence of tumour	T3: Tumour invading neighboring structures
T1: Superficial papillary tumour	
N: Regional lymph nodes (RLN)	
N0: No evidence of RLN involvement	N2: RLN and juxta RLN involved
N1: RLN involved	
M: Distant metastasis	
M0: No evidence of distant metastasis	M1: Distant metastasis detected
TNM roups	Clinical stage
T1 or T2, N0, M0	I
T1 or T2, N1, M0	II
T1 or T2, N2 or N3, M0; T3 or T4, any N, M0	III
Any TN, M1	IV

cystectomy (Kropp et al. 1996). Morbidity associated with this approach is low in healthy dogs; however, in tumor-bearing dogs (with incomplete resections), the graft can serve as a scaffold for tumor regrowth. No case series have described outcome associated with this or any other surgical approaches for subtotal cystectomy. While the more aggressive techniques are interesting, they are perhaps more applicable to cats who occasionally present with resectable tumors; the overwhelming number of dogs present with Stage III (nonresectable) disease and are thus not candidates for curative approaches.

Clinical symptoms seen in patients with advanced disease include pollakiuria, hematuria, urethral obstruction, and pain. Fortunately, there are a variety of approaches that can successfully address these symptoms. Historically, chemotherapy is the most widely used treatment for palliative therapy and has included doxorubicin, cyclophosphamide, carboplatin, cisplatin, taxol, mitomycin C, mitoxantrone, and gemcitabine (Moore et al. 1990; Helfand et al. 1994; Chun et al. 1996; Chun et al. 1997; Knapp et al. 2000a; Henry et al. 2003b; Kosarek et al. 2005). In many instances, these drugs have been used in intravenous systemic protocols and for intravesicular treatments. Of these agents, only intravenous cisplatin therapy has documented activity as a single agent with response rates up to 25% noted (Moore et al. 1990; Chun et al. 1996; Knapp et al. 2000a, 2000b; Mohammed et al. 2003). Objective responses, however, may not be appropriate measurement endpoints in palliative medicine. Amelioration of symptoms and improved quality of life measures are probably more important in palliative medicine but are difficult to objectively measure in veterinary patients.

Non-steroidal anti-inflammatory drugs (NSAIDs) are the most commonly used agent for palliation of symp-

toms in dogs with bladder tumors. In addition to effective analgesics, NSAIDs (cyclo-oxygenase (COX) inhibitors) appear to have antitumor properties with bladder tumors. On the basis of immunohistochemical studies, a high percentage (up to 100%) of canine transitional cell carcinomas have been shown to aberrantly express COX-1 and COX-2 enzymes (Knottenbelt et al. 2006), making them attractive targets for therapy. Several studies have examined antitumor activity of the NSAID, piroxicam (0.3 mg/kg per day in dogs), and response rates of 18–33% have been noted (Knapp et al. 1994; Mohammed et al. 2002). More recently, investigators have examined usage of combination protocols involving piroxicam and cytotoxic chemotherapeutics such as mitoxantrone and cisplatin (Henry et al. 2003b; Mohammed et al. 2003). Combinations are well tolerated with dose-limiting toxicities of azotemia and myelosuppression. Evidence from these studies suggests a synergistic combination with response rates of 33–75%. Furthermore, there is at least initial evidence suggesting a survival benefit for dogs treated with combination of piroxicam and chemotherapy.

Other methods that have been described for palliation of bladder tumors directly address management of urine outflow obstruction and include permanent cystostomy catheter placement, urethral stent placement, and urethral dissection (Chapter 32). Permanent cystostomy tubes are the most common method used to relieve urine outflow obstructions (Figure 79.4).

Complications are minimal with the most frequent being urinary tract infection (Smith et al. 1995). Palliative stenting involves placement of expandable metallic stents in obstructed urethral segments. These are generally placed under fluoroscopic guidance and are associated with slightly higher complication rates compared to

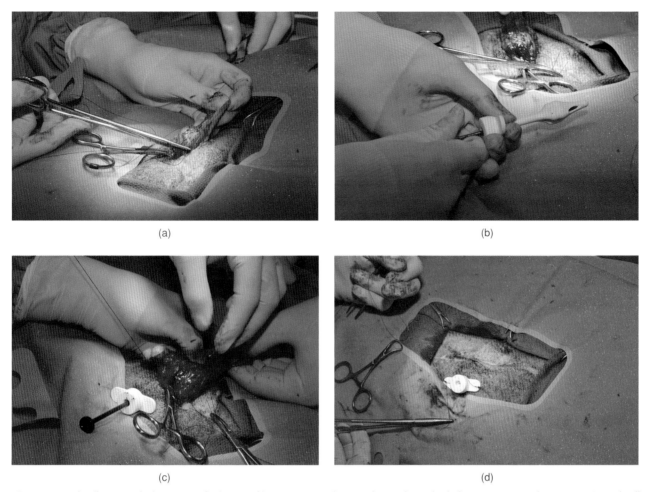

(a)

(b)

(c)

(d)

Figure 79.4 (a–d): Surgical placement of a low-profile cystotomy tube in a dog with urethral obstruction secondary to transitional cell carcinoma of the bladder and urethra. (Photographs courtesy of Dr. Karen Tobias.)

cystostomy tube placement, including recurrent obstruction, urethral tear, and recurrent infections (Weisse et al. 2006). Urethral dissection techniques involve surgically removing neoplastic tissue from the luminal aspect of the urethral obstruction (via electrocautery loops and other methods). One case series described outcome associated with this technique and suggested relatively high complication rates, especially in female dogs (Liptak et al. 2004).

Prognosis

Overall prognosis for dogs and cats diagnosed with bladder tumors is guarded. In select canine and feline patients with early stage disease, surgery may be considered. Median survival for dogs treated with partial cystectomy is approximately 1 year (Stone et al. 1996); however, most patients have advanced disease and are candidates for palliative therapy only. Reported median survival for patients treated with palliative protocols ranges from 132 days to approximately 1 year for dogs

and 261 days for cats (Rocha et al. 2000; Wilson et al. 2007). Objective responses and survival duration may not be the most appropriate measure of success in treated patients, especially in the palliative setting. Amelioration of symptoms is probably the most important measure and can be achieved in up to 75% of patients treated with combinations of chemotherapy and piroxicam for a median duration of 194 days (Henry et al. 2003b). Finally, prognostic factors associated with improved outcome in dogs include gender (spayed females Median Survival Time (MST) = 358 days versus neutered males MST = 145 days) and chemotherapy protocol (anthracycline plus platinum MST = 358 days versus platinum alone MST = 132 days). No prognostic factors have been identified in cats.

Mesenchymal tumors of the lower urinary tract

Mesenchymal bladder tumors are uncommon and account for approximately 10% of cases (Strafuss and

Dean 1975). In dogs, benign variants include leiomyoma and fibroma and malignant variants include leiomyosarcoma, fibrosarcoma, rhabdomyosarcoma, and rarely hemangiosarcoma. In cats, only smooth muscle variants (leiomyoma and leiomyosarcoma) have been described. Affected patients are typically middle-aged with no gender or breed predilection. Clinical symptoms include hematuria (>90% of cases), pollakiuria, and dysuria (Epslin 1987).

Fibroma and fibrosarcoma

Fibromas and fibrosarcomas are the most common benign and malignant mesenchymal tumors of the canine bladder. Tumors occur in various sites within the bladder while originating from the bladder wall. Fibromas expand between the muscle layers while fibrosarcomas invade between these tissues and can protrude into the lumen. In addition to being locally invasive, fibrosarcomas have been reported to metastasize, although the overall metastatic rate is unknown (Olausson et al. 2005).

Standard staging diagnostics are recommended as discussed for epithelial tumors. Following complete staging, treatment of choice in appropriate patients is surgical resection. Patients with advanced disease either locally or systemically can be treated with palliative chemotherapy agents such as doxorubicin, although benefit is unknown. Prognosis for dogs with benign tumors is excellent. In one case series of 51 dogs with fibromas treated surgically, 46 dogs had a complete resolution of symptoms with no reported tumor recurrence (Epslin 1987). Prognosis for dogs with fibrosarcomas is unknown due to paucity of reported cases.

Leiomyoma and leiomyosarcoma

Smooth muscle tumors of the urinary bladder are rare but have been described in cats and dogs (Burk et al. 1975; Strafuss and Dean 1975; Heng et al. 2006). As with other mesenchymal tumors, smooth muscle tumors involve primarily the bladder wall but can protrude into the lumen. Metastases have also been reported in dogs with leiomyosarcomas, but are thought to be rare. Staging diagnostics and treatment options are identical to those described for fibromas and fibrosarcomas. Prognosis for dogs and cats with smooth muscle tumors is unknown.

Rhabdomyosarcoma

Rhabdomyosarcomas are uncommon but have been reported in dogs and rarely in cats (Osborne et al. 1968; Strafuss and Dean 1975). They arise from skeletal muscle of the urethra and fundus or undifferentiated mes-

enchymal tissue within the bladder (Chapter 80). Rhabdomyosarcomas grow by local invasion into the bladder wall with extension into the luminal aspect. Gross appearance of the luminal growths often resemble grape-like bunches; giving rise to the term "botyroid" tumors. In addition to being locally invasive, rhabdomyosarcomas appear to have moderate to high metastatic rates based on case reports, although similar to other mesenchymal tumors the true metastatic rate is unknown (Stamps and Harris 1968; Halliwell and Ackerman 1974; Pletcher and Dalton 1981; Kim et al. 1996; Kuwamura et al. 1998; Takiguchi et al. 2002; Bae et al. 2007).

Affected patients are young with all reported dogs being <2 years old at time of diagnosis. Older reports suggested a breed predilection among Basset Hounds and Saint Bernards; however, reports over the last 10 years have failed to support this and describe a wide variety of breeds. A strong gender preference does appear to exist with females being affected more than twice as often as males. Common clinical signs include hematuria and hypertrophic osteopathy. A presumptive diagnosis can often be made based on signalment, clinical signs, and imaging results.

Staging diagnostics include standard recommendations described for other lower urinary tract tumors. Following complete staging treatment options include either surgical resection or palliative therapy. Because of the anatomic localization within the urethra, surgical resection is often not feasible; however, successful resection has been described for tumors within the bladder itself (Takiguchi et al. 2002). Because of the presumed moderate-high metastatic rate, chemotherapy is indicated following surgery with doxorubicin being a reasonable choice. Recommendations for palliative therapy are identical to those described for other bladder tumors with the goal of alleviating symptoms; however, no information is available regarding efficacy of these palliative approaches. Prognosis for dogs with rhabdomyosarcomas of the urinary bladder is unknown. No information is available regarding the treatment of these tumors in cats.

Secondary tumors of the lower urinary tract

Unlike secondary renal tumors, secondary or metastatic tumors to the bladder and urethra occur uncommonly. The most common secondary tumors include lymphoma and extension of tumors originating from surrounding organs such as the prostate, uterus, and rectum.

Lymphoma of the lower urinary tract

Primary lymphoma involving the urinary bladder and/or prostate has been described, but in general most cases represent part of a more generalized lymphoma (Struble et al. 1997; van Noort 1997; Maiolino and DeVico 2000; Benigni et al. 2006; Winter et al. 2006). On the basis of the few reported cases and in the author's experience, there is no specific age, gender, or signalment that is predisposed to have lower urinary tract involvement with lymphoma. Patients typically present symptomatic from systemic involvement or typical lower urinary tract signs with obstruction being most common. A presumptive diagnosis can be made based on systemic involvement, imaging findings, and urine sediment analysis for neoplastic cells. In general, fine-needle aspiration should be avoided due to risk of bladder rupture; also, without a priori knowledge of diagnosis (carcinoma versus sarcoma versus lymphoma), there is a small but real risk of needle-track tumor implantation that is associated with solid tumors.

Complete staging diagnostics are recommended to fully evaluate extent of disease including complete bloodwork, urinalysis, thoracic and abdominal imaging, ±bone marrow analysis, and peripheral lymph node aspirate. Following complete staging, traditional multiagent doxorubicin-based protocols are the standard treatment regimen. If urinary obstruction is present, a urethral catheter can be placed for palliation while pursuing therapy. On the basis of the author's experience and reported cases in the literature, prognosis for dogs with lymphoma involving the urinary bladder is guarded. The longest reported survival was 6 months in a dog treated with a multiagent protocol (Benigni et al. 2006).

Prostatic tumors

Prostatic carcinoma

Prostatic tumors (excluding transitional cell carcinoma) are uncommon in dogs, with a prevalence of less than 0.6% in necropsy studies, and virtually nonexistent in cats (Chapter 78) (Weaver 1981). Tumor histology is equally split between adenocarcinomas arising from glandular epithelium and mixed tumors including glandular and urothelial components (Cornell et al. 2000; Bryan et al. 2007). Regardless of histology, most canine prostate tumors do not express androgen receptors. Mesenchymal tumor histologies are rare and will not be discussed.

Average age of onset for dogs affected by prostatic carcinoma is 10 years with a median body weight of 20.5 kg (Cornell et al. 2000). Initial evidence suggests there may be an increased risk for prostatic carcinoma in certain breeds including Doberman pinschers, Shetland sheepdogs, Scottish terriers, Beagles, German shorthaired pointers, Airedale terriers, and Norwegian elkhounds (Bryan et al. 2007). Several papers also describe increased risk of tumor development in neutered males, with risk

ratios of up to 2.12 reported (Teske et al. 2002b; Bryan et al. 2007).

Prostatic carcinomas are locally invasive and highly metastatic. Metastatic rates as high as 80% have been reported and commonly involve pelvic and sublumbar lymph nodes and neighboring bone (Cornell et al. 2000). In general, metastatic sites include bone (22%), lymph nodes (50%), lungs (50%), and other sites (40%) (Cornell et al. 2000). Clinical signs are often referable to the urinary tract and include hematuria, stranguria, dysuria, and incontinence. Tenesmus due to prostatic enlargement can be seen in up to 30% of patients (Cornell et al. 2000). Other signs include pain due to bony involvement (36%) and signs of systemic disease such as weight loss and anorexia (42%).

Recommended staging diagnostics are similar to those described for bladder tumors while being careful to fully evaluate for bony metastatic lesions. A presumptive diagnosis of prostatic carcinoma is made based on signalment, imaging results, and cytologic evaluation of tumor samples. Cytologic samples can be obtained from urine sediment, traumatic catheter washes, or occasionally through fine needle aspiration (acknowledging the risk of needle track tumor implantation). Cytologic differentiation between different histologies, however, is difficult.

Following complete staging, treatment options for dogs with prostatic carcinoma include surgery, radiation, photodynamic therapy, and chemotherapy. Hormone antagonists, such as the antiandrogens used to treat humans, have not been shown to be effective. Surgical options that have been described include total prostatectomy, subtotal intracapsular prostatectomy, radiofrequency ablation, and Nd:YAG laser prostatectomy (Cromeens et al. 1993; Vlasin et al. 2006; Liu et al. 2008). These surgical approaches are reserved typically for patients whose tumors are confined to the prostate. Urinary incontinence is the most common complication of these procedures and is seen most often following total prostatectomy. While these approaches are generally successful at removing gross tumor and palliating symptoms, there has been no documented survival benefit.

Radiation therapy has been utilized for intraoperative treatment and standard teletherapy treatment of canine prostatic carcinoma. Only one case series describes outcome for dogs following radiotherapy (Turrel 1987). In this report, ten dogs were treated with intraoperative radiotherapy. Total intraoperative dosage ranged between 15 and 30 Gray (Gy), with one dog receiving an additional 40 Gy postoperatively. While objective response rate was extremely high (50%), there appeared to be no significant survival benefit in treated dogs (MST = 114 days). Incidence of side effects from a standard course of radiotherapy is also high and includes effects such as colitis (56%), cystitis (30%), and colonic perforation (18%) (Anderson et al. 2002). Because of the incidence of side effects and lack of discernible benefit, palliative use of radiotherapy is questionable.

Photodynamic therapy (PDT) is another local therapeutic modality that utilizes a photochemical reaction to kill cancer cells. This modality has been widely used to treat superficial epithelial malignancies in human and veterinary medicine. With respect to prostatic carcinoma, two reports have described this therapy as a sole modality or as an adjuvant to surgical resection. As an adjuvant to surgical resection (subcapsular prostatectomy), PDT was not successful at resolving signs or controlling the tumor. This approach resulted in a median survival of only 41 days in a group of 6 affected dogs (L'eplattenier et al. 2007). As a sole modality, a single dog has been described in the literature (Lucroy et al. 2003). Following treatment, this dog had an immediate resolution of lower urinary tract signs and had stable disease for a period of 34 weeks. These disparate results suggest further studies are warranted to fully evaluate the role of PDT in treatment of prostatic carcinoma.

Traditionally, cytotoxic chemotherapy has been considered inactive for treatment of prostatic cancer in dogs and humans (LeRoy and Northrup 2008). Drugs that have been evaluated in humans with prostatic cancer include taxanes, anthracyclines, and platinum drugs. On the basis of current literature, taxanes appear to be the most efficacious (Savarese et al. 2001). Unfortunately, there are no case series in dogs that have evaluated use of chemotherapy for treatment of prostatic tumors. NSAIDs have been suggested as palliative agents for dogs with prostatic carcinoma (Sorenmo et al. 2004). In one study evaluating the use of "NSAIDs" (piroxicam or carprofen), a significant survival benefit was noted for dogs receiving NSAIDs versus those who did not (6.9 months versus 0.7 months, $p < 0.0001$) (Sorenmo et al. 2004). These initial results suggest further investigation into NSAID therapy as sole agents and in combinations are warranted. Combination protocols using NSAIDs and other modalities have not been described.

Prognosis

Prognosis for dogs with prostatic carcinoma is guarded to grave. Reported median survival ranges from 2 to 6 months; survivals for >1 year are extremely rare. The majority of patients (60–80%) present with advanced local disease and overt gross metastatic disease. Local treatment options to remove the primary tumor are complicated by the invasive nature of the tumor and high complication rates. Systemic therapy to treat and/or prevent metastatic spread has no proven efficacy. Further

efforts are needed to explore roles of PDT, chemotherapy, and NSAIDs in dogs with prostatic cancer.

Summary

Tumors of the lower urinary tract account for >95% of all tumors in the urinary system, with the urinary bladder being the most common site. Of the urinary bladder malignancies, 80–90% arise from the urothelium while 10–20% originate from other epithelial and mesenchymal tissues. Treatment of choice for these tumors is surgical resection but is hindered by anatomic localization (trigonal) and in some cases advanced tumor stage. Novel surgical approaches have been described; however, further studies are needed to clarify their role. Thus, the primary treatment modality has become palliative therapy with combinations of chemotherapy and NSAIDs. These combinations appear to be highly successful in ameliorating tumor-related symptoms but have questionable survival benefit.

References

Anderson, C., E. McNiel, et al. (2002). Late complications of pelvic irradiation in 16 dogs. *Vet Radiol Ultrasound* **43**(2): 187–192.

Bae, I., Y. Kim, et al. (2007). Genitourinary rhabdomyosarcoma with systemic metastases in a young dog. *Vet Pathol* **44**(4): 518–520.

Benigni, L., C. Lamb, et al. (2006). Lymphoma affecting the urinary bladder in three dogs and a cat. *Vet Radiol Ultrasound* **47**(6): 592–596.

Billet, J., A. Moore, et al. (2002). Evaluation of a bladder tumor antigen test for the diagnosis of lower urinary tract malignancies in dogs. *Am J Vet Res* **63**(3): 370–373.

Bryan, J., M. Keeler, et al. (2007). A population study of neutering status as a risk factor for canine prostate cancer. *Prostate* **67**(11): 1174–1181.

Burk, R., E. Meierhenry, et al. (1975). Leiomyosarcoma of the urinary bladder in a cat. *J Am Vet Med Assoc* **167**(8): 749–751.

Caywood, D., C. Osborne, et al. (1980). Neoplasms of the canine and feline urinary tracts. In: *Current Veterinary Therapy VIII*. Philadelphia, PA: WB Saunders, pp. 1203–1212.

Chun, R., D. Knapp, et al. (1996). Cisplatin treatment of transitional cell carcinoma of the urinary bladder in dogs: 18 cases. *J Am Vet Med Assoc* **209**(9): 1588–1591.

Chun, R., D. Knapp, et al. (1997). Phase II clinical trial of carboplatin in canine transitional cell carcinoma of the urinary bladder. *J Vet Intern Med* **11**(5): 279–283.

Cornell, K., D. Bostwick, et al. (2000). Clinical and pathologic aspects of spontaneous canine prostate carcinoma: a retrospective analysis of 76 cases. *Prostate* **45**(2): 173–183.

Cromeens, D., D. Johnson, et al. (1993). Transurethral canine prostatectomy with the ND:YAG laser. *J Invest Surg* **6**(1): 97–103.

DeLuca, A., P. Johnstone, et al. (1994). Tolerance of the bladder to intraoperative radiation in a canine model: a five-year follow-up. *Int J Rad Oncol Biol Phys* **30**(2): 339–345.

Epslin, D. (1987). Urinary bladder fibromas in dogs: 51 cases. *J Am Vet Med Assoc* **190**(4): 440–444.

Glickman, L., F. Schofer, et al. (1989). Epidemiologic study of insecticide exposures, obesity, and risk of bladder cancer in household dogs. *J Toxicol Environ Health* **28**(4): 407–414.

Glickman, L., M. Raghavan, et al. (2004). Herbicide exposure and the risk of transitional cell carcinoma of the urinary bladder in Scottish Terriers. *J Am Vet Med Assoc* **224**(8): 1290–1297.

Halliwell, W. and N. Ackerman (1974). Botryoid rhabdomyosarcoma of the urinary bladder and hypertrophic osteoarthropathy in a young dog. *J Am Vet Med Assoc* **165**(10): 911–913.

Hayes, H. (1976). Canine bladder cancer: epidemiologic features. *Am J Epidemiol* **104**(6): 673–677.

Helfand, S., T. Hamilton, et al. (1994). Comparison of three treatments for transitional cell carcinoma of the bladder in the dog. *J Am Anim Hosp Assoc* **30**: 270–275.

Heng, H., J. Lowry, et al. (2006). Smooth muscle neoplasia of the urinary bladder wall in three dogs. *Vet Radiol Ultrasound* **47**(1): 83–86.

Henry, C., J. Tyler, et al. (2003a). Evaluation of a bladder tumor antigen test as a screening test for transitional cell carcinoma of the lower urinary tract in dogs. *Am J Vet Res* **64**(8): 1017–1020.

Henry, C., D. McCaw, et al. (2003b). Clinical evaluation of mitoxantrone and piroxicam in a canine model of human invasive urinary bladder carcinoma. *Clin Can Res* **9**(2): 906–911.

Kim, D., E. Hodgin, et al. (1996). Juvenile rhabdomyosarcomas in two dogs. *Vet Pathol* **33**(4): 447–450.

Knapp, D., R. Richardson, et al. (1994). Piroxicam therapy in 34 dogs with transitional cell carcinoma of the urinary bladder. *J Vet Intern Med* **8**(4): 273–278.

Knapp, D., N. Glickman, et al. (2000a). Naturally occuring canine transitional cell carcinoma of the urinary bladder. *Urol Oncol* **5**: 47–59.

Knapp, D., N. Glickman, et al. (2000b). Cisplatin versus cisplatin combined with piroxicam in a canine model of human invasive urinary bladder cancer. *Can Chemother Pharmacol* **46**(3): 221–226.

Knottenbelt, C., D. Mellor, et al. (2006). Cohort study of COX-1 and COX-2 expression in canine rectal and bladder tumors. *J Small Anim Pract* **47**(4): 196–200.

Kosarek, C., W. Kisseberth, et al. (2005). Clinical evaluation of gemcitabine in dogs with spontaneously occurring malignancies. *J Vet Intern Med* **19**(1): 81–86.

Kropp, B., M. Rippy, et al. (1996). Regenerative urinary bladder augmentation using small intestinal submucosal: urodynamic and histopathologic assessment in long-term canine bladder augmentations. *J Urol* **155**(6): 2098–2104.

Kuwamura, M., H. Yoshida, et al. (1998). Urinary bladder rhabdomyosarcoma (sarcoma botryoides) in a young Newfoundland dog. *J Vet Med Sci* **60**(5): 619–621.

L'eplattenier, H., B. Klem, et al. (2007). Preliminary results of intraoperative photodynamic therapy with 5-aminolevulinic acid in dogs with prostate carcinoma. *Vet J* **178**: 202–207.

LeRoy, B. and N. Northrup (2008). Prostate cancer in dogs: comparative and clinical aspects. *Vet J* **180**: 149–162.

Liptak, J., S. Brutscher, et al. (2004). Transurethral resection in the management of urethral and prostatic neoplasia in 6 dogs. *Vet Surg* **33**(5): 505–516.

Liu, J., G. Wansaicheong, et al. (2008). Canine prostate: contrast-enhanced US-guided radiofrequency ablation with urethral and neurovascular cooling-initial experience. *Radiology* **247**(3): 717–725.

Lucroy, M., M. Bowles, et al. (2003). Photodynamic therapy for prostatic carcinoma in a dog. *J Vet Intern Med* **17**(2): 235–237.

Maiolino, P. and G. DeVico (2000). Primary epitheliotrophic T-cell lymphoma of the urinary bladder in a dog. *Vet Pathol* **37**(2): 184–186.

Martinez, I., J. Mattoon, et al. (2003). Polypoid cystitis in 17 dogs (1978–2001). *J Vet Intern Med* **17**(4): 499–509.

Meuten, D. (2002). Tumors of the urinary system. In: *Tumors in Domestic Animals*, Chapter 10, 4th edition. Ames, IA: Iowa State Press, pp. 509–546.

Mohammed, S., P. Bennett, et al. (2002). Effects of the cyclooxygenase inhibitor, piroxicam, on tumor response, apoptosis, and angiogenesis in a canine model of human invasive urinary bladder cancer. *Can Res* **62**(2): 356–358.

Mohammed, S., B. Craig, et al. (2003). Effects of the cyclooxygenase inhibitor, piroxicam, in combination with chemotherapy on tumor response, apoptosis, and angiogenesis in a canine model of human invasive urinary bladder cancer. *Mol Can Ther* **2**(2): 183–188.

Moore, A., A. Cardona, et al. (1990). Cisplatin for the treatment of transitional cell carcinoma of the urinary bladder or urethra. A retrospective study of 15 dogs. *J Vet Intern Med* **4**(3): 148–152.

Moore, A.S., G.H. Theilen, et al. (1991). Preclinical study of sequential tumor necrosis factor and interleukin 2 in the treatment of spontaneous canine neoplasms. *Can Res* **51**(1): 233–238.

Murphy, S., A. Gutiérrez, et al. (2008). Laparoscopically implanted tissue expander radiotherapy in canine transitional cell carcinoma. *Vet Radiol Ultrasound* **49**(4): 400–405.

Norris, A., E. Laing, et al. (1992). Canine bladder and urethral tumors: a retrospective study of 115 cases (1980–1985). *J Vet Intern Med* **6**(3): 145–153.

Nseyo, U., R. Whalen, et al. (1993). Canine bladder response to red and green light whole bladder photodynamic therapy. *Urology* **41**(4): 392–396.

Nyland, T., S. Wallack, et al. (2002). Needle-tract implantation following us-guided fine-needle aspiration biopsy of transitional cell carcinoma of the bladder, urethra, and prostate. *Vet Radiol Ultrasound* **43**(1): 50–53.

Olausson, A., S. Stieger, et al. (2005). A urinary bladder fibrosarcoma in a young dog. *Vet Radiol Ultrasound* **46**(2): 135–138.

Osborne, C., D. Low, et al. (1968). Neoplasms of the canine and feline urinary bladder: incidence, etiologic factors, occurrence, and pathological features. *Am J Vet Res* **29**: 2041–2055.

Owen, L.N. (1980). *TNM Classification of Tumors in Domestic Animals*, 1st edition. Geneva: World Health Organization.

Patrick, D., S. Fitzgerald, et al. (2006). Classification of canine urinary bladder urothelial tumours based on the World Health Organization/International Society of Urological Pathology consensus classification. *J Comp Pathol* **135**(4): 190–199.

Pletcher, J. and L. Dalton (1981). Botryoid rhabdomyosarcoma in the urinary bladder of a dog. *Vet Pathol* **18**(5): 695–697.

Poirier, V., L. Forrest, et al. (2004). Piroxicam, mitoxantrone, and coarse fraction radiotherapy for the treatment of transitional cell carcinoma of the bladder in 10 dogs: a pilot study. *J Am Anim Hosp Assoc* **40**(2): 131–136.

Pope, J., M. Davis, et al. (1997). The ontogeny of canine small intestinal submucosal regenerated bladder. *J Urol* **158**(3 Pt 2): 1105–1110.

Raghavan, M., D. Knapp, et al. (2004). Topical flea and tick pesticides and the risk of transitional cell carcinoma of the urinary bladder in Scottish Terriers. *J Am Vet Med Assoc* **225**(3): 389–394.

Rocha, T., G. Mauldin, et al. (2000). Prognostic factors in dogs with urinary bladder carcinoma. *J Vet Intern Med* **14**(5): 486–490.

Sapierzynski, R., E. Malicka, et al. (2007). Tumors of the urogenital system in dogs and cats. Retrospective review of 138 cases. *Polish J Vet Sci* **10**(2): 97–103.

Savarese, D., S. Halabi, et al. (2001). Phase II study of doxetaxel, estramustine, and low-dose hydrocortisone in men with hormone-refractory prostate cancer: a final report of CALGB 9780. Cancer and Leukemia Group B. *J Clin Oncol* **19**(9): 2509–2516.

Smith, J., E. Stone, et al. (1995). Placement of a permanent cystostomy catheter to relieve urine outflow obstruction in dogs with transitional cell carcinoma. *J Am Vet Med Assoc* **206**(4): 496–499.

Sorenmo, K., M. Goldschmidt, et al. (2004). Evaluation of cyclooxygenase-1 and cyclooxygenase-2 expression and the effect of cyclooxygenase inhibitors in canine prostatic carcinoma. *Vet Comp Oncol* **2**(1): 13–23.

Stamps, P. and D. Harris (1968). Botryoid rhabdomyosarcoma of the urinary bladder of a dog. *J Am Vet Med Assoc* **153**(8): 1064–1068.

Stone, E., S. Withrow, et al. (1988). Ureterocolonic anastomosis in ten dogs with transitional cell carcinoma. *Vet Surg* **17**(3): 147–153.

Stone, E., T. George, et al. (1996). Partial cystectomy for urinary bladder neoplasia: surgical technique and outcome in 11 dogs. *J Small Anim Pract* **37**(10): 480–485.

Strafuss, A. and Dean, M. (1975). Neoplasms of the canine urinary bladder. *J Am Vet Med Assoc* **166**(12): 1161–1163.

Struble, A., G. Lawson, et al. (1997). Urethral obstruction in a dog: an unusual presentation of T-cell lymphoma. *J Am Anim Hosp Assoc* **33**(5): 423–426.

Takiguchi, M., T. Watanabe, et al. (2002). Rhabdomyosarcoma (botryoid sarcoma) of the urinary bladder in a Maltese. *Small Anim Pract* **43**(6): 269–271.

Teske, E., E. Naan, et al. (2002b). Canine prostate carcinoma: epidemiological evidence of an increased risk in castrated dogs. *Mol Cell Endocrinol* **197**(1–2): 251–255.

Turrel, J. (1987). Intraoperative radiotherapy of carcinoma of the prostate gland in ten dogs. *J Am Vet Med Assoc* **190**(1): 48–52.

Upton, M., C. Tangner, et al. (2006). Evaluation of carbon dioxide laser ablation combined with mitoxantrone and piroxicam treatment in dogs with transitional cell carcinoma. *J Am Vet Med Assoc* **228**(4): 549–552.

van Noort, R. (1997). 4 unusual cases of malignant lymphoma in the dog and cat. *Tijdschrift voor diergeneeskunde* **122**(18): 502–505.

Vignoli, M., F. Rossi, et al. (2007). Needle-tract implantation after fine-needle aspiration biopsy of transitional cell carcinoma of the urinary bladder and adenocarcinoma of the lung. *Schweizer Archiv fur Tierheilkunde* **149**(7): 314–318.

Vlasin, M., P. Rauser, et al. (2006). Subtotal intracapsular prostatectomy as a useful treatment for advanced-stage prostatic malignancies. *J Small Anim Pract* **47**(9): 512–516.

Weaver, A. (1981). Fifteen cases of prostatic carcinoma in the dog. *Vet Rec* **109**(4): 71–75.

Weisse, C., A. Berent, et al. (2006). Evaluation of palliative stenting for management of malignant urethral obstructions in dogs. *J Am Vet Med Assoc* **229**(2): 226–234.

Wilson, H., R. Chun, et al. (2007). Clinical signs, treatments, and outcome in cats with transitional cell carcinoma of the urinary bladder: 20 cases (1990–2004). *J Am Vet Med Assoc* **231**(1): 101–106.

Winter, M., J. Locke, et al. (2006). Imaging diagnosis—urinary obstruction secondary to prostatic lymphoma in a young dog. *Vet Radiol Ultrasound* **47**(6): 597–601.

Withrow, S., E. Gillette, et al. (1989). Intraoperative irradiation of 16 spontaneously occurring canine neoplasms. *Vet Surg* **18**(1): 7–11.

80

Congenital diseases of the lower urinary tract

Joe Bartges and John M. Kruger

Urinary tract disorders occurring in young animals may result from heritable (genetic) or acquired processes that affect differentiation and growth of the developing urinary tract. Formation of the urinary system depends on sequential and coordinated development and interaction of multiple embryonic tissues (Noden and deLahunta 1985; Kruger et al. 1995). Over 400 regulatory genes are believed to be involved in the embryogenesis of the urinary system (Glassberg 2002; Haraguchi et al. 2007; Schedl 2007). The urinary bladder and urethra are formed by subdivision of the cloaca, the caudal portion of the embryonic hindgut. Formation of the urorectal septum divides the cloaca into the rectum positioned dorsally and the urogenital sinus positioned ventrally. The urogenital sinus communicates caudally with the amniotic cavity via the urogenital orifice and cranially with the allantois (a portion of the placenta) via the urachus and allantoic stalk. The urinary bladder eventually develops from the proximal urachus and the cranial portion of the urogenital sinus. The caudal portion of the urogenital sinus differentiates into the urethra; the remainder of the urachus narrows and closes functionally by birth. With embryonic development, the mesonephric ducts and embryonic ureters (ureteral buds) establish separate openings in the caudal portion of the urogenital sinus. Initially, the ureteral orifice is located caudal to the opening of the mesonephric duct, but as the urinary bladder develops, positions of the embryonic ureter and the mesonephric ducts are transposed so that the ureter opens cranially in the neck of the bladder and the mesonephric duct opens in the cranial urethra. In male dogs and cat, the mesonephric ducts differentiate into components of the male reproductive system. In females,

the mesonephric ducts contribute to formation of the vagina.

Although the mesonephros and metanephros produce urine, maintenance of fetal homeostasis is primarily the responsibility of the placenta. Varying quantities of urine formed by the fetal kidneys pass from the developing urinary bladder through the urachus to the placenta, where unwanted waste products are absorbed by the maternal circulation and subsequently excreted in the mother's urine (Noden and deLahunta 1985). Fetal urine also passes through the urethra into the amniotic cavity where urine forms one of the major constituents of amniotic fluid. Normal patterns of urine storage and bladder emptying are evident during the latter part of gestation in human and ovine fetuses. Most newborn puppies and kittens void urine shortly after birth; however, micturition is rarely observed in most neonates because of maternal hygiene and caring of the neonate.

Urinary bladder

Urinary bladder agenesis and hypoplasia

Complete agenesis of the urinary bladder is rare, but has been reported in a 4-month-old, female, mixed breed dog with urinary incontinence (Pearson et al. 1965). Hypoplasia has been reported in dogs and cats and often associated with ectopic ureters (Holt and Gibbs 1992; Holt and Moore 1995; Agut et al. 2002). Embryonic maldevelopment may result in a hypoplastic bladder; however, disruption of urinary bladder function may be associated with potentially reversible reduction in bladder capacity (Schmaelzle et al. 1969). Small bladder capacity associated with ectopic ureters may contribute to urinary incontinence even with surgical correction, but bladder capacity may increase over time (Archibald and Owen 1974; Holt and Moore 1995).

Nephrology and Urology of Small Animals. Edited by Joe Bartges and David J. Polzin. © 2011 Blackwell Publishing Ltd.

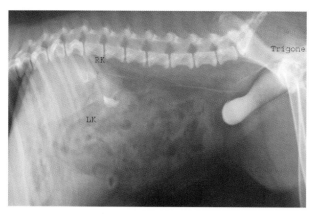

Figure 80.1 Lateral abdominal radiograph of an excretory urogram in a dog with a pelvic bladder and pyelonephritis. Pyelectasia is present bilaterally. The dog had urinary incontinence and recurrent bacterial urinary tract infections. RK, right kidney; LK, left kidney; Trigone, trigone of bladder located in pelvic canal.

Pelvic bladder

Pelvic bladder refers to urinary bladders that have a blunt-shaped trigone, which is located in an intrapelvic location associated with a shortened urethra (Figure 80.1) (Adams and DiBartola 1983). The role of pelvic bladder with urinary incontinence is controversial and dogs with pelvic bladder may be continent (Adams and DiBartola 1983; Mahaffey et al. 1984; Johnston et al. 1986). Normally, the trigone tapers and connects to the urethra in an intraabdominal location. The degree of distention of the bladder affects location of the trigone; therefore, the bladder should be adequately distended during contrast urethrocystography before diagnosing pelvic bladder (Chapter 15). Pelvic bladder has also been associated with urinary tract infection (Adams and DiBartola 1983). Although some dogs with pelvic bladders are continent, other dogs with pelvic bladders have refractory urinary incontinence without any other identifiable cause (Chapter 76) (Adams and DiBartola 1983; Lane and Lappin 1995). A diagnosis of pelvic bladder is established by contrast radiography. If pelvic bladder is associated with urinary incontinence, pharmacologic management with estrogens and/or alpha-adrenergic agonists should be tried prior to more invasive interventions. If urinary incontinence is refractory to medical therapy, urethral bulking with collagen or surgery (urethropexy or colposuspension) may be attempted (Rawlings et al. 2001; White 2001; Barth et al. 2005).

Exstrophy

Exstrophy refers to eversion of the urinary bladder, and often the intestines and external genitalia, due to absence of a portion of the ventral abdominal wall (Caione et al.

2005). This is a rare disorder being reported in an 8-month-old, female, English bulldog with urinary incontinence and pyelonephritis (Hobson and Ader 1979). Treatment involves managing-associated conditions and reconstructive surgery (Shimada et al. 2002).

Urinary bladder herniation

Exteriorization of the urinary bladder through an inguinal hernia has been described in a two-year-old cat (Zulauf et al. 2007). Clinical signs included chronic lower urinary tract signs and a soft mass was palpated in the region. Radiography revealed the urinary bladder to be extraabdominal. Treatment consisted of repositioning of the urinary bladder in the abdominal cavity with an incisional cystopexy and partial closure of the enlarged inguinal canals.

Urachal anomalies

Urachal anomalies occur commonly in dogs and cats. The urachus is a fetal connection allowing urine to pass between the developing urinary bladder and the placenta. It undergoes complete atrophy and is nonfunctional at birth. If it fails to completely atrophy, macroscopic or microscopic remnants may remain and result in persistent urachal patency or formation of urachal cysts or diverticula (Osborne et al. 1987; Bartges 2000).

A persistent urachus occurs when the urachal canal remains functionally patent between the urinary bladder and the umbilicus (Figure 80.2). It is characterized by inappropriate urine loss through the umbilicus (Osborne et al. 1966; Greene and Bohning 1971; Pearson and Gibbs 1971; Cornell 2000; Laverty and Salisbury 2002). A patent urachus is often accompanied by omphalitis, ventral dermatitis, and urinary tract infections. Rarely, uroabdomen may occur when a persistent urachus terminates in the abdominal cavity (Hanson 1972). A urachal cyst may develop if the urachal epithelium in an isolated segment of a persistent urachus continues to secrete fluid (Figure 80.3; Archibald and Owen 1974; Osborne et al. 1987).

A vesicourachal diverticulum occurs when a portion of the urachus located at the bladder vertex fails to close, resulting in a blind diverticulum that protrudes from the bladder apex (Figure 80.4). Vesicorachal diverticula may be microscopic or macroscopic. Microscopic vesicourachal diverticula are microscopic lumens lined by transitional epithelium that may persist at the bladder vertex from the level of the submucosal to the subserosa (Osborne et al. 1987). Approximately 40% of bladders from 80 cats had microscopic diverticula in one study (Wilson et al. 1983). Usually, microscopic diverticula are insignificant clinically; however, they may become macroscopic when acquired bladder and/or urethral

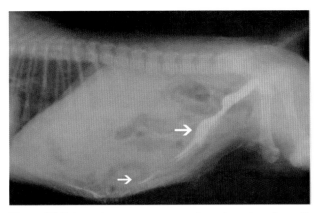

Figure 80.2 Lateral contrast cystogram in an immature dog with a patent urachus (arrows).

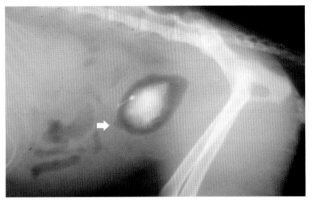

Figure 80.4 Lateral double contrast cystogram showing a urachal diverticulum (arrow) in a 3-year-old, castrated male, domestic shorthair cat with idiopathic cystitis.

diseases develop (e.g., urinary tract infections, urolithiasis, or idiopathic cystitis) (Lulich et al. 1989; Osborne et al. 1989; Scheepens and L'Eplattenier 2005). A microscopic diverticulum may "open" due to inflammation and/or increased intraluminal pressure from an acquired disease. Many of these macroscopic diverticula disappear within 2–3 weeks following treatment of the acquired disease and resolution of clinical signs (Osborne et al. 1987; Osborne et al. 1989). Congenital macroscopic vesicourachal diverticula are thought to be caused by urine

outflow obstruction and develop before or shortly after birth. These diverticula increase risk of bacterial urinary tract infection and associated clinical signs of lower urinary tract disease (Gotthelf 1981).

Vesicourachal diverticula may be visualized by contrast urethrocystography, ultrasonography, or cystoscopy. Treatment of vesicourachal diverticula depends on their size and association with clinical disease. Many macroscopic diverticula associated with active lower urinary tract disease regress with successful treatment of the acquired disease; therefore, documentation of regression of diverticulum following treatment is important (Lulich et al. 1989; Osborne et al. 1989). If the diverticulum does not resolve and recurrent disease occurs, then diverticulectomy may be warranted (Lobetti and Goldin 1998; Scheepens and L'Eplattenier 2005).

Urinary bladder duplication

Complete and partial urinary bladder duplication with and without concurrent urethral duplication has been reported in dogs (Hoskins et al. 1982). Urinary bladder duplication may result from any alteration of normal development of the cloaca or its subdivision into the urogenital sinus and rectum (Abrahamson 1961). Clinical signs develop early in life and include lower urinary tract signs, incontinence, and distended abdomen. Diagnosis is made by physical examination and imaging studies. Treatment involves surgical correction; however, success depends on degree of malformation and presence of additional congenital anomalies.

Colovesical fistula and uterine–bladder communication

Rarely, the urinary bladder may communicate with the colon or uterine horn (van Schouwenburg and Louw

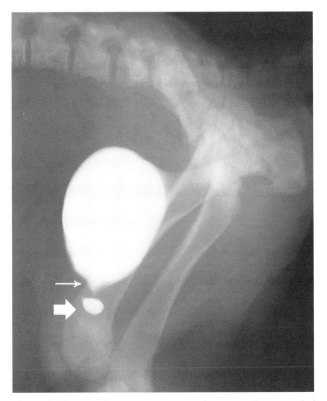

Figure 80.3 Lateral contrast cystogram demonstrating a urachal cyst (larger arrow) and urachal diverticulum (smaller arrow).

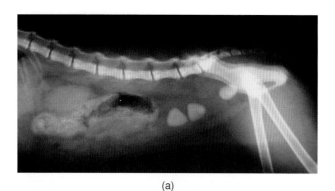

(a)

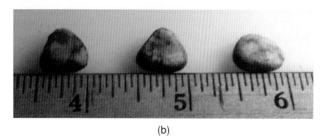

(b)

Figure 80.5 (a) Lateral abdominal radiograph of a kitten showing three radiodense uroliths. (b) The uroliths were composed of struvite that formed secondary to a infection with a urease-producing microbial organism (*Staphylococcus spp.*)

1982; Lawler and Monti 1984; Lulich et al. 1987). Clinical signs included urinary incontinence, lower urinary tract signs, and urinary tract infection. Treatment is limited to surgical correction.

Primary urinary bladder neoplasia

Urinary bladder neoplasia of immature dogs and cats are rare (Chapter 79) (Caywood et al. 1980). Botryoid rhabdomyosarcoma has been observed to occur in large breed dogs younger than 18 months, but can occur in other dogs (Osborne et al. 1968; Stamps and Harris 1968; Roszel 1972; Kelly 1973; Halliwell and Ackerman 1974; Pletcher and Dalton 1981; Stone et al. 1996 ; Takiguchi et al. 2002; Madarame et al. 2003; Bae et al. 2007). Botryoid rhabdomyosarcomas are embryonic mesenchymal tumors arising from pleuripotent stem cells originating from primitive urogenital ridge remnants. They are infiltrating tumors arising from the trigone and projecting into the bladder lumen as botryoid (resembling a cluster of grapes) masses (Kelly 1973). Clinical signs are consistent with lower urinary tract disease and the tumor may result in urinary outflow obstruction and hypertrophic osteoarthropathy (Kelly 1973; Halliwell and Ackerman 1974). Treatment includes surgery with or without additional chemotherapy (doxorubicin, cyclophosphamide, and vincristine sulfate) (Van Vechten et al. 1990; Senior et al. 1993). Metastases to local tissues (lymph nodes, mesentery, omentum, prostate) and distant organs (lung, liver, kidney, spleen) have been described with this tumor (Stamps and Harris 1968; Takiguchi et al. 2002; Bae et al. 2007).

Urocystolithiasis

Urocystolithiasis has been described in immature dogs and cats (Chapter 69). Most commonly, struvite secondary to infection with a urease-producing microbial organism and urate secondary to congenital hepatic disease occur (Figures 80.5 and 80.6; Kruger et al. 1995). Although certain breeds of dogs are prone to formation of metabolic uroliths, for example, Dalmatians and urate, and English bulldogs and urate or cystine, uroliths do not typically form in immature animals despite the metabolic abnormality relative to other breeds.

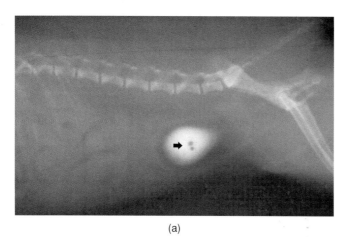

(a)

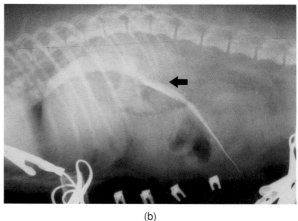

(b)

Figure 80.6 (a) Lateral double contrast cystogram of a 1-year-old, castrated male, Pomeranian showing urocystoliths (arrow) composed of ammonium urate that formed secondary to a congenital extrahepatic portovascular anomaly. (b) Lateral contrast portography of the dog described in (a) showing a single extrahepatic portovascular anomaly (arrow).

Urethra

Urethral aplasia and hypoplasia

Urethral aplasia is a rare congenital anomaly characterized by complete absence of a patent urethra. Incontinence occurs associated with ectopic location of the ureters (Chapter 58; Pearson and Gibbs 1971; Bargai and Bark 1982). Urethral hypoplasia described in immature female cats is associated with juvenile-onset urinary incontinence (Holt and Gibbs 1992; Baines et al. 1999). Diagnosis is based on clinical signs and imaging studies. Radiographic features include urethral shortening and vaginal aplasia. Urethral hypoplasia may be associated with other congenital anomalies and bacterial urinary tract infection. Surgical reconstruction of the bladder neck may improve or resolve clinical signs.

Epispadias and hypospadias

Epispadias refers to congenital defects in the dorsal aspect of the distal urethra, and hypospadias refers to anomalous ventral malposition of the urethral meatus (Hayes and Wilson 1986). Epispadias has been associated with exstrophy of the urinary bladder in an 8-month-old, female, English bulldog (Hobson and Ader 1979). Hypospadias occurs more commonly and usually in male dogs; Boston terriers and Dalmatians have been described as having an increased risk (Figure 80.7; Hayes and Wilson 1986; Cassata et al. 2008). It has been described in a Himalayan cat (King and Johnson 2000). In affected male dogs, an abnormal ventral urethral meatus may be located anywhere along the shaft of the penis, scrotum, or perineum. It is usually associated with malformation of the prepuce and penis (Ader and Hobson 1978; Grieco et al. 2008). Hypospadias has been described in female dogs in associated with concurrent disorders of intersexuality. Embryonically, hypospadias results from incomplete fusion of the urogenital fold. Affected dogs present at various ages and may asymptomatic or have clinical signs of urinary incontinence, peri-urethral dermatitis, or bacterial urinary tract infection (Ader and Hobson 1978). Diagnosis is often based on physical examination. The presence of an *os penis* in male dogs precludes surgical reconstruction in most cases. Scrotal or perineal urethrostomy combined with castration and removal of vestigial prepucial and penile tissues may be of cosmetic value. Shortening of the penis, amputation, and urethral reconstruction has also been described (Rawlings 1984; Lefebvre and Lussier 2005; Pavletic 2007; Galanty et al. 2008).

Urethrogenital malformations

Urethrogenital malformations associated with diseases of intersexuality, especially pseudohermaphroditism is

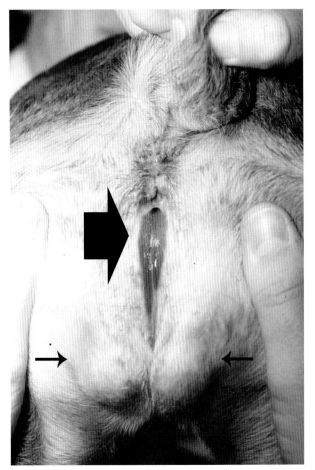

Figure 80.7 Perineal hypospadias (larger arrow) in a 6-month-old, male English bulldog. Smaller arrows designate position of the testicles.

often associated with urinary incontinence (Holt et al. 1983). Pseudohermaphrodites have gonads of one sex and external genitalia resembling those of the opposite sex (Jackson 1980). It occurs in both sexes as a result of simultaneous development of Mullerian duct derivatives (oviduct, uterus, and portions of the vagina) and masculinization of the urogenital sinus. The phenotypic appearance of the animal depends on the degree of masculinization of the urogenital sinus. Incontinence develops early in life and may be accompanied by signs of lower urinary tract disease due to a bacterial urinary tract infection. Urinary incontinence likely results from retention of urine in anomalous communications between the urethra and the genital tract and subsequent passive leakage (Jackson et al. 1978). Diagnosis is based on clinical signs and imaging studies. Urinary incontinence may resolve with surgical correction (Holt et al. 1983).

Urethral duplication

Urethral duplication is an uncommon congenital anomaly only described in immature dogs (Wolff and

Radecky 1973; Johnston et al. 1989; Longhofer et al 1991; Tobias and Barbee 1995; Duffey et al. 1998). Because of the close association between embryonic development of the urogenital and gastrointestinal system, urethral duplication is almost always accompanied by other duplication anomalies. These anomalies result from abnormal sagittal midline division and subsequent parallel development of the embryonic hindgut, cloaca, rectum, or urogenital sinus (Abrahamson 1961). Associated anomalies accompanying urethral duplication depends on stage at which dysmorphogenesis occurs. Examination of affected animals may reveal anatomic abnormalities, urinary incontinence, or clinical signs associated with secondary bacterial urinary tract infection. Diagnosis is based on physical examination, imaging studies, and exploratory surgery. Urethral duplication may in some cases be amenable to surgical extirpation of the duplicated structure; however, surgical reconstruction has rarely been attempted with extensive duplication.

Ectopic urethra

Ectopic urethra is characterized by abnormal position of the external urethral orifice. Embryonically, urethral ectopia results from anomalous morphogenesis of the urogenital sinus, paramesonephric ducts (Mullerian ducts), or mesonephric ducts (Noden and deLahunta 1985). Clinical signs depend on the site of the termination of the abnormal urethra and other concurrent urogenital anomalies. Lifelong urinary incontinence was the predominant clinical feature in a 21-month-old female English bulldog with unilateral ureteral ectopia and an ectopic urethra terminating in the distal vagina (Osborne and Hanlon 1967). In contrast, a 2-month-old, female, domestic shorthair cat with ectopic urethra terminating in the ventral rectum did not have urinary incontinence, but did void urine through the anus (Lulich et al. 1987).

Urethrorectal, urethrovaginal, and urethroperineal fistula and urethral diverticula

Fistulas connecting the urethral lumen with the large bowel, vagina, and perineal region have been described in dogs and cats (Gray 1968; Osborne et al. 1975; Miller 1980; Whitney and Schrader 1988; Osuna et al. 1989; Tobias and Barbee 1995; Foster et al. 1999; Lautzenhiser and Bjorling 2002; Agut et al. 2006). Fistula may be congenital or may be acquired due to traumatic, inflammatory, or neoplastic processes (Osborne 1977). Male dogs appear to be affected more frequently and English bulldogs appear to have a predilection for urethrorectal fistula (Osborne 1977). Clinical signs are due to abnormal passage of urine from the fistula during uri-

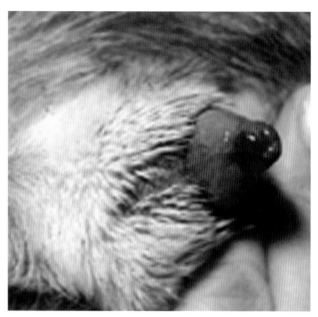

Figure 80.8 Urethral prolapse in a 2-year-old, intact male, English bulldog.

nation. Additional signs may include diarrhea, perineal dermatitis, and signs associated with secondary bacterial urinary tract infections. Fistulas have been associated with infection-induced struvite urolithiasis (Miller 1980; Osuna et al. 1989; Agut et al. 2006). Diagnosis is based on clinical signs and imaging studies. Treatment involves surgical correction or surgical urinary diversion. In one dog with a urethrorectal fistula secondary to a prostatic abscess, conservative therapy using an indwelling urinary catheter, low residue diet, and antibiotics was successful (Agut et al. 2006).

Urethral prolapse

Prolapse of the urethral mucosal lining through the external urethral orifice occurs primarily in male dogs under 5 years of age (Figure 80.8; Ragni 2007). English bulldogs and Boston terriers appear to have a predilection (Sinibaldi and Green 1973; Osborne and Sanderson 1995; Kirsch et al. 2002). Urethral prolapse may not be associated with clinical signs or owners may only notice a red to purple "mass" at the tip of the penis during urination; however, it may be associated with dripping of blood, licking of the prepuce or penis, or signs of lower urinary tract disease. Diagnosis is based on physical examination. If urethral prolapse is associated with no to minimal clinical signs, treatment may not be necessary (Osborne and Sanderson 1995). If associated with clinical signs, manual reduction if small or surgical correction if large may be done (Sinibaldi and Green 1973; Kirsch et al. 2002).

Urethral stricture and hypoplasia

Presumed congenital urethral strictures and hypoplasia have been described in young dogs and cats (Breitschwerdt et al. 1982; Holt 1990; 1993). Clinical signs relate to partial or complete urethral obstruction. Systemic signs, bladder distention or rupture, overflow incontinence, secondary bacterial urinary tract infection, and hydronephrosis occurs secondary to the urinary outflow obstruction. Urinary incontinence and bilateral hydroureter and hydronephrosis were observed in an 8-month-old, male, German shepherd with congenital mid-urethral stricture (Breitschwerdt et al. 1982). Treatment involves surgery. If the stricture occurs in the extrapelvic urethra, urethrostomy may be performed; if it occurs in the intrapelvic or intraabdominal urethra, then urethral resection and anastomosis or prepubic urethrostomy may be indicated (Baines et al. 2001; Bernarde and Viguier 2004). Dilation of the urethral stricture may also be attempted with balloon or bougienage catheters. In cats, urinary incontinence secondary to urethral hypoplasia may be treated surgically with variable success (Holt 1993).

Urethroliths

Urethroliths represent passage of urocystoliths and may or may not cause clinical signs of urethral obstruction (Chapter 69).

Congenital urinary incontinence

Many congenital disorders are associated with congenital urinary incontinence (Chapter 76). In addition to those described in the preceding sections, spinal dysraphism is associated with urinary and fecal incontinence. Spinal dysraphism refers to cleft-like malformations of the spine and spinal cord resulting from incomplete closure of the neural tube. Congenital urethral sphincter mechanism incompetency has been described in dogs and cats associated with urethral hypoplasia (Holt 1993); however, ectopic ureter is most commonly associated with juvenile urinary incontinence (McLoughlin and Chew 2000; Silverman and Long 2000; Berent et al. 2008).

References

Abrahamson, J. (1961). Double bladder and related anomalies: clinical and embryological aspects and a case report. *Br J Urol* **33**: 195–214.

Adams, W.M. and S.P. DiBartola (1983). Radiographic and clinical features of pelvic bladder in the dog. *J Am Vet Med Assoc* **182**(11): 1212–1217.

Ader, L. and H.P. Hobson (1978). Hypospadias: a review of the veterinary literature and a report of three cases in the dog. *J Am Anim Hosp Assoc* **14**: 721–727.

Agut, A., M.J. Fernandez del Palacio, et al. (2002). Unilateral renal agenesis associated with additional congenital abnormalities of the urinary tract in a Pekingese bitch. *J Small Anim Pract* **43**(1): 32–35.

Agut, A., X. Lucas, et al. (2006). A urethrorectal fistula due to prostatic abscess associated with urolithiasis in a dog. *Reprod Domest Anim* **41**(3): 247–250.

Archibald, J. and R.R. Owen (1974). Urinary system. In: *Canine Surgery*, edited by J. Archibald. Santa Barbara, CA: American Veterinary Publications, pp. 627–701.

Bae, I.H., Y. Kim, et al. (2007). Genitourinary rhabdomyosarcoma with systemic metastasis in a young dog. *Vet Pathol* **44**(4): 518–520.

Baines, S.J., A.J. Speakman, et al. (1999). Genitourinary dysplasia in a cat. *J Small Anim Pract* **40**(6): 286–290.

Baines, S.J., S. Rennie, et al. (2001). Prepubic urethrostomy: a long-term study in 16 cats. *Vet Surg* **30**(2): 107–113.

Bargai, U. and H. Bark (1982). Multiple congenital urinary tract abnormalities in a bitch: a case history report. *Veterinary Radiology & Ultrasound* **23**(1): 10–12.

Bartges, J.W. (2000). Diseases of the urinary bladder. In: *Saunders Manual of Small Animal Practice*, edited by S.J. Birchard and R.G. Sherding. Philadelphia, PA: WB Saunders, pp. 943–957.

Barth, A., I.M. Reichler, et al. (2005). Evaluation of long-term effects of endoscopic injection of collagen into the urethral submucosa for treatment of urethral sphincter incompetence in female dogs: 40 cases (1993–2000). *J Am Vet Med Assoc* **226**(1): 73–76.

Berent, A.C., P.D. Mayhew, et al. (2008). Use of cystoscopic-guided laser ablation for treatment of intramural ureteral ectopia in male dogs: four cases (2006–2007). *J Am Vet Med Assoc* **232**(7): 1026–1034.

Bernarde, A. and E. Viguier (2004). Transpelvic urethrostomy in 11 cats using an ischial ostectomy. *Vet Surg* **33**(3): 246–252.

Breitschwerdt, E.B., N.B. Olivier, et al. (1982). Bilateral hydronephrosis and hydroureter in a dog associated with congenital urethral stricture. *J Am Anim Hosp Assoc* **18**: 799–803.

Caione, P., N. Capozza, et al. (2005). Anterior perineal reconstruction in exstrophy-epispadias complex. *Eur Urol* **47**(6): 872–877; discussion 877–878.

Cassata, R., A. Iannuzzi, et al. (2008). Clinical, cytogenetic and molecular evaluation in a dog with bilateral cryptorchidism and hypospadias. *Cytogenet Genome Res* **120**(1–2): 140–143.

Caywood, D.D., C.A. Osborne, et al. (1980). Neoplasia of the canine and feline urinary tracts. In: *Current Veterinary Therapy VII*, edited by R.W. Kirk. Philadelphia, PA: WB Saunders, pp. 1203–1212.

Cornell, K.K. (2000). Cystotomy, partial cystectomy, and tube cystostomy. *Clin Tech Small Anim Pract* **15**(1): 11–16.

Duffey, M.H., M.D. Barnhart, et al. (1998). Incomplete urethral duplication with cyst formation in a dog. *J Am Vet Med Assoc* **213**(9): 1287–1289, 1279.

Foster, S.F., G.B. Hunt, et al. (1999). Congenital urethral anomaly in a kitten. *J Feline Med Surg* **1**(1): 61–64.

Galanty, M., P. Jurka, et al. (2008). Surgical treatment of hypospadias. Techniques and results in six dogs. *Pol J Vet Sci* **11**(3): 235–243.

Glassberg, K.I. (2002). Normal and abnormal development of the kidney: a clinician's interpretation of current knowledge. *J Urol* **167**: 2339–2351.

Gotthelf, L.N. (1981). Persistent urinary tract infection and urolithiasis in a cat with a urachal diverticulum. *Vet Med Small Anim Clin* **76**(12): 1745–1747.

Gray, L.A. (1968). Urethrovaginal fistulas. *Am J Obstet Gynecol* **101**(1): 28–36.

Greene, R.W. and R.H. Bohning, Jr. (1971). Patent persistent urachus associated with urolithiasis in a cat. *J Am Vet Med Assoc* **158**(4): 489–491.

Grieco, V., E. Riccardi, et al. (2008). Evidence of testicular dysgenesis syndrome in the dog. *Theriogenology* **70**(1): 53–60.

Halliwell, W.H. and N. Ackerman (1974). Botryoid rhabdomyosarcoma of the urinary bladder and hypertrophic osteoarthropathy in a young dog. *J Am Vet Med Assoc* **165**(10): 911–913.

Hanson, J.S. (1972). Patent urachus in a cat. *Vet Med Small Anim Clin* **67**: 379–381.

Haraguchi, R., J. Motoyama, et al. (2007). Molecular analysis of coordinated bladder and urogenital organ formation by hedgehog signalling. *Development* **134**: 525–533.

Hayes, H.M., Jr. and G.P. Wilson (1986). Hospital incidence of hypospadias in dogs in North America. *Vet Rec* **118**(22): 605–607.

Hobson, H.P. and P.L. Ader (1979). Exstrophy of the bladder in a dog. *J Am Anim Hosp Assoc* **15**: 103–107.

Holt, P.E. (1990). Urinary incontinence in dogs and cats. *Vet Rec* **127**(14): 347–350.

Holt, P.E. (1993). Surgical management of congenital urethral sphincter mechanism incompetence in eight female cats and a bitch. *Vet Surg* **22**(2): 98–104.

Holt, P.E. and C. Gibbs (1992). Congenital urinary incontinence in cats: a review of 19 cases. *Vet Rec* **130**(20): 437–442.

Holt, P.E., S.E. Long, et al. (1983). Disorders of urination associated with canine intersexuality. *J Small Anim Pract* **24**: 475–487.

Holt, P.E. and A.H. Moore (1995). Canine ureteral ectopia: an analysis of 175 cases and comparison of surgical treatments. *Vet Rec* **136**(14): 345–349.

Hoskins, J.D., Y.Z. Abdelbaki, et al. (1982). Urinary bladder duplication in a dog. *J Am Vet Med Assoc* **181**(6): 603–604.

Jackson, D.A. (1980). Pseudohermaphroditism. In: *Current Veterinary Therapy VII*, edited by R.W. Kirk. Philadelphia, PA: WB Saunders, pp. 1241–1243.

Jackson, D.A., C.A. Osborne, et al. (1978). Nonneurogenic urinary incontinence in a canine female pseudohermaphrodite. *J Am Vet Med Assoc* **172**(8): 926–930.

Johnston, G.R., C.A. Osborne, et al. (1986). Effects of urinary bladder distention on location of the urinary bladder and urethra of healthy dogs and cats. *Am J Vet Res* **47**(2): 404–415.

Johnston, S.D., N.C. Bailie, et al. (1989). Diphallia in a mixed-breed dog with multiple anomalies. *Theriogenology* **31**: 1253–1260.

Kelly, D.F. (1973). Rhabdomyosarcoma of the urinary bladder in dogs. *Vet Pathol* **10**: 375–384.

King, G.J. and E.H. Johnson (2000). Hypospadias in a Himalayan cat. *J Small Anim Pract* **41**(11): 508–510.

Kirsch, J.A., J.G. Hauptman, et al. (2002). A urethropexy technique for surgical treatment of urethral prolapse in the male dog. *J Am Anim Hosp Assoc* **38**(4): 381–384.

Kruger, J.M., C.A. Osborne, et al. (1995). Inherited and congenital disease of the lower urinary tract. In: *Canine and Feline Nephrology and Urology*, edited by C.A. Osborne and D.R. Finco. Baltimore, MD: Williams & Wilkins, pp. 681–692.

Lane, I.F. and M.R. Lappin (1995). Urinary incontinence and congenital urogenital anomalies in small animals. In: *Current Veterinary Therapy XII*, edited by J.D. Bonagura and R.W. Kirk. Philadelphia, PA: WB Saunders, pp. 1022–1026.

Lautzenhiser, S.J. and D.E. Bjorling (2002). Urinary incontinence in a dog with an ectopic ureterocele. *J Am Anim Hosp Assoc* **38**(1): 29–32.

Laverty, P.H. and S.K. Salisbury (2002). Surgical management of true patent urachus in a cat. *J Small Anim Pract* **43**(5): 227–229.

Lawler, D.V. and K.L. Monti (1984). Morbidity and mortality in neonatal kittens. *Am J Vet Res* **45**: 1455–1459.

Lefebvre, R. and B. Lussier (2005). A clinical case of hypospadias in a dog. *Can Vet J* **46**(11): 1022–1025.

Lobetti, R.G. and J.P. Goldin (1998). Emphysematous cystitis and bladder trigone diverticulum in a dog. *J Small Anim Pract* **39**(3): 144–147.

Longhofer, S.L., R.K. Jackson, et al. (1991). Hindgut and bladder duplication in a dog. *J Am Vet Med Assoc* **64**: 520–523.

Lulich, J.P., C.A. Osborne, et al. (1987). Urologic disorders of immature cats. *Vet Clin North Am Small Anim Pract* **17**(3): 663–696.

Lulich, J.P., C.A. Osborne, et al. (1989). Non-surgical correction of infection-induced struvite uroliths and a vesicourachal diverticulum in an immature dog. *J Small Anim Pract* **30**: 613–617.

Madarame, H., A. Ito, et al. (2003). Urinary bladder rhabdomyosarcoma (Botryoid Rhabdomyosarcoma) in a labrador retriever dog. *J Toxicol Pathol* **16**: 279–281.

Mahaffey, M.B., J.A. Barsanti, et al. (1984). Pelvic bladder in dogs without urinary incontinence. *J Am Vet Med Assoc* **184**(12): 1477–1479.

McLoughlin, M.A. and D.J. Chew (2000). Diagnosis and surgical management of ectopic ureters. *Clin Tech Small Anim Pract* **15**(1): 17–24.

Miller, C.F. (1980). Urethrorectal fistula with concurrent urolithiasis in a dog. *Vet Med Small Anim Clin* **75**(1): 73–76.

Noden, D.A. and A. deLahunta (1985). The Embryology of Domestic Animals. Baltimore: Williams & Wilkins.

Osborne, C.A. (1977). Urethrorectal fistulas. In: *Current Veterinary Therapy VI*, edited by R.W. Kirk. Philadelphia, PA: WB Saunders, pp. 985–986.

Osborne, C.A. and G.F. Hanlon (1967). Canine congenital ureteral ectopia: case report and review of literature. *J Am Anim Hosp Assoc* **3**: 111–122.

Osborne, C.A. and S.L. Sanderson (1995). Medical management of urethral prolapse in male dogs. In: *Current Veterinary Therapy XII*, edited by J.D. Bonagura and R.W. Kirk. Philadelphia, PA: WB Saunders, pp. 1027–1029.

Osborne, C.A., J.D. Rhoades, et al. (1966). Patent urachus in the dog. *J Am Anim Hosp Assoc* **2**: 245–250.

Osborne, C.A., D.G. Low, et al. (1968). Neoplasms of the canine and feline urinary bladder: incidence, etiologic factors, occurrence and pathologic features. *Am J Vet Res* **29**(10): 2041–2055.

Osborne, C.A., M.H. Engen, et al. (1975). Congenital urethrorectal fistula in two dogs. *J Am Vet Med Assoc* **166**(10): 999–1002.

Osborne, C.A., G.R. Johnston, et al. (1987). Etiopathogenesis and biological behavior of feline vesicourachal diverticula. Don't just do something—stand there. *Vet Clin North Am Small Anim Pract* **17**(3): 697–733.

Osborne, C.A., R.A. Kroll, et al. (1989). Medical management of vesicourachal diverticula in 15 cats with lower urinary tract disease. *J Small Anim Pract* **30**(11): 608–612.

Osuna, D.J., E.A. Stone, et al. (1989). A urethrorectal fistula with concurrent urolithiasis in a dog. *J Am Anim Hosp Assoc* **25**: 35–39.

Pavletic, M.M. (2007). Reconstruction of the urethra by use of an inverse tubed bipedicled flap in a dog with hypospadias. *J Am Vet Med Assoc* **231**(1): 71–73.

Pearson, H. and C. Gibbs (1971). Urinary tract abnormalities in the dog. *J Small Anim Pract* **12**(2): 67–84.

Pearson, H., C. Gibbs, et al. (1965). Some abnormalities of the canine urinary tract. *Vet Rec* **77**: 775–780.

Pletcher, J.M. and L. Dalton (1981). Botryoid rhabdomyosarcoma in the urinary bladder of a dog. *Vet Pathol* **18**(5): 695–697.

Ragni, R.A. (2007). Urethral prolapse in three male Yorkshire terriers. *J Small Anim Pract* **48**(3): 180.

Rawlings, C.A. (1984). Correction of congenital defects of the urogenital system. *Vet Clin North Am Small Anim Pract* **14**(1): 49–60.

Rawlings, C., J.A. Barsanti, et al. (2001). Evaluation of colposuspension for treatment of incontinence in spayed female dogs. *J Am Vet Med Assoc* **219**(6): 770–775.

Roszel, J.F. (1972). Cytology of urine from dogs with botryoid sarcoma of the bladder. *Acta Cytol* **16**(5): 443–446.

Schedl, A. (2007). Renal abnormalities and their developmental origin. *Nat Rev Gen* **8**: 791–802.

Scheepens, E.T. and H. L'Eplattenier (2005). Acquired urinary bladder diverticulum in a dog. *J Small Anim Pract* **46**(12): 578–581.

Schmaelzle, J.F., A.S. Cass, et al. (1969). Effect of disuse and restoration of function on vesical capacity. *J Urol* **101**(5): 700–705.

Senior, D.F., D.T. Lawrence, et al. (1993). Successful treatment of boytroid rhabdomyosarcoma in the bladder of a dog. *J Am Anim Hosp Assoc* **29**: 386–390.

Shimada, K., F. Matsumoto, et al. (2002). Surgical management of urinary incontinence in children with anatomical bladder-outlet anomalies. *Int J Urol* **9**(10): 561–566.

Silverman, S. and C.D. Long (2000). The diagnosis of urinary incontinence and abnormal urination in dogs and cats. *Vet Clin North Am Small Anim Pract* **30**(2): 427–448.

Sinibaldi, K.R. and R.W. Green (1973). Surgical correction of prolapse of the male urethra in three English bulldogs. *J Am Anim Hosp Assoc* **9**: 450–453.

Stamps, P. and D.L. Harris (1968). Botryoid rhabdomyosarcoma of the urinary bladder of a dog. *J Am Vet Med Assoc* **153**(8): 1064–1068.

Stone, E.A., T.F. George, et al. (1996). Partial cystectomy for urinary bladder neoplasia: surgical technique and outcome in 11 dogs. *J Small Anim Pract* **37**(10): 480–485.

Takiguchi, M., T. Watanabe, et al. (2002). Rhabdomyosarcoma (botryoid sarcoma) of the urinary bladder in a Maltese. *J Small Anim Pract* **43**(6): 269–271.

Tobias, K.S. and D. Barbee (1995). Abnormal micturition and recurrent cystitis associated with multiple congenital anomalies of the urinary tract in a dog. *J Am Vet Med Assoc* **207**(2): 191–193.

van Schouwenburg, S.J. and G.J. Louw (1982). A case of dysuria as a result of a communication between the urinary bladder and corpus uteri in a Cairn Terrier. *J S Afr Vet Assoc* **53**(1): 65–66.

Van Vechten, M., M.H. Goldschmidt, et al. (1990). Embryonal rhabdomyosarcoma of the urinary bladder in dogs. *Compend Contin Educ Vet* **12**: 783–793.

White, R.N. (2001). Urethropexy for the management of urethral sphincter mechanism incompetence in the bitch. *J Small Anim Pract* **42**(10): 481–486.

Whitney, W.O. and L.A. Schrader (1988). Urethrorectal fistulectomy in a dog, using a perineal approach. *J Am Vet Med Assoc* **193**(5): 568–569.

Wilson, G.P., L.S. Dill, et al. (1983). The relationship of urachal defects in the feline urinary bladder to feline urological syndrome. Proc 7th Kal Kan Symposium, Vernon, CA.

Wolff, A. and M. Radecky (1973). Anomaly in a poodle puppy. *Vet Med Small Anim Clin* **68**: 732–733.

Zulauf, D., K. Voss, et al. (2007). Herniation of the urinary bladder through a congenitally enlarged inguinal canal in a cat. *Schweiz Arch Tierheilkd* **149**(12): 559–562.

81

Inappropriate urination

Elizabeth A. Shull

Prevalence and etiology

Inappropriate urination is a frequent client behavioral complaint concerning both dogs and cats that are presented to veterinary behaviorists (Landsberg 1991; Denenberg et al. 2005) and a major reason for relinquishment of pets to animal shelters. In a multicenter study at 12 animal shelters, dogs and cats urinating inappropriately at least once a week were, respectively, 2–4 and 2–6 times more likely to be relinquished than were pets that only occasionally or never urinated inappropriately (Patronek et al. 1996a, 1996b; New et al. 2000).

The three major causes of inappropriate urination in dogs and cats are behavioral inappropriate urination, scent marking, and medically related inappropriate urination.

Despite owner's interpretations to the contrary, neither dogs nor cats urine mark or inappropriately urinate *out of spite*; to conclude, this is counterproductive to identifying the actual cause(s) and to resolving the problem.

Because the dissimilarities and idiosyncrasies of the diagnosis, management, and prognosis of inappropriate urination in the two species are greater than their similarities, each will be discussed separately.

Prevalence and etiology of inappropriate urination in cats

Inappropriate urination is the most common of all behavior problems in cats (Hart and Hart 1985; Landsberg 1991; Borchelt and Voith 1996; Salman et al. 2000; Denenberg et al. 2005) and is a major reason that cats are relinquished to animal shelters (Patronek et al.

1996b; Salman et al. 2000). Inappropriate urination may involve either depositing urine outside the litterbox for the purpose of elimination or depositing urine for the purpose of scent marking. It is possible for a cat to exhibit both inappropriate micturition and spraying. A variety of household surfaces may either be urinated or sprayed upon, resulting in objectionable odors, stains, and contamination of surfaces, which can lead to exclusion or removal of the cat from the household, or even euthanasia unless the behavior can be improved.

Urinating out of the litterbox for urine elimination will be referred to as inappropriate micturition, and depositing urine for scent marking will be referred to as spraying.

Inappropriate micturition accounts for over half of the cases of inappropriate urination in cats (Bamberger and Houpt 2006). Behavioral inappropriate micturition is primarily due to an aversion to something associated with the litter or litterbox or due to an attraction or preference for something outside the litterbox (Borchelt and Voith 1996; Neilson 2003, 2004).

Cats can have an aversion to the litter, the litterbox, and/or the location of the litterbox. Inadequate cleaning is a common cause of litter aversion. Different cats have different requirements for litter hygiene. Fastidious cats may seek alternative surfaces when the litter is even slightly dirty. In addition to an inadequately maintained litterbox, the texture and fragrance of the litter, the presence or absence of a litter deodorizer, the depth of litter in the box, or previous negative experiences, such as pain or fear, associated with the litter are also possible causes of litter aversion.

Litterbox aversion may be related to the type of box (open, covered, self-cleaning), inadequate size of the box, location of the box (high traffic, isolated, poor accessibility, or vulnerability e.g., surprise attacks by other cats), presence or absence of a litter liner, type or scent of the

Nephrology and Urology of Small Animals. Edited by Joe Bartges and David J. Polzin. © 2011 Blackwell Publishing Ltd.

agent used to clean the box, and previous negative litter-box experiences.

Cats that have been frightened or threatened by a person or another pet while in the box or that have experienced painful elimination in the litterbox can avoid using it. Cats that have had lower urinary tract disease may exhibit inappropriate micturition as a long-term sequelae (Neilson 2003), presumably due to a conditioned association of the litterbox with pain.

Alternatively, cats may seek other surfaces and locations for urination, either because they have a primary individual preference for a particular surface or because they have come to associate a particular type of surface or a certain location with the act of urinating (Borchelt and Voith 1996). This is not surprising given that free-ranging cats have an infinite choice of locations and surfaces from which to choose, while household cats are expected to use the litterbox, the litter, and the location that is selected by the care-giver.

Separation anxiety and other fears or anxieties may result in inappropriate micturition, which may or may not be accompanied by inappropriate defecation.

Medical abnormalities are important causes of inappropriate micturition as number of systemic and urinary disorders may lead to changes in micturition. Metabolic, endocrine, and renal diseases may cause inappropriate micturition due to polyuria, pollakiuria, or other mechanisms. Neurological, musculoskeletal, and lower urinary tract abnormalities may be responsible for inappropriate micturition as a result of pain, decreased mobility, weakness, decreased control, or decreased awareness, for example, cognitive dysfunction.

Lower urinary tract disease, especially feline idiopathic cystitis (FIC), is of special interest because of the inter-relationships between stress and FIC. On the one hand, cats suffering from FIC frequently urinate outside the litterbox and therefore may be presented for inappropriate urination. On the other hand, stress associated with factors in the cat's behavioral and environmental management has been shown to play a role in the development of FIC (Westropp and Buffington 2004; Houstuler et al. 2005) (see chapter on FIC in this text).

Spraying is a normal communication behavior that is objectionable inside the home. The scent of the urine and the posture assumed by the cat during spraying provide an olfactory and a visual communication signals, respectively.

Contrary to popular belief, spraying does not function to repel other cats from a resident cat's territory. Rather, it provides information about the individual that is spraying, such as its sex, reproductive status, and the length of time since it was at that location. Consequently, spraying may serve as an advertisement for breeding individuals and may facilitate temporal spacing of cats within their home range. Nonbreeding free-living intact males spray an average of 12 times an hour and breeding males spray an average of 22 times an hour, up to a maximum rate of 62 times an hour. Free-living intact female cats may spray 6 times per hour (Turner and Bateson 1988; Houpt 2005).

The likelihood that a household cat will spray is influenced by the cat's sex and sexual status. Intact males spray most frequently, followed by neutered males, then intact females and spayed females. Male cats living in the same household with female cats are more likely to spray than male cats not living with female cats; female cats in estrus are more likely to spray than nonestrus females and the greater the number of cats in the household the greater the probability that spraying will occur in the household. When there were ten or more cats living in a household, the probability of spraying in the household was 100% (Jemmette and Skeritt 1979).

Sexual, territorial, or conflict situations, often involving other cats, and heightened levels of arousal, and anxiety are associated with an increased incidence of spraying. Spraying can also be triggered by environmental factors such as residual urine odors, unfamiliar odors, or the presence of unfamiliar animals or people. Outside intruding cats may stimulate spraying around doors, windows, air vents, electrical receptacles, and fireplaces by the inside cat(s).

Clinical signs and diagnosis of inappropriate urination in cats

A medical history, physical examination, and baseline laboratory evaluation should be included in the diagnostic work-up of cats with inappropriate urination, even if the history is not necessarily suggestive of a medical cause. Additional laboratory tests, radiographs, and other imaging procedures may be necessary depending on the initial findings (see chapter on "Diagnostic Testing" in this text).

Once medical etiologies are excluded, the diagnosis of behavioral inappropriate urination is based on a careful, detailed behavioral history. A client-completed questionnaire and a simple diagram of the home's floor plan, indicating the locations of doors, windows, food, water, litter boxes, perches/resting sites, and the sites of inappropriate urination, are helpful in discriminating between inappropriate micturition and spraying and in beginning to elucidate their causes.

Inappropriate micturition is discriminated from spraying based on the cat's posture, the surface (horizontal or vertical) on which the urine is deposited, the volume of urine that is deposited, and by considering the context in which the urine is deposited.

Behavioral-inappropriate micturition involves depositing urine, while in a squatting posture on to a horizontal surface outside the litterbox for the purpose of urine elimination. The typical micturition behavioral sequence involves digging a hole, urinating in the hole, turning, sniffing, then earth-raking over the hole, and perhaps sniffing and earth-raking some more. Many deviations from the typical sequence are possible. The deviations may reflect normal variation in behavior, but in cats with inappropriate micturition, the deviations may provide clues to the cause of the problem. For example, cats that dig or earth-rake very little or not at all and cats that spray while in the litterbox may have an aversion to the litter or the litterbox. Others that "earth-rake" on surfaces other than the litter, for example the sides of the box, the bath tub beside the box, or a throw rug close to the box, may have or may be developing a preference for or an association with other surfaces with urination.

Cats with behavioral inappropriate micturition may also exhibit inappropriate defecation, but do not necessarily do so. Cats with inappropriate micturition may urinate out of the litterbox all of the time or only part of the time.

During spraying, a cat typically deposits a small amount of urine onto a vertical surface at a height that is conducive for olfactory investigation of the urine. In typical spraying, the cat is in a standing posture, the tail is held erect and quivered, and the hindquarters are held high. It is possible for a cat to exhibit only the visual signal of a spraying posture without expressing urine. Spraying may also be done in a squatting posture (Turner and Bateson 1988), but is less common than erect spraying. Urine is often sprayed on established marking posts and/or sites or objects that have social or conflict significance, for example, a cat that is motivated to go outside but is blocked from doing so may spray near exit doors.

In multiple-cat households, behavioral and environmental manipulations may be necessary to identify which cat(s) is(are) responsible. Several methods have been described for determining which cat(s) in a multi-cat house is responsible for inappropriate micturition or spraying, and each has advantages and limitations (Neilson 2003).

Systematic isolation of the cats may help; however, it may also change the behavior through changing the social relationships among the cats or by preventing the cat's access to urination sites.

Video recording has the advantage of potentially identifying the responsible cat(s) with certainty; however, the monitoring requires time, expense, and some technical ability, and the presence of the equipment may interfere with the cat's behavior. If the behavior only occurs sporadically and not at a consistent location, the behavior may be difficult to capture on video.

Fluorescein dye may be systematically administered to each cat to increase the fluorescence of the treated cat's urine (Hart and Leedy 1982). All urine fluoresces under UV light, but the urine of cats treated with fluorescein fluoresces more brightly for 24 hours. The fluorescein (50 mg of fluorescein per cat) may be administered orally in a capsule or may be administered subcutaneously (0.3 mL of 10% Fluorescite Injection per cat). The oral fluorescein can be prepared by a compounding pharmacist or can be made by inserting 9 fluorescein ophthalmic strips into a gelatin capsule that is then administered orally to the cat (Hart 1982). New urine spots should be checked with a portable, handheld, battery-powered UV light to determine the degree of fluorescence in order to incriminate or exonerate the fluorescein-treated cat. A reported important limitation of this identification method is that is works most effectively in an alkaline urine, thereby restricting its use only to cats with alkaline urine (Houpt 2005; Horwitz and Nielson 2007).

Establishing a functional diagnosis of inappropriate micturition helps identify the contributing factors and is determined through a comprehensive history and descriptions of the cat's behavior in and around the litterbox and at the inappropriate location.

Litter/litterbox aversion is suggested by any of the following behaviors: approaching the box hesitantly, perching on the edge of the box, not scratching in the litter, spraying while in the litterbox, urinating outside the box, running away from the box, and paw shaking or vocalizing upon exiting the box.

A surface preference is suggested when a cat predominantly selects a particular type of surface for inappropriate micturition.

A location preference is suggested when the cat predominantly selects one room or region of a room when it urinates outside the litterbox.

Inappropriate micturition due to separation anxiety is suspected when the elimination occurs in the owner's absence. Urinating on the owner's bed is a common manifestation of separation anxiety (Schwarz 2003). Cats may not exhibit inappropriate micturition for many hours following separation from the owner, as opposed to within the first 30 minutes of departures, which is often the case in dogs.

Inappropriate micturition due to other fears or anxieties is suggested when inappropriate micturition occurs in association with stimuli or circumstances to which the cat exhibits fear or anxiety, for example, aggression between cats or the presence of a visitor of whom the cat is fearful.

Spraying is diagnosed by either observing the cat in a spraying posture or observing urine on vertical surfaces. Infrequently, urine may be sprayed by a cat in a squatting posture, which can make the distinction between spraying and inappropriate micturition somewhat more difficult; however, even when a cat squat-sprays, its tail quivers and it makes treading movements with its back legs. In contrast to the behavior sequence when voiding, a spraying cat does not sniff or earthrake the site after depositing urine (Turner and Bateson 1988).

Treatment of inappropriate micturition

Enticing the cat to consistently use a litterbox involves changing the features and the maintenance of the litter and litterbox to accommodate the cat's behavioral needs and preferences, while concurrently modifying the behavioral and environmental management of the cat to make the inappropriate sites of inappropriate micturition less attractive and/or less accessible.

Because inadequate cleaning of the litterbox is a common reason for inappropriate elimination, scooping the litter at least once daily and, even more often for cats that are fastidious, is recommended. Litterboxes containing traditional litter should be emptied, and washed with fragrance-free soap and hot water at least once a week. Litterboxes containing clumpable litter should be completely emptied and washed every two weeks.

The odor of excreta and its breakdown products is presumably aversive to cats. One study demonstrated that a spray product (Zero-odor®) designed to reduce litterbox odors increased the use of the litterbox and decreased the frequency of inappropriate elimination (Cottam and Dodman 2007). Other investigations have shown that litter with activated carbon for odor control is used more frequently than both identical litter without activated carbon and another brand of litter that contains sodium bicarbonate for odor control (Neilson 2009).

Litter with no fragrance is frequently recommended, although results of studies have conflicting results (Horwitz 1997; Sung and Crowell-Davis 2006). A recent pilot study of scent preferences in cats demonstrated that cats in the study avoided floral and citrus scents (Neilson 2007). Based on this, litters with either floral or citrus fragrances are not recommended. In fact, clinical experience has shown that placement of citrus-scented air fresheners at inappropriate urination sites has been beneficial in deterring cats from returning to those sites.

In general, cats prefer clumpable, finely grained litter more than coarse, non-clumpable litter (Borchelt 1991).

However, cats can have unique preferences and providing a smorgasbord of litter choices may be necessary to identify the type of litter most appealing to an individual cat.

Trimming hair between footpads, under the tail, and in the perineal region of longhaired cats helps prevent litter and stool from attaching to the hair, which may be uncomfortable and result in the cat avoiding litter.

It is sometimes helpful to reinforce the cat's use of the litterbox by offering it a very palatable treat immediately after the litterbox is used. Care must be taken not to disturb the cat, while it is actually using the box or to be intrusive in any way, as this would only reinforce the cat's aversion to the litter. The treat should be offered only after the cat has taken a couple of steps away from the box. With some cats, the opportunity to play with a toy or catnip may be more rewarding than a food treat. This method does not always achieve the desired results; one of the author's patients that was highly motivated by food treats, learned to enter and exit the litterbox, and then approach the owner and solicit the treat.

The number of litterboxes in the household should equal the number of cats plus one. Boxes should be dispersed throughout the home and be easily accessible. Locations where the cat may be startled by household activities or other pets should be avoided.

Larger litterboxes (22 × 15 × 6.5 in) tend to be used more than identical smaller litterboxes (14 × 10 × 3.3 in) (Neilson 2009). Clinical experience suggests that the litterbox should be large enough to allow the cat to enter, turn around, and fully stand without contacting the box. Large plastic storage boxes rather than commercial litterboxes best accommodate large and overweight cats.

Open boxes are recommended because odors are less likely to be retained than in covered boxes and because owners may scoop more often when the excreta is visible.

When there is an aversion to the litterbox or the location of the litterbox, providing additional boxes at alternative locations or providing a different type of box may be necessary. If the cat has acquired a fear or aversion of litterboxes in general, it may be necessary to desensitize the cat to litterboxes. This can be done by replacing the box with a tray and rewarding the cat for using the tray. When the cat accepts using the tray and uses it consistently for at least 2 weeks, it can be replaced with a shallow box. This process can be continued, gradually returning to a litterbox with sides of adequate height to prevent litter from being scattered during digging.

For inappropriate micturition due to a substrate preference, for example carpet, the treatment strategy involves providing the preferred substrate in the litterbox and/or making the inappropriate surface outside of the litterbox less attractive.

Methods of modifying the litterbox to provide the cat's substrate preference are limited only by one's imagination and ingenuity. Some commonly used modifications include, placing carpet remnants on the floor of the litterbox or attaching strips of carpet to the interior upright sides of the litterbox with double-sided sticky tape for cats that are attracted to carpet, placing disposable diapers in the bottom of the litterbox for cats that are attracted to soft, plush substrates, and for cats that prefer smooth surfaces, litter can temporarily be left out of the box. Once the modified box is being consistently used, litter can be gradually reintroduced and the alternate substrate gradually replaced or withdrawn.

To make the substrate outside the litterbox less accessible or less attractive, it can be covered with other substrates that have a different or even aversive texture such as painter's plastic drop cloth, plastic carpet runner turned upside down with the hard nubs facing upward, aluminum foil, and double-sided sticky tape among many other possibilities. Alternatively, the significance of the region can be changed by placing food and water bowls over the area, or an odor that is unattractive to cats, such as strong floral or citrus scents may be placed in the area.

For a location preference, the litterbox may temporarily be placed at the preferred location until the cat reestablishes use of the box, then the litterbox may be gradually moved to a more acceptable location. Alternatively, the cat's access to the location may be physically blocked, or the location may be made less attractive in the same manner as described above for making a preferred substrate less attractive.

If the inappropriate micturition is due to fear, anxiety, or intercat conflict, those behavioral issues must be addressed in order to get the cat back in the litterbox. Changes in behavioral and environmental management to minimize the cat's exposure to a fearful-eliciting stimulus, desensitization and counterconditioning to reduce the cat's response to the fear stimulus and in some instances antianxiety medication may be necessary (See Table 81.1). A discussion of the diagnosis and management of anxiety and aggression problems and the use of behavior-modifying drugs in cats is beyond the scope of this chapter, and the reader is referred to a number of excellent references including but not limited to Voith and Borchelt (1996), Beaver (2003), Landsberg et al. (2003), Simpson and Papich (2003), Houpt (2005), and Horwitz and Neilson (2007) for a more complete treatment of these topics. It is important to note that no drugs have been approved for the treatment of behavioral problems in cats.

Sites of inappropriate micturition should be treated with an effective enzymatic odor eliminator and repeat applications should be done until urine odor is not renewed by a fresh application of the odor eliminator. Ammonia-based cleaners should be avoided.

Multimodal environmental modification (MEMO; Buffington et al. 2006) should be included in the treatment as well as the prevention of inappropriate micturition in cats with FIC as a contributing factor (Chapter 75).

Punishment is never helpful. Scolding, punishing, or rubbing the cat's nose in its mess, then putting it in the litterbox is especially detrimental and increases the likelihood that the cat will permanently avoid the litterbox in the future.

Many cases of inappropriate micturition could be avoided by adherence to basic principles for managing litterboxes and guidelines for preventing the development of behavioral inappropriate micturition are given in Table 81.2.

Treatment of spraying

The internal/endogenous motivational factors and the social and environmental triggers must be identified in order to develop a specific treatment plan for spraying.

Neutering decreases spraying in 90% of intact males and 95% of intact females, and is an absolute requisite

Table 81.1 Guidelines for preventing elimination problems in cats

A. Litter box location
   Easily accessible
   Quiet and away from traffic, but not isolated
   Away from food and water
   Accommodate physical limitations and personality

B. Litter
   Scoop at least once a day
   Change traditional litter once a week
   Change scoopable litter every two weeks
   Finely granular (clumpable, scoopable) usually preferred
   Offer smorgasbord to determine cat's preference

C. Type of box
   Open preferred most often
   Size accommodation, sweater storage box for larger cats

D. Minimum of one box for each cat

E. Avoid fear and pain in box

F. Never scold or punish for inappropriate elimination

G. Prevent other animals and people from disturbing cat in litter box

H. NEVER place or force into box associated with scolding!

I. Softly praise and occasionally reinforce with treat for use of litter box

J. Make any and all litterbox changes gradually

Table 81.2 Guidelines for house-training

- Provide constant supervision when the dog is loose and observe for signals (restlessness, sniffing, circling, etc.) that it is preparing to eliminate. Take outside to a designated area. Pair a cue work with elimination; later the cue can be used to trigger eliminations.
- Use "umbilical cord" method of tethering the dog to a person to prevent the dog from wandering away and eliminating.
- Take dog out at least every 1 to 2 hours when awake. Puppies younger than 3–4 months of age urinate frequently when they are awake.
- Encouraged the dog to eliminate in various locations in the yard and on walks to avoid elimination from becoming contextualized to one location.
- Eating, drinking, playing, and awakening stimulate elimination. Walk puppies within one minute or even less, and juveniles and adults within 5 minutes of these activities.
- Confine when supervision is not possible. This utilizes a dog's natural tendency to keep its "nest" clean. For puppies and small dogs, a crate is adequate for confinement no more than 2 or 3 hours. For longer periods and for larger dogs, a X pen will provide space for separate sleeping, water, and elimination area, out of the immediate vicinity of the "nesting" area. House-training will become a difficult and arduous task if the inhibition of soiling the nest is lost.
- Praise and sometimes provide a small treat for eliminating at an appropriate location.
- Go outside with the dog during house-training. Putting the dog outside, but not going with it to assure it eliminated and to praise it for appropriate elimination often leads to house-training failure.
- Feed meals on a regular schedule to regulate eliminations.
- Scolding and correction are only helpful if the dog is observed eliminating. The intensity of the correction should only be enough to interrupt the elimination behavior, then the dog should be taken outside, allowed to calm down, and encouraged to finish eliminating at a correct location. Harsh scolding or punishment will teach the dog to avoid eliminating in the owner's presence. Scolding after the fact by taking the dog to the spot and pointing out what it did wrong or rubbing its nose in its mess is totally ineffective and only confuses the dog.
- Block the dog's access to a preferred location or substrate, until a consistent habit of eliminating in the correct location has been established.
- When elimination occurs inside urine should be soaked up with an absorbent cloth, and feces should be picked up as soon as possible, then the area thoroughly cleaned with plain soap and water. If the elimination occurred on a carpeted area or upholstered object, an enzymatic odor eliminator should be applied after the area has dried from the cleaning. For urination sites, reapplication of the odor eliminator may be necessary until a new application does not refresh the urine odor.

for successfully treating spraying in intact cats, although it may not completely eliminate the problem. There may be a delay of several weeks to a few months in reduction of spraying after neutering.

For cats that are already neutered and/or cats in which neutering is not adequately successful, the cat's exposure to identified triggering stimuli can be minimized and/or the cats response to those factors reduced using desensitization methods. Triggers from outside cats may be reduced by blocking the inside cat's view of the outside and by discouraging the presence of outside cats by removing attractants such as outside food and water, bird feeders, etc., and employing repellents such as *The Scarecrow*®, a motion-activated water sprinkler.

In multi-cat households, reducing the number of cats may also decrease the incidence of spraying; however, this is often an unacceptable solution to many owners. Alternatively, minimizing the distress some cats experience as a result of being in a multicat household by employing environmental and cognitive enrichment techniques and, if indicated, addressing inter-cat aggression between specific cats are often beneficial. The diagnosis and treat-

ment of inter-cat aggression is beyond the scope of this chapter and the reader is referred to other texts for a more complete discussion.

Environmental enrichment provides inside cats with more choices and a degree of control of their environment, as well as segregating resources in order to limit competition and congregation of cats around resources. There should be several sites of food, water, resting perches, hiding boxes, climbing structures, and increased access to vertical space throughout the living space. Cognitive enrichment can be achieved through play and interaction with the owners that occurs regularly and predictably and through activities, such as clicker training, and foraging games.

Urine odor should be removed by the application of an enzymatic urine odor eliminator. When areas have been repeatedly sprayed and become saturated with urine it may not be possible to get rid of the odor unless the objects are removed from the home.

The cat's access to spraying posts may be blocked or the site made less attractive by placing aversive scents, for example floral potpourri or citrus scent in the vicinity or changing the significance from a spraying post to a feeding or play station. Alternatively, the cat may be encouraged to scent mark with cheek glands or by scratching by providing cat combs (Mr. Spats®, Cat-a-Combs®, Levine) or scratching posts. *Feliway® (a synthetic facial pheromone)*, may have the dual benefit of inducing a cat to mark by facial rubbing rather than spraying and may also function to help reduce anxiety.

One study (Pryor year) demonstrated that cleaning urine marks with an enzymatic odor neutralizer and improved management of litterboxes, that is adding more boxes, and increasing the frequency of litterbox cleaning decreased the frequency of spraying.

In the author's experience, anti-anxiety medication is frequently the first treatment that is considered by many veterinarians and that owners request for urine marking. Anti-anxiety medication is in fact beneficial in some cases of urine marking to reduce the spraying cat's arousal level and response to triggering stimuli; however, it should be used as an adjunctive treatment to changes in the cat's environmental and behavioral management.

Before a behavioral drug is prescribed, a thorough knowledge of its actions, side-effect profile, and drug interactions should be understood, and the cat should have routine laboratory work performed. Owners must be informed that no drugs have been approved by the FDA for treatment of spraying or any behavior problems in cats.

Selective serotonin reuptake inhibitors and tricyclic antianxiety medications are the currently preferred medications based on their efficacy and how they are tolerated. Medications and dosages for anxiety-related inappropriate micturition and spraying are given in Table 81.2.

The reader is encouraged to consult other references for more complete discussion of behavioral drugs and their use in cats.

Punishment is counterproductive and only increases the cat's anxiety, which has the potential of increasing spraying.

Prevalence and etiology of inappropriate urination in dogs

House-soiling, in general, is reported to be either the most common or one of the most common reasons that dogs are relinquished to animal shelters (Salman et al. 2000; Scarlett 2003), and it is one of the top four reasons that dogs are presented to veterinary behaviorists Bamberger and Houpt 2006).

The major causes of inappropriate urination in dogs include incomplete house-training, which involves both urination and defecation, urine marking, anxiety dis-

orders, for example separation anxiety and noise phobia, which also usually involve both inappropriate urination and defecation, submissive urination, excitement/greeting urination, and inappropriate urination due to underlying medical disorders.

Incomplete house-training is a very common cause of house-soiling. In one retrospective study at a veterinary teaching hospital of 105 dogs diagnosed with house-soiling, 84% were diagnosed with incomplete house-training. Dogs that are incompletely house-trained deposit urine and/or stool at inappropriate locations within the home for the purpose of ridding the body of waste. Incomplete house-training is especially typical of puppies and young dogs, but it may turn into a long-term problem and continue into adulthood if it is not properly addressed in a timely manner, before the dog develops elimination preferences and habits.

Urine marking is a normal behavior that is an important mode of communication in dogs. Chemical or olfactory communication is thought to be more important for domestic dogs than are visual signals (Serpell). Dogs can identify species, sex, and even individuals from urine odors (Houpt 2005) and also use urine to indicate home ranges and territories. Estrus females advertise by urine marking and the pheromone in estrus female urine aids males in locating and identifying estrus females. Consequently, urine marking often occurs in territorial, sexual, and conflict situations.

Intact males, and estrus females mark most frequently; however, other intact females, and neutered males and females may also urine mark. Urine marking typically develops between one and two years of age; however, in one report, 10% of dogs that presented for a problem of urine marking began exhibiting urine marking at 3 months of age (Voith and Borchelt 1996). Dogs may urine mark inside the home despite being otherwise well house-trained.

Dogs with separation anxiety and noise phobias may exhibit inappropriate elimination as part of their anxiety response. Anxiety disorders are the second most common reason that dogs are presented for behavior problems, less common only than aggression. Dogs with separation anxiety and noise phobia are often well house-trained except when they are anxious. The inappropriate elimination of dogs with separation anxiety is often misinterpreted by owners as spiteful behavior for being left home alone when in fact it is a reflection of the physiological arousal that accompanies the dog's anxiety.

Submissive urination is manifested by submissive dogs in response to perceived threats or dominance signals from other dogs or from humans. It is normal in puppies and is most common in female and excessively submissive dogs.

Excitement/greeting urination is urination that occurs when the dog is very excited, oftentimes by owners returning home and when greeting new individuals. Similar to submissive urination, this occurs most frequently in young dogs and female dogs.

Any systemic or urinary disorder, which results in pollakiuria, polyuria, or dysuria, may present as inappropriate urination. Additionally, disorders that interfere with the dog's mobility (musculoskeletal or neurological disorders, systemic weakness, and painful conditions), or voluntary control or cognitive awareness of micturition may result inappropriate urination (Chapter 47).

Clinical signs

Incomplete house-training usually involves both urination and defecation and is related to normal patterns of elimination. The character and the volume of urine and stool are normal and the eliminations occur in association with eating, drinking, and other predictable patterns of activity. The occurrence of inappropriate elimination due to incomplete house-training is typically correlated to the length of time since the dog had access to an appropriate site for eliminating. The longer the length of time since the dog has had access to an appropriate outside location for eliminating, the greater the likelihood that it will eliminate inside. House-soiling due to incomplete house-training may occur whether or not the owner is home, and it is not associated with fear or anxiety, or other arousing circumstances as are urine marking, and submissive and excitement/greeting urination. The dog may have a substrate and/or location preferences within the home, always returning to a specific area or always seeking certain surfaces on which to eliminate.

Anxiety disorders may result in inappropriate elimination, often both urination and defecation, when the dog is experiencing fear or anxiety. Dogs with separation anxiety and noise phobias are frequently well house-trained at other times. In addition to the inappropriate urination, these dogs typically also exhibit other symptoms of anxiety, including frantic/panicked attitude, destructive behavior, excessive vocalization, and evidence of autonomic arousal, that is panting, salivating, and trembling. Urine marking typically involves raised-leg urination onto a vertical surface, although there are many variations of urine-marking postures in male dogs in response to arousing social stimuli such as female dogs in estrus, unfamiliar dogs, strange odors, human visitors, and even anxiety (Landsberg 1991). There may be established marking posts that are regularly marked. The volume of urine is usually smaller than the volume that is deposited when emptying the bladder for voiding. Marking is unrelated to the length of time since the dog has had an opportunity to go outside to eliminate.

Female urine marking

Submissive urination is voiding of a relatively small amount of urine by a dog in a submissive posture (lowered head and neck, ears back, averted gaze, and low to crouched body posture, or rolling over on its side to expose its inguinal area) in the context of the dog perceiving a threat or having a dominance signal directed toward it. Submissive urination has a communication function of inhibiting aggression from the challenging/threatening dog. People may trigger this behavior in submissive dogs by approaching, or leaning over them, speaking loudly to, staring at, picking up, scolding, or punishing the dog. This type of urination is not related to house-training.

Excitement/greeting urination is voiding of a small amount of urine while standing, walking, or jumping in the context of being very excited. This seems to occur most when the dog is excitedly greeting owners on their return from an absence. It is most common in puppies and young females. Excitement/greeting urination is not related to inadequate house-training.

Medically related inappropriate urination is suggested by loss of house-training in a previously well-trained dog. There is often a change in the frequency of elimination, the character and/or volume of the urine that is deposited, or evidence of loss of control of eliminations. Weakness, discomfort, or other symptoms of illness may also be evident.

Diagnosis

An accurate behavioral diagnosis of the type of inappropriate urination is necessary for successful treatment. The diagnosis is based on the age and sex of the dog, a description of the inappropriate urination, and the circumstances in which it occurs. The possibility of an underlying medical problem must also be considered and ruled out before a strictly behavioral diagnosis is made. A medical history, physical examination, baseline laboratory evaluation, including a CBC, serum chemistries, urinalysis, and possibly a urine culture and sensitivity will often be necessary in the evaluation of inappropriate urination.

Depending on the history and initial physical examination and results of the baseline laboratory tests, other medical tests may be indicated. If the use of behavioral medication is being considered in the therapeutic plan, baseline laboratory testing should be done, even if a contributing medical disorder is not suspected.

Treatment

The ideal treatment for incomplete house-training is prevention. *House-training is based on the principle that dogs learn where to eliminate rather than where NOT to eliminate.* Never giving a dog an opportunity to eliminate in the house is the best method of training it to only urinate outside. When a new puppy or dog is brought into the household, a house-training program should be instituted as soon as the dog arrives. A successful house-training program consists of taking the dog to an appropriate location for elimination on a regular schedule, positive reinforcement for eliminating at an acceptable location, constant supervision when the dog is loose in the house, and confinement when supervision is not possible.

Inappropriate urination due to anxiety is treated by managing the underlying anxiety. However, when a dog eliminates inappropriately as a result of being anxious, it may lose its inhibitions for eliminating inside and may secondarily learn to associate locations within the house with eliminating. If this happens, in addition to treating the anxiety disorder, remedial house-training will be required.

Urine marking

- Neuter intact dogs. Castration results in improvement in 70% of intact male dogs, and spaying will resolve heat-related urine marking in female dogs. The decline in urine marking may be delayed for several weeks to several months following neutering.
- If possible, either identify and remove arousing stimuli or minimize the dog's exposure to the stimuli; if that is not possible, institute supervision and confinement, as with incomplete house-training. If there are only one or two stimuli that elicit the marking, for example strangers coming to the home, desensitization training may be beneficial in decreasing the dog's arousal to the triggering stimuli.
- If the dog only marks at one or two marking posts, the significance of those sites may be changed by turning them into water and feeding stations.
- Clean and apply an enzymatic urine odor eliminator to the marked surfaces, to remove odor cues in the urine that may trigger additional marking.
- Dog belly bands for male dogs, available as many different commercial brands, or easily made, will absorb urine when it is expressed and prevent it from hitting surfaces and may even inhibit a dog from marking while it is being worn.
- Startling or scolding the dog when caught in the act may interrupt the behavior, but will probably not prevent the dog from marking again. If the correction is too harsh, the dog will just learn to not mark in the owner's presence, and the dog may become fearful of the person.
- DAP® synthetic dog appeasing pheromone may be helpful in some dogs to decrease anxiety and subsequently decrease the dog's arousal level in response to triggering stimuli.
- In difficult cases, anti-anxiety medication may be prescribed as an adjunctive treatment to the changes in behavioral and environmental management and the behavioral modification training (see Appendix).

Submissive urination

Inappropriate management of this type of elimination in puppies and adults frequently makes it worse. In general, the adult dog with this disorder is excessively submissive.

- In many cases, this type of urination will spontaneously resolve with maturity.
- The behavior should be *ignored*! The dog should not be punished or "reassured." Punishment will elicit more submission and consequently more urination. Reassurance by petting or talking to the dog while it is urinating submissive will reinforce the behavior.
- Avoid threatening and dominance gestures.
  - Instead of making direct eye contact, look at the dog with an averted gaze.
  - Squat down beside the dog rather leaning over it.
  - Petting the dog on the side or under the chin is less threatening than petting on the top of the head or the back.
  - Use a quiet tone of voice and avoid speaking loudly.
  - Desensitization to triggers of submissive behavior may be necessary if management changes are not adequate.
- In difficult cases, anti-anxiety medication may be prescribed to decrease the dog anxiety.

If the behavior doesn't spontaneously resolve with maturity or respond to behavior modification changes in management, the possibility of weak urethral tone or control should be considered. Medications that increase urethral tone may be prescribed in those instances.

Excitement/greeting urination

Greeting is a very important part of dog's social behavior and should not be eliminated. However, the greeting routine can be changed to reduce the consequences of the excitement/greeting urination.

- Make inside greetings low-key and calm.
- If possible, instead of greeting the dog inside the house, call the dog outside and greet there. The excitement and

exuberance of the greeting can be redirected to running and playing.

- As with submissive urination, excitement/greeting urination often resolves with maturity, if it does not specific desensitization training, may be necessary and the possibility of inadequate urethral tone or control should be considered.
- Anti-anxiety medication or medication to increase urethral tone may be considered in cases that do not resolve or respond to behavioral methods.
- Scolding and punishment is not helpful.

Prognosis

The prognosis for many inappropriate problems in dogs is good as long as the correct diagnosis is determined and appropriate treatment is implemented. The longer the duration of inappropriate urination, the more difficult it will be to completely resolve it.

House-training will be most successful when appropriate measures are used and the problem is addressed before long-standing habits and preferences have been established. Urine marking significantly improves with neutering in the majority of dogs. Submissive and excitement/greeting urination generally spontaneously resolve as maturity is reached and the object of treatment is to find a method of managing the urination until the dog matures. Those cases that do not resolve with maturity are challenging and may require additional medical evaluation. Inappropriate elimination due to anxiety disorders is more problematic, because, permanently resolving separation anxiety and noise phobia is unlikely, and the inappropriate elimination associated with those disorders can be expected to persist until the anxiety is adequately managed.

References

Bamberger, M. and K. Houpt (2006). Signalment factors, comorbidity and trends in behavioral diagnosis in cats 736 cases (1991–2001). *J Am Vet Med Assoc* **229**(10): 1602–1606.

Borchelt, P.L. (1991). Cat elimination problems, edited by A.R. Marder and V.L. Voith. *Vet Clin North Am: Small Anim Pract* **21**(2): 247–256.

Borchelt, P.L. and V.L. Voith (1996). Elimination behavior problems in cats. In: *Readings in Companion Animal Behavior*, edited by Victoria L. Voith and Peter L. Borchelt. Trenton: Veterinary Learning Systems Co., Inc, pp. 179–190.

Buffington, C.A.T., J.L. Westropp, et al. (2006). Clinical evaluation of multimodal environmental modification (MEMO) in management of cats with idiopathic cystitis. *J Feline Med Surg* **8**: 261–268.

Cottam, N. and N. Dodman (2007). Effect of an odor eliminator on feline litterbox behavior. *Journal of Feline Medicine and Surgery* **9**: 44–50.

Denenberg, S., G.M. Landsberg, et al. (2005). A comparison of cases referred to behviorists in three different countries. In: *Current Issues and Research in Veterinary Behavioral Medicine*, edited by D. Mills, E. Levine, et al. Lafayette: Purdue University, pp. 56–62.

Hart, B.L. and M. Leedy (1982). Identification of source of urine stains in multi-cat households. *J Am Vet Med Assoc* **180**: 77–78.

Hart, B., et al. (2006). *Canine and Feline Behavioral Therapy*, 2nd edition. Ames, IA: Blackwell Publishing.

Horwitz, D.F. (1997). Behavioral and environmental factors associated with elimination behavior problems in cats: a retrospective study. *Appl Anim Behav Sci* **52**: 129–137.

Horwitz, D.F. and J.C. Neilson (2007). *Canine and Feline Behavior*. Ames, IA: Blackwell Publishing, p. 508.

Houpt, K.A. (2005). *Domestic Animal Behavior for Veterinarians and Animal Scientists*, 4th edition. Ames, IA: Blackwell Publishing, pp. 24–27.

Houstuler, R.A., D.F. Chew, et al. (2005). Recent concepts in feline lower urinary tract disease. *Vet Clin Small Anim* **35**: 147–170.

Jemmette, J.E. and G. Skeritt (1979). Poster display, Annual Meeting of the American Veterinary Medical Association. Cited in D.C. Turner and P. Bateson. 1988. *The Domestic Cat: Tthe Biology of its Behaviour*. Cambridge: Cambridge University Press, p. 187.

Landsberg, G.M. (1991). The distribution of canine behavior cases at three behavior referral practices. *Vet Med* **86**: 1011–1018.

Neilson, J.C. (2003). Feline house-soiling: elimination and marking behaviors. *Vet Clin N Am: Small Anim Pract* **33**(2): 287–301.

Neilson, J.C. (2004). Thinking outside the box. *J Feline Med Surg* **6**: 5–11.

Neilson, J.C. (2007). Scent preferences in the domestic cat. In: *Proc 6th International Veterinary Behavior Meeting and the European College of Veterinary Behavioural Medicine —Companion Animals European Society of Veterinary Clinical Ethology*.

Neilson, J.C. (2009). The latest scoop on litter. *Vet Med* **104**: 140–144.

New, J.C., M.D. Salman, et al. (2000). Shelter relinquishment: characteristics of shelter-relinquished animals and their owners compared with animals and their owners in U.S. pet-owning households. *J Appl Anim Welfare Sci* **3**(3): 179–201.

Patronek, G.J., L.T. Glickman, et al. (1996a). Risk factors for relinquishment of dogs to an animal shelter. *J Am Vet Med Assoc* **209**: 572–581.

Patronek, G.J., L.T. Glickman, et al. (1996b). Risk factors for relinquishment of cats to an animal shelter. *J Am Vet Med Assoc* **209**: 582–588.

Salman, M.D., J.G. New Jr, et al. (1998). Human and animal factors related to relinquishment of dogs and cats in 12 selected animal shelters in the United States. *J Appl Anim Welfare Sci* **1**(3): 207–226.

Salman, M.D., J.M. Hutchinson, et al. (2000). Behavioral reasons for relinquishment of dogs and cats to 12 shelters. *J Appl Anim Welfare Sci* **3**(2): 93–106.

Schwarz, S. (2003). Separation anxiety syndrome in dogs and cats. *J Am Vet Med Assoc* **222**(11): 1526–1531.

Sung, W. and S.L. Crowell-Davis (2006). Elimination behavior patterns of domestic cats (*Felis catus*) with and without elimination behavior problems. *Am J Vet Res* **67**(9): 1500–1504.

Turner, D.C. and P. Bateson (1988). *The Domestic Cat: The Biology of its Behaviour*. Cambridge: Cambridge University Press.

Westropp, J.L. and C.A.T. Buffington (2004). Feline idiopathic systitis: current understanding of pahtophysiology and management. *Vet Clin Small Anim* **34**: 1043–1055.

82

Lower urinary tract trauma

Patricia Sura

Lower urinary tract trauma is frequently recognized in veterinary patients and is the most common cause of uroperitoneum in cats, dogs, and humans (Aumann et al. 1998; Gannon and Moses 2002; Rieser 2005). It is estimated that 10% of adult humans with external trauma sustain urinary tract injury (Tezval et al. 2007). The majority of specific information regarding lower urinary tract injuries in companion animals exists as isolated case reports or small case series; therefore, true incidence rates and absolute treatment recommendations and prognoses are not available. Of 600 consecutive dogs injured in motor vehicle accidents, 2.5% had urinary tract trauma (Kolata and Johnston 1975). Additionally, a study of 100 consecutive dogs sustaining pelvic fractures found that 39% had urinary tract injury detected with contrast radiography. The incidence of injury did not correlate with the severity of fracture (Selcer 1982).

Multiple organ injury is common with abdominal trauma (Selcer 1982; Weisse et al. 2002). In a study of 1,000 consecutive veterinary trauma patients evaluated at a single hospital, approximately 12% had significant abdominal injury (Kolata et al. 1974). On presentation of the acute trauma patient, stabilization of life-threatening injuries is of paramount importance. Evidence of urinary tract injury may not be apparent initially, and development of clinical signs can be protracted (Bjorling 1984; McLoughlin 2000; Rieser 2005). In the 100 dogs with pelvic fractures, 1/3 of those with urinary tract injury were clinically silent (Selcer 1982).

Urine can collect in the peritoneum, retroperitoneum, and subcutaneous dependent tissues (McLoughlin 2000). Retroperitoneal fluid accumulates due to damage to the kidneys, proximal ureter, or distal urethra, while

peritoneal leakage indicates ureteral, urinary bladder, or proximal urethral trauma (Gannon and Moses 2002). Urine extravasation into the subcutaneous tissues presents as bruised, edematous, painful, necrotic areas of dependent skin (Holt 1989; Rieser 2005). Extensive areas of skin loss have been reported, requiring advanced reconstructive procedures for closure (Holt 1989).

While blunt and penetrating trauma can lead to urinary tract rupture, iatrogenic damage via urethral catheterization, cystocentesis, bladder expression, and cystoscopic injury cannot be overlooked (Hay and Rosin 1997; McLoughlin 2000; Gannon and Moses 2002). Presence of sterile urine in the abdomen results in chemical peritonitis, while infected urine may lead to systemic sepsis (McLoughlin 2000; Rieser 2005).

Clinical signs associated with uroperitoneum include pain on abdominal palpation, dehydration, ballotment of a fluid wave, hematuria, dysuria, progressive depression, hypothermia, and other signs of external trauma (Burrows 1974; Pechman 1982; Gannon and Moses 2002). Delayed signs are those of uremia and peritonitis and may be nonspecific or suggestive of other organ systems. In 26 cats with uroperitoneum, the most common historical complaints other than anuria were vomiting and lethargy (Aumann 1998). Vomiting may begin approximately 24 hours prior to detection of severe azotemia (Burrows 1974). Presence or absence of hematuria, ability to void voluntarily, and presence of a palpable bladder do not predict urinary tract integrity (Burrows 1974; Rieser 2005).

Often, animals with uroabdomen present with significant metabolic compromise due to latency in clinical signs following urinary leakage (Bjorling 1984; McLoughlin 2000; Rieser 2005); therefore, medical stabilization is required before reparative intervention is attempted. Common clinicopathological changes with uroperitoneum are azotemia, hyperkalemia,

Nephrology and Urology of Small Animals. Edited by Joe Bartges and David J. Polzin. © 2011 Blackwell Publishing Ltd.

hypernatremia, hyperphosphatemia, and metabolic acidosis (Gannon and Moses 2002; Rieser 2005). Intravascular volume loss and collapse occurs due to third spacing of water into the peritoneal cavity as it is drawn into the hyperosmolar urine (Burrows 1974; Rawlings 1976; Gannon and Moses 2002; Rieser 2005).

Early stabilization includes administration of intravenous crystalloids and colloids to address systemic shock and initiation of peritoneal drainage (McLoughlin 2000; Gannon and Moses 2002). Treatment for severe hyperkalemia may be required especially if bradycardia or electrocardiographic abnormalities are noted.

Delay in diagnosis of urinary tract trauma increases mortality rate. Death occurs 47–90 hours after experimental urinary bladder rupture (Burrows 1974), although in traumatic cases, mortality is typically from associated sustained injuries (Aumann 1989). Abdominocentesis is necessary to definitively diagnose a uroabdomen. Routine paracentesis can be employed, but large volumes of fluid are necessary for a diagnostic sample (5–25 mL/kg) (Crowe 1976; Kolata 1976). Diagnostic peritoneal lavage may also be used, in which 20 mL/kg of sterile isotonic saline is infused into the abdomen and retrieved. This technique can detect 0.8–4.4 mL/kg of free abdominal fluid (Crowe 1976; Kolata 1976; Saxon 1994), but cannot detect retroperitoneal fluid (Saxon 1994). The focused assessment for abdominal trauma (FAST) technique may also be useful, which allows for ultrasonographic localization of small amounts of free fluid and directed centesis (Helling 2007).

Small molecules such as urea nitrogen diffuse readily across the peritoneum and equilibrate rapidly (Gannon and Moses 2002). Comparison of the larger creatinine molecule and potassium concentrations in centesis fluid compared with serum yields a definitive diagnosis (Chapter 11). In dogs, a fluid to serum creatinine concentration ratio of greater than 2:1 and a fluid to serum potassium concentration ratio greater than 1.4:1 are predictive of uroperitoneum (Schmiedt 2001). In cats, mean fluid to serum creatinine concentration ratio of 2:1 and mean fluid to serum potassium concentration ratio of 1.9:1 are predictive of uroabdomen (Aumann 1998).

Urinary drainage and diversion is essential in treating urinary tract trauma. If a urinary catheter can be passed, it should be left indwelling within the urinary bladder. If catheterization is impossible, drainage can be achieved via cystocentesis, cystostomy tube placement, or urinary bladder marsupialization (Chapter 32; Bjorling 1984). Cystostomy and marsupialization require general anesthesia; intermittent cystocentesis may be preferred in the severely compromised animal. To address urine accumulation in the peritoneal cavity, a peritoneal catheter can be placed to lavage and evacuate it (McLoughlin 2000).

Less ideal is placement of multiple Penrose drains covered with sterile bandage.

Peritoneal catheter placement also permits dialysis and treatment of hypothermia (Dzyban 2000). Median as well as paramedian catheter placement has been described (Dzyban 2000; McLoughlin 2000). The catheter is placed using a trocar or manual entry through a small stab incision. The catheter is secured, bandaged, and attached to a sterile collection system. Dialysis fluid is usually comprised of a dextrose solution, which can be heparinized to prevent catheter occlusion with clots (Carter 1989; Crisp 1989; Dzyban 2000). The dialysate is instilled at 38–42°C depending on heat requirements with a 30–40 minute dwell time. Most of the fluid should be retrieved and the time to next instillation of dialysate tailored on an individual case basis. Complications of peritoneal dialysis include catheter obstruction, peritonitis, hypoalbuminemia, overhydration, and electrolyte disturbances (Carter 1989; Crisp 1989; Dzyban 2000).

When considering dialysis for patients with severe azotemia due to urinary tract rupture, lower percent dextrose solutions (1.5%) are used to minimize loss of free water, which is contraindicated in dehydrated animals (Carter 1989). As many of these animals are presented after sustaining blunt trauma, extreme caution and close monitoring of the patient is essential, as a previously unsuspected diaphragmatic defect may become apparent (Carter 1989; Dzyban 2000). In a study of dogs in renal failure, peritoneal dialysis significantly lowered blood urea nitrogen concentration in 19/25 dogs and creatinine concentration in 20/25 dogs (Crisp 1989). In this study, hypoalbuminemia occurred in 11/25 (41%), obstruction in 8/25 (30%), and peritonitis in 6/25 (22%) (Crisp 1989).

Following rehydration and stabilization, perform radiographic contrast studies to localize the site of leakage (McLoughlin 2000). Survey thoracic and abdominal radiography are obtained in all cases of trauma to evaluate diaphragmatic integrity, identify pneumothorax, hemothorax, and pulmonary contusions, and pertinent fractures. Radiographic evidence of urinary tract trauma includes loss of abdominal or retroperitoneal detail, lack of a distinct urinary bladder, and displacement or nonvisualization of a kidney (Pechman 1982). Prolonged uroabdomen can lead to marked fluid accumulation, ileus, abdominal adhesions, and peritonitis (Burrows 1974).

The most reliable noninvasive means of detecting urinary tract trauma is via contrast radiography (Chapter 15; Pechman 1982; McLoughlin 2000). Urethral tears and bladder rupture can be visualized by urethrocystography, although complete filling of the urinary bladder is required to demonstrate small defects (McLoughlin

2000). In a study of experimental urinary tract rupture in 14 dogs, contrast cystography diagnosed 100% of cases (Burrows 1974). Similarly, positive contrast urethrocystography delineated all cases of urinary bladder and urethral trauma in dogs with pelvic fractures (Selcer 1982).

Excretory urography is used to evaluate kidneys and ureters, which are generally not easily assessed by survey radiography (Chapter 15; Feeney et al. 1982). Intravenous administration of contrast material may cause acute systemic hypotension and collapse, as well as acute renal failure; therefore, it is not recommended in dehydrated or azotemic patients (Feeney et al. 1982; McLoughlin 2000; Gannon and Moses 2002). As contrast media can alter urine specific gravity, this should be assessed prior to contrast study (Feeney et al. 1982). The kidneys are best demonstrated immediately and 5 minutes postinjection. The renal pelves are identified at 10 and 20 minutes postinjection and the ureters at 5, 10, and 20 minutes (Feeney 1979).

Ureteral injury

Ureteric injury is relatively rare due to their position beneath thick epaxial musculature and their relative mobility in the retroperitoneal space (Palmer 1999; Brandes 2004). Approximately 25% of ureteral injuries in humans are from blunt or penetrating trauma (Tezval 2007). Blunt trauma can lead to ureteric injury from rapid deceleration or hyperextension (Brandes 2004). Penetrating trauma, such as gunshot wounds, knife wounds, and dog fight wounds in companion animals, may result in ureteral injury. Penetrating injury is responsible for 75–96% of traumatic ureteral injuries in humans (DiGiacomo 2001), and exploratory celiotomy is warranted in animals with penetrating abdominal wounds (Fullington 1997; Davidson 1998).

Excretory urography remains the imaging modality of choice to assess ureters (Chapter 15). In a study of 10 animals with ureteric rupture, excretory urography demonstrated ureteral leakage in all cases. Unfortunately, the extent of damage (partial versus complete transection) could not be determined (Weisse 2002). In human trauma centers, excretory urography can be unreliable, as can contrast computed tomography. Surgical exploration is considered an acceptable means for evaluating the ureters for trauma (DiGiacomo 2001; Brandes 2004).

Ureteric rupture, both unilateral and bilateral, has been described as a result of trauma in companion animals (Weisse 2002; Hamilton 2006). In addition to urinary diversion procedures discussed previously, nephrostomy catheters (Chapter 32) have been used to stabilize

animals in which both ureters have been affected, either to aid in the resuscitative effort or to manage postoperative drainage (Kyles 1998; Nwadike 2000). These can be placed percutaneously with fluoroscopic or ultrasound guidance or surgically.

Surgical intervention should be performed as soon as possible following diagnosis and stabilization (Thornhill 1981; Brandes 2004). Ureteronephrectomy, ureterostomy, or ureteroneocystostomy can be considered in these cases, based on the location and degree of injury (Chapter 61; Weisse 2002; Mehl 2003; Hamilton 2006).

With primary ureteral repair, the ureter must be repaired without tension, with an adequate blood supply and without accumulation of urine at the anastomotic site (Thornhill 1981; Bellah 1989). As watertight anastomoses are rarely performed, urinary diversion is recommended (Caywood 1986). A ureteral catheter or nephrostomy tube may be used as a stent (Chapter 32). Ureteroscopy and ureteral stenting has been described in dogs and cats and is expected to receive wider attention as interventional techniques become increasingly available (Berent 2008; Weisse 2008). Typically, hydroureter and hydronephrosis are noted following ureteral transection. Marked improvement in these qualities was noted 10 weeks after repair in one dog (Chambers 1987).

In humans, iatrogenic ureteral injuries occur in 0.5–1% of abdominal and pelvic surgery patients and are the leading cause of ureteral damage (Selzman 1996; Brandes 2004). Unfortunately, iatrogenic ureteral damage also occurs during routine surgical procedures in companion animals. Proximal and distal ureteral ligation and transection have occurred during ovariohysterectomy (Okkens 1981; Tidwell 1990; Nwadike 2000; Mehl 2003). Ovariectomy may lessen this risk as distal ligation is not performed (van Goethem 2006). In dogs, 65% of renal filtration is achievable if ligation is relieved within the first week of ureteral obstruction. This drops to 46% after 14 days of ligation (Wilson 1977). The canine ureter has been subjected experimentally to crush injury, which causes focal devascularization. Crush injuries have been applied to the ureter lasting up to 60 minutes and result in a fulminate periureteral scar. Function resolves by 12 weeks postinjury (Brodsky 1977).

Post-traumatic complications from ureteral damage include urinomas or periureteral pseudocysts, which represent urine encased in fibrous tissue (Chapter 59). These have been described in companion animals and are amenable to resection and drainage (Tidwell 1990; Moores 2002; Worth 2004). In addition, ureteral stricture and fistulation has been described (Rawlings 1976; Palmer 1999; Brandes 2004).

Urinary bladder rupture

Of 600 dogs injured in motor vehicle accidents, nine had confirmed urinary bladder trauma (Kolata 1975). Urinary bladder rupture is the most common traumatic urinary injury in dogs and cats (Thornhill 1981). It is more common in male dogs due to less urethral compliance and dilation in response to increased intravesicular pressure (Thornhill 1981).

Eighty percent of urinary bladder perforations in people are associated with pelvic fractures (Tezval 2007). Mechanisms for rupture include direct penetration by fracture fragments or sudden increase in intravesicular pressure (Selcer 1982). Between 1966–1971, ruptured urinary bladder was confirmed in 26 dogs and 14 cats at one institution; 84.6% were due to trauma and 46.2% had associated pelvic fractures (Burrows 1974). Urinary bladder rupture has been reported in 1/119 cats and 3/132 cats with high-rise syndrome (Whitney 1987; Vnuk 2003). Undifferentiated abdominal injury has been reported in 12/81 dogs injured by this same mechanism (Gordon 1993).

In clinical and experimental studies of urinary bladder rupture, the earliest clinical sign noted is abdominal tenderness and pain. After approximately 12 hours, vomiting commences and increases in frequency. Progressive dehydration and uremia eventually culminates in death within 72 hours (Chapter 71; Meynard 1961; Burrows 1974).

Urinary bladder rupture is confirmed with radiographic contrast studies, as described previously. Ultrasound-assisted contrast cystography, in which microbubbled saline is injected into the bladder and observed to migrate into the tissues around the bladder, has also been described (Cote 2002).

Opinion has changed regarding surgical management of urinary bladder rupture. Initially, speed was considered of optimum concern due to rapid deterioration of patient status (Meynard 1961). As early and active stabilization has been proven to improve mortality rates, the concept of conservative management of urinary bladder ruptures has emerged. In a study of experimental urinary bladder perforation, three dogs survived without any adjunctive therapy (Burrows 1974). Current principles of medical management of urinary bladder rupture include lack of an underlying cause for rupture, lack of hypotonicity of the bladder, no evidence of devitalization, no urosepsis, and no other reason for celiotomy (Osborne 1996). Should conservative management be chosen, careful observation is necessary. Nonsurgical management of traumatically ruptured urinary bladder has also been reported in children, resulting in a shorter hospital stay and equivalent outcome to those surgically managed (Osman 2005).

An indwelling urinary catheter is placed and maintained with a sterile collection system (Chapters 32 and 36). It is essential that the catheter is not placed through the rent into the abdominal cavity as this will prevent mucosal apposition and healing. After 3–5 days of catheterization, a contrast cystourethrogram is performed. If urinary leakage is still present, catheterization may be continued. An abdominal drainage catheter may also be used in conjunction with urethral catheter. Once cystourethrography has proven that leakage has ceased, the catheters are removed and the animal is monitored for voluntary urination. All catheters should be submitted for bacterial culture at time of removal, as the odds ratio for development of a urinary tract infection increases approximately 27% for each day of catheterization (Bubenik 2007).

Should urine leakage persist despite appropriate management or should patient status decline during medical therapy, surgical correction is indicated. A midline celiotomy is performed, the defect in the bladder wall is located, debrided, and closed with fine absorbable suture. Care is taken to ensure continued patency of the ureteral openings (Bjorling 1984).

Urethral tears

In addition to blunt trauma (Jones 1981; Goldman 1989), urethral rupture may also occur from bite wounds, gunshot wounds, and fractures of the os penis (Thornhill 1981). In a study of 20 dogs and 29 cats with urethral rupture, presence of multiple concurrent injuries was the only factor statistically associated with a poor outcome. Laboratory findings, timing and type of surgical correction, and timing and type of urinary diversion had no apparent effect on outcome (Anderson 2006). In this study, the most common cause of urethral trauma in dogs was automobile collision, with 12 of 14 sustaining concurrent pelvic fractures (Anderson 2006). In cats, iatrogenic trauma during catheterization attempts was the most common cause of urethral rupture (Anderson 2006).

Iatrogenic urethral damage is common in cats and dogs. Catheter-induced damage from therapy for feline lower urinary tract disease is a major etiology for urethrostomy in cats (Aumann 1998; Anderson 2006; Corgozinho 2007; Meige 2008). Urethral entrapment has been reported secondary to pelvic fracture repair in a dog (Messmer 2001), as well as presumed impingement by bilateral triple pelvic osteotomy (Dudley 2004). The author has observed a kitten with a complete urethral transection secondary to ovariohysterectomy. Urethral injury has also been described in cats with pelvic trauma (Fearnside 2003). Another means of reported iatrogenic urethral trauma is inadvertent prostatectomy and urethral transection during cryptorchidectomy or perineal hernia surgery (Bellah et al. 1989; Schulz 1996; Sereda 2002).

Contrast cystourethrography (Chapter 15) is the imaging modality of choice to evaluate urethral disruption. The normal luminal diameter in an animal can vary with amount of contrast material as well as the pressure at which it is administered. This high-yield procedure can clinically demonstrate urethral transaction, urethral laceration and bladder rupture, and urethral stricture (Ticer 1980).

Principles of urethral trauma management include accurate patient assessment and stabilization, urinary diversion, and conservative management or definitive repair (Chapter 83; Boothe 2000). If a urinary catheter is placed, it is secured in position with suture. A contrast cystourethrogram is used to document extent and location of urine leakage.

Since urinary diversion favors wound healing, cystostomy tubes can be used either for preoperative stabilization or postoperative diversion (Caywood 1986; Williams 1991; Beck 2007). Following placement in 10 dogs and 1 cat, micturition returned to normal after tube removal with leakage from the stoma expected for up to 4 days while granulation occurs (Williams 1991). Common complications of tube cystostomy include urinary tract infection, inadvertent tube removal, and stomal infection or inflammation (Williams 1991; Beck 2007).

As with urinary bladder rupture, conservative management of urethral tears is possible. Urethral healing relies on mucosal continuity and lack of significant urine extravasation (Bellah 1989). A small, persistent strip of mucosa is all that is necessary to allow urethral healing, generally without stricture formation (Robertson 1984; Waldron 1985; Bellah 1989). Primary alignment has been described in 10 cats in which a urinary catheter was used to span the ruptured area for 5–14 days. A 100% success rate for urethral healing was reported, with a single case of urethral stricture (Meige 2008). An appropriate-sized catheter approximates the urethral diameter without exerting outward pressure as this may slow wound healing.

If a retrograde catheter cannot be passed, a laparotomy may be useful to pass a urinary catheter from inside the bladder through the urethra. A second urinary catheter can then be attached to the end of the first and pulled into the bladder (Rawlings 1976; Fearnside 2003; Meige 2008).

Urethral tears and transections can be surgically managed either by primary apposition and repair or via bypass of the ruptured area through performance of a urethrostomy. A degree of stricture occurs whether primary repair or conservative management over a catheter is chosen in cases of complete urethral transection (Layton 1987). When urinary diversion techniques in cases of urethral resection and anastomosis in dogs were compared, no outcome difference was noted between a urethral catheter only, cystostomy tube only, or both (Cooley 1999).

Infection rates following permanent urethrostomy can approach 53% (Corgozinho 2007). In a study of 59 cats that had undergone perineal urethrostomy, there was a 25% complication rate within the first month of surgery, including stricture formation, urinary tract infection, and perineal urine leakage (Bass 2005). Complications from urethrostomy include stricture formation, urine leakage into the subcutaneous space, chronic urinary tract infection, perineal hernia, and possible incontinence (Bass 2005; Phillips 2006). In cats with perineal urethrostomy, complete dissection to the level of the bulbourethral glands prevents stricture formation. In a study of failed urethrostomies, 8/11 cats with stricture formation had evidence of incomplete dissection and improper surgical technique (Phillips 2006). Other causes of stricture formation are inappropriate apposition of the mucosa to the skin, resulting in scarring and self-mutilation (Bilbrey 1991; Phillips 2006). A study evaluating long-term outcome of scrotal urethrostomies in dogs found a 15% infection rate (Bilbrey 1991). Treatment is directed via culture and sensitivity results.

References

Anderson, R.B., L.R. Aronson, et al. (2006). Prognostic factors for successful outcome following urethral rupture in dogs and cats. *J Am Anim Hosp Assoc* **42**(2): 136–146.

Aumann, M., L.T. Worth, et al. (1998). Uroperitoneum in cats: 26 cases (1986–1995). *J Am Anim Hosp Assoc* **34**(4): 315–324.

Bass, M., J. Howard, et al. (2005). Retrospective study of indications for and outcome of perineal urethrostomy in cats. *J Small Anim Pract* **46**(5): 227–231.

Beck, A.L., J.M. Grierson, et al. (2007). Outcome of and complications associated with tube cystostomy in dogs and cats: 76 cases (1995–2006). *J Am Vet Med Assoc* **230**(8): 1184–1189.

Bellah, J.R. (1989). Wound healing in the urinary tract. *Sem Vet Med Surg (Small Anim)* **4**(4): 294–303.

Bellah, J.R., C.P. Spencer, et al. (1989). Hemiprostatic urethral avulsion during cryptorchid orchiectomy in a dog. *J Am Anim Hosp Assoc* **25**(5): 553–556.

Berent, A. (2008). Ureteral interventions: a minimally invasive approach to diagnosis and treatment of ureteral disease. Proceedings of the 26th Annual ACVIM Forum, June 4–7, San Antonio, TX.

Bilbrey, S.A., S.J. Birchard, et al. (1991). Scrotal urethrostomy: a retrospective review of 38 dogs (1973 through 1988). *J Am Anim Hosp Assoc* **27**(5): 560–564.

Bjorling, D.E. (1984). Traumatic injuries of the urogenital system. *Vet Clin N Am: Small Anim Pract* **14**(1): 61–76.

Boothe, H.W. (2000). Managing traumatic urethral injuries. *Clin Tech Small Anim Pract* **15**(1): 35–39.

Brandes, S., M. Coburn, et al. (2004). Consensus on genitourinary trauma: diagnosis and management of ureteric injury: an evidence-based analysis. *BJU Int* **94**(3): 277–289.

Brodsky, S.L., P.D. Zimskind, et al. (1977). Effects of crush and devascularizing injuries to the proximal ureter: an experimental study. *Invest Urol* **14**(5): 361–365.

Bubenik, L.J., G.L. Hosgood, et al. (2007). Frequency of urinary tract infection in catheterized dogs and comparison of bacterial culture and susceptibility testing results for catheterized and noncatheterized dogs with urinary tract infections. *J Am Vet Med Assoc* **231**(6): 893–899.

Burrows, C.F. and K.C. Bovee (1974). Metabolic changes due to experimentally induced rupture of the canine urinary bladder. *Am J Vet Res* **35**(8): 1083–1088.

Carter, L.J., W.E. Wingfield, et al. (1989). Clinical experience with peritoneal dialysis in small animals. *Compend Contin Educ Pract Vet* **11**(11): 1335–1343.

Caywood, D.D. and C.A. Osborne (1986). Surgical removal of canine uroliths. *Vet Clin N Am: Small Anim Pract* **16**(2): 389–407.

Chambers, J.N., B.A. Selcer, et al. (1987). Recovery from severe hydroureter and hydronephrosis after ureteral anastomosis in a dog. *J Am Vet Med Assoc* **191**(12): 1589–1592.

Cooley, A.J., D.R. Waldron, et al. (1999). The effects of indwelling transurethral catheterization and tube cystotomy on urethral anastomoses in dogs. *J Am Anim Hosp Assoc* **35**(4): 341–347.

Corgozinho, K.B., H.J.M. de Souza, et al. (2007). Catheter-induced urethral trauma in cats with urethral obstruction. *J Feline Med Surg* **9**(6): 481–486.

Cote, E., M.C. Carroll, et al. (2002). Diagnosis of urinary bladder rupture using ultrasound contrast cystography: in vitro model and two case-history reports. *Vet Radiol Ultrasound* **43**(3): 281–286.

Crisp, M.S., D.J. Chew, et al. (1989). Peritoneal dialysis in dogs and cats: 27 cases (1976–1987). *J Am Vet Med Assoc* **195**(9): 1262–1266.

Crowe, D.T. and S.W. Crane (1976). Diagnostic abdominal paracentesis and lavage in the evaluation of abdominal injuries in dogs and cats: clinical and experimental investigations. *J Am Vet Med Assoc* **168**(8): 700–705.

Davidson, E.B. (1998). Managing bite wounds in dogs and cats—part I. *Compend Contin Educ Small Anim Pract* **20**(7): 811–820.

DiGiacomo, J.C., H. Frankel, et al. (2001). Preoperative radiographic staging for ureteral injuries is not warranted in patients undergoing celiotomy for trauma. *Am Surg* **67**(10): 969–973.

Dudley, R.M. and B.E. Wilkens (2004). Urethral obstruction as a complication of staged bilateral triple pelvic osteotomy. *J Am Anim Hosp Assoc* **41**(5): 162–164.

Dzyban, L.A., M.A. Labato, et al. (2000). Peritoneal dialysis: a tool in veterinary critical care. *J Vet Emerg Crit Care* **10**(2): 91–106.

Fearnside, S.M., R.D. Eaton-Wells, et al. (2003). Surgical management of urethral injury following pelvic trauma in three cats. *Aus Vet Pract* **33**(1): 2–7.

Feeney, D.A., D.E. Thrall, et al. (1979). Normal canine excretory urogram: effects of dose, time and individual dog variation. *Am J Vet Res* **40**(11): 1596–1604.

Feeney, D.A., D.L. Barber, et al. (1982). The excretory urogram: part I. Techniques, normal radiographic appearance, and misinterpretation. *Compend Cont Educ Small Anim Pract* **4**(3): 233–240.

Feeney, D.A., D.L. Barber, et al. (1982). The excretory urogram: part II. Interpretation of abnormal findings. *Compend Contin Educ Small Anim Pract* **4**(4): 321–329.

Fullington, R.J. and C.M. Otto (1997). Characteristics and management of gunshot wounds in dogs and cats: 84 cases (1986–1995). *J Am Vet Med Assoc* **210**(5): 658–662.

Gannon, K.M. and L. Moses (2002). Uroabdomen in dogs and cats. *Comp Contin Educ Pract Vet* **24**(8): 604–612.

Goldman, A.L. and S.L. Beckman (1989). Traumatic urethral avulsion at the preputial fornix in a cat. *J Am Vet Med Assoc* **194**(1): 88–90.

Gordon, L.E., C. Thacher, et al. (1993). High-rise syndrome in dogs: 81 cases (1985–1991). *J Am Vet Med Assoc* **202**(1): 118–122.

Hamilton, M.H., T.R. Sissener, et al. (2006). Traumatic bilateral ureteric rupture in two dogs. *J Small Anim Pract* **47**(12): 737–740.

Hay, C.W. and E. Rosin (1997). Repair of an intrapelvic urethral tear in a bitch caused by iatrogenic trauma. *Vet Rec* **140**(2): 48–49.

Helling, T.S., J. Wilson, et al. (2007). The utility of focused abdominal ultrasound in blunt abdominal trauma: a reappraisal. *Am J Surg* **194**(6): 728–733.

Holt, P.E. (1989). Hindlimb skin loss associated with urethral rupture in two cats. *J Small Anim Pract* **30**(7): 406–409.

Jones, G.H., W.T. Testerman, et al. (1981). Ruptured urethra caused by trauma in a dog. *Vet Med Small Anim Clin* **76**(5): 672–673.

Kolata, R.J., N.H. Kraut, et al. (1974). Patterns of trauma in urban dogs and cats: a study of 1,000 cases. *J Am Vet Med Assoc* **164**(5): 499–502.

Kolata, R.J. and D.E. Johnston (1975). Motor vehicle accidents in urban dogs: a study of 600 cases. *J Am Vet Med Assoc* **167**(10): 938–941.

Kolata, R.J. (1976). Diagnostic peritoneal paracentesis and lavage: experimental and clinical evaluations in the dog. *J Am Vet Med Assoc* **168**(8): 697–699.

Kyles, A.E., E.A. Stone, et al. (1998). Diagnosis and surgical management of obstructive ureteral calculi in cats: 11 cases (1993–1996). *J Am Vet Med Assoc* **213**(8): 1150–1156.

Layton, C.E., H.R. Ferguson, et al. (1987). Intrapelvic urethral anastomosis: a comparison of three techniques. *Vet Surg* **16**(2): 175–182.

McLoughlin, M.A. (2000). Surgical emergencies of the urinary tract. *Vet Clin N Am: Small Anim Pract* **30**(3): 581–602.

Mehl, M.L. and A.E. Kyles (2003). Ureteroureterostomy after proximal ureteric injury during an ovariohysterectomy in a dog. *Vet Rec* **153**(15): 469–470.

Meige, F., S. Sarrau, et al. (2008). Management of traumatic urethral rupture in 11 cats using primary alignment with a urethral catheter. *Vet Comp Orthopaed Traumatol* **21**(1): 76–84.

Messmer, M., U. Rytz, et al. (2001). Urethral entrapment following pelvic fracture fixation in a dog. *J Small Anim Pract* **42**(7): 341–344.

Meynard, J.A. (1961). Traumatic rupture of the bladder in the dog—a clinical study of nine cases. *J Small Anim Pract* **2**(1–4): 131–134.

Moores, A.P., A.M.D. Bell, et al. (2002). Urinoma (para-ureteral pseudocyst) as a consequence of trauma in a cat. *J Small Anim Pract* **43**(5): 213–216.

Nwadike, B.S., L.P. Wilson, et al. (2000). Use of bilateral temporary nephrostomy catheters for emergency treatment of bilateral ureter transaction in a cat. *J Am Vet Med Assoc* **217**(12): 1862–1865.

Okkens, A.C., I. van de Gaag, et al. (1981). Urological complications following ovariohysterectomy in dogs. *Tijdschrift voor Diergeneeskunde* **106**(23): 1189–1198.

Osborne, C.A., S.L. Sanderson, et al. (1996). Medical management of iatrogenic rents in the wall of the feline urinary bladder. *Vet Clin N Am: Small Anim Pract* **26**(3): 551–562.

Osman, Y., N. El-Tabey, et al. (2005). Nonoperative treatment of isolated posttraumatic intraperitoneal bladder rupture in children—is it justified? *J Urol* **173**(3): 955–957.

Palmer, L.S., R.R. Rosenbaum, et al. (1999). Penetrating ureteral trauma at an urban trauma center: 10 year experience. *Urology* **54**(1): 34–36.

Pechman, R.D. (1982). Urinary trauma in dogs and cats: a review. *J Am Anim Hosp Assoc* **18**(1): 33–40.

Phillips, H. D.E. Holt (2006). Surgical revision of the urethral stoma following perineal urethrostomy in 11 cats:(1998–2004). *J Am Anim Hosp Assoc* **42**(3): 218–222.

Rawlings, C.A. and W.E. Wingfield (1976). Urethral reconstruction in dogs and cats. *J Am Anim Hosp Assoc* **12**(6): 850–860.

Rieser, T.M. (2005). Urinary tract emergencies. *Vet Clin N Am: Small Anim Pract* **35**(2): 359–373.

Robertson, J.J. and M.J. Bojrab (1984). Subtotal intracapsular prostatectomy results in normal dogs. *Vet Surg* **13**(1): 6–10.

Saxon, W.D. (1994). The acute abdomen. *Vet Clin N Am: Small Anim Pract* **24**(6): 1207–1224.

Schmiedt, C., K.M. Tobias, et al. (2001). Evaluation of abdominal fluid: peripheral blood creatinine and potassium ratios for diagnosis of uroperitoneum in dogs. *J Vet Emerg Crit Care* **11**(4): 275–280.

Schulz, K.S., D.R. Waldron, et al. (1996). Inadvertent prostatectomy as a complication of cryptorchidectomy in four dogs. *J Am Anim Hosp Assoc* **32**(3): 211–214.

Selcer, B.A. (1982). Urinary tract trauma associated with pelvic trauma. *J Am Anim Hosp Assoc* **19**(5): 785–793.

Selzman, A.A. and J.P. Spirnak (1996). Iatrogenic ureteral injuries: a 20 year experience in treating 165 injuries. *J Urol* **155**(3): 878–881.

Sereda, C., D. Fowler, et al. (2002). Iatrogenic proximal urethral obstruction after inadvertent prostatectomy during bilateral perineal herniorrhaphy in a dog. *Can Vet J* **43**(4): 288–290.

Tezval, H., M. Tezval, et al. (2007). Urinary tract injuries in patients with multiple trauma. *World J Urol* **25**(2): 177–184.

Thornhill, J.A. and P.E. Cechner (1981). Traumatic injuries to the kidney, ureter, bladder and urethra. *Vet Clin N Am: Small Anim Pract* **11**(1): 157–169.

Ticer, J.W., C.P. Spencer, et al. (1980). Positive contrast retrograde urethrography: a useful procedure for evaluating urethral disorders in the dog. *Vet Radiol Ultrasound* **21**(1): 2–11.

Tidwell, A.S., S.L. Ullman, et al. (1990). Urinoma (para-ureteral pseudocyst) in a dog. *Vet Radiol Ultrasound* **31**(4): 203–206.

Van Goethem, B., A. Schaefers-Okkens, et al. (2006). Making a rational choice between ovariectomy and ovariohysterectomy in the dog: a discussion of the benefits of either technique. *Vet Surg* **35**(2): 136–143.

Vnuk, D., B. Pirkic, et al. (2003). Feline high-rise syndrome: 119 cases (1998–2001). *J Feline Med Surg* **6**(5): 305–312.

Waldron, D.R., C.S. Hedlund, et al. (1985). The canine urethra: a comparison of first and second intention healing. *Vet Surg* **14**(3): 213–217.

Weisse, C., L.R. Aronson, et al. (2002). Traumatic rupture of the ureter: 10 cases. *J Am Anim Hosp Assoc* **38**(2): 188–192.

Weisse, C., A.C. Berent, et al. (2008). Potential applications of interventional radiology in veterinary medicine. *J Am Vet Med Assoc* **233**(10): 1564–1574.

Whitney, W.O. and C.J. Mehlhaff (1987). High-rise syndrome in cats. *J Am Vet Med Assoc* **191**(11): 1399–1403.

Williams, J.M. and R.A.S. White (1991). Tube cystostomy in the dog and cat. *J Small Anim Pract* **32**(12): 598–602.

Wilson, D.R. (1977). Renal function during and following obstruction. *Ann Rev Med* **28**: 329–339.

Worth, A.J. and S.C. Tomlin (2004). Post-traumatic paraureteral urinoma in a cat. *J Small Anim Pract* **45**(8): 413–416.

83

Surgery of the lower urinary tract

Karen Tobias

Because of rich blood supply and rapid rate of healing, the bladder and distal urethra respond well to surgical procedures, as long as a proper technique is used. Lower urinary tract procedures such as cystotomy and urethrostomy are commonly performed by general practitioners. Patients requiring urethral anastomosis and other more advanced techniques are usually referred to an experienced surgeon.

Healing of the lower urinary tract

Like other organs, healing of the bladder occurs in stages. Initially, the margins of a bladder incision are held in apposition by the applied suture material and, subsequently, a fibrin seal. Gradually, fibrous tissue ingrowth strengthens the wound. Collagen synthesis peaks by day 5 in dogs and then rapidly decreases until day 14. By 14–21 days after surgery, the bladder has regained 100% of its original strength. Sutures that penetrate the bladder lumen are covered by mucosa 3–4 days after surgery. By one month, a denuded bladder will be completely reepithelialized with mucosa from the urethra, ureters, and any uninjured bladder remnant (Bellah 1989).

Healing of the urethra is dependent on urethral continuity and local urine extravasation (Bellah 1989). If a strip of urethra remains intact and urine is diverted from the site, the urethral mucosa can seal the wound in 1 week. Regeneration of the remaining urethral layers depends on the location of the defect; for instance, corpus spongiosum may regenerate within a month. If the urethra is completely transected, the mucosal ends will retract. Fibrous tissue fills the intervening gap, producing a scar that eventually obstructs the urethral lumen.

Primary repair is therefore required with complete urethral transection (Bellah 1989).

Urethral injuries heal best when urine is diverted from tears or surgical sites (Bellah 1989). Urethral mucosa can seal wounds as early as 3 days after injury. Periurethral urine leakage delays wound healing and increases periurethral fibrosis, particularly if the urine is infected. Excessive fibrosis from urine leakage can lead to urethral stricture. Urine diversion can be performed with transurethral catheters or cystostomy tubes. Either method will decrease the risk of stricture compared to primary anastomosis alone. Risk of urethral stricture formation is increased with tension on the anastomosis or use of oversized urethral catheters (Bellah 1989).

Perioperative management

Lower urinary tract surgery may be required in patients with cystic or urethral trauma (Chapters 82), obstruction (Chapter 77), or neoplasia (Chapter 79). Lower urinary tract procedures may also be recommended when animals have not responded to medical management or when additional samples are needed for culture (Chapter 9 and 71) or histopathology.

Diagnostic tests

In general, most patients with lower urinary tract disease are evaluated for hematologic and biochemical abnormalities before surgery. Obstructed patients (Chapters 70) may be severely hyperkalemic, which can lead to bradycardia and predispose the animal to arrhythmias. Azotemia from obstruction or renal dysfunction may interfere with platelet function, increasing the risk of intraoperative and postoperative hemorrhage (Mische and Schulze 2004). A buccal mucosal bleeding time can be performed to assess platelet function in azotemic animals with thrombocytopenia. If possible, urine should be

Nephrology and Urology of Small Animals. Edited by Joe Bartges and David J. Polzin. © 2011 Blackwell Publishing Ltd.

obtained by cystocentesis for analysis and culture (Chapter 7 and 9). If a large prostatic cyst or abscess is suspected, urine samples should be obtained under ultrasound guidance or by urethral catheterization to reduce the risk of cyst or abscess rupture. Patients with lower urinary tract trauma, obstruction, or neoplasia or prostatic disorders usually undergo plain or contrast abdominal radiography or ultrasonography to diagnose the underlying condition and determine the extent of disease. Thoracic radiographs should be performed in patients with suspected neoplasia or that have suffered vehicular trauma. Patients with urinary trauma should be evaluated for other injuries such as fractures or abdominal hernias. If free fluid is noted within the abdomen, a sample should be obtained for cytology and culture. If uroperitoneum is suspected, potassium or creatinine concentrations of abdominal fluid and peripheral blood should be compared (Chapter 11). With uroperitoneum, creatinine concentrations of abdominal fluid will be at least twice serum concentrations, and abdominal fluid potassium concentrations will be at least 1.9 and 1.4 times that of serum in cats and dogs, respectively (Aumann et al. 1998; Schmiedt et al. 2001).

Preoperative care

Azotemia, dehydration, and severe electrolyte disturbances should be corrected if possible before surgery. Patients with packed cell volume <25% should be cross-matched for a red cell transfusion. Urinary tract obstructions should be relieved by retrograde urethral catheterization. If a catheter cannot be passed, the bladder should be drained by percutaneous cystocentesis every 4–6 hours until the patient is considered stable for surgery. In animals with uroabdomen that are unstable, a multifenestrated abdominocentesis catheter can be placed into the peritoneal cavity and connected to a closed collection system. The abdomen can be drained for 6–12 hours while the patient receives fluids and supportive care.

Patients with urinary tract trauma and obstruction are painful and should receive appropriate analgesics. Narcotics, such as hydromorphone or buprenorphine, can be administered by intermittent intravenous bolus or, in the case of fentanyl, as a continuous rate infusion. Epidural administration of analgesics provides excellent intraoperative and postoperative pain relief in animals undergoing lower urinary tract procedures. Epidural morphine should be used with caution since it may cause bladder atony and urine retention (Herperger 1998).

Bladder and urethral surgeries are classified as clean-contaminated if urinary spillage is controlled and contaminated if infected urine spills from the site. Prophylactic antibiotics are recommended for animals in which intraoperative contamination or surgical duration >60 minutes is expected. Therapeutic antibiotics should be administered if infection is present at any site in the body. First-generation cephalosporins provide broad-spectrum coverage for common urinary tract pathogens. If needed, culture samples should be obtained before antibiotic therapy is initiated.

Surgical principles

When lower urinary tract surgeries are performed through an abdominal approach, the incision usually extends along the caudal abdominal midline. In male dogs, the prepuce should be clipped and flushed with antiseptic solution during the prep. The prepuce should be left within the surgical field to permit intraoperative retrograde urethral catheterization. The skin incision will deviate around the base of the prepuce, resulting in transection the ipsilateral preputial muscle. This muscle should be reapposed at the time of subcutaneous closure. Branches of the external pudendal artery and vein should be ligated along the prepuce before they are transected.

The proximal urethra can often be reached through a caudal abdominal incision. Approach to the midportion of the urethra may require pelvic osteotomy or ostectomy. Pelvic ostectomy can be partial or complete. If a complete ostectomy is performed, bone removal should be limited to the pelvic symphysis and the medial portions of the pubis and ischium so that the obturator nerves are not damaged as they pass through the obturator foramina. The osseous gap can be closed by reapposing the elevated margins of the adductor muscles over the midline.

For abdominal procedures, the bladder, prostate, or urethra should be isolated with moistened laparotomy sponges to reduce contamination. Suction should be available to remove urine, blood, and exudate from surgical sites. The suction tip should be kept away from mucosa to reduce tissue damage. Forceps and gauze sponges can also traumatize bladder and urethral mucosa and should therefore be used gently and judiciously. Many surgeons manipulate urinary tract tissues with stay sutures to avoid excessive handling. Because of hemorrhage and tissue retraction, urethral mucosa can be difficult to identify during surgery. Surgical loupes or $1.0\times$ reading glasses may improve visualization. Fine-tipped needle holders (e.g., Derf), atraumatic thumb forceps (e.g., Debakey), and iris scissors are helpful for urethral surgeries.

A variety of suture materials have been evaluated for use in the urinary tract. Because the bladder and urethra heal rapidly, absorbable suture is recommended. Polyglycolic acid, polyglactin 910, glycomer 631, poliglecaprone 25, polyglyconate, and polydioxanone all provide sufficient strength for closure. Compared with polyglactin

910, polyglycolic acid suture loses tensile strength more quickly in alkaline or neutral urine. Sutures are covered rapidly by mucosa in most animals; therefore, exposure of the material to urine is limited. Monofilament sutures are often used because of reduced drag. Taper or taper-cut needles are preferred to reduce the tissue trauma. Sutures should incorporate the submucosal layer of the bladder or urethra to provide sufficient holding strength.

If lower urinary tract surgery is performed to biopsy or remove cystic or urethral neoplasia, instruments, gloves, and drapes should be changed before abdominal closure to reduce the risk of tumor seeding (Gilson and Stone 1990; Cornell 2000).

Postoperative care

Hemorrhage is expected after bladder and urethral surgery. Because blood clots can obstruct the lower urinary tract, most animals are kept on intravenous fluids for 12–36 hours. Analgesics will be required for several days. Nonsteroidal anti-inflammatory drugs should be avoided in patients with renal dysfunction. In patients with infection, duration of antibiotic therapy depends on the underlying condition. Animals with recurrent urinary tract infections may require several weeks of antibiotic treatment. Urine cultures should be reassessed 1 week after therapeutic antibiotics are discontinued.

Surgery of the bladder

Cystotomy

Introduction

Indications for cystotomy include removal of cystic calculi, polyps, or foreign bodies; intraluminal mass biopsy; ureteral reconstruction; or antegrade urethral catheterization. Incisions are usually made over the apex or ventral midline of the bladder to avoid damaging the ureteral openings. Ventral cystotomy improves exposure to the trigone and does not increase the risk of postoperative adhesions (Crowe 1986). Two layer appositional or inverting closures are stronger than single layer interrupted appositional patterns immediately after placement; however, no difference in strength is seen 3 or more hours after surgery. In properly apposed bladders, rupture after 24 hours usually occurs at sites other than the incision line (Radasch et al. 1990).

Cystotomy is performed with the patient in dorsal recumbency. Male cats can be positioned with their rear legs pulled cranially to expose the preputial area. In this position, a perineal urethrostomy can be performed simultaneously as needed. In female dogs and cats, the perivulvar region should be prepped to reduce the risk

of contamination in the event that antegrade urethral catheterization is required during surgery.

Technique

Make a caudal midline abdominal incision. Place Balfour retractors to improve visualization. Isolate the bladder with moistened laparotomy pads. If desired, place full thickness stay sutures at the apex or along the ventrolateral aspects of the bladder to provide retraction. Make a stab incision into the bladder and remove any residual urine with a Poole suction tip. Extend the bladder incision as needed with Metzenbaum or Mayo dissecting scissors. Obtain a piece of the incision margin for culture or biopsy. If inflammatory polyps are present, clamp the base of the polyps with hemostats for several minutes, then transect the polypoid tissue above the hemostat (Lipscombe 2003). Alternatively, transect the base of the polyp with a laser or cautery but do not damage the bladder submucosa. Remove any calculi with forceps or a bladder spoon. Avoid traumatizing the ureteral openings and bladder mucosa. Catheterize the urethra retrograde in male dogs or antegrade in cats or female dogs to verify patency. Appose bladder incisions with 3-0 or 4-0 absorbable monofilament material (e.g., poliglecaprone 25 or glycomer 631). Close thick bladder walls or trigonal incisions with a simple continuous or interrupted appositional pattern. Close thin bladders with a single or double layer continuous, appositional, or inverting pattern (Figure 83.1). If contamination occurs, lavage the peritoneal cavity with sterile saline before abdominal wall closure.

Complications

Hematuria and pollakiuria usually persist for several days after surgery. Potential complications include recurrent obstruction secondary to calculi, blood clots, swelling,

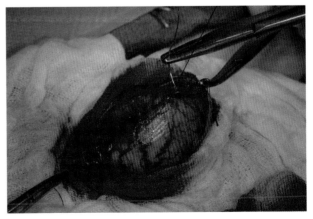

Figure 83.1 Using stay sutures to manipulate the bladder, close the cystotomy with a simple continuous pattern of absorbable monofilament.

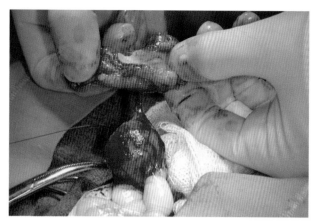

Figure 83.2 Patent urachus in a cat. The skin was incised around the fistula during the initial surgical approach and was excised during partial cystectomy.

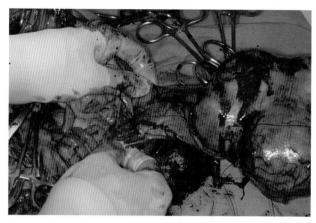

Figure 83.3 Leiomyosarcoma of the bladder apex in a dog. The ureters (within the surgeon's hands) were identified and spared during resection.

or mass regrowth, and uroabdomen from bladder rupture or incisional leakage. In animals with cystic calculi, postoperative radiographs are recommended to confirm removal of all stones (Cornell 2000).

Partial cystectomy

Introduction

Indications for partial cystectomy include removal of cystic neoplasia, granulomas, and urachal diverticulum (Figure 83.2) or devitalized or traumatized tissue. Resection may also be required if the bladder adheres to other abdominal structures that require excision because of neoplasia or infection. Dogs and cats can tolerate extensive resection of the bladder wall. After 75% resection, the remaining bladder regenerates through a combination of epithelial proliferation, fibrous tissue synthesis and remodeling, hypertrophy, and expansion. Additionally, a limited amount of smooth muscle may regenerate. Expansion of the bladder remnant relies on stretching from retained urine. Good function is expected within 3 months after subtotal cystectomy (Bellah 1989).

When tumors are present, resection with 2 cm margins of healthy tissue is recommended, since neoplastic tissue often extends beyond the visible mass (Stone et al. 1996). Partial cystectomy is therefore usually limited to lesions of the cranial two-thirds of the bladder (Figure 83.3), since most owners will not tolerate incontinence resulting from trigonal resection. Transitional cell carcinomas exfoliate easily and the abdominal cavity and body wall must be protected from inadvertent seeding of tumor cells during surgery (Gilson and Stone 1990). Total cystectomy with ureterocolonic anastomosis is not recommended for treatment of cystic neoplasia because of severe physiologic side effects and morbidity.

Animals with bladder rupture may require partial cystectomy to remove devitalized tissue (Cornell 2000). If viability of the incision line or remaining bladder wall is questionable, the bladder can be reinforced with omentum (Figures 83.4 and 83.5) or sutured to loops of small intestines ("serosal patch") (Pozzi et al. 2006). In animals with questionable bladder viability or extensive resection, a cystostomy tube or Foley catheter is left in place for 3–5 days to maintain decompression while the bladder heals.

Technique

Isolate the bladder with moistened laparotomy pads. If the bladder is ruptured, place stay sutures in the healthy tissue and debride nonviable tissue with Metzenbaum or Mayo scissors. If the bladder is intact, place two or more stay sutures in healthy bladder tissue several centimeter from the proposed resection site. If a tumor is present,

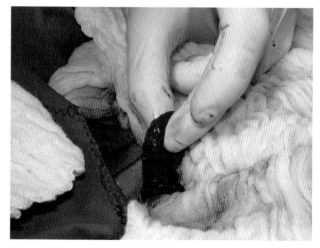

Figure 83.4 Rupture bladder with devitalized wall.

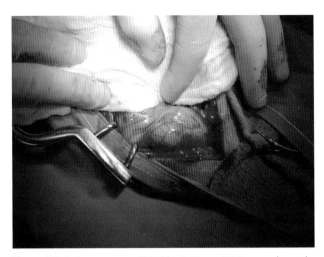

Figure 83.5 Appearance of bladder in Figure 83.3 several months after bladder repair and omentalization.

palpate the bladder to identify the tumor location. Make the initial incision approximately 1 cm beyond the margin of the palpable mass. Suction urine from the bladder before extending the incision. Extend the resection to include tissues up to 2 cm from the visible tumor base. If the ureters are included in the resection, perform a ureteroneocystostomy (Chapter 60). Close the incision with 3-0 or 4-0 absorbable monofilament material (e.g., poliglecaprone 25 or glycomer 631). If minimal bladder tissue has been resected, appose the wound edges with a single or double layer appositional or inverting pattern. If the bladder is thick, the resection includes a portion of the trigone, or a large amount of bladder has been removed, close the incision with a single layer continuous appositional pattern. If needed, drape the omentum over the bladder and tack it at several sites to the bladder wall with interrupted sutures of absorbable material.

Complications

If a large portion of the bladder has been resected, animals will be pollakiuric for weeks to months after the surgery until the bladder regenerates. Ureteral or urethral obstruction may occur, particularly if inverting patterns are used near the ureteral openings or urethra, respectively (Crowe 1986; Pozzi et al. 2006). If the bladder is devitalized, urine may leak from the bladder wall as the bladder stretches. Severely traumatized bladders may temporarily lose contractile function.

Cystostomy tube placement

Introduction

Urine diversion may be necessary in patients with urethral or cystic injury, resection, or obstruction or blad-

der atony. Options for diversion include transurethral catheters or cystostomy tubes (Chapter 32). Cystostomy tubes are most frequently placed in animals with urethral or trigonal neoplasia, bladder dysfunction (e.g., spinal cord trauma or detrussor atony), or urinary tract rupture (Beck et al. 2007). Types of cystostomy tubes include Foley, mushroom tip, and low profile catheters. Tube sizes are based on the size of the animal and the bladder and range from 8–24 Fr. Low profile tubes are preferred for chronic diversion because they are more difficult to accidently dislodge. They can be inserted surgically or used as a replacement tube for preexisting Foley or mushroom-tipped cystostomy catheters. For patients with preexisting tubes, the Foley or mushroom tipped catheter is pulled 2–4 weeks after placement. The low profile tube is inserted immediately through the same stoma, using a stylet to straighten the mushroom tip during passage within the fistula. Appropriate positioning can be confirmed by contrast radiography.

Although percutaneous placement has been described, most cystostomy tubes are placed surgically. Usually, a midline abdominal incision is performed, and the tube is inserted through a separate incision in the ventrolateral abdominal wall and into the ventral midbody of the bladder. The bladder is then secured (pexied) to the body wall to decrease the risk of urine leakage into the abdomen. To facilitate placement, the bladder can be partially pexied to the abdominal wall before inserting a low profile tube (Figure 83.6).

Tubes can be removed percutaneously in healthy animals as early as 7 days after surgical placement. Tubes should be left in longer in patients with immunosuppression, delayed wound healing, or leakage of urine around the tube. Once the tube is removed, the stoma will usually close within 3 days unless the urethra or trigone is obstructed.

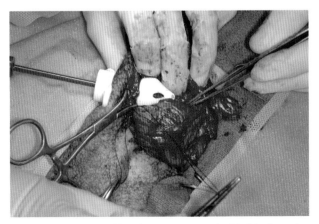

Figure 83.6 Low profile tube cystostomy. The bladder lateral to the purse string suture is pexied to the body wall dorsal to the cystostomy tube before the tube is inserted into the bladder.

Technique

Isolate the bladder with moistened laparotomy pads. If a Foley catheter is used, test the balloon for leaks. Force a hemostat from the peritoneal surface outward through the abdominal musculature of the ventrolateral body wall parallel to the level of the bladder. Incise the skin over the forceps to expose the tips. Grasp the tube end with the forceps and pull it into the peritoneal cavity. Place a purse string suture of 2-0 or 3-0 monofilament absorbable material in the ventral midbody of the bladder, penetrating the submucosa with each suture bite. Make a stab incision through the bladder wall within the purse string suture. Suction out any urine. Flatten the cystostomy tube tip with forceps or a stylet and insert the tube into the bladder. Tighten the purse string to appose the bladder wall around the tube and tie the suture without necrosing the enclosed tissue. Place a towel clamp on the edge of the abdominal wall and evert the incision edge to expose the peritoneum. Place 4 or 5 interrupted mattress sutures between the bladder and abdominal wall around the tube, starting with the dorsal most sutures. Use monofilament absorbable suture and include bladder submucosa in each bite. Secure the tube to the skin with a finger trap or other pattern and close the abdomen routinely.

Complications

Urinary tract infections are expected in most animals that have cystostomy tubes. Urine should be cultured after tube removal. Major complications include inadvertent tube removal (16%), uroperitoneum, tube breakage, and obstruction. Minor complications include stomal irritation and urine leakage around the tube. Complications are not correlated with species, age, body weight, or tube type (Beck et al. 2007).

Surgery of the prostate

Prostatic biopsy

Introduction

Prostatic disease may result in recurrent urinary tract infections, dysuria, or stranguria. Tentative diagnosis of the underlying condition is usually based on digital rectal examination; results of digital imaging; and cytology and culture of ejaculate, prostatic washes, or aspirates. Unfortunately, percutaneous prostatic aspirates and needle biopsies may provide insufficient samples for diagnosis in 50–75% of dogs (Barsanti et al. 1980; Powe et al. 2004). Surgical prostatic biopsy is recommended if diagnostic results are equivocal, particularly in dogs that are undergoing laparotomy for other reasons.

If possible, wedge biopsy of the prostate should be limited to the ventrolateral or lateral surfaces of the gland. The hypogastric and pelvic nerves are closely associated with the prostatic vessels dorsal and dorsolateral to the prostate gland. The urethra, which passes along the midline through the gland just dorsal to its center, can be avoided more easily if a urethral catheter is left in place during the procedure.

Technique

Approach the prostate through a caudal midline abdominal incision. If the prostate is small, place stay sutures in the bladder apex and retract the bladder cranially to expose the gland. If the prostate gland is diffusely affected, use a scalpel blade to take a wedge biopsy of the ventrolateral aspect of the gland. Remove the tissue sample by transecting the base with the blade; if thumb forceps must be used to grasp the sample, handle only the capsule. Appose the incised edges with interrupted, mattress, or cruciate sutures of 3-0 absorbable monofilament material. Include capsule and parenchyma in each bite. If the prostate is focally affected, obtain biopsies in a similar fashion, avoiding large vessels, or use a Tru-cut or other needle biopsy instrument to obtain multiple samples.

Complications

Excessive traction on the prostate or dorsal dissection could result in urinary incontinence. Major complications such as significant hemorrhage or urine leakage are uncommon when appropriate technique is used.

Prostatic omentalization

Introduction

Prostatic cysts or abscesses that do not respond to castration, percutaneous drainage, and appropriate medical management are usually treated by omentalization (Bray et al. 1997; White and Williams 1995). Insertion of the omentum into the prostate gland provides vasculature to improve delivery of antimicrobials, white blood cells, and angiogenic factors. The omentum also serves as a physiologic drain. Because abscesses are suctioned and flushed during the procedure, omentalization does not increase the risk of sepsis or peritonitis (Freitag et al. 2007).

Prostatic cysts and abscesses are approached through a caudal midline incision. A urinary catheter can be left in place during surgery to facilitate urethral identification during surgery. The cyst or abscess wall should be opened ventrally or ventrolaterally to avoid damage to bladder and urethral innervation and blood supply. After the cavity is drained, samples are obtained for biopsy and culture, and the cavity is omentalized. In most dogs,

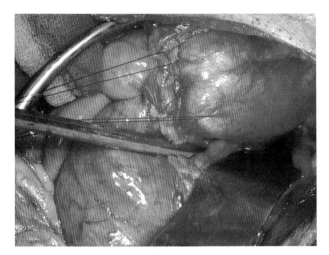

Figure 83.7 Stay sutures in the prostatic cyst.

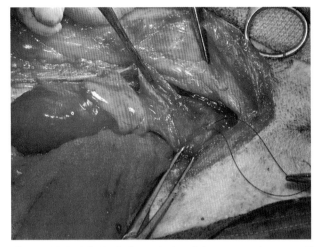

Figure 83.8 If desired, the majority of the cyst or abscess wall can be resected before omentalization. The urethra should be catheterized during resection.

omentum easily reaches the cyst cavity. Occasionally, the omentum must be transected along its dorsal attachment to lengthen the pedicle. If peritonitis is present, continuous suction drainage of the abdominal cavity may be required. The dog should be castrated at the end of the procedure if it is intact.

Technique

Isolate the prostate with moistened laparotomy pads. If necessary, place stay sutures in the bladder or prostate capsule and retract them cranially to improve prostatic exposure (Figure 83.7). Make a 1–2 cm incision in the ventrolateral surface of the cyst or abscess wall and insert a Poole suction tip into the incision. Suction the cavity and then extend the incision with scissors. Insert an index finger into the cavity and digitally break down any septa within the site. With Metzenbaum or Mayo scissors, resect a portion of the incised wall for culture and histologic evaluation (Figure 83.8). Flush the cavity with sterile saline and then remove the laparotomy pads. Insert the free edge of the omentum into the cavity (Figure 83.9). Tack the omentum to the edges of the prostate incision with interrupted sutures of 3-0 absorbable monofilament (e.g., poliglecaprone 25 or glycomer 631). If the cavity extends around the urethra, make a second ventrolateral incision on the opposite side of the prostate. Insert omentum into the site and tack in place. If an abscess is present, change gloves and instruments. If peritoneal contamination has occurred, flush the abdomen before closure.

Complications

Vomiting or urine retention is reported in 7% of dogs after recovery. Up to 20% of dogs may have transient urinary incontinence after prostatic omentalization. Incon-

tinence may be secondary to cystitis, continued prostatic enlargement, or neurologic damage from excessive dissection or traction during surgery (Freitag et al. 2007).

Subtotal prostatectomy

Introduction

Prostatectomy has been recommended for treatment of advanced prostatic neoplasia in dogs without evidence of metastases. Total prostatectomy, however, is likely to result in severe complications, including urinary incontinence, uroperitoneum, urethral stenosis, hemorrhage, and death. Compared to total prostatectomy, subtotal prostatectomy significantly decreases postoperative

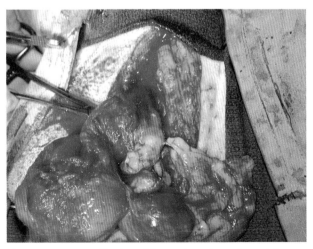

Figure 83.9 Ometalization of the cystic cavity. A Carmalt forceps has been inserted through the cyst and the omentum is pulled into the cavity and tacked in place.

complication rates and increases lifespan by over 400% (Vlasin et al. 2006).

Technique

Place a urinary catheter to facilitate urethral identification during the procedure. Make a caudal midline abdominal incision. Place umbilical tape ribbons around the urethra proximal and distal to the prostate to provide retraction and improve exposure. Incise the ventral prostatic sulcus with electrocautery. Remove about 85% of the parecnchyma within both lobes with the cautery, preserving the dorsal prostatic capsule and at least 2 mm of underlying prostatic tissue. If the prostatic urethra is penetrated, leave at least the dorsal half of the urethra intact. Appose the remaining prostatic capsule and parenchyma ventrally with simple interrupted or continuous sutures of monofilament absorbable material. Leave the urethral catheter in place for 3–5 days.

Complications

Complications that result in death or euthanasia of the patients are noted in 18% of dogs undergoing subtotal prostatectomy (Vlasin et al. 2006). These may include shock, uncontrollable hemorrhage, or irresolvable damage to the prostatic urethra. Minor complications such as transient dysuria or dyschezia and occasional urine leakage may be seen in some dogs. Mean postoperative survival is 112 days, with some dogs living up to 7 months after the procedure (Vlasin et al. 2006).

Urethral anastomosis

Introduction

Urethral tears and lacerations are usually secondary to trauma, urethral catheterization, or calculi (Anderson et al. 2006). The urethra can also be inadvertently damaged during surgery. If a strip of the urethral wall remains intact, most patients can be treated with urinary diversion by cystostomy tube or urethral catheterization. If the urethra is completed transected, primary repair is required. Urethral resection and anastomosis is occasionally performed to resolve strictures or remove tumors. In male dogs undergoing intrapelvic urethral resection and anastomosis, there was no significant difference in urethral healing in those that had an indwelling urethral catheter, cystostomy tube, or a combination of both after surgery (Cooley et al. 1999). Urinary diversion should be maintained for a minimum of 3–5 days, depending on the health of the urethral tissues and the amount of tension on the anastomosis. Urine should be cultured after catheters are removed.

Proximal urethral tears can be exposed through a caudal midline abdominal incision. The bladder is retracted cranially to improve exposure. Urethral tears within the pelvic canal may require pubic osteotomy or ostectomy. Pubic osteotomy alone will expose the cranial half of the intrapelvic urethra. Adductor muscular attachments are left in place along the caudal edge of the pubis to improve blood supply and stability. If possible, a portion of the prepubic tendon can also be left attached to the pubic flap. The bone flap is reflected ventrally and caudally during surgery. If a wider exposure is required, a bilateral pubic and ischial osteotomy or symphyseal ostectomy can be performed. With bilateral pubic and ischial osteotomy, muscular attachments are left in place along one lateral margin of the bone flap, and the flap is reflected laterally along these attachments. To facilitate closure of osteotomies, holes can be drilled in the pubis and ischium before osteotomy to facilitate repair. The prepubic tendon can be secured to the bone fragment through additional drill holes or reapposed along its midline and sutured caudally to the adductors.

Pubic ostectomy can be performed with rongeurs. The cranial half of the pubis can be removed to expose the urethra immediately caudal to the prostate and trigone. If more extensive exposure is required, the entire pubic and ischial symphysis can be removed (Figure 83.10) to produce a gap that is 2–3 cm wide, depending on the size of the animal. A portion of the cranial (acetabular) branch of the pubis medial to the iliopubic eminence should be left intact with the attached prepubic tendons.

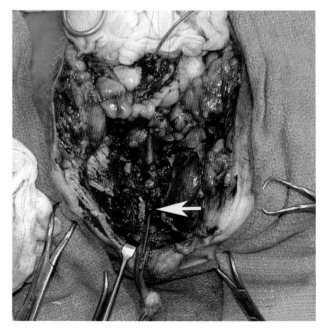

Figure 83.10 Traumatic separation of the urethra in a cat. The midurethral tear (arrow) was exposed through a pubic ostectomy.

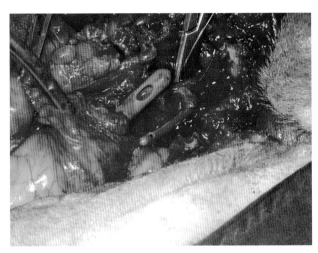

Figure 83.11 Resection and anastomosis of a urethral stricture secondary to pubic fractures. Red rubber catheters were advanced antegrade and retrograde to identify the ends of the urethra. A cranial pubic ostectomy was performed to improve exposure.

During closure, the prepubic tendon and adductors are apposed along the midline, and the tendon is sutured caudally to the cranial edge of the adductors.

Technique

Expose the urethra through a midline caudal abdominal incision. Perform a pelvic osteotomy or ostectomy as needed to increase exposure. Advance a distal urethral catheter (preferably, a Foley catheter) retrograde to the level of the transection. If the proximal urethral end cannot be identified, make a stab incision into the bladder and insert another urinary catheter antegrade into the proximal urethral segment (Figure 83.11). Limit dissection around the urethra to minimize the risk of neurogenic or vascular trauma to the urethra and bladder. If resection is required, place stay sutures of 3-0 monofilament through the proximal and distal segments of the urethra abaxial to the proposed sites of transection. If a stricture is present, transect the urethral segments close to the stricture. If a tumor is present, take 1–2 cm margins, if possible, but leave sufficient urethral length to provide a tension-free anastomosis. If the urethra is ruptured or traumatized, resect any unhealthy tissue from the urethral ends. Advance the distal urethral catheter retrograde into the bladder so that it bridges the urethral gap. Identify the urethral mucosa, which will normally retract into the urethral lumen. Wear magnification glasses or loupes to improve visualization. Place 6–8 interrupted sutures of 4-0 or 5-0 absorbable monofilament suture (e.g., poliglecaprone 25 or glycomer 631). Include mucosa and submucosa in each bite. If desired, preplace all sutures before tying. Remove any stay sutures. If a catheter was placed through the bladder, remove the catheter and close the stab incision with interrupted sutures of 3-0 absorbable monofilament, or place a cystostomy tube through the site to divert urine. Flush the abdomen and pelvic canal before closure.

Complications

Urinary tract infections are common when urethral or cystostomy catheters are left in place for several days (Cooley et al. 1999). Urethral stricture is likely to occur if urine is not diverted from the repair site (Layton et al. 1987). The urethra can also be narrowed by fibrous tissue adhesions at symphysiotomy or symphysiectomy sites. Subcutaneous, scrotal, or hind limb edema may occur if lymphatic or venous drainage is affected. Urine leakage may occur with tension or vascular injury along the anastomosis, particularly if urine diversion is inadequate.

Prescrotal urethrotomy

Introduction

Under general anesthesia, most urethral calculi can be retropulsed into the urinary bladder. Those that cannot be shifted are usually lodged within the urethra at the caudal end of the os penis. Many of these calculi become embedded within the mucosa and are not easily removed, even through a urethrotomy. In these dogs, scrotal urethrostomy is usually performed. In a few dogs, the calculus can be dislodged through a prescrotal urethral incision. Prescrotal urethrotomies are usually closed primarily to reduce postoperative hemorrhage. Urethral incisions that are left open to heal by second intention will bleed for 3–14 days, particularly when animals are excited (Waldron et al. 1985; Weber et al. 1985).

Technique

Make a 2–3 cm ventral midline incision through skin and subcutis, centering the incision over the obstruction. Excise the retractor penis muscle or elevate and retract it laterally. Stabilize the penile body between thumb and forefingers and, with a small blade, incise through urethra on midline over the calculus (Figure 83.12). Extend the incision as needed with fine scissors. Remove the calculus with forceps. Advance a urethral catheter retrograde through the penile urethra to verify all calculi have been removed. Leave the urethral catheter in place during urethrotomy closure. Close the urethrotomy with 5-0 absorbable monofilament suture (e.g., poliglecaprone 25 or glycomer 631) in a simple continuous pattern. Close the subcutaneous tissues and skin routinely.

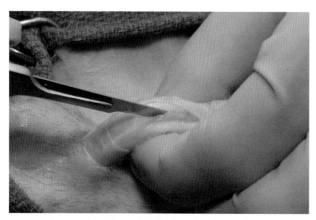

Figure 83.12 Prescrotal urethrotomy. The subcutaneous tissues and retractor penis muscle have been elevated and lateralized to expose the urethra, which usually has a pale blue or purple color.

Complications

Dogs may hemorrhage during urination or excitement; sedation may reduce bleeding. Complications are rare when tissues are handled gently and apposed appropriately. Narrowing of the urethral lumen may occur at the site, particularly if urine leaks subcutaneously. If urine leakage is suspected based on peri-incisional bruising or cellulitis, a urethral catheter should be left in place for 3–5 days to divert urine. If cellulitis occurs, the skin and subcutaneous sutures can be removed to permit drainage and the site is left to heal by second intention.

Scrotal urethrostomy in dogs

Introduction

Scrotal urethrostomy is most commonly performed in dogs with irresolvable distal urethral obstruction or recurrent cystic and urethral calculi. Compared with the perineal urethra, the scrotal urethra is wide, distensible, and superficial, making it the preferred site for permanent urethrostomy. Scrotal urethrostomy also reduces the risk of urine scald of the inner thighs or perineum. In dogs with distal penile trauma or tumors, a penile amputation can be performed concurrently.

In intact dogs, a scrotal ablation is performed to remove the testicles and expose the underlying penile body. In unobstructed dogs, the urethra can be catheterized during surgery to facilitate identification. Scrotal urethrostomies are centered over the curve of the penile body where it changes direction from vertical to horizontal. Although the urethra is superficial at this point, hemorrhage from the corpus spongiosum surrounding the urethra is expected during surgery. Postoperative hemorrhage can be reduced by apposing the urethral mucosa to the skin with a simple continuous pattern (Newton

and Smeak 1996). Mucocutaneous anastomosis can be performed with rapidly absorbable sutures; these sutures will slough from the site after several weeks and therefore do not need to be removed. If cystic calculi are present and the distal urethra is obstructed, scrotal urethrostomy and cystotomy are performed simultaneously. The urethra is catheterized retrograde through the urethrostomy to permit urethral and cystic lavage. Calculi distal to the urethrostomy site can be left in place. Dogs should wear Elizabethan collars or side bars for at least a week after the surgery to prevent self-trauma.

Technique

If the dog has previously been castrated, incise the skin of the scrotal remnant. If the dog is intact, perform a scrotal ablation and castration. Gently dissect the subcutaneous fat to expose the penile body. Elevate and excise or retract the retractor penis muscle. If possible, pass a urethra catheter retrograde into the perineal urethra. Identify the urethra: it may look like a large blue vein in some dogs (Figure 83.13). With a no. 11 or 15 blade, make a small incision on the urethra midline. Extend the incision with iris scissors until it is 2–3 cm in length, centering the incision over the curve of the penile body between the perineum and os penis. Control hemorrhage with digital pressure. Identify the urethral mucosa, which usually retracts away from the incised edge. Use magnifying glasses or loupes to facilitate visualization. Along one side of the incision, appose the skin to the urethral mucosa with a simple continuous pattern of 4-0 monofilament

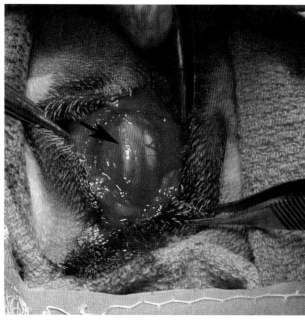

Figure 83.13 In the scrotal region, the urethra (arrow) may have the appearance of a large vein.

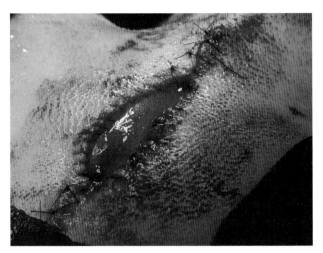

Figure 83.14 Scrotal urethrostomy. Urethral mucosa has been sutured to skin with a simple continuous pattern of 4-0 poligle-caprone 25.

absorbable suture (e.g., poliglecaprone 25 or glycomer 631) on a taper or taper-cut needle (Figure 83.14). Space suture bites 2–4 mm apart and tighten the suture so that the tissues are apposed but not compressed. Tie off the suture once the first side is completed. Appose the opposite side similarly. If needed, place a simple interrupted or mattress suture to appose the apex of the skin and urethral incisions caudally. Close any remaining subcutaneous and skin defects routinely.

Complications

Hemorrhage with urination is expected for several days after surgery. Persistent or severe hemorrhage and dehiscence are uncommon when the urethrocutaneous apposition is performed with a continuous pattern, suture bites include mucosa, and postoperative self-mutilation is prevented. Intermittent urine scald has been reported in 10% of dogs after scrotal urethrostomy with simple continuous closure (Newton and Smeak 1996). Dogs may develop recurrence of clinical signs because of calculus formation and urinary tract infections (Bilbrey et al. 1991).

Perineal urethrostomy in cats

Introduction

In cats, surgical widening of the distal urethra increases the risk of urinary tract infections (Bass et al. 2005). Resolvable urethral obstructions are therefore usually managed medically. For cats that have recurrent or irresolvable obstruction or irreparable distal urethral injury, perineal urethrostomy is recommended. Perineal urethrostomy can be performed with the cat in dorsal recum-

bency or in a perineal position, with the rear legs hanging over the end of a padded table. Dorsal recumbency permits simultaneous cystotomy if cystic calculi are present. The perineum is clipped and prepped, and a purse string suture is placed in the anus to reduce intraoperative contamination. The tail is pulled dorsally and cranially; if the cat is placed in dorsal recumbency, the rear legs are also pulled cranially.

During surgery, the penile body must be completely freed from its ventral and ventrolateral ischial attachments to reduce the risk of stricture (Phillips and Holt 2006). Dorsal and lateral dissection is limited to prevent damage to local innervation. The urethra should be opened to the level of the bulbourethral glands to ensure that stomal size is adequate. Stomal size should be large enough to permit insertion of a 6 or 8 Fr red rubber catheter or a Kelly or Halsted hemostatic forceps to the level of the box locks. In cats that require proximal perineal urethrostomy, the ischial symphysis can be removed with rongeurs to improve penile body exposure and decrease tension on the surgery site (Bernarde and Viquier 2004). To reduce postoperative hemorrhage and subcutaneous urine leakage, the urethral mucosa is apposed to the skin with a simple continuous pattern (Agrodnia et al. 2004). Magnification may be necessary to visualize the mucosal edge, which usually retracts 1 or more mm from the cut edge of the urethra.

Cats with proximal perineal urethrostomies or preoperative urethral trauma from catheterization or calculi may require urine diversion for 1–3 days with a Foley catheter to prevent subcutaneous urine leakage. Cats should wear Elizabethan collars for at least a week after the procedure to prevent self-mutilation. Suture removal is usually not required when mucocutaneous apposition is performed with rapidly absorbable suture material.

Technique

Make an elliptical incision through the skin and subcutis around the prepuce. If the cat is intact, castrate it through a scrotal incision or scrotal ablation. Wipe the penile body toward the ischium with a dry gauze sponge to remove any remaining subcutaneous attachments. With the tip of an index finger, palpate the ventral penile ligament between the penile body and ischial symphysis. Transect the ligament with Metzenbaum scissors (Figure 83.15). With an index finger, gently disrupt additional ventral midline attachments. Identify the ischiocavernosus and ischiourethralis muscles. Transect the muscles at their ischial attachments with Metzenbaum or Mayo scissors (Figure 83.16). With digital palpation, verify that ventral and ventral lateral attachments of the penile body have been severed from the ischium. If present, resect

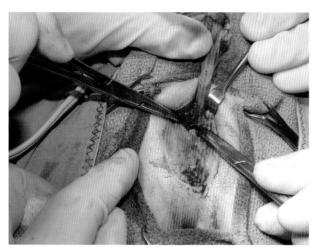

Figure 83.15 Perineal urethrostomy, perineal position. The ventral penile ligament has been transected with scissors. The muscular attachments to the ischium are visible near the tips of the hemostat.

the retractor penis muscle from the dorsal urethra. With Mayo scissors, cut open the prepuce dorsally to expose the penile tip. Insert one blade of an iris scissors into the urethral opening and incise the urethra on its dorsal midline (the side closest to the anus) to the level of the bulbourethral glands. Verify that the urethral stoma is adequate by inserting a 6 or 8 Fr red rubber catheter or Kelly or Halsted forceps to its box locks. Suture the urethral mucosa to the skin with 4-0 or 5-0 monofilament rapidly absorbable suture on a taper or taper-cut needle. Preplace interrupted sutures between the skin and mucosa at the 10 o'clock, 12 o'clock, and 2 o'clock positions. Place a slightly open hemostat in the urethral lumen to facilitate passage of the 12 o'clock suture. Include mucosa in each bite. Tie the sutures and cut the ends short. Anastomose the remaining mucosa to the skin along one side with a simple continuous pattern (Figure 83.17). Space bites 2

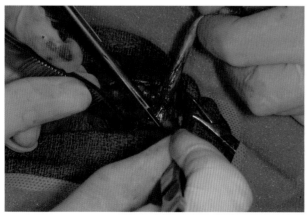

Figure 83.16 Perineal urethrostomy, dorsal recumbancy. Transect the muscles near their ischial attachments.

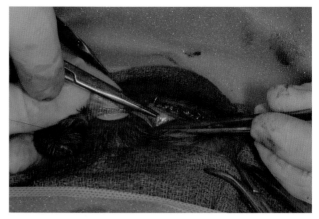

Figure 83.17 Suture mucosa to skin with a continuous pattern.

and 3 mm apart and take mucosal bites that include less than one-third of the urethral diameter. End the first continuous pattern near the distal urethra. Ligate and transect the distal penile body before apposing the mucosa and skin on the opposite side. Close any remaining skin defects.

Complications

Hemorrhage or subcutaneous urine leakage (Figure 83.18) may occur if gaps are present along the mucocutaneous suture line or the mucosa was not included in suture bites. Hemorrhage is more likely to occur with urination or excitation; cats may require sedation for several days after the surgery. Urine may also leak subcutaneously if preoperative urethral catheterization was traumatic or postoperative swelling is significant. Occasionally, cats will be unable to urinate after the procedure, despite an adequate stomal size. Functional obstruction occurs

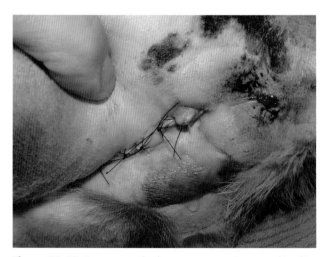

Figure 83.18 Because urethral mucosa was not apposed to skin, this cat developed subcutaneous urine leakage, azotemia, hyperkalemia, and skin bruising and necrosis and bruising.

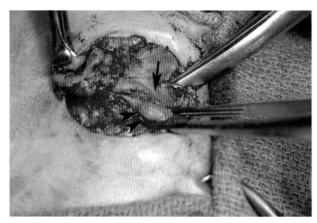

Figure 83.19 Stricture repair, dorsal recumbancy. Urethrostomy stenosis resulted from inadequate dissection of the muscular ischial attachments (arrowheads) and insufficient ostium size. Arrow indicates penile body.

more commonly with proximal perineal urethrostomy or excessive swelling; the skin along the proximal urethrocutaneous anastomosis inverts into the lumen of the urethra and acts as a one-way valve. These cats will require urine diversion with a Foley catheter for 1–3 days until the swelling resolves and the mucosa has sealed. Strictures may occur from urine extravasation but are more likely caused by inadequate dissection (Figure 83.19) (Phillips and Holt 2006). Bacterial cystitis occurs as a late complication of perineal urethrostomy in 17–40% of cats with an underlying uropathy; therefore, periodic urinalysis and culture are recommended (Bass et al. 2005; Corgozinho et al. 2007).

Prepubic urethrostomy

Introduction

Indications for prepubic urethrostomy include urethral neoplasia, stricture, and extensive trauma (Baines et al. 2001; Risselada et al. 2006). Prepubic urethrostomy is considered a salvage procedure because of the high rate of postoperative complications and should be avoided if possible.

Technique

Make a caudal midline incision, extending the incision over the pubis. Retract the bladder cranially with stay sutures. Identify the urethra and gently dissect the distal portion of the exposed urethra from the surrounding periurethral fat. Avoid traumatizing the nerves and vessels dorsally. If further exposure is required, perform a pubic or pubic and ischial osteotomy or symphysiectomy. Place a moistened umbilical tape around the distal extent of the urethra to elevate it. Ligate the most distal portion

of the healthy urethra with 3-0 monofilament suture. Transect the urethra immediately cranial to the suture and insert a red rubber catheter into the new opening. Incise the ventral surface of the transected urethral end to make a 1 cm spatulated opening. If large inguinal fat pads or skin folds are present, resect them before proceeding to urethrocutaneous anastomosis. Exteriorize the urethra through the caudal end of the celiotomy incision. Alternatively, place a stay suture in the end of the urethra, temporarily remove the urinary catheter, and pull the urethra through a separate abdominal incision 2–3 cm lateral to midline. Close the linea routinely without kinking the urethra. Place one or two interrupted sutures between the urethral wall and the external rectus sheath to reduce tension. Include submucosa in the suture bites but do not occlude the lumen. To form the stoma, place interrupted sutures cranially and caudally between the urethral mucosa and the skin. Use absorbable or nonabsorbable monofilament on a taper or taper-cut needle. Complete the urethrocutaneous anastomosis with simple interrupted sutures or a simple continuous pattern on each side of the new stoma. Remove the urethral catheter and close subcutaneous tissues and skin routinely.

Complications

Skin irritation and necrosis from urine scald or leakage is noted in 44% of cats undergoing prepubic urethrostomy. Urinary incontinence is reported in 38% (Baines et al. 2001). Stricture or dehiscence may occur with urine leakage, excessive tension, or postoperative self-mutilation. Prepubic urethrostomy can predispose animals to recurrent bacterial cystitis.

Urethral prolapse repair

Introduction

Urethral prolapse is an uncommon condition that is reported primarily in intact male brachycephalic dogs. Proposed etiologies include urethritis, cystitis, preputial inflammation, or sexual activity (Kirsch et al. 2002; Lipscomb 2004). The prolapse appears as a reddish mass protruding from the penile tip (Figure 83.20), particularly with urination or excitation. Because of environmental exposure and excessive trauma, affected dogs may have significant hemorrhage. Surgical treatments include urethral resection and anastomosis, urethropexy, or penile amputation and scrotal urethrostomy. Affected dogs should be castrated to reduce sexual activity, and underlying conditions such as balanoposthitis or cystitis should be treated. Activity, grooming, and excitement must be limited after surgery to reduce postoperative hemorrhage and recurrence.

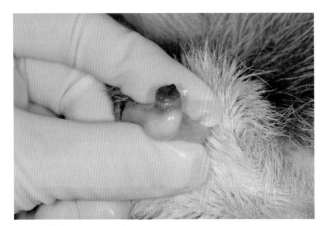

Figure 83.20 Urethral prolapse in a dog.

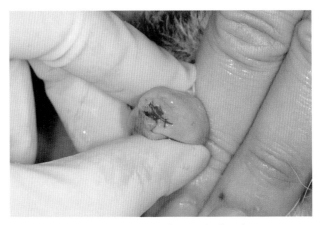

Figure 83.22 Final appearance after urethral prolapse resection.

Technique

Retract the prepuce with a Penrose drain to expose the penile body. To perform a urethral resection and anastomosis, pass a lubricated red rubber catheter into the urethra. With fine scissors, incise the urethral perpendicular to the edge of the prolapse to the level of the penile tip, then incise one-third of the circumference of the prolapsed tissue along the penile tip. Anastomose the transected urethral mucosa to the penile mucosa with a simple continuous pattern using 4-0 or 5-0 monofilament absorbable suture (e.g., poliglecaprone 25 or glycomer 631) on a taper or taper-cut needle. Place bites about 2 mm apart. Using a cut-and-sew technique, continue the urethral prolapse transection, and anastomosis circumferentially (Figure 83.21) until the anastomosis is complete (Figure 83.22).

To perform a urethropexy (Kirsch et al. 2002), insert a groove director into the urethral lumen and reduce the urethral prolapse. Use 2-0 or 3-0 absorbable monofilament suture on a taper or taper-cut needle for the pexy. Pass the needle full thickness through the penile wall at the level of the os penis and out the urethral lumen; use the groove director to control the needle passage in the urethra and direct it out of the lumen (Figure 83.23). Reverse the needle and pass it through the urethral lumen and out the penile body about 5 mm distal to the initial suture bite. Tie the suture snuggly without crushing the tissue. Place 1–3 additional sutures, spacing them evenly around the penile body (Figure 83.24). Pass a red rubber catheter to verify that the urethra is patent.

Complications

Hemorrhage may occur for up to 7 days after urethral prolapse resection and anastomosis. Swelling is expected with both techniques and can be reduced by preventing self-trauma and administering sedatives. Recurrence can be a problem after resection and anastomosis, particularly if the dog was not castrated, the underlying etiology was not treated, or the dog was not appropriately managed after surgery. Urethropexy has been used successfully in dogs with recurrence (Kirsch et al. 2002). If the

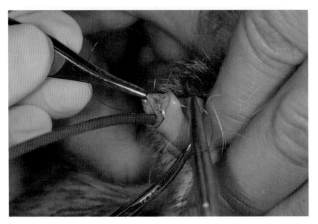

Figure 83.21 Suture the penile and urethral mucosa together with a continuous pattern.

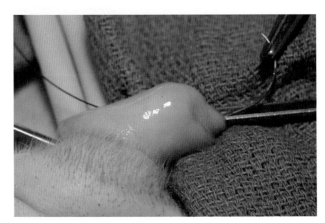

Figure 83.23 Using a groove director to guide the needle, pass suture from the external surface of the penis into the urethral lumen, then reverse the needle and pass it back out of the penis.

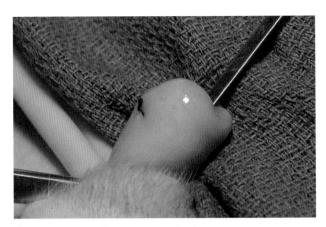

Figure 83.24 Urethropexy suture in place.

condition persists, penile amputation and scrotal urethrostomy are recommended.

Penile amputation in dogs

Introduction

Indications for penile amputation include penile or preputial neoplasia, hypospadias, irresolvable paraphimosis or priapism, recurrent urethral prolapse, penile necrosis, or severe trauma (Papazoglou and Kazakos 2002). If a small amount of the penile tip is affected, a partial amputation (Figure 83.25) can be performed with anastomosis of the urethral mucosa to the remaining penile body. If a large section of the penis must be removed, the urethra can be anastomosed to the preputial mucosa (Pavletic and O'Bell 2007). Preputial urethrostomy has been recommended to reduce the risk of urine scald associated with scrotal urethrostomy. If the entire glans penis must be removed, a scrotal urethrostomy is performed concurrently. To reduce hemorrhage during

and after penile amputation, transection of cavernous tissues can be performed with a carbon dioxide laser. Alternatively, bleeding can be controlled intraoperatively with a penile tourniquet. Sedation and Elizabethan collars or side bar restraints are recommended after surgery to reduce postoperative complication.

Technique

To perform a partial penile amputation, retract or incise the prepuce to expose the penis. Place a Penrose drain or Rümel tourniquet around the base of the glans. Insert a urethral catheter and tighten the drain or tourniquet to provide hemostasis. Incise the dorsal penile body at a 45° angle down to the os penis or urethra. Incise the ventral penile body similarly, leaving the urethra intact. If needed, elevate the urethra from the groove in the os penis and remove the distal end of the os penis with rongeurs. Dissect the penile tissue from the urethra, leaving at least 3 mm of urethral length beyond the transected cavernous tissue, and remove the penile tissue. Close the penile stump with simple continuous or interrupted sutures of 3-0 or 4-0 absorbable monofilament (e.g., poliglecaprone 25 or glycomer 631) medially and laterally. Spatulate the urethra and suture the urethral mucosa to the penile body with interrupted sutures at three sites, spacing the bites evenly. Use 4-0 or 5-0 absorbable monofilament suture. Complete the urethral apposition with an interrupted or continuous suture pattern (Figure 83.26).

To perform a subtotal penile amputation and preputial urethrostomy (Pavletic and O'Bell 2007), incise through the central third of the prepuce along the ventral midline. This will expose the penis and preputial cavity. If possible, catheterize the urethra before proceeding. Incise the penis to the level of the urethra with a carbon dioxide laser. Alternatively, place a tourniquet around the penile body and transect the penile tissue to the level of

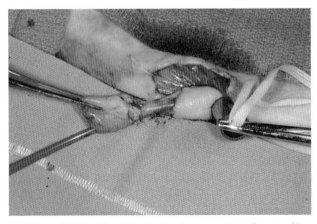

Figure 83.25 Partial penile amputation. A portion of urethral has been dissected from the remaining penile tissue. In this dog, the prepuce was incised to improve exposure.

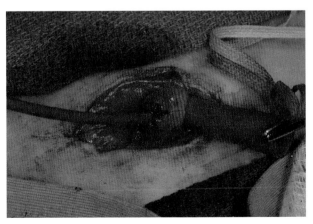

Figure 83.26 Final appearance after partial penile amputation and before preputial closure.

the urethra with a blade. If possible, leave at least 3 mm of urethra beyond the transected cavernous tissue. If not already in place, insert a urethral catheter. Spatulate the urethral end and suture it to adjacent preputial mucosa with 4-0 monofilament absorbable suture. To reduce tension during anastomosis, make a 2 cm releasing incision cranial to the prepuce. Once the anastomosis is complete, remove the urethral catheter. If desired, insert a Foley catheter through the original preputial opening and into the preputial urethrostomy site to temporarily divert urine. Close the remaining preputial mucosa with 4-0 monofilament in a simple interrupted or simple continuous pattern. Close the subcutis and skin of the prepuce and releasing incision routinely.

To amputate the entire penis ("phallectomy"), make an elliptical incision around the prepuce. Ligate any large preputial and dorsal penile vessels. Perform a scrotal urethrostomy as previously described. Ligate the penile body cranial to the scrotal urethrostomy site with encircling and transfixing sutures. Transect the penis cranial to the ligatures. Appose the tunica albuginea over the transected penile end with 3-0 absorbable monofilament suture in a continuous or interrupted pattern. Close the subcutaneous tissues and skin routinely.

Complications

Potential complications include hemorrhage, swelling, or infection. Animals undergoing partial penile amputation could develop urethral obstruction if improper technique is used.

Surgical treatments for urinary incontinence

Introduction

A variety of methods have been proposed to reduce or correct urinary incontinence. Some methods alter bladder position or lengthen the urethra, while others increase urethral resistance. Outcomes of these procedures are variable, depending on the underlying cause of incontinence and, in some instances, the experience of the surgeon. Deterioration of continence may occur over time as sphincter function decreases or the surgical repair stretches or breaks down.

Colposuspension increases urethral pressure and repositions the bladder neck into the abdomen. In one study (Marchevsky et al. 1999), outcome was excellent in 68% and 32% of dogs with acquired and congenital sphincter mechanism incompetence, respectively. Most of the remaining dogs were continent or improved immediately after colposuspension; however, continence deteriorated in these dogs 1–11 months after surgery. In another study (Rawlings et al. 2001), 55% of dogs were completely con-

tinent 2 months after colposuspension. One year after surgery, only 14% were continent, while 33% were considered greatly improved by their owners. When medical management was added, 38% of dogs were completely continent and 43% were greatly improved 1 year after surgery.

Transpelvic sling will increase pressure on the midpelvic urethra, increasing urethral resistance (Nikel et al. 1998). A synthetic material such as polyester ribbon is placed around the midportion of the pelvic urethra and exited from the obturator foramina. The ribbon is tightened to compress the urethra and secured to itself ventral to the pubis. Long-term continence is reported in 46% of dogs that undergo sling urethroplasty alone and 54% of dogs that undergo sling urethroplasty and colposuspension, simultaneously (Nikel et al. 1998). Some of the incontinent dogs improved with additional medical management.

Urethropexy relocates the bladder neck into an intraabdominal position and locally increases resistance by altering the shape of the urethra. In one study (White 2001), the ventral urethral wall was pexied to the abdominal wall just cranial to the pubic brim. Continence was noted in 73 of 100 dogs 1 year after surgery. Of those available for follow-up longer than 3 years, 48% remained continent. Eight of 100 dogs showed initial improvement and then gradually relapsed. Six of these dogs underwent a second urethropexy and four of these were continent more than 1 year later. In another study (Massat 1993), mattress sutures were placed between the lateral walls of the urethra and trigone and the ventral abdominal wall musculature ("cystourethropexy"). Continence was achieved in 90% of dogs immediately after surgery; however, 80% of dogs were incontinent within 5 months.

Sphincter mechanism incontinence is uncommon in male dogs. Ductus deferens and prostatic pexy have been used to relocate the bladder neck into the abdomen. Pexy of the ductus deferens to the abdominal wall resulted in long-term continence in 43% of male dogs and improvement in 43% (Weber et al. 1997). Prostatopexy to the prepubic tendon resulted in complete continence in 11% and improvement in 44% (Holt et al. 2005).

Dogs with recessed or infantile vulvas (Figure 83.27) may develop urinary incontinence from recurrent vaginitis, cystitis, and urine pooling. Clinical signs caused by skin-fold obstruction of the external genital opening will resolve with vulvoplasty (Lightner et al. 2001). Dogs that have concurrent vestibulovaginal stenosis will require vaginectomy or resection and anastomosis to resolve clinical signs (Crawford and Adams 2002). In dogs with perivulvar dermatitis, surgery should be delayed while the dermatitis is treated with appropriate topical and systemic therapy. If incontinence persists after surgery, the

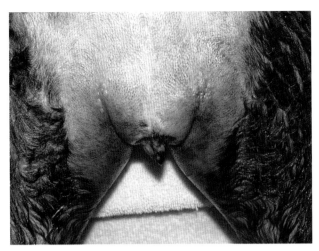

Figure 83.27 Recessed vulva causing chronic recurrent vaginitis, cystitis, and incontinence.

dog should be evaluated for other etiologies (Hammel and Bjorling 2002).

Techniques

Colposuspension

Prep the caudal abdomen to include perivulvar and vestibular regions. Expose the bladder through a midline caudal abdominal incision. Retract the bladder cranially to expose the bladder neck. Identify the vagina; if desired, insert closed Carmalt forceps through the vestibule into the vagina to facilitate identification. With Babcock or Allis tissue forceps or stay sutures, grasp the vaginal wall as far caudally as possible on either side of the urethra. Remove the Carmalt forceps and discard them from the surgical area to prevent contamination. Preplace two full-thickness mattress sutures of 0 monofilament nonabsorbable material through the vaginal wall and pubic tendon on each side of the urethra. Catheterize the urethra, or lay a urinary catheter of appropriate diameter alongside the proximal urethra and tighten the sutures. Check the urethra to verify that it is not strangulated between the pubis and vagina. Close the abdomen routinely.

Urethropexy

Perform a caudal midline celiotomy, extending the incision to the pubic brim. Place a stay suture in the bladder and retract it cranially. Identify the urethra by palpation. Bluntly dissect the overlying tissues to expose the ventral aspect of the urethra at the level of the cranial pubic brim. Just cranial to the pubic brim, pass a 2-0 or 0 polypropylene suture 1 cm lateral to the incised edge of the prepubic tendon and into the caudal abdominal cav-

ity. With the bladder retracted cranially, pass the suture through the muscularis of the ventral urethral wall. Pass the suture out of the prepubic tendon on the opposite site. Secure the suture with hemostats. Place a second suture 3–5 mm cranial to the first. Remove the bladder stay suture. Tighten each urethropexy suture; this will simultaneously appose the caudal midline abdominal incision (White 2001). Close the remaining abdomen routinely.

Vulvoplasty

Clip and prep the perineum and place a purse string suture in the anus. Place the dog in a perineal position over the padded end of a raised table with the tail pulled cranially. Grasp the entire width of the redundant vulvar fold with Allis tissue forceps and crush it along its base at several sites. This will provide a guide for resection. Make a horseshoe-shaped incision around the vulva along the outer row of crush marks. The incision should start and end at the level of the ventral vulvar commissure on each side. It will be closer to the vulva ventrally and ventrolaterally and farther from the vulva dorsally. To determine how much tissue to remove, pull the ventral edge of the skin incision upward so that it overlaps the dorsal edge of the skin incision. The remaining inner row of crush marks should not overlap with the dorsal skin edge, since the skin retracts after cutting. Make a second horseshoe-shaped incision, using the inner crush marks as a guide. Bluntly and sharply dissect subcutaneous tissue attachments to excise the redundant skin (Figure 83.28). Appose the skin edges at 10 o'clock, 12 o'clock, and 2 o'clock with simple interrupted skin sutures. Check the skin position before tightening each suture to make sure that the vulva is appropriately positioned and the incision line will not have gaps or dog ears.

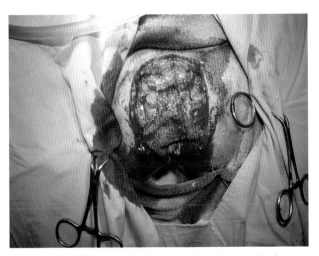

Figure 83.28 Skin resection for correction of recessed vulva.

Add absorbable, buried interrupted sutures to appose the subcutis if desired. Complete the skin closure.

Complications

Postoperative complications of colposuspension, urethropexy, and urethral sling techniques include dysuria, stranguria, urethral obstruction, or persistent or recurrent incontinence. Transpelvic slings have been associated with fistula formation (Nikel et al. 1998). Animals with obstruction may require urethral catheterization for up to 5 days after surgery until swelling resolves. If incontinence persists or reoccurs, the animals should be evaluated for cystitis or other etiologies. Medical management of sphincter mechanism incompetence should be attempted (Chapter 76) before considering surgical revision. Swelling is common after vulvoplasty, and some animals may have bruising or pain for several days after the surgery.

References

Agrodnia, M.D., J.G. Hauptman, et al. (2004). A simple continuous pattern using absorbable suture for perineal urethrostomy in the cat: 18 cases (2000–2002). *J Am Anim Hosp Assoc* **40**: 479–483.

Anderson, R.B., L.R. Aronson, et al. (2006). Prognostic factors for successful outcome following urethral rupture in dogs and cats. *J Am Anim Hosp Assoc* **42**: 136–146.

Aumann, M., L.T. Worth, et al. (1998). Uroperitoneum in cats: 26 cases (1986–1995). *J Am Anim Hosp Assoc* **34**: 315–324.

Baines, S.J., S. Rennie, et al. (2001). Prepubic urethrostomy: a long-term study in 16 cats. *Vet Surg* **30**: 107–113.

Barsanti, J.A., E.B. Shotts, et al. (1980). Evaluation of diagnostic techniques for canine prostatic diseases. *J Am Vet Med Assoc* **177**: 160–163.

Bass, M., J. Howard, et al. (2005). Retrospective study of indications for and outcome of perineal urethrostomy in cats. *J Small Anim Pract* **46**: 227–231.

Beck, A.L., J.M. Grierson, et al. (2007). Outcome of and complications associated with tube cystostomy in dogs and cats: 76 cases (1995–2006). *J Am Vet Med Assoc* **230**: 1184–1189.

Bellah, J.R. (1989). Wound healing in the urinary tract. *Semin Vet Med Surg Small Anim* **4**: 294–303.

Bernarde, A. and E. Viguier (2004). Transpelvic urethrostomy in 11 cats using an ischial ostectomy. *Vet Surg* **33**: 246–252.

Bilbrey, S.A., S.J. Birchard, et al. (1991). Scrotal urethrostomy: a retrospective review of 38 dogs (1973 through 1988). *J Am Anim Hosp Assoc* **27**: 561–564.

Bray, J.P., R.A.S. White, et al. (1997). Partial resection and omentalization: a new technique for management of prostatic retention cysts in dogs. *Vet Surg* **26**: 202–209.

Cooley, A.J., D.R. Waldron, et al. (1999). The effects of indwelling transurethral catheterization and tube cystostomy on urethral anastomosis in dogs. *J Am Anim Hosp Assoc* **35**: 341–347.

Corgozinho, K.B., H.J.M. De Souza, et al. (2007). Catheter-induced urethral trauma in cats with urethral obstruction. *J Feline Med Surg* **9**: 481–486.

Cornell, K.K. (2000). Cystotomy, partial cystectomy, and tube cystostomy. *Clin Tech Small Anim Pract* **15**: 11–16.

Crawford, J.T. and W.M. Adams (2002). Influence of vestibulovaginal stenosis, pelvic bladder, and recessed vulva on response to treatment for clinical signs of lower urinary tract disease in dogs:38 cases (1990–1999). *J Am Vet Med Assoc* **221**: 995–999.

Crowe, D.T. (1986). Ventral versus dorsal cystotomy: an experimental investigation. *J Am Anim Hosp Assoc* **22**: 382–386.

Freitag, T., R.M. Jerram, et al. (2007). Surgical management of common canine prostatic conditions. *Compend Contin Educ Pract Vet* **29**: 656–672.

Gilson, S.D. and E.A. Stone (1990). Surgically induced tumor seeding in eight dogs and two cats. *J Am Vet Med Assoc* **196**: 1811–1815.

Hammel, S.P. and D.E. Bjorling (2002). Results of vulvoplasty for treatment of recessed vulva in dogs. *J Am Anim Hosp Assoc* **38**: 79–83.

Herperger, L.J. (1998). Postoperative urinary retention in a dog following morphine with bupivicaine epidural analgesia. *Can Vet J* **39**: 650–652.

Holt, P.E., R.J. Coe, et al. (2005). Prostatopexy as a treatment of urethral sphincter mechanism incompetence in male dogs. *J Small Anim Pract* **46**: 567–570.

Kirsch, J.A., J.G. Hauptman, et al. (2002). A urethropexy technique for surgical treatment of urethral prolapse in the male dog. *J Am Anim Hosp Assoc* **38**: 381–384.

Layton, C.E., H.R. Ferguson, et al. (1987). Intrapelvic urethral anastomosis. A comparison of three techniques. *Vet Surg* **16**: 175–182.

Lightner, B.A., M.A. McLoughlin, et al. (2001). Episioplasty for the treatment of perivulvar dermatitis or recurrent urinary tract infections in dogs with excessive perivulvar skin folds: 31 cases (1983–2000). *J Am Vet Med Assoc* **219**: 1577–1581.

Lipscomb, V. (2003). Surgery of the lower urinary tract in dogs: 1. Bladder surgery. *In Pract* **25**: 597–605.

Lipscomb, V. (2004). Surgery of the lower urinary tract in dogs: 2. Urethral surgery. *In Pract* **26**: 13–19.

Marchevsky, A.M., G.A. Edwards, et al. (1999). Colposuspension in 60 bitches with incompetence of the urethral sphincter mechanism. *Aust Vet Pract* **29**: 2–8.

Mische, R. and U. Schulze (2004). Studies on platelet aggregation using the Born method in normal and uraemic dogs. *Vet J* **168**: 270–275.

Newton, J. and D. Smeak (1996). Simple continuous closure of canine scrotal urethrostomy: results in 20 cases. *J Am Anim Hosp Assoc* **32**: 531–534.

Nikel, R.F., U. Wiegand, et al. (1998). Evaluation of a transpelvic sling procedure with and without colposuspension for treatment of female dogs with refractory urethral sphincter mechanism incompetence. *Vet Surg* **27**: 94–104.

Papazoglou, L.G. and G.M. Kazakos (2002). Surgical conditions of the canine penis and prepuce. *Compend Contin Educ Pract Vet* **24**: 204–218.

Pavletic, M.M. and S.A. O'Bell (2007). Subtotal penile amputation and preputial urethrostomy in a dog. *J Am Vet Med Assoc* **230**: 375–377.

Phillips, H. and D.E. Holt (2006). Surgical revision of the urethral stoma following perineal urethrostomy in 11 cats: (1998–2004). *J Am Anim Hosp Assoc* **42**: 218–222.

Powe, J.R., P.J. Caqnfield, et al. (2004). Evaluation of the cytologic diagnosis of canine prostatic disorders. *Vet Clin Path* **33**: 150–154.

Pozzi, A., D.D. Smeak, et al. (2006). Colonic seromuscular augmentation cystoplasty following subtotal cystectomy for treatment of bladder necrosis caused by bladder torsion in a dog. *J Am Vet Med Assoc* **229**: 235–239.

Radasch, R.M., D.F. Merkley, et al. (1991). Cystotomy closure. A comparison of the strength of appositional and inverting suture patterns. *Vet Surg* **20**: 283–288.

Rawlings, C., J.A. Barsanti, et al. (2001). Evaluation of colposuspension for treatment of incontinence in spayed female dogs. *J Am Vet Med Assoc* **219**: 770–775.

Risselada, M., H. Rooster, et al. (2006). A prepubic urethrostomy in a bitch after resection of the vagina and distal part of the urethra. *Vlaams Diergeneeskundig Tijd* **75**: 35–40.

Schmiedt, C., K.M. Tobias, et al. (2001). Evaluation of abdominal fluid: peripheral blood creatinine and potassium ratios for diagnosis of uroperitoneum in dogs. *J Vet Emerg Crit Care* **11**: 275–280.

Stone, E.A., T.F. George, et al. (1996). Partial cystectomy for urinary bladder neoplasia: surgical technique and outcome in 11 dogs. *J Small Anim Pract* **37**: 480–485.

Vlasin, M., P. Rauser, et al. (2006). Subtotal intracapsular prostatectomy as a useful treatment for advanced-stage prostatic malignancies. *J Small Anim Pract* **47**: 512–516.

Waldron, D.R., C.S. Hedlund, et al. (1985). The canine urethra. A comparison of first and second intention healing. *Vet Surg* **14**: 213–217.

Weber, W.J., H.W. Boothe, et al. (1985). Comparison of the healing of prescrotal urethrotomy incisions in the dog: sutured versus nonsutured. *Am J Vet Res* **46**: 1309–1325.

Weber, U.T., S. Arnold, et al. (1997). Surgical treatment of male dogs with urinary incontinence due to urethral sphincter mechanism incompetence. *Vet Surg* **26**: 51–56.

White, R.A.S. and J.M. Williams (1995). Intracapsular prostatic omentalization: a new technique for management of prostatic abscesses in dogs. *Vet Surg* **24**: 390–395.

White, R.N. (2001). Urethropexy for the management of urethral sphincter mechanism incompetence in the bitch. *J Small Anim Pract* **42**: 481–486.

Section 10

Urinary disorders of avian and exotic companion animals

84

Avian and exotic companion animals

Cheryl B. Greenacre

Avian urology

Overview

Avian species in this text will refer to commonly seen pet exotic birds, including parrots, canaries, and finches. There are over 8,000 species of birds and the order Psittaciformes (parrots) alone consists of over 350 species and subspecies that are as diverse as a parakeet at 30 g and a blue and gold macaw at 1,000 g. Differences between the species not only includes size, but also country and climate of origin, and physiology. Some parrots are from rain forest climates and some are from desert (xerophilic) climates. It is known that some species within an order can metabolize drugs differently than other birds within the same order. For example, macaws often regurgitate on "regular" avian doses of trimethoprim-sulfa, and African grey parrots often become profoundly depressed on "regular" avian doses of itraconazole. Recently it has been shown that Old World Gyps Vultures are extremely sensitive to the nonsteroidal anti-inflammatory drug (NSAID) diclofenac compared to turkey vultures, with development of visceral gout, renal necrosis, and death a few days after exposure to relatively small doses of diclofenac. The median lethal dose in Gyps Vultures is 0.1–0.2 mg/kg, which is low enough to allow exposure to lethal doses by ingesting tissues of cattle given diclofenac just prior to death, whereas turkey vultures receiving doses of up to 25 mg/kg had no ill effects recognized either clinically or histologically (Rattner et al. 2008). Recent pharmacokinetic studies showed meloxicam, another NSAID, to be safe for use in several species of Gyps Vultures (Naidoo et al. 2008). Basically, there is no generic bird, or generic parrot

for that matter, and exotic animal formularies should be consulted prior to prescribing any drug.

Anatomy and physiology

Paired kidneys lay in a depression (Figure 84.1) of the fused synsacrum in birds, essentially surrounding the avian kidneys by bone on three sides.

Since spinal nerves of the lumbar and sacral plexus course through the kidney in birds, swelling of the kidney can cause pressure on these nerves and subsequent paresis and lameness (Figure 84.2; King and McLelleand 1984).

The avian kidneys generally have three (parrots) or two (canaries and finches) divisions: the cranial, middle, and caudal. The divisions are areas of the kidney and are not separate lobes. The external iliac vein courses ventrally between the cranial and middle divisions. Birds lack a diaphragm; therefore, ascites may cause a bird to present with dyspnea.

Urine and urates from each kidney travel through a ureter to the urodeum, an area of the vestibule-like cloaca that is an endpoint of the urologic, reproductive, and gastrointestinal systems. This unique arrangement allows urine to pass retrograde from the cloaca into the colon for further resorption of fluid. In dehydrated birds, up to 15% of urine water can be reabsorbed by the colon (Lumeij 1994). Renal output can decrease from the average 100–200 mL/kg/day down to 25 mL/kg/day during dehydaration (Lumeij 1994).

Birds possess both mammalian and reptilian type nephrons. Mammalian-type nephrons possess a relatively short loop of Henle and reside within the medulla and produce urine that is hypertonic to plasma, but not as concentrated as mammalian urine. Reptilian-type nephrons are the most numerous in birds, do not possess a loop of Henle, reside within the relatively large cortex of the kidney, and produce uric acid (Lumeij 1994). Uric acid is synthesized in the liver and 90% excreted

Nephrology and Urology of Small Animals. Edited by Joe Bartges and David J. Polzin. © 2011 Blackwell Publishing Ltd.

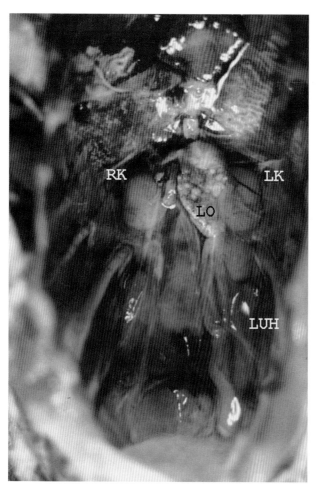

Figure 84.1 Paired kidneys (RK, right kidney; LK, left kidney) lay in a depression of the fused synsacrum of a female psittacine bird. The left ovary (LO) with opaque follicles is between the cranial divisions of both kidneys. The left uterine horn (LUH) is seen coursing ventral to the left kidney. Note the pale color of the cranial, middle, and the cranial part of the caudal divisions of this kidney. Also note the right external iliac vein coursing between the right cranial and middle divisions of the kidney.

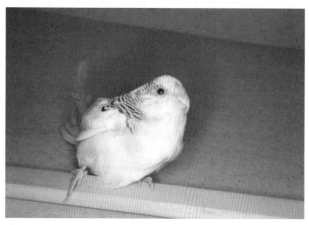

Figure 84.2 Budgerigar exhibiting right leg paresis secondary to a renal carcinoma creating pressure on the nerves of the lumbar plexus.

via tubular secretion from the reptilian-type nephrons. Uric acid production is independent of urine flow rate, and therefore independent of tubular water resorption (Lumeij 1994). Uric acid and its salts, urates, are a nonsoluble form of nitrogenous waste that allows development within an egg. The embryo can develop next to its own nitrogenous waste in the presence of a limited water supply within the egg (King and McLelland 1984).

Birds possess a renal portal system regulated by a conical valve in the common iliac vein. When this valve is closed, under stimulation by acetylcholine, blood flows toward the liver, essentially acting as an artery by supplying blood to the renal tubules. When this valve is open, under inhibition by adrenalin as in times of exercise or escape, blood can be shunted from the caudal half of the body away from kidney tissues and directly to the caudal vena cava (King and McLelland 1984; Lumeij 1994). The importance of this mechanism is to realize that substances injected into the caudal half of the body may go directly to the kidneys before going through the general circulation, causing damage to renal tissue. Intramuscular injections, especially with potentially renal toxic medications, should be given in the pectoral muscles in birds.

Diagnostic tests

Determining plasma or serum uric acid concentration is the most widely used method for determining the presence of renal disease in birds. Uric acid levels greater than 10 mg/dL are generally considered elevated for most species, but refer to species-specific reference ranges on individual cases. Hyperuricemia is a good indicator of renal disease; however, normal uric acid concentrations do not necessarily rule-out renal disease, and a profound hyperuricemia can be present postprandially in healthy raptors.

Radiography may be helpful in cases of renalmegaly, neprocalcinosis, ureteral stones, or severe gout. In psittacine birds, a rim of air, part of the abdominal air sac, should be visualized dorsal to the kidneys on a properly aligned lateral view, and its absence may signify pathologic swelling of the kidneys. An excretory urogram may be helpful in determining function of one kidney and ureter versus the other, and renal scintigraphy has been performed to evaluate glomerular filtration rate in birds. A 15-minute dynamic study was performed using 99mTc-diethylenetriamine pentaacetic acid (DTPA) to assess renal function in birds given a toxic dose of gentamycin (Marshall et al. 2003). Ultrasound of the kidneys in birds is not practical because of interference from the air in the air sacs surrounding the kidneys.

The most common "next step" in attempting to definitively diagnose renal disease in a bird is to perform an exploratory endoscopy with a rigid endoscope placed through the abdominal or caudal thoracic air sac. Courses are offered through national and regional conferences to train veterinarians in this technique that is common practice in exotic animal medicine. The kidneys can be directly visualized and a 3.5 or 5 Fr biopsy forceps can be used to obtain samples for histopathologic examination and culture.

Cloacoscopy using a rigid endoscope with a flush port can be used to visualize urine and urates exiting the ureteral papillae and entering the urodeum. The best visualization is achieved when the cloaca has been flushed clean and is filled with fluid by digitally preventing fluid from escaping the vent during cloacoscopy.

Urinalysis in birds is limited to evaluating specific gravity and for the presence of casts because of the inherent fecal and urate contamination. Wax paper can be used to obtain a minimally contaminated specimen. The presence of casts is strongly suggestive of renal disease. Proteinuria, and glucosuria without hyperglycemia, can also be present with renal disease. The specific gravity should be approximately 1.005–1.020 g/mL (Pollack et al. 2005). Porphyrinuria in Amazon parrots has been associated with lead toxicosis. Oftentimes, a bird is stressed when visiting the veterinary hospital causing an evacuation of the cloaca before colonic resorption of fluid has occurred, giving the appearance of polyuria and or diarrhea. Green urates, called biliverdinuria, are indicative of liver disease in birds (Figure 84.3).

Birds are unable to produce bilirubin due to the lack of biliverdin reductase.

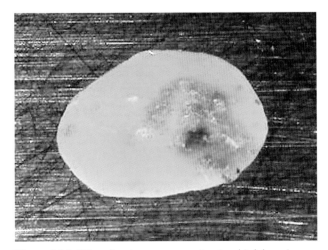

Figure 84.3 Biliverdinuria, or green urates, in a bird dropping are indicative of renal disease.

Common diseases

Bacterial nephritis

Gram-negative organisms can spread hematogenously during sepsis or can ascend from the cloaca causing a bacterial nephritis. Younger birds are more susceptible. The following bacteria have been associated with nephritis in birds: Staphylococcus, Streptococcus, Listeria, E. coli, Klebsiella, Salmonella, Yersinia, Proteus, Citrobacter, Edwardsiella, Enterobacter, Morganella, Providencia, Serratia, Pasteurella, and Mycobacteria (Lumeij 1994). A CBC profile including uric acid, a urinalysis, radiograph, fecal Gram's stain and culture, ± biopsy and culture of the kidney are commonly employed to aggressively workup renal disease. In cases of an ascending infection from the cloaca, a fecal Gram's stain showing more than 10% Gram-negative organisms in a psittacine bird is suggestive of enteritis, and a fecal culture may be a noninvasive method of diagnosing the causative organism. A broad spectrum, bactericidal antibiotic such as enrofloxacin, trimethoprim-sulfa (not macaws), or cephalosporin is recommended. Fluid therapy, at maintenance of 50 mL/kg/day, plus more for any losses, via the SC, IV, or intraosseous route for several days, is usually necessary.

Polyomavirus

Polyomavirus is a fatal disease of young birds, but it can also affect adult birds. There is a licensed vaccine (Psittimmune) available by Biomune (Lenexa, KS) to prevent the disease. Many aviary birds are subclinically affected and are a constant source of infection in the aviary and a particular danger for young birds, therefore all birds should be vaccinated. The virus is nonenveloped and therefore can remain viable in the environment for possibly years. Transmission of polyomavirus is through exposure to excretion and secretions, especially urine. Acute disease occurs in young birds with an approximate mortality rate of 27–41%, and includes 12–48 hours of depression, anorexia, delayed crop emptying, regurgitation, diarrhea, dehydration, SQ hemorrhage, dyspnea, and polyuria (Ritchie 1995). The SQ hemorrhages are most easily seen over the crop, carpi, or cranium. Typically, during an acute outbreak, approximately 30% of birds between 28 and 48 days of age die within a 6-week period (Ritchie 1995). Chronic disease is associated with weight loss, intermittent anorexia, polyuria, renal failure, and poor feather growth, as well as signs of immunosuppression, such as secondary bacterial or fungal infections. It seems the chronic disease occurs in immunosuppressed adults that cannot overcome the clinical signs of infection. There is no treatment for the disease. The prognosis is grave if clinical signs are present in a young bird. Disinfection of the environment is imperative and includes the use of a synthetic phenol, sodium hypohlorite (bleach), stabilized chlorine dioxide, or 70% ethanol. A PCR test can be done on a swab of the environment to evaluate the efficacy of the disinfection process. A PCR test can be used to evaluate tissues or feces for the virus.

Parasitic infections

Parasitic infections involving the urinary tract are not common in pet birds, although renal coccidiosis in geese due to *Eimeria truncata* is well known, and adult trematodes (*Tanaisia bragai*) in chickens, turkeys, and pigeons have been described in the collecting ducts (Lumeij 1994).

Fungal infections

Although aspergillosis infection with *Aspergillus flavus* or *A. funigatus* most commonly affects the caudal thoracic air sacs, the tracheal bifurcation or the sinuses, the infection can sometimes spread through the thin air sacs to a nearby kidney. One such aspergillosis infection spread not only to the kidney but also to the nerves of the lumbar plexus result in lameness (Greenacre et al. 1992). Immunosuppression, hypovitaminosis A, or massive exposure to fungal organisms is usually the inciting cause. Aspergillosis is more common in African Grey parrots, macaws, and raptors. A suggestive diagnosis is based on a heterophilic and monocytic leukocytosis, elevated enzymes (AST, LDH, CK) suggesting tissue destruction, an elevated aspergillus antigen and/or body, an elevated galactomannan level (through University of Miami Pathology Laboratory), plasma electrophoresis pattern suggestive of infection, and radiographs suggesting granulomatous masses in the air sacs. A definitive diagnosis is based on direct visualization with endoscopy and histopathologic examination and fungal culture of biopsy samples. An aspergilloma, or fungal ball, can be present in severe cases. Treatement consists of antifungals such as the conazoles, including ketaconazole, itraconazole, and fluconazole. Itraconazole is the best, but should not be used in African grey parrots (or used at very low doses). Also, amphotericin-B is good, but can only be given IV, or through nebulization, and it is quickly renal-toxic. Months of treatment are necessary, so diagnose early and treat for a month past resolution of clinical signs. Also, correct any underlying cause of immunosupression or overexposure. Again, fluid therapy is beneficial initially for several days.

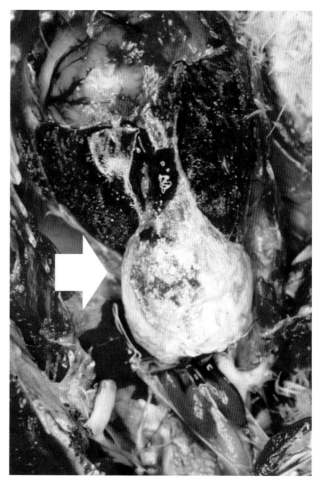

Figure 84.4 Visceral gout (uric acid deposition) in the pericardial sac (arrow) of a bird.

Gout

Gout is defined as uric acid deposition in tissues. Birds commonly present with renal, visceral, or articular gout due to hyperuricemia secondary to renal disease of various causes, including dehydration (Figure 84.4).

A sample of the white material can be examined under the microscope and appears as round crystals. Allopurinol has been used in some parrot species to successfully decrease blood uric acid levels, but a study in red-tailed hawks showed allopurinol-caused hyperuricemia (Lumeij and Redig 1992). A postprandial hyperuricemia is common and normal in hawks and should not be confused with renal disease, so recheck levels after fasting. Allopurinol inhibits xanthine oxidase, the enzyme that forms xanthine, which in turn forms uric acid (Lumeij 1994). Gout is painful; therefore, an analgesic should be administered. Most NSAIDs are renally excreted and can cause further renal damage; therefore, some clinicians use tramadol, but its use in psittacine birds has not yet been studied. Large pockets of uric acid, usually found on the dorsal surface of the tarsometatarsus, can be lanced and drained, but be ready for more hemorrhage than expected since the overlying tissues are inflamed. Again, fluid therapy is given to reestablish hydration.

Hypervitaminosis D

Hypervitaminosis D can cause gout. Inappropriate diets are the usual cause, for example, a blue and gold macaw neonate was hand-fed dog food causing hypervitaminosis D, leading to articular gout involving both carpi and metstarsi, visceral gout, and death. Renal calcinosis has been associated with hypervitaminosis D.

Renal calcinosis

Renal calcinosis can be seen radiographically in clinically normal African grey parrots and is considered an incidental finding, but in other species has been associated with hypervitaminosis D.

Urolithiasis

Ureteroliths secondary to severe dehydration and their surgical removal have been described (Figures 84.5a and b).

Cloacoliths secondary to poor emptying of the cloaca due to papillomatous lesions has also been seen (Figure 84.6).

Toxins

Aminoglycosides can cause renal tubular necrosis and are not recommended for use in birds. Heavy metals, aflatoxins, and salty food also can cause acute renal failure in birds. Lead and zinc toxicosis is common in pet birds and clinical signs include neurological signs, regurgitation, and depression. Amazon parrots can present with porphyrinuria. Diagnosis is based on visualizing heavy metal particles on radiographs or documenting elevated blood lead or serum zinc levels. The University of Louisiana Toxicology Laboratory has a graphite furnace to evaluate lead and zinc levels using just 0.1 mL of blood or serum. Treatment for lead or zinc toxicosis in birds is Ca EDTA (30 mg/kg IM q12h × 5 d) or dimercaptosuccinic acid (DMSA at 30 mg/kg PO q12h × 30 d), or both. Again, fluid therapy is beneficial, as is supportive care for the liver with lactulose (Duphulac 1 mL/kg PO q24h). Aflatoxicosis is more hepatotoxic than renal toxic; therefore, besides fluid therapy, supportive care is aimed toward the liver. Salt toxicosis can lead to urate impaction of the ureters and neurological signs. Elevated plasma sodium levels with a history of salt intake, and concurrent neurological signs, is highly suggestive. Sea birds have a special

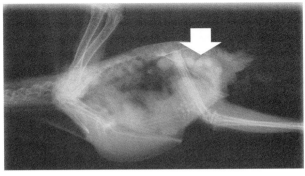

(a)

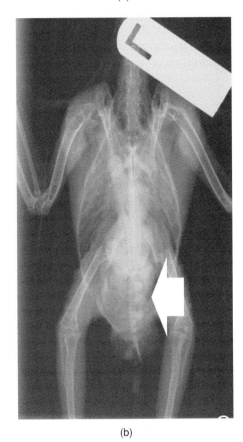

(b)

Figure 84.5 (a, b) Lateral and ventrodorsal radiographs of an adult umbrella cockatoo with multiple ureteroliths (arrows).

nasal salt gland to secrete a 5% salt solution so they can drink sea water (3% salt).

Neoplasia

Common tumors of the urogenital system of pet birds include nephroblastoma, adenocarcinoma, carcinoma, and adenomas (Latimer 1994; Reavill 2004). Renal carcinomas are most frequently reported in budgerigars greater than 5 years of age with a 3-week to 6-month disease course. Common presenting signs include coelomic enlargement, weight loss, vomiting or regurgitation, and

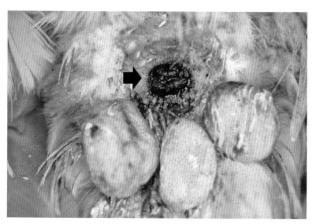

Figure 84.6 Three cloacoliths removed from the cloaca of an Amazon parrot. A cloacal papillomatous mass (arrow) was causing physical obstruction at the vent and accumulation of urates.

unilateral leg lameness caused by pressure on the nerves of the lumbar plexus. Most tumors occur in the cranial division and do not seem to impair function. Metastasis is rare. A radiograph often confirms a mass in the coelomic cavity. There is no treatment and surgical attempts result in massive hemorrhage.

Reptile urology

Overview

There are over 7,000 species of reptiles. There are four orders: Squamata (including the snakes and lizards), Rhynchocephala (the tuataras), Testudines (including the turtles and tortoises), and Crocodilia (the crocodiles). Commonly kept reptiles include extremely diverse species and vary not only in size, but also country and climate of origin, and physiology. It is known that some species of reptiles can metabolize drugs differently than others. For example, tortoises die after administration of ivermectin, but most other reptiles do not. It is hypothesized that tortoises have GABA receptors peripherally or that the ivermectin passes the blood–brain barrier. Death is usually due to paralysis of respiratory muscles. Therefore, it must be taken into account that there is no generic reptile and exotic animal formularies that should be consulted prior to prescribing any drug.

Anatomy and physiology

The urinary anatomy of reptiles is quite diverse and this text will include a brief description of snakes, turtles/tortoises, and lizards. For a more detailed description, the reader is directed to Dr. Mader's book for species-specific descriptions with color plates (Holz 2006). The elongated body of snakes makes for elongated kidneys with the right cranial to the left, located approximately in the caudal third of the body, extending 10–15% of the body length (Holz 2006). The kidneys have the shape of a stack of coins that has fallen over in an overlapping fashion, representing the 25–30 lobules that typically constitute a snake kidney. Snakes do not possess a urinary bladder, therefore urine and urates pass from the ureters into the urodeum, a portion of the cloaca, much the way it occurs in birds.

Most lizards possess a urinary bladder, and iguanas possess a urethra that extends from the bladder to the urodeum. The urine travels from the kidneys through the ureter to the urodeum, where it can be become contaminated with feces and bacteria and then is retropulsed into the bladder and colon. The paired kidneys in lizards are generally located within the pelvic canal and base of the tail, and because of this location, severe renalmegaly can lead to constipation (Figure 84.7).

It is possible in large iguanas to perform a digital rectal examination through the cloaca. The kidneys should not

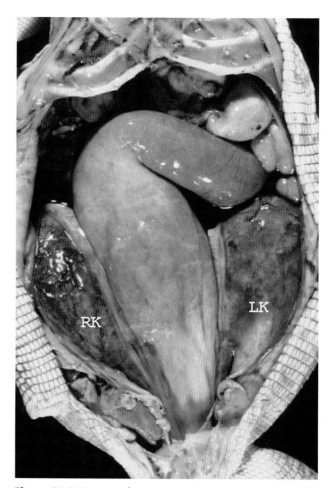

Figure 84.7 Necropy of an iguana with severe renalmegaly (RK, right kidney; LK, left kidney) and secondary constipation. Note how the enlarged kidneys obstruct the pelvic canal inhibiting defecation.

extend much past the pelvic canal into the celomic cavity, nor should they be visible cranial to the pelvic canal radiographically. Cloacal palpation can also be used in large lizards to evaluate kidney size and shape. Intraoperatively, do not confuse the bilateral lobe-shaped fat pads for kidneys or uterine horns.

Turtles and tortoises also possess paired kidneys, but they are located in the dorsal caudal celomic cavity just ventral to the carapace. Turtles and tortoises also possess a urinary bladder and urethra, and ureters that connect to the neck of the bladder, but the urinary bladder may be divided into three sections, a main bladder and two accessory bladders (Holz 2006).

The reptilian nephron does not possess a loop of Henle; therefore, reptile urine is not hypertonic. The major form of nitrogenous waste in reptiles is uric acid bound to protein and sodium or potassium to form a suspension called urates. The urine is retropulsed from the cloaca to the colon for further water resorption and further precipitation of uric acid (Holz 2006). Reptiles with a urinary bladder also retropulse urine from the cloaca to the colon for further resorption, but the bladder resorbs some water as well and acidifies the urine to precipitate uric acid (Holz 2006). Reptiles also can take in fluid from the environment through the cloaca and into the colon; therefore, an enema of physiologic saline is an excellent method of providing fluids to a reptile. Never use castile soap enemas in reptiles. Besides SC, IV, intraosseous, and via enema, fluids can also be given intracoelomically. Tilting the reptile so the celomic contents fall away from the side of needle penetration usually prevents puncturing of an internal organ (Hernandez-Divers and Innis 2006; Sykes and Greenacre 2006). Usually, no more than 3% of body weight in fluids is given at one time to a reptile.

Reptiles possess a renal portal system similar to that described in birds. For years, the general rule was to inject all drugs in the cranial half of the body to avoid undiluted drug exposure to the kidneys, but recent studies in red-eared sliders and carpet pythons show this rule may be unfounded. If using amikacin, a potentially nephrotoxic drug, it is still recommended that it be given in the cranial half of the body and most importantly to a hydrated animal and/or give concurrently with fluids.

Diagnostic tests

Acute renal failure presents as acute depression, anorexia, decreased to no fecal/urinary output, and usually a heterophilic, azurophilic leukocytosis. Chronic renal failure presents with depression, anorexia, severe weight loss, and usually a regenerative anemia.

Although uric acid is the major nitrogenous waste in reptiles, blood uric acid levels do not seem to increase until after renal failure has occurred. If phlebotomy is contaminated by urates, say if the sample was acquired from a tail vein with urates on the skin, then very high, untrue blood uric acid levels may be obtained. Oftentimes, in iguanas, the best initial indicator of possible renal disease is hyperphosphotemia. A phosphorus level greater than 5 mg/dL should stimulate further diagnostic tests. An excellent source of published species-specific reference values exists in Dr. Carpenter's Exotic Animal Formulary (Diethelm 2005). Commonly, elevated enzymes (AST, LDH, CK), suggesting tissue destruction, are present.

Radiography may be helpful in cases of renalmegaly, neprocalcinosis, ureteral stones, or severe gout. Normal-sized iguana kidneys are not visible past the pelvic inlet on either the ventrodorsal or the lateral view. In all reptiles, the lateral view should be taken with a horizontal beam for better visualization. Oftentimes with renalmegaly, especially in iguanas, constipation is seen radiographically, due to physical obstruction by the kidney in the pelvic canal. Intravenous injection of 800–1,000 mg/kg of iohexol, an aqueous-iodinated contrast medium, and taking serial radiographs at 0, 0.5, 2, 5, 15, 30, and 60 minutes post administration may be helpful in outlining the kidneys and evaluating function of the kidneys or ureters (Hernandez-Divers and Innis 2006). If the contrast medium is injected in the cranial half of the body, then essentially an excretory urogram is obtained, but if the contrast medium is injected into the tail vein, then, because of the renal portal system, an outline of the kidney may be visible. Renal scintigraphy has been performed to evaluate glomerular filtration rate in iguanas (Greer et al. 2005). Ultrasound of the kidneys is helpful in iguanas and snakes and can be used to perform an ultrasound guided biopsy.

The most common "next step" in attempting to definitively diagnose renal disease in any reptile is to perform an exploratory endoscopy with a rigid endoscope placed into the caudal aspect of the coelomic cavity. Sometimes, mild insufflation is necessary to adequately visualize and access structures. Courses are offered through national and regional conferences to train veterinarians in this technique that is common practice in exotic animal medicine. The kidneys can be directly visualized and a 3.5 or 5 Fr biopsy forcep can be used to obtain samples for histopathologic examination and culture.

Urinalysis in reptiles is limited to evaluating for the presence of casts and evaluating for large numbers of leucocytes, erythrocytes, epithelial cells, or a monomorphic population of bacteria. Small numbers of a mixed population of bacteria is expected, even if a cytocentesis is done in a species with a urinary bladder, because of fecal contamination that occurs in the urodeum. Proteinuria, glucosuria, and blood are not normal findings and are suggestive of renal disease, although blood could have arisen from anywhere in the gastrointestinal, urinary, or reproductive tracts. Protozoan parasites can be found in reptile, especially tortoise, urine.

Common diseases

Glomerulonephrosis

The most common renal disease seen in captive reptiles is glomerulonephrosis and tubulonephrosis of iguanas. The most common inciting cause is a diet high in animal proteins at any stage of life. Even a young iguana fed animal protein can develop glomerulonephrosis later in life. The iguana presents with signs of chronic renal disease, including severe weight loss, anorexia, depression, and lack of fecal or urine production. Usually, renomegaly is palpated, but in end stages, small kidneys may be present. Oftentimes, iguanas present after several weeks of clinical signs, and there is little, if any, renal function remaining; therefore, this disease generally has a poor prognosis. Hyperuricemia is usually present, but not always, and hyperphosphotemia of greater than 5 mg/dL is usually present. Sometimes, the phosphorus level is higher than the calcium level in the blood, a calcium:phosphorus inversion, sometimes leading to concurrent renal calcinosis. Concurrent gout is also seen. Oftentimes the ionized calcium is also low, below 1.3 mg/dL. Fluid therapy, preferably intravenous, is paramount. Some veterinarians administer oral calcium and oral phosphorus binders (to bind dietary phosphorus in the gastrointestinal tract only, not blood), but these treatments are controversial due to lack of scientific studies. Some believe calcium supplementation in the presence of hyperphosphatemia encourages renal calcinosis. If after several days of intensive IV fluid therapy, an iguana is not responding by lower uric acid or lower phosphorus levels, then euthanasia is recommended. Some dedicated iguana owners have given oral fluids, calcium, and phosphorus binders daily for years to manage chronic renal disease, but eventually their iguanas succumb to multiple organ dysfunction with ascites.

Gout

Gout is the deposition of uric acid in tissues. Common factors that contribute to gout in reptiles include dehydration, misuse of aminoglycoside antibiotics, renal disease of any kind but especially tubular disease, and high protein diets in herbivorous reptiles (Mader 2006a). Diagnosis is based on demonstrating uric acid crystals from a white mass in tissues usually found near a joint. Treatment is aimed at decreasing blood uric acid levels, decreasing inflammation and managing the pain. Allopurinol, colchicine, fluid therapy to reestablish hydration, NSAIDs, and opiates can be given, but relay to the client that many dosages are empirical in reptile medicine. Prognosis is poor unless caught early and treated aggressively.

Urinary calculi

Urinary calculi are usually composed of uric acid and are commonly diagnosed in lizards and tortoises (Figure 84.8).

Renal calculi have not been described in reptiles. A common theme is chronic dehydration form either a dry environment or lack of access to adequate amounts of water, but a diet high in protein or oxalates (found

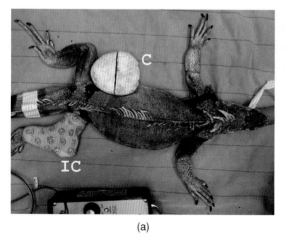
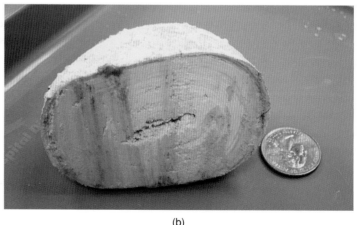

(a)   (b)

Figure 84.8 (a) A very large cystic calculi, C, composed of 100% uric acid removed from an iguana is placed next to the iguana immediately postoperatively. Note the prominent pelvic bones consistent with emaciation. The iguana was being administered fluids via an intraosseous catheter (IC) placed in the right femur. (b) Close up of cystic calculi cut in half showing the laminar appearance.

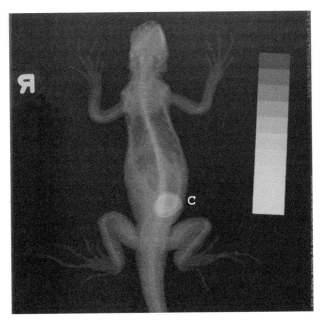

Figure 84.9 Ventrodorsal radiograph of an iguana with a cystic calculus, C. Analysis showed it was 100% uric acid.

in spinach) has also been suggested (Mader 2006b). All reptiles should have access to a large, shallow pan of fresh water. A common history in iguanas with urinary calculi is an owner that was told years previously to just spray the leaves with water and not offer a bowl of water. Urinary calculi can usually be palpated just cranial to the pelvis and tilting a tortoise side to side may facilitate palpation (or eggs can be palpated in this way as well). Radiographs are very helpful in demonstrating the urinary calculi, which are oftentimes very large (Figure 84.9).

Surgical removal is recommended (Figure 84.10).

A paramedian incision is used in lizards to avoid the ventral abdominal vein. A plastronotomy, a bone flap in

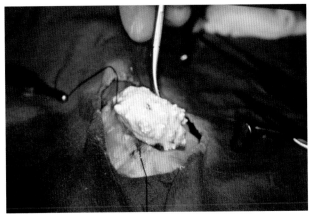

Figure 84.10 Cystic calculus being removed surgically from an iguana. Sometimes, the calculi can have an irregular surface as in this case.

the plastron, or a prefemoral celiotomy is used to access the bladder in tortoises.

Prolapsed tissue

Any tissue protruding from the vent must be identified prior to correction and possibilities include penis (turtles and tortoises), hemipenes (snakes and lizards), bladder in those species with a bladder, cloaca, or distal intestinal tract. A hemipene everts on either side of the vent during copulation or excitation, but should return to its inverted position in the anal gland momentarily. Penile prolapse is most common in turtles and tortoises and can be replaced and secured at the vent with stay sutures for a few weeks, or if severely damaged, can be amputated since they are not needed for urination.

Neoplasia

The most common tumors of the urological system of reptiles include renal adenocarcinoma, mostly of snakes, renal tubular adenoma of snakes and iguanas, and nephroblastomas. Renal adenocarcinomas are the most common and present most commonly in colubrid snakes such as the king snake, and present with a large, unilateral mass. Metastasis is rare and a nephrectomy may be useful in treatment (Garner et al. 2004).

Rabbit urology
Anatomy and physiology

The anatomy of a rabbit kidney is very similar to a cat kidney. The kidneys are easily palpable once the rabbit relaxes and are more ventral and free-floating than one would expect. Obese rabbits can have a very large retroperitoneal fat pad that can cause the kidneys to be almost ventral on radiographs or during palpation. Like horses, rabbits excrete calcium carbonate in the urine, giving it a cloudy appearance. Normal daily water intake for a rabbit is relatively high at approximately 120 mL/kg. Urine output is approximately 130 mL/kg/day. The color of rabbit urine may vary greatly and is influenced by diet and stress. Urine can be cloudy or clear and range in color from pale yellow to orange-red. Red urine in rabbits may not necessarily be hematuria but the more common, and normal, porphyrinuria pigments (Figure 84.11).

A urine dipstick is an easy method to differentiate porphyrinuria from hematuria. Possibilities for hematuria include cystic calculi, blood of renal origin, or in female rabbits, of uterine origin, such as with cystic endometrial hyperplasia and/or uterine adenocarcinoma. Rabbit urine has an average pH of 8.2, which can easily lead to

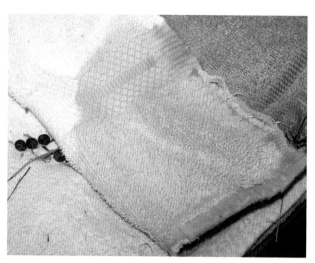

Figure 84.11 Porphyrinuria, a reddish-orange urine commonly seen in rabbits has discolored the white towel placed in the cage bottom. No blood was present in this rabbit's urine.

urine scalding of thin inguinal skin in incontinent rabbits.

Diagnostic tests

Blood urea nitrogen (published reference range 13–29 mg/dL) and creatinine (published reference range 0.5–2.5) are used to evaluate for evidence of renal disease (Mader 2004). Increases in BUN and creatinine are not expected to increase until 50–70% of nephrons are lost (Jenkins 2008).

Urinalysis is a useful tool and may be obtained by free catch, manual expression, catheterization, or cystocentesis. Care must be taken to avoid the large cecum of rabbits during cystocentesis by inserting the needle quite caudally. The published reference range for urine specific gravity is 1.003–1.036, with an average of 1.015 (Mader 2004; Jenkins 2008). Small amounts of protein may be found in the urine of young, healthy rabbits and even normal adults can have trace levels of protein (Mader 2004; Jenkins 2008). Although glucose is not normally found in rabbit urine, rabbits easily develop a stress hyperglycemia that may spill over into the urine. Spontaneous diabetes mellitus has been described in New Zealand white rabbits, but is not commonly seen. Many calcium carbonate crystals are expected in rabbit urine. The fractional excretion of calcium in urine of most mammals is 2%, whereas in a rabbit, it can reach 60% (Pare and Paul-Murphy 2004; Jenkins 2008). Same as other mammals, casts, epithelial cells, and bacteria should not be present in urine, and red and white blood cells should only be seen occasionally.

Radiographically, rabbits are similar to cats, except the kidneys can occur more ventrally and it is a common incidental finding to visualize some calcium carbonate

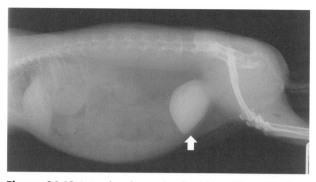

Figure 84.12 Lateral radiograph of rabbit with a significant amount of "sand," or "sludge" in the urinary bladder (arrow). More appropriately, "sand" is multiple, small calcium carbonate stones creating a toothpaste-like consistency to the urine. Also note in this obese rabbit, the large retroperitoneal fat pad displacing the kidneys ventrally.

in the bladder called "sludge" because of its consistency. Ultrasound, excretory urogram, intravenous pyelography, and other diagnostic modalities would be similar to a cat.

Common diseases

Lower urinary tract disease

This condition is lumped to together as cystitis, urine "sludging," and incontinence because it is a common presentation (Figure 84.12).

The cause of these symptoms is unknown, but anecdotally, there are some common factors such as a high-calcium diet (as found with alfalfa hay and alfalfa hay-based pellets), inactivity, obesity, large skin folds, and chronic lumbosacral subluxation. Most rabbits have a concurrent disease condition, including bacterial cystitis, infection with *Encephalitozooan cuniculi*, cystic endometrial hyperplasia, cystic calculi, uterine/ovarian adenocarcinoma, or spinal disease. Therefore, any rabbit presenting with inappropriate urination, dysuria, depression, hunched posture, teeth grinding, perineal scalding, or polyuria/polydipsia should have the following tests: CBC, chemistry profile, urinalysis, urine culture, radiograph, ± contrast radiography, ultrasound, and *E. cuniculi* titer. First, treat any underlying disease (Harcourt-Brown 2002), That is aggressive early treatment with a broad-spectrum, bactericidal antibiotic that rabbits tolerate, such as enrofloxacin or trimethoprim-sulfa. If the culture shows no evidence of a bacterial cystitis and no dermatitis is present, then antibiotics can be discontinued. If cystitis is present, the usual bacterial culprit is *Pseudomonas* spp. or *E. coli* (Pare and Paul-Murphy 2004). Fluid therapy to reestablish hydration, analgesics, ± flushing the bladder of sludge under anesthesia may be necessary. Long-term treatment can focus on changing the diet to a timothy hay based pellet, timothy hay, and green leafy vegetables. Diligent and frequent cleaning, and flushing and minimal application of zinc oxide ointment is necessary to treat concurrent urine scald. If the rabbit is suspected of having encephalitozooanosis, then albendazole at 30 mg/kg PO daily for 30 days or more may be necessary.

Urinary calculi

Calculi can occur in the kidney, ureter, bladder, or urethra commonly in rabbits. Renal calculi often take on a "staghorn" appearance. The composition is almost always calcium carbonate and the cause is usually high dietary calcium. Other processes that can contribute to stone formation include neurological disease from *E. cuniculi* or spinal disease, obesity, and rarely, cystitis. Radiographs are usually confirmatory since calcium carbonate is radio-opaque. If large cystic calculi are present, then surgical removal is best. Small calculi can pass, especially in female rabbits. Some urethral calculi can be retropulsed back into the bladder and then a cystotomy performed. Ureteral calculi that are not moving and are causing obstruction need to be removed surgically. Renal calculi are difficult and risky to remove surgically because they often have a staghorn shape. A nephrectomy or pyelolithotomy may be necessary. Surprisingly, the rabbit is the animal model of choice for lithotripsy research, and many reports of lithotripsy and the new laser lithotripsy technique have been described, but no clinical use has yet been recorded (Zörcher et al. 1999). There is a concern for collateral tissue damage.

Encephalitozoonosis

Encephalitozooan cuniculi is a coccidian parasite that is spread via the doe's urine to her offspring usually in the first few days of the kit's life. Most rabbits have been exposed and have an antibody titer, but rarely show any clinical signs. Pitted kidneys are a common incidental finding at necropsy. Old age or immunosuppression can sometimes cause clinical signs to surface, such as neurological signs including torticollis, hind limb paresis or paralysis, and incontinence. Sometimes, ocular signs alone are present as a phacoclastic uveitis that looks like a granuloma in the anterior chamber of the eye, but the lesion is originating from the lens capsule. An antibody titer can be run at Sound Diagnostics (in the state of Washington) but the titer is not indicative of infection (meaning a higher or rising titer does not suggest active disease). The treatment in humans with *E. intestinalis* is with albendazole, and the same is true for rabbits at 30 mg/kg PO q24h long-term; usually 30 days past clinical resolution. More frequent dosing resulted in

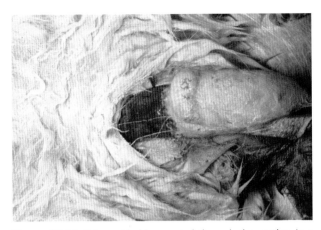

Figure 84.13 Urinary bladder everted through the urethra in a young rabbit.

subclinical renal calcinosis (author's unpublished research). Urinary signs are treated as described above for lower urinary tract disease.

Neoplasia

Benign embryonal nephroma is the third most frequent tumor of rabbits and is usually an incidental finding at necropsy. Any age rabbit can be affected. Renal carcinomas are rarely reported.

Bladder eversion

Urinary bladder eversion secondary to stretching of tissues after parturition in young does has been recorded (Figure 84.13).

The bladder everts through the urethra. Surgical repair is possible. Ectopic urinary bladder, through a rent in the abdominal wall, has been seen in a rabbit (Figure 84.14).

Ferret urology
Anatomy and physiology

The anatomy and physiology of the urinary system is much the same as a dog. The kidneys are very easy to palpate. The male has a prostate, an os penis, and a bend in the urethra very similar to a dog. The os penis is curved into a hook at the end and extends beyond the penis distally (Figure 84.15).

The urethral opening is not distinct, but a flap of tissue, and can be found ventrally where the penile tissue ends. Typically, a 3.5 Fr red rubber catheter is used for urethral catheterization and a video demonstrating the technique is available at the following website (Greenacre 1999): http://www.vet.uga.edu/vpp/ivcvm/1999/index.php.

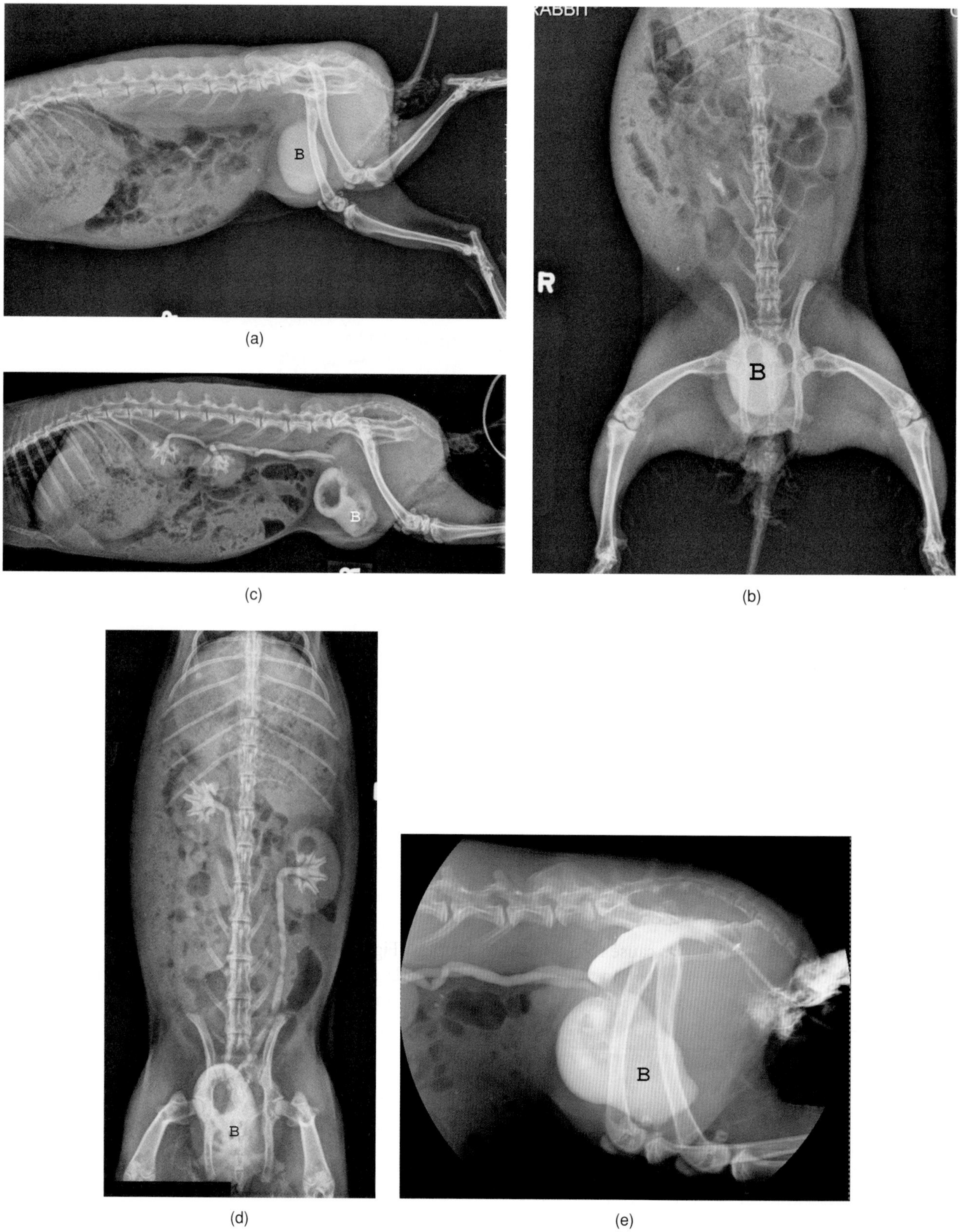

Figure 84.14 (a–e) Survey radiographs (a and b), excretory urogram (c and d), and contrast urethrogram (e) of a female rabbit with an ectopic bladder, B.

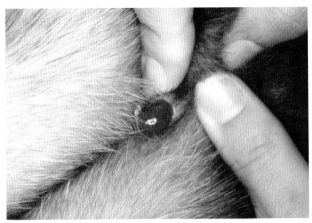

Figure 84.15 Normal ferret penis exposed from the sheath. The dark color of the penile tissue is normal. The os penis is curved into a hook at the end and extends beyond the penis distally.

Diagnostic tests

Diagnostic tests are very similar to those done in dogs and cats, including CBC, chemistry profile, urinalysis, radiography, contrast radiography, ultrasound, and culture.

A 25-gauge needle is recommended for cystocentesis due to the relatively thin wall of the bladder. The pH of ferret urine is generally 6.5–7.5, but on a high-quality meat-based diet, the pH can be 6.0 (Gamble and Morrisey 2005). Ferrets generally only produce on average about 26 mL of urine daily. Water intake is approximately 75–100 mL daily (Fox 1998).

Common diseases

Adrenal gland disease leading to prostatic disease

The most common disease of middle age to older ferrets is adrenal gland disease. Adrenal gland adenocarcinoma is the most common manifestation, followed by adrenal gland adenoma or hyperplasia. The cause is most likely due to spaying or neutering a ferret of any age, which stimulates metaplasia of undifferentiated gonadal cells left over embryologically in the adrenal capsule (Quesenberry and Rosenthal 2004). The most common clinical sign is a bilateral symmetrical alopecia, and females commonly present with vulvar enlargement. Less commonly, males develop prostatic hyperplasia, cysts, and abscesses with a concurrent urinary tract infection and small urethral or cystic calculi. Clinical signs then also include stranguria and dysuria. Prostatic enlargement is due to elevation of the hormones estradiol, testosterone, 17-B-hydroxyprogesterone produced by the neoplastic adrenal cortex from an adrenal gland tumor. Urethral blockages are commonly due to sloughed proteinaceous debris from squamous metaplasia of prostatic tissue and

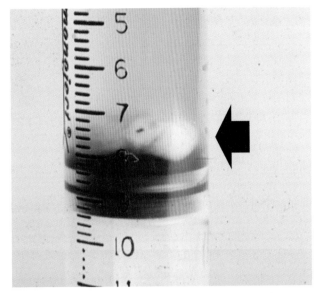

Figure 84.16 Urine removed from a male ferret through a 3.5 Fr urethral catheter containing proteinaceous debris (arrow) due to prostatitis secondary to adrenal disease.

small struvite calculi from the rise in pH due to bacterial cystitis (Figure 84.16).

The usual initial course of action is to administer an opiate pain reliever such as butorphanol, anesthetize the ferret with isoflurane, relieve some of the pressure on the bladder, obtain a urine sample for urinalysis and culture by performing a cystocentesis, and obtain blood for a CBC, chemistry profile, and adrenal hormone panel. While the ferret is under anesthesia, place a urethral catheter. An ultrasound of the abdomen including the adrenal glands, and bladder and prostate can be done during the initial anesthetic episode or later when the ferret is better stabilized. The prostate is normally approximately 10 mm wide and the adrenal glands are generally 3 × 5 mm (Figure 84.17).

Fluids to re-establish hydration are administered as well as antibiotics. The adrenal gland disease must be addressed soon by either hormonal treatment (leuprolide acetate, melatonin implants, or deslorelin) or surgery, or both, to resolve the underlying stimulus to the prostate. If "sand" or multiple small calculi cannot be flushed from the urethra, a perineal urethrostomy can be done to allow urine exit before the narrow areas of the bend or tip of the urethra (Figure 84.18).

Long-term antibiotics based on urine culture are needed to resolve the probable concomitant bacterial cystitis. Within several days of removing the neoplastic adrenal gland, the prostatic cysts begin to resolve. Cysts can sometimes be larger than the bladder itself (Figures 84.19 and 84.20).

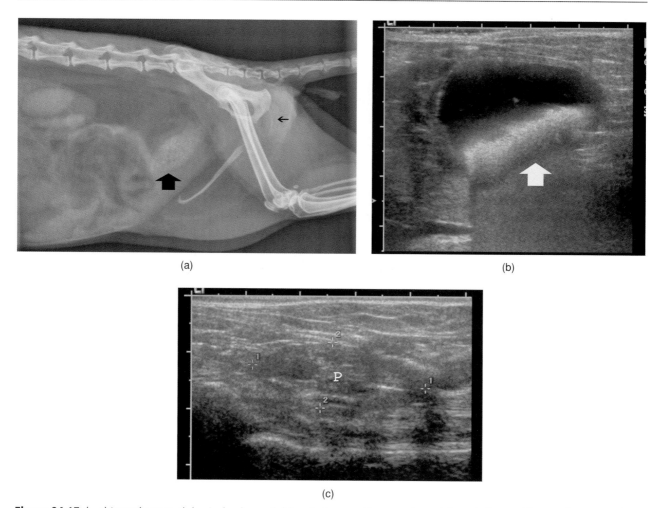

(a)

(b)

(c)

Figure 84.17 (a–c) Lateral survey abdominal radiograph (a) and ultrasound images of an adult, male ferret with cystic (large arrow) and urethral (small arrow) calculi (b), and an abnormal prostate (P) (c) secondary to adrenal disease.

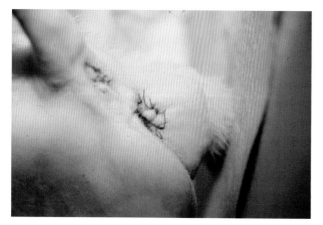

Figure 84.18 Ferret post-perineal urethrostomy. The surgery was done to allow ease of urine flow at a point before the narrowing of the urethra in a ferret with proteineaceous sludge and small urethral calculi obstruction secondary to adrenal disease.

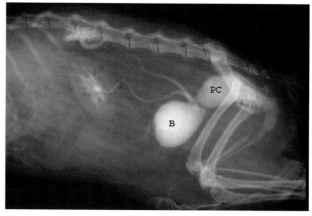

Figure 84.19 Bladder (B) and prostatic cyst (PC) outlined with contrast media after IV injection in a ferret. Prostatic cysts can be as large as, or larger than, the bladder.

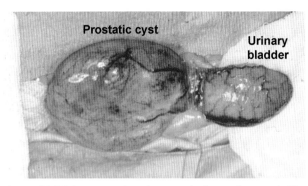

Figure 84.20 Intraoperative photograph of same ferret as in Figure 84.19 showing the size of the prostatic cyst (left) in comparison to the bladder (right).

Cysts can be drained with a 25-gauge needle. Some sources recommend flushing and marsupializing large abcesses with omentum, but in this author's experience, it is best to leave the abcesses unopened and treat with long-term antibiotics rather than risk peritonitis, no matter how carefully the surgery is performed (Ludwig and Aiken 2004).

Urolithiasis

Other than underlying adrenal disease, the other cause of urinary calculi in ferrets is a diet of vegetable protein origin. Ferrets have a higher protein and fat requirement than cats. Recommended levels in ferrets for dietary protein are 30–40%, and fat are 20–30%. Ferrets lack a cecum and have a relatively short gastrointestinal (GI) tract; in fact, it is half the length of a cat's. The GI transit time in ferrets is 3–4 hours. Vegetable-based protein diets increase urine pH, leading to struvite stone formation (Figure 84.21; Fox et al. 1998; Pollack 2004).

Clinical signs include stranguria and dysuria. The usual course of action is to administer an opiate pain reliever such as butorphanol, anesthetize the ferret with isoflurane, relieve some of the pressure on the bladder and obtain a urine sample for urinalysis and culture by performing a cystocentesis, and obtain blood for a CBC, chemistry profile, and adrenal hormone panel (just in case there is adrenal disease without alopecia). Flushing can be performed to remove small calculi, or a cystotomy can be performed to remove large cystic calculi. Long-term appropriate antibiotics are usually needed for the probably concurrent cystitis, and a change in diet to a ferret appropriate meat-based chow is mandatory.

Renal cysts

Small or large, usually multiple, renal cysts are common in ferrets with a reported incidence of 10–15% of ferrets at necropsy (Figure 84.22; Pollack 2004).

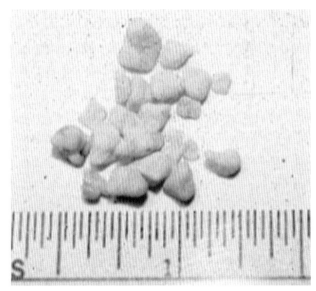

Figure 84.21 Struvite cystic calculi removed from an adult ferret. The vegetable-based, dry dog food diet the ferret was eating was a contributory factor.

Cyst resection or nephrectomy is limited to very large cysts causing significant pathology.

Neoplasia

Renal adenocarcinoma has been described in one ferret presenting with unilateral hydronephrosis with subsequent metastasis to the lumber spine several months after nephrectomy (Figure 84.23; Volgenaeu et al. 1998).

Transitional cell carcinoma has also been described in the bladder of ferrets. Hematuria is the presenting complaint. Contrast radiography or ultrasonography is used to diagnose this disease.

Guinea pig urology

Anatomy and physiology

Male guinea pigs have an os penis.

Diagnostic tests

Guinea pigs have alkaline urine with many crystals. The urine is think and cloudy and white to pale yellow.

Common diseases

Urolithiasis

Urolithiasis is very common in guinea pigs, especially females greater than three years of age. The cause is unknown, but researchers at the University of California, Davis, have collected data from multiple institutions and

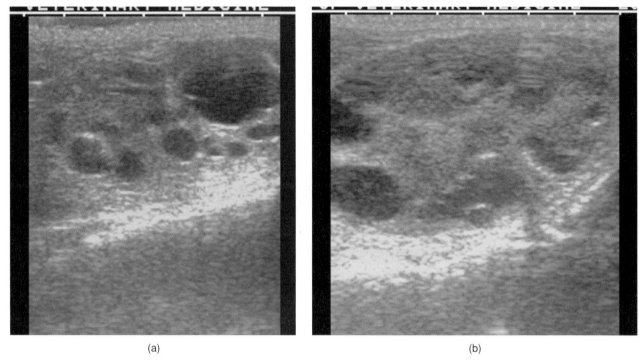

(a)   (b)

Figure 84.22 Ultrasonagraphic images of a ferret with bilateral polycystic renal disease (a, right kidney; b, left kidney).

will report their findings soon. Calculi can be renal, ureteral, cyctic, or urethral (Figure 84.24).

Calculi composition is typically calcium carbonate, but calcium oxalate has also been documented. Generally, affected guinea pigs present with depression, anorexia, and dysuria with occasional hematuria. The workup and treatment is the same as for urolithiasis in rabbits, except *Streptococcus pyogenes* is commonly cultured (O'Rourke 2004).

Chronic interstitial nephritis (CIN)

CIN is a common incidental finding at necropsy in guinea pigs greater than 3 years of age (O'Rourke 2004). It can occur secondary to the very common chronic staphylococcal pododermatitis creating a chronic renal amyloidosis.

Renal coccidiosis

The coccidian parasite *Klossiella cobayae* can be found in the epithelial cells lining the renal tubules in guinea pigs (Harkness et al. 2002; O'Rourke 2004). There are no clinical sings unless there is a heavy infestation, then the surface of the kidney is irregular with gray mottling (Harkness et al. 2002).

Chinchilla urology

Anatomy and physiology

Female chinchillas have a large urinary papillae (has also been called urethral cone or clitoris) that can easily be mistaken for a penis. Males can be distinguished from females by the greater distance between the anus and the ureteral papilla.

Common diseases

Urolithiasis

Urolithiasis has been described in chinchillas, but it is not common. Most involve male chinchillas with calcium carbonate calculi, but there is a report of six adult females spontaneously developing calcium oxalate urolithiasis with no known exposure to toxins (Donnelley 2004a). The workup and treatment is the same as for urolithiasis in rabbits.

Rat urology

Anatomy and physiology

Rats produce approximately 13–23 mL of urine per 24-hour period with a pH range of 6–7.8 depending on strain and gender (Kohn and Clifford 2002; Bihun 2004).

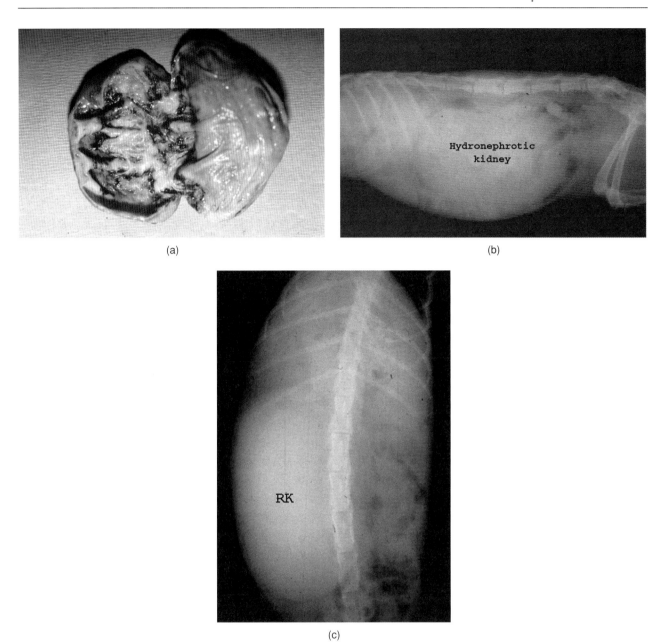

(a)

(b)

(c)

Figure 84.23 (a–c) – Right renal pelvis of a hydronephrotic kidney removed from a ferret with renal adenocarcinoma. Ventrodorsal and lateral radiographs of the same ferret with severe right hydronephrosis (RK, right kidney).

Diagnostic tests

The specific gravity of rat urine is 1.022–1.050 (Bihun 2004).

Common diseases

Chronic progressive nephrosis

The most common renal disease in rats is their most common age-related disease, chronic progressive nephrosis (CPN). It is usually an incidental finding at necropsy, but the disease occurs earlier, more severely, and more com-

monly in males than females (Kohn and Clifford 2002; Donnelley 2004b). A progressively worsening proteinuria is the most common finding. Feeding a low-protein diet and reducing any excess weight is the only method to manage this disease.

Mouse urology

Anatomy and physiology

Mice produce approximately 0.5–2.5 mL of urine per 24-hour period with a pH range of approximately 5 (Kohn

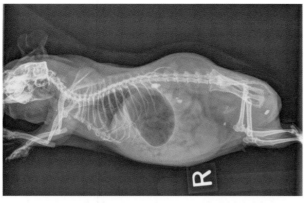

(a)

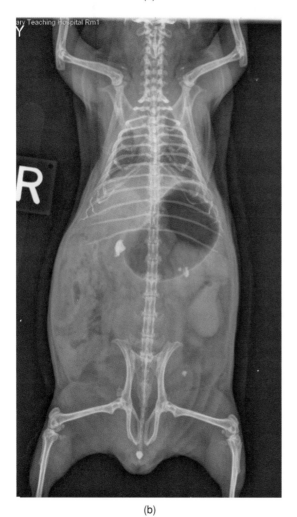

(b)

Figure 84.24 (a) Lateral and (b) ventrodorsal radiograph of an adult, male guinea pig with renal, ureteral, cystic, and urethral calculi composed of calcium carbonate.

and Clifford 2002; Bihun 2004). The glomeruli of mice are relatively small at 74 μm in diameter compared to rat glomeruli, which are almost twice as large, but the mouse has 4.8 times more glomeruli with twice the filtering surface per gram of tissue compared to rats. Therefore, the urine of mice is very concentrated (Jacoby et al. 2002).

Diagnostic tests

The specific gravity of mouse urine is approximately 1.034 (Bihun 2004). Male mice are normally proteinuric.

Common diseases

Urethral obstruction

Urethral obstruction is very common in male mice 1.5–2.5 years of age secondary to bacterial infection of the preputial gland or bulbourethral gland by *Staphylococcus* spp. or *Pasteurella* spp., respectively (Donnelley 2004b). Males will commonly mutilate their penis with this disease. Treatment consists of topical and parenteral antibiotics.

Hamster urology

Anatomy and physiology

Hamsters produce approximately 5.1–8.4 mL of urine per 24-hour period with a pH range of approximately 8.5 (Kohn and Clifford 2002; Bihun 2004).

Diagnostic tests

The specific gravity of mouse urine is approximately 1.060 (Bihun 2004). Hamsters will commonly urinate when restrained, so be prepared to catch a voided sample by holding them over a clean stainless steel table.

Common diseases

No urinary-specific diseases are common in hamsters other than diabetes is common in dwarf hamsters and the most common method of appreciating this disease is to document a glucosuria.

Sugar glider urology

Anatomy and common disease

Sugar gliders are a marsupial and like most marsupials, males have a forked penis. They commonly present for self-mutilation of the penis. The forked portion of the penis can be amputed without disturbance of urine flow since they urinate from the base of the forked area. Castration may help this condition since reproductive frustration is thought to be the cause (Ness and Booth 2004).

References

Bihun, C. (2004). Basic anatomy, physiology, husbandry, and clinical techniques. In: *Ferrets, Rabbits, and Rodents—Clinical Medicine and Surgery*, edited by K.E. Quesenberry and J.W. Carpenter, 2nd edition. St. Louis, MO: WB Saunders, pp. 286–298.

Diethelm, G. (2005). Reptiles. In: *Exotic Animal Formulary*, edited by J.W. Carpenter, 3rd edition. St. Louis, MO: Elsevier, pp. 55–134.

Donnelley, T.M. (2004a). Disease problems of chinchillas. In: *Ferrets, Rabbits, and Rodents—Clinical Medicine and Surgery*, edited by K.E. Quesenberry and J.W. Carpenter, 2nd edition. St. Louis, MO: WB Saunders, pp. 255–265.

Donnelley, T.M. (2004b). Disease problems of small rodents. In: *Ferrets, Rabbits, and Rodents—Clinical Medicine and Surgery*, edited by K.E. Quesenberry and J.W. Carpenter, 2nd edition. St. Louis, MO: WB Saunders, pp. 299–315.

Fox, J.G. (1998). Normal clinical parameters. In: *Biology and Diseases of the Ferret*, edited by J.G. Fox, 2nd edition. Baltimore, MD: Williams and Wilkens, pp. 183–210.

Fox, J.G., R.C. Pearson, et al. (1998). Diseases of the genitourinary system. In: *Biology and Diseases of the Ferret*, edited by J.G. Fox, 2nd edition. Baltimore: Williams and Wilkens, pp. 247–272.

Gamble, C. and J.K. Morrisey (2005). Ferrets. In: *Exotic Animal Formulary*, edited by J.W. Carpenter, 3rd edition. St. Louis, MO: Elsevier, pp. 447–478.

Garner, M.M., S.M. Hernandez-Divers, et al. (2004). Reptile neoplasia: a retrospective study of case submissions to a specialty diagnostic service. *Vet Clin N Am* **7**(3): pp. 653–671.

Greenacre, C.B., K.S. Latimer, et al. (1992). Leg paresis in a black palm cockatoo (Probosciger aterrimus). *J Zoo Wildl Med* **23**(1): 122–126.

Greenacre, C.B. (1999). Technique for urethral catheterization of the male domestic ferret (Mustela putorius furo). Website Proceedings of the International Virtual Conferences in Veterinary Medicine, Diseases of Exotic Animals and Wildlife. Available at: http://www.vet.uga.edu/vpp/ivcvm/1999/index.php.

Greer, L.L., G.B. Daniel, et al. (2005). Evaluation of the use of technetium Tc 99m diethylenetriamine pentaacetic acid and Tc 99m dimercaptosuccinic acid for scintographic imaging of the kidneys in green iguanas (Iguana iguana). *Am J Vet Res* **66**: 87–92.

Harcourt-Brown, F. (2002). Urogenital diseases. In: *Textbook of Rabbit Medicine*, edited by F. Harcourt-Brown. Oxford: Butterworth-Heinemann, pp. 335–351.

Harkness, J.E., K.A. Murray, et al. (2002). Biology and diseases of guinea pigs. In: *Laboratory Animal Medicine*, edited by J.G. Fox, L.C. Anderson, F.M. Loew, and F.W. Quimby, 2nd edition. San Diego: Academic Press, pp. 203–246.

Hernandez-Divers, S.J. and C.J. Innis (2006). Renal disease in reptiles: diagnosis and clinical treatment. In: *Reptile Medicine and Surgery*, edited by D.R. Mader, 2nd edition. St. Louis, MO: Elsevier, pp. 878–892.

Holz, P. (2006). Renal anatomy and physiology. In: *Reptile Medicine and Surgery*, edited by D.R. Mader, 2nd edition. St. Louis, MO: Elsevier, pp. 135–144.

Jacoby, R.O., et al. (2002). Biology and Diseases of Mice. In: *Laboratory Animal Medicine*, edited by J.G. Fox, L.C. Anderson, F.M. Loew, and F.W. Quimby, 2nd edition. San Diego: Academic Press, pp. 35–120.

Jenkins, J.R. (2008). Rabbit diagnostic testing. *J Exot Pet Med* **17**(1): 4–15.

King, A.S. and J. McLelland (1984). Urology. In: *Birds—Their Structure and Function*, 2nd edition. Philadelphia, PA: Bailliere Tindall, pp. 175–186.

Kohn, D.F. and C.B. Clifford (2002). Biology and diseases of rats. In: *Laboratory Animal Medicine*, edited by J.G. Fox, L.C. Anderson, F.M. Loew, and F.W. Quimby, 2nd edition. San Diego: Academic Press, pp. 121–165.

Latimer, K.S. (1994). Oncology. In: *Avian Medicine: Principles and Application*, edited by B.W. Ritchie, G.J. Harrison, and L.R. Harrison. Lake Worth: Wingers Publishing, pp. 640–672.

Ludwig, L. and S. Aiken (2004). Soft tissue surgery. In: *Ferrets, Rabbits, and Rodents—Clinical Medicine and Surgery*, edited by K.E. Quesenberry and J.W. Carpenter, 2nd edition. St. Louis, MO: WB Saunders, pp. 121–134.

Lumeij, J.T. (1994). Nephrology. In: *Avian Medicine: Principles and Application*, edited by B.W. Ritchie, G.J. Harrison, and L.R. Harrison. Lake Worth: Wingers Publishing, pp. 538–555.

Lumeij, J.T. and P.T. Redig (1992). Hyperuricemia and visceral gout induced by allopurinol in red-tailed hawks (Buteo jamaicensis). *Proc Tagung Vogelkrankheiten der Deutche Veterinarmedizinische Gesellschaft e.V.*, Munich.

Mader, D.R. (2004). Basic approach to veterinary care. In: *Ferrets, Rabbits, and Rodents—Clinical Medicine and Surgery*, edited by K.E. Quesenberry, J.W. Carpenter, 2nd edition. St. Louis, MO: WB Saunders, pp. 147–154.

Mader, D.R. (2006a). Gout. In: *Reptile Medicine and Surgery*, edited by D.R. Mader, 2nd edition. St. Louis, MO: Elsevier, pp. 793–800.

Mader, D.R. (2006b). Calculi: urinary. In: *Reptile Medicine and Surgery*, edited by D.R. Mader, 2nd edition. St. Louis, MO: Elsevier, pp. 763–771.

Marshall, K.L., L.E. Craig, et al. (2003). Quantitative renal scintigraphy in domestic pigeons (Columba livia domestica) exposed to toxic doses of gentamycin. *Am J Vet Res* **64**(4): 453–462.

Naidoo, V., K. Wolter, et al. (2008). The pharmacokinetics of meloxicam in cultures. *J Vet Pharmacol Ther* **31**(2): 128–134.

Ness, R.D. and R. Booth (2004). Sugar gliders. In: *Ferrets, Rabbits, and Rodents—Clinical Medicine and Surgery*, edited by K.E. Quesenberry and J.W. Carpenter, 2nd edition. St. Louis, MO: WB Saunders, pp. 330–338.

O'Rourke, D.P. (2004). Disease problems of guinea pigs. In: *Ferrets, Rabbits, and Rodents—Clinical Medicine and Surgery*, edited by K.E. Quesenberry and J.W. Carpenter, 2nd edition. St. Louis, MO: WB Saunders, pp. 245–254.

Pare, J.A. and J. Paul-Murphy (2004). Disorders of the reproductive and urinary systems. In: *Ferrets, Rabbits, and Rodents—Clinical Medicine and Surgery*, edited by K.E. Quesenberry and J.W. Carpenter, 2nd edition. St. Louis, MO: WB Saunders, pp. 183–193.

Pollack, C.G. (2004). Urogenital diseases. In: *Ferrets, Rabbits, and Rodents—Clinical Medicine and Surgery*, edited by K.E. Quesenberry and J.W. Carpenter, 2nd edition. St. Louis, MO: WB Saunders, pp. 41–49.

Pollack, C., J.W. Carpenter, et al. (2005). *Birds*. In: *Exotic Animal Formulary*, edited by J.W. Carpenter, 3rd edition. St. Louis, MO: Elsevier, pp. 135–346.

Quesenberry, K.E. and K.L. Rosenthal (2004). Endocrine diseases. In: *Ferrets, Rabbits, and Rodents—Clinical Medicine and Surgery*, edited by K.E. Quesenberry and J.W. Carpenter, 2nd edition. St. Louis, MO: WB Saunders, pp. 79–90.

Rattner, B.A., M.A. Whitehead, et al. (2008). Apparent tolerance of turkey vultures (Cathartes aura) to the non-steroidal anti-inflammatory drug diclofenac. *Environ Toxicol Chem*, 2008, May 13:1 (Epub ahead of print).

Reavill, D.R. (2004). Tumors of pet birds. *Vet Clin N Am—Exotic Anim Pract* **7**(3): 537–560.

Ritchie, B.W. (1995). Papoviviridae. In: *Avian Viruses—Function and Control*, edited by B.W. Ritchie. Lake Worth: Winger's, pp. 127–170.

Sykes, J.M. and C.B. Greenacre. (2006). Techniques for drug delivery in reptiles and amphibians. *J Exot Pet Med* **15**(3): 210–217.

Volgenaeu, T., C.B. Greenacre, et al. (1998). Challenging cases in internal medicine: what's your diagnosis? *Vet Med* **9**(93): 797–804.

Zörcher, T., J. Hochberger, et al. (1999). In vitro study concerning the efficiency of the frequency-doubled double-pulse Neodymium:YAG laser (FREDDY) for lithotripsy of calculi in the urinary tract. *Lasers Surg Med* **25**(1): 38–42.

Section 11

Counseling clients

85

Counseling clients

Elizabeth Strand

This chapter is designed to provide helpful and practical information for counseling clients who are caring for animals with acute and chronic urinary and kidney diseases. It will review basic and more complex client communication skills and issues. Basic skills include open-ended and close-ended questions, reflective listening, empathy, nonjudgmental attitude, and nonanxious presence. More complex skills that build on the basic skills include seeking informed consent and treatment decision-making, gaining medical compliance, discussing and negotiating money, and discussing and implementing the euthanasia process. The content for this chapter is largely based on Bayer Animal Health Communication Project Veterinary Communication Modules (https://www.healthcarecomm.org/bahcp/).

Open- and close-ended questions

Open-ended questions are questions that cannot be answered with "yes" or "no," but require a story or several consecutive details and opinions from clients. For instance, "Why do you think Frances was vomiting?" is an open-ended question that allows the client to tell a story. A close-ended question requires a yes, a no, a specific quantity, or a choice. "How many times did Francis vomit last night?" is an example of a close-ended question.

Many veterinarians interrupt clients after only a few seconds of listening to the patient history. This behavior cannot only disrupt the rapport with clients but also cause the veterinarian to miss important details of the history that are salient to the case. Clients who ask questions of the veterinarian after being allowed to fully share what they see as important to the visit feel more

empowered in the veterinary–client–patient relationship (https://www.healthcarecomm.org/bahcp/).

Reflective listening

The ability to accurately repeat back what clients are saying and feeling (reflective listening) helps clients trust that the veterinarian is seeing and considering their perspective in medical care recommendations for their pet. This important communication skill also helps clients to clarify what they are meaning to say by allowing them to know what the veterinarian has heard from their statements. Additionally, if a client is experiencing high emotion, reflective listening can significantly decrease the emotion because clients know the veterinarian is aware and respects their emotional experience, alleviating the client of the effort to "convince" the veterinarian how they are feeling. This form of reflective listening begins to focus on the skill of exhibiting empathy (https://www.healthcarecomm.org/bahcp/).

Empathy

Expressing empathy gives the message to clients that the veterinarian has care, concern, understanding, and respect for them as human beings. Empathy is exhibited by using feeling words to restate clients' stories and concerns. For instance, "I can see you are very sad hearing that Sadie is in kidney failure." Empathy can also be expressed by exhibiting empathic nonverbal behavior such as nodding the head, making eye contact, sitting at the same level as clients, and matching the volume and pace of their speech.

Nonjudgmental attitude

Along with empathy is the ability to help clients feel that the veterinarian accepts them. Clients who are afraid that

Nephrology and Urology of Small Animals. Edited by Joe Bartges and David J. Polzin. © 2011 Blackwell Publishing Ltd.

the veterinarian is judging their feelings, thoughts about or behaviors with their pets are less likely to tell the truth or feel trust with their veterinarian. If a veterinarian is feeling judgmental toward a client (which is normal and expected at times during a veterinary career), it can be useful for the veterinarian pose to him or herself the following question, "What must be true in the way this client views the world that would cause him or her to behave in this way?" Reflecting on this question can help the veterinarian re-establish positive feelings and more understanding for a challenging client. Expressing non-judgmental statements such as, "I can understand why you feel that way," or "It is OK to have trouble deciding what to do. Making these decisions can be very hard," is also very helpful in letting clients know they are accepted (https://www.healthcarecomm.org/bahcp/).

Nonanxious presence

Nonanxious presence (NAP) is a veterinarian's ability to remain internally calm, flexible, and appropriately responsive during moment-to-moment interpersonal interactions. This is especially important during tense moments in veterinarian–client relations. NAP also refers to the ability to disagree agreeably. These two aspects of NAP are extremely helpful in obtaining informed consent and in counseling clients around difficult treatment decisions, financial choices, and the euthanasia decision process. Clients very often become emotional facing urinary and kidney diseases in their animals, and it is important for the veterinarian to be both empathic by showing care and emotion, and also calm by not becoming as or more emotional than the client. Additionally, if a client desires something for his or her animal that is against the veterinarian's judgment, it is important that the veterinarian be able to disagree with the client in a way that respects and supports the rapport between them—disagreeing in agreeable and respectful ways. Developing NAP is a lifelong practice that is directed toward developing precise control over one's emotional, cognitive, and physiological responses in the veterinary–client relationship. The strategies that promote NAP are emotional self-awareness, reflective and logical thinking habits, and the ability to engage the physiological relaxation response as needed (Strand 2006).

Informed consent and treatment decision-making

Informed consent is more than a fine print form clients sign when they come to seek care for their animals. True informed consent demands an ongoing dialogue between clients and veterinarians where information is exchanged and shared understanding is achieved. Some clients like for veterinarians to make decisions for the care of the animal, that is "Whatever you think, Doc." However, clients are increasingly informed about the medical options for their animals and want to feel *they* are the experts for their own animal's care.

Describing and writing, in simple concrete terms, the scope of all treatment options from the least expensive to the most expensive and the least invasive to the most invasive is an initial step in obtaining informed consent. Next is inquiring what the client feels and thinks regarding these options and if the client has any questions. Through a dialogue in which the veterinarian uses reflective listening, empathic and nonjudgmental statements, and a nonanxious presence, the client may come to 2–4 treatment options that fit into his or her comfort zone of care. The veterinarian may then suggest that the client talk it over with loved ones who will influence the decision. If the client is socially isolated, offering a mental health counselor for the client to connect with to discuss treatment options can be helpful. If there is disparity between family members about what level of care is desired, it is best to talk with both parties at the same time or at the very least get agreement about who has ultimate decision-making responsibility and converse directly with that individual.

Set a time for the client to inform the veterinarian which treatment option is preferred. If the same client questions are repeated many times, it may be an indicator that there is something missing or misunderstood in the veterinary–client relationship. For instance, clients may be afraid to tell the veterinarian the truth about what they would like to do because of a fear of being judged by the veterinarian. In this case use an open-ended question like "What is the hardest thing about this decision for you?" (https://www.healthcarecomm.org/bahcp/).

Gaining medical adherence

Adherence is the degree to which a client's behavior corresponds with agreed on recommendations from the veterinarian. Gaining adherence to the veterinary recommendations for medical care involves (a) having a veterinary–client relationship that encompasses feelings of trust, care, credibility, and concern; (b) having recommendations that are understandable by the client; and (c) follow through from the veterinary team.

Developing a good client–veterinarian relationship with trust and credibility occurs through reflective listening, exhibiting empathy, tailoring treatment to unique needs of the client, and acknowledging when there may be a problem in the client–veterinarian relationship. If a problem arises, the veterinarian needs to ask an open-ended question such as, "You seem concerned. Is there anything that doesn't make sense or feels wrong about this to you?"

After recommendations, the veterinarian needs to assess client understanding and confidence. For instance, "What do you understand the course of treatment will look like at home?" To assess clients feelings of confidence, treatment scaling questions are useful. "On a scale of 1–10 with 10 being the most confident and 1 being the least, how confident are you that you can give this medication as prescribed?" or ". . .that this treatment will work." This helps the veterinarian know what worries or problems there may be in obtaining the best adherence to the treatment protocol so these problems can be addressed (https://www.healthcarecomm.org/bahcp/).

Considering and discussing money

Generally, neither clients nor veterinarians like or find it comfortable to discuss money. This dislike can cause many problems in the veterinary–client relationship. Clients may experience "sticker shock" when they get the bill if finances have not been discussed and agreed upon. On the other hand, veterinarians may give away treatment and feel taken advantage of, which is unwise and will eventually contribute to veterinarian burn out.

The reason it is difficult to discuss money in the veterinary–client relationship is because both clients and veterinarians make assumptions about each other's behavior regarding decision-making involving money. The assumptions can lead to misunderstanding, which can eventually lead to conflict in the relationship. Costs of treatment must be discussed at each decision point in the veterinary–client interaction. Each treatment option may have both short-term and long-term costs associated with it, which should be estimated for clients so they can make informed decisions. These costs must be described to the client and become an integral part of the informed consent and treatment decision-making process. The nonjudgmental attitude and NAP skills are particularly important in discussing money (https://www.healthcarecomm.org/bahcp/).

The euthanasia decision and process

For some clients deciding to euthanize their animal is impossible. For others, it is simple although very painful.

In acute situations, being clear with clients about prognosis and helping them connect with other people in their lives to support them in making the decision, or a counselor if supportive individuals do not exist, is very important. In chronic cases where the animal may have a slow decline, it is helpful for the client to write down quality of life parameters for the animal and the client. Record these in the medical record as well so when these parameters are broken, the veterinarian can remind clients of their decisions when emotions were not so high. Lastly, if a client is not responding to suggestions that it may be time to euthanize the animal, assess what the client's opinions and past experiences are regarding euthanasia. There may be a fear that is driving their resistance or there may be religious reasons.

If the client and veterinarian agree that the animal must be euthanized, it is very important that this be handled in ways that promote clients' emotional healing. Facilitating this means assessing clients' desires about the euthanasia process and doing the best to meet them. There is a wide degree of needs, feelings, and thoughts that are considered "normal" for clients preparing for the euthanasia process. Some clients really just want to say goodbye and have the veterinarian euthanize, some clients want to be present during the process, and some clients want to spend time with the body. It is normal for some clients to want the veterinarian to dispose of the body, others want the body cremated, others want to bury the animal's body themselves, and some clients even want the body to be preserved in some way. Some clients want to have some form of a religious ceremony before, during, or after the euthanasia (https://www.healthcarecomm.org/bahcp/).

For more information and training in client communication and counseling skills, contact Bayer Animal Health Communication Project. Another source for client counseling consultation is Veterinary Social Work, University of Tennessee College of Veterinary Medicine (865-755-8839; http://www.utk.vet.edu).

References

Institute for Healthcare Communication (2008). Bayer Animal Health Communication Project, New Haven, CT. Available at: https://www.healthcarecomm.org/bahcp/.

Strand, E.B. (2006). Nonanxious presence: a key attribute of the successful veterinarian. *J Vet Med Educ* **33**(1): 65–70.

Appendix: Physiology of the lower urogenital tract

Thomas F. Fletcher and Christina E. Clarkson

The urinary bladder and pelvic urethra have a common embryonic origin and operate as a functional unit to store and void urine. The unit consists of three components arranged in series: detrusor smooth muscle, smooth muscle sphincter (internal urethral sphincter), and striated muscle sphincter (urethralis muscle; external urethral sphincter).

The detrusor muscle, smooth muscle of the apex and body of the urinary bladder, acts to expel urine when contracted by parasympathetic innervation via pelvic nerves (Figure A.1). The smooth muscle sphincter, located in the bladder neck and proximal urethra, provides involuntary tonic resistance when contracted by sympathetic innervation via hypogastric nerves. (Sympathetic innervation also inhibits detrusor activity.) The striated urethralis muscle, located distally in the pelvic urethra and innervated by pudendal nerves, opposes sudden increases in bladder pressure and is employed for voluntary continence (Fletcher et al. 2008).

Each of the three components has a distinct peripheral innervation and all are controlled by the central nervous system, so they work synergistically to store and void urine. The forebrain is responsible for deciding when urination is appropriate. The pons has micturition and continence centers. Sphincter resistance is effected by spinal reflexes.

Normal micturition is a voluntary act. It entails coordinated actions of detrusor and sphincter musculature to produce virtually complete emptying of the urinary bladder at appropriate times. (Voluntary urination can also be emotionally motivated, e.g., marking territory, dispensing pheromones. In such cases, complete bladder emptying is not a goal and would be a disadvantage.)

In neonatal kittens (<4 weeks), a micturition reflex can be triggered by licking the perineum. Later in life, urination becomes subject to brain coordination and voluntary control (Blok and Holstege 2001). In view of such extensive brain involvement, the phrase "micturition reflex" is misleading and inappropriate.

Bladder compliance and wall tension

The normal urinary bladder exhibits high compliance. It is able to undergo large volume increases with only minor elevations in intravesical pressure over a wide range of filling. Bladder compliance is a consequence of wall tension interacting with viscoelastic properties of the bladder wall. Tension, initially taken up by elastic elements, is transferred to viscous elements that elongate and thereby moderate the tension. The wall is reshaped as tension stretches lumen epithelium and wall connective tissue; the latter rearranges muscle fascicles and elongates individual myocytes. At some point, viscoelastic accommodation and thus bladder compliance approaches a limit. Thereafter, wall tension and intravesical pressure rapidly rise with additional filling (Figure A.2).

According to physics (Law of Laplace), lumen pressure (P) is related to wall tension (T) and container radius (R) such that $P = f^* T / R$, where $f = 2$ for a sphere (balloon/basketball) but is unknown for the bladder (and ignored in this discussion). Stored urine volume exerts a pressure (force/area) on the bladder wall that tends to expand the wall. The expansive internal pressure (P) is opposed by wall tension (T) at each bladder volume (R) (Zinner et al. 1977).

During voiding, the detrusor must generate sufficient lumen pressure (P) to overcome sphincter resistance. Because of the $P = T / R$ relationship, a bladder containing a larger volume (R) will require a higher wall tension (T) to generate the necessary intravesical pressure (P). In other words, wall tension is at a mechanical disadvantage in regard to generating lumen pressure as the bladder expands. This is so because detrusor fascicles shift from an encircling orientation toward a tangential one as the bladder enlarges.

883

Canine lower urinary tract

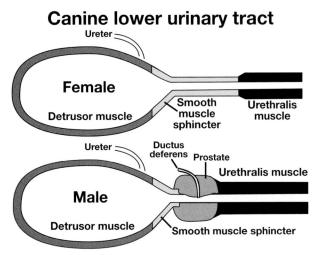

Figure A.1 Drawing of the three functional components of the canine lower urinary tract. The detrusor, which expels urine, the smooth muscle sphincter, and striated muscle sphincter (urethralis muscle) are arranged in series.

Urine flow normally improves as a greatly distended detrusor recovers mechanical advantage during voiding. Decreased urine flow that persists is a sign of excess urethral resistance. The detrusor responds to elevated outlet resistance by contracting more slowly (Nitti and Kim 2001).

The $T = P * R$ relationship applies more or less to the urethra (and ureter) as well as the bladder. To ensure continence, a timely sphincter reflex must generate sufficient wall tension (T) to combat the effects of both P and R when a bolus of urine enters the urethra.

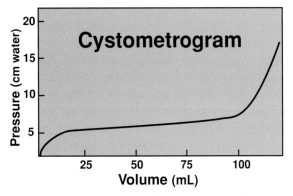

Figure A.2 Drawing of a normal cystometrogram (intravesical pressure vs bladder volume plot during urine storage). Following an initial pressure rise, the plateau of relatively low pressure despite the considerable increase in bladder volume reflects bladder compliance. As wall accommodation approaches its limit, wall tension greatly increases and consequently lumen pressure abruptly rises.

Bladder filling

Urine enters the renal pelvis continuously but exits the ureter periodically, as peristaltic waves propel urine boluses into the bladder. Urine drains into the renal pelvis from papillary ducts that open onto the renal medullary surface. Accumulated urine stretches smooth muscle pacemaker cells in the wall of the renal pelvis, triggering them to fire action potentials that result in increased intracellular $[Ca^{2+}]$.

Via gap junctions, increased intracellular $[Ca^{2+}]$ spreads among smooth muscle cells of the renal pelvis and ureter. This leads to a peristaltic wave of smooth muscle contraction that forces a bolus of urine along the ureter and into the bladder. Bladder filling requires sufficient peristaltic force to open the terminal intramural ureter, normally held closed by intravesical pressure and wall tension to preclude urine reflux into the ureter.

Urinary continence

Urinary continence, the ability to store urine without leakage, requires that outlet resistance exceed intravesical pressure. Initially, when bladder volume and pressure are low, passive viscoelastic resistance offered by the urethral wall provides adequate resistance to maintain closure (Figure A.3). Passive resistance is enhanced by mucosal enfolding and by elastic fibers and stratum spongiosum within the submucosa.

In quadrupeds, passive resistance is augmented when urine weight pulls the bladder cranially into the abdomen away from the urethra, which is simultaneously elongated. (Squatting to urinate shifts urine weight caudally against the urethral opening.) In bipeds (humans), urine weight is continuously impacting the urethra and continence demands more active resistance and more continuous support than is the case for quadrupeds (Schmidt 2001).

As bladder volume approaches half-full, continued continence requires spinal sympathetic reflexes that contract the smooth muscle sphincter and inhibit spontaneous contractions of the detrusor (Vaughan and Satchell 1992). These reflexes involve bladder afferent axons that run through the pelvic nerve to sacral spinal segments and efferent axons that come from lumbar spinal segments and travel though hypogastric nerves to reach the bladder and urethra.

To halt urine leakage when the tonic smooth muscle sphincter is breached during abrupt increases in intravesical pressure, the striated urethral sphincter (urethralis muscle) contracts in a spinal reflex triggered by urine flow into the urethra. Afferent axons run through the pudendal nerve to enter the sacral spinal cord; efferent axons

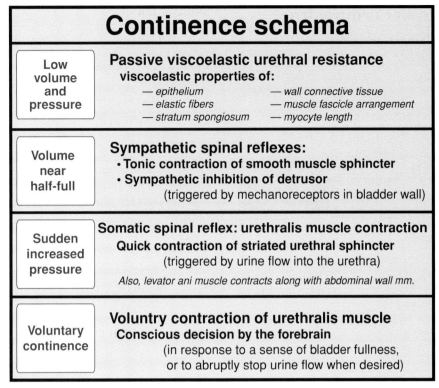

Figure A.3 Continence schema. Continence involves different mechanisms depending on pressure conditions within the urinary bladder.

also run through the pudendal nerve. The urethralis muscle, which has relatively fast twitch muscle fibers (Bowen et al. 1976), is also used for voluntary continence, including retrograde closure during abrupt cessation of urine flow. Finally, the urethralis muscle contracts during male ejaculation.

Continence is also facilitated by striated muscles comprising the pelvic diaphragm. The levator ani muscle reflexly contracts to support pelvic viscera when muscles of the abdominal wall contract and cause increased intra-abdominal pressure during running, jumping, etc. Pelvic diaphragm muscles are innervated by axons from the sacral part of the lumbosacral plexus. (In bipedal humans, in contrast to quadrupeds, the pelvic diaphragm is horizontally oriented, and it continuously supports the bladder and urethra, contributing tonically to continence.)

Micturition

As volume expands, there is an increase in afferent nerve activity generated by tonic mechanoreceptors sensitive to bladder wall tension. When spontaneous detrusor contractions occur, afferent activity is further increased. The afferent axons travel through the pelvic plexus and pelvic nerve to enter the sacral spinal cord. There they synapse on interneurons and on projection neurons. The

interneurons generate continence-related spinal reflexes; they also produce feeble contractions of the detrusor. The projection neurons relay wall tension status to the brain.

In the forebrain, a sense of bladder awareness/fullness/urgency is detected along with cognitive interpretation of surroundings and consideration of emotional status as it relates to urination. All of these perceptions are factored into a decision either to inhibit or to initiate micturition. The latter involves onset of behavior that facilitates micturition (movement, posture, abdominal press) and instructions to the midbrain and pons (Figure A.4).

The pons switches from continence to micturition by deactivating a pontine continence center and activating a pontine micturition center (Holstege et al. 1986). Descending tracts from the pontine micturition center inhibit neurons to smooth and striated sphincters and excite parasympathetic preganglionic neurons to the detrusor.

Following voluntary relaxation of the striated sphincter, detrusor contraction boosts wall tension and intravesical pressure within the closed bladder. The detrusor pulls open the bladder neck and intravesical pressure forces urine into the relaxed bladder neck and urethra. Eventually, wall tension and mechanoreceptor activity decline along with bladder volume, but brain facilitation sustains detrusor contraction until the bladder is

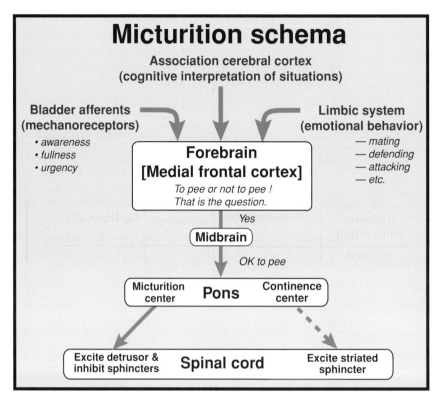

Figure A.4 Micturition schema. Micturition is a voluntary act initiated by the forebrain. Effective implementation involves pontine descending tracts to spinal cord neurons. The net effect is detrusor excitation and sphincter inhibition.

virtually empty (except when urination is motivated by a need to mark territory or dispense pheromones rather than empty the bladder).

Spinal lesions that damage descending tracts from the pons impair normal micturition by diminishing sustained detrusor contraction and by producing detrusor-sphincter dyssynergy (failure to inhibit sphincter spinal reflexes during detrusor contraction). Dyssynergy impedes attempts to manually empty the bladder in paraplegic patients and chronically results in detrusor hypertrophy and predisposition to cystitis (Amarenco et al. 2001).

Smooth muscle properties

On a phasic–tonic (contraction rate) axis and a unitary–multiunit (innervation dependency) axis, smooth muscles across the body exhibit a continuum of values. Smooth muscle of the ureter is regarded as unitary because only a few pacemaker muscle cells in the renal pelvis are innervated and excitation spreads among individual myocytes by gap junctions. In contrast, detrusor contraction is innervation dependent; cell to cell coupling is limited to small collections of muscle cells. Also, the contraction rate for bladder smooth muscle is relatively fast among smooth muscles. Thus, the detrusor muscle

is characterized as a multiunit, phasic type of smooth muscle (Andersson and Arner 2004). Bladder neck and urethral smooth muscles appear similar in nature to the detrusor.

Detrusor myocytes have resting transmembrane potentials that range from 35 to 70 mV (Turner 2001). Depolarization increases the frequency of spontaneous action potentials in myocytes, while hyperpolarization has the opposite effect. The rising phase of the myocyte action potential (AP) is due to Ca^{2+} influx through voltage gated ion channels; the AP fall is driven by K+ efflux. The Ca^{2+} influx associated with an AP leads to additional Ca^{2+} release from sarcoplasmic reticulum. The combined increased cytoplasmic $[Ca^{2+}]$ initiates smooth muscle contraction via a complex series of events involving Ca^{2+}-calmodulin formation, myosin-II phosphorylation, and myosin–actin interaction.

Neurotransmitters and receptors

Somatic efferent neurons release acetycholine (ACh) at neuromuscular synapses in striated muscles. Autonomic preganglionic neurons also release ACh at synapses with postganglionic neurons. In both cases, ACh targets nicotinic ion channel receptors that generate depolarization via enhanced cation permeability.

Figure A.5 Table of neurotransmitters and myocyte receptors for the lower urinary tract. Acetylcholine elicits smooth and striated muscle contraction by different mechanisms. The effect of norepinephrine depends on the receptors expressed by the myocytes being innervated.

Postganglionic neurons release neurotransmitters from synaptic vesicles contained within preterminal and terminal varicosities (swellings) along axonal terminal branches. The neurotransmitters diffuse variable distances to bind with receptors on myocytes, generating either excitatory or inhibitory junction potentials. Excitatory potentials lead to myocyte APs and contraction. Inhibitory potentials produce hyperpolarization and myocyte relaxation. Myocyte receptors are generally associated with G proteins and second messengers (metabotropic) (Figure A.5).

Detrusor contraction is produced by ACh released from postganglionic parasympathetic axons. ACh increases AP frequency in myocytes. Contraction is mediated mainly through M_3 muscarinic receptors. The receptors are linked to G_q proteins that generate IP_3 second messengers which drive Ca^{2+} release from sarcoplasmic reticulum (Andersson and Arner 2004). The elevated $[Ca^{2+}]$ initiates the myocyte contraction process.

In cats and rodents, it has been shown that some detrusor contraction results from ATP co-released with ACh from postganglionic parasympathetic axons (Turner 2001). The ATP neurotransmitter leads to Ca^{2+} influx through an ionotropic purinergic receptor (P_{2X}).

Detrusor relaxation results from norepinephrine released by sympathetic postganglionic axons either within the bladder or within parasympathetic gan-glia supplying the bladder. Within the detrusor, norepinephrine binds to β_3 adrenergic receptors that are linked to G_s proteins that elevate levels of the second messenger cAMP (Andersson and Arner 2004). (Depending on species, β_2 adrenergic receptors linked to G_i proteins may be chiefly responsible for detrusor relaxation.) The other mechanism for producing detrusor relaxation involves norepinephrine binding to α_2 receptors on postganglionic neurons in pelvic and vesical ganglia. The effect is inhibition of parasympathetic synaptic transmission in the ganglia (Janig and McLachlan 1987).

Norepinephrine released by sympathetic postganglionic axons in the bladder neck and proximal urethra produces contraction of the smooth muscle sphincter. The norepinephrine binds to α_1 adrenergic receptors linked to G_q proteins that generate IP_3 second messengers, which drive Ca^{2+} release from sarcoplasmic reticulum. The elevated $[Ca^{2+}]$ initiates the myocyte contraction.

Role of the pelvic urethra in ejaculation

In addition to its urinary function, the male urethra conveys ejaculate. Urination requires a low resistance tube able to accommodate a large volume propelled by low pressure. In contrast, ejaculation involves a small volume accelerated to considerable velocity by abrupt episodes of high pressure. Thus ejaculation requires a small urethral lumen with stiff walls and rapid contraction of the thick striated musculature surrounding the urethra.

Parasympathetic-induced erection includes engorgement of the stratum spongiosum within the submucosa of the postprostatic urethra as well as engorgement of the corpus spongiosum penis that immediately surrounds the penile urethra and forms the bulb of the penis. These vascular changes reduce lumen size and make the urethral wall more rigid.

Sympathetic innervation initiates ejaculation (Janig and McLachlan 1987). Peristaltic waves in the ductus deferens convey spermatozoa into the lumen of the prostatic urethra. Prostatic secretion and contraction of smooth muscle surrounding prostate lobules adds prostatic secretion to the ejaculate. The smooth muscle sphincter situated in the bladder neck and proximal urethra contract to preclude ejaculation into the urinary bladder and minimize urine contamination of the ejaculate.

Somatic innervation completes ejaculation. Innervated by the pudendal nerve, both the urethralis muscle and the bulbospongiosus muscle are engaged in propelling ejaculate along the urethra.

Based on anatomical evidence, the prostatic urethra has a passive, elastic role during ejaculation (Cullen et al. 1981). Except at its cranial extent, smooth muscle does not encircle the prostatic urethral submucosa, which is rich in elastic fibers (Cullen et al. 1981).

The wall of the urethral lumen is passively stretched when sperm and prostatic fluid are added under pressure, the ejaculate being temporarily trapped by contractions of the smooth muscle sphincter cranially and the urethralis muscle caudally.

An ejaculation event would be initiated by relaxation of the urethralis muscle, allowing ejaculate to enter the postprostatic urethra, followed by urethralis muscle peristalsis to propel the ejaculate bolus.

References

Amarenco, G., S.S. Ismael, et al. (2001). The dyssynergic sphincter. In: The Urinary Sphincter, edited by J. Corcos and E. Schick. New York: Marcel Dekker, Inc, pp. 223–230.

Andersson, K.E. and A. Arner (2004). Urinary bladder contraction and relaxation: physiology and pathophysiology. Physiol Rev 84: 935–986.

Blok, B.F.M. and G. Holstege (2001). The neural control of micturition and urinary continence. In: The Urinary Sphincter, edited by J. Corcos and E. Schick. New York: Marcel Dekker, Inc, pp. 89–99.

Bowen, J.M., G.W. Timm, et al. (1976). Some contractile and electrophysiological properties of the periurethral striated muscle of the cat. Invest Urol 13: 327–330.

Cullen, W.C., T.F. Fletcher, et al. (1981). Histology of the canine urethra. II. Morphometry of the male pelvic urethra. Anat Rec 199: 187–195.

Fletcher, T.F., J. Lulich, et al. (2008). Lower Urinary Tract Web Site: http://vanat.cvm.umn.edu/lut/.

Holstege, G., D. Griffiths, et al. (1986). Anatomical and physiological observations on supraspinal control of bladder and urethral sphincter muscles in the cat. J Comp Neur 250: 449–461.

Janig W. and E.M. McLachlan (1987). Organization of Lumbar Spinal Outflow to distal colon and pelvic organs. Physiol Rev 67(4): 1332–1404.

Nitti, V.W. and Y.H. Kim. (2001). Multichannel urodynamic and videourodynamic testing. In: The Urinary Sphincter, edited by J. Corcos and E. Schick. New York: Marcel Dekker, Inc, pp. 311–334.

Schmidt, R.A. (2001). The pelvic floor: lessons from out past. In: The Urinary Sphincter, edited by J. Corcos and E. Schick. New York: Marcel Dekker, Inc, pp. 43–70.

Turner, W.H. (2001). Physiology of the smooth muscles of the bladder and urethra. In: The Urinary Sphincter, edited by J. Corcos and E. Schick. New York: Marcel Dekker, Inc, pp. 43–70.

Vaughan, C.W. and Satchell P.M. (1992). Role of sympathetic innervation in the feline continence process under natural filling conditions. J Neurophysiol 68(5): 1842–1849.

Zinner, N.R., R.C. Ritter, et al. (1977). The physical basis of some urodynamic measurements. J Urol 117: 682–689.

Index